Fifth Edition

Pharmacology

H. P. Rang MB BS MA DPhil FMedSci FRS

Senior Research Associate, Novartis Institute for Medical Sciences, London;
Emeritus Professor of Pharmacology, University College, London

M. M. Dale MB BCh PhD

Senior Teaching Fellow, Department of Pharmacology, University of Oxford;
Honorary Lecturer, Department of Pharmacology, University College, London

J. M. Ritter MA DPhil FRCP FMedSci

Professor of Clinical Pharmacology, The Guy's, King's College
and St Thomas' Hospitals' Medical and Dental School, King's College, London

P. K. Moore BSc PhD

Professor of Pharmacology, National University of Singapore

Illustrations by Peter Lamb

Fifth Edition

Pharmacology

CHURCHILL LIVINGSTONE
An Imprint of Elsevier

Pharmacology 5/e
Rang

CHURCHILL LIVINGSTONE
An imprint of Elsevier

Previous editions 1987, 1991, 1995, 1999, 2003

Original ISBN 0443 071454

First Printed In India 2005

Indian Reprint ISBN : 81-8147-917-3

Notice
Medical knowledge is constantly changing. Standard safety precautions must be followed, but as new research and clinical experience broaden our knowledge, changes in treatment and drug therapy may become necessary or appropriate. Readers are advised to check the most current product information provided by the manufacturer of each drug to be administered to verify the recommended dose, the method and duration of administration, and contraindications. It is the responsibility of the practitioner, relying on experience and knowledge of the patient, to determine dosages and the best treatment for each individual patient. Neither the Publisher nor the authors assume any liability for any injury and/or damage to persons or property arising from this publication.

Published by Elsevier, a division of Reed Elservier India Private Limited,
17-A/1, Main Ring Road, Lajpat Nagar-IV, New Delhi - 110 024, INDIA

Printed and bound at International Print-O-Pac Limited
C/4-11, Phase-II Extn., NOIDA - 201 301 (U.P.)

Preface

For this fifth edition, as in the previous four, our approach has been not just to describe what drugs do, but to emphasise the *mechanisms* by which they act — where possible at the cellular and molecular level. Therapeutic agents have a high rate of obsolescence and new ones appear each year. An appreciation of the mechanisms of action of the class of drugs to which a new agent belongs provides a good starting point for understanding and using the new compound intelligently.

Pharmacology is a lively scientific discipline in its own right, with an importance beyond that of providing a basis for the use of drugs in therapy. We have therefore, where appropriate, included brief coverage of the use of drugs as probes for elucidating cellular and physiological functions, even when the compounds have no clinical uses.

We have retained the short summaries of relevant physiological and biochemical processes, placed at the beginning of most chapters, to form a basis for the subsequent discussion of pharmacological actions. As before, short sets of key points are placed in boxes throughout the text. These are not intended as comprehensive summaries but rather to highlight pharmacological information that we consider important. Factual knowledge in pharmacology is so extensive and expanding so rapidly that students can easily find the information load daunting, and these key points are intended to make it easier for students to gets to grips with the essentials of the subject. And as in the fourth edition, the therapeutic use of drugs has been given prominence by setting it out in easily identified 'clinical boxes'.

In this edition, as will already be apparent to the astute observer, we have gone into riotous colour. Most diagrams have been updated, all have been redrawn in colour, and many new figures have been added. Continuing the approach used in earlier editions, we have, wherever feasible, used real data in our diagrams rather than notional information. As previously, we have put emphasis on the chemical structures of drugs where this information helps in understanding how the drugs act, and we have omitted many chemical structures that do not add to pharmacological understanding in favour of diagrams that do.

All chapters have been updated and an 'overview' section has been introduced at the beginning of each to help the reader get a flying start on that topic. In including new material, we have taken into account not only new agents but also recent extensions of basic knowledge which presage further drug development, and, where possible, we have given a brief outline of new treatments in the pipeline. New 'small print' sections have been included in many chapters. These contain more detailed, sometimes speculative material, which can be skipped by the reader in a hurry without losing the main thread, but will be of interest to readers wishing to go into greater depth.

As before, we have included fairly extensive sections on 'References and further reading' at the end of each chapter. Because the medical curriculum stresses project work and the preparation of special study modules, references have been annotated to emphasise the main aspects of their coverage and so make the Reference section easier for students to use.

Section 1 now includes a new introductory chapter, and two new chapters on the cellular mechanisms that are affected by many important drugs described in later parts of the book. Chapter 4 deals with mechanisms involved in short term reactions such as excitation, contraction and secretion, which underlie the rapid actions of many drugs that affect the cardiovascular, nervous, respiratory and endocrine systems. Chapter 5 deals with cell proliferation and apoptosis: reactions that occur rather more slowly and are involved in more gradually developing phenomena, such as inflammation, immune responses, tissue repair and malignancies, and are affected by drugs used for these conditions. These chapters bring together, update and extend information that was previously scattered throughout the book, and are intended to establish the common ground on which many, at first sight very different, drug effects are based, not only drugs in use but drugs in development or being planned.

A new chapter on 'Drug discovery' looks at the rapid progress that is occurring in this field, driven by advances in molecular biology. It contains a brief account of the regulatory controls involved in putting a new drug on the market.

In addition to these new chapters, and extensive updating throughout, the following new information has been included.

- The use of disease models, including transgenic animal models, in drug testing (Ch. 6).
- The role of innate immunity and of the significance of the two wings of the adaptive immune response—new knowledge likely to be important for drug treatment in the future (Ch. 15).
- The molecular control of nitric oxide biosynthesis, and the more controversial issues of transport and export of biologically active nitric oxide by red blood cells (Ch. 14).
- Endothelium-derived mediators, including endothelin and the elusive endothelium-derived hyperpolarising factor (Ch. 18).

- Recent advances in the treatment of cardiac failure (Ch. 17).
- Statins — now very important in clinical practice — are further emphasised in the chapter on 'Atherosclerosis and lipoprotein metabolism', and the many pharmacological effects of these drugs that are not direct consequences of their action on LDL-cholesterol and which are the focus of much current interest are discussed (Ch. 19).
- Thiazolidinediones (currently in widespread use for treating diabetes), including their mechanism of action via nuclear PPAR-gamma receptors (Ch. 25).
- The chapter on 'Obesity' that many were surprised to see in our 4th edition, now justifies its inclusion with coverage of new anti-obesity drugs. The 'new drug' pipeline is expected to disgorge many more such agents — as horizontally-challenged individuals will be pleased to learn. The coverage of the biology of obesity is updated and pointers given to the targets for the development of new drugs (Ch. 26).
- A new section on erectile dysfunction, which has taken a recent leap from charlatanry to medical orthodoxy (Ch. 29).
- New approaches to the treatment of neurodegenerative disorders (Ch. 34).
- New information on the interaction of the osteoclast and osteoblast; the role of osteoprotegerin ligand and osteoprotegerin, and potential new anti- osteoporosis therapies are discussed (Ch. 32).
- The burgeoning understanding of the pathogenesis of cancer is discussed and its significance for the development of new anticancer drugs is stressed. Included in the chapter is coverage of new drugs that are based on this understanding which are already in clinical use (Ch. 45).
- In the 'Antiviral drugs' chapter, new information on host/viral interactions and the mechanisms of action of antivirals is included, and also new approaches to therapy of HIV infection (Ch. 47).

The section on 'Chemotherapy of infectious and malignant disease' has been renamed 'Drugs used in the treatment of infections and cancer'. The opening chapter on the 'Basic principles of chemotherapy' gives an overview of the basic mechanisms of drug action common both to agents acting on various parasitic infections and to anti-cancer drugs. It is aimed primarily at non-medical students studying pharmacology who need a birds-eye view of this topic but do not have sufficient background in microbiology, parasitology and cancer pathology to be able to cope with the more detailed chapters in the rest of the section on 'Selective toxicity'. Since such students have found this approach useful, this introductory chapter has been retained and updated.

We are grateful to the readers who have taken the trouble to write to us with constructive comments and suggestions; we have done our best to incorporate these. Comments on the new edition will be welcome.

ACKNOWLEDGEMENTS

We would like to thank the following for their help and advice in the preparation of this edition: Professor J. H. Abramson, Professor J. Mandelstam, Dr M. Weber, Professor R. J. P. Williams, Sir John Vane and the staff of the Royal Society of Medicine Library.

London 2003

H. P. Rang
M. M. Dale
J. M. Ritter
P. K. Moore

Contents

SECTION 1

GENERAL PRINCIPLES

1. What is pharmacology? 2
Pharmacology in the 20th century 3

2. How drugs act: general principles 7
The binding of drug molecules to cells 7
Desensitisation and tachyphylaxis 19

3. How drugs act: molecular aspects 22
Targets for drug action 22
Receptor proteins 26
Ion channels as drug targets 45
Control of receptor expression 47
Receptors and disease 48

4. Cellular mechanisms: excitation, contraction and secretion 51
Regulation of intracellular calcium levels 51
Excitation 55
Muscle contraction 62
Release of chemical mediators 64
Epithelial ion transport 66

5. Cellular mechanisms: cell proliferation and apoptosis 69
Cell proliferation 69
Angiogenesis 74
Apoptosis and cell removal 74
Pathophysiological implications 77
Therapeutic implications 77

6. Method and measurement in pharmacology 80
Bioassay 80
Animal models of disease 84
Clinical trials 86
Balancing benefit and risk 89

7. Absorption and distribution of drugs 91
Translocation of drug molecules 91
Drug disposition 97
Drug absorption 98
Special drug delivery systems 104

8. Drug elimination and pharmacokinetics 106
Drug metabolism 106
Renal excretion of drugs and drug metabolites 111
Biliary excretion and enterohepatic circulation 113
Pharmacokinetics 114

SECTION 2

CHEMICAL MEDIATORS

9. Chemical mediators and the autonomic nervous system 122
Historical aspects 122
The peripheral nervous system 123
Some general principles of chemical transmission 126
Basic steps in neurochemical transmission: sites of drug action 133

10. Cholinergic transmission 136
Muscarinic and nicotinic actions of acetylcholine 136
Acetylcholine receptors 137
Physiology of cholinergic transmission 139
Effects of drugs on cholinergic transmission 143

11. Noradrenergic transmission 161
Classification of adrenoceptors 161
Physiology of noradrenergic transmission 164
Drugs acting on adrenoceptors 168
Drugs that affect noradrenergic neurons 176

12. Other peripheral mediators: 5-hydroxytryptamine and purines 184
5-hydroxytryptamine 184
Purines 192

13. Peptides and proteins as mediators 198
General principles of peptide pharmacology 198
Biosynthesis and regulation of peptides 202
Peptide antagonists 204
Proteins and peptides as drugs 205
Concluding remarks 206

14. Nitric oxide 208
Biosynthesis of nitric oxide and its control 209
Degradation and carriage of nitric oxide 210
Effects of nitric oxide 212
Therapeutic approaches 213
Clinical conditions in which nitric oxide may play a part 214

15. Local hormones, inflammation and immune reactions 217
The components of the acute inflammatory reaction 217
The outcome of the inflammatory response 228
Mediators of inflammation and immune reactions 229
Current therapies based on manipulation of the immune response 241
Potential new therapies 241

16. Anti-inflammatory and immunosuppressant drugs 244
Non-steroidal anti-inflammatory drugs 244
Antagonists of histamine 252
Drugs used in gout 254
Antirheumatoid drugs 255
Immunosuppressant drugs 257
Possible future developments 260

SECTION 3

DRUGS AFFECTING MAJOR ORGAN SYSTEMS

17. The heart 264
Physiology of cardiac function 264
Drugs that affect cardiac function 272

18. The vascular system 285
Vascular structure and function 285
Control of vascular smooth muscle tone 286
Vasoactive drugs 292
Clinical uses of vasoactive drugs 298

19. Atherosclerosis and lipoprotein metabolism 306
Atherogenesis 306
Lipoprotein transport in the blood 307
Lipid-lowering drugs 309

20. Haemostasis and thrombosis 314
Blood coagulation 315
Drugs that act on the coagulation cascade 317
Platelet adhesion and activation 323
Fibrinolysis (thrombolysis) 327

21. The haemopoietic system 330
The haemopoietic system 330
Haematinic agents 331
Haemopoietic growth factors 336

22. The respiratory system 340
The regulation of respiration 340
Disorders of respiration and the drugs used in treatment 341

23. The kidney 352
Outline of renal function 352
The structure and function of the nephron 352
Drugs acting on the kidney 362
Drugs which alter the pH of the urine 365
Drugs which alter the excretion of organic molecules 365

24. The gastrointestinal tract 367
The innervation and the hormones of the gastrointestinal tract 367
Gastric secretion 368
Vomiting 372
The motility of the gastrointestinal tract 375
Drugs for chronic inflammatory bowel disease 377
Drugs affecting the biliary system 378

25. The endocrine pancreas and the control of blood glucose 380
Pancreatic islet hormones 380
Control of blood glucose 385
Diabetes mellitus and the drugs used in treatment 385

26. Obesity 394
The homeostatic mechanisms controlling energy balance 394
Obesity as a health problem and possible treatments 397

27. The pituitary and adrenal cortex 404
The pituitary and drugs used in therapy 404
The adrenal cortex and drugs used in therapy 411

28. The thyroid 421
Synthesis, storage and secretion of thyroid hormones 421
Regulation of thyroid function 422
Actions of the thyroid hormones 423
Transport and metabolism 424
Abnormalities of thyroid function 424
Drugs used in diseases of the thyroid 425

29. The reproductive system 429
Endocrine control of reproduction and modulating drugs 429
Drugs used for contraception 439
The uterus 441
Erectile dysfunction 443

30. Bone metabolism 446
Bone structure and composition 446
Bone remodelling 446
Disorders of bone and the drugs used in treatment 451

SECTION 4

THE NERVOUS SYSTEM

31. Chemical transmission and drug action in the central nervous system 456
Chemical signalling in the nervous system 457
Targets for drug action 458
Drug action in the central nervous system 459
The classification of psychotropic drugs 460

32. Amino acid transmitters 462
Excitatory amino acids 462
Glutamate 463
Gamma-aminobutyric acid 470
Glycine 473

33. Other transmitters and modulators 474
Noradrenaline 475
Dopamine 476
5-Hydroxytryptamine 480
Acetylcholine 483
Purines 485
Histamine 485
Other CNS mediators 485
A final message 488

34. Neurodegenerative disorders 490
Mechanisms of neuronal death 490
Ischaemic brain damage 493
Alzheimer's disease 494
Parkinson's disease 497
Huntington's disease 501
Neurodegenerative prion diseases 501

35. General anaesthetic agents 503
Mechanism of action of anaesthetic drugs 504
The effects of anaesthetics on nervous system 505
Effects on the cardiovascular respiratory systems 506
Inhalation anaesthetics 506
Individual inhalation anaesthetics 509
Intravenous anaesthetic agents 511

36. Anxiolytic and hypnotic drugs 515
The nature of anxiety and measurement of anxiolytic activity 515
Classification of anxiolytic and hypnotic drugs 516
Benzodiazepines 517
Benzodiazepine antagonists 523
Buspirone 523
Barbiturates 523
Other potential anxiolytic drugs 524

37. Antipsychotic drugs 525
The nature of schizophrenia 525
Antipsychotic drugs 528

38. Drugs used in affective disorders 535
The nature of depression 535
Theories of depression 536
Antidepressant drugs 538
Electroconvulsive therapy 547
Clinical effectiveness of antidepressant treatments 548
Mood-stabilising drugs 548

39. Antiepileptic drugs 550
The nature of epilepsy 550
Mechanism of action of antiepileptic drugs 553
Antiepileptic drugs 554
Muscle spasm and centrally acting muscle relaxants 559

40. Analgesic drugs 562
Neural mechanisms of pain 562
Analgesic drugs 572
New approaches 583

41. CNS stimulants and psychotomimetic drugs 585
Convulsants and respiratory stimulants 585
Psychomotor stimulants 587
Psychotomimetic drugs 591

42. Drug dependence and drug abuse 594
The nature of drug dependence 595
Nicotine and tobacco 598
Ethanol 603
Cannabis 608

43. Local anaesthetics 612
Local anaesthetics 612
Other drugs that affect sodium channels 616

SECTION 5

DRUGS USED IN THE TREATMENT OF INFECTIONS AND CANCER

44. Basic principles of chemotherapy 620
The molecular basis of chemotherapy 620
Resistance to antibacterial drugs 629

45. Antibacterial drugs 635
Antimicrobial agents that interfere with the synthesis or action of folate 637
Beta-lactam antibiotics 639
Antimicrobial agents affecting bacterial protein synthesis 643
Antimicrobial agents affecting topoisomerase II 647
Miscellaneous antibacterial agents 648
Antimycobacterial agents 649
Possible new antibacterial drugs 652

46. Antiviral drugs 654
Background information about viruses 654
The host–virus interaction 655
HIV and AIDS 657
Antiviral drugs 659

47. Antifungal drugs 666
Fungal infections 666
Drugs used for fungal infections 666
Potential new antifungal therapies 670

48. Antiprotozoal drugs 672
Host–parasite interactions 672
Malaria 673
Pneumocystis pneumonia and its treatment 682
Amoebiasis and amoebicidal drugs 682
Leishmaniasis and leishmanicidal drugs 683
Trypanosomiasis and trypanosomicidal drugs 684
Trichomoniasis and trichomonicidal drugs 684
Toxoplasmosis and toxoplasmocidal drugs 684
New approaches to antiprotozoal therapy 685

49. Anthelminthic drugs 687
Helminth infections 687
Anthelminthic drugs 688
Resistance to anthelminthic drugs 691
New approaches to anthelminthic therapy 691

50. Cancer chemotherapy 693
The pathogenesis of cancer 693
General principles of action of cytotoxic anticancer drugs 696
Drugs used in cancer chemotherapy 698
Resistance to anticancer drugs 706
Treatment schedules 707
Techniques for dealing with emesis and myelosuppression 707
Possible future strategies for cancer chemotherapy 707

SECTION 6

SPECIAL TOPICS

51. Individual variation and drug interaction 712
Effects of ethnicity 712
Effects of age 713
Effects of pregnancy 714
Genetic factors 714
Idiosyncratic reactions 716
Effects of disease 717
Drug interactions 718

52. Harmful effects of drugs 724
Types of adverse drug reaction 724
Drug toxicity 725

53. Gene therapy 738
Technical aspects 739
Safety 743
Therapeutic aspects 743

54. Drug discovery and development 747
The preclinical stages 747
Clinical development 749
Commercial aspects 750
A final note 750

APPENDIX 753

INDEX 761

SECTION

1

GENERAL PRINCIPLES

1 What is pharmacology?

Overview 2
— Origins and antecedents 2

Pharmacology in the 20th century 3
— Alternative therapeutic principles 4
— The emergence of biotechnology 4
— Pharmacology today 4

OVERVIEW

In this introductory chapter, we explain how pharmacology came into being and evolved as a scientific discipline, and describe the present day structure of the subject and its links to other biomedical sciences. The structure that has emerged forms the basis of the organisation of the rest of the book. Readers in a hurry to get to the here-and-now of pharmacology can safely skip this chapter.

ORIGINS AND ANTECEDENTS

Pharmacology can be defined as the study of the effects of chemical substances on the function of living systems. As a science, it was born in the mid-19th century, one of a host of new biomedical sciences based on principles of experimentation rather than dogma that came into being in that remarkable period. Long before that—indeed from the dawn of civilisation—herbal remedies were widely used, pharmacopoeias were written and the apothecaries' trade flourished, but nothing resembling scientific principles was applied to therapeutics. Even Robert Boyle, who laid the scientific foundations of chemistry in the middle of the 17th century, was content, when dealing with therapeutics (A Collection of Choice Remedies, 1692), to recommend concoctions of worms, dung, urine and the moss from a dead man's skull. The impetus for pharmacology came from the need to improve the outcome of therapeutic intervention by doctors, who were at that time skilled at clinical observation and diagnosis, but broadly ineffectual when it came to treatment.* Until the late 19th century, knowledge of the normal and abnormal functioning of the body was too rudimentary to provide even a rough basis for understanding drug effects; at the same time, disease and death were regarded as semi-sacred subjects, appropriately dealt with by authoritarian, rather than scientific, doctrines. Clinical practice often displayed an obedience to authority and ignored what appear to be easily ascertainable facts. For example, cinchona bark was recognised as a specific and effective treatment for malaria, and a sound protocol for its use was laid down by Lind in 1765. In 1804, however, Johnson declared it to be unsafe until the fever had subsided, and he recommended instead the use of large doses of calomel in the early stages—a murderous piece of advice, which was slavishly followed for the next 40 years.

The motivation for pharmacology came from clinical practice, but the science could only be built on the basis of secure foundations in physiology, pathology and chemistry. It was not until 1858 that Virchow proposed the cell theory. The first use of a structural formula to describe a chemical compound was in 1868. Bacteria as a cause of disease were discovered by Pasteur in 1878. Previously, pharmacology hardly had the legs to stand on, and we may wonder at the bold vision of Rudolf Buchheim, who created the first pharmacology institute (in his own house) in Estonia in 1847.

In its beginnings, before the advent of synthetic organic chemistry, pharmacology concerned itself exclusively with understanding the effects of natural substances, mainly plant extracts. An early development in chemistry was the purification of active compounds from plants. Friedrich Sertürner, a young German apothecary, purified morphine from opium in 1805. Other substances quickly followed, and, even though their structures were unknown, these compounds showed that chemicals, not magic or vital forces, were responsible for the effects that plant extracts produced on living organisms. Early pharmacologists focussed most of their attention on such plant-derived drugs as quinine, digitalis, atropine, ephedrine, strychnine and others (many of which are still used today and will have become old friends by the time you have finished reading this book).**

*Oliver Wendell Holmes, an eminent physician, wrote in 1860: '...firmly believe that if the whole materia medica, as now used, could be sunk to the bottom of the sea, it would be all the better for mankind—and the worse for the fishes.' (see Porter, 1997).

**A handful of synthetic substances achieved pharmacological prominence long before the era of synthetic chemistry began. Diethyl ether, first prepared as 'sweet oil of vitriol' in the 16th century, and nitrous oxide, prepared by Humphrey Davy in 1799, were used to liven up parties before

PHARMACOLOGY IN THE 20TH CENTURY

Beginning in the 20th century, the fresh wind of synthetic chemistry began to revolutionise the pharmaceutical industry, and with it the science of pharmacology. New synthetic drugs, such as barbiturates and local anaesthetics, began to appear, and the era of antimicrobial chemotherapy began with the discovery by Paul Ehrlich in 1909 of arsenical compounds for treating syphilis. Further breakthroughs came when the sulphonamides, the first antibacterial drugs, were discovered by Gerhard Domagk in 1935, and with the development of penicillin by Chain and Florey during World War II, based on the earlier work of Fleming.

These few well-known examples show how the growth of synthetic chemistry, and the resurgence of natural product chemistry, caused a dramatic revitalisation of therapeutics in the first half of the 20th century. Each new drug class that emerged gave pharmacologists a new challenge, and it was then that pharmacology really established its identity and its status among the biomedical sciences.

In parallel with the exuberant proliferation of therapeutic molecules—driven mainly by chemistry—which gave pharmacologists so much to think about, physiology was also making rapid progress, particularly in relation to chemical mediators, which are discussed in depth elsewhere in this book. Many hormones, neurotransmitters and inflammatory mediators were discovered in this period, and the realisation that chemical communication plays a central role in almost every regulatory mechanism that our bodies possess immediately established a large area of common ground between physiology and pharmacology, for interactions between chemical substances and living systems were exactly what pharmacologists had been preoccupied with from the outset. The concept of 'receptors' for chemical mediators, first proposed by Langley in 1905, was quickly taken up by pharmacologists such as Clark, Gaddum, Schild and others and is a constant theme in present-day pharmacology (as you will soon discover as you plough through the next two chapters). The receptor concept, and the technologies developed from it, have had a massive impact on drug discovery and therapeutics. Biochemistry also emerged as a distinct science early in the 20th century, and the discovery of enzymes and the delineation of biochemical pathways provided yet another framework for understanding drug effects. The picture of pharmacology that emerges from this brief glance at history (Fig. 1.1) is of a subject evolved from ancient prescientific therapeutics, involved in commerce from the 17th century onwards and which gained respectability by donning the trappings of science as soon as this became possible in the mid-19th century. Signs of its carpetbagger past still cling to pharmacology, for the pharmaceutical industry has become very big business and much pharmacological research nowadays takes place in a commercial environment, a rougher and more pragmatic place than the glades of academia.* No other biomedical 'ology' is so close to Mammon.

ALTERNATIVE THERAPEUTIC PRINCIPLES

Modern medicine relies heavily on drugs as the main tool of therapeutics. Other therapeutic procedures such as surgery, diet, exercise, etc. are also important, of course, as is deliberate non-intervention, but none is so widely applied as drug-based therapeutics.

Before the advent of science-based approaches, repeated attempts were made to construct systems of therapeutics, many of which produced even worse results than pure empiricism. One of these was allopathy, espoused by James Gregory (1735–1821). The favoured remedies included blood-letting, emetics and purgatives, which were used until the dominant symptoms of the disease were suppressed. Many patients died from such treatment, and it was in reaction against it that Hahnemann introduced the practice of homœopathy in the early 19th century. The guiding principles of homœopathy are:

- like cures like
- activity can be enhanced by dilution.

The system rapidly drifted into absurdity: for example, Hahnemann recommended the use of drugs at dilutions of 1:1060, equivalent to 1 molecule in a sphere the size of the orbit of Neptune.

Many other systems of therapeutics have come and gone, and the variety of dogmatic principles that they embodied have tended to hinder rather than advance scientific progress. Currently, therapeutic systems that have a basis which lies outside the domain of science are actually gaining ground under the general banner of 'alternative' or 'holistic' medicine. Mostly, they reject the 'medical model', which attributes disease to an underlying derangement of normal function that can be defined in biochemical or structural terms, detected by objective means, and influenced beneficially by appropriate chemical or physical interventions. They focus instead mainly on subjective malaise, which may be disease associated or not. Abandoning objectivity

being introduced as anaesthetic agents in the mid-19th century (see Ch. 35). Amyl nitrite (see Ch. 17) was made in 1859 and can claim to be the first 'rational' therapeutic drug; its therapeutic effect in angina was predicted on the basis of its physiological effects—a true 'pharmacologist's drug' and the smelly fore-runner of the nitro-vasodilators that are widely used today. Aspirin (Ch. 16), the most widely used therapeutic drug in history, was first synthesised in 1853, with no pharmacological application in mind. It was rediscovered in 1897 in the laboratories of the German company Bayer, who were seeking a less toxic derivative of salicylic acid. Bayer commercialised aspirin in 1899 and made a fortune.

*Some of our most distinguished pharmacological pioneers made their careers in industry: for example, Henry Dale, who laid the foundations of our knowledge of chemical transmission and the autonomic nervous system; George Hitchings and Gertrude Elion, who described the antimetabolite principle and produced the first effective anticancer drugs; and James Black, who introduced the first β-adrenoceptor and histamine H_2-receptor antagonists. It is no accident that in this book, where we focus on the scientific principles of pharmacology, most of our examples are products of industry, not of nature.

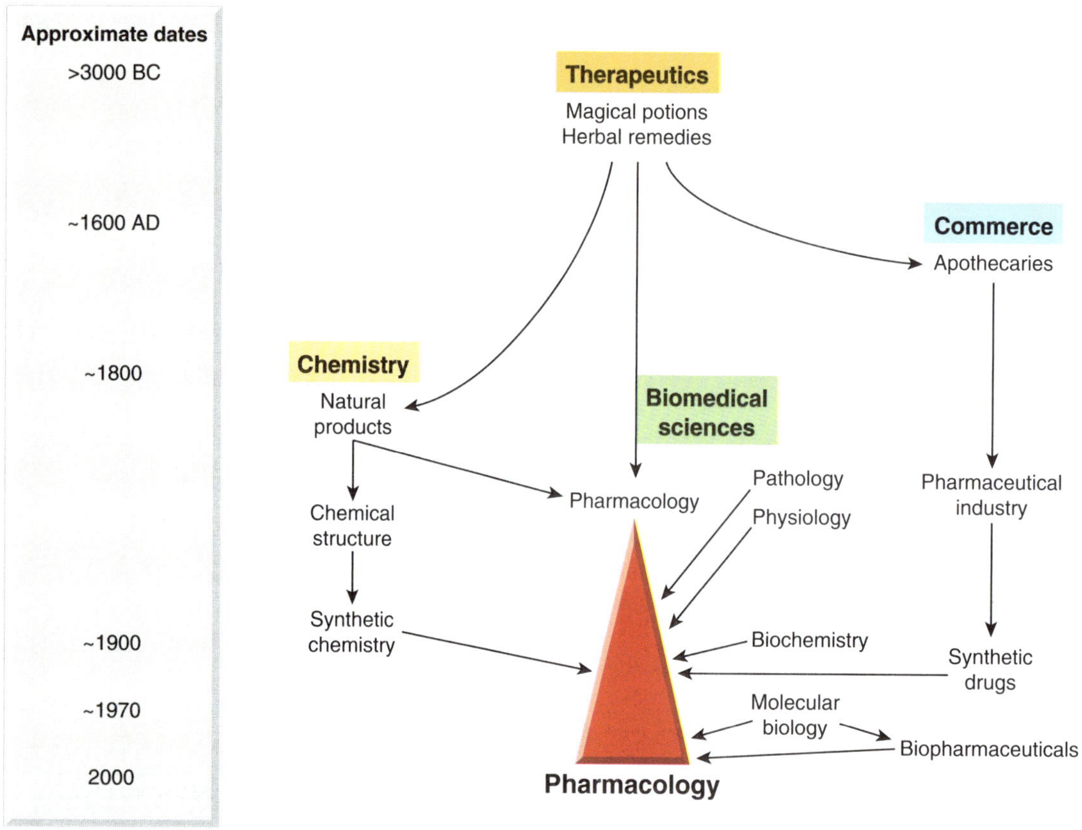

Fig. 1.1 The development of pharmacology.

in defining and measuring disease goes along with a similar departure from scientific principles in assessing therapeutic efficacy, with the result that principles and practices can gain acceptance without satisfying any of the criteria of validity that would convince a critical scientist, and that are required by law to be satisfied before a new drug can be introduced into therapy. Public acceptance, alas, has little to do with demonstrable efficacy.

THE EMERGENCE OF BIOTECHNOLOGY

In recent years, biotechnology has emerged as a major source of new therapeutic agents in the form of antibodies, enzymes and various regulatory proteins, including hormones, growth factors and cytokines (see Buckel, 1996). Though such products (known as biopharmaceuticals) are generally produced by genetic engineering rather than by synthetic chemistry, the pharmacological principles are essentially the same as for conventional drugs. Looking further ahead, gene- and cell-based therapies (Ch. 51), though still in their infancy, will take therapeutics into a new domain. The principles governing the design, delivery and control of functioning artificial genes introduced into cells, or of engineered cells introduced into the body, are very different from those of drug-based therapeutics and will require a different conceptual framework, which texts such as this will increasingly need to embrace if they are to stay abreast of modern medical treatment.

PHARMACOLOGY TODAY

As with other biomedical disciplines, the boundaries of pharmacology are not sharply defined nor are they constant. Its exponents are, as befits pragmatists, ever ready to poach on the territory and techniques of other disciplines. If it ever had a conceptual and technical core that it could really call its own, this has now dwindled almost to the point of extinction, and the subject is defined by its purpose—to understand what drugs do to living organisms, and more particularly how their effects can be applied to therapeutics—rather than by its scientific coherence.

Figure 1.2 shows the structure of pharmacology as it appears today. Within the main subject fall a number of compartments (neuropharmacology, immunopharmacology, pharmacokinetics, etc.), which are convenient, if not watertight, subdivisions. These topics form the main subject matter of this book. Around the edges are several interface disciplines, not covered in this book, which form bridges between pharmacology and other fields of biomedicine. Pharmacology tends to have more of these than other disciplines. Recent arrivals on the fringe are subjects such as pharmacogenomics, pharmacoepidemiology and pharmacoeconomics.

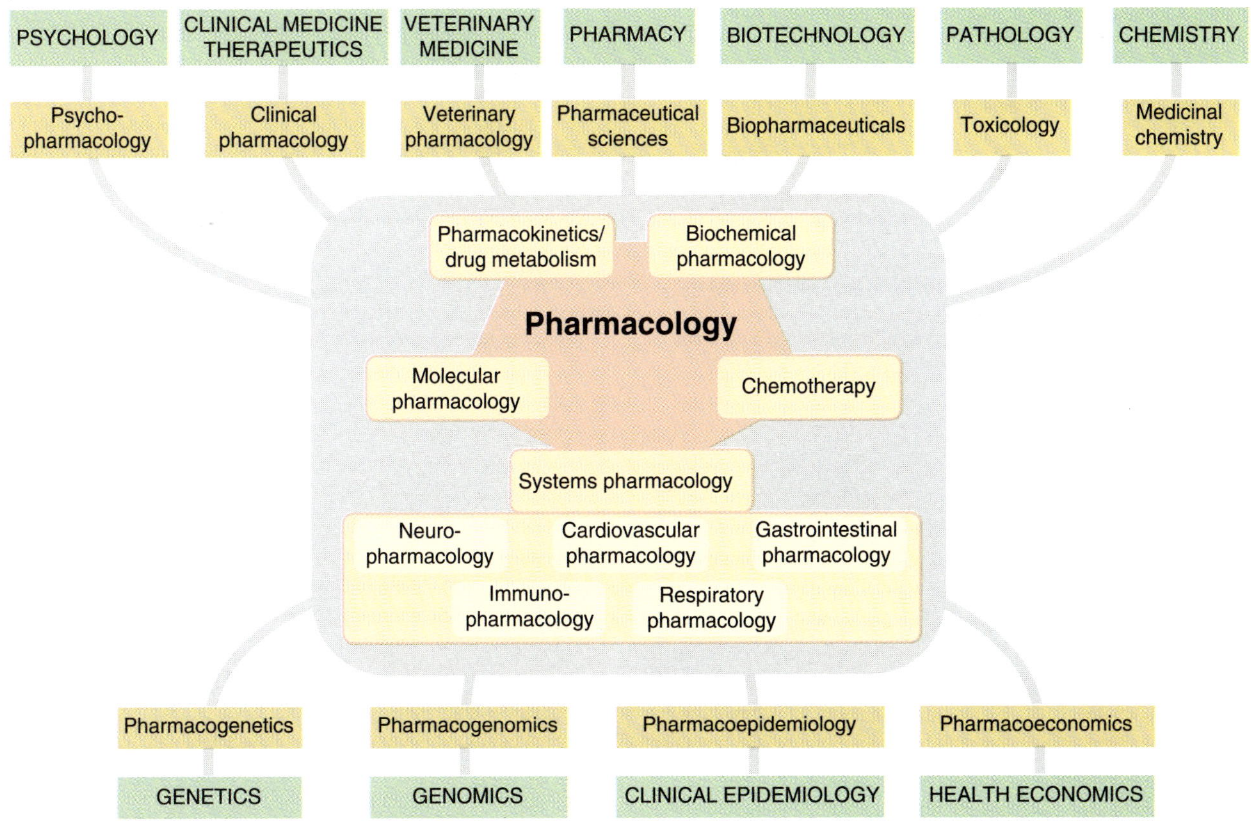

Fig. 1.2 Pharmacology today with its various subdivisions. Interface disciplines (brown boxes) link pharmacology to other mainstream biomedical disciplines (green boxes).

Biotechnology Originally, this was the production of drugs or other useful products by biological means (e.g. antibiotic production from microorganisms or production of monoclonal antibodies). Currently in the biomedical sphere, biotechnology refers mainly to the use of recombinant DNA technology for a wide variety of purposes, including the manufacture of therapeutic proteins, diagnostics, genotyping, production of transgenic animals, etc. The many non-medical applications include agriculture, forensics, environmental sciences, etc.

Pharmacogenetics This is the study of genetic influences on responses to drugs. Originally, pharmacogenetics focussed on familial idiosyncratic drug reactions, where affected individuals show an abnormal—usually adverse—response to a class of drug (see Nebert & Weber, 1990). It now covers broader variations in drug response, where the genetic basis is more complex.

Pharmacogenomics This recent term overlaps with pharmacogenetics, describing the use of genetic information to guide the choice of drug therapy on an individual basis. The underlying assumption is that differences between individuals in their response to therapeutic drugs can be predicted from their genetic make-up. On this principle, discovering which specific gene variations are associated with a good or poor therapeutic response to a particular drug should enable individual tailoring of therapeutic choices on the basis of an individual's genotype. Pharmacogenomics is, in essence, a branch of pharmacogenetics, with a good deal of 'spin'. So far, the concept is largely theoretical, but if it proves valid, the consequences for therapeutics will be far reaching.

Pharmacoepidemiology This is the study of drug effects at the population level (see Strom, 1994). It is concerned with the variability of drug effects between individuals in a population, and between populations. It is an increasingly important topic in the eyes of the regulatory authorities who decide whether or not new drugs can be licensed for therapeutic use. Variability between individuals or populations has an adverse effect on the utility of a drug, even though its mean effect level may be satisfactory. Pharmacoepidemiological studies also take into account patient compliance and other factors that apply when the drug is used under real-life conditions.

Pharmacoeconomics This branch of health economics aims to quantify in economic terms the cost and benefit of drugs used therapeutically. It arose from the concern of many governments to provide for healthcare from tax revenues, raising questions of what therapeutic procedures represent the best value for money. This, of course, raises fierce controversy, since it ultimately comes down to putting monetary value on health and longevity. As with pharmacoepidemiology, regulatory authorities are increasingly requiring economic analysis, as well as evidence of individual benefit, when making decisions on licensing. For more information on this complex subject, see Drummond et al. (1997).

REFERENCES AND FURTHER READING

Buckel P 1996 Recombinant proteins for therapy. Trends Pharmacol Sci 17: 450–456 (*Thoughtful review of the status of, and prospects for, protein-based therapeutics*)

Drews J 1998 In quest of tomorrow's medicines. Springer-Verlag, New York (*An excellent account of the past, present and future of the drug discovery process, emphasising the growing role of biotechnology*)

Drummond M F, O'Brien B, Stoddart G I, Torrance G W (1997) Methods for the economic evaluation of healthcare programmes. Oxford University Press, Oxford (*Coverage of the general principles of evaluating the economic costs and benefits of healthcare, including drug-based therapeutics*)

Evans W E, Relling M V 1999 Pharmacogenomics: translating functional genomics into rational therapeutics. Science 286: 487–501 (*A general overview of pharmacogenomics*)

Nebert D W, Weber W W 1990 Pharmacogenetics. In: Pratt W B, Taylor P (eds) Principles of drug action, 3rd edn. Churchill-Livingstone, New York (*A detailed account of genetic factors that affect responses to drugs, with many examples from the pre-genomic literature*).

Porter R 1997 The greatest benefit to mankind. Harper-Collins, London (*An excellent and readable account of the history of medicine, with good coverage of the early development of pharmacology and the pharmaceutical industry*)

Strom B L (ed) 1994 Pharmacoepidemiology. Wiley, Chichester (*A multi-author book covering all aspects of a newly emerged discipline, including aspects of pharmacoeconomics*)

2 How drugs act: general principles

Overview 7

The binding of drug molecules to cells 7
- Protein targets for drug binding 8
- Drug specificity 8
- Receptor classification 9
- Drug–receptor interactions 9
- Drug antagonism 17

Desensitisation and tachyphylaxis 19

OVERVIEW

The emergence of pharmacology as a science came when the emphasis shifted from describing what drugs do to explaining how they work. In this chapter, we set out some general principles underlying the interaction of drugs with living systems (Ch. 3 goes into the molecular aspects in more detail). The interaction between drugs and cells is described followed by a more detailed examination of different types of drug–receptor interaction. We are still far from the holy grail of being able to predict the pharmacological effects of a novel chemical substance, or to design *ab initio* a chemical to produce a specified therapeutic effect; nevertheless, we can identify some important general principles, which is our purpose in this chapter.

THE BINDING OF DRUG MOLECULES TO CELLS

To begin with, we should gratefully acknowledge Paul Ehrlich for insisting that drug action must be explicable in terms of conventional chemical interactions between drugs and tissues, and for dispelling the idea that the remarkable potency and specificity of action of some drugs put them somehow out of reach of chemistry and physics and required the intervention of magical 'vital forces'. Although many drugs produce effects in extraordinarily low doses and concentrations, low concentrations still involve very large numbers of molecules. One drop of a solution of a drug at only 10^{-10} mol/l still contains about 10^{10} drug molecules, so there is no mystery in the fact that it may produce an obvious pharmacological response. Some bacterial toxins (e.g. diphtheria toxin) act with such precision that a single molecule taken up by a target cell is sufficient to kill it.

One of the basic tenets of pharmacology is that drug molecules must exert some chemical influence on one or more constituents of cells in order to produce a pharmacological response. In other words, drug molecules must get so close to these constituent cellular molecules that the function of the latter is altered. Of course, the molecules in the organism vastly outnumber the drug molecules and if the drug molecules were merely distributed at random, the chance of interaction with any particular class of cellular molecule would be negligible. Pharmacological effects, therefore, require, in general, the non-uniform distribution of the drug molecule within the body or tissue, which is the same as saying that drug molecules must be 'bound' to particular constituents of cells and tissues in order to produce an effect. Ehrlich summed it up thus: 'Corpora non agunt nisi fixata' (in this context, 'A drug will not work unless it is bound').*

Understanding the nature of these binding sites, and the mechanisms by which the association of a drug molecule with a binding site leads to a physiological response, constitutes the major thrust of pharmacological research. Most drugs produce their effects by binding, in the first instance, to protein molecules (often called 'targets', an obvious allusion to Ehrlich's famous phrase 'magic bullets' describing the potential of antimicrobial drugs). Even general anaesthetics (see Ch. 35), which were long thought to produce their effects by an interaction with membrane lipid, now appear to interact mainly with membrane proteins (see Franks & Lieb, 1994). All rules need exceptions, and many antimicrobial and antitumour drugs (Chs 44 and 50), as well as mutagenic and carcinogenic agents (Ch. 51), interact directly

*There are, if one looks hard enough, exceptions to Ehrlich's dictum, drugs that act without being bound to any tissue constituent (for example osmotic diuretics, osmotic purgatives, antacids, heavy metal chelating agents). Nonetheless, the principle remains true for the great majority.

with DNA rather than protein; bisphosphonates, used to treat osteoporosis (Ch. 30), bind to calcium salts in the bone matrix, rendering it toxic to osteoclasts, much like rat poison.

PROTEIN TARGETS FOR DRUG BINDING

Four kinds of regulatory protein are commonly involved as primary drug targets, namely:

- enzymes
- carrier molecules
- ion channels
- receptors.

A few other types of protein (e.g. structural proteins such as tubulin, which specifically binds colchicine; Ch. 16) are known to function as drug targets, and it must be remembered that there exist many drugs with sites of action that are not yet known. Furthermore, many drugs are known to bind (in addition to their primary targets) to plasma proteins (see Ch. 5), as well as to cellular constituents, without producing any obvious physiological effect. Nevertheless, the generalisation that most drugs act on one or other of the four types of protein listed above serves as a good starting point.

Further discussion of the mechanisms by which such binding leads to cellular responses is given in Chapters 3–5.

A NOTE ON TERMINOLOGY

▼ The term *receptor* tends to be used loosely and can cause confusion. Some authors use it to mean any target molecule with which a drug molecule has to combine in order to elicit its specific effect, which can include any of the four types listed. Thus, the voltage-sensitive sodium channel of excitable membranes is sometimes referred to as the 'receptor' for local anaesthetics (see Ch. 43), or the enzyme dihydrofolate reductase as the 'receptor' for methotrexate (Ch. 16). In each case the drug molecule combines with and affects the function of the protein molecule, thus producing its effect. In contrast, adrenaline affects the heart by binding to a receptor protein that has as its primary function the role of recognition site for catecholamines. When adrenaline binds to the receptor, a train of reactions is initiated (see Ch. 3) leading to an increase in force and rate of the heartbeat. In the absence of adrenaline, the receptor is functionally silent.* This, in general, is true of all receptors for endogenous mediators (hormones, neurotransmitters, cytokines, etc.). There is a distinction between *agonists*, which 'activate' the receptors, and *antagonists*, which may combine at the same site without causing activation. Receptors of this type form a key part of the system of chemical communication that all multicellular organisms use to coordinate the activities of their cells and organs. Without them we would be no better than a bucketful of amoebae. The distinction between agonists and antagonists only exists for receptors with this type of physiological regulatory role; we cannot usefully speak of 'agonists' for the noradrenaline carrier, for the voltage-sensitive sodium channel or for dihydrofolate reductase. In pharmacology, it is best to reserve the term 'receptor' for interactions of the regulatory type, where the small molecule (ligand) may function either as an agonist or as an antagonist; in practice this limits use of the term to receptors that have a physiological regulatory function, and this usage will be observed in this book.** More details about the molecular nature of receptors, and the ways in which they influence cell function, are given in Chapter 3.

DRUG SPECIFICITY

For a drug to be useful as either a therapeutic or a scientific tool, it must act selectively on particular cells and tissues. In other words, it must show a high degree of binding-site specificity. Conversely, proteins that function as drug targets generally show a high degree of ligand specificity; they will recognise only ligands of a certain precise type and ignore closely related molecules.

These principles of binding-site and ligand specificity can be clearly recognised in the actions of a mediator such as angiotensin (Ch. 18). This peptide acts strongly on vascular smooth muscle, and on the kidney tubule, but has very little effect on other kinds of smooth muscle or on the intestinal epithelium. Other mediators affect a quite different spectrum of cells and tissues, the pattern in each case being determined by the specific pattern of expression of the protein receptors for the various mediators. A small chemical change, such as conversion of one of the amino acids in angiotensin from L- to D-form or removal of one amino acid from the chain, can inactivate the molecule altogether, since the receptor fails to bind the altered form. The complementary specificity of ligands and binding sites, which gives rise to the very exact molecular recognition properties of proteins, is central to explaining many of the phenomena of pharmacology. It is no exaggeration to say that the ability of proteins to interact in a highly selective way with other molecules—including other proteins—is the basis of living

Targets for drug action

- A drug is a chemical that affects physiological function in a specific way.
- With few exceptions, drugs act on target proteins, namely:
  —enzymes
  —carriers
  —ion channels
  —receptors.
- Specificity is reciprocal: individual classes of drug bind only to certain targets, and individual targets recognise only certain classes of drug.
- No drugs are completely specific in their actions. In many cases, increasing the dose of a drug will cause it to affect targets other than the principal one, and this can lead to side-effects.

*Actually some receptors, such as the benzodiazepine receptor (Ch. 36), show resting activity, which can be either increased or decreased when a ligand molecule binds (see p. 520).

**We break our own rule in Chapter 19 by referring to the 'LDL receptor', a term in common usage to describe a macromolecule—not strictly a receptor according to our definition—that plays a key role in lipoprotein metabolism.

machines. Its relevance to the understanding of drug action will be a recurring theme in this book.

Finally, it must be emphasised that no drug acts with complete specificity. Thus tricyclic antidepressant drugs (Ch. 38) act by blocking monoamine transporters but are notorious for producing side-effects (e.g. dry mouth) related to their ability to block various receptors. In general, the lower the potency of a drug, and the higher the dose needed, the more likely it is that sites of action other than the primary one will assume significance. In clinical terms, this is often associated with the appearance of unwanted side-effects, of which no drug is free.

Since the 1970s, pharmacological research has succeeded in identifying the protein targets of many different types of drug. Drugs such as opiate analgesics (Ch. 40), cannabinoids (Ch. 42), and benzodiazepine tranquillisers (Ch. 36), with actions that were described in exhaustive detail for many years, are now known to target well-defined receptors, which have been fully characterised by gene-cloning techniques (see Ch. 3).

RECEPTOR CLASSIFICATION

▼ Where the action of a drug can be associated with a particular receptor, this provides a valuable means for classification and refinement in drug design. For example, pharmacological analysis of the actions of histamine (see Ch. 15) showed that some of its effects (the H_1 effects, such as smooth muscle contraction) were strongly antagonised by the competitive histamine antagonists then known. Black and his colleagues suggested in 1970 that the remaining actions of histamine, which included its stimulant effect on gastric secretion, might represent a second class of histamine receptor (H_2). Testing a number of histamine analogues, they found that some were selective in producing H_2 effects, with little H_1 activity. By analysing which parts of the histamine molecule conferred this type of specificity, they were able to develop selective antagonists, which proved to be potent in blocking gastric acid secretion, a development of major therapeutic significance (Ch. 24). Two further types of histamine receptor (H_3 and H_4) were recognised later.

Receptor classification based on pharmacological responses continues to be a valuable and widely used approach. Newer experimental approaches have produced other criteria on which to base receptor classification. The direct measurement of ligand binding to receptors (see p. 10) has allowed many new receptor subtypes to be defined: subtypes that could not easily be distinguished by studies of drug effects. Molecular cloning (see Ch. 3) provided a completely new basis for classification at a much finer level of detail than can be reached through pharmacological analysis. Finally, analysis of the biochemical pathways that are linked to receptor activation (see Ch. 3) provides yet another basis for classification. The result of this data explosion has been that receptor classification has suddenly become very much more detailed, with a proliferation of receptor subtypes for all of the main types of ligand; more worryingly, alternative molecular and biochemical classifications began to spring up that were incompatible with the accepted pharmacologically defined receptor classes. Responding to this growing confusion, the International Union of Pharmacological Sciences (IUPHAR) convened expert working groups to produce agreed receptor classifications for the major types, taking into account the pharmacological, molecular and biochemical information available.* These wise people have a hard task; their conclusions will be neither perfect nor final but are essential to ensure a consistent terminology. To the student, this may seem an arcane exercise in taxonomy, generating much detail but little illumination. There is a danger that the tedious lists of drug names, actions and side-effects that used to burden the subject will be replaced by exhaustive tables of receptors, ligands and transduction pathways. In this book, we have tried to avoid detail for its own sake and include only such information on receptor classification as seems interesting in its own right or is helpful in explaining the actions of important drugs. A useful summary of known receptor classes is now published annually (Trends in Pharmacological Sciences, Receptor Supplement).

*Published as The IUPHAR compendium of receptor characterization and classification 1998. IUPHAR Media, London.

DRUG–RECEPTOR INTERACTIONS

Occupation of a receptor by a drug molecule may or may not result in *activation* of the receptor. By activation, we mean that the receptor is affected by the bound molecule in such a way as to elicit a tissue response. The molecular mechanisms associated with receptor activation are discussed in Chapter 3. Binding and activation represent two distinct steps in the generation of the receptor-mediated response by an agonist (Fig. 2.1). If a drug binds to the receptor without causing activation and thereby prevents the agonist from binding, it is termed a *receptor antagonist.* The tendency of a drug to bind to the receptors is governed by its *affinity*, whereas the tendency for it, once bound, to activate the receptor is denoted by its *efficacy*. These terms are defined more precisely below (pp. 15–17). Drugs of high potency will generally have a high affinity for the receptors and thus occupy a significant proportion of the receptors even at low concentrations. Agonists will also possess high efficacy, whereas antagonists will, in the simplest case, have zero efficacy. Drugs with intermediate levels of efficacy, such that even when 100% of the receptors are occupied the tissue response is submaximal, are known as *partial agonists*, to distinguish them from *full agonists*, the efficacy of which is sufficient that they can elicit a maximal tissue response. These concepts, even though we now see them as

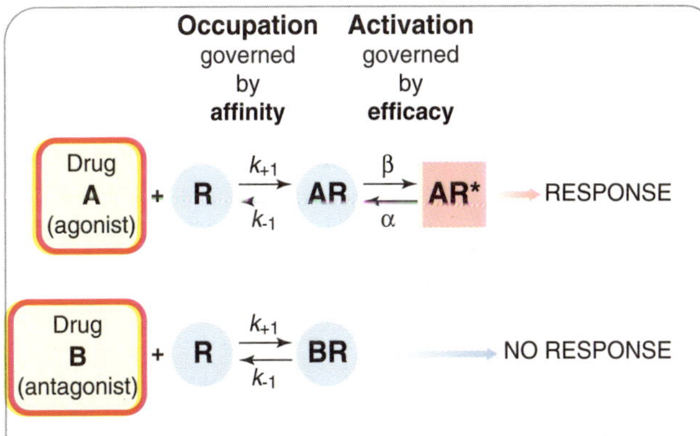

Fig. 2.1 The distinction between drug binding and receptor activation. The rate constants k_{+1}, k_{-1}, β and α, which apply to the binding and activation reactions, respectively are referred to in the text (p. 17). Ligand A is an agonist, since it leads to activation of the receptor, whereas ligand B is an antagonist.

an over-simplified description of events at the molecular level (see Ch. 3), provide a useful basis for characterising drug effects.

We now discuss certain aspects in more detail, namely drug binding, agonist concentration–effect curves, competitive antagonism, partial agonists and the nature of efficacy and spare receptors. Understanding these concepts at a qualitative level is sufficient for many purposes, but for more detailed analysis a quantitative formulation is needed (see pp. 15–17).

THE BINDING OF DRUGS TO RECEPTORS

The binding of drugs to receptors can often be measured directly by the use of radioactive drug molecules (usually with ^3H, ^{14}C or ^{125}I). The main requirements are that the radioactive ligand (which may be an agonist or antagonist) must bind with high affinity and specificity, and that it can be labelled to a sufficient specific radioactivity to enable minute amounts of binding to be measured. The usual procedure is to incubate samples of the tissue (or membrane fragments) with various concentrations of radioactive drug until equilibrium is reached. The tissue is then removed, or the membrane fragments separated by filtration or centrifugation, and dissolved in scintillation fluid for measurement of its radioactive content.

In such experiments, there is invariably a certain amount of 'non-specific binding' (i.e. drug taken up by structures other than receptors), which obscures the specific component and needs to be kept to a minimum. The amount of non-specific binding is estimated by measuring the radioactivity taken up in the presence of a saturating concentration of a (non-radioactive) ligand that inhibits completely the binding of the radioactive drug to the receptors, leaving behind the non-specific component. This is then subtracted from the total binding to give an estimate of specific binding (Fig. 2.2). The *binding curve* (Fig. 2.2B) defines the relationship between concentration and the amount of drug bound (*B*), and in most cases it fits well to the relationship predicted theoretically (see Fig. 2.8, below), allowing the *affinity* of the drug for the receptors to be estimated, as well as the *binding capacity* (B_{max}), representing the density of receptors in the tissue.

Autoradiography can also be used to investigate the distribution of receptors in structures such as the brain, and direct labelling with ligands containing positron-emitting isotopes is now used to obtain images by positron-emission tomography (PET) of receptor distribution in humans. This technique has been used, for example, to measure the degree of dopamine receptor blockade produced by antipsychotic drugs in the brains of schizophrenic patients (see Ch. 37). When combined with pharmacological studies, binding measurements have proved very valuable. It has, for example, been confirmed that the spare receptor hypothesis (p. 15) for muscarinic receptors in smooth muscle is correct; agonists are found to bind, in general, with rather low affinity, and a maximal biological effect occurs at low receptor occupancy. It has also been shown, in skeletal muscle and other tissues, that denervation leads to an increase in the number of receptors in the target cell, a finding that accounts, at least in part, for the phenomenon of denervation supersensitivity. More generally, it appears that receptors tend to increase in number, usually over the course of a few days, if the relevant hormone or transmitter is absent or scarce, and to decrease in number if it is in excess, a process of adaptation to drugs or hormones resulting from continued administration (see p. 19).

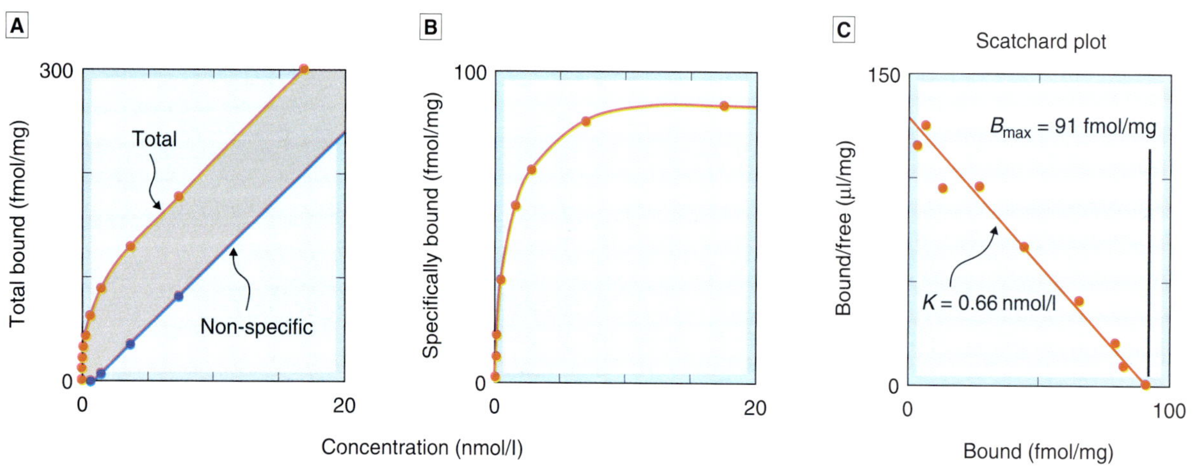

Fig. 2.2 Measurement of receptor binding (β-adrenoceptors in cardiac cell membranes). The ligand was [^3H]-cyanopindolol, a derivative of pindolol (see Ch. 11). **A** Measurements of total and non-specific binding at equilibrium. Non-specific binding is measured in the presence of a saturating concentration of a non-radioactive β-adrenoceptor agonist, which prevents the radioactive ligand from binding to β-adrenoceptors. The difference between the two lines represents specific binding. **B** Specific binding plotted against concentration. The curve is a rectangular hyperbola (equation 2.5). **C** Scatchard plot (equation 2.7, p. 16). This gives a straight line from which the binding parameters *K* and B_{max} can be calculated.

Binding curves with agonists are more difficult to interpret than those with antagonists, since they often reveal an apparent heterogeneity among receptors. For example, agonist binding to muscarinic receptors (Ch. 10) and also to β-adrenoceptors (Ch. 11) suggests at least two populations of binding sites with different affinities. This may be because the receptors can exist either unattached or coupled within the membrane to another macromolecule, the G-protein (see Ch. 3), which constitutes part of the transduction system through which the receptor exerts its regulatory effect. Antagonist binding does not show this complexity, probably because antagonists, by their nature, do not lead to the secondary event of G-protein coupling. Agonist affinity has proved to be an elusive concept, a fact that has generated an algebraic paperchase in the pharmacological literature, with many enthusiastic followers.

AGONIST CONCENTRATION-EFFECT CURVES

Though binding can be measured directly, it is usually a biological response, such as a rise in blood pressure, contraction or relaxation of a strip of smooth muscle in an organ bath, or the activation of an enzyme, that we are interested in, and this is often plotted as a *concentration–effect* or *dose–response curve*, as in Figure 2.3. Such curves allow us to estimate the maximal response that the drug can produce (E_{max}), and the concentration or dose needed to produce a 50% maximal response (EC_{50} or ED_{50}), parameters, which are useful for comparing the potencies of different drugs that produce qualitatively similar effects (see Ch. 4). Though they look similar to the binding curves in Figure 2.2, concentration–effect curves cannot be used to measure the affinity of agonist drugs for their receptors, since the physiological response produced is not, as a rule, directly proportional to occupancy. For an integrated physiological response, such as a rise in arterial blood pressure produced by adrenaline (epinephrine), many factors interact. Adrenaline (see Ch. 11) increases cardiac output and constricts some blood vessels while dilating others, and the change in arterial pressure itself evokes a reflex response that modifies the primary response to the drug. The final effect will clearly not be a direct measure of receptor occupancy in this instance, and the same is true of most drug-induced effects.

In interpreting concentration–effect curves, it must be remembered that the concentration of the drug at the receptors may differ from the known concentration in the organ bath. Agonists may be subject to rapid enzymic degradation or uptake by cells as they diffuse from the surface towards their site of action, and a steady state can be reached in which the agonist concentration at the receptors is very much less than the concentration in the bath. In the case of acetylcholine, for example, which is hydrolysed by cholinesterase present in most tissues (see Ch. 10), the concentration reaching the receptors can be less than 1% of that in the bath, and an even bigger difference has been found with noradrenaline (norepinephrine), which is avidly taken up by sympathetic nerve terminals in many tissues (Ch. 11). Thus, even if the concentration–effect curve looks just like a facsimile of the binding curve, as in Figure 2.3, it cannot be used directly to determine the affinity of the agonist for the receptors.

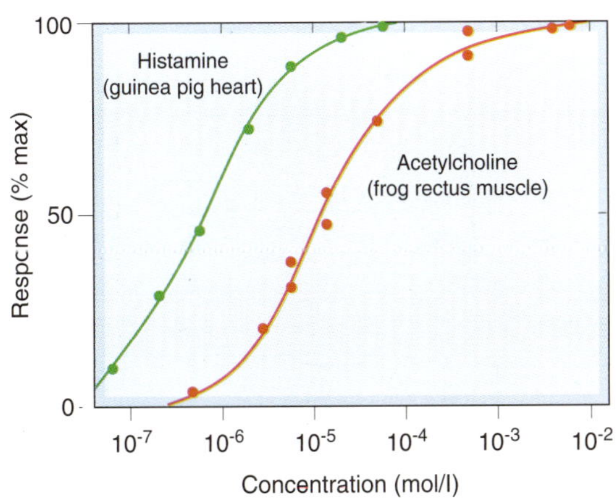

Fig. 2.3 Experimentally observed concentration–effect curves. Though the lines, drawn according to the binding equation 2.5, fit the points well, such curves do not give correct estimates of the affinity of drugs for receptors. This is because the relationship between receptor occupancy and response is usually non-linear.

COMPETITIVE ANTAGONISM

Competitive antagonism describes the common situation whereby a drug binds selectively to a particular type of receptor without activating it, but in such a way as to prevent the binding of the agonist. There is often some similarity between the chemical structures of the agonist and antagonist molecules. The two drugs compete with each other, since the receptor can bind only one drug molecule at a time. At a given agonist concentration, the agonist occupancy will be reduced in the presence of the antagonist. However, because the two are in competition, raising the agonist concentration can restore the agonist occupany (and hence the tissue response). The antagonism is, therefore, said to be *surmountable*, in contrast to

Binding of drugs to receptors

- Binding of drugs to receptors necessarily obeys the Law of Mass Action.
- At equilibrium, receptor occupancy is related to drug concentration by the Hill–Langmuir equation (2.7).
- The higher the affinity of the drug for the receptor, the lower the concentration at which it produces a given level of occupancy.
- The same principles apply when two or more drugs compete for the same receptors; each has the effect of reducing the apparent affinity for the other.

other types of antagonism (see below) where increasing the agonist concentration fails to overcome the blocking effect. A simple theoretical analysis (see p. 17) predicts that, in the presence of a fixed concentration of the antagonist, the log concentration–effect curve for the agonist will be shifted to the right, without any change in slope or maximum—the hallmark of competitive antagonism. The shift is expressed as a *dose ratio* (the ratio by which the agonist concentration has to be increased in the presence of the antagonist in order to restore a given level of response). Theory predicts that the dose ratio increases linearly with the concentration of the antagonist (see p. 17). These predictions are often borne out in practice (see Fig. 2.4), and examples of competitive antagonism are very common in pharmacology. The surmountability of the block by the antagonist may be important in practice, since it allows the functional effect of the agonist to be restored by an increase in concentration. With other types of antagonism (see below), the block is usually insurmountable.

The salient features of competitive antagonism are:

- shift of the agonist log concentration–effect curve to the right, without change of slope or maximum
- linear relationship between dose ratio and antagonist concentration
- evidence of competition from binding studies.

Competitive antagonism is the most direct mechanism by which one drug can reduce the effect of another (or of an endogenous mediator), and several examples are listed in Table 3.1; other mechanisms that are commonly encountered are discussed below (p. 18).

Competitive antagonism

- Reversible competitive antagonism is the commonest and most important type of antagonism; it has two main characteristics:
  —in the presence of the antagonist, the agonist log concentration–effect curve is shifted to the right without change in slope or maximum, the extent of the shift being a measure of the dose ratio
  —the dose ratio increases linearly with antagonist concentration; the slope of this line is a measure of the affinity of the antagonist for the receptor.
- Antagonist affinity, measured in this way, is widely used as a basis for receptor classification.

PARTIAL AGONISTS AND THE CONCEPT OF EFFICACY

So far, we have considered drugs either as agonists, which in some way 'activate' the receptor when they occupy it, or as antagonists, which cause no activation. However, the ability of a drug molecule to activate the receptor is actually a graded, rather than an all-or-nothing, property. If a series of chemically related agonist drugs acting on the same receptors is tested on a given biological system, it is often found that the maximal response (the largest response that can be produced by that drug in high concentration) differs from one drug to another. Some compounds (known as *full agonists*) can produce a maximal response (the largest response that the tissue is capable of giving), whereas others (*partial agonists*) can only produce a submaximal response (Fig. 2.5). The difference between full and

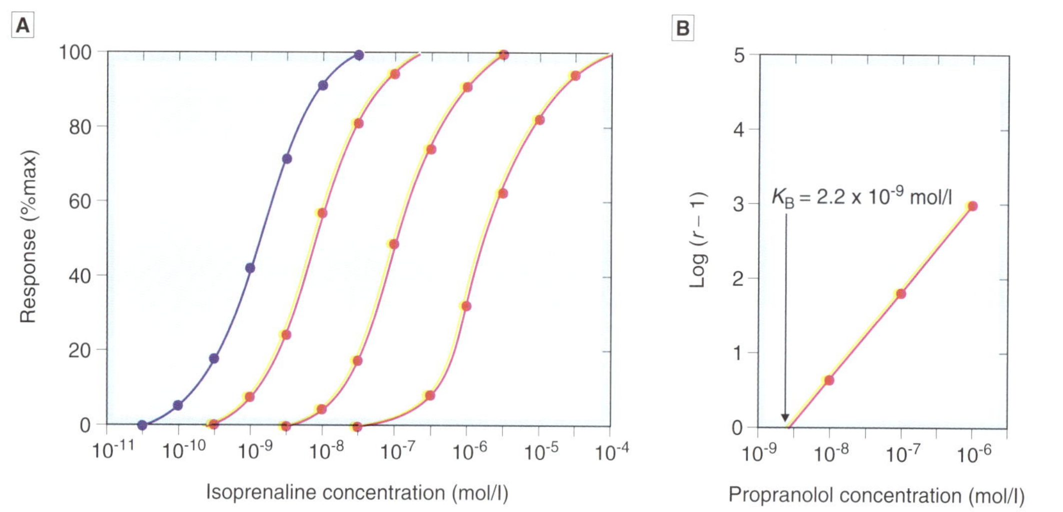

Fig. 2.4 Competitive antagonism of isoprenaline by propranolol measured on isolated guinea-pig atria. A Concentration–effect curves at various propranolol concentrations (indicated on the curves). Note the progressive shift to the right without a change of slope or maximum. B Schild plot (equation 2.10). The equilibrium constant (K) for propranolol is given by the abscissal intercept 2.2 × 10^{-9} mol/l. (Results from: Potter L T 1967 J Pharmacol 155: 91.)

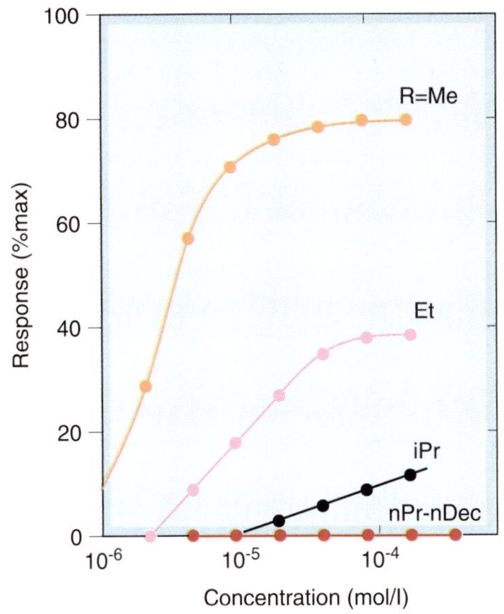

Fig. 2.5 Partial agonists. Concentration–effect curves for substituted methonium compounds on frog rectus abdominis muscle. The compounds were members of the decamethonium series (Ch. 7), $RMe_2N^+(CH_2)_{10}N^+Me_2R$. The maximum response obtainable decreases (i.e. efficacy decreases) as the size of R is increased. With R = nPr or larger, the compounds cause no response and are pure antagonists. (Results from: Van Rossum J M 1958 Pharmacodynamics of cholinometic and cholinolytic drugs. St Catherine's Press, Bruges.)

partial agonists lies in the relationship between occupancy and response.

Figure 2.6 shows the relationship between occupancy and concentration for drugs with equilibrium constants of 1.0 μmol/l. Drug **a** is a full agonist, producing a maximal response at about 0.2 μmol/l, the relationship between response and occupancy being shown by the steep curve in B. Comparable plots for a partial agonist (**b**) are shown as the shallow curves in A and B, the essential difference being that the response at any given occupancy is much smaller for the partial agonist, which cannot produce a maximal response even at 100% occupancy. This can be expressed quantitatively in terms of *efficacy*, a parameter originally defined by Stephenson (1956) that describes the 'strength' of a single drug–receptor complex in evoking a response of the tissue.

▼ Subsequently, it was appreciated that characteristics of the tissue (e.g. the number of receptors that it possesses and the nature of the coupling between the receptor and the response; see Ch. 3), as well as of the drug itself, were important, and the concept of intrinsic efficacy was developed (see Jenkinson 1996, Kenakin 1997). The relationship between occupancy and response can thus be represented:

$$\text{Response} = f\left(\frac{\varepsilon N_{tot} x_A}{x_A + K_A}\right)$$

In this equation, f (the transducer function) and N_{tot} (the total number of receptors) are characteristics of the tissue; ε (the intrinsic efficacy) and K_A (the equilibrium constant) are characteristics of the agonist. The importance of this formal representation is that it explains how differences in the transducer function and the density of receptors in different tissues can result in the same agonist, acting on the same receptor, appearing as a full agonist in one tissue and as a partial agonist in another. By the same token, the relative potencies of two agonists may be different in different tissues, even though the receptor is the same.

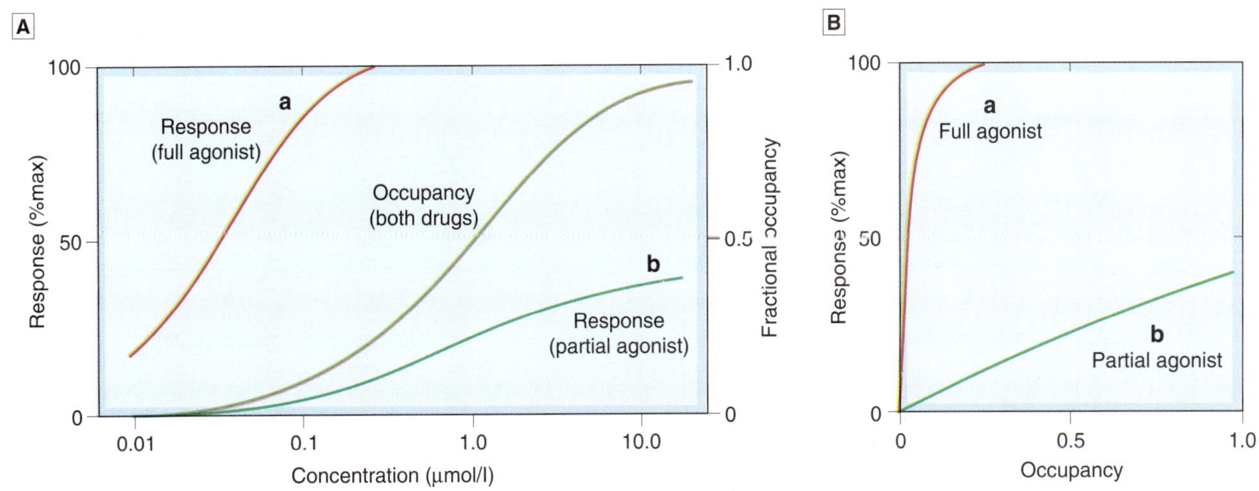

Fig. 2.6 Theoretical occupancy and response curves for full and partial agonists. A The occupancy curve is for both drugs, the response curves a and b are for full and partial agonist, respectively. B The relationship between response and occupancy for full and partial agonist, corresponding to the response curves in A. Note that curve a produces maximal response at about 20% occupancy, while curve b produces only a submaximal response even at 100% occupancy.

For a more detailed discussion of drug–receptor interactions, see Jenkinson (1996) and Kenakin (1997).

It would be nice to be able to explain what efficacy means in physical terms, and to understand why one drug may be an agonist while another, chemically very similar, is an antagonist. We are beginning to understand the molecular events underlying receptor activation (described in Ch. 3) but can still give no clear answer to the question of why some ligands are agonists and some are antagonists, though the simple theoretical two-state model described below (p. 17) provides a useful starting point.

Despite its uncertain theoretical status, efficacy is a concept of great practical importance. Adrenaline (epinephrine) and propranolol have comparable affinities for the β-adrenoceptor but differ in efficacy. Woebetide the doctor—and the student, for that matter—who confuses them. Efficacy matters!

CONSTITUTIVE RECEPTOR ACTIVATION AND INVERSE AGONISTS

▼ Though we are accustomed to thinking that receptors are activated only when an agonist molecule is bound, there are examples (see de Ligt et al., 2000) where an appreciable level of activation may exist even when no ligand is present. These include receptors for benzodiazepines (see Ch. 36), cannabinoids (Ch. 52), dopamine (Ch. 33) and several other mediators. Furthermore, receptor mutations occur—either spontaneously, in some disease states or experimentally created (see Ch. 4)—that result in appreciable activation in the absence of any ligand (*constitutive activation*). Simply overexpressing β-adrenoceptors in an engineered cell line can result in their constitutive activation (Bond et al., 1995), a result that may prove to have major pathophysiological implications. Under these conditions, it may be possible for a ligand to *reduce* the level of constitutive activation; such drugs are known as *inverse agonists* (Fig. 2.7; see de Ligt et al., 2000) to distinguish them from simple competitive antagonists, which do not by themselves affect the level of activation. Inverse agonists can be regarded as drugs with negative efficacy, to distinguish them from agonists, (positive efficacy) and competitive antagonists (zero efficacy). New examples of constitutively active receptors and inverse agonists are emerging with increasing frequency (mainly among G-protein-coupled receptors; see Daeffler & Landry, 2000; Seifert & Wenzel-Seifert, 2002), and it is likely that future drugs based on the inverse agonist principle will be developed for clinical use. The two-state model described below explains these operational distinctions in terms of the relative affinity of different ligands for the resting and activated states of the receptor. Most receptors—like cats—seem to have a strong preference for the inactive state; for these, there is no practical difference between a competitive antagonist and an inverse agonist. Constitutive activation is a relatively recent discovery, however, and may prove to be of greater pharmacological significance than is realised at present (see Milligan et al., 1995).

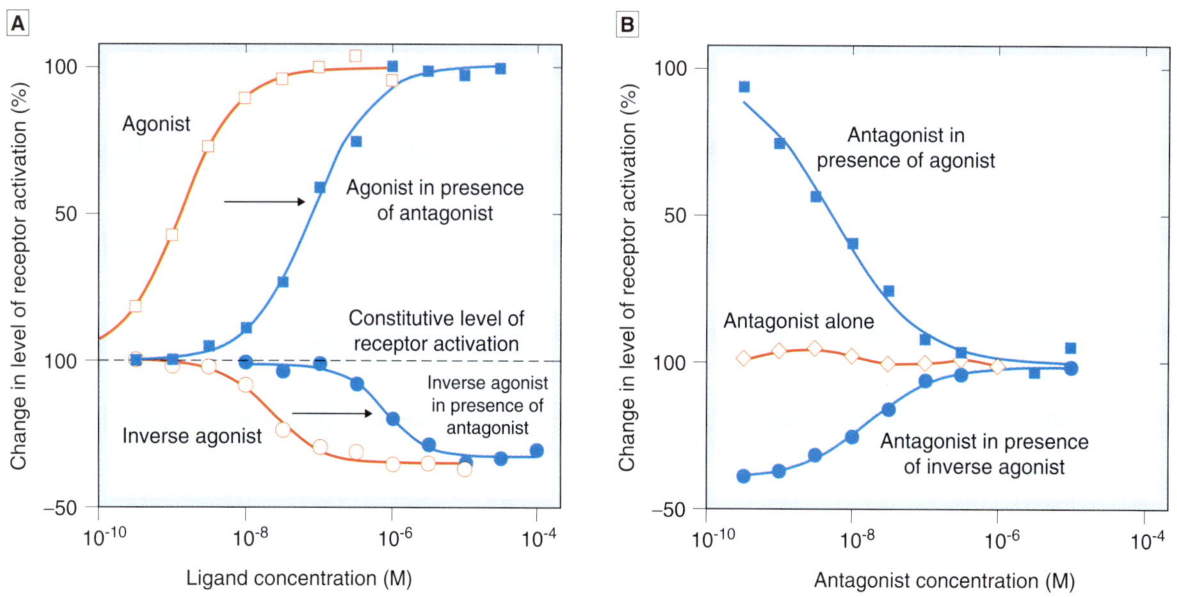

Fig. 2.7 The interaction of a competitive antagonist with normal and inverse agonists in a system that shows receptor activation in the absence of any added ligands (constitutive activation). A The degree of receptor activation (vertical scale) increases in the presence of an agonist (open squares) and decreases in the presence of an inverse agonist (open circles). Addition of a competitive antagonist shifts both curves to the right (closed symbols). B The antagonist on its own does not alter the level of constitutive activity (open symbols) since it has equal affinity for the active and inactive states of the receptor. In the presence of an agonist (closed squares) or an inverse agonist (closed circles), the antagonist restores the system towards the constitutive level of activity. These data (reproduced with permission from Newman-Tancredi A et al. 1997 Br J Pharmacol 120: 737–739) were obtained with cloned human 5-hydroxytryptamine (5-HT) receptors expressed in a cell line. (Agonist, 5-carboxamidotryptamine; inverse agonist, spiperone; antagonist, WAY 100635; ligand concentration (M = mol/l); see Ch. 9 for information on 5-HT receptor pharmacology.)

SPARE RECEPTORS

▼ Stephenson (1956), studying the actions of acetylcholine analogues in isolated tissues, found that many full agonists were capable of eliciting maximal responses at very low occupancies, often less than 1%. This means that the mechanism linking the response to receptor occupancy has a substantial reserve capacity. Such systems may be said to possess *spare receptors*, or a *receptor reserve*. This is common with drugs that elicit smooth muscle contraction but less so for other types of receptor-mediated response, such as secretion, smooth muscle relaxation or cardiac stimulation, where the effect is more nearly proportional to receptor occupancy. The existence of spare receptors does not imply any functional subdivision of the receptor pool, but merely that the pool is larger than the number needed to evoke a full response. This surplus of receptors over the number actually needed might seem a wasteful biological arrangement. It means, however, that a given number of agonist–receptor complexes, corresponding to a given level of biological response, can be reached with a lower concentration of hormone or neurotransmitter than would be the case if fewer receptors were provided. Economy of hormone or transmitter secretion is thus achieved at the expense of providing more receptors.

QUANTITATIVE ASPECTS OF DRUG–RECEPTOR INTERACTIONS

Here we present some aspects of so-called *receptor theory*, which is based on applying the Law of Mass Action to the drug–receptor interaction and which has served well as a framework for interpreting a large body of quantitative experimental data.

The binding reaction

▼ The first step in drug action on specific receptors is the formation of a reversible drug–receptor complex, the reactions being governed by the law of mass action. Suppose that a piece of tissue, such as heart muscle or smooth muscle, contains a total number of receptors, N_{tot}, for an agonist such as adrenaline. When the tissue is exposed to adrenaline at concentration x_A and allowed to come to equilibrium, a certain number, N_A, of the receptors will become occupied, and the number of vacant receptors will be reduced to $N_{tot} - N_A$. Normally, the number of adrenaline molecules applied to the tissue in solution greatly exceeds N_{tot}, so that the binding reaction does not appreciably reduce x_A. The magnitude of the response produced by the adrenaline will be related (even if we do not know exactly how) to the number of receptors occupied, so it is useful to consider what quantitative relationship is predicted between N_A and x_A. The reaction can be represented by:

$$\underset{(x_A)}{\underset{\text{drug}}{A}} + \underset{(N_{tot} - N_A)}{\underset{\text{free receptor}}{R}} \underset{k_{-1}}{\overset{k_{+1}}{\rightleftharpoons}} \underset{(N_A)}{\underset{\text{complex}}{AR}}$$

The Law of Mass Action (which states that the rate of a chemical reaction is proportional to the product of the concentrations of reactants) can be applied to this reaction.

$$\text{Rate of forward reaction} = k_{+1}x_A(N_{tot} - N_A) \quad (2.1)$$

$$\text{Rate of backward reaction} = k_{-1}N_A \quad (2.2)$$

At equilibrium, the two rates are equal:

$$k_{+1}x_A(N_{tot} - N_A) = k_{-1}N_A \quad (2.3)$$

The proportion of receptors occupied or 'occupancy', (p_A) is N_A/N_{tot}, which is independent of N_{tot} and is given by:

$$p_A = \frac{x_A}{x_A + k_{-1}/k_{+1}} \quad (2.4)$$

Defining the equilibrium constant for the binding reaction, $K_A = k_{-1}/k_{+1}$, equation 2.4 can be written:

$$p_A = \frac{x_A/K_A}{x_A/K_A + 1} \quad (2.5)$$

This important result is known as the Hill–Langmuir equation*.

The equilibrium constant,** K_A, is a characteristic of the drug and of the receptor; it has the dimensions of concentration and is numerically equal to the concentration of drug required to occupy 50% of the sites at equilibrium. (Verify from equation 2.5 that when $x_A = K_A$, $p_A = 0.5$.) The higher the affinity of the drug for the receptors, the lower will be the value of K_A. Equation 2.5 describes the relationship between occupancy and drug concentration and generates a characteristic curve known as a rectangular hyperbola, as shown in Figure 2.8A. It is common in pharmacological work to use a logarithmic scale of concentration; this converts the hyperbola to a symmetrical sigmoid curve (Fig. 2.8B).

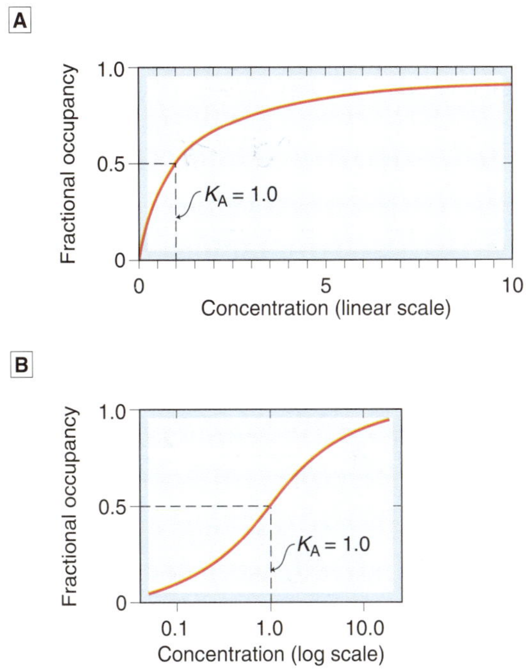

Fig. 2.8 Theoretical relationship between occupancy and ligand concentration. The relationship is plotted according to equation (2.5). **A** Plotted with a linear concentration scale, this curve is a rectangular hyperbola. **B** Plotted with a log concentration scale, it is a symmetrical sigmoid curve.

*A. V. Hill first published it in 1909, when he was still a medical student. Langmuir, a physical chemist working on gas adsorption, derived it independently in 1916. Both subsequently won Nobel prizes. Until recently, it was known to pharmacologists as the Langmuir equation, even though Hill deserves the credit.

**The equilibrium constant is sometimes called the *dissociation constant*. Some authors prefer to use the reciprocal of K_A, referred to as an *affinity constant*, in these expressions, which can cause confusion to the unwary.

The same approach is used to analyse data from experiments in which drug binding is measured directly (see p. 10). In this case, the relationship between the amount bound (B) and ligand concentration (x_A) should be:

$$B = B_{max} x_A/(x_A + K_A) \tag{2.6}$$

where B_{max} is the total number of binding sites in the preparation (often expressed as picomoles per milligram protein). To display the results in linear form, equation 2.6 may be rearranged to:

$$B/x_A = B_{max}/K_A - B/K_A \tag{2.7}$$

A plot of B/x_A against B (known as a Scatchard plot; Fig. 2.2C) gives a straight line from which both B_{max} and K_A can be estimated. Statistically, this procedure is not without problems, and it is now usual to estimate these parameters from the untransformed binding values by an iterative non-linear curve-fitting procedure.

To this point our analysis has considered the binding of one ligand to a homogeneous population of receptors. To get closer to real-life pharmacology, we must consider (a) what happens when more than one ligand is present, and (b) how the tissue response is related to receptor occupancy.

Binding when more than one drug is present

▼ Suppose that two drugs, A and B, which bind to the same receptor with equilibrium constants K_A and K_B, respectively, are present at concentrations x_A and x_B. If the two drugs *compete* (i.e. the receptor can accommodate only one at a time), then, by application of the same reasoning as for the one-drug situation described above, the occupancy by drug A is given by:

$$p_A = \frac{x_A/K_A}{x_A/K_A + x_B/K_B + 1} \tag{2.8}$$

Comparing this result with equation 2.5 shows that adding drug B, as expected, reduces the occupancy by drug A. Figure 2.9A shows the predicted binding curves for A in the presence of increasing concentrations of B, demonstrating the shift without any change of slope or maximum that characterises the pharmacological effect of a

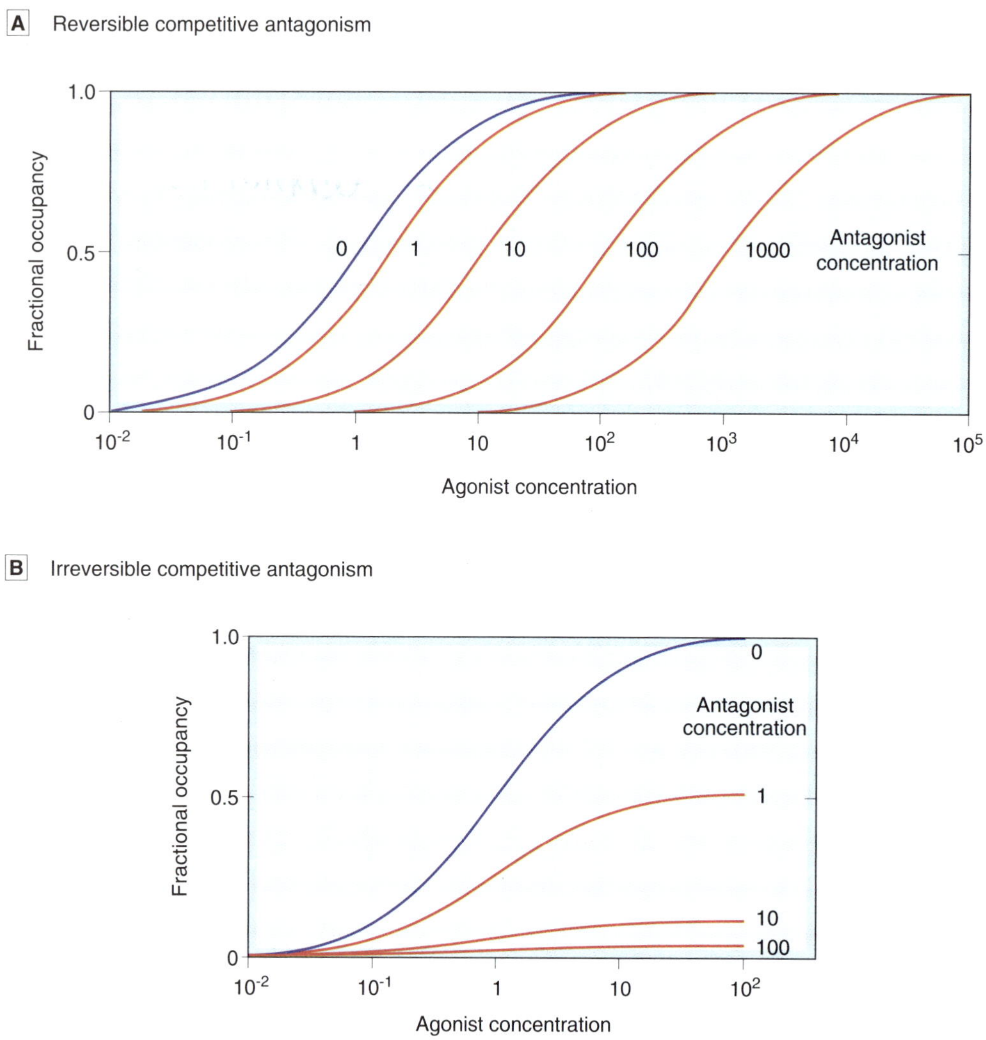

Fig. 2.9 Hypothetical agonist concentration–occupancy curves in the presence of reversible and irreversible competitive antagonists. The concentrations are normalised with respect to the equilibrium constants (K, i.e. 1.0 corresponds to a concentration equal to K, and results in 50% occupancy). **A** Reversible competitive antagonism. **B** Irreversible competitive antagonism.

competitive antagonist (see Fig. 2.4). The extent of the rightward shift, on a logarithmic scale, represents the *ratio* (r_A, given by x_A'/x_A where x_A' is the increased concentration of A) by which the concentration of A must be increased to overcome the competition by B. Rearranging 2.8 shows that

$$r_A = (x_B/K_B) + 1 \qquad (2.9)$$

Thus r_A depends only on the concentration and equilibrium constant of the competing drug B, not on the concentration or equilibrium constant of A.

If A is an agonist, and B is a competitive antagonist, and we assume that the response of the tissue will be a function of p_A (not necessarily a linear function), then the value of r_A determined from the shift of the agonist concentration–effect curve at different antagonist concentrations can be used to estimate the equilibrium constant K_B for the antagonist. Such pharmacological estimates of r_A are commonly termed *agonist dose ratios*. This simple and very useful equation (2.9) is known as the *Schild equation*, after the pharmacologist who first used it to analyse drug antagonism.

Equation (2.9) can be expressed logarithmically in the form:

$$\log(r - 1) = \log x_B - \log K_B \qquad (2.10)$$

Thus a plot of $\log(r - 1)$ against $\log x_B$, usually called a Schild plot (as in Fig. 2.4), should give a straight line with unit slope and an abscissal intercept equal to $\log K_B$. Following the pH and pK notation, antagonist potency can be expressed as a pA_2 value; under conditions of competitive antagonism $pA_2 = -\log K_B$. Numerically, pA_2 is defined as the negative logarithm of the molar concentration of antagonist required to produce an agonist dose ratio equal to 2. As with pH notation, its principal advantage is that it produces simple numbers, a pA_2 of 6.5 being equivalent to a K_B of 3.2×10^{-7} mol/l.

This analysis of competitive antagonism shows the following characteristics of the dose ratio *r*:

- it depends only on the concentration and equilibrium constant of the antagonist and not on the sise of response that is chosen as a reference point for the measurements
- it does not depend on the equilibrium constant for the agonist
- it increases linearly with x_B, and the slope of a plot of $(r - 1)$ against x_B is equal to $1/K_B$; this relationship, being independent of the characteristics of the agonist, should be the same for all agonists that act on the same population of receptors.

These predictions have been verified for many examples of competitive antagonism (Fig. 2.4).

Receptor activation and the nature of efficacy

▼ As illustrated in Figure 2.1, agonists and antagonists both bind to receptors, but only agonists activate them. How can we express this difference in theoretical terms? The simplest formulation (see Fig. 2.1) envisages that the occupied receptor can switch from its 'resting' (R) state to an activated (R*) state, R* being favoured by binding of an agonist but not an antagonist molecule.

The tendency for the occupied receptor, AR, to convert to the activated form, AR*, will depend on the equilibrium constant for this reaction, β/α.

For a pure antagonist, $\beta/\alpha = 0$, implying that there is no conversion to the activated state, whereas for an agonist, β/α has a finite value, which will be different for different drugs. Suppose that for drug X, β/α is small, so that only a small proportion of the occupied receptors will be activated even when the receptor occupancy approaches 100%, whereas for drug Y, β/α is large and most of the occupied receptors will be activated. The constant β/α is, therefore, a measure of efficacy (see p. 13). As we now know (see p. 14), receptors may show constitutive activation (i.e. the R* conformation can exist without any ligand being bound, so the added drug encounters an equilibrium mixture of R and R* (Fig. 2.10). If it has a higher affinity for R* than for R, the drug will cause a shift of the equilibrium towards R* (i.e. it will promote activation and be classed as an agonist). If its preference for R* is very large, nearly all of the occupied receptors will adopt the R* conformation, and the drug will be a full agonist (positive efficacy); if it shows no preference, the prevailing R:R* equilibrium will not be disturbed, and the drug will be a competitive antagonist (zero efficacy), whereas if it prefers R it will shift the equilibrium towards R, and be an inverse agonist (negative efficacy). We can, therefore, think of efficacy as a property determined by the relative affinity of a ligand for R and R*: a formulation known as the *two-state hypothesis*, which is useful in that it puts a physical interpretation on the otherwise mysterious meaning of efficacy.

In this section we have avoided going into great detail and have oversimplified the theory considerably. As we learn more about the actual molecular details of how receptors work to produce their biological effects (see Ch. 3), the shortcomings of this theoretical treatment become more obvious. Particular complications arise when we include the involvement of G-proteins (see Ch. 3) in the reaction scheme, and when we allow for the fact that receptor 'activation' is not a simple on–off switch, as the two-state model assumes, but may take different forms. It is as though the same receptor can turn on a tap or a light bulb, depending on which agonist does the talking. Attempts by theoreticians to allow for such possibilities lead to some unwieldy algebra and fancy three-dimensional graphics, but somehow the molecules always seem to remain one step ahead. Nevertheless, the two-state model remains a useful basis for developing quantitative models of drug action. The book by Kenakin (1997) is recommended as an introduction.

DRUG ANTAGONISM

Frequently, the effect of one drug is diminished or completely abolished in the presence of another. One mechanism,

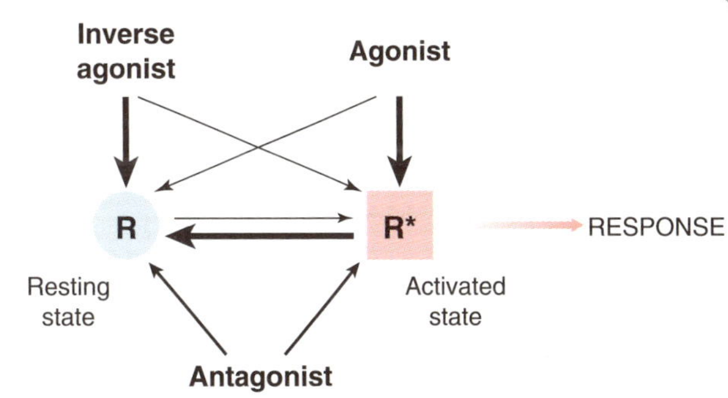

Fig. 2.10 The two-state model. The receptor is shown in two conformational states, 'resting' (R) and 'activated' R*, which exist in equilibrium. Normally, when no ligand is present, the equilibrium lies far to the left, and few receptors are found in the R* state. For constitutively active receptors, an appreciable proportion of receptors adopt the R* conformation in the absence of any ligand. Agonists have higher affinity for R* than for R, so shift the equilibrium towards R*. The greater the relative affinity for R* with respect to R, the greater the efficacy of the agonist. An inverse agonist has higher affinity for R than for R* and so shifts the equilibrium to the left. A 'neutral' antagonist has equal affinity for R and R* so does not by itself affect the conformational equilibrium but reduces by competition the binding of other ligands.

Agonists, antagonists and efficacy

- Drugs acting on receptors may be *agonists* or *antagonists*.
- Agonists initiate changes in cell function, producing effects of various types; antagonists bind to receptors without initiating such changes.
- Agonist potency depends on two parameters: *affinity* (i.e. tendency to bind to receptors) and *efficacy* (i.e. ability, once bound, to initiate changes that lead to effects).
- For antagonists, efficacy is zero.
- Full agonists (which can produce maximal effects) have high efficacy; partial agonists (which can produce only submaximal effects) have intermediate efficacy.
- According to the two-state model, efficacy reflects the relative affinity of the compound for the resting and activated states of the receptor. Agonists show selectivity for the activated state; antagonists show no selectivity.
- Inverse agonists show selectivity for the resting state of the receptor, this being of significance only in unusual situations where the receptors show constitutive activity.

competitive antagonism, was discussed earlier; a more complete classification includes the following mechanisms:

- chemical antagonism
- pharmacokinetic antagonism
- antagonism by receptor block
- non-competitive antagonism, i.e. block of receptor–effector linkage
- physiological antagonism.

CHEMICAL ANTAGONISM

Chemical antagonism refers to the uncommon situation where the two substances combine in solution; as a result, the effect of the active drug is lost. Examples include the use of chelating agents (e.g. **dimercaprol**) that bind to heavy metals and thus reduce their toxicity, and the use of neutralising antibodies against protein mediators, such as cytokines and growth factors, a strategy recently applied for therapeutic use (see Ch. 13).

PHARMACOKINETIC ANTAGONISM

Pharmacokinetic antagonism describes the situation in which the 'antagonist' effectively reduces the concentration of the active drug at its site of action. This can happen in various ways. The rate of metabolic degradation of the active drug may be increased (e.g. the reduction of the anticoagulant effect of **warfarin** when an agent that accelerates its hepatic metabolism, such as **phenobarbital**, is given; see Chs 6 and 50). Alternatively, the rate of absorption of the active drug from the gastrointestinal tract may be reduced, or the rate of renal excretion may be increased. Interactions of this sort can be important in the clinical setting and are discussed in more detail in Chapter 51.

ANTAGONISM BY RECEPTOR BLOCK

Receptor-block antagonism involves two important mechanisms:

- reversible competitive antagonism
- irreversible, or non-equilibrium, competitive antagonism.

Reversible competitive antagonism was described earlier (pp. 11, 17), its key features being the parallel shift of the agonist log concentration–effect curve without any reduction in the maximal response, and the linear Schild plot. These characteristics reflect the fact that the rate of dissociation of the antagonist molecules is sufficiently high that a new equilibrium is rapidly established on addition of the agonist. In effect, the agonist is able to displace the antagonist molecules from the receptors, although it cannot, of course, evict a bound antagonist molecule. Displacement occurs because, by occupying a proportion of the vacant receptors, the agonist reduces the rate of association of the antagonist molecules; consequently, the rate of dissociation temporarily exceeds that of association, and the overall antagonist occupancy falls.

Irreversible, or non-equilibrium, competitive antagonism occurs when the antagonist dissociates very slowly, or not at all, from the receptors, with the result that no change in the antagonist occupancy takes place when the agonist is applied.*

If the antagonist occupies a fraction p_B of the receptors, then no matter how high the agonist concentration, the agonist occupancy cannot exceed $(1 - p_B)$, so the antagonism is non-surmountable. The predicted effects of reversible and irreversible antagonists are compared in Figure 2.9.

▼ In some cases (Fig. 2.11A), the theoretical effect is accurately reproduced, but the distinction between reversible and irreversible competitive antagonism (or even non-competitive antagonism; see p. 19) is not always so clear. This is because of the phenomenon of spare receptors (see p. 15); if the agonist occupancy required to produce a maximal biological response is very small (say 1% of the total receptor pool), then it is possible to block irreversibly nearly 99% of the receptors without reducing the maximal response. The effect of a lesser degree of antagonist occupancy will be to produce a parallel shift of the log concentration–effect curve that is indistinguishable from reversible competitive antagonism (Fig. 2.11B). In fact, it was the finding that an irreversible competitive antagonist of histamine was able to reduce the sensitivity of a smooth muscle preparation to histamine nearly 100-fold without reducing the maximal response that first gave rise to the spare receptor hypothesis.

Irreversible competitive antagonism occurs with drugs that possess reactive groups which form covalent bonds with the receptor. These are mainly used as experimental tools for

*This type of antagonism is sometimes called non-competitive, but that term is best reserved for antagonism that does not involve occupation of the receptor site (see p. 19).

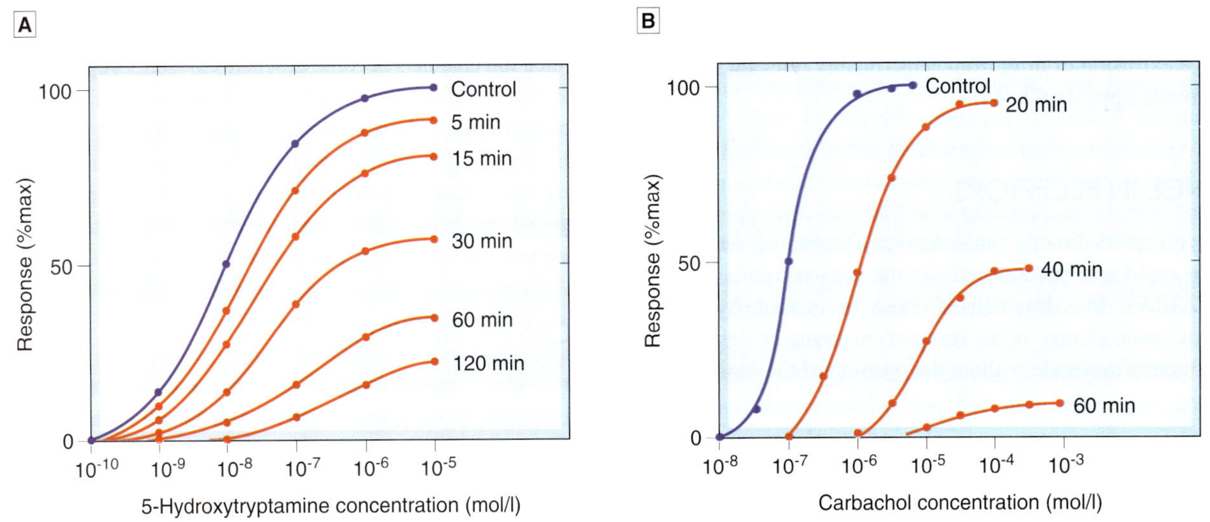

Fig. 2.11 Effects of irreversible competitive antagonists on agonist concentration–effect curves. A Rat stomach smooth muscle responding to 5-hydroxytryptamine at various times after addition of methysergide (10^{-9} mol/l). B Rabbit stomach responding to carbachol at various times after addition of dibenamine (10^{-5} mol/l). (After: (A) Frankhuijsen A L, Bonta I L 1974 Eur J Pharmacol 26: 220; (B) Furchgott R F 1965 Adv Drug Res 3: 21.)

investigating receptor function, and few are used clinically. Irreversible enzyme inhibitors that act similarly are clinically used, however, and include drugs such as aspirin (Ch. 16), omeprazole (Ch. 24) and monoamine oxidase inhibitors (Ch. 38).

NON-COMPETITIVE ANTAGONISM

Non-competitive antagonism describes the situation where the antagonist blocks at some point the chain of events that leads to the production of a response by the agonist. For example, drugs such as verapamil and nifedipine prevent the influx of calcium ions through the cell membrane (see Ch. 18) and thus block non-specifically the contraction of smooth muscle produced by other drugs. As a rule, the effect will be to reduce the slope and maximum of the agonist log concentration–response curve as in Figure 2.11B, though it is quite possible for some degree of rightward shift to occur as well.

> **Drug antagonism**
>
> Drug antagonism occurs by various mechanisms:
> - chemical antagonism (interaction in solution)
> - pharmacokinetic antagonism (one drug affecting the absorption, metabolism or excretion of the other)
> - competitive antagonism (both drugs binding to the same receptors); the antagonism may be reversible or irreversible
> - non-competitive antagonism (the antagonist interrupts receptor–effector linkage)
> - physiological antagonism (two agents producing opposing physiological effects).

PHYSIOLOGICAL ANTAGONISM

Physiological antagonism is a term used loosely to describe the interaction of two drugs whose opposing actions in the body tend to cancel each other. For example, histamine acts on receptors of the parietal cells of the gastric mucosa to stimulate acid secretion, while omeprazole blocks this effect by inhibiting the proton pump; the two drugs can be said to act as physiological antagonists.

DESENSITISATION AND TACHYPHYLAXIS

Often, the effect of a drug gradually diminishes when it is given continuously or repeatedly. Desensitisation and tachyphylaxis are synonymous terms used to describe this phenomenon, which often develops in the course of a few minutes. The term *tolerance* is conventionally used to describe a more gradual decrease in responsiveness to a drug, taking days or weeks to develop, but the distinction is not a sharp one. The term *refractoriness* is also sometimes used, mainly in relation to a loss of therapeutic efficacy. *Drug resistance* is a term used to describe the loss of effectiveness of antimicrobial or antitumour drugs (see Chs 44 and 50). Many different mechanisms can give rise to this type of phenomenon. They include:

- change in receptors
- loss of receptors
- exhaustion of mediators

3 How drugs act: molecular aspects

Overview 22

Targets for drug action 22

Receptor proteins 26
- Type 1: ligand-gated ion channels 29
- Type 2: G-protein-coupled receptors 32
- Type 3: kinase-linked and related receptors 42
- Type 4: nuclear receptors 44

Ion channels as drug targets 45

Control of receptor expression 47

Receptors and disease 48

OVERVIEW

In this chapter, we move from the general principles of drug action outlined in Chapter 2 to the molecules that are involved in recognising chemical signals and translating them into cellular responses. Molecular pharmacology has advanced rapidly in recent years. This new knowledge can seem impenetrably complex when couched in the terminology and style of modern molecular biology, but it actually provides a simpler and more coherent framework for understanding drug action than existed previously. It is this aspect, rather than the molecular detail, on which we focus here. Advances in molecular pharmacology are not only changing our understanding of drug action; they are also opening up many new therapeutic possibilities, further discussed in other chapters.

First, we consider the types of target protein on which drugs act. Next, we describe the main families of receptors and ion channels that have been revealed by cloning and structural studies. Finally, we discuss the various forms of receptor–effector linkage (signal transduction mechanisms) through which receptors are coupled to the regulation of cell function. The relationship between the molecular structure of a receptor and its functional linkage to a particular type of effector system is a principal theme. In the next two chapters, we see how these molecular events alter important aspects of cell function—a useful basis for understanding the effects of drugs on intact living organisms. We go into more detail than is necessary for understanding today's pharmacology at a basic level, intending that students can, if they wish, skip or skim these chapters without losing the thread; however, we are confident that tomorrow's pharmacology will rest solidly on the advances in cellular and molecular biology that are discussed here.

TARGETS FOR DRUG ACTION

The protein targets for drug action on mammalian cells (Fig. 3.1) that are described in this chapter can be broadly divided into:

- receptors
- ion channels
- enzymes
- carrier molecules.

The great majority of important drugs act on one or other of these types of protein, but there are exceptions. For example **colchicine** (Ch. 16) interacts with the structural protein tubulin, while several immunosuppressive drugs (e.g. **ciclosporin**, Ch. 16) bind to cytosolic proteins known as immunophilins. Therapeutic antibodies that act by sequestering cytokines (protein mediators involved in inflammation, see Ch. 15) are also used. Targets for chemotherapeutic drugs (Chs 44–50), where the aim is to suppress invading microorganisms or cancer cells, include DNA and cell wall constituents as well as other proteins.

Receptors

Receptors (Fig. 3.1A) are the sensing elements in the system of chemical communications that coordinates the function of all the different cells in the body, the chemical messengers being the various hormones, transmitters and other mediators discussed in Section 2. Many therapeutically useful drugs act, either as agonists or antagonists, on receptors for known endogenous mediators. Some examples are given in Table 3.1. In most cases, the endogenous mediator was discovered before—often many

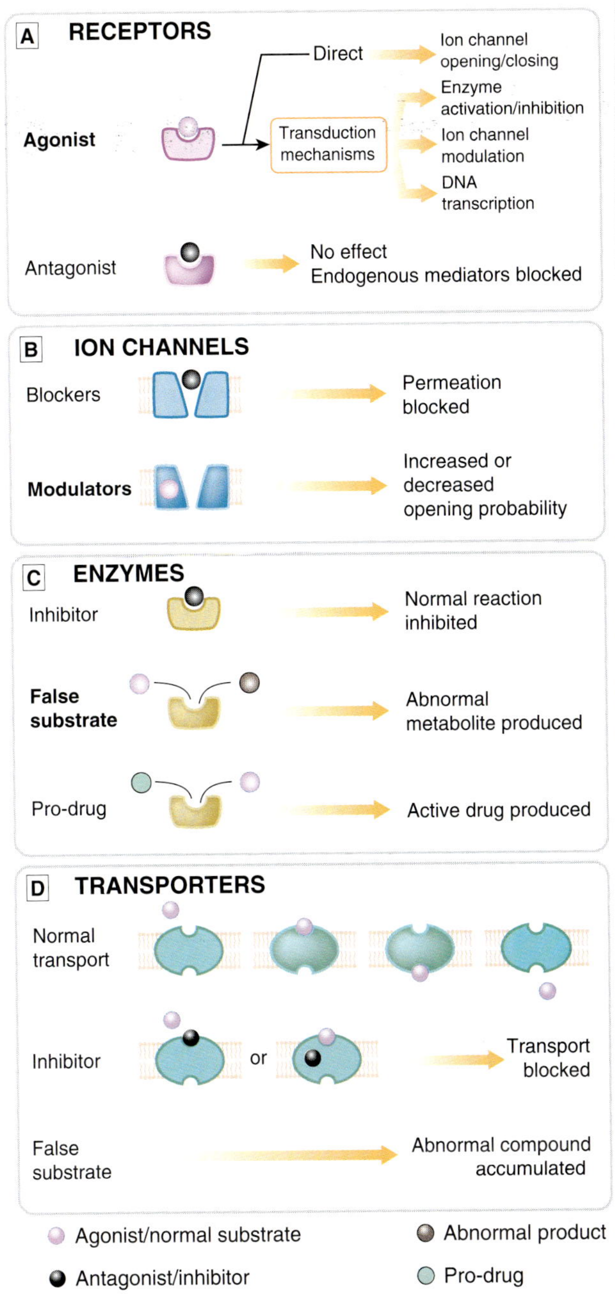

Fig. 3.1 Types of target for drug action.

years before—the receptor was characterised pharmacologically and biochemically, but there are examples of receptors for synthetic drug molecules (e.g. **benzodiazepines**, Ch. 36, and **sulfonylureas**, Ch. 25) for which no endogenous mediator has been identified. Receptors are discussed in more detail below (p. 26).

Ion channels

Some ion channels (known as *ligand-gated ion channels* or *ionotropic receptors*) incorporate a receptor and open only when the receptor is occupied by an agonist; others (see p. 46) are gated by different mechanisms, *voltage-gated ion channels* being particularly important. In general, drugs can affect ion channel function by interacting either with the receptor site of ligand-gated channels or with other parts of the channel molecule. The interaction can be indirect, involving a G-protein and other intermediaries (see below), or direct, where the drug itself binds to the channel protein and alters its function. In the simplest case, exemplified by the action of local anaesthetics on the voltage-gated sodium channel (see Ch. 43), the drug molecule plugs the channel physically (Fig. 3.1B) blocking ion permeation.

Examples of drugs that bind to accessory sites on the channel protein and thereby affect channel gating include:

- vasodilator drugs of the *dihydropyridine* type (see Ch. 18): these inhibit the opening of L-type calcium channels (see p. 52)
- *benzodiazepine tranquillisers* (see Ch. 36): these bind to a region of the gamma-aminobutyric acid (GABA) receptor/chloride channel complex (a ligand-gated channel; see above) that is distinct from the GABA-binding site; most benzodiazepines facilitate the opening of the channel by the inhibitory neurotransmitter GABA (see Ch. 32), but some *inverse agonists* are known that have the opposite effect, causing anxiety rather than tranquillity
- *sulfonylureas* (see p. 47 and Ch. 25): these are used in treating diabetes mellitus and act on ATP-sensitive potassium channels of pancreatic B-cells and thereby enhance insulin secretion.

A summary of the different ion channel families and their functions is given below (p. 45)

Enzymes

Many drugs target enzymes (Fig. 3.1C), examples being given in Table 3.1. Often the drug molecule is a substrate analogue that acts as a competitive inhibitor of the enzyme, either reversibly (e.g. **neostigmine**, acting on acetylcholinesterase; Ch. 10) or irreversibly (e.g. **aspirin**, acting on cyclooxygenase; Ch. 16). The immunophilin to which ciclosporin binds (see above) has enzymic activity as an isomerase that catalyses the *cis–trans* isomerisation of proline residues in proteins, a reaction that is important in allowing expressed proteins to fold correctly. Inhibition of this enzymic activity is one of the mechanisms by which ciclosporin causes immunosuppression. Drugs may also act as *false substrates*, where the drug molecule undergoes chemical transformation to form an abnormal product that subverts the normal metabolic pathway. An example is the anticancer drug **fluorouracil**, which replaces uracil as an intermediate in purine biosynthesis but cannot be converted into thymidylate, thus blocking DNA synthesis and preventing cell division (Ch. 50).

It should also be mentioned that drugs may require enzymic degradation to convert them from an inactive form, the *pro-drug* (see Ch. 8), to an active form. Examples are given in Table 8.3. Furthermore, as discussed in Chapter 52, drug toxicity often results from the enzymic conversion of the drug molecule to a reactive metabolite. As far as the primary action of the drug is concerned, this is an unwanted side reaction, but it is of major importance as a mechanism of drug toxicity.

Carrier molecules

The transport of ions and small organic molecules across cell membranes generally requires a carrier protein, since the permeating molecules are often too polar (i.e. insufficiently lipid soluble) to penetrate lipid membranes on their own. There are many examples of such carriers (Fig. 3.1D), including those responsible for the transport of glucose and amino acids into cells, the transport of ions and many organic molecules by the renal tubule, the transport of Na^+ and Ca^{2+} out of cells and the uptake of neurotransmitter precursors (such as choline) or of neurotransmitters themselves (such as noradrenaline, 5-hydroxytryptamine (5-HT), glutamate and peptides) by nerve terminals. These transporters belong to a well-defined structural family, distinct from the corresponding receptors (see Giros & Caron, 1993). The carrier proteins embody a recognition site that makes them specific for a particular permeating species, and these recognition sites can also be targets for drugs that block the transport system. Some examples are given in Table 3.1.

Table 3.1 Some examples of targets for drug action

Type of target	Effectors		Refer to
Receptors	**Agonists**	**Antagonists**	
Nicotinic ACh receptor	Acetylcholine Nicotine	Tubocurarine α-Bungarotoxin	Ch. 10
Beta-adrenoceptor	Noradrenaline (norepinephrine) Isoprenaline	Propranolol	Ch. 11
Histamine (H_1-receptor)	Histamine	Mepyramine	Ch. 17
Histamine (H_2-receptor)	Impromidine	Ranitidine	Ch. 24
Opiate (μ-receptor)	Morphine	Naloxone	Ch. 40
5-HT_2-receptor	5-Hydroxytryptamine	Ketanserin	Ch. 12
Dopamine (D_2 receptor)	Dopamine Bromocriptine	Chlorpromazine	Chs 34, 37
Insulin receptor	Insulin	Not known	Ch. 25
Oestrogen receptor	Ethinylestradiol	Tamoxifen	Ch. 29
Progesterone receptor	Norethisterone	Danazol	Ch. 29
Ion channels	**Blockers**	**Modulators**	
Voltage-gated sodium channels	Local anaesthetics Tetrodotoxin	Veratridine	Ch. 43
Renal tubule sodium channels	Amiloride	Aldosterone	Ch. 23
Voltage-gated calcium channels	Divalent cations (e.g. Cd^{2+})	Dihydropyridines Beta-adrenoceptor agonists	Chs 17,18 Ch. 11
Voltage-gated potassium channels	4-Aminopyridine	Many neuromodulators	Chs 9, 40
ATP-sensitive potassium channels	ATP	Cromokalim Sulphonylureas	Ch. 18 Ch. 25
GABA-gated chloride channels	Picrotoxin	Benzodiazepines	Ch. 32
Glutamate-gated (NMDA) cation channels	Dizocilpine, Mg^{2+} Ketamine	Glycine	Ch. 32

Table 3.1 Continued

Enzymes	Inhibitors	False substrates	
Acetylcholinesterase	Neostigmine Organophosphates		Ch. 10
Choline acetyltransferase		Hemicholinium	Ch. 10
Cyclooxygenase	Aspirin		Ch. 16
Xanthine oxidase	Allopurinol		Ch. 16
Angiotensin-converting enzyme	Captopril		Ch. 18
Carbonic anhydrase	Acetazolamide		Ch. 23
HMG-CoA reductase	Simvastatin		Ch. 19
Dopa decarboxylase	Carbidopa	Methyldopa	Ch. 11
Monoamine oxidase-A	Iproniazid		Ch. 38
Monoamine oxidase-B	Selegiline	MPTP	Ch. 34
Dihydrofolate reductase	Trimethoprim Methotrexate		Ch. 52 Chs 16, 50
DNA polymerase	Cytarabine	Cytarabine	Ch. 50
Enzymes involved in DNA synthesis	Azathiaprine		Ch. 16
Enzymes of blood clotting cascade	Heparin		Ch. 20
Plasminogen[a]			Ch. 20
Thymidine kinase	Aciclovir		Ch. 46
HIV protease	Saquinavir		Ch. 46
Reverse transcriptase	Didanosine, zidovudine		Ch. 46
Carriers	**Inhibitors**	**False substrates**	
Choline carrier (nerve terminal)	Hemicholinium		Ch. 10
Noradrenaline uptake 1	Tricyclic antidepressants Cocaine	 Amphetamine Methyldopa	Ch. 38 Chs 11, 52 Chs 11, 41 Ch. 18
Noradrenaline uptake (vesicular)	Reserpine		Ch. 11
Weak acid carrier (renal tubule)	Probenecid		Ch. 23
$Na^+/K^+/Cl^-$ co-transporter (loop of Henle)	Loop diuretics		Ch. 23
Na^+/K^+ pump	Cardiac glycosides		Ch. 18
Proton pump (gastric mucosa)	Omeprazole		Ch. 24
Others			
Immunophilins	Ciclosporin, tacrolimus		Ch. 16
Tubulin	Colchicine Taxol		Ch. 16 Ch. 50

HMG-CoA, 3-hydroxy-3-methylglutaryl-coenzyme A; HIV, human immunodeficiency virus; other biochemical targets for drugs used in chemotherapy are discussed in Chapters 43–50.
[a]Plasminogen activators: tissue plasminogen activator (tPA), APSAC (Ch. 20)

RECEPTOR PROTEINS

ISOLATION AND CLONING OF RECEPTORS

In the 1970s, pharmacology entered a new phase when receptors, which had until then been theoretical entities, began to emerge as biochemical realities, following the development of receptor labelling techniques (see Ch. 2), which made it possible to extract and purify the radioactively labelled receptor material. This approach was first used successfully on the nicotinic acetylcholine receptor (see Ch. 10), where advantage was taken of two natural curiosities. The first is that the electric organs of many fish, such as rays (*Torpedo* sp.) and electric eels (*Electrophorus* sp.) consist of modified muscle tissue in which the acetylcholine-sensitive membrane is extremely abundant, and these organs contain much larger amounts of acetylcholine receptor than any other tissue. Secondly, the venom of snakes of the cobra family contains polypeptides that bind with very high specificity to nicotinic acetylcholine receptors. These substances, known as α-toxins, can be labelled and used to assay the receptor content of tissues and tissue extracts. The best-known is **α-bungarotoxin**, which is the main component of the venom of the Malayan banded krait (*Bungarus multicinctus*).* Treatment of muscle or electric tissue with non-ionic detergents renders the membrane-bound receptor protein soluble. It can then be purified by the technique of affinity chromatography in which a receptor ligand, bound covalently to the matrix of a chromatography column, is used to adsorb the receptor and separate it from other substances in the extract. The receptor can then be eluted from the column by flushing it through with a solution containing an antagonist, such as **gallamine**. Similar approaches have now been used to purify a great many hormone and neurotransmitter receptors, as well as ion channels, carrier proteins and other kinds of target molecule.

Once receptor proteins were isolated and purified, it was possible to analyse the amino acid sequence of a short stretch, allowing the corresponding base sequence of the mRNA to be deduced. Oligonucleotide probes were then synthesised and used to extract the full-length DNA sequence by conventional complimentary DNA (cDNA) cloning methods, starting from a cDNA library obtained from a tissue source rich in the receptor of interest. The first receptor clones were obtained in this way, but now there are alternative strategies for *expression cloning*, which do not require prior isolation and purification of the receptor protein.

Much information has been gained by introducing the cloned DNA encoding individual receptors into cell lines by transfection, producing cells that express the foreign receptors in a functional form. Such engineered cells allow much more precise control of the expressed receptors than is possible with natural cells or intact tissues, and the technique is widely used to study the binding and pharmacological characteristics of cloned receptors.

▼ Cloning strategies that require neither protein purification nor expression systems, but only faith, are being used increasingly as more sequence information becomes available. These are based on anticipated sequence homologies between the receptor that is sought and those already known. A region of sequence homology allows, by the use of PCR (polymerase chain reaction) and RACE (rapid amplification of cDNA ends), replication of DNA molecules that contain that sequence. If the chosen sequence is, for example, one that is conserved in several dopamine receptors, what is amplified may well turn out to be another (novel) dopamine receptor, or it may turn out to be something quite different. Unexpected receptors (e.g. the cannabinoid receptor; see Ch. 53) are sometimes found by accident in this way, and there are many examples of 'orphan receptors'**—receptor-like structures for which no functional ligand is known.

The cloning of receptors often reveals molecular variants (subtypes) of known receptors that had not been evident from pharmacological studies. This tends to produce some taxonomic confusion, but in the long term, molecular characterisation of receptors is essential. Barnard, one of the high priests of receptor cloning, is undaunted by the proliferation of molecular subtypes among receptors which pharmacologists had thought that they understood. He quotes Thomas Aquinas: 'Types and shadows have their ending, for the newer rite is here'. The newer rite, he confidently asserts, is molecular biology.

TYPES OF RECEPTOR

Receptors elicit many different types of cellular effect. Some of them are very rapid, such as those involved in synaptic transmission, operating within milliseconds, whereas other receptor-mediated effects, such as those produced by thyroid hormone or various steroid hormones, occur over hours or days. There are also many examples of intermediate timescales; catecholamines, for example, usually act in a matter of seconds, whereas many peptides take rather longer to produce their effects. Not surprisingly, very different types of linkage between the receptor occupation and the ensuing response are involved. Based on molecular structure and the nature of this linkage (the transduction mechanism), we can distinguish four receptor types, or superfamilies (see Figs 3.2 and 3.3 and Table 3.2).

Type 1: ligand-gated ion channels

The ligand-gated ion channels are also known as *ionotropic receptors*.*** These are membrane proteins with a similar structure to other ion channels but incorporating a ligand-binding (receptor) site, usually in the extracellular domain. Typically, these are the receptors on which fast neurotransmitters act. Examples include the nicotinic acetylcholine receptor (see Ch. 10), $GABA_A$ receptor (see Ch. 32), and glutamate receptors of the

*Nature has had the good sense to keep these heavily armed fishes and snakes well apart. Ironically enough, *B. multicinctus* is now officially an endangered species, threatened by scientists' demand for its venom. Evolution for survival can go one step too far.

**An oddly Dickensian term that seems inappropriately condescending since we can assume that these receptors play defined roles in physiological signalling—their 'orphanhood' reflects our ignorance, not their status.

***Here, focussing on receptors, we consider ligand-gated ion channels as an example of a receptor family. Other types of ion channels are described later (p. 45); many of them are also drug targets, though not receptors in the strict sense.

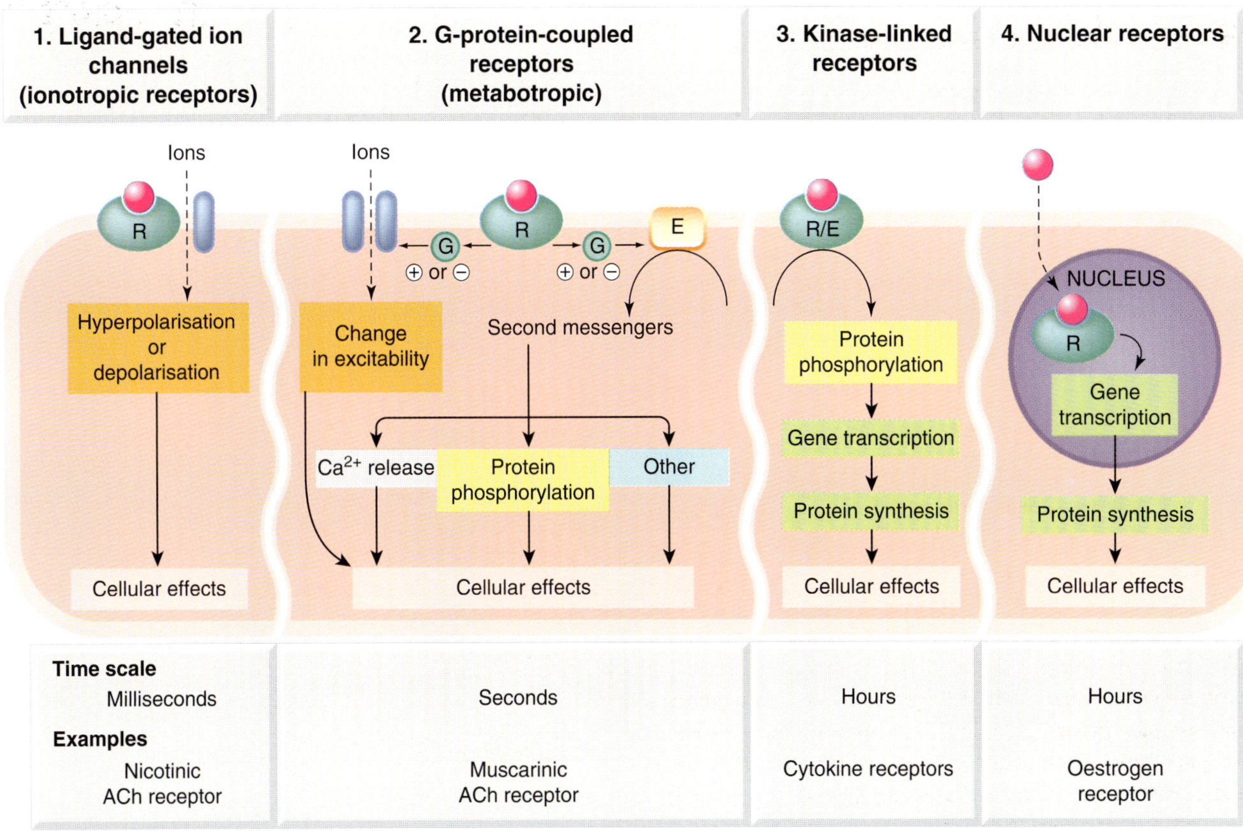

Fig. 3.2 **Types of receptor–effector linkage.** (R, receptor; G, G-protein; E, enzyme; ACh, acetylcholine.)

Table 3.2 The four main types of receptor

	Type 1 Ligand-gated ion channels	Type 2 G-protein-coupled receptors	Type 3 Kinase-linked receptors	Type 4 Nuclear receptors
Location	Membrane	Membrane	Membrane	Intracellular
Effector	Ion channel	Channel or enzyme	Enzyme	Gene transcription
Coupling	Direct	G-protein	Direct	Via DNA
Examples	Nicotinic acetylcholine receptor (nAChR), gamma-aminobutyric acid type A ($GABA_{A)}$)	Muscarinic acetylcholine receptor (mAChR), adrenoceptors	Insulin, growth factor, cytokine receptors	Steroid, thyroid hormone receptors
Structure	Oligomeric assembly of subunits surrounding central pore	Monomeric (occasionally dimeric) structure comprising seven transmembrane helices	Single transmembrane helix linking extracellular receptor domain to intracellular kinase domain	Monomeric structure with separate receptor and DNA-binding domains

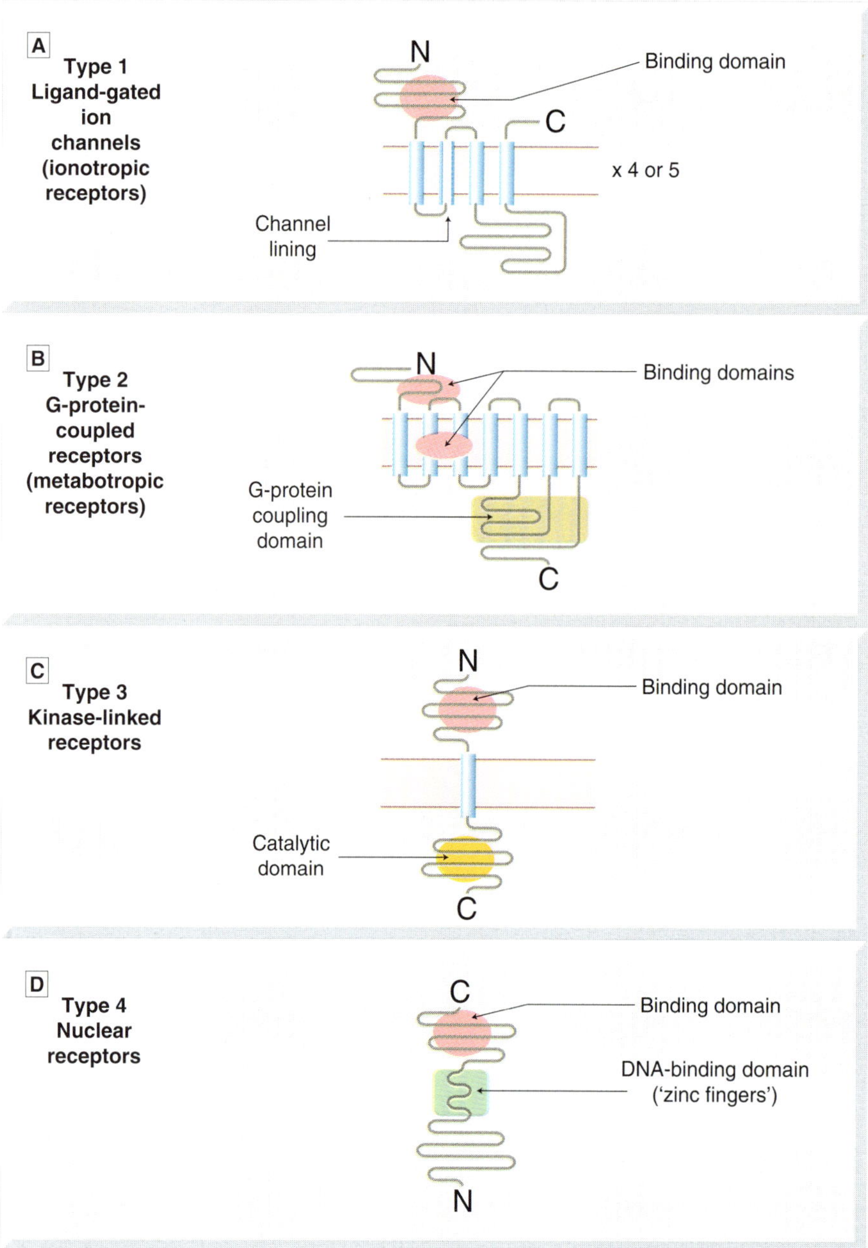

Fig. 3.3 General structure of four receptor families. The rectangular segments represent hydrophobic α-helical regions of the protein comprising approximately 20 amino acid residues, which form the membrane-spanning domains of the receptors. Receptors coupled directly to ion channels comprise four or five subunits of the type shown, the whole complex containing 16–20 membrane-spanning segments surrounding a central ion channel. [A] Type 1: ligand-gated ion channels; [B] type 2: G-protein-coupled receptors; [C] type 3: kinase-linked receptors; [D] type 4: nuclear receptors that control gene transcription.

NMDA (*N*-methyl-D-aspartate), AMPA (α-amino-3-hydroxy-5-methyl-4-isooxazolepropionate) and kainate types (see Ch. 32).

Type 2: G-protein-coupled receptors

The G-protein-coupled receptors (GPCRs) are also known as *metabotropic receptors* or *seven–transmembrane-spanning (heptahelical) receptors*. They are membrane receptors that are coupled to intracellular effector systems via a G-protein (see below). They constitute the largest family* and include receptors

*In the nematode *Caenorhabditis elegans*, approximately 5% of its 19 000 genes encode for GPCRs, 90% of which are 'orphans' (Bergmann, 1998). There are probably more than 1000 GPCRs in the human genome—enough to keep pharmacologists busy for some time yet.

for many hormones and slow transmitters, e.g. the muscarinic acetylcholine receptor (see Ch. 10), adrenoceptors (see Ch. 11) and chemokine receptors (see Ch. 15).

Type 3: kinase-linked and related receptors

There is a large and heterogeneous group of membrane receptors responding to protein mediators. They comprise an extracellular ligand-binding domain linked to an intracellular domain by a single transmembrane helix. In many cases, the intracellular domain is enzymic in nature (with protein kinase or guanylate cyclase activity). Type 3 receptors include those for insulin and various cytokines and growth factors, (see Chs 15 and 25); the receptor for atrial natriuretic factor (Chs 17 and 18) is the main example of the guanylate cyclase type. The two kinds are very similar structurally, even though their transduction mechanisms differ.

Type 4: nuclear receptors

The nuclear receptors regulate gene transcription. The term nuclear receptors is something of a misnomer since some are actually located in the cytosol and migrate to the nuclear compartment when a ligand is present. They include receptors for steroid hormones (see Ch. 27), thyroid hormone (Ch. 30) and other agents such as retinoic acid and vitamin D.

MOLECULAR STRUCTURE OF RECEPTORS

The molecular organisation of typical members of each of these four receptor superfamilies is shown in Figure 3.3. Though individual receptors show considerable sequence variation in particular regions, and the lengths of the main intracellular and extracellular domains also vary from one to another within the same family, the overall structural patterns and associated signal transduction pathways are very consistent. The realisation that just four receptor superfamilies provide a solid framework for interpreting the complex welter of information about the effects of a large proportion of the drugs that have been studied has been one of the most refreshing developments in modern pharmacology.

Receptor heterogeneity and subtypes

As sequence data have accumulated, it has become clear that receptors within a given family generally occur in several molecular varieties, or subtypes, with similar architecture but significant differences in their sequences, and often in their pharmacological properties.* Nicotinic acetylcholine receptors are typical in this respect; distinct subtypes occur in different brain regions, and these differ from the muscle receptor. Some of the known pharmacological differences (e.g. sensitivity to blocking agents) that are known to exist between muscle and brain acetylcholine receptors are now known to correlate with specific sequence differences; however, as far as we know, all nicotinic acetylcholine receptors respond to the same physiological mediator and produce the same kind of synaptic response, so why many variants should have evolved is still a puzzle.

▼ Much of the sequence variation that accounts for receptor diversity arises at the genomic level, i.e. distinct genes give rise to distinct receptor subtypes. Additional variation arises from *alternative mRNA splicing*, which means that a single gene can give rise to more than one receptor *isoform*. After translation from genomic DNA, the mRNA normally contains non-coding regions (*introns*) that are excised by mRNA splicing before the message is translated into protein. Depending on the location of the splice sites, splicing can result in insertion or deletion of one or more of the mRNA coding regions, giving rise to long or short forms of the protein. This is an important source of variation, particularly for GPCRs (see Kilpatrick et al., 1999), which produces receptors with different binding characteristics and different signal transduction mechanisms, though its pharmacological relevance remains to be clarified. Another process that can produce different receptors from the same gene is *mRNA editing*, which involves the mischievous substitution of one base in the mRNA for another, and hence a small variation in the amino acid sequence of the receptor.

Molecular heterogeneity of this kind is a feature of all kinds of receptor—indeed of functional proteins in general. New receptor subtypes and isoforms are continually being discoverd, and a regular update of the catalogue is available (Trends in Pharmacological Sciences Receptor and Ion Channel Nomenclature Supplement). The problems of classification, nomenclature and taxonomy resulting from this flood of data have been mentioned above. From the pharmacological viewpoint, where our concern is to understand individual drugs and what they do to living organisms, and to devise better ones, it is important that we keep molecular pharmacology in perspective. The 'newer rite' has proved revelatory in many ways, but the sheer complexity of the ways in which molecules behave means that we have a long way to go before reaching the reductionist Utopia that molecular biology promises. When we do, this book will get much shorter. In the meantime, we try to pick out the general principles without getting too bogged down in detail. We will now describe the characteristics of each of the four receptor superfamilies.

TYPE 1: LIGAND-GATED ION CHANNELS

MOLECULAR STRUCTURE

The ligand-gated ion channels have structural features in common with other ion channels (described on p. 46; see Ashcroft, 2000). The nicotinic acetylcholine receptor (Fig. 3.3A), the first to be cloned, has been studied in great detail (see Karlin, 1993). It is assembled from four different types of subunit, termed α, β, γ, δ each of molecular mass 40–58 kDa. The four subunits show marked sequence homology, and analysis of the hydrophobicity profile, which determines which sections of the chain are likely to form membrane-spanning α-helices, suggests that they are inserted into the membrane as shown in Figure 3.4. The oligomeric structure (α_2, β, γ, δ) possesses two acetylcholine-binding sites, each lying at the interface between one of the two α-subunits and its neighbour. Both must bind

*Receptors for 5-HT (see Ch. 12) are currently the champions with respect to diversity, with 14 cloned subtypes.

acetylcholine molecules in order for the receptor to be activated. This receptor is sufficiently large to be seen in electron micrographs, and Figure 3.4 shows its structure, based mainly on a high-resolution electron diffraction study (Unwin 1993, 1995). Each subunit spans the membrane four times, so the channel comprises no less than 20 membrane-spanning helices surrounding a central pore.

▼ The two acetylcholine-binding sites lie on the N-terminal regions of the two α-subunits. One of the transmembrane helices (M2) from each of the five subunits forms the lining of the ion channel (Fig. 3.4). The five M2 helices that form the pore are sharply kinked inwards halfway through the membrane, forming a constriction, and are believed to swivel out of the way when acetylcholine is bound, thus opening the channel.

The use of site-directed mutagenesis, which enables short regions or single residues of the amino acid sequence to be altered, has shown that a mutation of a critical residue in the M2 helix changes the channel from being cation selective (hence excitatory, in the context of synaptic function) to being anion selective (typical of receptors for inhibitory transmitters, such as GABA) (see Galzi & Changeux 1994). Other mutations affect properties such as gating and desensitisation of ligand-gated channels.

Receptors for some other fast transmitters, such as the $GABA_A$ receptor (Ch. 32), the $5\text{-}HT_3$–receptor (Ch. 12) and the glycine receptor (Ch. 32) are built on the same pattern, and some show considerable sequence homology with the nicotinic acetylcholine receptor; the number of subunits that go to make up a functional receptor varies somewhat but is usually four or five. However, other ligand-gated ion channels have a somewhat different architecture, in which the pore is built from loops rather than transmembrane helices (see Fig. 3.16, below), in common with many other (non-ligand-gated) ion channels. ATP receptors of the P_{2X} type (see Ch. 12) and glutamate receptors (see Ch. 32), the structures of which are shown in Fig. 3.16 below, are of this type.

THE GATING MECHANISM

Receptors of this type control the fastest synaptic events in the nervous system, in which a neurotransmitter acts on the postsynaptic membrane of a nerve or muscle cell and transiently increases its permeability to particular ions. Most excitatory neurotransmitters such as acetylcholine at the neuromuscular junction (Ch. 10) or glutamate in the central nervous system (CNS; Ch. 32) cause an increase in Na^+ and K^+ permeability. This results in a net inward current carried mainly by Na^+, which depolarises the cell and increases the probability that it will generate an action potential. The action of the transmitter reaches a peak in a fraction of a millisecond and usually decays within a few milliseconds. The sheer speed of this response implies that the coupling between the receptor and the ionic channel is a direct one, and the molecular structure of the receptor–channel complex (see above) agrees with this. It is known that purified acetylcholine receptors can function as ionic gates in completely artificial membranes, which rules out the involvement of any biochemical intermediates (in the cell or within the membrane) in the transduction process.

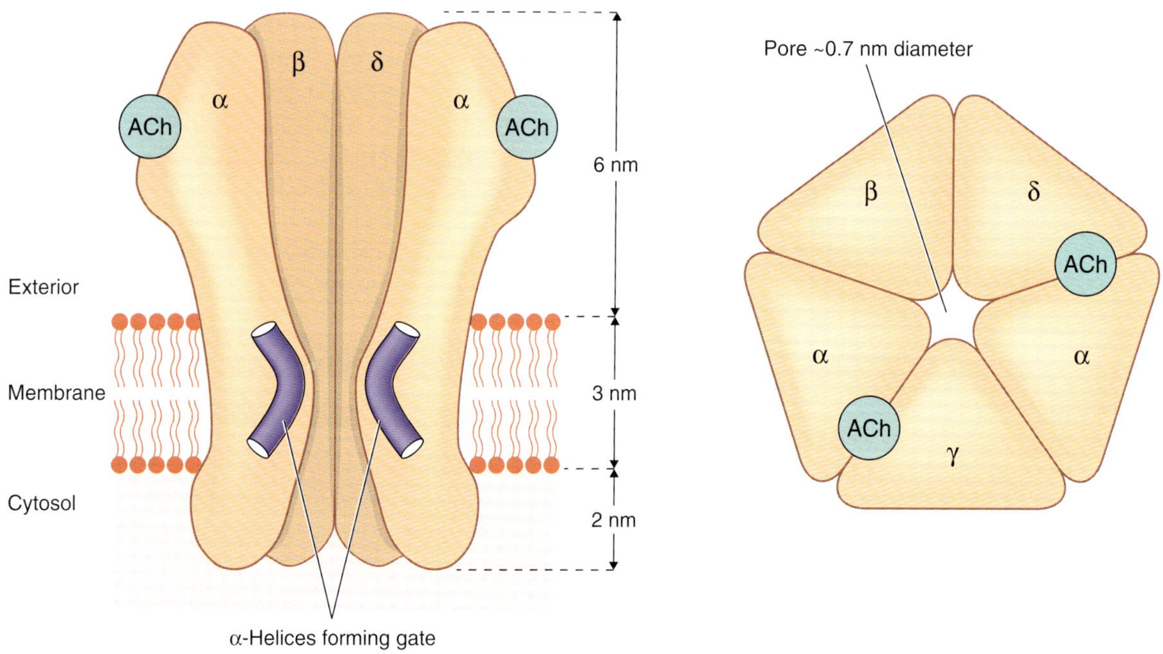

Fig. 3.4 Structure of the nicotinic acetylcholine receptor (a typical ligand-gated ion channel) in side-view (left) and plan-view (right). The five receptor subunits (α_2, β, γ, σ) form a cluster surrounding a central transmembrane pore, the lining of which is formed by the M2 helical segments of each subunit. These contain a preponderance of negatively charged amino acids, which makes the pore cation selective. There are two acetylcholine (ACh)-binding sites in the extracellular portion of the receptor, at the interface between the α- and the adjoining subunits. When acetylcholine binds, the kinked α-helices swing out of the way, thus opening the channel pore. (Based on Unwin 1993, 1995.)

▼ A breakthrough by Katz & Miledi in 1972 made it possible for the first time to study the properties of individual receptor-operated ionic channels by the use of *noise analysis*. Studying the action of acetylcholine at the motor endplate they observed that small random fluctuations of membrane potential were superimposed on the steady depolarisation produced by acetylcholine (Fig. 3.5A). These fluctuations arise because, in the presence of an agonist, there is a dynamic equilibrium between open and closed ion channels. In the steady state, the rate of opening balances the rate of closing, but from moment to moment the number of open channels will show random fluctuations about the mean. By measuring the amplitude of these fluctuations, the conductance of a single ion channel can be calculated, and by measuring their frequency (usually in the form of a spectrum in which the noise power of the signal is plotted as a function of frequency; Fig. 3.5B) the average duration for which a single channel stays open (mean open time) can be calculated. In the case of acetylcholine acting at the endplate, the channel conductance is about 20 picosiemens (pS), which is equivalent to an influx of about 10^7 ions per second through a single channel under normal physiological conditions, and the mean open time is 1–2 milliseconds. The magnitude of the single channel conductance confirms that permeation occurs through a physical pore through the membrane, since the ion flow is too large to be compatible with a carrier mechanism. The channel conductance produced by different acetylcholine-like agonists is the same, whereas the mean channel lifetime varies.

The simple scheme shown in Figure 2.1 is a useful model for ion channel gating. The conformation R*, representing the open state of the ion channel, is thought to be the same for all agonists, accounting for the finding that the channel conductance does not vary. Kinetically, the mean open time is determined mainly by the closing rate constant, α, and this varies from one drug to another. As explained in Chapter 2, an agonist of high efficacy that activates a large proportion of the receptors that it occupies will be characterised by $\beta/\alpha \gg 1$, whereas for a drug of low efficacy β/α has a lower value.

The patch-clamp recording technique, devised by Neher and Sakmann, allows the very small current flowing through a single ionic channel to be measured directly (Fig. 3.6), and the results have fully confirmed the interpretation of channel properties based on noise analysis. This technique, introduced in 1976, provides a view, unique in biology, of the physiological behaviour of individual protein molecules in real time and has given many new insights into the gating reactions and permeability characteristics of both ligand-gated and voltage-gated channels. Single-channel recording has shown that many transmitters cause individual channels to open to any one of several distinct conductance levels, a finding that clearly necessitates some revision of the simple scheme of Figure 2.1 in which only a single open state, R*, is represented. It is uncertain how this comes about, and what its physiological significance may be, but it is an example of the way in which the actual behaviour of receptors makes our theoretical models look a little threadbare.

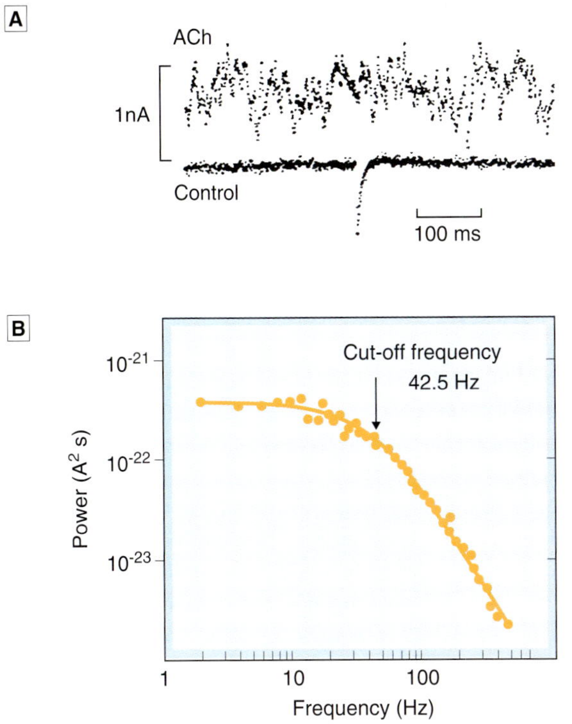

Fig. 3.5 Acetylcholine-induced noise at the frog motor endplate. [A] Records of membrane current recorded at high gain under voltage-clamp. The upper noise record was recorded during the application of acetylcholine (ACh) from a micropipette. The lower record was obtained in the absence of ACh, the blip in the middle being caused by the spontaneous release of a packet of ACh from the motor nerve. The steady (DC) component of the ACh signal has been removed by electronic filtering, leaving the high-frequency noise signal. [B] Power spectrum of ACh-induced noise recorded in a similar experiment to that shown above. The spectrum is calculated by Fourier analysis and fitted with a theoretical (Lorentzian) curve that corresponds to the expected behaviour of a single population of channels with lifetimes varying randomly. The cut-off frequency (at which the power is half of its limiting low-frequency value) enables the mean channel lifetime to be calculated. (From: (A) Anderson C R, Stevens C F 1973 J Physiol 235: 655; (B) Ogden D C et al. 1981 Nature 289: 596.)

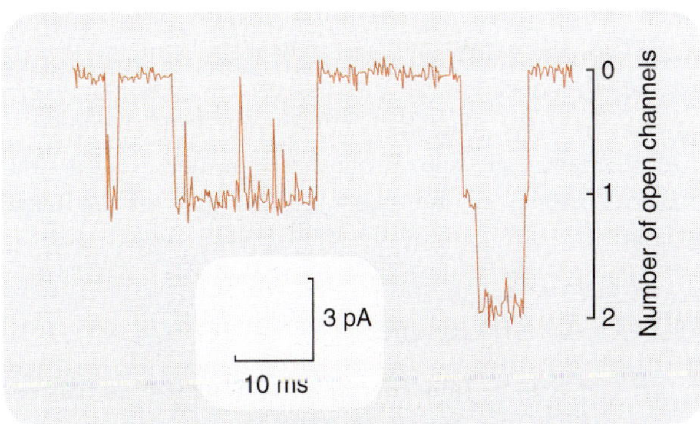

Fig. 3.6 Single acetylcholine-operated ion channels at the frog motor endplate recorded by the patch-clamp technique. The pipette, which was applied tightly to the surface of the membrane, contained 10 mmol/l acetylcholine (ACh). The downward deflections show the currents flowing through single ion channels in the small patch of membrane under the pipette tip. Towards the end of the record, two channels can be seen to open simultaneously. The conductance and mean lifetime of these channels agrees well with indirect estimates from noise analysis (see Fig. 3.5).
(Figure courtesy of D Colquhoun and D C Ogden.)

Ligand-gated ion channels

- These are sometimes called ionotropic receptors.
- They are involved mainly in fast synaptic transmission.
- There are several structural families, the commonest being heteromeric assemblies of 4–5 subunits, with transmembrane helices arranged around a central aqueous channel.
- Ligand binding and channel opening occur on a millisecond timescale.
- Examples include the nicotinic acetylcholine, gamma-aminobutyric acid type A ($GABA_A$) and 5-hydroxytryptamine type 3 ($5\text{-}HT_3$) receptors.

TYPE 2: G-PROTEIN-COUPLED RECEPTORS

The abundant GPCR family comprises many of the receptors that are familiar to pharmacologists, such as muscarinic acetylcholine receptors, adrenoceptors, dopamine receptors, 5-HT receptors, opiate receptors, receptors for many peptides, purine receptors and many others, including the chemoreceptors involved in olfaction (see Dryer & Berghard, 1999) and pheromone detection, and also many 'orphans' (see Marchese et al., 1999). For most of these, quantitative pharmacological studies with different agonists and antagonists have revealed a variety of subtypes. Many GPCRs have been cloned, revealing a strikingly coherent pattern of their molecular structure. Like Greek amphitheatres, they are all very similar in their basic architecture.

Most neurotransmitters, apart from peptides, can interact with both GPCRs and with ligand-gated channels, allowing the same molecule to produce a wide variety of effects. Individual peptide hormones, however generally act either on GPCRs or on kinase-linked receptors (see below), but rarely on both, and a similar choosiness applies to the many ligands that act on nuclear receptors.*

MOLECULAR STRUCTURE

The first GPCR to be fully characterised was the β-adrenoceptor (Ch. 11), which was cloned in 1986. Subsequently molecular biology caught up very rapidly with pharmacology, and most of the receptors that had been identified by their pharmacological properties have now been cloned; what seemed revolutionary in 1986 is now commonplace. Nowadays, any aspiring receptor has to be cloned before it is taken seriously.

GPCRs consist of a single polypeptide chain of up to 1100 residues; their general anatomy is shown in Figure 3.3B. Their characteristic structure comprises seven transmembrane α-helices, similar to those of the ion channels discussed above, with an extracellular N-terminal domain of varying length and an intracellular C-terminal domain. GPCRs are divided into three distinct families (see Schwartz, 1996). There is considerable sequence homology between the members of one family, but none between different families. They share the same heptahelical structure but differ in other respects, principally in the length of the N-terminus and the location of the agonist-binding domain (Table 3.3). Family A, related to rhodopsin (see below), is by far the largest, comprising most monoamine and neuropeptide receptors. Family C is the smallest, its main members being the metabotropic glutamate receptors (Ch. 32) and the Ca^{2+}-sensing receptors** (see Ch. 30).

The understanding of the function of receptors of this type owes much to studies of a closely related protein, rhodopsin, which is responsible for transduction in retinal rods. This protein is abundant in the retina and is much easier to study than receptor proteins (which are anything but abundant); it is built on an identical plan to that shown in Figure 3.3 (see Stryer, 1986) and also produces a response in the rod (hyperpolarisation, associated with a switching off of a Na^+ conductance) through a mechanism involving a G-protein (see below). The most obvious difference is that a photon, rather than an agonist molecule, produces the response. In effect, rhodopsin can be regarded as incorporating its own inbuilt agonist molecule, namely retinal, which isomerises from the *trans* (inactive) to the *cis* (active) form when it absorbs a photon.

Site-directed mutagenesis experiments show that the long third cytoplasmic loop is the region of the molecule that couples to the G-protein, since deletion or modification of this section results in receptors that still bind ligands but cannot associate with G-proteins or produce responses. Usually, a particular receptor subtype couples selectively with a particular G-protein; swapping parts of the cytoplasmic loop between different receptors alters their G-protein selectivity.

For small molecules, such as noradrenaline, the ligand-binding domain appears to reside not on the extracellular N-terminal region, as with the ion channel-coupled receptors, but buried in the cleft between the α-helical segments within the membrane (Fig. 3.3B), similar to the slot occupied by retinal in the rhodopsin molecule (see review by Hibert et al., 1993). Peptide ligands, such as substance P (Ch. 13), bind more superficially to the extracellular loops, as shown in Figure 3.3B (see Schwartz &

*Examples of promiscuity are increasing, however. Steroid hormones, normally faithful to nuclear receptors, make the occasional pass at ion channels and other targets (see Falkenstein et al., 2000), and some eicosanoids act on nuclear receptors as well as GPCRs. Nature is quite open-minded, though such examples are liable to make pharmacologists frown, and students despair.

**The Ca^{2+}-sensing receptor (see Conigrave et al., 2000) is an unusual GPCR that is activated not by conventional mediators but by extracellular Ca^{2+} in the range 1–10 mmo/l: an extremely low affinity in comparison with other GPCR agonists. It is expressed by cells of the parathyroid gland and serves to regulate the extracellular Ca^{2+} concentration by controlling parathyroid hormone secretion. This homeostatic mechanism is quite distinct from the mechanisms for regulating *intracellular* Ca^{2+} discussed in Chapter 4.

Table 3.3 G-protein-controlled receptor families

Family	Receptors[a]	Structural features
A. Rhodopsin family	The largest group; receptors for most amine neurotransmitters, many neuropeptides, purines, prostanoids, cannabinoids, etc.	Short extracellular (N-terminal) tail; ligand binds to transmembrane helices (amines) or to extracellular loops (peptides)
B. Secretin/glucagon receptor family	Receptors for peptide hormones, including secretin, glucagon, calcitonin	Intermediate extracellular tail, incorporating ligand-binding domain
C. Metabotropic glutamate receptor/calcium sensor family	Small group; metabotropic glutamate receptors, $GABA_B$ receptors, calcium-sensing receptors	Long extracellular tail, incorporating ligand binding domain

[a]For full lists, see Wess (1998).
Note: A fourth distinct family includes many receptors for pheromones, but no pharmacological receptors.

Rosenkilde, 1996). By single-site mutagenesis experiments, it is possible to map the ligand-binding domain of these receptors, and the hope is that it may soon be possible to design synthetic ligands based on knowledge of the structure of the receptor site—an important milestone for the pharmaceutical industry, which has relied up to now mainly on the structure of endogenous mediators (such as histamine) or plant alkaloids (such as morphine) for its chemical inspiration.* So far, GPCRs cannot be obtained in crystalline form, so the powerful technique of X-ray crystallography cannot yet be used to define the molecular structure of these receptors in detail. Until then, designing new GPCR ligands will remain a somewhat hit-or-miss business.

ALTERNATIVE MECHANISMS OF RECEPTOR ACTIVATION

Though activation of GPCRs is normally the consequence of agonist binding, it can occur by other mechanisms. Rhodopsin, mentioned earlier, is activated by light-induced *cis–trans* isomerisation of prebound retinal. Another example is that of the protease-activated receptors, of which four have so far been identified (see Vergnolle et al., 2001). It has been known for a long time that thrombin, a protease involved in the blood clotting cascade (see Ch. 20), also initiates a variety of cellular response by binding to a GPCR. Its protease activity is essential for this activity, and it works by snipping off a length of 41 amino acid residues from the extracellular N-terminal tail of the receptor (Fig. 3.7; see Hollenberg, 1996; Dery et al., 1998). The exposed N-terminal residues then bind to receptor domains in the extracellular loops, functioning as a 'tethered agonist'. Receptors of this type occur in many tissues, and it is likely that proteases other than thrombin can function as agonists.** One consequence of this type of activation is that the receptor can only be activated once, since the cleavage cannot be reversed, so continuous resynthesis of receptor protein is necessary. Inactivation occurs by desensitisation, involving phosphorylation (see below), after which the receptor is internalised and degraded, to be replaced by newly synthesised protein.

GPCRs may also be constitutively active, in the absence of any agonist (see Ch. 2). This was first shown for the β-adrenoceptor (see Ch. 11), where mutations in the third intracellular loop, or simply overexpression of the receptor, result in constitutive receptor activation. Several human disease states have been described (see below) that are associated either with spontaneous receptor mutations which result in constitutive activation of receptors or with the production of autoantibodies directed against the extracellular domain of receptors, which mimic the effect of agonists.

SIGNAL TRANSDUCTION BY GPCRs

GPCRs control many different aspects of cell function, discussed in more detail in Chapters 4 and 5, by acting on a variety of different signal transduction mechanisms. The link between the membrane receptor and the first stage of the signal transduction cascade is established through the G-proteins.

G-proteins and their role

G-proteins represent the level of middle management in the organisational hierarchy, intervening between the receptors—choosy mandarins alert to the faintest sniff of their own particular hormone—and the effector enzymes or ion channels—the blue collar brigade that gets the job done without needing to know which hormone authorised the process. They are the go-between proteins but were actually called G-proteins because of their interaction with the guanine nucleotides GTP and GDP. They are

*Increasingly, nowadays, the pharmaceutical industry finds lead structures by screening huge chemical libraries (see Ch. 54). No inspiration is required, just robust assays and efficient robotics.

**One of the family of protease-activated receptors, PAR-2, is activated by a protease released from mast cells and is expressed on sensory neurons. It is thought to play a role in inflammatory pain (see Ch. 40)

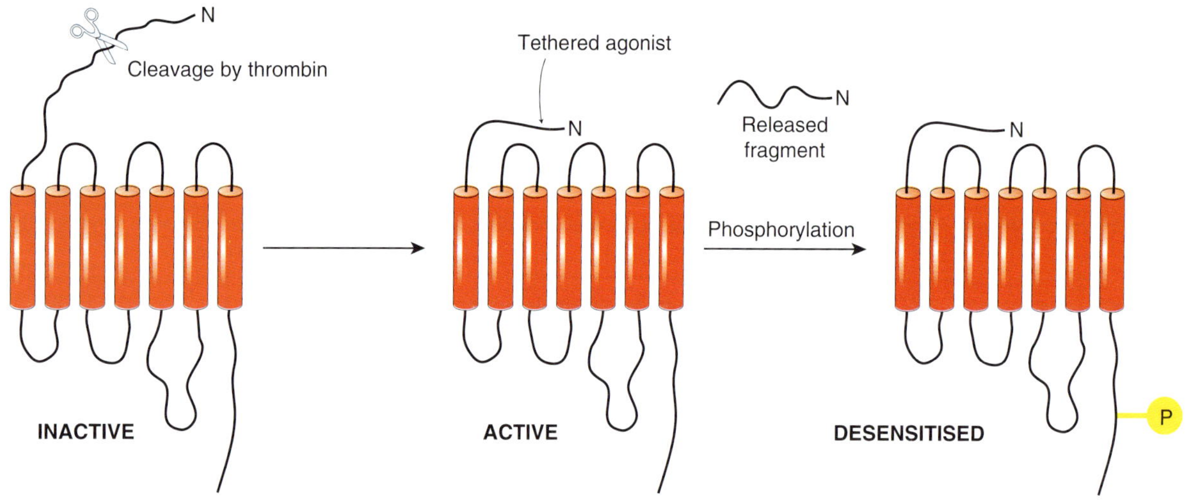

Fig. 3.7 Activation of the thrombin receptor by proteolytic cleavage of the N-terminal extracellular domain. Inactivation occurs by phosphorylation. Recovery requires resynthesis of the receptor.

currently the object of much interest (for reviews, see Dolphin, 1996; Gudermann et al., 1996; Schoenberg et al., 1999).

G-proteins consist of three subunits, α, β and γ (Fig. 3.8). Guanine nucleotides bind to the α-subunit, which has enzymic activity, catalysing the conversion of GTP to GDP. The β- and γ-subunits remain together as a βγ-complex. All three subunits are anchored to the membrane through a fatty acid chain, coupled to the G-protein through a reaction known as *prenylation*. G-proteins appear to be freely diffusible in the plane of the membrane; consequently, a single pool of G-protein in a cell can interact with several different receptors and effectors in an essentially promiscuous fashion. In the 'resting' state (Fig. 3.8), the G-protein exists as an unattached αβγ-trimer, with GDP occupying the site on the α-subunit. When a GPCR is occupied by an agonist molecule, a conformational change occurs, involving the cytoplasmic domain of the receptor (Fig. 3.3B), causing it to acquire high affinity for the αβγ-trimer. Association of αβγ-trimer with the receptor causes the bound GDP to dissociate and to be replaced with GTP (GDP/GTP exchange), which in turn causes dissociation of the G-protein trimer, releasing α-GTP and βγ-subunits; these are the 'active' forms of the G-protein, which diffuse in the membrane and can associate with various enzymes and ion channels, causing activation or inactivation as the case may be (Fig. 3.8).* The process is terminated when the hydrolysis of GTP to GDP occurs through the GTPase activity of the α-subunit. The resulting α-GDP then dissociates from the effector and reunites with the βγ-complex, completing the cycle. Attachment of the α-subunit to an effector molecule actually increases its GTPase activity, the magnitude of this increase being different for different types of effector. Since GTP hydrolysis is the step that terminates the ability of the α-subunit to produce its effect, regulation of its GTPase activity by the effector protein means that the activation of the effector tends to be self-limiting. The mechanism results in *amplification* because a single agonist–receptor complex can activate several G-protein molecules in turn, and each of these can remain associated with the effector enzyme for long enough to produce many molecules of product. The product (see below) is often a second messenger, and further amplification occurs before the final cellular response is produced.

How is specificity achieved so that each kind of receptor produces a distinct pattern of cellular responses? With a common pool of promiscuous G-proteins linking the various receptors and effector systems in a cell it might seem that all specificity would be lost, but this is clearly not the case. For example, muscarinic acetylcholine receptors and β-adrenoceptors, both of which occur in cardiac muscle cells, produce opposite functional effects (Chs 10 and 11). The main reason is molecular variation within the G-protein family (see Wess, 1998).** These variants give rise to

*Until recently it was thought that G-protein signalling occurred only through the α-subunit, and that the βγ-complex served merely as a chaperone to keep the flighty α-subunits out of range of the various effector proteins to which they might otherwise snuggle up. However, the βγ-complexes actually make assignations of their own, and control effectors in much the same way as the α-subunits (see Clapham & Neer, 1997). In general, it appears that higher concentrations of βγ-complex than of α-subunits are needed, so βγ-mediated effects occur at higher levels of receptor occupancy than α-mediated effects. The control of ion channels by G-proteins (p. 47) exemplifies the dual role of the α- and βγ-subunits.

**There are, to date, more than 20 known subtypes of the α-subunit, six of the β-subunit and 12 of the γ-subunit of G-protein providing, in theory, about 1500 variants of the trimer. From what we know so far, specificity seems to depend mainly on the α-subunit; even so, the 20 subtypes give ample scope for specific linkages between receptors and their effectors (and we certainly should not assume that the βγ-complex variations are functionally irrelevant). By now, you will be unsurprised (even if somewhat bemused) by such a display of molecular heterogeneity, for it is the way of evolution.

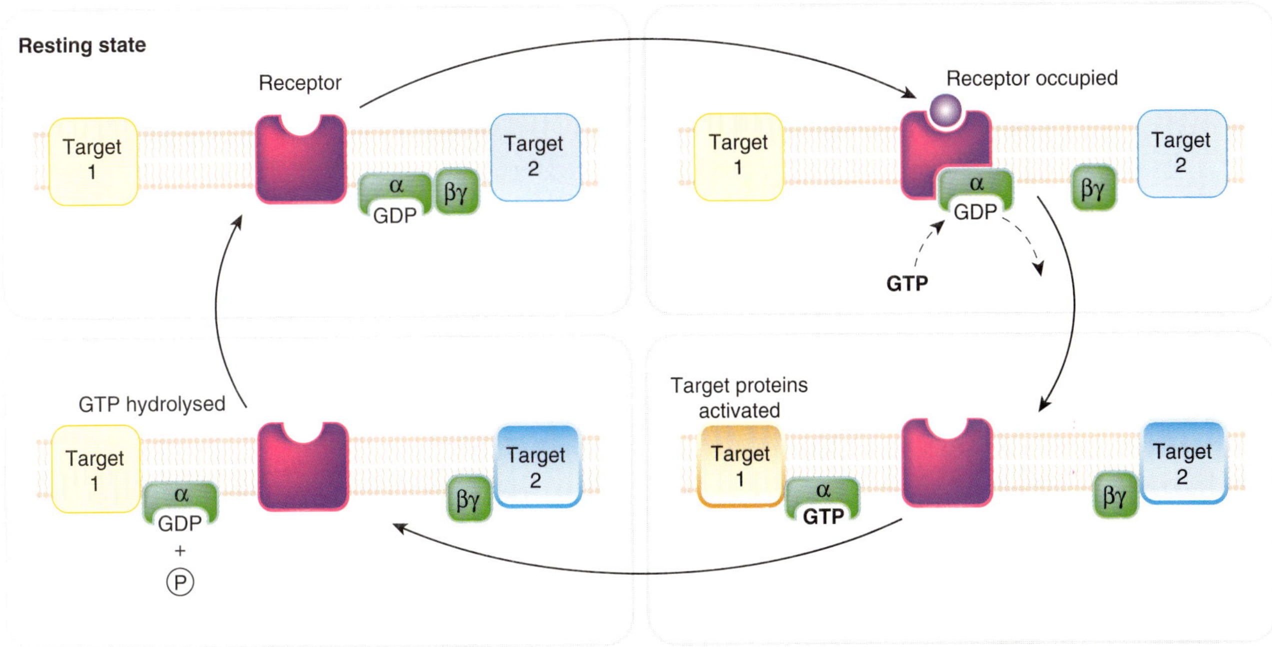

Fig. 3.8 The function of the G-protein. The G-protein consists of three subunits (α, β, γ), which are anchored to the membrane through attached lipid residues. Coupling of the α-subunit to an agonist-occupied receptor causes the bound GDP to exchange with intracellular GTP; the α-GTP complex then dissociates from the receptor and from the βγ-subunit complex and interacts with a target protein (target 1, which may be an enzyme such as adenylate cyclase or an ion channel). The βγ-complex may also activate a target protein (target 2). The GTPase activity of the α-subunit is increased when the target protein is bound, leading to hydrolysis of the bound GTP to GDP, whereupon the α-subunit reunites with the βγ-complex. The activated state of the target proteins is shown in colour.

G-protein-coupled receptors

- These are sometimes called metabotropic receptors.
- All are monomers comprising seven membrane-spanning segments (recent evidence for dimeric structures in some cases).
- One of the intracellular loops is larger than the others and interacts with the G-protein.
- The G-protein is a membrane protein comprising three subunits (αβγ), the α-subunit possessing GTPase activity.
- When the trimer binds to antagonist-occupied receptor, the α-subunit dissociates and is then free to activate an effector (a membrane enzyme or ion channel). In some cases the βγ-subunit may be the activator species.
- Activation of the effector is terminated when the bound GTP molecule is hydrolysed, which allows the α-subunit to recombine with βγ.
- There are several types of G-protein, which interact with different receptors and control different effectors.
- Examples include the muscarinic acetylcholine receptor, adrenoceptors and neuropeptide receptors.

three main classes of G-protein (G_s, G_i and G_q), which show selectivity with respect to both the receptors and the effectors with which they couple, having specific recognition domains in their structure complementary to specific G-protein-binding domains in the receptor and effector molecules. G_s and G_i produce, respectively, stimulation and inhibition of the enzyme adenylate cyclase (Fig. 3.9), and a similar bidirectional control operates on other effectors, such as phospholipase C (PLC; see Gudermann et al., 1996). The G-proteins can be thought of as the intramembrane gophers, bustling between receptors and effectors, controlling this microcosm but communicating very little with the world outside.

The α-subunits of these G-proteins differ in structure. One functional difference, which has been useful as an experimental tool to distinguish which type of G-protein is involved in different situations, concerns the action of two bacterial toxins, cholera toxin and pertussis toxin. These toxins, which are enzymes, catalyse a conjugation reaction (ADP-ribosylation) on the α-subunit of G-proteins. Cholera toxin acts only on G_s, and it causes persistent activation. Many of the symptoms of cholera, such as the excessive secretion of fluid from the gastrointestinal epithelium, are the result of the uncontrolled activation of adenylate cyclase that occurs. Pertussis toxin acts on G_i in a similar way.

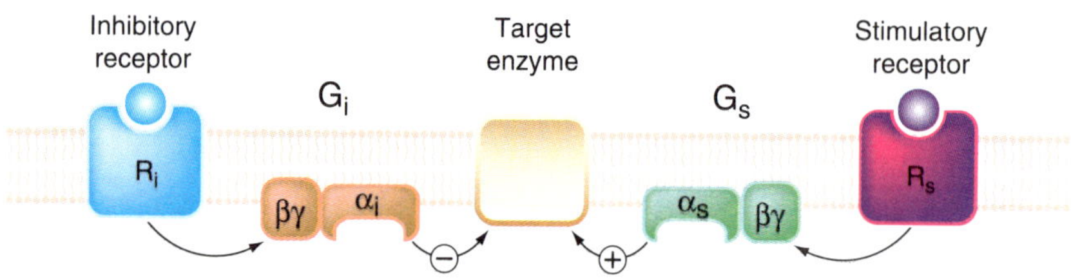

Fig. 3.9 Bidirectional control of a target enzyme by G-protein varients. Heterogeneity of G-proteins allows different receptors to exert opposite effects on a target enzyme, e.g. G_s and G_i on adenylate cyclase.

TARGETS FOR G-PROTEINS

The main targets for G-proteins, through which GPCRs control different aspects of cell function (see Milligan, 1995; Gudermann et al., 1996), are:

- *adenylate cyclase:* the enzyme responsible for cAMP formation
- *phospholipase C:* the enzyme responsible for inositol phosphate and diacylglycerol formation
- *ion channels*: particularly calcium and potassium channels.

The adenylate cyclase/cAMP system

The discovery by Sutherland and his colleagues of the role of cAMP (cyclic 3′,5′-adenosine monophosphate) as an intracellular mediator demolished at a stroke the barriers that existed between biochemistry and pharmacology and introduced the concept of second messengers in signal transduction. cAMP is a nucleotide synthesised within the cell from ATP by the action of a membrane-bound enzyme, adenylate cyclase. cAMP is produced continuously and inactivated by hydrolysis to 5′-AMP through the action of a family of enzymes known as *phosphodiesterases*. Many different drugs, hormones and neurotransmitters act on GPCRs and produce their effects by increasing or decreasing the catalytic activity of adenylate cyclase, thus raising or lowering the concentration of cAMP within the cell. There are several different molecular isoforms of the enzyme, some of which respond selectively to G_s or G_i (see Simonds, 1999).

cAMP regulates many aspects of cellular function including, for example, enzymes involved in energy metabolism, cell division and cell differentiation; ion transport; ion channels; and the contractile proteins in smooth muscle. These varied effects are, however, all brought about by a common mechanism, namely the activation of *protein kinases* by cAMP. Protein kinases regulate the function of many different cellular proteins by catalysing the phosphorylation of serine and threonine residues, using ATP as a source of phosphate groups. Phosphorylation can either activate or inhibit target enzymes or ion channels. Figure 3.10 shows the ways in which increased cAMP production in response to β-adrenoceptor activation affects enzymes involved in glycogen and fat metabolism in liver, fat and muscle cells. The result is a coordinated response in which stored energy in the form of glycogen and fat is made available as glucose to fuel muscle contraction.

Other examples of regulation by cAMP-dependent protein kinases include the increased activity of voltage-activated calcium channels in heart muscle cells (see Ch. 17); phosphorylation of these channels increases the amount of Ca^{2+} entering the cell during the action potential and, thus, increases the force of contraction of the heart.

In smooth muscle, cAMP-dependent protein kinase phosphorylates (thereby inactivating) another enzyme, myosin-light-chain kinase, which is required for contraction. This accounts for the smooth muscle relaxation produced by many drugs that increase cAMP production in smooth muscle (see Ch. 18).

As mentioned above, receptors linked to G_i rather than G_s inhibit adenylate cyclase and thus reduce cAMP formation. Examples include certain types of muscarinic acetylcholine receptor (e.g. the M_2-receptor of cardiac muscle; see Ch. 10), α_2-adrenoceptors in smooth muscle (Ch. 11) and opioid receptors (see Ch. 40). Adenylate cyclase can be activated directly by certain agents, including forskolin and fluoride ions; these agents are used experimentally in studies on the role of the cAMP system.

cAMP is hydrolysed within cells by phosphodiesterases, a family of enzymes that is inhibited by drugs such as methylxanthines (e.g. **theophylline, caffeine**; see Chs 22 and 41) and **sildenafil** (better known as Viagra). The similarity of some of the actions of these drugs to those of catecholamines probably reflects their common property of increasing the intracellular concentration of cAMP. Various tissue-specific isoforms of phosphodiesterase exist, and selective inhibitors of this enzyme have applications in cardiovascular and respiratory diseases (Chs 18 and 22).

The phospholipase C/inositol phosphate system

The phosphoinositide system, an important intracellular second messenger system, was first discovered by Hokin and Hokin in the 1950s, whose recondite interests centred on the mechanism of salt secretion by the nasal glands of seabirds. They found that secretion was accompanied by increased turnover of a minor class of membrane phospholipids known as *phosphoinositides* (collectively known as PI*; Fig. 3.11). Subsequently, Michell and

*Alternative abbreviations for these mediators are: PtdIns for PI; PtdIns(4,5)-P_2 for PIP_2; Ins(1,4,5)-P_3 for IP_3; Ins(1,3,4,5)-P_4 for IP_4.

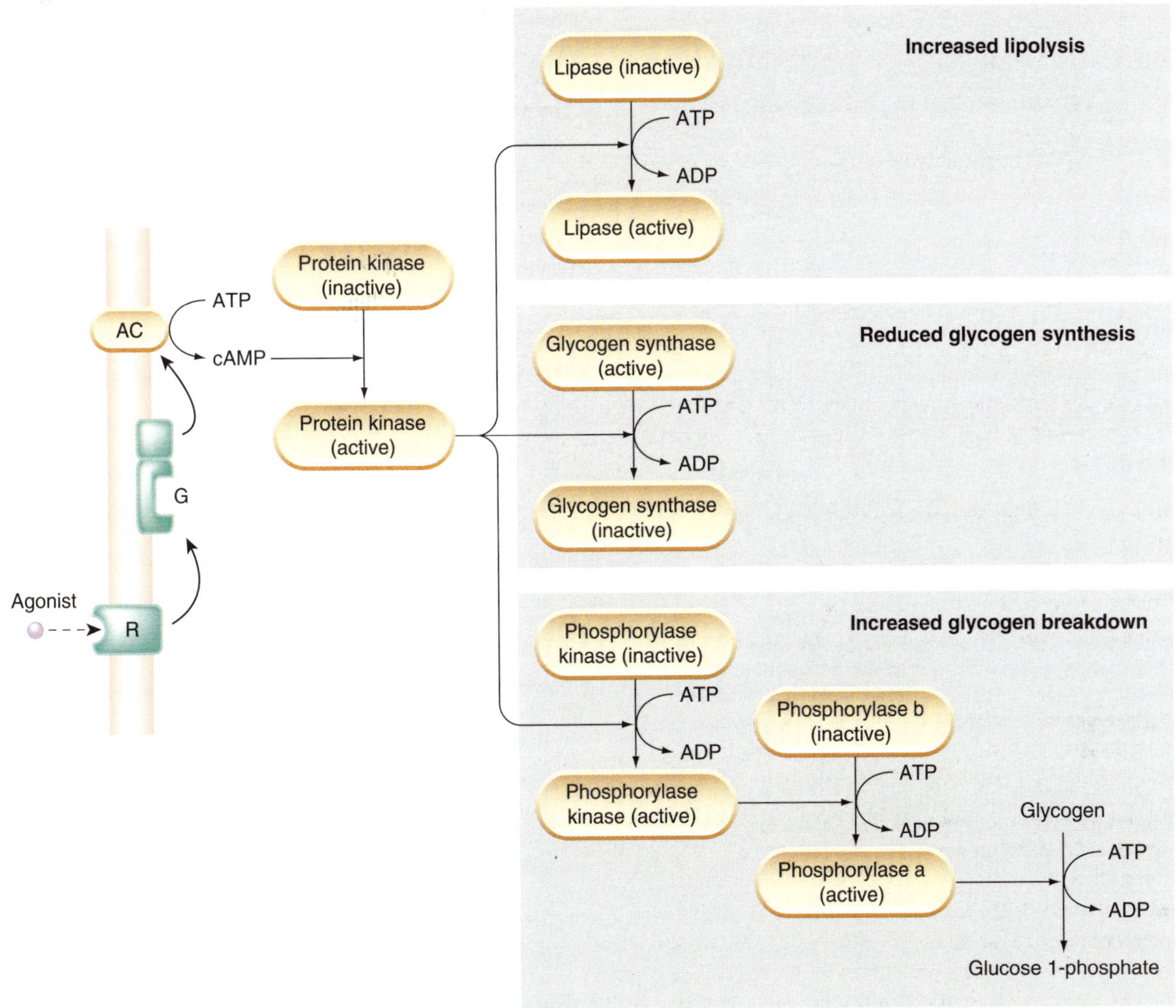

Fig. 3.10 Regulation of energy metabolism by cAMP. (AC, adenylate cyclase.)

Berridge found that many hormones which produce an increase in free intracellular Ca^{2+} concentration (which include, for example, muscarinic agonists and α-adrenoceptor agonists acting on smooth muscle and salivary glands, and antidiuretic hormone (vasopressin) acting on liver cells) also increase PI turnover. Subsequently it was found that one particular member of the PI family, namely phosphatidylinositol 4,5-bisphosphate (PIP_2), which has additional phosphate groups attached to the inositol ring, plays a key role. PIP_2 is the substrate for a membrane-bound enzyme, $PLC_β$, which splits it into diacylglycerol (DAG) and inositol 1,4,5-trisphosphate (IP_3; Fig. 3.12), both of which function as second messengers as discussed below. The activation of $PLC_β$ by various agonists is mediated through a G-protein in just the same way as adenylate cyclase, described above, though different G-protein subtypes are involved. After cleavage of PIP_2 the status quo is restored, as shown in Figure 3.12, DAG being phosphorylated to form phosphatidic acid, while the IP_3 is dephosphorylated and then recoupled with phosphatidic acid to form PIP_2 once again. **Lithium**, an agent used in psychiatry (see Ch. 38), blocks this recycling pathway (see Fig. 3.12).

Inositol phosphates and intracellular calcium

IP_3 is water-soluble mediator that is released into the cytosol and acts on a specific receptor—the IP_3 receptor—which is a ligand-gated calcium channel present on the membrane of the endoplasmic reticulum. The main role of IP_3, described in more detail in Chapter 4, is to control the release of Ca^{2+} from intracellular stores. Since many drug and hormone effects involve intracellular Ca^{2+}, this pathway is particularly important and has attracted much attention. IP_3 is converted inside the cell to the 1,3,4,5-tetraphosphate, IP_4, by a specific kinase. The exact role of

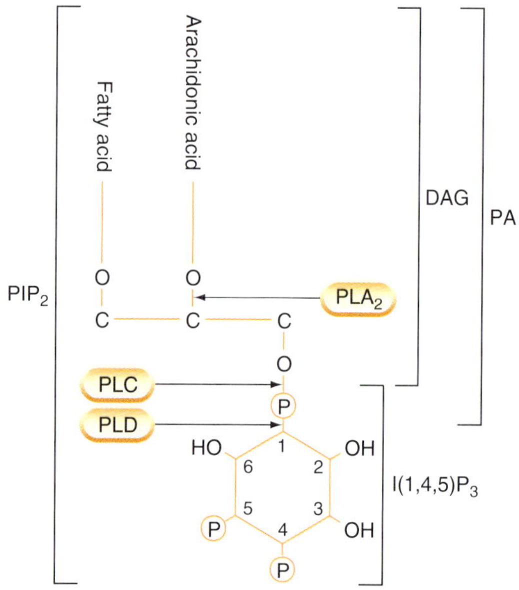

Fig. 3.11 Structure of phosphatidylinositol bisphosphate (PIP_2), showing sites of cleavage by different phospholipases to produce active mediators. Cleavage by phospholipase A_2 (PLA_2) yields arachidonic acid. Cleavage by phospholipase C (PLC) yields inositol trisphosphate ($I(1,4,5)P_3$) and diacylglycerol (DAG). (PA, phosphatidic acid; PLD, phospholipase D.) Note that the inositol ring is a hexose structure: substituent groups project above or below the plane of the ring and, therefore, the 3 and 5 positions are not equivalent.

IP_4 remains unclear (see Irvine et al., 1999), but there is evidence that it too is involved in Ca^{2+} signalling. One possibility (see Clapham, 1995) is that it facilitates Ca^{2+} entry through the plasma membrane, thus avoiding depletion of the intracellular stores as a result of the action of IP_3.

Diacylglycerol and protein kinase C

DAG is produced as well as IP_3 whenever receptor-induced PI hydrolysis occurs. The main effect of DAG is to activate a membrane-bound protein kinase, *protein kinase C* (PKC), which catalyses the phosphorylation of a variety of intracellular proteins (see Nishizuka, 1988; Walaas & Greengard, 1991; Parker & Dekker, 1996). DAG, unlike the IPs, is highly lipophilic and remains within the membrane. It binds to a specific site on the PKC molecule, which migrates from the cytosol to the cell membrane in the presence of DAG, thereby becoming activated. There are at least 12 different PKC subtypes (see Toker, 1998), which have distinct cellular distributions and phosphorylate different proteins. Most are activated by DAG and raised intracellular Ca^{2+} levels, both of which are produced by activation of GPCRs. PKCs are also activated by **phorbol esters** (highly irritant, tumour-promoting compounds produced by certain plants), which has been extremely useful in studying the functions of PKC. One of the subtypes is activated by the lipid mediator arachidonic acid (see Ch. 15), which is generated by the action of phospholipase A_2 on membrane phospholipids, so PKC activation can also occur with agonists that activate this enzyme. The various PKC isoforms, like the tyrosine kinases discussed below (p. 42), act on many different functional proteins, such as ion channels, receptors, enzymes (including other kinases) and cytoskeletal proteins. Kinases, in general, play a central role in signal transduction and control many different aspects of cell function. The DAG–PKC link provides a mechanism whereby GPCRs can mobilise this army of control freaks.

Ion channels as targets for G-proteins

GPCRs can control ion channel function directly by mechanisms that do not involve second messengers such as cAMP or IPs. This was first shown for cardiac muscle, but it now appears that direct G-protein–channel interaction may be quite general (see Wickham & Clapham, 1995). Early examples came from studies on potassium channels. In cardiac muscle, for example, muscarinic acetylcholine receptors are known to enhance K^+ permeability (thus hyperpolarising the cells and inhibiting electrical activity; see Ch. 17). Similar mechanisms are believed to operate in neurons, where opiate analgesics reduce excitability by opening potassium channels (see Ch. 40). These actions are produced by direct interaction between the G-protein subunit and the channel, without the involvement of second messengers. As shown in Figure 3.8, either the free α-subunit, or the $\beta\gamma$-subunit complex of the G-protein may be the mediator that controls the channel.

The postulated roles of G-protein-coupled receptors in controlling enzymes and ion channels are summarised in Figure 3.13.

Agonist specificity

▼ The linkage of a particular GPCR to a particular signal transduction pathway depends mainly on the structure of the receptor, particularly in the region of the third intracellular loop, which confers specificity for a particular G-protein, from which the rest of the signal transduction pathway follows. Mutations in this region, which do not affect the ligand-binding specificity of the receptor, can cause it to switch from one pathway (e.g. cAMP) to another (e.g. the PI pathway) that it would not normally activate. In general, the nature of the agonist does not alter the signal transduction pathway, so all agonists acting on a particular receptor produce basically the same type of cellular response. Complications are beginning to appear, however, and there is now evidence (see Kenakin, 1995) that different agonists may produce different activated forms of the receptor, and hence different cellular responses—a phenomenon termed *agonist trafficking*. Examples are rare, and the idea is currently controversial—indeed heretical to many pharmacologists, who are accustomed to think of agonists in terms of their affinity and efficacy and nothing else. If substantiated, it will add a new dimension to the way in which we think about drug specificity.

Desensitisation

▼ As described in Chapter 2, desensitisation is a feature of most GPCRs, and the mechanisms underlying it have been extensively studied. Two main processes are involved (see Koenig & Edwardson, 1997; Krupnik & Benovic, 1998; Ferguson, 2001):

- receptor phosphorylation
- receptor internalisation (endocytosis).

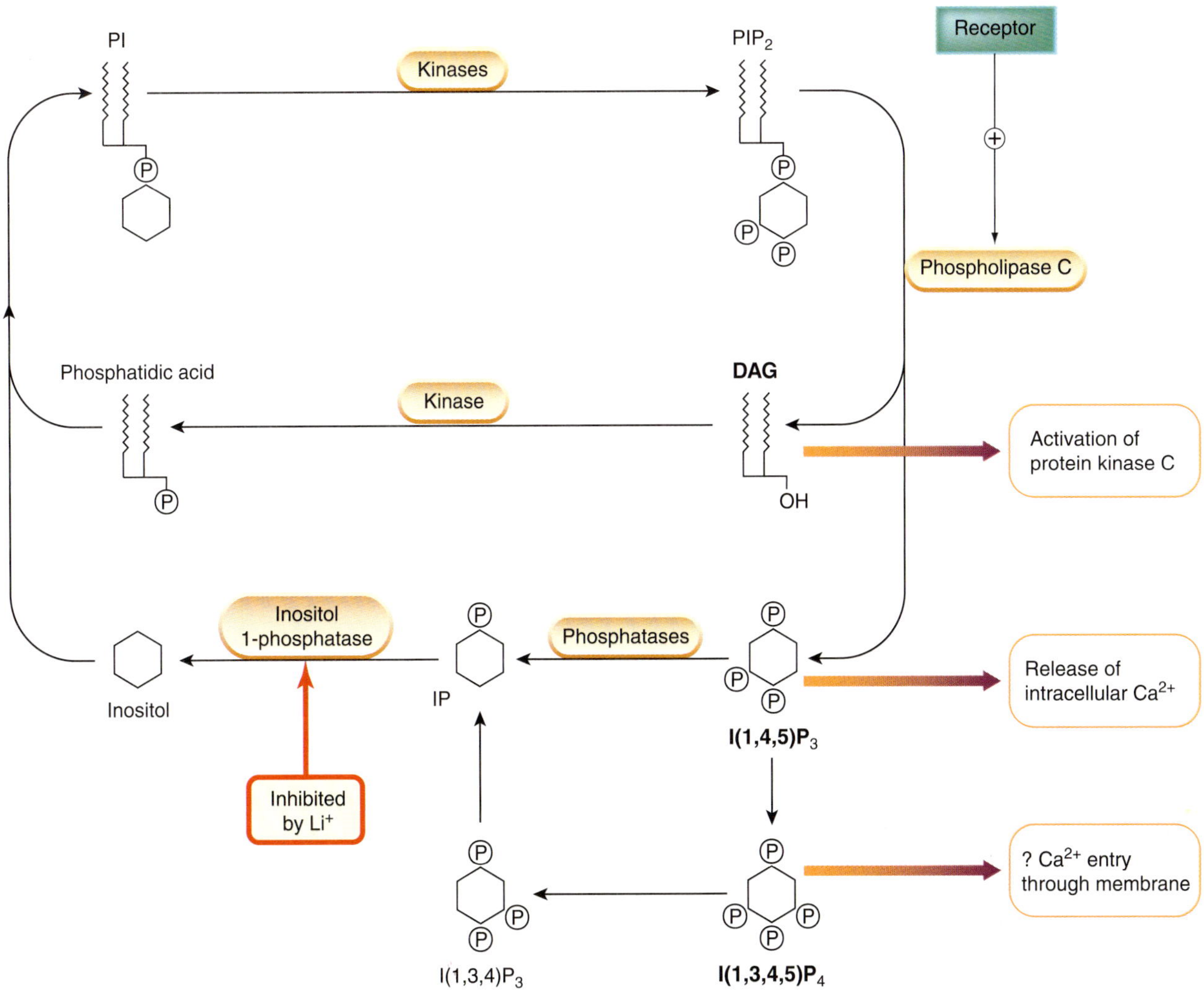

Fig. 3.12 The phosphatidylinositol (PI) cycle. Receptor-mediated activation of phospholipase C results in the cleavage of phosphatidylinositol biophosphate (PIP_2), forming diacylglycerol (DAG), which activates protein kinase C, and inositol trisphosphate (IP_3), which releases intracellular Ca^{2+}. The role of inositol tetraphosphate (IP_4), which is formed from IP_3 and other inositol phosphates, is unclear, but it may facilitate Ca^{2+} entry through the plasma membrane. IP_3 is inactivated by dephosphorylation to inositol. DAG is converted to phosphatidic acid, and these two products are used to regenerate PI and PIP_2.

The sequence of GPCRs includes certain residues (serine and threonine), mainly in the C-terminal cytoplasmic tail, that can be phosphorylated by kinases, such as protein kinase A, PKC and specific membrane-bound GPCR kinases (GRKs).

Phosphorylation by PKA and PKC, which are activated by many GPCRs, generally leads to impaired coupling between the activated receptor and the G-protein, so the agonist effect is reduced. These kinases are not very selective, so receptors other than that for the desensitising agonist will also be affected. This effect, whereby one agonist can desensitise other receptors, is known as *heterologous desensitisation* and is generally weak and short lasting (see Fig. 3.14).

Phosphorylation by GRKs (see Krupnick & Benovic, 1998; Fig. 3.14) is receptor-specific to a greater or lesser degree and affects mainly receptors in their activated (i.e. agonist-bound) state, resulting in *homologous desensitisation*. The residues that GRKs phosphorylate are different from those targeted by other kinases; the phosphorylated receptor serves as a binding site for *arrestins,* intracellular proteins that block the interaction of the receptor with G-proteins, and also is targeted for endocytosis, producing a more profound and long-lasting desensitisation. The first GRK to be identified was the β-adrenoceptor kinase, BARK, but several others have since been discovered, and this type of desensitisation seems to occur with most GPCRs.

SOME RECENT SURPRISES

Here we describe some recent developments in the field of GPCR biology that, though yet to be fully explored, are likely to have important implications for pharmacology in the future.

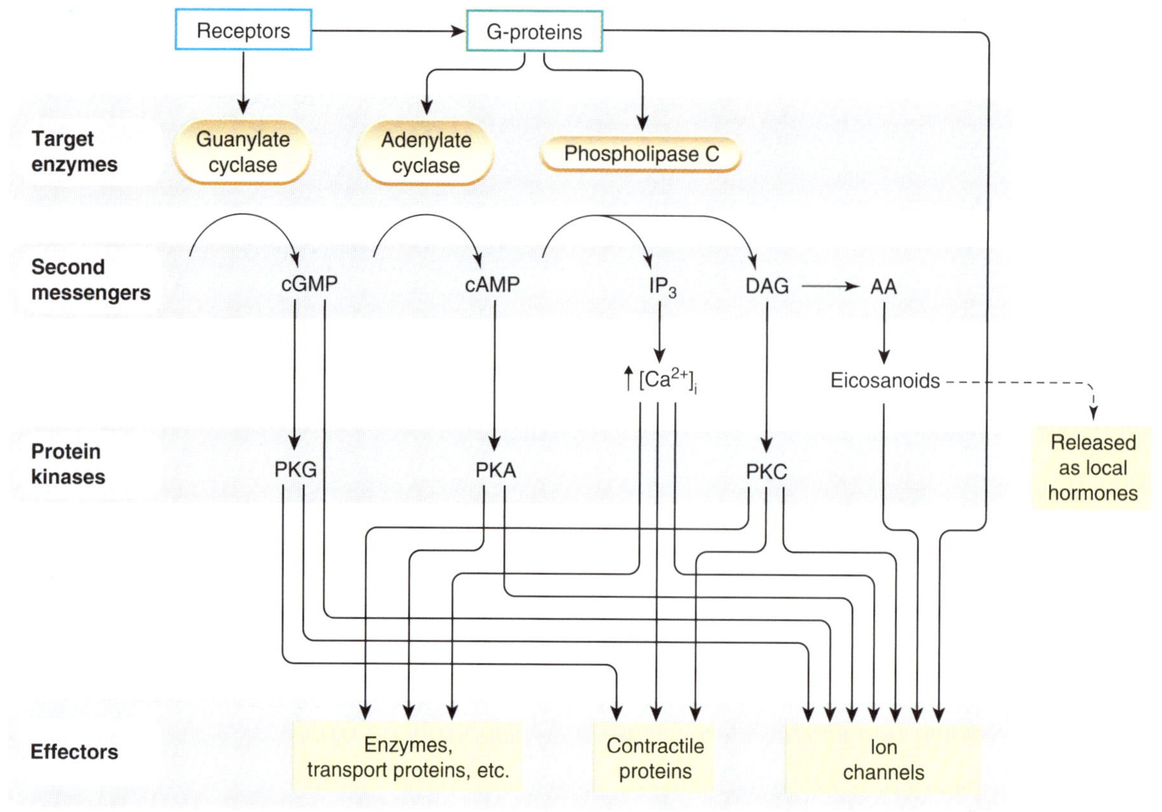

Fig. 3.13 G-protein and second messenger control of cellular effector systems. (IP_3, inositol trisphosphate; DAG, diacylglycerol; AA, arachidonic acid.)

GPCR dimerisation

▼ The conventional view that GPCRs exist and function as monomeric proteins (in contrast to ion channels, which generally from multimeric arrays, see p. 29), was upset by work on the $GABA_B$ receptor, a GPCR first cloned in 1997 (see Marshall et al., 1999). Two subtypes of this receptor exist, encoded by different genes, and the functional receptor consists of a heterodimer of the two. Other examples of GPCR oligomerisation are reviewed by Bouvier (2001). Within the opioid receptor family (see Ch. 40), stable and functional dimers of κ- and δ-receptors have been found, the pharmacological properties of which differ from those of either parent. More diverse GPCR combinations have also been found, such as that between dopamine (D_2) and somatostatin receptors, on which both ligands act with increased potency. Roaming even further afield in search of functional assignations, the dopamine (D_5) receptor can couple directly with a ligand-gated ion channel, the $GABA_A$ receptor, inhibiting the function of the latter without the intervention of any G-protein (Liu et al., 2000). These interactions have so far been studied mainly in engineered cell lines, and evidence that they are important in native cells remains fragmentary.* It is too early to say what impact this newly discovered versatility of GPCRs in linking up with other receptors to form functional combinations will have on conventional pharmacology and therapeutics, but it could be considerable.

*A recent study (AbdAlla et al., 2001) has shown that functional dimeric complexes between angiotensin (AT_1) and bradykinin (B_2) receptors occur in human platelets and show increased sensitivity to angiotensin compared with 'pure' AT_1 receptors. In pregnant women suffering from hypertension (pre-eclamptic toxaemia), the number of these dimers increases owing to increased expression of B_2-receptors, resulting—paradoxically—in increased sensitivity to the vasoconstrictor action of angiotensin. This is the first instance of the role of dimerisation in human disease.

Receptor activity modifying proteins

▼ Receptor activity modifying proteins (RAMPs) are a family of membrane proteins that associate with GPCRs and alter their functional characteristics. They were discovered by McLatchie et al. (1998) during attempts to clone the receptor for a neuropeptide: calcitonin gene-related peptide (CGRP; see Ch. 13). It was found that the functionally active CGRP receptor consisted of a complex of a GPCR (called CRLR, or calcitonin receptor-like receptor) that by itself lacked activity with another membrane protein (RAMP1). More surprisingly, CRLR when coupled with another RAMP (RAMP2) showed a quite different pharmacology, being activated by another peptide, adrenomedullin. In other words, the agonist specificity is conferred by the associated RAMP rather than by the GPCR itself. Other examples in the peptide receptor field are now emerging, but it is not known how widespread this phenomenon may be. It is another example where interactions at the molecular level influence the pharmacological behaviour of the receptors in an unexpected way.

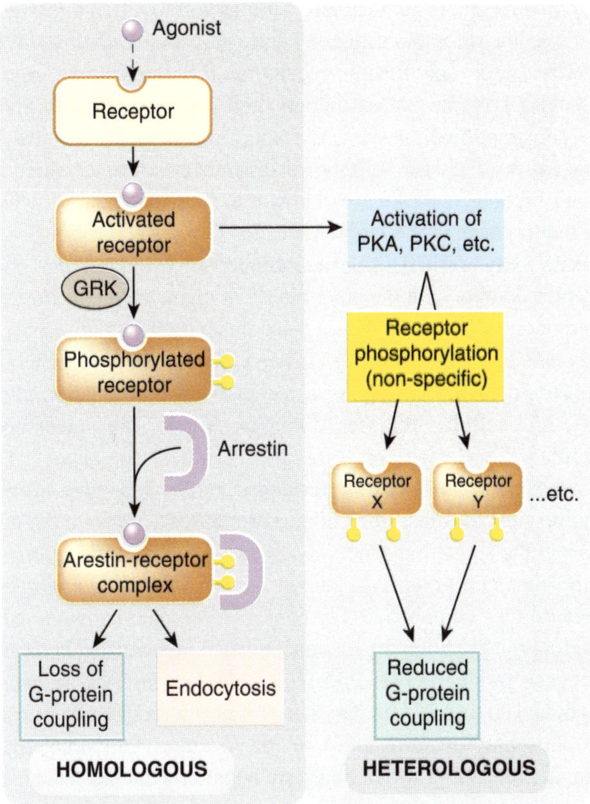

Fig 3.14 Desensitisation of G-protein-coupled receptors. Homologous (agonist-specific) desensitisation involves phosphorylation of the activated receptor by a specific kinase (GRK). The phosphorylated receptor (P-R) then binds to arrestin, causing the receptors to lose its ability to associate with a G-protein, and undergoes endocytosis, which removes the receptor from the membrane. Heterologous (cross-) desensitisation occurs as a result of phosphorylation of one type of receptor through activation of kinases by another. (PKA and PKC, protein kinase A and C, respectively.)

Effectors controlled by G-proteins

- Two key pathways are controlled by receptors, via G-proteins. Both can be activated or inhibited by pharmacological ligands, depending on the nature of the receptor and G-protein.
- Adenylate cyclase (AC)/cAMP:
  —AC catalyses formation of the intracellular messenger cAMP
  —cAMP activates various protein kinases, which control cell function in many different ways by causing phosphorylation of various enzymes, carriers and other proteins.
- Phospholipase C/inositol trisphosphate (IP_3)/diacylglycerol (DAG)
  —catalyses the formation of two intracellular messengers, IP_3 and DAG, from membrane phospholipid
  —IP_3 acts to increase free cytosolic Ca^{2+} by releasing Ca^{2+} from intracellular compartments
  —increased free Ca^{2+} initiates many events, including contraction, secretion, enzyme activation and membrane hyperpolarisation
  —DAG activates protein kinase C, which controls many cellular functions by phosphorylating a variety of proteins.
- Receptor-linked G-proteins also control:
  —phospholipase A (and thus the formation of arachidonic acid and eicosanoids)
  —ion channels (e.g. potassium and calcium channels, thus affecting membrane excitability, transmitter release, contractility, etc.).

G-protein-independent signalling

▼ In using the term 'G-protein-coupled receptor' to describe the class of receptors characterised by their seven-helical structure, we are following conventional textbook dogma, but neglecting the fact that G-proteins are not the only link between GPCRs and the various effector systems that they regulate. The example of direct linkage between GPCRs and ion channels was mentioned above. There are also many examples where the various 'adapter proteins' which link receptors of the tyrosine kinase type to their effectors (see below) can also interact with GPCRs (see Brzostowski & Kimmel, 2001), allowing the same effector systems to be regulated by receptors of either type. In this context, the GRKs, which are involved in desensitisation (see above), may also contribute to signal transduction, since phosphorylation of the C-terminal region of the GPCR produces a recognition site for molecules of the signal transduction pathway, analogous to the functioning of the kinase-linked receptors (see below; review by Bockaert & Pin, 1999).

SUMMARY

The simple dogma that underpins much of our current understanding of GPCRs, namely:

One GPCR gene—one GPCR protein—
one functional GPCR—one G-protein

is beginning to show signs of wear. In particular:

- one gene, through alternative splicing, RNA editing, etc. can give rise to more than one protein
- one GPCR protein can associate with others to produce more than one type of functional receptor
- the signal transduction pathway does not invariably require G-proteins.

GPCRs seem to have a particularly adventurous streak, and nobody imagines that we have reached the end of the story.

TYPE 3: KINASE-LINKED AND RELATED RECEPTORS

The kinase-linked receptors are quite different in structure and function from either the ligand-gated channels or the GPCRs. They mediate the actions of a wide variety of protein mediators, including growth factors and cytokines (see Ch. 15), and hormones such as insulin (see Ch. 25) and leptin (Ch. 26). For more detail, see reviews by Barbacid (1996), Ihle (1995), Schenk & Snaar-Jakelska (1999). Reflecting their inherent enzymic properties, growth factor receptors are often referred to as *receptor tyrosine kinases*. Guanylate-cyclase-linked receptors (see Lucas et al., 2000) are much less numerous and mediate the actions of certain peptides such as atrial natriuretic peptide (see Ch. 17). They can be considered as a separate superfamily, but we lump them together with growth factor receptors on account of their close structural relationship.

The basic structure of type 3 receptors is shown in Figure 3.3C. They comprise very large extracellular (ligand-binding) and intracellular (effector) domains, with about 400–700 residues in each. In the case of the insulin receptor, the extracellular domain consists of a separate polypeptide, which is linked to the rest of the molecule by disulfide bonds. In contrast, the growth factor receptors consist of a single long chain of over 1000 residues. Cytokine receptors are generally similar but are often dimeric. In all cases, the receptors trigger a kinase cascade (see below). With growth factor and insulin receptors, the intracellular region possesses tyrosine kinase activity and incorporates both ATP- and substrate-binding sites. Cytokine receptors do not usually have intrinsic kinase activity but associate, when activated by ligand binding, with kinases known as Jaks (see below), which are the first step in the kinase cascade.

With only a single transmembrane helix linking the outer receptor domain with the inner kinase domain, a simple allosteric interaction seems unlikely as a mechanism by which the kinase is activated by ligand binding. Instead, ligand binding generally leads to *dimerisation* of pairs of receptors. The association of the two intracellular kinase domains allows an incestuous autophosphorylation of tyrosine residues to occur. The autophosphorylated tyrosine residues then serve as high-affinity binding sites for other intracellular proteins, which form the next stage in the signal transduction cascade. One important group of such 'adapter' proteins is known as the *SH2-domain proteins* (because they contain a highly conserved domain known as SH2 standing for 'src homology', since it was first identified in the Src oncogene product). These possess a highly conserved sequence of about 100 amino acid residues forming a recognition site for the phosphotyrosine residues of the receptor. Individual SH2-domain proteins, of which many are now known, bind selectively to particular receptors, so the pattern of events triggered by particular growth factors is highly specific. The mechanism is summarised in Figure 3.15.

Kinase-linked receptors

- Receptors for various hormones (e.g. insulin) and growth factors incorporate tyrosine kinase in their intracellular domain.
- Cytokine receptors have an intracellular domain that binds and activates cytosolic kinases when the receptor is occupied.
- The receptors all share a common architecture, with a large extracellular ligand-binding domain connected via a single α-helix to the intracellular domain.
- Signal transduction generally involves dimerisation of receptors, followed by autophosphorylation of tyrosine residues. The phosphotyrosine residues act as acceptors for the SH2 domains of a variety of intracellular proteins, thereby allowing control of many cell functions.
- They are involved mainly in events controlling cell growth and differentiation; they also act indirectly by regulating gene transcription.
- Two important pathways are:
  - —the Ras/Raf/MAP kinase pathway, which is important in cell division, growth and differentiation
  - —the Jak/Stat pathway, which is activated by many cytokines and which controls the synthesis and release of many inflammatory mediators.
- A few hormone receptors (e.g. atrial natriuretic factor) have a similar architecture and are linked to guanylate cyclase.

PROTEIN PHOSPHORYLATION AND KINASE CASCADE MECHANISMS

What happens when the SH2-domain containing protein binds to the phosphorylated receptor varies greatly according to the receptor that is involved; many SH2-domain proteins are enzymes, such as protein kinases or phospholipases. Some growth factors activate a specific subtype of PLC, PLC_{γ}, thereby causing phospholipid breakdown, IP_3 formation and Ca^{2+} release (see above). Other SH2-containing proteins couple phosphotyrosine-containing proteins with a variety of other functional proteins, including many that are involved in the control of cell division and differentiation, the end result being to stimulate transcription of particular genes.

▼ Two well-defined signal transduction pathways are summarised in Figure 3.15. The Ras/Raf pathway (Fig. 3.15A) mediates the effect of many growth factors and mitogens. Ras, which is a proto-oncogene product, functions like a G-protein and conveys the signal (by GDP/GTP exchange) from the SH2-domain protein Grb, which is phosphorylated by the receptor tyrosine kinase. Activation of Ras, in turn, activates Raf, which is the first of a sequence of serine/threonine kinases, each of which phosphorylates, and activates, the next in line. The last of these, MAP (mitogen-activated protein) kinase, phosphorylates one or more transcription factors that initiate gene expression, resulting in a variety of cellular responses, including cell division. Many cancers are associated with mutations in the genes coding for proteins involved in this cascade, leading to activation of the cascade in the absence of the growth factor

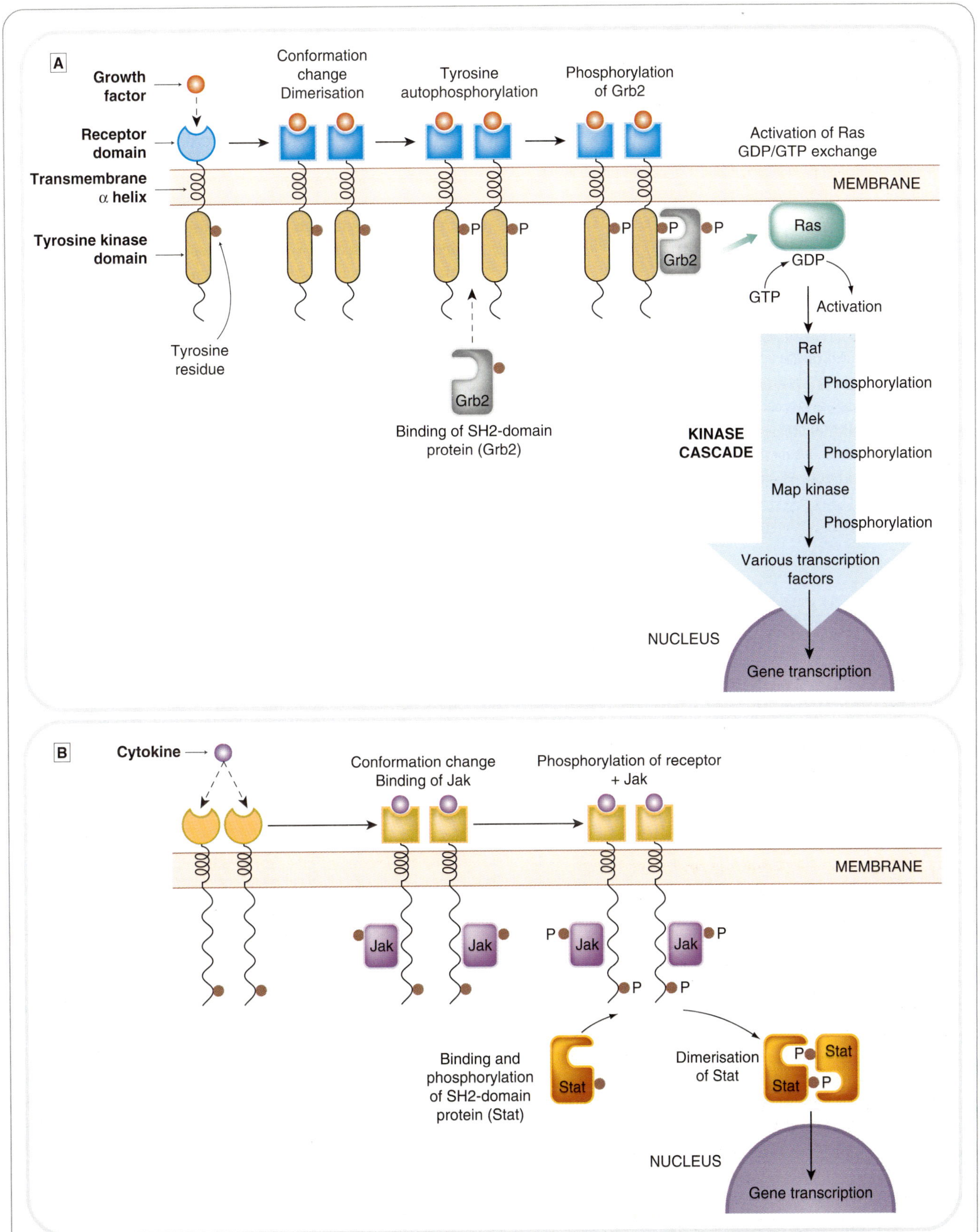

Fig 3.15 Transduction mechanisms of kinase-linked receptors. The first step following agonist binding is dimerisation, which leads to autophosphorylation of the intracellular domain of each receptor. SH2 domain proteins then bind to the phosphorylated receptor and are themselves phosphorylated. Two well-characterised pathways are shown. A The growth factor (Ras/Raf/MAP kinase) pathway (see also Ch. 5); B The cytokine (Jak/Stat) pathway (see also Ch. 15). Several other pathways exist, and these phosphorylation cascades interact with components of G-protein systems.

Protein phosphorylation in signal transduction

- Many receptor-mediated events involve protein phosphorylation, which controls the functioning and binding properties of intracellular proteins.
- Receptor-linked tyrosine kinases, cyclic nucleotide-activated tyrosine kinases, and intracellular serine/threonine kinases comprise a 'kinase cascade' mechanism that leads to amplification of receptor-mediated events.
- There are many kinases, with differing substrate specificities, allowing specificity in the pathways activated by different hormones.
- Desensitisation of G-protein-coupled receptors occurs as a result of phosphorylation by specific receptor kinases, causing the receptor to become non-functional and to be internalised.
- There is a large family of phosphatases that act to reverse the effects of kinases.

signal (see Ch. 5; for more details, see reviews by Avruch et al. (1994) Marshall (1996) Schenk & Snaar-Jakelska (1999)).

A second pathway, the Jak/Stat pathway (Fig. 3.15B), is involved in responses to many cytokines. Dimerisation of these receptors occurs when the cytokine binds, and this attracts a cytosolic tyrosine kinase unit (Jak) to associate with, and phosphorylate, the receptor dimer. Jaks belong to a family of proteins, different members having specificity for different cytokine receptors. Among the targets for phosphorylation by Jak are a family of transcription factors (Stats). These are SH2-domain proteins that bind to the phosphotyrosine groups on the receptor–Jak complex, and are themselves phosphorylated. Thus activated, Stat migrates to the nucleus and activates gene expression (see Ihle, 1995).

Recent work on signal transduction pathways has produced a bewildering profusion of molecular detail, often couched in a jargon that is apt to deter the faint-hearted. Perseverance will be rewarded, however, for there is no doubt that important new drugs, particularly in the areas of inflammation, immunology and cancer, will come from the targeting of these proteins (see Levitzki, 1996).*

The membrane-bound form of guanylate cyclase, the enzyme responsible for generating the second messenger cGMP in response to the binding of peptides such as atrial natriuretic peptide (see Chs 14 and 18), resembles the tyrosine kinase family and is activated in a similar way by dimerisation when the agonist is bound (see Lucas et al., 2000).

*A recent breakthrough in the treatment of chronic myeloid leukaemia was achieved with the introduction of **imatinib,** a drug that inhibits a specific tyrosine kinase involved in the pathogenesis of the disease (see Goldman & Melo, 2001).

TYPE 4: NUCLEAR RECEPTORS

The receptor-mediated regulation of DNA transcription is characteristic of steroid and thyroid hormones and is quite different from the mechanisms described so far (for reviews see Evans, 1988; Mangelsdorf et al., 1995). The work of Jensen in Chicago originally led to the recognition that the highly varied effects of different steroid drugs and hormones (which include numerous effects on the reproductive system, the kidney, the immune system, etc.) all operate through the same basic mechanism, namely by stimulating transcription of selected genes, leading to the synthesis of particular proteins and the production of cellular effects (see Chs 27 and 29). Most receptors are located in the nucleus, and the ligands are all lipophilic compounds that can readily cross the cell membrane. The basic structure of this family of receptors is shown in Fig. 3.3D. They possess a highly conserved region of about 60 residues in the middle of the molecule that constitutes the DNA-binding domain of the receptor. It contains two loops of about 15 residues each (zinc fingers), knotted together by a cluster of four cysteine residues surrounding a zinc atom; these structures occur in many proteins that regulate DNA transcription, and the fingers are believed to wrap around the DNA helix. The hormone-binding domain lies downstream of this central region, while upstream lies a variable region that is responsible for controlling gene transcription (see Bourguet et al., 2000).

On binding a steroid molecule, the receptor changes its conformation, which facilitates the formation of receptor dimers. These dimers bind to specific sequences of the nuclear DNA, known as *hormone-responsive elements*, which lie about 200 base pairs upstream from the genes that are regulated. An increase in RNA polymerase activity and the production of specific mRNA occur within a few minutes of adding the steroid, though the physiological response may take hours or days to develop. The different steroid hormones are able to induce or repress specific genes, and thus initiate completely different patterns of protein synthesis and produce different physiological effects. For example, glucocorticoids inhibit transcription of the gene for cyclooxygenase-2 (COX-2), which may account for their anti-inflammatory properties (see Ch. 16), whereas mineralocorticoids stimulate the production of various transport proteins that are involved in renal tubular function (see Ch. 23). Specificity at the DNA level is a function of the N-terminal and DNA-binding domain of the receptor rather than of the hormone-binding domain; thus chimeric receptors consisting of the N-terminus/DNA-binding part of one receptor (A) coupled to the hormone-binding part of another (B) will respond to hormone B but produce the effects associated with hormone A. More detail is given in the reviews mentioned above. Nuclear receptors form a large and ever-growing family, currently with more than 150 members, many of which belong to the class of 'orphan receptors' (see above) for which the physiological ligand remains to be identified (Laudet & Adelmant, 1995).

Other ligands that act on nuclear receptors of this family include thyroid hormones (Ch. 28), vitamin D (Ch. 30) and retinoic acid. Retinoic acid is an important regulator of embryonic development, and gradients of this substance arising

Receptors that control gene transcription (nuclear receptors)

- Ligands include steroid hormones, thyroid hormones, vitamin D and retinoic acid, as well as certain lipid-lowering and antidiabetic drugs.
- Receptors are intracellular proteins, so ligands must first enter cells.
- Receptors consist of a conserved DNA-binding domain attached to variable ligand-binding and transcriptional control domains.
- DNA-binding domain recognises specific base sequences, thus promoting or repressing particular genes.
- Pattern of gene activation depends on both cell type and nature of ligand, so effects are highly diverse.
- Effects are produced as a result of altered protein synthesis and, therefore, are slow in onset.
- One type of nuclear receptor is responsible for the increased expression of drug-metabolising enzymes induced by many therapeutic agents.

during development play a key role in controlling the development of limbs and organs.

Many drugs and other foreign molecules produce changes in the activity of drug-metabolising enzymes and drug transporters, thereby affecting the body's response to drugs that are eliminated by these mechanisms (see Chs 8 and 50). The class of nuclear receptors known as PXR (or SXR) responds to a wide range of foreign molecules and regulates the expression of these 'drug-handling' proteins (see Synold et al., 2001). PXR is akin to the airport security officer, who picks up the phone and summons the bomb disposal specialists when suspicious luggage is detected.

Recently, considerable attention has been focused on *PPARs* (*peroxisome proliferation-activated receptors*). Despite its clumsy name, this family of nuclear receptors, discovered in the early 1990s, has emerged as a key player in the control of lipid metabolism, and in the pathogenesis of various forms of metabolic and cardiovascular disease (see Kersten et al., 2000; Murphy & Holder, 2000). Of three known subtypes, PPARα is the target for drugs such as **clofibrate**, used to reduce plasma cholesterol (Ch. 19), while PPARγ is the target for the recently introduced thiazolidinedione class of drugs (e.g. **troglitazone**) used to treat diabetes (Ch. 25). All of the PPARs respond to a variety of endogenous lipids. Among the lipid mediators that affect nuclear receptors are some prostaglandins and leukotrienes (see Ch. 15), the main actions of which are mediated through GPCRs.

ION CHANNELS AS DRUG TARGETS

We have discussed ligand-gated ion channels as one of the four main types of drug receptor. There are many other types of ion channel that represent important drug targets, even though they are not generally classified as 'receptors' since they are not the immediate targets of fast neurotransmitters.* Here we discuss the structure and function of ion channels at the molecular level; their role as regulators of cell function is described in Chapter 4.

Ions are unable to penetrate the lipid bilayer of the cell membrane and can get across only with the help of membrane-spanning proteins in the form of channels or transporters. The concept of ion channels was developed more than 50 years ago on the basis of electrophysiological studies on the mechanism of membrane excitation (see below), and electrophysiology, particularly the *voltage-clamp* technique (see Ch. 4), remains an essential tool for studying the physiological and pharmacological properties of ion channels. Since the mid-1980s, when the first ion channels were cloned by Numa in Japan, a highly productive collaboration between electrophysiologists and molecular biologists has revealed many details about the structure and function of these complex molecules. The use of tight-seal ('patch clamp') recording, which allows the behaviour of individual channels to be studied in real time, has been particularly valuable in distinguishing channels on the basis of their conductance and gating characteristics. Accounts by Hille (1992), Ashcroft (2000) and Catterall (2000) give more information.

Ion channels consist of protein molecules designed to form water-filled pores that span the membrane, and they can switch between open and closed states. The rate and direction of ion movement through the pore is governed by the electrochemical gradient for the ion in question, which is a function of its concentration on either side of the membrane, and of the membrane potential. Ion channels are characterised by:

- their *selectivity* for particular ion species, which depends on the size of the pore and the nature of its lining
- their *gating* properties (i.e. the mechanisms that controls the transition between open and closed states of the channel)
- their molecular architecture.

SELECTIVITY

Channels are generally either cation or anion selective. Cation-selective channels may be selective for Na^+, Ca^{2+} or K^+ or may be non-selective and permeable to all three. Anion channels are mainly permeable to Cl^-, though other types also occur. The effect of modulation of ion channels on cell function is discussed in Ch. 4.

*In truth, the distinction between ligand-gated channels and other ion channels is an arbitrary one. In grouping ligand-gated channels with other types of receptor in this book, we are respecting the historical tradition established by Langley and others, who first defined receptors in the context of the action of acetylcholine at the neuromuscular junction. The advance of molecular biology may force us to reconsider this semantic issue in the future, but for now we make no apology for upholding the pharmacological tradition.

GATING

Voltage-gated channels

Most voltage-gated channels open when the cell membrane is depolarised. They form a very important group because they underly the mechanism of membrane excitability (see Ch. 4). The most important channels in this group are selective sodium, potassium or calcium channels.

Commonly, the channel opening *(activation)* induced by membrane depolarisation is short-lasting, even if the depolarisation is maintained. This is because, with some channels, the initial activation of the channels is followed by a slower process of *inactivation* (see below).

The role of voltage-gated channels in the generation of action potentials and in controlling other cell functions is described in Chapter 4.

Ligand-gated channels

The ligand-gated channels (see above) are activated by binding of a chemical ligand to a site on the channel molecule. Fast neurotransmitters, such as glutamate, acetylcholine, GABA and ATP (see Chs 10, 12, 32) act in this way, binding to sites on the outside of the membrane. Some ligand-gated channels in the plasma membrane respond to intracellular, rather than extracellular, signals, the most important being:

- Ca^{2+}-activated potassium channels, which occur in most cells and open, thus hyperpolarising the cell, when intracellular Ca^{2+} levels increases
- ATP-sensitive potassium channels, which open when the intracellular ATP concentration falls because the cell is short of nutrients; these channels, which are quite distinct from those mediating the excitatory effects of extracellular ATP, occur in many nerve and muscle cells, and also in insulin-secreting cells (see Ch. 25), where they are part of the mechanism linking insulin secretion to blood glucose concentration
- the vanilloid receptor, for which the binding site for capsaicin (and possibly endogenous mediators, see Piomelli (2000)) resides on the cytoplasmic part of the molecule.

Calcium release channels

Calcium release channels are present on the endoplasmic or sarcoplasmic reticulum, rather than the plasma membrane. The main ones, IP_3 and ryanodine receptors (see Ch. 4), are a special class of ligand-gated calcium channels that controls the release of Ca^{2+} from intracellular stores.

Store-operated calcium channels

When the intracellular Ca^{2+} stores are depleted, channels in the plasma membrane open to allow Ca^{2+} entry. The mechanism by which this linkage occurs is poorly understood (see Barritt, 1999), but these store-operated channels (SOCs) are important in the mechanism of action of many GPCRs that elicit Ca^{2+} release. The opening of SOCs allows intracellular Ca^{2+} to remain elevated even when the stores are running low, and they also provide a route through which the stores can be replenished (see Ch. 4).

MOLECULAR ARCHITECTURE

▼ Ion channels are large and elaborate molecules. Their characteristic structural motifs have been revealed as knowledge of their sequence and structure has accumulated since the mid-1980s, when the first ligand-gated channel (the nicotinic acetylcholine receptor) and the first voltage-gated sodium channel were cloned. The main structural subtypes are shown in Figure 3.16. All consist of several (often four) domains, which are similar or identical to each other, organised either as an oligomeric array of separate subunits, or as a one large protein. Each subunit or domain contains a bundle of two to six membrane-spanning helices. Most ligand-gated channels have the basic structure shown in Figure 3.16A, comprising a pentameric array of non-identical subunits, each consisting of four transmembrane helices, of which one—the M2 segment—from each subunit lines the pore. The large extracellular N-terminal region contains the ligand-binding region (see p. 30). Several exceptions to this simple design for ligand-gated channels have emerged recently, amid a flurry of initial disbelief. They include (see Fig. 3.16) the *glutamate NMDA receptor* (Ch. 32), the *purine* P_{2X} *receptor* (Ch. 12) and the *vanilloid receptor* (a channel which responds not only to chemicals of the vanilloid class but also to heat and protons; see Ch. 40). In these, as in many other types of channel, the pore-forming part of the molecule consists of a hairpin loop—the P-loop—between two of the helices. Voltage-gated channels generally include one transmembrane helix that contains an abundance of basic (i.e. positively charged) amino acids. When the membrane is depolarised, so that the interior of the cell becomes less negative, this region—the voltage sensor—moves slightly towards the outer surface of the membrane, which has the effect of opening the channel. Many voltage-activated channels also show inactivation, which happens when one of the intracellular domains shifts in such a way as to block the channel from the inside, in the manner of a self-clogging drainpipe. Voltage-gated sodium and calcium channels are remarkable in that the whole structure with four six-helix domains consists of a single huge protein molecule, the domains being linked together by intracellular loops of varying length. Potassium channels constitute the most numerous and heterogeneous class.* Voltage-gated potassium channels resemble sodium channels, except that they are made up of four subunits rather than a single long chain. The class of potassium channels known as 'inward rectifier channels' because of their biophysical properties has the two-helix structure shown in Figure 3.16C, whereas others are classed as two-pore domain channels, because each subunit contains two P-loops.

The various architectural motifs shown in Figure 3.16 only scrape the surface of the molecular diversity of ion channels. In all cases the individual subunits come in several molecular varieties, and these can unite in different combinations to form functional channels as hetero-oligomers (as distinct from homo-oligomers built from identical subunits). Furthermore, the channel-forming structures described are usually associated with other membrane proteins, which significantly affect their functional properties. For example, the ATP-gated potassium channel exists in association with the *sulfonylurea receptor* (SUR), and it is through this linkage that various drugs (including antidiabetic drugs of the sulfonylurea class; see Ch. 25) regulate the channel (see Ashcroft & Gribble, 2000). Determined efforts are under way to understand the relation between molecular structure and ion channel function, and good progress is being made, but we still have only a fragmentary

*The genome of the worm *Caenorhabditis elegans* encodes no fewer than 60 distinct potassium-channel subtypes, and mammals undoubtedly possess even more. Either a nightmare or a golden opportunity for the pharmacologist depending on one's perspective.

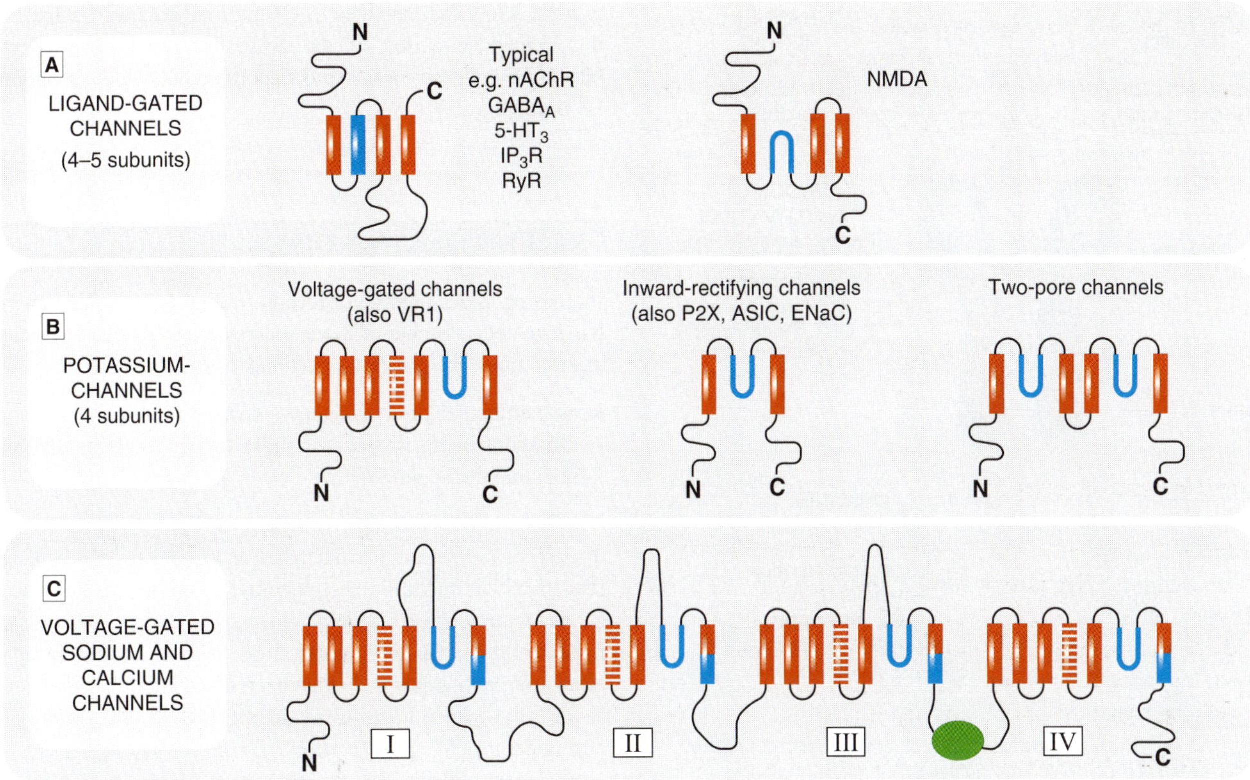

Fig 3.16 Molecular architecture of ion channels. Red and blue rectangles represent membrane-spanning α-helices. Blue hairpins are pore-loop (P) domains, present in many channels, blue rectangles being the pore-forming regions of the membrane-spanning α-helices. Cross-shaded rectangles represent the voltage-sensing regions of voltage-gated channels. (nAchR, nicotinic acetylcholine receptor; GABA$_A$, gamma-aminobutyric acid type A; 5-HT$_3$, 5-hydroxytryptamine type 3; IP$_3$R, inositol trisphosphate receptor; RyR, ryanodine receptor; NMDA, *N*-methyl-D-aspartate.)

understanding of the physiological role of many of these channels. Many important drugs exert their effects by influencing channel function, either directly or indirectly.

PHARMACOLOGY OF ION CHANNELS

▼ Many drugs and physiological mediators described in this book exert their effects by altering the behaviour of ion channels. A comprehensive review would be long and repetitive, so here we outline the general mechanisms as exemplified by the pharmacology of voltage-gated sodium channels (Fig. 3.17). Ion channel pharmacology is likely to be a fertile source of future new drugs (see Triggle, 1999; Clare et al., 2000).

The gating and permeation of both voltage- and ligand-gated ion channels is modulated by many factors.

- Ligands that bind directly to various sites on the channel protein. These include many neurotransmitters, as already discussed (p. 30), and also a variety of drugs and toxins that act in different ways, for example, by blocking the channel or by affecting the gating process, thereby either facilitating or inhibiting the opening of the channel.
- Mediators and drugs that act indirectly, mainly by activation of GPCRs. The latter produce their effects mainly by affecting the state of phosphorylation of individual amino acids located on the intracellular region of the channel protein. As described above, this modulation involves the production of second messengers that activate protein kinases. The opening of the channel may be facilitated or inhibited, depending on which residues are phosphorylated. Drugs such as opioids (Ch. 40) and β-adrenoceptor agonists (Ch. 11) affect calcium and potassium channel function in this way, producing a wide variety of cellular effects.
- Intracellular signals, particularly Ca^{2+} and nucleotides such as ATP and GTP (see Ch. 4). Many ion channels possess binding sites for these intracellular mediators. Increased intracellular Ca^{2+} levels open certain types of potassium channels and inactivates voltage-gated calcium channels. As described in Chapter 4, intracellular Ca^{2+} is itself affected by the function of ion channels and GPCRs. Drugs of the sulfonylurea class (see Ch. 25) act selectively on ATP-gated potassium channels.

Figure 3.17 summarises the main sites and mechanisms by which drugs affect voltage-gated sodium channels, a typical example of this type of drug target.

CONTROL OF RECEPTOR EXPRESSION

Receptor proteins are synthesised by the cells that express them, and the level of expression is itself controlled, via the pathways

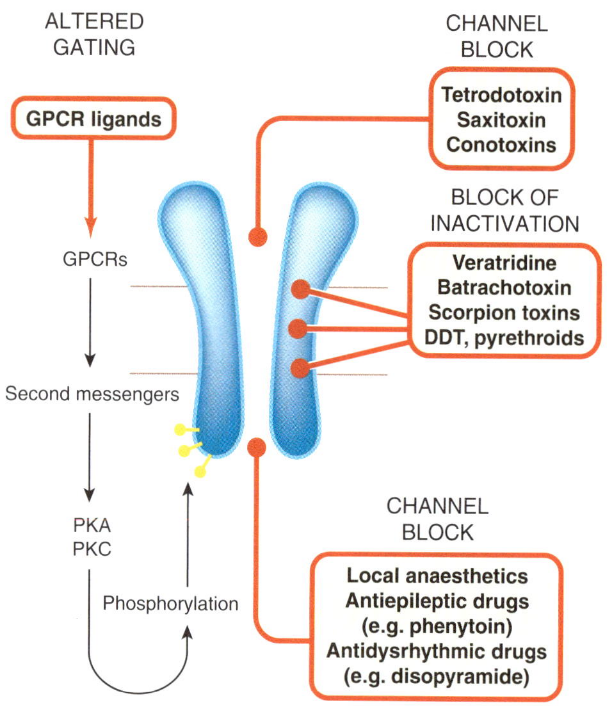

Fig 3.17 Drug-binding domains of voltage-gated sodium channels (see Ch. 43). The multiplicity of different binding sites and effects appears to be typical of many ion channels. (GPCR, G-protein-controlled receptor; PKA, protein kinase A; PKC, protein kinase C; DDT, dichlorodiphenyltrichloroethane (dicophane, a well-known insecticide).)

discussed above, by receptor-mediated events. We can no longer think of the receptors as the fixed elements in cellular control systems, responding to changes in the concentration of ligands and initiating changes via signal transduction pathways—they are themselves subject to regulation. Short-term regulation of receptor function generally occurs through desensitisation, as discussed above. Long-term regulation occurs through an increase or decrease of receptor expression. Examples of this type of control (see review by Donaldson et al., 1997) include the proliferation of various postsynaptic receptors after denervation (see Ch. 9), the upregulation of various GPCRs and cytokine receptors in response to inflammation (see Ch. 15) and the induction of growth factor receptors by certain tumour viruses (see Ch. 44). Adaptive responses to long-term drug treatment are very common, particularly with drugs that act on the CNS. They may take the form of a very slow onset of the therapeutic effect (e.g. with antidepressant drugs; see Ch. 38) or the development of drug dependence (Ch. 52). Though the details are not yet clear, it is most likely that changes in receptor expression, secondary to the immediate action of the drug, are involved—a kind of 'secondary pharmacology' the importance of which is only now becoming clearer.

RECEPTORS AND DISEASE

Increasing understanding of receptor function in molecular terms has revealed a number of disease states directly linked to receptor malfunction. The principal mechanisms involved are:

- autoantibodies directed against receptor proteins
- mutations in genes encoding receptors and proteins involved in signal transduction.

An example of the former is *myasthenia gravis* (see Ch. 10), a disease of the neuromuscular junction caused by autoantibodies that inactivate nicotinic acetylcholine receptors. Autoantibodies can also mimic the effects of agonists, as in many cases of thyroid hypersecretion caused by activation of thyrotrophin receptors. Activating antibodies have also been discovered in patients with severe hypertension (α-adrenoceptors), cardiomyopathy (β-adrenoceptors) and certain forms of epilepsy and neurodegenerative disorder (glutamate receptors). The list is growing steadily.

Inherited mutations of genes encoding GPCRs account for various disease states (see Birnbaumer, 1995). Mutated receptors for vasopressin and adrenocorticotrophic hormone (see Chs 23 and 27) can result in resistance to these hormones. Conditions in which receptor mutations result in permanently switched-on effector mechanisms in the absence of agonist have also been described (see Lefkowitz, 1993). One of these involves the receptor for thyrotrophin, producing continuous oversecretion of thyroid hormone; another involves the receptor for luteinising hormone and results in precocious puberty. Adrenoceptor polymorphisms are common in humans, and recent studies suggest that certain mutations of the β_2-adrenoceptor, though they do not directly cause disease, are associated with a reduced efficacy of β-adrenoceptor agonists in treating asthma (Ch. 22), and a poor prognosis in patients with cardiac failure (Ch. 17). Mutations in G-proteins can also cause disease (see Farfel et al., 1999). For example, mutations of a particular α-subunit cause one form hypoparathyroidism, while mutations of a β-subunit result in hypertension.

Mutations of the genes encoding growth factor receptors and many other proteins involved in signal transduction can result in malignant transformation of cells (see Ch. 5).

REFERENCES AND FURTHER READING

AbdAlla S, Lother H, El Massiery A, Quitterer U 2001 Increased AT_1 receptor heterodimers in preeclampsia mediate enhanced angiotensin II responsiveness. Nat Med 7: 1003–1009 (*The first instance of disturbed GPCR heterodimerisation in relation to human disease*)

Ashcroft F M 2000 Ion channels and disease. Academic Press, London (*A useful textbook covering all aspects of ion channel physiology and its relevance to disease, with a lot of pharmacological information for good measure*)

Ashcroft F M, Gribble F M 2000 New windows on the mechanism of action of K_{ATP} channel openers. Trends Pharmacol Sci 21: 439–445

Avruch J, Zhang X-F, Kyriakis J M 1994 Raf meets Ras: completing the framework of a signal transduction pathway. Trends Biochem Sci 19: 277–283 (*Review focusing on the linkage between two important pathways that link membrane receptors to intracellular events*)

Barbacid M 1996 Neurotrophic factors and their receptors. Curr Biol 7: 148–155 (*Useful review of neural growth factors and their associated tyrosine kinase–linked receptors*)

Barritt G J 1999 Receptor-activated Ca^{2+} inflow in animal cells: a variety of pathways tailored to meet different intracellular Ca^{2+} signalling requirements. Biochem J 337: 153–169 (*Useful overview of mechanisms involved in calcium signalling*)

Bergmann C I 1998 Neurobiology of the *Caenorhabditis elegans* genome. Science 282: 2028–2033 (*Analysis of the genes of the nematode* C. elegans; *the genome was fully sequenced in 1998 and a similar analysis of the human genome is in progress*)

Birnbaumer M 1995 Mutations and diseases of G-protein-coupled receptors. Recept Signal Transduct 15: 131–160 (*Focuses on the growing list of clinical disorders associated with receptor malfunction*)

Bockaert J, Pin J P 1999 Molecular tinkering of G protein-coupled receptors: an evolutionary success. EMBO J 18: 1723–1729 (*Short review covering some newer aspects of GPCR function*)

Bouvier M 2001 Oligomerization of G-protein-coupled transmitter receptors. Neuroscience 2: 274–286 (*Review of the unexpected behaviour of GPCRs in linking together as dimers*)

Bourguet W, Germain P, Gronemeyer H 2000 Nuclear receptor ligand-binding domains: three-dimensional structures, molecular interactions and pharmacological implications. Trends Pharmacol Sci 21: 381–388 (*Review concentrating on distinction between agonist and antagonist effects at the molecular level*)

Brzostowski J A, Kimmel A R 2001 Signaling at zero G: G-protein-independent functions for 7TM receptors. Trends Biochem Sci 26: 291–297 (*Review of evidence for GPCR signalling that does not involve G-proteins, thus conflicting with the orthodox dogma*)

Catterall W A 2000 From ionic currents to molecular mechanisms: the structure and function of voltage-gated sodium channels. Neuron 26: 13–25 (*General review of sodium channel structure, funtion and pharmacology*)

Clapham D E 1995 Calcium signaling. Cell 80: 259–268 (*Excellent general review*)

Clapham D, Neer E 1997 G-protein $\beta\gamma$ subunits. Annu Rev Pharmacol Toxicol 37: 167–203 (*On the diversity and role in signalling of G-protein $\beta\gamma$-subunits—the poor relations of the α-subunits*)

Clare J J, Tate S N, Nobbs M, Roamnos M A 2000 Voltage-gated sodium channels as therapeutic targets. Drug Discov Today 5: 506–520 (*Useful review dealing at a basic level with the therapeutic potential of dugs affecting Na channels*)

Conigrave A D, Quinn S J, Brown E M 2000 Cooperative multi-modal sensing and therapeutic implications of the extracellular Ca^{2+}-sensing receptor. Trends Pharmacol Sci 21: 401–407 (*Short account of the Ca^{2+}-sensing receptor, an anomalous type of GPCR*)

Dery O et al. 1998 Proteinase-activated receptors: novel mechanisms of signalling by serine proteases. Am J Physiol C 274: 1429–1452 (*Detailed review article*)

Dolphin A C 1996 G-proteins. In: Foreman J C, Johansen G (eds) Textbook of receptor pharmacology. CRC Press, Boca Raton, FL

Donaldson L F, Hanley M R, Villablanca A C 1997 Inducible receptors. Trends Pharmacol Sci 18: 171–181 (*Emphasises processes controlling receptor expression*)

Dryer L, Berghard A 1999 Odorant receptors: a plethora of G-protein-coupled receptors. Trends Pharmacol Sci 20 413–417.

Evans R M 1988 The steroid and thyroid hormone receptor superfamily. Science 240: 889–895 (*Excellent general review*)

Falkenstein E, Tillmann H-C, Christ M, Fuering M, Wehling M 2000 Multiple actions of steroid hormones—a focus on rapid, non-genomic effects. Pharmacol Rev 52: 513–553 (*comprehensive review article describing the non-classical effects of steroids*)

Farfel Z, Bourne H R, Iiri T 1999 The expanding spectrum of G protein diseases. N Engl J Med 340: 1012–1020 (*Review of recent work revealing how G-protein mutations lead to disease. Useful for reference*)

Ferguson S S G 2001 Evolving concepts in G protein-coupled receptor endocytosis: the role in receptor desensitization and signaling. Pharmacol Rev 53: 1–24 (*Detailed account of the role of phosphorylation of receptors in fast and slow desensitization mechanisms*)

Galzi J-L, Changeux J-P 1994 Neurotransmitter-gated ion channels as unconventional allosteric proteins. Curr Opin Struct Biol 4: 554–565 (*Review focusing on molecular mechanisms of channel activation*)

Giros B, Caron M G 1993 Molecular characteristics of the dopamine transporter. Trends Pharmacol Sci 14: 43–49

Goldman J M, Melo J V 2001 Targeting the BCR–ABL tyrosine kinase in chronic myeloid leukaemia. N Engl J Med 344: 1084–1086 (*Account of a significant new development in cancer treatment*)

Gudermann T, Kalkbrenner F, Schultz G 1996 Diversity and selectivity of receptor-G protein signalling. Annu Rev Pharmacol Toxicol 36: 429–459 (*Discusses how selectivity is achieved between many ligands, receptors and interlinking transduction pathways*)

Hibert M F, Trumpp-Kallmeyer S, Hoflack J, Bruinvels A 1993 This is not a G protein-coupled receptor. Trends Pharmacol Sci 14: 7–12 (*Discusses what can and cannot be inferred from molecular modelling of receptor structure and function*)

Hille B (1992) Ionic channels of excitable membranes. Sinauer, Sunderland, MA (*A clear and detailed account of the basic principles of ion channels, with emphasis on their biophysical properties*)

Hollenberg M D 1996 Protease-mediated signalling: new paradigms for cell regulation and drug development. Trends Pharmacol Sci 17: 3–6 (*Short review article by one of the pioneers in this field*)

Ihle J N 1995 Cytokine receptor signalling. Nature 377: 591–594

Irvine R F, McNulty T J, Schell M J 1999 Inositol 1,3,4,5–tetrakisphosphate as a second messenger—a special role in neurones? Chem Phys Lipids 98: 49–57 (*Discussion of possible second messenger roles of IP_4*)

Karlin A 1993 Structure of nicotinic acetylcholine receptors. Curr Opin Neurobiol 3: 299–309 (*Excellent general review*)

Kenakin, T 1995 Agonist–receptor efficacy II: agonist trafficking of receptor signals. Trends Pharmacol Sci 16: 232–238 (*Discusses whether and how different ligands acting on the same receptor might elicit different cellular responses*)

Kersten S, Desvergne B, Wahli W 2000 Roles of PPARs in health and disease. Nature 405: 421–424 (*General review of an important class of nuclear receptors*)

Kilpatrick G, Dautzenberg F M, Martin G R, Eglen R M 1999 7TM receptors: the splicing on the cake. Trends Pharmacol Sci 20: 294–301 (*Review of the importance of mRNA splicing as a source of variation among GPCRs— a salutary reminder that cloning genes is not the last word in defining receptor diversity*)

Koenig J A, Edwardson J M 1997 Endocytosis and recycling of G protein-coupled receptors. Trends Pharmacol Sci 18: 276–287 (*Excellent review of the complex life cycle of a receptor molecule*)

Krupnick J G, Benovic J L 1998 The role of receptor kinases and arrestins in G protein coupled receptor regulation. Annu Rev Pharmacol Toxicol 38: 298–319 (*Review on GPCR phosphorylation, arrestins and desensitisation*)

Laudet V, Adelmant G 1995 Lonesome receptors. Curr Biol 5: 124–127 (*Short review of 'orphan' receptors*)

Lefkowitz R J 1993 Turned on to ill effect. Nature 365: 603–605 (*Discussion of the pathological consequences of β-adrenoceptors that are activated without agonists being present*)

Levitzki A 1996 Targeting signal transduction for disease therapy. Curr Opin Cell Biol 8: 239–244 (*Points out therapeutic opportunities for targeting components of signal transduction pathways*)

Liu F, Wan Q, Pristupa Z, Yu X-M, Wang Y T, Miznik H B 2000 Direct protein–protein coupling enables cross-talk between dopamine D_5 and γ-aminobutyric acid A receptors. Nature 403: 274–280 (*The first demonstration of direct coupling of a GPCR with an ion channel. Look, no G-protein!*)

Lucas K A, Pitari J M, Kazerounian S et al. 2000 Pharmacol Rev 52:

376–413 (*Detailed review of guanylate cyclase and its role in signalling. Covers both membrane receptors linked to GC, and soluble GCs which respond to nitric oxide etc.*)
Mangelsdorf D J, Thummel C, Beato M et al. 1995 The nuclear receptor superfamily: the second decade. Cell 83: 835–839
Marchese A, George S R, Kolakowski L F, Lynch K R, O'Dowd B F 1999 Novel GPCRs and their endogenous ligands: expanding the boundaries of physiology and pharmacology. Trends Pharmacol Sci 20: 370–375 (*Short review, which emphasises the abundance of GPCRs, and the number of orphans which may prove valuable as drug targets in the future*)
Marshall C J 1996. Ras effectors. Curr Opin Cell Biol 8: 197–204 (*Account of one of the most important signal transduction pathways*)
Marshall F H, Jones K A, Kaupmann K, Bettler B 1999 $GABA_B$ receptors—the first 7TM dimers (*Short report of recent surprising findings about GPCR dimerisation, with references to original studies*)
McLatchie L M, Fraser N J, Main M J et al. 1998 RAMPs regulate the transport and ligand specificity of the calcitonin–receptor–like receptor. Nature 393: 333–339 (*First description of RAMPs—accessory proteins that alter the pharmacology of GPCRs*)
Milligan G 1995 Signal sorting by G-protein-linked receptors. Adv Pharmacol 32: 1–29 (*More on the selectivity problem*)
Murphy G J, Holder J C 2000 PPAR-γ agonists: therapeutic role in diabetes, inflammation and cancer. Trends Pharmacol Sci 21: 469–474 (*Account of the emerging importance of nuclear receptors of the PPAR family as therapeutic targets*)
Nishizuka Y 1988 The molecular heterogeneity of protein kinase C and its implications for cellular regulation. Nature 334: 661–665 (*As above*)
Parker P J, Dekker L (eds) 1996 Protein kinase C. Springer, Berlin (*Authoritative reviews for PKC aficionados*)
Piomelli D 2000. The ligand that came from within. Trends Pharmacol Sci 22:17–19 (*Speculative review article about the ability of intracellular lipid mediators to act on ligand–gated ion channels*)
Schenk P W, Snaar-Jakelska B E 1999 Signal perception and transduction: the role of protein kinases. Biochem Biophys Acta 1449: 1–24 (*General review of receptor–protein kinase interactions*)
Schoneberg T, Schultz G, Gudermann T 1999 Structural basis of G protein-coupled receptor function. Mol Cell Endocrinol 151: 181–193 (*Review of recent developments in GPCR signal transduction mechanisms*)
Schwartz T W 1996 Molecular structure of G-protein-coupled receptors. In: Foreman J C, Johanesen T (eds) Textbook of receptor pharmacology. CRC Press, Boca Raton, FL (*Useful account without unnecessary detail*)
Schwartz T W, Rosenkilde M M 1996 Is there a 'lock' for all agonist 'keys' in 7TM receptors? Trends Pharmacol Sci 17: 213–216 (*More on the selectivity problem*)
Simonds W F 1999 G-protein regulation of adenylate cyclase. Trends Pharmacol Sci 20: 66–72 (*Review of mechanisms by which G-proteins affect adenylate cyclase at the level of molecular structure*)
Stryer L 1986 Cyclic GMP cascade of vision. Annu Rev Neurosci 6: 87–119 (*Review by one of the pioneers, showing similarities of visual transduction and chemical receptor mechanisms*)
Synold T W, Dussault I, Forman B M 2001 The orphan nuclear receptor SXR coordinately regulates drug metabolism and efflux. Nature Med 7: 584–590
Toker A 1998 Signalling through protein kinase C. Front Biosci D 3: 1134–1147 (*Description of the various members of the PKC family, how they are reguated and what they do*)
Trends Pharmacol Sci 2000 Receptor and ion channels nomenclature supplement (*Annual catalogue of cloned receptor and ion channel families—useful source of reference*)
Triggle D J 1999 The pharmacology of ion channels: with particular reference to voltage-gated Ca^{2+} channels. Eur J Pharmacol 375: 311–325 (*Basic information about ion channels, plus a good summary of calcium channel pharmacology*)
Unwin N 1993 Nicotinic acetylcholine receptor at 9 Å resolution. J Mol Biol 229: 1101–1124 (*The first structural study of a channel–linked receptor*)
Unwin N 1995 Acetylcholine receptor channel imaged in the open state. Nature 373: 37–43 (*Refinement of 1993 paper, showing for the first time how channel opening occurs—a technical tour de force*)
Vergnolle N, Wallace J L, Bunnett N W, Hollenberg M D 2001 Protease-activated receptors in inflammation, neuronal signalling and pain. Trends Pharmacol Sci 22: 146–152 (*Short review article on this recently discovered family of GPCRs*)
Walaas S I, Greenglard P 1991 Protein phosphorylation and neuronal function. Pharmacol Rev 43: 299–349 (*Excellent general review*)
Wess J 1998 Molecular basis of receptor/G-protein-coupling selectivity. Pharmacol Ther 80: 231–264 (*Detailed review of molecular biology of GPCRs and G-proteins, emphasising what is known about the thorny question of how selectivity is achieved*)
Wickham K D, Clapham, D E 1995 G-protein regulation of ion channels. Curr Opin Neurobiol 5: 278–285 (*Discusses direct and indirect regulation of ion channels by G-protein-coupled receptors*)

4 Cellular mechanisms: excitation, contraction and secretion

Overview 51

Regulation of intracellular calcium levels 51
- Calcium entry mechanisms 52
- Calcium extrusion mechanism 54
- Calcium release mechanisms 54
- Calmodulin 55

Excitation 55
Channel function 56

Muscle contraction 62

Release of chemical mediators 64

Epithelial ion transport 66

OVERVIEW

The link between a drug interacting with a molecular target and its effect at the pathophysiological level, such as a change in blood glucose concentration or the shrinkage of a tumour, involves events at the cellular level. Whatever their specialised physiological function, cells generally deploy much the same repertoire of signalling mechanisms. In the next two chapters, we describe the parts of this repertoire that are of particular significance in understanding drug action at the cellular level. In this chapter we describe mechanisms that operate mainly over a short timescale (milliseconds to hours), particularly *excitation*, *contraction* and *secretion*, which account for many physiological responses.

The short-term regulation of cell function depends mainly on the following components and mechanisms, which regulate, or are regulated by, the free concentration of Ca^{2+} in the cytosol $[Ca^{2+}]_i$:

- **ion channels and transporters in the plasma membrane**
- **the storage and release of Ca^{2+} by intracellular organelles**
- **Ca^{2+}-dependent regulation of enzymes, contractile proteins and vesicle proteins.**

Because $[Ca^{2+}]_i$ plays such a key role in cell function, a wide variety of drug effects results from interference with one more of these mechanisms. If love makes the human world go round, $[Ca^{2+}]_i$ does the same for cells. Knowledge of the molecular and cellular details has expanded remarkably during the 1990s, and here we focus on the aspects that help to explain drug effects.

REGULATION OF INTRACELLULAR CALCIUM LEVELS

Ever since the famous accident by Sidney Ringer's technician, which showed that using tap water rather than distilled water to make up the bathing solution for isolated frog hearts would allow them to carry on contracting, the role of Ca^{2+} as the most important regulator of cell function has never been in question. Many drugs and physiological mechanisms operate, directly or indirectly, by influencing the free intracellular concentrations of Ca^{2+}, $[Ca^{2+}]_i$. Here we consider the main ways in which it is regulated, and below (p. 62) we describe some of the ways in which $[Ca^{2+}]_i$ controls cell function. Details of the molecular components and drug targets were presented in Chapter 3, and descriptions of drug effects on integrated physiological function are given in later chapters. More detailed coverage of the topics presented in this chapter can be found in Aidley (1998), Kandel et al. (2000), Nicholls et al. (2000).

The study of Ca^{2+} regulation took a big step forward in the 1970s with the development of fluorescent techniques based on the Ca^{2+}-sensitive photoprotein aequorin, and dyes such as Fura-2, which allowed free $[Ca^{2+}]_i$ to be continuously monitored in living cells with a high level of temporal and spatial resolution for the first time.

Most of the Ca^{2+} in a resting cell is sequestered in organelles, particularly the endoplasmic or sarcoplasmic reticulum (ER or SR) and the mitochondria, and the free $[Ca^{2+}]_i$ is kept to a low level, about 10^{-7} mol/l. The Ca^{2+} concentration in tissue fluid $[Ca^{2+}]_o$, is about 2.4 mmol/l so there is a large concentration gradient favouring Ca^{2+} entry. $[Ca^{2+}]_i$ is kept low by (a) the operation of active transport mechanisms which eject Ca^{2+} through the plasma membrane, and pump it into the ER, and (b) the normally low Ca^{2+} permeability of the plasma and ER

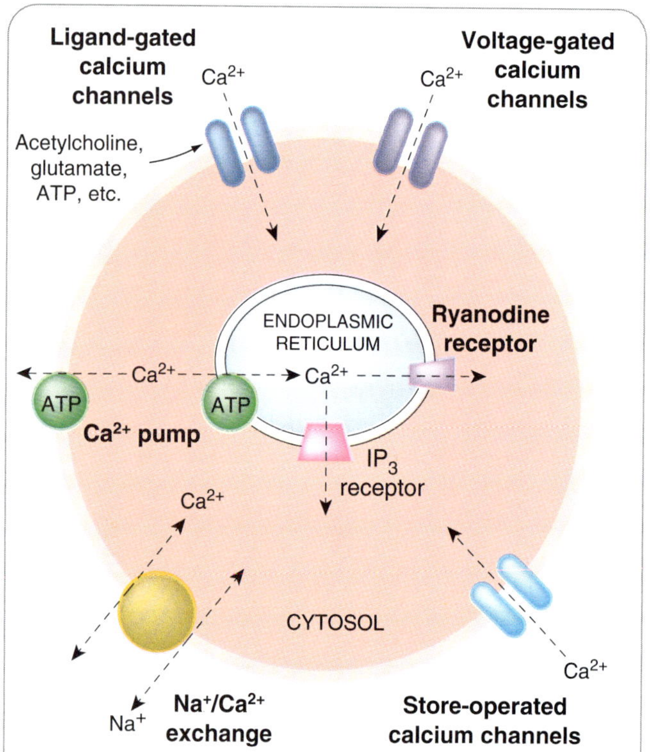

Fig. 4.1 Regulation of intracellular calcium. The main routes of transfer of Ca^{2+} into, and out of, the cytosol and endoplasmic reticulum are shown for a typical cell (see text for details). Most of the channels and transporters have been characterised at the molecular level, but the nature of the store-operated channels in the plasma membrane, and the mechanism by which they are linked to the state of the intracellular Ca^{2+} store, are uncertain. Normally $[Ca^{2+}]_i$ is regulated to about 10^{-7} mol/l in a 'resting' cell.

membranes. Regulation of $[Ca^{2+}]_i$ involves three main mechanisms:

- control of Ca^{2+} entry
- control of Ca^{2+} extrusion
- exchange of Ca^{2+} between the cytosol and the intracellular stores.

These are described in more detail below and are summarised in Figure 4.1.

CALCIUM ENTRY MECHANISMS

There are four main routes by which Ca^{2+} enters cells across the plasma membrane:

- voltage-gated calcium channels
- ligand-gated calcium channels
- Na^+–Ca^{2+} exchange (see above)
- store-operated calcium channels (SOCs).

VOLTAGE-GATED CALCIUM CHANNELS

The pioneering work of Hodgkin and Huxley on the ionic basis of the nerve action potential (see below) identified voltage-dependent Na^+ and K^+ conductances as the main participants. It was later found that some invertebrate nerve and muscle cells could produce action potentials that depended on Ca^{2+} rather than Na^+, and improved voltage clamp methods revealed that vertebrate cells also possess voltage-activated calcium channels capable of allowing substantial amounts of Ca^{2+} to enter the cell when the membrane is depolarised. These voltage-gated channels are highly selective for Ca^{2+} (though they also conduct Ba^{2+}, which is often used as a substitute in electrophysiological experiments) and do not conduct Na^+ or K^+; they are also ubiquitous in excitable cells and allow Ca^{2+} to enter the cell whenever the membrane is depolarised, for example by a conducted action potential.

A combination of electrophysiological and pharmacological criteria suggests that there are five distinct subtypes of voltage-gated calcium channels: L, T N, P and R.* The subtypes vary with respect to their activation and inactivation kinetics, their voltage threshold for activation, their conductance, and their sensitivity to blocking agents, as summarised in Table 4.1. The molecular basis for this heterogeneity has been worked out in some detail. The main pore-forming subunits (termed $\alpha1$, see Fig. 3.4) occur in at least 10 molecular subtypes, and they are associated with other subunits (β, γ, δ) which also exist in different forms. Though some details remain uncertain, it is clear that distinct combinations of these subunits give rise to the different physiological subtypes. In general, L-channels are particularly important in regulating contraction of cardiac and smooth muscle (see below); N channels (and also P/Q) are involved in neurotransmitter and hormone release, while T channels mediate Ca^{2+} entry into neurons, and thereby control various Ca^{2+}-dependent functions such as regulation of other channels, enzymes, etc. With the exception of the group of 'Ca^{2+} antagonists' consisting of dihydropyridines (e.g. **nifedipine**), **verapamil** and **diltiazem** (see Chs 17 and 18), relatively few clinically used drugs affect these channels directly, though many do so indirectly by acting on G-protein-coupled receptors (see Ch. 3). A number of toxins have been discovered that act selectively on one or other type of calcium channel (Table 4.1), and these are used as experimental tools.

LIGAND-GATED CHANNELS

Most ligand-gated cation channels (see Ch. 3) that are activated by excitatory neurotransmitters are relatively non-selective, and conduct Ca^{2+} as well as other cations. Most important in this respect is the glutamate receptor of the *N*-methyl-D-aspartate (NMDA) type (Ch. 32), which has a particularly high

*A sixth (Q) has also been found, but its properties so closely resemble those of P that they usually get considered together. The terminology is less than poetic: L stands for *long-lasting*; T stands for *transient*; N stands for *neither* long-lasting nor transient; P, Q and R carry on alphabetically from N, with O (of course) *omitted*.

Table 4.1 Types and functions of calcium channels

Gated by	Main types	Characteristics	Location and function	Drug effects
Voltage	L	High activation threshold; slow inactivation	Plasma membrane of many cells; main Ca^{2+} source for contraction in smooth and cardiac muscle	Blocked by dihydropyridines, **verapamil**, **diltiazem**; activated by **BayK 8644**
	N	Low activation threshold; slow inactivation	Main Ca^{2+} source for transmitter release by nerve terminals	Blocked by **ω-conotoxin** (component of *Conus* snail venom)
	T	Low threshold; fast inactivation	Widely distributed; important in cardiac pacemaker and atria (role in dysrhythmias)	Blocked by **mibefradil**
	P/Q	Low activation threshold; slow inactivation	Nerve terminals; transmitter release	Blocked by ω-agatoxin (component of funnel web spider venom)
	R	Low threshold; fast inactivation	?	
Inositol trisphosphate	IP_3 receptor		Located in ER/SR; mediates Ca^{2+} release in response to IP_3 produced by GPCR activation	Not directly targeted by drugs; some experimental blocking agents known; responds to GPCR agonists and antagonists in many cells
Calcium ions	Ryanodine receptor	Directly activated in striated muscle via dihydropyridine receptor of T-tubules	Located in ER/SR; mediates Ca^{2+}-evoked Ca^{2+} release in muscle; also activated by the second messenger cADP-ribose	Activated by **caffeine** (high concentrations), blocked by **ryanodine**; mutations may lead to drug-induced malignant hypothermia
Store depletion	Store-operated channels	Indirectly coupled to ER/SR Ca^{2+} stores	Located in plasma membrane	Activated indirectly by agents that deplete intracellular stores (e.g. GPCR agonists, **thapsigargin**); not directly targeted by drugs

ER/SR, endoplasmic reticulum/sarcoplasmic reticulum; GPCR, G-protein-coupled receptor.

permeability to Ca^{2+} and is a major contributor to Ca^{2+} uptake by postsynaptic neurons (and also glial cells) in the central nervous system. Activation of this receptor can readily cause so much Ca^{2+} entry that the cell dies, mainly through activation of Ca^{2+}-dependent proteases, but also by triggering apoptosis (see Ch. 5). This mechanism, termed *excitotoxicity*, probably plays a part in various neurodegenerative disorders (see Ch. 34).

For many years there has been dispute about the existence of 'receptor-operated channels' in smooth muscle, responding directly to mediators such as adrenaline, acetylcholine and histamine. Now it seems (see Kuriyama et al., 1998) that the P_{2X} receptor (see Ch. 3), activated by ATP, is the only example of a true ligand-gated channel in smooth muscle, and this constitutes an important route of entry for Ca^{2+}. Other mediators, acting on G-protein-coupled receptors, affect Ca^{2+} entry indirectly, mainly by regulating voltage-gated calcium channels or potassium channels.

'STORE-OPERATED' CALCIUM CHANNELS

SOCs are channels that occur in the plasma membrane and open to allow Ca^{2+} entry when the ER stores are depleted. They are distinct from other membrane calcium channels, and remain somewhat mysterious, since it is unclear what kind of linkage couples them to the ER (see Berridge, 1997; Barritt, 1999). Like the ER and SR channels, they can serve to amplify the rise in $[Ca^{2+}]_i$ resulting from Ca^{2+} release from the stores. So far, only experimental compounds are known to block these channels, but efforts are being made to develop specific blocking agents for therapeutic use as relaxants of smooth muscle.

CALCIUM EXTRUSION MECHANISMS

Active transport of Ca^{2+} outwards across the plasma membrane, and inwards across the membranes of the ER or SR, depends on the activity of a Ca^{2+}-dependent ATPase, similar to the Na^+/K^+-dependent ATPase that pumps Na^+ out of the cell in exchange for K^+. Several subtypes of the Ca^{2+}-dependent ATPase have been cloned, but the physiological significance of this heterogeneity remains unclear. They have not been implicated in pharmacological responses, with the exception that **thapsigargin** (derived from a Mediterranean plant, *Thapsia garganica*) specifically blocks the ER pump, causing loss of Ca^{2+} from the ER. It is a useful experimental tool but has no therapeutic significance.

Calcium is also extruded from cells in exchange for Na^+, by Na^+–Ca^{2+} exchange. The transporter that does this has been fully characterised and cloned and (as you would expect) comes in several molecular subtypes, the significance of which remain to be worked out. The exchanger transfers three Na^+ for one Ca^{2+} and, therefore, produces a net hyperpolarising current when it is extruding Ca^{2+}. The energy for Ca^{2+} extrusion comes from the electrochemical gradient for Na^+, not directly from ATP hydrolysis. This means that a reduction in the Na^+ concentration gradient resulting from Na^+ entry will reduce Ca^{2+} extrusion by the exchanger, causing a secondary rise in $[Ca^{2+}]_i$, a mechanism that is particularly important in cardiac muscle (see Ch. 17). The exchanger can actually function in reverse if $[Na^+]_i$ rises excessively, resulting in increased Ca^{2+} entry into the cell. The effect of **digoxin** on cardiac muscle (Ch. 17) involves this mechanism.

CALCIUM RELEASE MECHANISMS

There are two main types of calcium channel in the ER and SR membrane, which play an important part in controlling the release of Ca^{2+} from these stores.

The inositol trisphosphate receptor (IP_3R). This is activated by IP_3, a second messenger produced by the action of many ligands on G-protein-coupled receptors (see Ch. 3). IP_3R is a ligand-gated ion channel, though its molecular structure differs from that of ligand-gated channels in the plasma membrane. This is the main mechanism by which activation of G-protein-coupled receptors causes an increase in $[Ca^{2+}]_i$.

The ryanodine receptor (RyR) is so-called because it was first identified through the specific blocking action of the plant alkaloid **ryanodine**. It is particularly important in skeletal muscle, where there is direct coupling between the RyRs of the sarcoplasmic reticulum and the dihydropyridine receptors of the T-tubules (see below); this coupling results in Ca^{2+} release following the action potential in the muscle fibre. RyRs are also present in other types of cell that lack T-tubules; here they are activated by *ADP-ribose (cADPR)*, a recently discovered intracellular messenger the synthesis of which is linked by poorly understood mechanisms to activation of cell surface receptors (see Guse, 2000). There are close parallels between cADPR and IP_3, both of which release Ca^{2+} by binding to receptors on the ER or SR, but we know much less about the role of the former system.

Both IP_3Rs and RyRs are also sensitive to Ca^{2+} and open more readily if $[Ca^{2+}]_i$ is increased. This means that release tends to be regenerative, since an initial puff of Ca^{2+} releases more, resulting in localised 'sparks' or 'waves' of Ca^{2+} release. Fluorescence imaging techniques have revealed a remarkable level of complexity and spatio-temporal patterning of Ca^{2+} signals (see Petersen et al., 1996; Berridge, 1997), and much remains to be discovered about the importance of this patterning in relation to pharmacological mechanisms. The Ca^{2+} sensitivity of RyRs is increased by **caffeine**, causing Ca^{2+} release from the SR even at resting levels of $[Ca^{2+}]_i$. This is used experimentally but rarely happens in humans, since the other pharmacological effects of caffeine (see Ch. 31), occur at much lower doses. The blocking effect of **dantrolene**, a compound related to ryanodine, is used therapeutically to relieve muscle spasm in the rare condition of *malignant hyperthermia* (see Ch. 35), which is associated with inherited abnormalities in the RyR protein. There are, as yet, few other examples of drugs that directly affect these Ca^{2+} release mechanisms.

A typical $[Ca^{2+}]_i$ signal resulting from activation of a G-protein-coupled receptor is shown in Figure 4.2. The response produced in the absence of extracellular Ca^{2+} represents release of

Calcium regulation

- Intracellular calcium concentration $[Ca^{2+}]_i$ is critically important as a regulator of cell function.
- Intracellular calcium is determined by (a) Ca^{2+} entry, (b) Ca^{2+} extrusion and (c) Ca^{2+} exchange between the cytosol, endoplasmic reticulum and mitochondria.
- Calcium entry occurs by various routes, including Ca^{2+} channels and Na^+/Ca^{2+} exchange.
- Calcium extrusion depends mainly on an ATP-driven Ca^{2+} pump.
- Calcium release from the endoplasmic reticulum is controlled partly by the membrane potential, and partly by the second messenger, IP_3, which is produced by many agonists acting on G-protein coupled receptors.
- Calcium affects many aspects of cell function by binding to proteins such as calmodulin, which in turn bind other proteins and regulate their function.

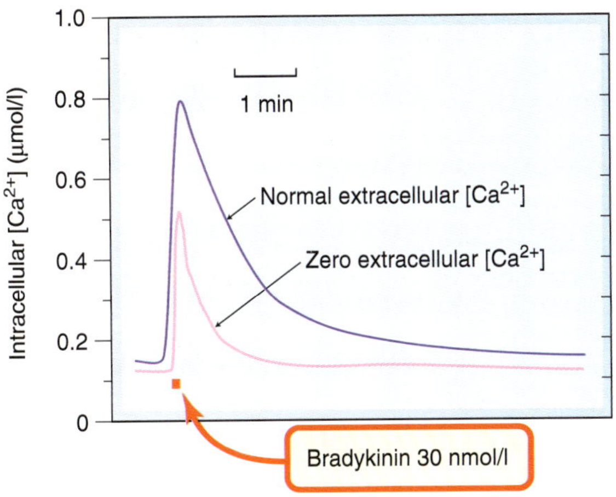

Fig. 4.2 Increase in intracellular calcium concentration in response to receptor activation. The records were obtained from a single rat sensory neuron grown in tissue culture. The cells were loaded with the fluorescent Ca^{2+} indicator Fura-2, and the signal from a single cell monitored with a fluorescence microscope. A brief exposure to the peptide bradykinin, which causes excitation of sensory neurons (see Ch. 40) causes a transient increase in $[Ca^{2+}]_i$ from the resting value of about 150 nmol/l. When Ca^{2+} is removed from the extracellular solution, the bradykinin-induced increase in $[Ca^{2+}]_i$ is still present but is smaller and briefer. The response in the absence of extracellular Ca^{2+} represents the release of stored intracellular Ca^{2+}, resulting from the intracellular production of inositol trisphosphate. The difference between this and the larger response when Ca^{2+} is present extracellularly is believed to represent Ca^{2+} entry through receptor-operated ion channels in the cell membrane. (Figure kindly provided by G M Burgess and A Forbes, Novartis Institute for Medical Research.)

intracellular Ca^{2+}. The larger and more prolonged response when extracellular Ca^{2+} is present shows the contribution of SOC-mediated Ca^{2+} entry.

CALMODULIN

Calcium exerts its control over cell functions by virtue of its ability to regulate the activity of many different proteins, including enzymes (particularly kinases and phosphatases), channels, transporters, transcription factors, etc. In most cases, a Ca^{2+}-binding protein serves as an intermediate between Ca^{2+} and the regulated functional protein. Several such go-between proteins exist, the best known being *calmodulin*, an ubiquitous and much-studied protein with the ability to regulate at least 40 different functional proteins—indeed a powerful fixer. Calmodulin is a dimeric protein, with four Ca^{2+}-binding sites. When all are occupied, it undergoes a conformational change, exposing a 'sticky' hydrophobic domain that lures many proteins into association, thereby affecting their functional properties.

EXCITATION

Excitability describes the ability of a cell to show a regenerative all-or-nothing electrical response to depolarisation of its membrane, this membrane response being known as an *action potential*. It is a characteristic of most neurons and muscle cells (including striated, cardiac and smooth muscle), and of many endocrine gland cells. In neurons and muscle cells, the ability of the action potential, once initiated, to propagate to all parts of the cell membrane, and often to spread to neighbouring cells, explains the importance of membrane excitation in intra- and intercellular signalling. In the nervous system, and in striated muscle, action potential propagation is the mechanism responsible for communication over long distances at high speed, indispensable for large, fast-moving creatures. In cardiac and smooth muscle, as well as in some central neurons, spontaneous rhythmic activity occurs. In gland cells, the action potential, where it occurs, serves not so much to propagate as to amplify the signal, which causes the cell to secrete. In each type of tissue, the properties of the excitation process reflect the special characteristics of the ion channels that underly the process. The molecular nature of ion channels, and their importance as drug targets, is considered in Chapter 3; here we discuss the cellular processes that depend primarily on ion channel function.

THE 'RESTING' CELL

The 'resting' cell is not resting at all but is very busy controlling the state of its interior, and it requires a continuous supply of energy to do so. In relation to the topics discussed in this chapter, the following characteristics are particularly important:

- membrane potential
- permeability of the plasma membrane to different ions
- intracellular ion concentrations, especially $[Ca^{2+}]_i$.

Under 'resting' conditions, all cells maintain a negative internal potential between about –30 and –80 mV, depending on the cell type. This arises because (a) the membrane is relatively impermeable to Na^+, and (b) Na^+ is actively extruded from the cell in exchange for K^+ by an energy-dependent transporter, the sodium pump (or Na^+-K^+-ATPase). The result is that the intracellular K^+ concentration $[K^+]_i$ is higher, and $[Na^+]_i$ is lower, than the respective extracellular concentrations. In many cells, other ions, particularly Cl^-, are also actively transported and unequally distributed across the membrane. In many cases (e.g. neurons), the membrane permeability to K^+ is relatively high, and the membrane potential settles at a value of –60 to –80 mV, close to the equilibrium potential for K^+ (Fig. 4.3). In other cells (e.g. smooth muscle), anions play a larger part, and the membrane potential is generally lower (–30 to –50 mV) and less dependent on K^+.

ELECTRICAL AND IONIC EVENTS UNDERLYING THE ACTION POTENTIAL

Our present understanding of electrical excitability rests firmly on the work of Hodgkin, Huxley and Katz on squid axons,

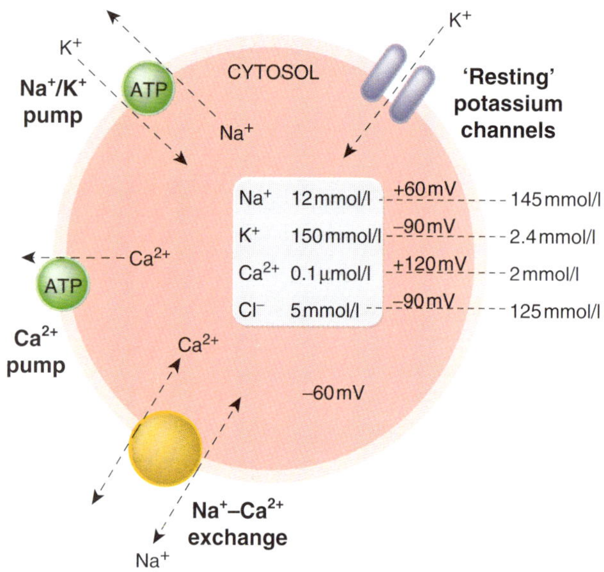

Fig. 4.3 Simplified diagram showing the ionic balance of a typical 'resting' cell. The main transport mechanisms that maintain the ionic gradients across the plasma membrane are the ATP-driven Na^+/K^+ and Ca^{2+} pumps and the Na^+–Ca^{2+} exchange transporter. The membrane is relatively permeable to K^+, because potassium channels are open at rest but impermeable to other cations. The unequal ion concentrations on either side of the membrane give rise to the 'equilibrium potentials' shown. The resting membrane potential, typically about –60 mV but differing between different cell types, is determined by the equilibrium potentials and the permeabilities of the various ions involved, and by the 'electrogenic' effect of the transporters. For simplicity, anions and other ions such as protons are not shown, though these play an important role in many cell types.

published in 1949–1952. Their experiments revealed the existence of voltage-gated ion channels (see above) and showed that the action potential is generated by the interplay of two processes.

1. A rapid, transient increase in Na^+ permeability, which occurs when the membrane is depolarised beyond about –50 mV
2. A slower, sustained increase in K^+ permeability.

Because of the inequality of Na^+ and K^+ concentrations on the two sides of the membrane, an increase in Na^+ permeability causes an inward current of Na^+, whereas an increase in K^+ permeability causes an outward current. The separate nature of these two currents can be most clearly demonstrated by the use of drugs blocking sodium and potassium channels, as shown in Figure 4.4. During the physiological initiation or propagation of a nerve impulse, the first event is a small depolarisation of the membrane, produced either by transmitter action or by the approach of an action potential passing along the axon. This opens sodium channels, allowing an inward current of Na^+ to flow, which depolarises the membrane still further. The process is thus a regenerative one, and the increase in Na^+ permeability is enough to bring the membrane potential close to the equilibrium potential E_{Na}. The increased Na^+ conductance is transient, since the channels inactivate rapidly, and the membrane returns to its resting state.

In many types of cell, including most nerve cells, repolarisation is assisted by the opening of voltage-dependent potassium channels. These function in much the same way as sodium channels but their activation kinetics are about 10 times slower; they do not inactivate appreciably. This means that the potassium channels open later than the sodium channels, and they contribute to the rapid termination of the action potential. The behaviour of the sodium and potassium channels during an action potential is shown in Figure 4.5.

The foregoing account, based on Hodgkin and Huxley's work 50 years ago, involves only sodium and potassium channels. Subsequently (see p. 52), voltage-gated calcium channels were discovered. These function in basically the same way as sodium channels; they contribute to action potential generation in many cells, particularly cardiac and smooth muscle cells, but also in neurons and secretory cells.

CHANNEL FUNCTION

The discharge patterns of excitable cells vary greatly. Skeletal muscle fibres are quiescent unless stimulated by the arrival of a nerve impulse at the neuromuscular junction. Cardiac muscle fibres discharge spontaneously at a regular rate (see Ch. 17). Neurons may be normally silent, or they may discharge spontaneously, either regularly or in bursts; smooth muscle cells show a similar variety of firing patterns. The frequency at which different cells normally discharge action potentials also varies greatly, from several hundred hertz for fast-conducting neurons, down to about 1 Hz for cardiac muscle cells. These very pronounced functional variations reflect the different characteristics of the ion channels expressed in different cell types.

Drugs that alter channel characteristics, either by interacting directly with the channel itself or by acting indirectly through second messengers, affect the function of many organ systems, including the nervous, cardiovascular, endocrine, respiratory and reproductive systems, and are a frequent theme in this book. Here we describe some of the key mechanisms involved in the regulation of excitable cells.

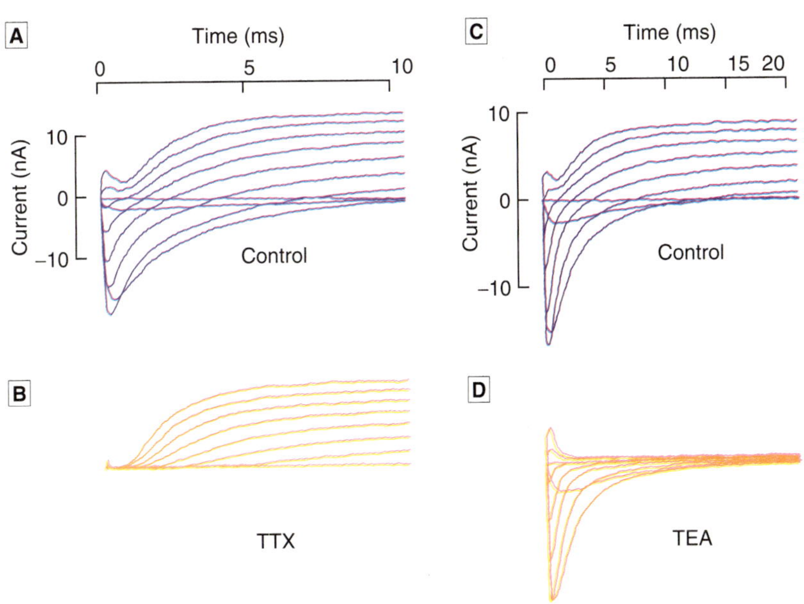

Fig. 4.4 Separation of sodium and potassium currents in the nerve membrane. Voltage clamp records from the node of Ranvier of a single frog nerve fibre. At time 0, the membrane potential was stepped to a depolarised level, ranging from −60 mV (lower trace in each series) to +60 mV (upper trace in each series) in 15 mV steps. A, C Control records from two fibres. B Effect of tetrodotoxin (TTX), which abolishes Na^+ currents. D Effect of tetraethylammonium (TEA), which abolishes K^+ currents. (From: Hille B 1970 Prog Biophys 21:1.)

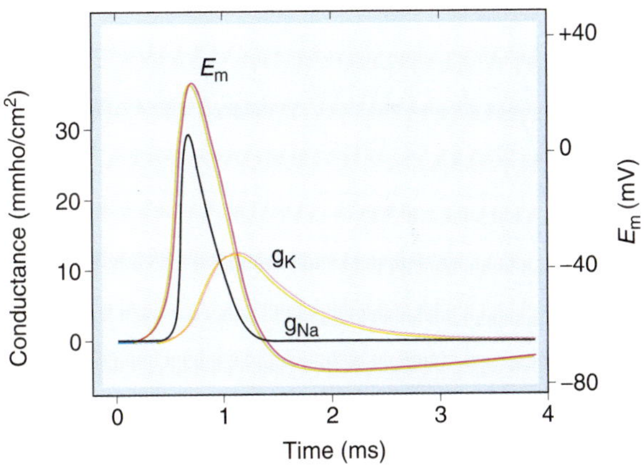

Fig. 4.5 Behaviour of sodium and potassium channels during a conducted action potential. Rapid opening of sodium channels occurs during the action potential upstroke. Delayed opening of potassium channels, and inactivation of sodium channels, causes repolarisation.

In general, action potentials are initiated by membrane currents that cause depolarisation of the cell. These currents may be produced by synaptic activity, by an action potential approaching from another part of the cell, by a sensory stimulus or by spontaneous *pacemaker* activity. The tendency of such currents to initiate an action potential is governed by the *excitability* of the cell, which depends mainly on the state of (a) the voltage-gated sodium and/or calcium channels, and (b) the potassium channels of the resting membrane. Anything that increases the number of available sodium or calcium channels, or reduces their activation threshold, will tend to increase excitability, whereas increasing the resting K^+ conductance reduces it. Agents that do the reverse, by blocking channels or interfering with their opening, will have the opposite effect. Some examples are shown in Figures 4.6 and 4.7 and Tables 4.1 and 4.2.

USE-DEPENDENCE AND VOLTAGE-DEPENDENCE

▼ Voltage-gated channels can exist in three functional states, (Fig. 4.8): *resting* (the closed state which prevails at the normal resting potential), *activated* (the open state favoured by brief depolarisation) and *inactivated* (blocked state resulting from a trapdoor-like occlusion of the channel by a floppy part of the intracellular region of the channel protein, see Ch. 2). After the action potential has passed, many sodium channels are in the inactivated state; after the membrane potential returns to its resting value, the inactivated channels revert to the resting state and thus become available for activation once more. In the meantime, the membrane is temporarily *refractory*. Each action potential causes the channels to cycle through these states. The duration of the refractory period, which determines the maximum frequency at which action potentials can occur, depends on the rate of recovery from inactivation. Drugs that block sodium channels (particularly local anaesthetics, antidysrhythmic drugs and antiepileptic drugs) commonly show a selective affinity for one or other of these functional states of the channel, and in their presence the proportion of channels in the high-affinity state is increased. Of particular importance are drugs that bind most strongly to the inactivated state of the channel and thus favour the adoption of this state and prolong the refractory period, thereby reducing the maximum frequency at which action potentials can be generated. This type of block is called *use-*

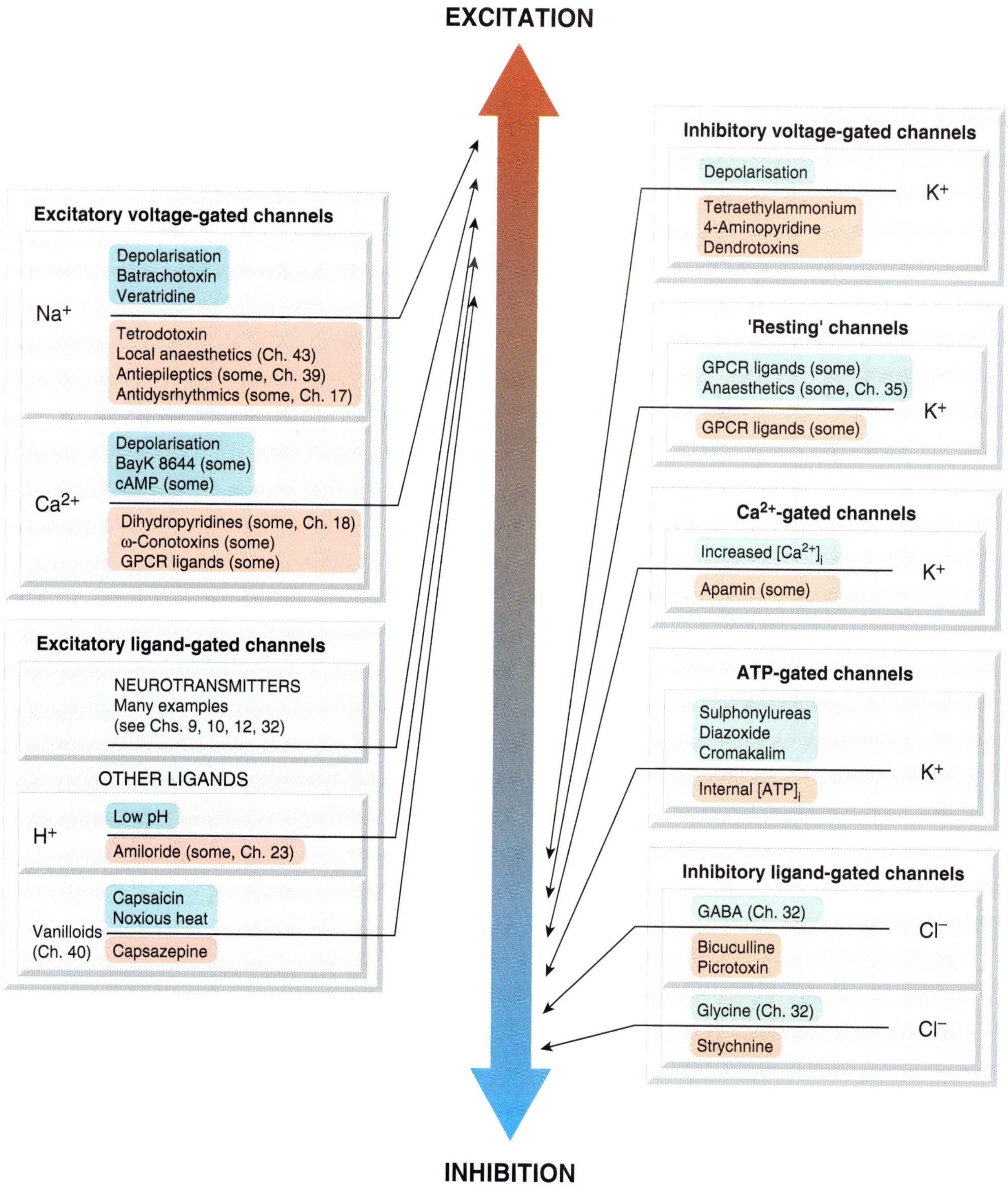

Fig. 4.6 Examples of drugs and endogenous mediators that act on membrane ion channels to produce excitatory or inhibitory effects. Activators are shown in green: inhibitors in pink. (GPCR, G-protein-controlled receptors; GABA, gamma-aminobutyric acid.)

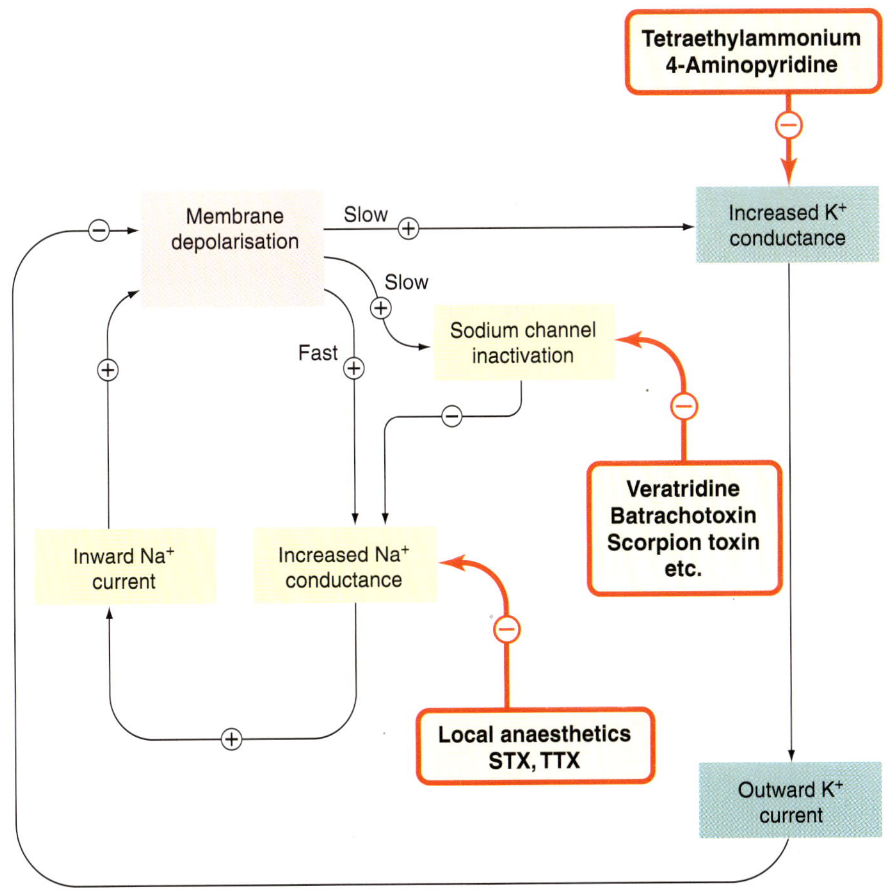

Fig. 4.7 Sites of action of drugs and toxins that affect channels involved in action potential generation. Many other mediators affect these channels indirectly via membrane receptors, through phosphorylation or altered expression. (STX, saxitoxin; TTX, tetrodotoxin.)

dependent, because the binding of such drugs increases as a function of the rate of action potential discharge, which governs the rate at which inactivated—and, therefore, drug-sensitive—channels are generated. This is important for some antidysrhythmic drugs (see Ch. 17), and for antiepileptic drugs (Ch. 39), since high-frequency discharges can be inhibited without affecting excitability at normal frequencies. Drugs that readily block sodium channels in their resting state (e.g. local anaesthetics, Chapter 43) prevent excitation at low as well as high frequencies.

Most drugs blocking sodium channels are cationic at physiological pH and are, therefore, affected by the voltage gradient across the cell membrane; consequently, their blocking action is favoured by depolarisation. This phenomenon, known as *voltage-dependence,* is also of relevance to the action of antidysrhythmic and antiepileptic drugs, since the cells that are the seat of dysrhythmias and seizure activity are generally somewhat depolarised and, therefore, more strongly blocked than 'healthy' cells. Similar considerations apply also to drugs that block potassium or calcium channels, but we know less about the importance of use- and voltage-dependence than we do for sodium channels.

SODIUM CHANNELS

▼ In most excitable cells, the regenerative inward current that initiates the action potential results from activation of voltage-gated sodium channels. The early voltage clamp studies by Hodgkin and Huxley on the squid giant axon, described above, revealed the essential functional properties of these channels. Later, advantage was taken of the potent and highly selective blocking action of **tetrodotoxin** (TTX; see Ch. 43) to label and purify the channel protein, and subsequently to clone it, revealing the complex structure shown in Figure 3.16, with four similar domains each comprising six membrane-spanning helices (reviewed by Catterall, 2000). One of these helices, S4, contains several basic amino acids and forms the voltage sensor; this moves outwards, thus opening the channel, when the membrane is depolarised. One of the intracellular loops is designed to swing across and block the channel when S4 is displaced, thus inactivating the channel.

It was known from physiological studies that the sodium channels of heart and skeletal muscle differ in various ways from those of neurons. In particular, cardiac sodium channels are relatively insensitive to TTX, and

Table 4.2 Types and functions of potassium channel

Structural class[a]	Functional subtypes[b]	Functions	Drug effects	Notes
Voltage-gated: 6T 1P	Voltage-gated	Action potential repolarisation; limits maximum firing frequency	Blocked by **tetraethylammonium**, **4-aminopyridine**; certain subtypes blocked by **dendrotoxins** (from mamba snake venom)	Subtypes in the heart include HERG and LQT channels, which are involved in congenital and drug-induced dysrhythmias; other subtypes may be involved in inherited forms of epilepsy
	Ca^{2+}-activated	Inhibition following stimuli that increase $[Ca^{2+}]_i$	Certain subtypes blocked by apamin (from bee venom) and **charybdotoxin** (from scorpion venom)	Important in many excitable tissues to limit repetitive discharges, also in secretory cells
Inward rectifying: 2T 1P	G-protein-activated	Mediate effects of many GPCRs, which cause inhibition by increasing K^+ conductance	GPCR agonists and antagonists; no important direct interactions	Other inward rectifying potassium channels important in kidney
	ATP-sensitive	Found in many cells; channels open when [ATP] is low, causing inhibition; important in control of insulin secretion	Association of one subtype with the sulfonylurea receptor (SUR) results in modulation by sulfonylureas (e.g. **glibenclamide**), which close channel, and by potassium channel openers (e.g. **diazoxide**, **pinacidil**), which relax smooth muscle	
Two-pore domain: 4T 2P	Several subtypes identified (TWIK, TRAAK, TREK, TASK, etc.)	Most are voltage insensitive; some are normally open and contribute to the 'resting' K^+ conductance; modulated by GPCRs	Certain subtypes are activated by volatile anaesthetics (e.g. **halothane**); no selective blocking agents; modulation by GPCR agonists and antagonists	Recently discovered, so knowledge is fragmentary as yet

GPCR, G-protein-controlled receptor.
[a]Potassium channel structures (see Fig. 3.16) are defined according to the number of transmembrane helices (T) and the number of pore-forming loops (P) in each α-subunit. Functional channels contain several subunits (often four), which may be identical or different, and they are often associated with accessory (β) subunits.
[b]Within each functional subtype, several molecular variants have been identified, often restricted to particular cells and tissues. The physiological and pharmacological significance of this heterogeneity is not yet understood.

slower in their kinetics (as are those of some sensory neurons), compared with most neuronal sodium channels. Eight distinct molecular subtypes have so far been identified, more than enough to explain the functional diversity.

Various experimental compounds affect sodium channel gating and inactivation, the most important being TTX (Ch. 42) and certain substances (e.g. **batrachotoxin**, **veratridine**) that prevent inactivation and, therefore, cause sodium channels to remain open after activation. Therapeutic agents that act by blocking sodium channels include local anaesthetic drugs (Ch. 42), antiepileptic drugs (Ch. 39) and antidysrhythmic drugs (Ch. 17). The sodium channel blocking actions of these drugs were in most cases discovered long after their clinical applications were recognised; many of them lack specificity and produce a variety of unwanted side-effects. The use of induced mutations affecting cloned sodium channels expressed in cell lines is now revealing which regions of the very large channel molecule are involved in the binding of particular agents, and it is hoped that this information will allow more specific drugs to be designed in the future.

POTASSIUM CHANNELS

In a typical resting cell (see above) the membrane is selectively permeable to K^+, and the membrane potential (about −60 mV) is

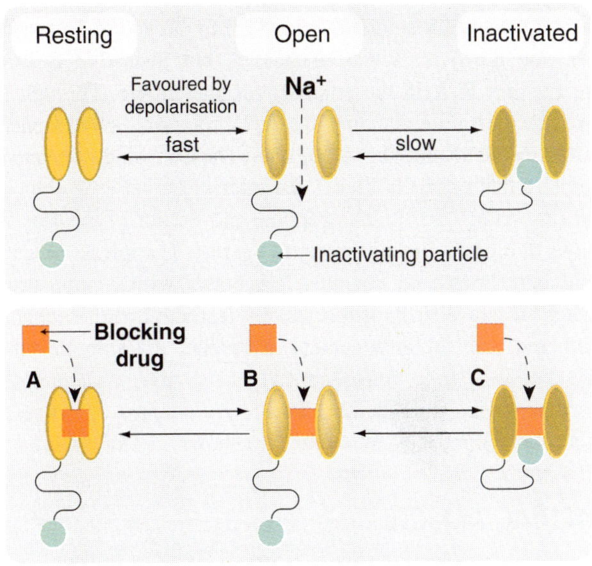

Fig. 4.8 Resting, activated and inactivated states of voltage-gated channels, exemplified by the sodium channel. Membrane depolarisation causes a rapid transition from the resting (closed) state to the open state. The inactivating particle (part of the intracellular domain of the channel protein) is then able to block the channel. Blocking drugs (e.g. local anaesthetics, antiepileptic drugs, etc.) often show preference for one of the three channel states and thus affect the kinetic behaviour of the channels, with implications for their clinical application.

somewhat positive to the K^+ equilibrium (about −90 mV). This resting permeability comes about because potassium channels are open. If more potassium channels open, the membrane hyperpolarises, and the cell is inhibited, whereas the opposite happens if potassium channels close. As well as affecting *excitability* in this way, potassium channels also play an important role in regulating the *duration* of the action potential and the *temporal patterning* of action potential discharges. Altogether, these channels play a central role in regulating cell function. As mentioned in Chapter 3, the number and variety of potassium channel subtypes is extraordinary, implying that evolution has been driven by the scope for biological advantage to be gained from subtle variations in the functional properties of these channels. A recent resumé lists over 60 different pore-forming subunits, plus another 20 or so auxiliary subunits. An impressive evolutionary display, maybe, but hard going for the reader. Here we outline the main types that are known to be important pharmacologically. For more details of the different drugs and toxins that affect potassium channels, see Shieh et al. (2000).

Classes of potassium channel

▼ Potassium channels fall into three main classes,* the structures of which are shown in Figure 3.16.

Voltage-gated potassium channels These possess six membrane-spanning helices, one of which serves as the voltage sensor, causing the channel to open when the membrane is depolarised. Included in this group are channels of the *shaker* family, accounting for most of the voltage-gated K^+ currents familiar to electrophysiologists and others such as the *Ca^{2+}-activated potassium channels* and two subtypes that are important in the heart, *HERG* and *LQT channels.* Disturbance of these channels, either by genetic mutations or by unwanted drug effects, are a major factor in causing cardiac dysrhythmias, which can cause sudden death (see Ch. 17). Many of these channels are blocked by drugs such as **tetraethylammonium** and **4-aminopyridine.**

Inwardly rectifying potassium channels These allow K^+ to pass inwards much more readily than outwards (see review by Reimann & Ashcroft, 1999). They have two membrane-spanning helices and a single pore-forming loop (P-loop). These channels are regulated by interaction with G-proteins (see Ch. 3) and mediate the inhibitory effects of many agonists acting on G-protein-coupled receptors. Certain types are important in the heart, particularly in regulating the duration of the cardiac action potential (Ch. 17); others are the target for the action of **sulfonylureas** (antidiabetic drugs that stimulate insulin secretion by blocking the potassium channels; see Ch. 25) and smooth muscle relaxant

Electrical excitability

- Excitable cells generate an all-or-nothing action potential in response to membrane depolarisation. This occurs in most neurons and muscle cells, and also in some gland cells. The ionic basis and time course of the response varies between tissues.
- The regenerative response results from the depolarising current associated with opening of voltage-dependent cation channels (mainly sodium and calcium). It is terminated by spontaneous closure of these channels, accompanied by opening of potassium channels
- The membrane of the 'resting' cell is relatively permeable to K^+, but impermeable to Na^+ and Ca^{2+}. Drugs or mediators which open potassium channels reduce membrane excitability, and vice versa. Inhibitors of sodium or calcium channel function have the same effect.
- Cardiac muscle cells, some neurons and some smooth muscle cells generate spontaneous action potentials whose amplitude, rate and rhythm is affected by drugs that affect ion channel function.

*Potassium channel terminology is confusing, to put it mildly. Electrophysiologists have christened K^+ *currents* prosaically on the basis of their functional properties (IK_V, IK_{Ca}, IK_{ATP}, IK_{IR}, etc.); geneticists have named genes somewhat fancifully according to the phenotypes associated with mutations (*shaker, ether-a-go-go*, etc.), while molecular biologists have introduced a rational but unmemorable nomenclature on the basis of sequence data (KCNK, KCNQ, etc., with numerical suffixes). The rest of us have to make what we can of the unlovely jargon of labels such as HERG (which—don't blink—stands for *human ether-a-go-go related gene*), TWIK, TREK and TASK.

drugs, such as **cromakalim** and **diazoxide,** which open the channels (see Ch. 18).

Two-pore domain potassium channels These have four helices and two P-loops (see review by Goldstein et al., 2001). They show outward rectification and, therefore, exert a strong repolarising influence, opposing any tendency to excitation. They may contribute to the 'resting' K^+ conductance in many cells and are susceptible to regulation via G-proteins; certain subtypes have been implicated in the action of volatile anaesthetics, such as halothane (Ch. 35).

Channelopathies

Inherited abnormalities of potassium channels (channelopathies; see Ch. 3) contribute to a rapidly growing number of cardiac, neurological and other diseases. These include the *long-QT syndrome*, associated with mutations affecting cardiac voltage-gated potassium channels; episodes of ventricular arrest occur that can result in sudden death. Certain familial types of deafness and epilepsy are associated with mutations affecting voltage-gated potassium channels. Mutations of inward-rectifing potassium channels can lead to a renal disorder (Bartter's syndrome) in which excessive K^+ excretion occurs, or to familial hypoglycaemia associated with excessive insulin secretion.

MUSCLE CONTRACTION

Effects of drugs on the contractile machinery of smooth muscle are the basis of many therapeutic applications, for smooth muscle is an important component of most physiological systems, including blood vessels, gastrointestinal and respiratory tracts. For many decades, smooth muscle pharmacology with its trademark technology—the isolated organ bath—held the centre of the pharmacological stage, and neither the subject nor the technology show any sign of flagging, even though the stage has become much more crowded. Cardiac muscle contractility is also the target of important drug effects, whereas striated muscle contractility is only rarely affected by drugs.

Though, in each case, the basic molecular basis of contraction is similar, namely an interaction between actin and myosin, fuelled by ATP and initiated by an increase in $[Ca^{2+}]_i$, there are differences between these three kinds of muscle that account for their different responsiveness to drugs and chemical mediators.

These differences (Fig. 4.9) involve (a) the linkage between membrane events and increase in $[Ca^{2+}]_i$, and (b) the mechanism by which $[Ca^{2+}]_i$ regulates contraction.

SKELETAL MUSCLE

Skeletal muscle possesses an array of transverse T-tubules extending into the cell from the plasma membrane. The action potential of the plasma membrane depends on voltage-gated sodium channels, as in most nerve cells, and propagates rapidly along the whole fibre. The T-tubule membrane contains a protein known as the *dihydropyridine receptor*, which is closely related to the L-type calcium channel. This protein responds to membrane depolarisation conducted passively along the T-tubule when the plasma membrane is invaded by an action potential. It does not, however, act as a channel, but instead it is linked directly to a RyR in the adjacent SR membrane. Through this link, depolarisation activates the RyR, releasing a short puff of Ca^{2+} from the SR into the sarcoplasm. The Ca^{2+} binds to *troponin*, a protein that normally blocks the interaction between actin and myosin. When Ca^{2+} binds, troponin moves out of the way and allows the contractile machinery to operate. The release of Ca^{2+} is rapid, and brief, and the muscle reponds with a short-lasting 'twitch' response. This is a relatively fast and direct mechanism compared with the arrangement in cardiac and smooth muscle (see below), and, consequently, it is less susceptible to pharmacological modulation. The few examples of drugs that affect skeletal muscle contraction are shown in Table 4.1.

CARDIAC MUSCLE

Cardiac muscle (see review by Bers, 2002) differs from skeletal muscle in several important respects. The nature of the cardiac action potential, the ionic mechanisms underlying its inherent rhythmicity, and the effects of drugs on the rate and rhythm of the heart are described in Chapter 17. Cardiac muscle cells lack T-tubules, and there is no direct coupling between the plasma membrane and the SR. The cardiac action potential varies in its configuration in different parts of the heart but commonly shows a 'plateau' lasting several hundred milliseconds following the initial rapid depolarisation. The plasma membrane contains many L-type calcium channels, which open during this plateau and allow Ca^{2+} to enter the cell, though not in sufficient quantities to activate the contractile machinery directly. Instead, this initial Ca^{2+} entry acts on RyR (a different molecular type from that of skeletal muscle) to release Ca^{2+} from the SR, producing a secondary and much larger wave of Ca^{2+} release. Because the RyR of cardiac muscle are themselves activated by Ca^{2+}, the $[Ca^{2+}]_i$ wave is a regenerative, all-or-nothing event. The initial Ca^{2+} entry that triggers this event is highly dependent on the action potential duration, and on the functioning of the membrane L-type channels. Some of the drugs that affect it are shown in Table 4.1. With minor differences, the mechanism by which the contractile machinery is activated by $[Ca^{2+}]_i$ is the same as in skeletal muscle.

SMOOTH MUSCLE

The properties of smooth muscle vary considerably in different organs, and the link between membrane events and contraction is less direct and less well understood than in other kinds of muscle. The action potential of smooth muscle is generally a rather lazy and vague affair compared with the more military behaviour of skeletal and cardiac muscle, and it propagates through the tissue much more slowly and uncertainly. The action potential is, in most cases, generated by L-type calcium channels rather than voltage-gated sodium channels, and this is one important route of Ca^{2+} entry. In addition, many smooth muscle cells possess ligand-gated cation channels, which allow Ca^{2+} entry when they respond

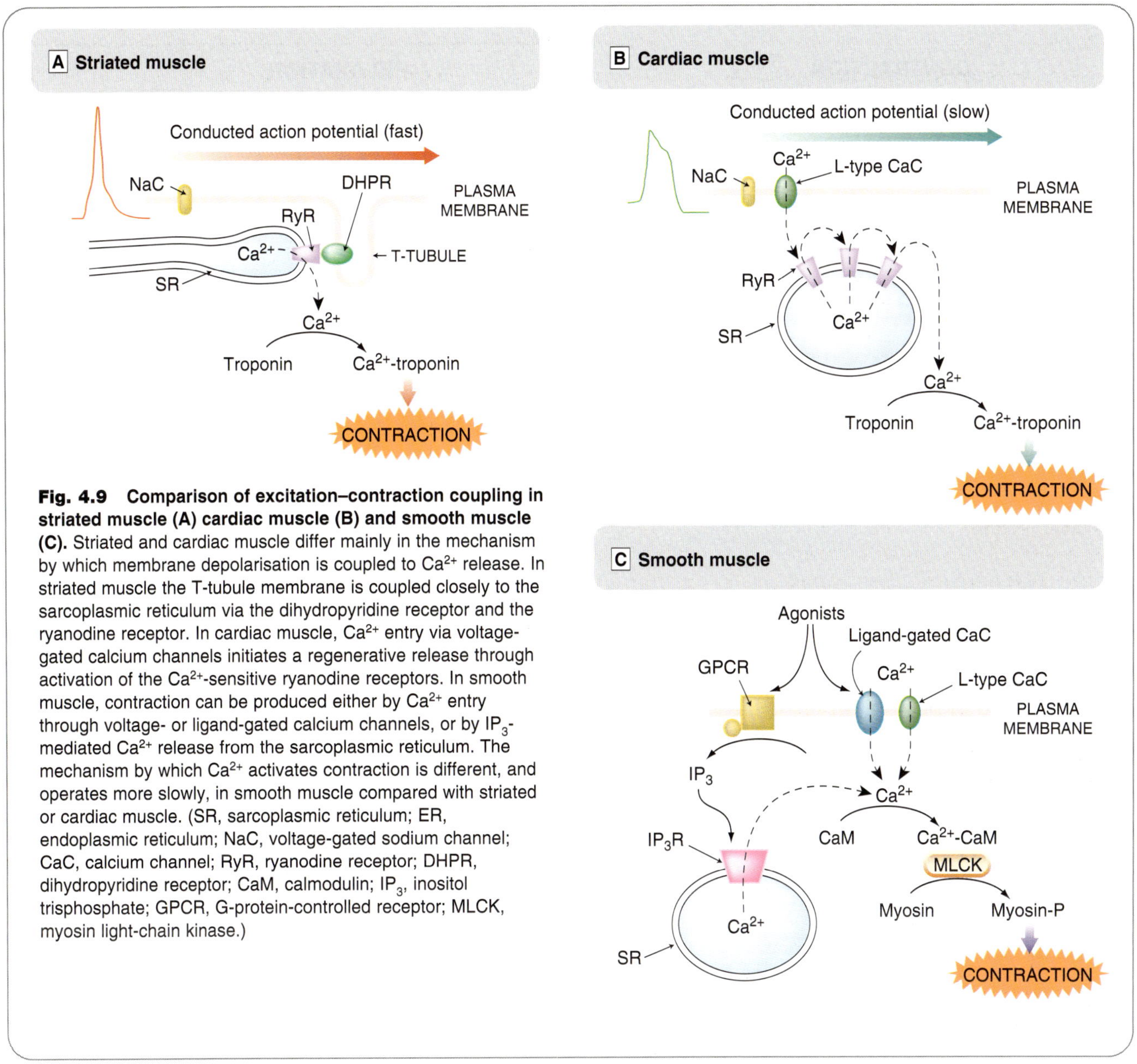

Fig. 4.9 Comparison of excitation–contraction coupling in striated muscle (A) cardiac muscle (B) and smooth muscle (C). Striated and cardiac muscle differ mainly in the mechanism by which membrane depolarisation is coupled to Ca^{2+} release. In striated muscle the T-tubule membrane is coupled closely to the sarcoplasmic reticulum via the dihydropyridine receptor and the ryanodine receptor. In cardiac muscle, Ca^{2+} entry via voltage-gated calcium channels initiates a regenerative release through activation of the Ca^{2+}-sensitive ryanodine receptors. In smooth muscle, contraction can be produced either by Ca^{2+} entry through voltage- or ligand-gated calcium channels, or by IP_3-mediated Ca^{2+} release from the sarcoplasmic reticulum. The mechanism by which Ca^{2+} activates contraction is different, and operates more slowly, in smooth muscle compared with striated or cardiac muscle. (SR, sarcoplasmic reticulum; ER, endoplasmic reticulum; NaC, voltage-gated sodium channel; CaC, calcium channel; RyR, ryanodine receptor; DHPR, dihydropyridine receptor; CaM, calmodulin; IP_3, inositol trisphosphate; GPCR, G-protein-controlled receptor; MLCK, myosin light-chain kinase.)

to transmitters. The best characterised of these are the receptors of the P_{2X} type (see Ch. 12), which respond to ATP released from autonomic nerves. Smooth muscle cells also store Ca^{2+} in the ER, from which it can be released when the IP_3R is activated by IP_3 (see Ch. 3). The IP_3 is generated by activation of many types of G-protein-coupled receptor. Thus, in contrast to skeletal and cardiac muscle, Ca^{2+} release and contraction can occur in smooth muscle when such receptors are activated without the involvement of electrical events and Ca^{2+} entry through the plasma membrane.

The contractile machinery of smooth muscle is activated when the *myosin light chain* (MLC) undergoes phosphorylation, allowing it to become detached from the actin filaments. This phosphorylation is catalysed by a kinase, *myosin-light-chain kinase* (MLCK), which is activated when it binds to Ca^{2+}-calmodulin (see Ch. 3). A second enzyme, *myosin phosphatase*, reverses the phosphorylation and causes relaxation. The activity of MLCK and myosin phosphatase thus exert a balanced effect, promoting contraction and relaxation, respectively. Both enzymes are regulated by cyclic nucleotides (cAMP and cGMP; see Ch. 3), and many drugs that cause smooth muscle contraction or relaxation mediated through G-protein-coupled receptors or through guanylate cyclase-linked receptors act in this way. Figure 4.10 summarises the main mechanisms by which drugs control smooth muscle contraction.

The complexity of these control mechanisms and interactions explains why pharmacologists have been entranced for so long by smooth muscle. Many therapeutic drugs work by contracting or relaxing smooth muscle, particularly those affecting the cardiovascular, respiratory and gastrointestinal systems, as

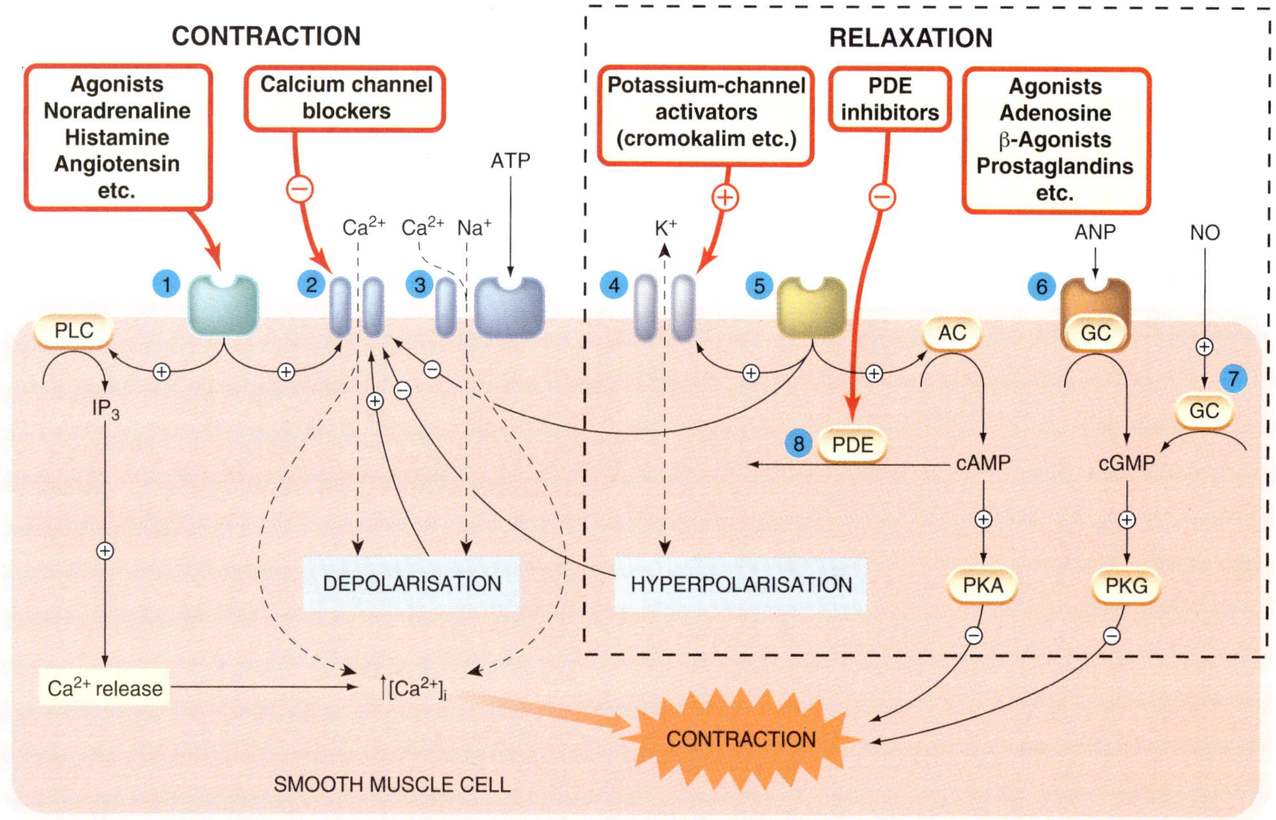

Fig. 4.10 Mechanisms controlling smooth muscle contraction and relaxation. 1. G-protein coupled receptors for excitatory agonists, mainly regulating inositol trisphosphate formation and calcium channel function. 2. Voltage-gated calcium channels. 3. Ligand-gated cation channels (P_{2X} receptor for ATP is the main example). 4. Potassium channels. 5. G-protein-coupled receptors for inhibitory agonists, mainly regulating cAMP formation, potassium and calcium channel function. 6. Receptor for atrial natriuretic peptide (ANP), coupled directly to guanylate cyclase (GC). 7. Soluble guanylate cyclase, activated by nitric oxide (NO). 8. Phosphodiesterase (PDE) is the main route of inactivation of cAMP and cGMP. (AC, adenylate cyclase; PKA, protein kinase A; PKG, protein kinase G; PLC, phospholipase C.)

discussed in later chapters, where details of specific drugs and their physiological effects are given.

RELEASE OF CHEMICAL MEDIATORS

Much of pharmacology is based on interference with the body's own chemical mediators, particularly neurotransmitters, hormones and inflammatory mediators. Here we discuss some of the common mechanisms involved in the release of such mediators, and it will come as no surprise that Ca^{2+} plays a central role. Drugs and other agents that affect the various control mechanisms which regulate $[Ca^{2+}]_i$ will, therefore, also affect mediator release, and this accounts for many of the physiological effects that they produce.

Chemical mediators that are released from cells fall into two main groups (Fig. 4.11).

- Mediators that are preformed and packaged in storage vesicles—sometimes called storage granules—from which they are released by *exocytosis*. This large group comprises all the conventional neurotransmitters and neuromodulators (see Chs 9 and 31) and many hormones. It also includes secreted proteins, such as cytokines (Ch. 15) and various growth factors (Ch. 13).
- Mediators that are produced on demand and are released by diffusion or by membrane carriers. This group includes nitric oxide (Ch. 14) and many lipid mediators (e.g. prostanoids, Ch. 15).*

Calcium ions play a key role in both cases, since a rise in $[Ca^{2+}]_i$ initiates exocytosis and is also the main activator of the enzymes responsible for the synthesis of diffusible mediators.

In addition to mediators that are released from cells, some are formed from precursors in the plasma, two important examples

*Carrier-mediated release can also occur with neurotransmitters that are stored in vesicles but is quantitatively less significant than exocytosis (see Ch. 9).

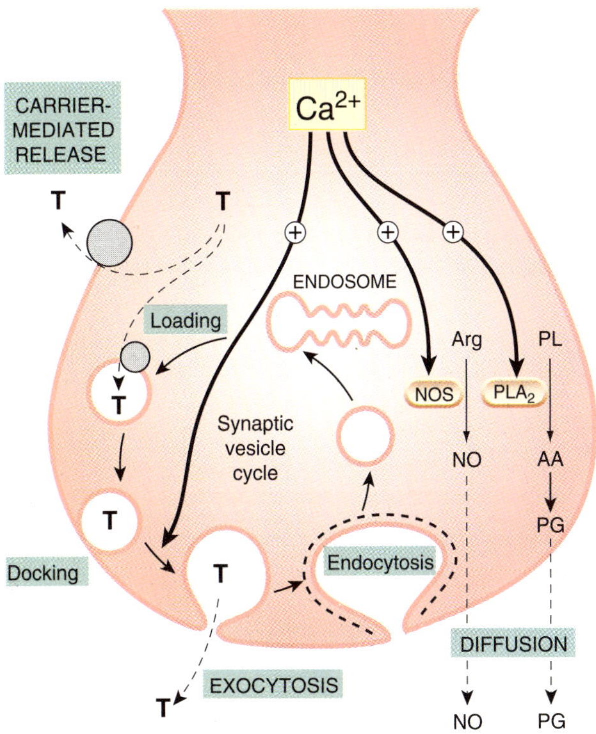

Fig. 4.11 Role of exocytosis, carrier-mediated transport and diffusion in mediator release. The main mechanism of release of monoamine and peptide mediators is by Ca^{2+}-mediated exocytosis, but carrier-mediated release from the cytosol also occurs. T represents a typical amine transmitter, such as noradrenaline or 5-hydroxytryptamine. Nitric oxide (NO) and prostaglandins (PGs) are released by diffusion as soon as they are formed, from arginine (Arg) and arachidonic acid (AA), respectively, through the action of Ca^{2+}-activated enzymes, nitric oxide synthase (NOS) and phospholipase A_2 (see Chs 13 and 14 for more details).

being *kinins* (Ch. 15) and *angiotensin* (Ch. 18), which are peptides produced by protease-mediated cleavage of circulating proteins.

EXOCYTOSIS

Exocytosis, occurring in response to an increase of $[Ca^{2+}]_i$, is the principal mechanism of transmitter release (see Fig. 4.11) in the peripheral and central nervous systems, as well as in endocrine cells and mast cells. The secretion of enzymes and other proteins by gastrointestinal and exocrine glands is also basically similar. Exocytosis involves fusion between the membrane of synaptic vesicles, which are pre-loaded with stored transmitter, and the inner surface of the plasma membrane. Release thus occurs in discrete packets, or *quanta*. The first evidence for this (see Nicholls et al., 2000) came from the work of Katz and his colleagues in the 1950s, who recorded spontaneous 'miniature endplate potentials' at the frog neuromuscular junction and showed that each resulted from the spontaneous release of a packet of the transmitter acetylcholine. They also showed that release evoked by nerve stimulation occurred by the synchronous release of several hundred such quanta; this was highly dependent on the presence of Ca^{2+} in the bathing solution. Unequivocal evidence that the quanta represented vesicles releasing their contents by exocytosis came from electron microscopic studies, in which the tissue was rapidly frozen in mid-release revealing vesicles in the process of extrusion, and from elegant electrophysiological measurements showing that membrane capacitance (reflecting the area of the presynaptic membrane) increased in a stepwise way as each vesicle fused and then gradually returned as the vesicle membrane was recovered from the surface. There is also biochemical evidence showing that, in addition to the transmitter, other constituents of the vesicles are released at the same time.

In nerve terminals specialised for fast synaptic transmission, Ca^{2+} enters through voltage-gated calcium channels, mainly of the N- and P-type (see p. 52), and the synaptic vesicles are 'docked' at *active zones*—specialised regions of the presynaptic membrane from which exocytosis occurs. These are situated close to the relevant calcium channels and opposite receptor-rich zones of the postsynaptic membrane (see Stanley, 1997). Elsewhere, where speed is less critical, Ca^{2+} may come from intracellular stores as described above, and the spatial organisation of active zones is less clear. It is common for individual nerve terminals to release both 'fast' and 'slow' neurotransmitters (see Ch. 9), e.g. glutamate plus a neuropeptide. Release of the fast transmitter, because of the tight spatial organisation, occurs as soon as the neighbouring calcium channels open, before the Ca^{2+} has a chance to diffuse throughout the terminal, whereas release of the slow transmitter requires the Ca^{2+} to diffuse more widely. As a result, release of fast transmitters occurs impulse by impulse, even at low

> **Muscle contraction**
>
> - Muscle contraction occurs in response to a rise in $[Ca^{2+}]_i$.
> - In skeletal muscle, depolarisation causes rapid Ca^{2+} release from the sarcoplasmic reticulum (SR). In cardiac muscle, Ca^{2+} enters through voltage-gated channels, and this initial entry triggers further release from the SR. In smooth muscle, the Ca^{2+} signal results partly from Ca^{2+} entry and partly from IP_3-mediated release from SR.
> - In smooth muscle, contraction can occur without action potentials, e.g. when agonists at G-protein-coupled receptors lead to IP_3 formation.
> - Activation of the contractile machinery in smooth muscle involves phosphorylation of the myosin light chain, a mechanism that is regulated by a variety of second messenger systems.

stimulation frequencies, whereas release of slow transmitters builds up only at higher stimulation frequencies. The release rates of the two, therefore, depend critically on the frequency and patterning of firing of the presynaptic neuron.

Exactly how Ca^{2+} causes exocytosis remains conjectural, but recent evidence suggests that it binds to a vesicle-bound protein, *synaptotagmin,* and that this favours association between a second vesicle-bound protein, *synaptobrevin,* and a related protein, *syntaxin,* on the inner surface of the plasma membrane. This association brings the vesicle membrane into close apposition with the plasma membrane, causing membrane fusion. These proteins, known as *SNAREs*, play a key role in exocytosis

Having undergone exocytosis, the empty vesicle* is recaptured by endocytosis and returns to the interior of the terminal, where it fuses with the larger endosomal membrane. The endosome buds off new vesicles, which take up transmitter from the cytosol by means of specific transport proteins and are again docked on the presynaptic membrane. This sequence, which typically takes several minutes, is controlled by various trafficking proteins associated with the plasma membrane and the vesicles, as well as cytosolic proteins. Further details about exocytosis and vesicle recycling are given by Südhof (1995), Calakos & Scheller (1996), Gerst (1999) and Nestler et al. (2001). So far, there are few examples of drugs that affect transmitter release by interacting with synaptic proteins, though the **botulinum neurotoxins** (see Ch. 10) produce their effects by proteolytic cleavage of certain components of this system.

NON-VESICULAR RELEASE MECHANISMS

If this neat and tidy picture of transmitter packets ready and waiting to pop obediently out of the cell in response to a puff of Ca^{2+} seems a little too good to be true, rest assured that the picture is no longer quite so simple. Acetylcholine, noradrenaline and other mediators can leak out of nerve endings from the cytosolic compartment, independently of vesicle fusion, by utilising carriers in the plasma membrane (Fig. 4.11). Drugs such as *amphetamines*, which release amines from central and peripheral nerve terminals (see Chs 11 and 31), displace the endogenous amine from storage vesicles into the cytosol, from where it escapes via the monoamine transporter in the plasma membrane, a mechanism that does not depend on Ca^{2+}.

Nitric oxide (see Jaffrey & Snyder, 1995; Yun et al., 1996; Ch. 14) and arachidonic acid metabolites (e.g. prostaglandins; see Piomelli, 1994; Ch. 18) are two important examples of mediators where release does not involve vesicles and exocytosis but relies on diffusion. The mediators are not stored but escape from the cell as soon as they are synthesised. In both cases, the synthetic enzyme is activated by Ca^{2+}, and the moment-to-moment control of the rate of synthesis depends on the intracellular $[Ca^{2+}]_i$. This kind of release is necessarily slower than the classical exocytotic mechanism but, in the case of nitric oxide, is fast enough for it to function as a true transmitter (see Ch. 14).

*The vesicle contents may not always be discharged completely. Instead, vesicles may fuse transiently with the cell membrane and release only part of their contents (see Neher, 1993) before becoming disconnected.

Mediator release

- Most chemical mediators are packaged into storage vesicles and released by exocytosis. Some are synthesised on demand and released by diffusion or the operation of membrane carriers.
- Exocytosis occurs in response to increased $[Ca^{2+}]_i$, as a result of a Ca^{2+}-mediated interaction between proteins of the synaptic vesicle and the plasma membrane, causing the membranes to fuse.
- Stored mediators (e.g. neurotransmitters) may be released directly from the cytosol independently of Ca^{2+} and exocytosis by drugs that interact with membrane transport mechanisms.
- Non-stored mediators, such as prostanoids and nitric oxide, are released by increased $[Ca^{2+}]_i$, which activates the enzymes responsible for their synthesis.

EPITHELIAL ION TRANSPORT

Fluid-secreting epithelia include the renal tubule, salivary glands, gastrointestinal tract and airways epithelia. In each case, epithelial cells are arranged in sheets, separating the interior (blood-perfused) compartment from the exterior lumen compartment, into which, or from which, secretion takes place. Fluid secretion involves two distinct mechanisms, which often coexist in the same cell and indeed interact with each other. Greger (2000) and Ashcroft (2000) give more detailed accounts. The two mechanisms (Fig. 4.12) are concerned, respectively, with Na^+ transport and Cl^- transport.

In the case of Na^+ transport, secretion occurs because Na^+ enters the cell passively at one end and is pumped out actively at the other, with water following passively. Critical to this mechanism is a class of highly regulated epithelial sodium channels (ENaCs), which allow Na^+ entry.

ENaCs (see de la Rosa et al., 2000) belong to the same structural class as the inward-rectifying potassium channels (Fig. 3.16) and they are widely expressed, not only in epithelial cells but also in neurons and other excitable cells, where their function is largely unknown. ENaCs are regulated mainly by *aldosterone,* a hormone produced by the adrenal cortex that enhances Na^+ reabsorption by the kidney (Ch. 23). Aldosterone, like other steroid hormones, exerts its effects by regulating gene expression (see Ch. 3) and causes an increase in ENaC expression, thereby increasing the rate of Na^+ and fluid transport. This takes a few hours. Aldosterone also affects ENaC function through other more rapid mechanisms, but the details are not well understood. ENaCs are selectively blocked by certain diuretic drugs, notably

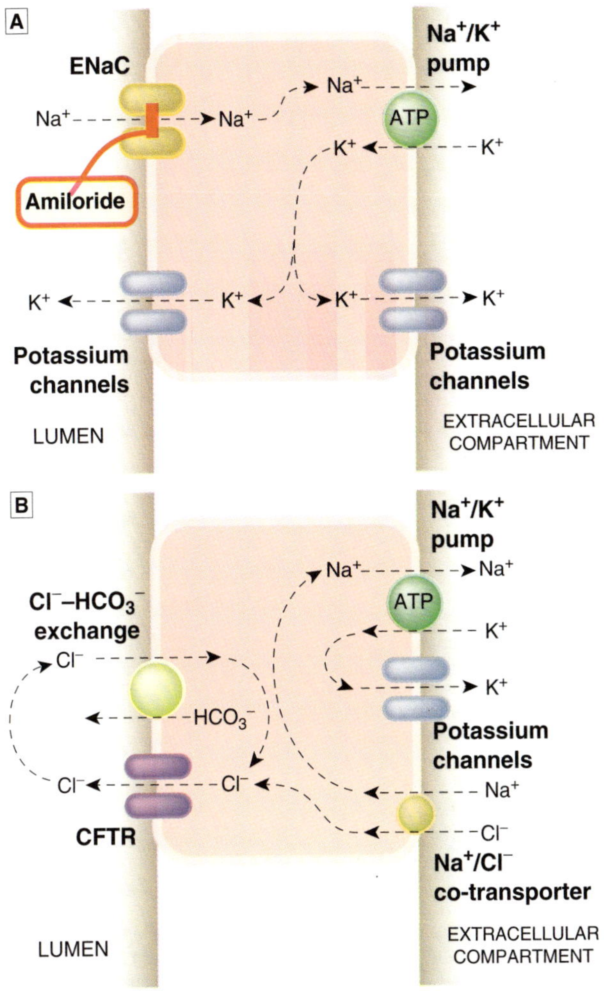

Fig. 4.12 Mechanisms of epithelial ion transport. Such mechanisms are important in renal tubules (see Ch. 23 for more details), and also in many other situations, such as the gastrointestinal and respiratory tracts. [A] Sodium transport. A special type of epithelial sodium channel (ENaC) controls entry of Na^+ into the cell from the lumenal surface, the Na^+ being actively pumped out at the apical surface by the Na^+/K^+ exchange pump. Potassium ions moves passively via potassium channels. [B] Chloride transport. Chloride leaves the cell via a special membrane channel, the 'cystic fibrosis transmembrane conductance regulator' (CFTR), after entering the cell either from the apical surface via the Na^+/Cl^- co-transporter, or at the lumenal surface via the Cl^-/HCO_3^- co-transporter.

amiloride (see Ch. 23), a compound that is widely used to study the functioning of ENaCs in different situations.

Chloride transport is particularly important in the airways and gastrointestinal tract. In the airways, it is essential for fluid secretion, whereas in the colon, it mediates fluid reabsorption, the difference being caused by the different arrangements of various transporters and channels with respect to the polarity of the cells. The simplified diagram in Figure 4.12B represents the situation in the pancreas, where secretion depends on Cl^- transport. The key molecule in Cl^- transport is the *cystic fibrosis transmembrane conductance regulator* (*CFTR*), so named because early studies on the inherited disorder cystic fibrosis showed it to be associated with impaired Cl^- conductance in the membrane of secretory epithelial cells. The gene *CFTR*, identified through painstaking genetic linkage studies and isolated in 1989, was found to encode a Cl^--conducting ion channel. Severe physiological consequences follow from the impairment of secretion, particularly in the airways, but also in many other systems, such as sweat glands and pancreas. Genetic studies of cystic fibrosis revealed mutations in *CFTR*; this knowledge has produced a flood of research on the molecular mechanisms involved in Cl^- transport, but so far no significant therapeutic advance. Pharmacological agents that affect CFTR directly are being sought (see Hwang & Sheppard, 1999), and this may well bear fruit in the future.

Both Na^+ and Cl^- transport are regulated by intracellular messengers, notably by Ca^{2+} and cAMP, the latter exerting its effects by activating protein kinases and thereby causing phosphorylation of channels and transporters. CFTR itself is activated by cAMP. In the gastrointestinal tract, increased cAMP formation causes a large increase in the rate of fluid secretion, an effect that leads to the copious diarrhoea produced by cholera infection (see Ch. 3) and also by inflammatory conditions in which prostaglandin formation is increased (see Ch. 15). Activation of G-protein-coupled receptors, which cause release of Ca^{2+}, also stimulates secretion, possibly also by activating CFTR. Many examples of therapeutic drugs that affect epithelial secretion by activating or blocking G-protein coupled receptors appear in later chapters.

Epithelial ion transport

- Many epithelia (e.g. renal tubules, exocrine glands, airways) are specialised to transport specific ions.
- This type of transport depends on a class of Na^+ channels known as ENaCs, which allow Na^+ entry into the cell at one surface, coupled to active extrusion of Na^+, or exchange for another ion, from the opposite surface.
- ENaC expression is increased by aldosterone.
- ENaCs are blocked by amiloride.
- The activity of channels, pumps and exchange transporters is regulated by various second messengers and nuclear receptors, which control the transport of ions in specific ways.

REFERENCES AND FURTHER READING

Aidley D J 1998 The physiology of excitable cells. Cambridge University Press, Cambridge (*Good general textbook, covering ion channels, Ca^{2+} regulation and contractile mechanisms*)

Ashcroft F M 2000 Ion channels and disease. Academic Press, San Diego, CA (*A very useful textbook which describes the physiology of different kinds of ion channels and relates it to their molecular structure. Emphasises the importance of 'channelopathies', genetic channel defects associated with disease states*)

Barritt G J 1999 Receptor-activated Ca^{2+} inflow in animal cells: a variety of pathways tailored to meet different intracellular Ca^{2+} signalling requirements. Biochem J 337: 153–169 (*Useful overview of mechanisms involved in calcium signalling*)

Berridge M J 1995 Capacitative calcium entry. Biochem J 312: 1–11 (*Clear description of an important mechanism that remains somewhat mysterious*)

Berridge M J 1997 Elementary and global aspects of calcium signalling. J Physiol 499: 291–306 (*Review of calcium signalling, emphasising the various intracellular mechanisms that produce spatial and temporal patterning: 'sparks', 'waves', etc.*)

Berridge M J 1998 Neuronal calcium signaling. Neuron 21: 13–26 (*Review article describing the mechanisms of Ca^{2+} regulation by neurons and their role in controlling excitability, transmitter release and plasticity*)

Bers D M 2002 Cardiac excitation–contraction coupling. Nature 415: 198–205 (*Short well illustrated review article*)

Bolton T B, Prestwich S A, Zholos A V, Gordienko D V 1999 Excitation–contraction coupling in gastrointestinal and other smooth muscles. Annu Rev Physiol 61: 85–115 (*Comprehensive review of the role of Ca^{2+} in controlling smooth muscle contraction*)

Calakos N, Scheller R H 1996 Synaptic vesicle biogenesis, docking and fusion: a molecular description. Physiol Rev 76: 1–29 (*Summarises recent advances in mechanism of exocytosis*)

Catterall W A 2000 From ionic currents to molecular mechanisms: the structure and function of voltage-gated sodium channels. Neuron 26: 13–25 (*Useful review article*)

de la Rosa D A, Canessa C M, Fyfe G K, Zhang P 2000 Structure and regulation of amiloride-sensitive sodium channels. Annu Rev Physiol 62: 573–594 (*General review on the nature and function of 'epithelial' sodium channels*)

Gerst J E 1999 SNAREs and SNARE regulators in membrane fusion and exocytosis. Cell Mol Life Sci 55: 707–734 (*Review of molecular events in exocytosis*)

Goldstein S A N, Bockenhauer D, Zilberberg N 2001 Potassium leak channels and the KCNK family of two-P-domain subunits. Nat Rev Neurosci 2: 175–184 (*Review on the current state of knowledge of a recently discovered class of potassium channels*)

Greger R 2000 The role of CFTR in the colon. Annu Rev Physiol 62: 467–491 (*A useful resume of information about CFTR and epithelial secretion, more general than its title suggests*)

Guse A H 2000 Cyclic ADP-ribose. J Mol Med 78: 26–35 (*Review article describing the role of cADPR, a recently discovered second messenger similar to IP_3*)

Hille B 1992 Ionic channels of excitable membranes. Sinauer, Sunderland, MA (*A clear and detailed account of the basic principles of ion channels with emphasis on their biophysical properties*)

Hwang T-C, Sheppard D N 1999 Molecular pharmacology of the CFTR channel. Trends Pharmacol Sci 20: 448–453 (*Description of approaches to find therapeutic drugs that alter the function of the CFTR channel*)

Jaffrey SR, Snyder SH 1995 Nitric oxide: a neural messenger. Annu Rev Cell Dev Biol 11: 417–440

Jentsch T J 2000 Neuronal KCNQ potassium channels: physiology and role in disease. Nat Rev Neurosci 1: 21–30 (*Review describing a subclass of potassium channels that have relevance to pathophysiology*)

Kandel E R, Schwartz J H, Jessell T M 2000 Principles of neural science. McGraw-Hill, New York (*Standard heavyweight textbook covering all aspects of neuroscience from molecules to brains*)

Kuriyama H, Kitamura K, Itoh T, Inoue R 1998 Physiological features of visceral smooth muscle cells, with special reference to receptors and ion channels. Physiol Rev 78: 811–920 (*Comprehensive review article*)

Neher E 1993 Secretion without full fusion. Nature 363: 497–498 (*Elegant techniques*)

Nestler E J, Hyman S E, Malenka R C 2001 Molecular neuropharmacology. McGraw-Hill, New York (*Excellent modern textbook*)

Nicholls J G, Fuchs P A, Martin A R, Wallace B G 2000 From neuron to brain. Sinauer, Sunderland, MA (*Excellent, well written textbook of neuroscience*)

Petersen O H, Petersen C C H, Kasai H 1996 Calcium and hormone action. In: Foreman J C, Johansen T (ed) Textbook of receptor pharmacology, Ch. 10. CRC Press, Boca Raton, FL (Useful general review article, not overdetailed)

Piomelli D 1994 Eicosanoids in synaptic transmission. Crit Rev Neurobiol 8: 65–83 (*Discusses role of arachidonic acid metabolites as neural mediators*)

Putney J W, McKay R R 1999 Capacitative calcium entry channels. Bioessays 21: 38–46 (*Review by a pioneer in this field*)

Reimann F, Ashcroft F M 1999 Inwardly rectifying potassium channels. Curr Opin Cell Biol 11: 503–508 (*Review describing the various mechanisms by which K_{IR} is modulated*)

Shieh C-C, Coghlan M, Sullivan J P, Gopalakrishnan M 2000 Potassium channels: molecular defects, diseases and therapeutic opportunities. Pharmacol Rev 52: 557–593 (*Comprehensive review of potassium channel pathophysiology and pharmacology*)

Stanley E E 1997 The calcium channel and the organization of the presynaptic transmitter release face. Trends Neurosci 20: 404–409 (*Discusses the microphysiology of vesicular release*)

Südhof T C 1995 The synaptic vesicle cycle: a cascade of protein–protein interactions. Nature 375: 645–653 (*Summarises recent advances in vesicular release at the molecular level*)

Triggle D J 1999 The pharmacology of ion channels: with particular reference to voltage-gated Ca^{2+} channels. Eur J Pharmacol 375: 311–325 (*Review focussing mainly on various types of calcium channel blockers, many of which are important therapeutically*)

Vandenberg J I, Walker B D, Campbell T J 2001 HERG potassium channels: friend and foe. Trends Pharmacol Sci 22: 240–246 (*Review on the function and pharmacology of an important class of potassium channels that are responsible for various adverse drug effects on cardiac function*)

Yun HY, Dawson VL, Dawson TM 1996 Neurobiology of nitric oxide. Crit Rev Neurobiol 10: 291–316 (*General review article*)

5 Cellular mechanisms: cell proliferation and apoptosis

Overview 69

Cell proliferation 69
— The cell cycle 69
— Interactions between cells, growth factors and the extracellular matrix 73

Angiogenesis 74

Apoptosis and cell removal 74
— Pathways to apoptosis 75

Pathophysiological implications 77

Therapeutic implications 77
— Targets for new drug development 77

OVERVIEW

This chapter deals with the slower mechanisms of cell responses (sometimes days or months), including *cell division, cell proliferation, tissue growth,* and *cell death*. In the adult body, about 10 billion new cells are manufactured daily through division of existing cells—a prodigious output that must be counter-balanced by the elimination of a similar number of cells. A balance between cell generation and cell removal is also critical during embryogenesis and development. This chapter covers the main elements involved in the processes of cell proliferation and cell removal. We consider the changes that occur within an individual cell when, after stimulation by growth factors, it gears up to divide into two daughter cells and describe the interaction of cells, growth factors and the extracellular matrix in cell proliferation. We consider the phenomenon of apoptosis—a programmed series of events leading to cell death—detailing the changes that occur in a cell preparing to die and describing the intracellular pathways that lead to its demise.

Lastly we briefly discuss the pathophysiological significance of the events we have described and their implications for the potential development of clinically useful drugs.

CELL PROLIFERATION

Cell proliferation is involved in many physiological and pathological processes including growth, healing, repair, hypertrophy, hyperplasia and the development of tumours. *Angiogenesis* (the development of new blood vessels) necessarily occurs during many of these processes.

Proliferating cells go through what is termed the *cell cycle*, during which the cell replicates all its components and then bisects itself into two identical daughter cells. Important components of the signalling pathways in proliferating cells are *receptor tyrosine kinases* or receptor-linked kinases and the *mitogen-activated kinase* cascade (see Ch. 3). In all cases, the pathways eventually lead to transcription of the genes that control the cell cycle.

THE CELL CYCLE

The cell cycle is an ordered series of events consisting of several sequential phases: G_1, S, G_2* and M (Fig. 5.1)

M is the phase of <u>m</u>itosis
S phase is the phase of DNA <u>s</u>ynthesis
G_1 is the gap between the mitosis that gave rise to the cell and the S phase; during G_1 the cell is preparing for DNA synthesis
G_2 is the gap between S phase and the mitosis that will give rise to two daughter cells; during G_2 the cell is preparing for the mitotic division into two daughter cells.

Cell division requires the controlled timing of two critical events of the cell cycle: S phase (DNA replication) and M phase (mitosis). Entry into each of these phases is carefully regulated and this gives rise to two 'check points' (restriction points) in the cycle: one at the start of S and one at the start of M. DNA damage results in the cycle being stopped at one or other of these. The integrity of the check points is critical for the maintenance of genetic stability (explained below).

In the adult, most cells do not constantly divide; most spend a varying amount of time in a quiescent phase *outside* the cycle as it were, in the phase termed G_0 (Fig. 5.1). (Note that G_0 means 'G nought' not the word 'Go'.) Neurons and skeletal muscle cells

*In cells that are dividing continuously, G_1, S and G_2 constitute 'interphase'—the phase between one mitosis and the next.

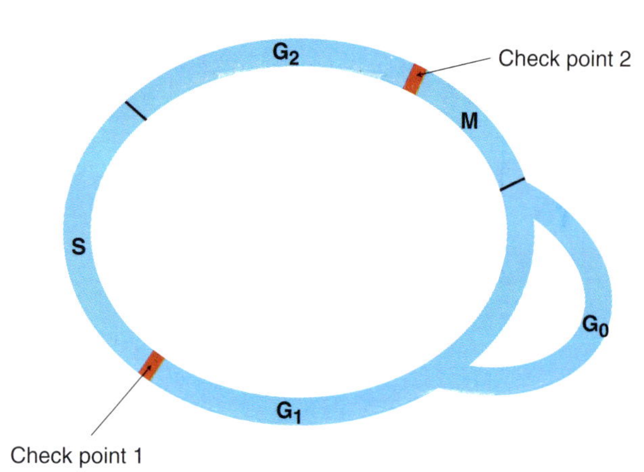

Fig. 5.1 The main phases of the cell cycle of dividing cells.

spend all their lifetime in G_0; bone marrow cells and the lining cells of the gastrointestinal tract divide daily.

Quiescent cells can be activated into G_1 by chemical stimuli associated with damage; for example, a quiescent skin cell can be stimulated by a wound into dividing and repairing the lesion. The impetus for a cell to start off on the cell cycle (i.e. to move from G_0 into G_1) can be provided by several stimuli, the most important being growth factor action.*

Growth factors stimulate the production of signal transducers of two types:

- positive regulators of the cell cycle that control the changes necessary for cell division
- negative regulators that control the positive regulators.

The maintenance of normal cell numbers in tissues and organs requires that there be a balance between the positive regulatory forces and the negative regulatory forces. *Apoptosis* also has a role in the control of cell numbers (see below).

POSITIVE REGULATORS OF THE CELL CYCLE

The cell cycle is initiated when a growth factor acts on a quiescent cell provoking it to divide. One of the main actions of a growth factor is to stimulate production of the cell cycle regulators, which are coded for by the delayed response genes (explained below).

The main components of the control system that determines progress through the cycle are two families of proteins: *cyclins*** and *cyclin-dependent kinases* (*cdks*).

The cdks phosphorylate various proteins (e.g. enzymes)—activating some and inhibiting others—to coordinate their activities.

Sequential functioning of several different cdks activates the processes that promote progress through the phases of the cycle. Each cdk is inactive until it binds to a cyclin, the binding enabling the cdk to phosphorylate the protein(s) necessary for a particular step in the cycle (Fig. 5.2). It is the cyclin that determines which protein(s) are phosphorylated. After the phosphorylation event has taken place, the cyclin is degraded (Fig. 5.2) by the ubiquitin/protease system. This involves several enzymes (E_1, E_2, E_3) acting sequentially to add small molecules of ubiquitin to the cyclin, with the resulting ubiquitin polymer acting as an 'address label' that directs the cyclin to the proteasome where it is degraded.

There are eight main groups of cyclins. Those important in the control of the cell cycle are cyclins A, B, D and E. Each cyclin is associated with and activates particular cdk(s). Cyclin A activates cdks 1 and 2; cyclin B, cdk 1; cyclin D, cdks 4 and 6; cyclin E,

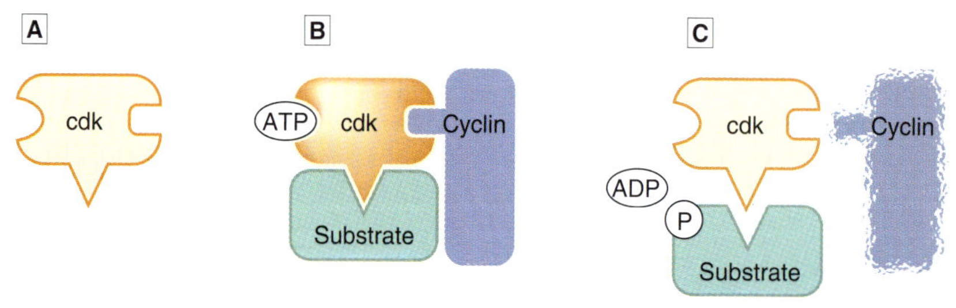

Fig. 5.2 Schematic representation of the activation of a cyclin-dependent kinase (cdk). A An inactive cdk. B The inactive cdk is activated by being bound to a cyclin; it can now phosphorylate a protein substrate (e.g. an enzyme). C After the phosphorylating event, the cyclin is degraded.

*G-protein-coupled receptors can also stimulate cell proliferation (Marinissen & Gutkind, 2001).

**The name 'cyclin' comes from the fact that these proteins undergo a cycle of synthesis and breakdown during each cell division.

cdk 2. Precise timing of each activity is essential and many cycle proteins are degraded after they have carried out their functions. The actions of the cyclin/cdk complexes in the cell cycle are depicted in Figure 5.3.

The activity of these cyclin/cdk complexes is modulated by various negative regulatory forces (considered below), most of which act at one or other of the two check points.

Cells in G_0

In quiescent G_0 cells, cyclin D is present in low concentration and an important regulatory protein—the Rb protein*—is hypophosphorylated.

Hypophosphorylated Rb holds the cell cycle in check at check point 1 by inhibiting the expression of several proteins critical for cell cycle progression. The Rb protein accomplishes this by binding to the E2F transcription factors, which control the expression of the genes that code for cyclins E and A, for DNA polymerase, for thymidine kinase, for dihydrofolate reductase, etc.—all essential for DNA replication during S phase.

Growth factor action on a cell in G_0 propels it into G_1 phase (Fig. 5.4).

*The Rb protein is coded for by the Rb gene. The Rb gene is so named because mutations of this gene are associated with retinoblastoma tumours.

Phase G_1

G_1 is the phase in which the cell is preparing for S phase by synthesising the messenger RNAs (mRNAs) and proteins needed for DNA replication. During G_1, the concentration of cyclin D increases and the cyclin D/cdk complex phosphorylates and activates the necessary proteins.

In mid-G_1, the cyclin D/cdk complex phosphorylates the Rb protein, releasing transcription factor E2F; this then activates the genes for the components specified above that are essential for the next phase—DNA synthesis—namely cyclins E and A, DNA polymerase and so on.

The action of the cyclin E/cdk complex is necessary for transition from G_1 to S phase, i.e. past check point 1. Once past

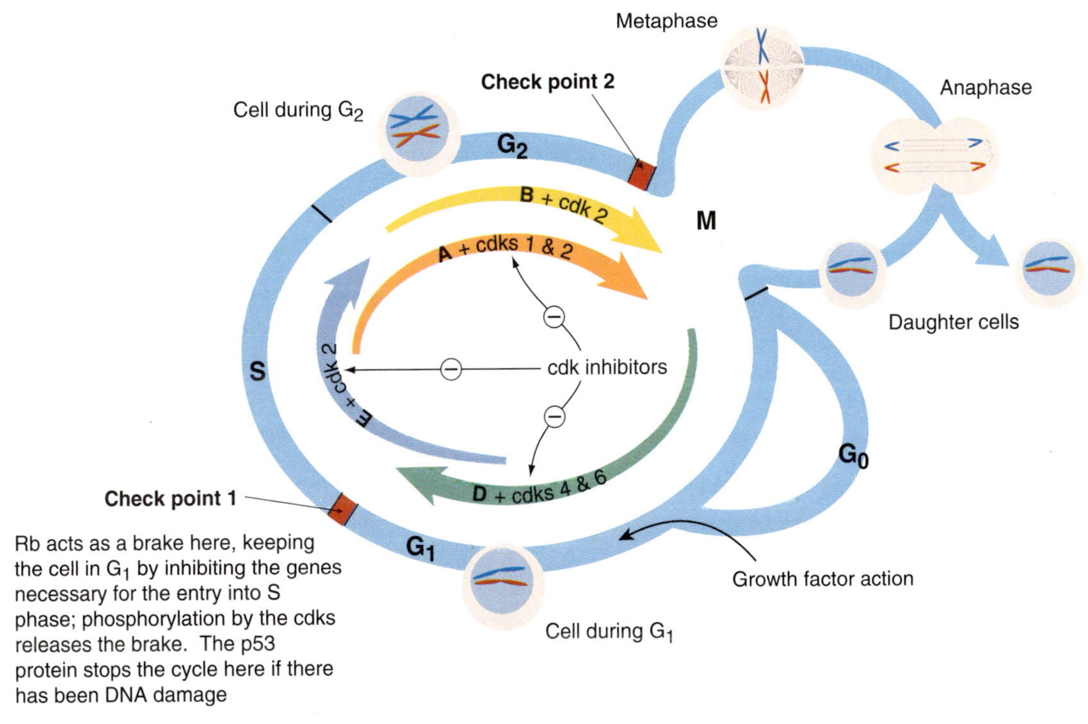

Fig. 5.3 Schematic diagram of the cell cycle showing the role of the cyclin/cdk complexes. The processes outlined in the cycle occur inside a cell such as the one shown in Figure 5.4. A quiescent cell (in G_0 phase), when stimulated to divide by growth factors, is propelled into G_1 phase and prepares for DNA synthesis. Progress through the cycle is determined by sequential action of the cyclin/cdk complexes—depicted here by coloured arrows, the arrows being given the names of the relevant cyclins: D, E, A and B. The cyclin-dependent kinase (cdks) are given next to the relevant cyclins. The thickness of each arrow represents the intensity of action of the cdk at that point in the cycle. The activity of the cdks is regulated by cdk inhibitors. At check point 1, Rb protein acts as a brake; phosphorylation by the cyclin D kinases releases the brake. If there is DNA damage, the products of the tumour suppressor gene p53 stop the cycle at check point 1, allowing for repair. If repair fails, apoptosis (see Fig. 5.5) is initiated. The state of the chromosomes is shown schematically in each G phase—as a single pair in G_1 and each duplicated and forming two daughter chromatids in G_2. Some changes that occur during mitosis (metaphase, anaphase) are shown in a subsidiary circle. After the mitotic division, the daughter cells may enter G_1 or G_0 phase. (Rb, retinoblastoma.)

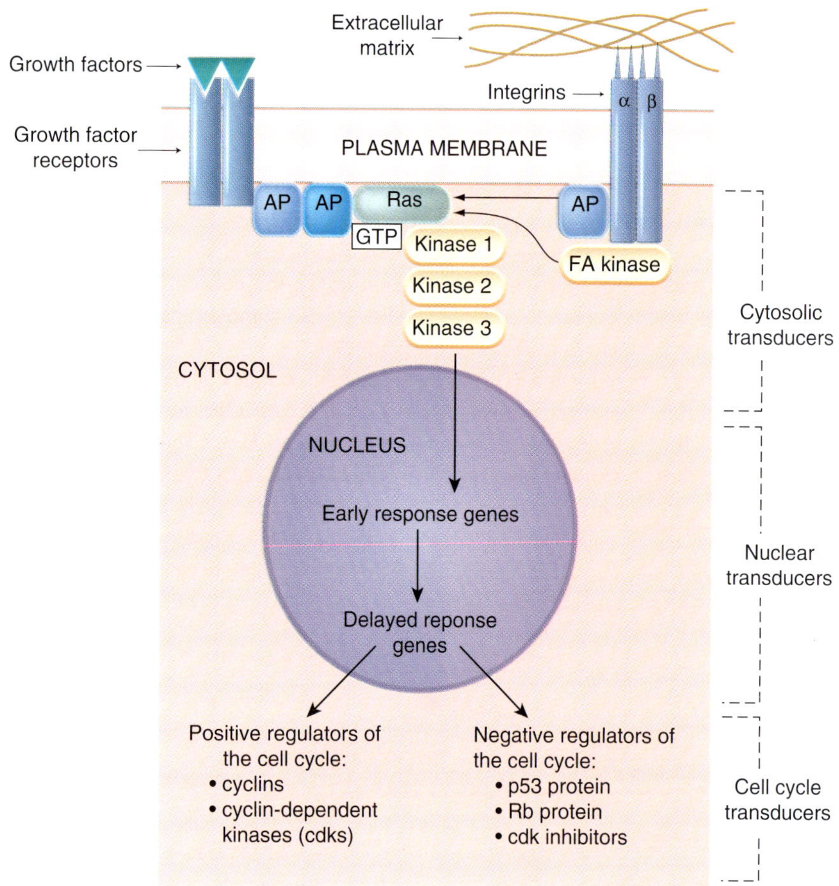

Fig. 5.4 Simplified diagram of the effect of growth factors on a cell in G_0. The overall effect of growth factor action is the generation of the cell cycle transducers. A cell such as the one depicted will then embark on G_1 phase of the cell cycle. Most growth factor receptors have integral tyrosine kinase (see Fig. 3.15). These receptors dimerise (form pairs), then phosphorylate each other's tyrosine residues. The early cytosolic transducers include proteins that bind to the phosphorylated tyrosine residues. Optimum effect requires cooperation with integrin action. Integrins (which have α- and β-subunits) connect the extracellular matrix with intracellular signalling pathways and also with the cell's cytoskeleton (not shown here). G-protein-coupled receptors can also stimulate cell proliferation because their intracellular pathways can connect with the Ras/kinase cascade (not shown). (AP, adapter proteins; Rb, retinoblastoma.)

check point 1, the processes that have been set in motion cannot be reversed and the cell is committed to continue with DNA replication and mitosis.

S phase

Cyclin E/cdk and cyclin A/cdk regulate progress through S phase, phosphorylating and thus activating proteins/enzymes involved in DNA synthesis.

G_2 phase

In G_2 phase, the cell, which now has double the number of chromosomes, must duplicate all other cellular components for allocation to the two daughter cells. Synthesis of the necessary mRNAs and proteins occurs.

Cyclin A/cdk and cyclin B/cdk complexes are active during G_2 phase and are necessary for entry into M phase, i.e. for passing check point 2. The presence of cyclinB/cdk complexes in the nucleus is required for mitosis to commence.

Unlike cyclins C, D and E, which are short lived, cyclins A and B remain stable throughout interphase but undergo proteolysis by a ubiquitin-dependent pathway during mitosis.

Mitosis

Mitosis is a continuous process but can be considered to consist of four stages.

Prophase The duplicated chromosomes (which have up to this point formed a tangled mass filling the nucleus) condense, each now consisting of two daughter chromatids, (the original chromosome and a copy). These are released into the cytoplasm as the nuclear membrane disintegrates.

Metaphase The chromosomes are aligned at the equator (Fig. 5.3)

Anaphase A specialised device, the *mitotic apparatus*, captures the chromosomes and draws them to opposite poles of the dividing cell (Fig. 5.3).

Telophase A nuclear membrane forms round each set of chromosomes. Finally the cytoplasm divides between the two forming daughter cells. Each daughter cell will be in G_0 phase and will remain there unless stimulated into G_1 phase as described above.

During metaphase, the cyclin A and B complexes phosphorylate cytoskeletal proteins, histones and possibly components of the spindle (the microtubules along which the chromatids are pulled during metaphase).

NEGATIVE REGULATORS OF THE CELL CYCLE

One of the main negative regulators has already been mentioned—the Rb protein that holds the cycle in check while it is hypophosphorylated. Another negative regulatory mechanism is the action of the inhibitors of the cdks. These bind to and inhibit the action of the complexes, their main action being at check point 1.

There are two families of inhibitors:

- the CIP family (cdk inhibitory proteins; also termed KIP or kinase inhibitory proteins): p21, p27 and p57
- the Ink family (inhibitors of kinases): p16, p19, p15.

The action of p21 (explained below) serves as an example of the role of a cyclin/cdk inhibitor. Protein p21 is under the control of the *p53* gene—a particularly important negative regulator that operates at check point 1.

Inhibition of the cycle at check point 1

The *p53* gene has been called the 'guardian of the genome'. It codes for a protein transcription factor—the p53 protein. In normal healthy cells, the steady-state concentration of p53 protein is low. But when there is DNA damage, the protein accumulates and activates the transcription of several genes, one of which codes for p21. Protein p21 inactivates cyclin/cdk complexes, thus preventing Rb phosphorylation, which means the cycle is arrested at check point 1. This allows for DNA repair. If the repair is successful, the cycle proceeds past check point 1 into S phase. If the repair is unsuccessful, the *p53* gene triggers apoptosis—cell suicide (see below).

Inhibition of the cycle at check point 2

There is evidence that DNA damage can result in the cycle being stopped at check point 2 but the mechanisms involved are less clear than those at check point 1. Inhibition of the accumulation of cyclinB/cdk complex in the nucleus seems to be a factor.

The cell cycle

- The term 'cell cycle' refers to the sequence of events that take place within a cell as it tools up for division.
- The phases of the cell cycle are:
  —G_1: preparation for DNA synthesis
  —S: DNA synthesis
  —G_2: preparation for division
  —mitosis: division into two daughter cells.
- Growth factor action stimulates a quiescent cell—said to be in G_0 (G nought)—to divide, i.e. to start on G_1 phase.
- In G_0 phase, a hypophosphorylated protein, coded for by the *Rb* gene, holds the cycle in check by inhibiting expression of critical factors necessary for DNA replication.
- Progress through the cycle is controlled by specific kinases (cyclin-dependent kinases; cdks) that are activated by binding to proteins termed cyclins.
- Four main cyclin/cdk complexes involving cyclins D, E, A and B drive the cycle; the first complex, cyclinD/cdk, releases the Rb protein-mediated inhibition.
- Various families of proteins act as cdk inhibitors. Important is protein p21 which is expressed when DNA damage causes transcription of gene p53. The p21 protein stops the cycle at check point 1.
- Growth factors act through receptor tyrosine kinases or receptor-coupled kinases to stimulate the production of the positive and negative regulators of the cell cycle.

INTERACTIONS BETWEEN CELLS, GROWTH FACTORS AND THE EXTRACELLULAR MATRIX

During cell proliferation, there is integrated interplay between growth factors, cells, the extracellular matrix and the matrix metalloproteinases. The extracellular matrix supplies the supporting framework for the cells of the body and is secreted by the cells themselves. It also profoundly influences cell behaviour through the cell's integrins (see below). Matrix expression is regulated by the action on the cell of growth factors and cytokines (see Haralson, 1993; Kresse & Schönherr, 2001). The activation status of some growth factors is, in turn, determined by the matrix since they are sequestered by interaction with matrix components and released by enzymes (e.g. metalloproteinases, see below) secreted by the cells.

It is clear that the action of growth factors—which act through receptor tyrosine kinases or receptor-coupled kinases (see Ch. 3) initiating the cell cycle (see above)—is a fundamental part of these processes.* There are numerous growth factors, important examples being fibroblast growth factor (FGF), epidermal growth factor (EGF), platelet-dependent growth factor (PDGF), vascular endothelial growth factor (VEGF) and transforming growth factor-β (TGF-β).

The main components of the extracellular matrix are:

Proteoglycans These have a growth-regulating role, in part by functioning as a reservoir of sequestrated growth factors (as specified above). Some proteoglycans are associated with the cell surface, where they help to bind cells to the matrix (Kresse & Schönherr, 2001).

Collagens These are the main proteins of the extracellular matrix.

Adhesive proteins (e.g. fibronectin) These link the various elements of the matrix together and also form links between the cells and the matrix through integrins on the cells (see below)

INTEGRINS

Integrins are transmembrane receptors with α- and β-subunits. On interaction with the extracellular matrix elements outside the cell (e.g. fibronectin), integrins mediate various cell responses

*But there is also a role for ligands acting on G-protein-coupled receptors in cell cycle initiation.

such as cytoskeletal rearrangement (not considered here) and coregulation of growth factor function. Intracellular signalling by both growth factor receptors and integrins is important for optimal cell proliferation (Fig. 5.4). Integrin stimulation activates an intracellular transduction pathway, which, through an adapter protein and an enzyme (focal adhesion kinase), can activate the kinase cascade that forms part of the growth factor signalling pathway (Fig. 5.4). Cross-talk between the integrin and growth factor pathways occurs by several other means as well. Autophosphorylation of growth factor receptors (Ch. 3) is enhanced by integrin activation; in addition integrin-mediated adhesion to the extracellular matrix (Fig. 5.4) not only suppresses the concentrations of cdk inhibitors p21 and p27 but also is required for the expression of cyclins A and D and, therefore, for the progression of the cell cycle. Furthermore, integrin action stimulates apoptosis-inhibiting signals (see below), further facilitating growth factor action. (See reviews by Howe et al., 1998; Schwartz et al., 1999; Dedhar, 2000; Eliceiri, 2001.)

MATRIX METALLOPROTEINASES

Degradation of the extracellular matrix by metalloproteinases is necessary during the growth, repair and remodelling of tissues. These enzymes are secreted as inactive precursors by local cells. When growth factors stimulate a cell to enter the cell cycle they also stimulate the secretion of metalloproteinases, which then sculpt the matrix, producing the local changes necessary for the resulting increase in cell numbers. Metalloproteinases, in turn, play a part in releasing growth factors from the matrix as described above and, in some cases (e.g. interleukin-1β), in processing them from precursor to active form.

The action of these enzymes is regulated by TIMPS (tissue inhibitors of metalloproteinases), which are also secreted by local cells.

Interactions between cells, growth factors and the matrix

- Cells are imbedded in the extracellular matrix (ECM), which is secreted by the cells themselves.
- The ECM profoundly influences the cells through the cells' integrins; it also forms a store of growth factors by sequestering them.
- Integrins are transmembrane receptors that, on interaction with elements of the ECM, cooperate with growth factor signalling pathways (this is necessary for optimum cell division) and also mediate cytoskeletal adjustments within the cell.
- On stimulation with growth factors, cells release metalloproteinases, which degrade the local matrix in preparation for the increase in cell numbers.
- Metalloproteinases release growth factors from the ECM and can activate some that are present in precursor form.

In addition to the physiological function outlined above, metalloproteinases are involved in the tissue destruction that occurs in various diseases such as rheumatoid arthritis, osteoarthritis, periodontitis, macular degeneration, myocardial restonosis, etc. They also have a critical role in the growth, invasion and metastasis of tumours. (See reviews by Chang & Werb, 2001; McCawley & Matrisian, 2001; Sternlicht & Werb, 2001.)

ANGIOGENESIS

Angiogenesis, which normally accompanies cell proliferation, is the formation of new capillaries from existing small blood vessels. Angiogenic stimuli, in the context of cell proliferation, include the action of various growth factors and cytokines, in particular VEGF. The sequence of events is as follows:

1. VEGF induces nitric oxide and also the expression of proteases (e.g. metalloproteinases). Nitric oxide (see Ch. 14) causes local vasodilatation and the proteases degrade the local basement membrane and the local matrix and also mobilise further growth factors from the matrix.
2. Endothelial cells migrate out forming a solid capillary sprout.
3. The endothelial cells behind the leading cells are activated by growth factors and start to divide.
4. A lumen forms in the sprout.
5. Local fibroblasts, activated by growth factors, proliferate and lay down matrix around the capillary sprout.
6. A process of 'maturation' occurs in which there is stabilisation of the endothelial layer through cell to cell binding by adherence proteins and integrin binding of the cells to the matrix.

APOPTOSIS AND CELL REMOVAL

Apoptosis is cell suicide by a built-in self-destruct mechanism; it consists of a genetically programmed sequence of biochemical events. It is, therefore, unlike necrosis, which is a disorganised disintegration of damaged cells resulting in products that trigger the inflammatory response.

Angiogenesis

- Angiogenesis is the formation of new capillaries from existing blood vessels, an important stimulus being vascular endothelial growth factor (VEGF).
- The sequence of events is as follows:
  1. The basement membrane is degraded locally by proteases
  2. Endothelial cells migrate out forming a sprout
  3. Endothelial cells following the leading cells proliferate under the influence of VEGF
  4. Matrix is laid down around the new capillary.

Apoptosis is the mechanism which each day unobtrusively removes 10 billion cells from the adult human body. It is involved in the shedding of the intestinal lining, the regression of mammary gland cells after lactation and the death of time-expired neutrophils. It is the basis for the development of self-tolerance in the immune system (Ch. 15) and is implicated in the pathophysiology of cancer, autoimmune diseases, neurodegenerative conditions (Ch. 31), cardiovascular diseases and the acquired immunodeficiency syndrome (AIDS). It plays an essential role in embryogenesis, helping to shape organs during development by eliminating cells that have become redundant. It has a role in the monitoring of cancerous change because it acts as a first-line defence against mutations—purging cells with abnormal DNA that could become malignant.

There is evidence that apoptosis is a default response (i.e. that continuous active signalling by tissue-specific trophic factors, cytokines, hormones and cell-to-cell contact factors (adhesion molecules, integrins, etc.) may be required for cell survival and viability) and that the self-destruct mechanism is automatically triggered unless it is actively and continuously inhibited by these anti-apoptotic factors. Different cell types require differing sets of survival factors, which function only locally. If a cell strays or is dislodged from the area where its paracrine survival signals operate, it will die.

Withdrawal of these cell survival factors—which has been termed 'death by neglect'—is not the only pathway to apoptosis (see Fig. 5.5). The death machinery can be activated by ligands that stimulate death receptors ('death by design') and by DNA damage.

MORPHOLOGICAL CHANGES IN APOPTOSIS

As the cell dies it rounds up, the chromatin in the nucleus condenses into dense masses and the cytoplasm shrinks. This is followed by blebbing of the plasma membrane and finally transformation of the cell into a cluster of membrane-bound entities, which are rapidly phagocytosed by macrophages. It is important to note that at no stage are the internal constituents (enzymes, mitochondrial components, DNA fragments, etc.) released into the cell's surroundings; thus there are no elements that could trigger an inflammatory reaction.

THE MAJOR PLAYERS IN APOPTOSIS

The major players are the caspases—a family of cysteine proteases present in the cell in inactive form. They do not perform generalised proteolysis; they undertake delicate protein surgery, selectively cleaving a specific set of target proteins (enzymes, structural components, etc.) inactivating some and activating others. A cascade of about nine different caspases take part in bringing about apoptosis, some functioning as *initiators* that transmit the initial apoptotic signals, and some being responsible for the final *effector* phase of cell death (Fig. 5.5).

The capases are not the only executors of apoptotic change. Various pathways that result in apoptosis without the action of the caspase fraternity have recently been described. One involves a protein termed AIF (apoptotic initiating factor), which is released from the mitochondria, enters the nucleus and triggers cell suicide.

Note that not all caspases are death-mediating enzymes; some, not specified here, have a role in the processing and activating of cytokines.

PATHWAYS TO APOPTOSIS

There are two main routes to cell death, one involving stimulation of death receptors by external ligands and one arising within the cell and involving the mitochondria. Both these routes activate initiator caspases and both converge on a final common effector caspase pathway.

THE DEATH RECEPTOR PATHWAY

Lurking in the plasma membrane of most cell types are members of the tumour necrosis factor (TNF) receptor (TNFR) family, which function as death receptors. Important family members are TNFR-1 and CD95 (aka Fas or Apo-1). Each receptor has a

Apoptosis

- Apoptosis is programmed cell death, essential in embryogenesis and tissue homeostasis; it is brought about principally by a cascade of proteases—the caspases. Two sets of initiator caspases converge on a set of effector caspases.
- There are two main pathways to activation of the effector caspases: the death receptor pathway and the mitochondrial pathway.
- The death receptor pathway involves stimulation of members of the tumour necrosis factor receptor (TNFR) family; and the main initiator caspase is caspase 8.
- The mitochondrial pathway is activated by internal factors such as DNA damage, which results in transcription of gene *p53*. The p53 protein activates a subpathway that results in release from the mitochondrion of cytochrome *c*. This, in turn, complexes with protein Apaf-1 and together they activate initiator caspase 9.
- In undamaged cells, survival factors (cytokines, hormones, cell-to-cell contact factors) continuously activate anti-apoptotic mechanisms. Withdrawal of survival factor stimulation causes cell death through the mitochondrial pathway.
- The effector caspases (e.g. caspase 3) start a pathway that results in cleavage of cell constituents: DNA, cytoskeletal components, enzymes, etc. This reduces the cell to a cluster of membrane-bound entities that are eventually phagocytosed by macrophages.

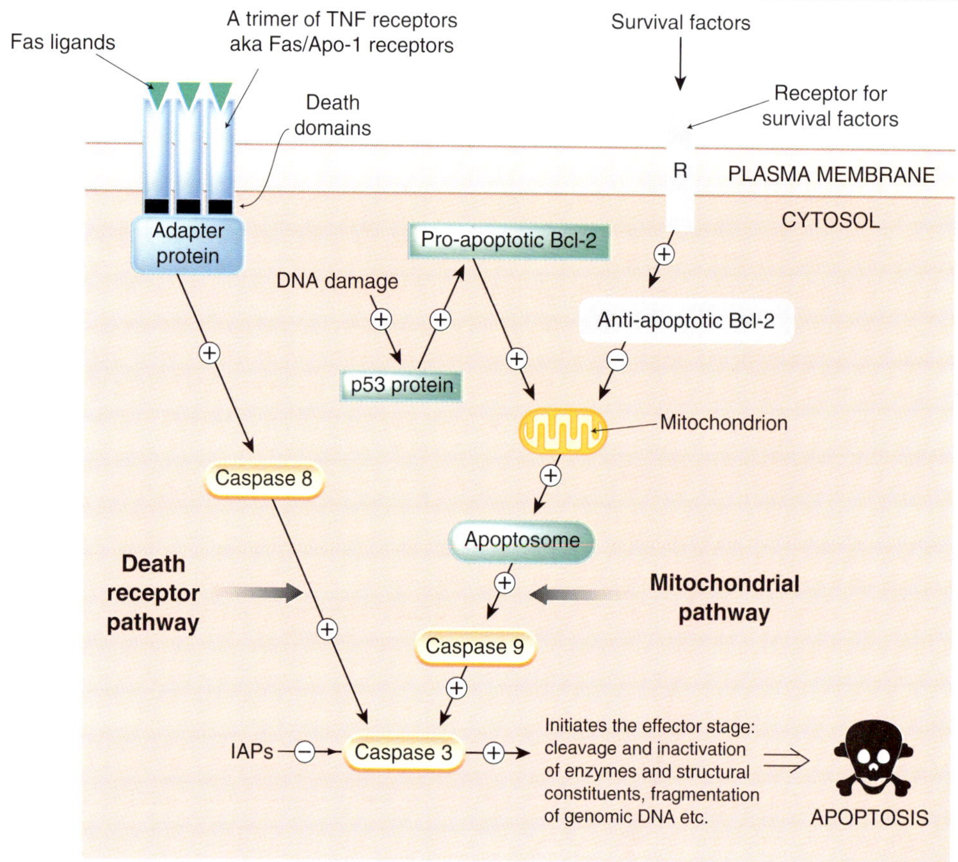

Fig. 5.5 Simplified diagram of the two main signalling pathways in apoptosis. The death receptor pathway is activated when death receptors such as members of the tumour necrosis factor (TNF) family are stimulated by specific death ligands. This recruits adapter proteins that activate initiator caspases (e.g. caspase 8), which in turn activate effector caspases, such as caspase 3. The mitochondrial pathway is activated by diverse signals, one being DNA damage. In the presence of DNA damage that cannot be repaired, the p53 protein (see text and Figs 5.3 and 5.4) activates a subpathway that results in release of cytochrome *c* from the mitochondrion, with subsequent involvement of the apotosome and activation of an initiator caspase, caspase 9. The apoptosome is a complex of procaspase 9, cytochrome *c* and apoptotic-activating protease factor-1 (Apaf-1). Both these pathways converge on the effector caspase (e.g. caspase 3), which bring about the demise of the cell. The survival factor subpathway (shown here in grey) normally holds apoptosis at bay by inhibiting the mitochondrion pathway through activation of an anti-apoptotic member of the Bcl-2 family. The receptor labelled 'R' represents the respective receptors for trophic factors, growth factors, cell-to-cell contact factors (adhesion molecules, integrins), etc. Continuous stimulation of these receptors is necessary for cell survival/proliferation. If this pathway is non-functional, this anti-apoptotic drive is withdrawn. (IAPs, inhibitor of apoptosis proteins.)

'death domain' in its cytoplasmic tail. Stimulation of the receptors by an external ligand such as TNF itself or TRAIL* causes them to get together in threes (trimerise) and recruit an adapter protein that complexes with the trimer by associating with the death domains. The resulting complex activates caspase 8, an initiator caspase that, in turn, activates the effector caspases.

THE MITOCHONDRIAL PATHWAY

The mitochondrial pathway can be called into action in two principal ways: by DNA damage and by withdrawal of the action of cell survival factors.

*TRAIL is tumour necrosis factor-α-related apoptosis-inducing ligand of course; what else?

DNA damage

In the presence of DNA damage that cannot be repaired, the p53 protein activates a subpathway involving p21 protein (see above) and pro-apoptotic members of the Bcl-2 protein family. In addition to these pro-apoptotic individuals, this family has anti-apoptotic members.** They meet at the surface of mitochondria and compete with each other. The pro-apoptotic branch of the family (e.g. Bax) promotes release of *cytochrome* c from the mitochondria; the anti-apoptotic branch inhibits this. The released cytochrome *c* complexes with a protein termed Apaf-1 (apoptotic protease-activating factor-1) and the two then combine with procaspase 9

**Another brake on the cell death mechanisms is a family of caspase-inhibiting proteins called, you will not be surprised to learn, IAPs (inhibitors of apoptosis proteins).

and activate it. This latter enzyme activates the effector caspase pathway. The three-party composite of cytochrome *c*, Apaf-1 and procaspase 9 is termed the apoptosome (Fig. 5.5).

Withdrawal of survival factors

In normal cells, survival factors (specified above) continuously activate anti-apoptotic mechanisms, and the withdrawal of survival factors can cause death in several different ways depending on the cell type. But a common mechanism is a tipping of the balance between Bcl-2 family members, leading to loss of the stimulation of anti-apoptotic Bcl-2 protein action with resultant unopposed action of the pro-apoptotic Bcl-2 proteins (Fig. 5.5).

THE EFFECTOR STAGE CASPASES

The effector stage caspases (e.g. caspase 3) cleave and inactivate cell constituents such as the DNA repair enzymes, protein kinase C, cytoskeletal components, etc. A DNAase is activated and cuts genomic DNA between the nucleosomes, generating DNA fragments of approximately 180 base pairs.

THE FINAL STAGE: DISPOSAL OF THE REMAINS

When the effector caspases have carried out their functions, the cell is reduced to a cluster of membrane-bound bodies, each containing a variety of organelles. The dying cell displays several 'eat-me' signals such as surface exposure of phosphatidylserine and changes in cell surface sugars, which can be detected by macrophages. The final stage of cells, removal then is phagocytosis by macrophages.

PATHOPHYSIOLOGICAL IMPLICATIONS

As outlined briefly above, cell proliferation and apoptosis are involved in many physiological and pathological processes:

- the growth of tissues and organs
- the replenishment of lost or time-expired cells such as leucocytes, gut epithelium, uterine endometrium, etc.
- healing and repair after injury or inflammation
- the hyperplasia (increase in cell number) associated with chronic inflammatory, hypersensitivity and autoimmune diseases (Ch. 15)
- the growth, invasion and metastasis of tumours.

The role of cell proliferation and apoptosis in the first two processes listed is self-evident and needs no further comment.

Healing and *repair* can be regarded as paradigms of the processes in the above list. In both, there is an ordered series of events involving cell migration, cell proliferation, synthesis of extracellular matrix and remodelling—all coordinated by the growth factors and cytokines that are relevant for the particular tissue involved. TGF-β is a key cytokine in many of these processes. Resolution of an inflammatory reaction and wound healing after injury follow this pattern.

Cell proliferation and matrix expansion are hall marks of *chronic inflammatory, hypersensitivity* and *autoimmune* diseases such as rheumatoid arthritis (Ch. 15), psoriasis, chronic ulcers, chronic obstructive lung disease, the processes underlying the bronchial hyper-reactivity of chronic asthma (Ch. 22), glomerular nephritis, etc.

Cell proliferation and apoptotic events are also implicated in atherosclerosis, restenosis, and myocardial repair after infarction.

As regards the *growth, invasion and metastasis of tumours*, one does not need to be a rocket scientist to be aware that tumour cells proliferate; what may not be so obvious is that perturbations in the growth factor signalling pathways, the anti-apoptotic pathways and the function of the cell cycle controllers have a role in the *pathogenesis* of malignancy. New understanding of this is leading to novel approaches to the treatment of cancer (see below and in Ch. 50).

THERAPEUTIC IMPLICATIONS

Considerable effort is being expended on finding compounds that will inhibit or modify the processes described in this chapter, most but not all work being aimed at developing new drugs for cancer therapy. Theoretically, all the processes could constitute targets for new drug development. Here we concentrate on those approaches that are proving to be most fruitful.

TARGETS FOR NEW DRUG DEVELOPMENT

ANGIOGENESIS

As specified above, angiogenesis has a critical role in numerous bodily processes, some physiological (e.g. growth, repair) some pathological (e.g. tumour growth, chronic inflammatory conditions).

Angiogenesis inhibitors

Angiogenesis inhibitors are being sought for use in pathological angiogenesis and there are currently 30 compounds in clinical trial (Griffioen & Molema, 2000). The approaches being used include:

- interference with endothelial cell growth, for example by the use of monoclonal antibodies that prevent the interaction of VEGF and FGF with their receptors
- interference with the necessary adherence of endothelial cells in the endothelial sprout to the matrix; an anti-integrin monoclonal antibody has shown promise
- interference with the necessary degradation of the matrix round the developing endothelial sprout; inhibitors of metalloproteinases (see below) are under test.

It should be noted that though anti-angiogenesis drugs may be helpful in some conditions (e.g. cancer) they could be harmful in others (e.g. heart disease).

Angiogenesis stimulators

Angiogenesis stimulators are also being investigated for use in various ischaemic conditions, for example coronary disease, limb ischaemia, and gastrointestinal ulcers associated with insufficient local perfusion. The main compound under investigation is VEGF. In pilot studies, naked DNA encoding the gene for VEGF has been injected directly into the relevant tissue along with a viral promoter.

APOPTOTIC MECHANISMS

Defective apoptosis is a factor in several diseases, and compounds that modify it are under investigation (Nicholson, 2000; Reed, 2002).

Examples of defective apoptosis include cancer cell proliferation, resistance to cancer chemotherapy (Ch. 50) and ineffective eradication of virus-infected cells (Ch. 46).

Examples of over-exuberant apoptosis include depletion of T cells in human immunodeficiency virus (HIV) infection (Ch. 46), allograft rejection (Ch. 15), loss of neurons in neurodegenerative diseases (Ch. 34) and loss of chondrocytes in osteoarthritis (Ch. 30).

Several anti-apoptosis compounds are in clinical trials for neurodegenerative and inflammatory diseases (Reed, 2002) and numerous pro-apoptosis compounds are in clinical trials for cancer. Various approaches to apoptosis-based therapies are being explored.

The Bcl-2 family

Since the balance between the pro- and anti-apoptotic members of the Bcl-2 family determines the sensitivity or resistance of a cell to apoptotic stimuli, strategies to develop compounds that could tip the balance in a required therapeutic direction are being actively sought.

Caspase inhibitors

The key players in apoptosis, the caspases, are controlled by endogenous inhibitors, the IAPs (see the footnote above). One of these, survivin, occurs in high concentration in certain tumours, its gene being one of the most cancer-specific genes in the genome. The possibility of developing compounds that inhibit this IAP is being pursued, the object being to free caspases to induce cancer cell suicide.

However, as with anti-angiogenesis compounds, drugs affecting apoptosis may be helpful in some conditions but could be harmful in others.

METALLOPROTEINASE ACTION

As outlined above, the metalloproteinases are implicated in many diseases. Inhibitors are actively being sought and numerous compounds—including marimastat—are in clinical trial (Nelson et al., 2000; Hoekstra et al., 2001; McCawley & Matrisian, 2001)

CELL CYCLE REGULATORS

The main endogenous positive regulators of the cell cycle are the cdks. During the 1990s, these were cloned and small molecule inhibitors sought (Senderowicz & Sausville, 2000). Several agents (e.g. flavopitridol) are undergoing clinical testing.

THE GROWTH FACTOR SIGNALLING PATHWAY

Of the various components of the growth factor signalling pathway, receptor tyrosine kinases, the Ras protein and cytoplasmic kinases have been the subjects of most interest and several new drugs have been developed. Their main use is in cancer therapy and details are given in Chapter 50 (p. 706) and in Figure 50.1 (p. 695).

REFERENCES AND FURTHER READING

Apoptosis

Desagher S, Martinou J-C 2000 Mitochondria as the central control point of apoptosis. Trends in Cell Biol 10: 369–377 (*Lucid review of the mitochondrial mechanisms involved in cell death, with simple clear diagrams*)

Hengartner M O 2000 The biochemistry of apoptosis. Nature 407: 770–776 (*Excellent review article, very clearly written, with exceptionally clear diagrams*)

Kaufman S H, Kengartner M O 2001 Programmed cell death: alive and well in the new millenium. Trends in Cell Biol 11: 526–534 (*Review summarising the information on apoptosis and outlining questions that might lead to future therapies*)

Mallat Z, Tedgui K 2000 Apoptosis in the vasculature: mechanisms and functional importance. Br J Pharmacol 130: 947–962 (*Adroit coverage of the molecular mechanisms of apoptosis. Stresses apoptosis of endothelial cells, vascular smooth muscle cells and the role of apoptosis in normal vessel development and in vascular pathology*)

Nicholson D W 2000 From bench to clinic with apoptosis-based therapeutic agents. Nature 407: 810–816 (*Useful review that covers the potential of apoptosis modulation for the treatment of human disease*)

Reed J C 2001 Apoptosis-regulating proteins as targets for drug discovery. Trends Mol Med 7: 314–319 (*Discusses caspases, caspase inhibitors, Bcl-2 proteins and protein kinases as targets for future new drug development*)

Reed J C 2002 Apoptosis-based therapies. Nat Rev Drug Discov 1: 111–121 (*Excellent coverage, useful tables good diagrams*)

Renehan A G, Booth C, Potten C S 2001 What is apoptosis, and why is it important? Br Med J 322: 1536–1538 (*Simple exposition of apoptosis covering briefly: biological mechanisms, physiological role and pathological significance. Very simple diagram but caspases 3 and 8 should be transposed, and caspase 9 should act on caspase 3!)*)

Rich T, Allen R L, Wyllie A H 2000 Defying death after DNA damage. Nature 407: 777–783 (*Comprehensive coverage of the sequence of changes involved in the response to DNA damage*)

Salveson G S, Duckett C S 2002 IAP proteins: blocking the road to death's door. Nat Rev: Mol Cell Biol 3: 401– 410 (*Review covering the molecular biology of IAP proteins and their functions*)

Savill J, Fadok V 2000 Corpse clearance defines the meaning of cell death. Nature 407: 784–788 (*A review article setting out the factors involved in phagocytosis of apoptotic cells and the relationship to inflammation and*

the regulation of the immune response)
Song Z, Steller H 1999 Death by design: mechanism and control of apoptosis. Trends Biochem Sci (Millennium issue) 24: M49–M52 (*Brief succinct article with clear coverage of topic*)
Strasser A, O'Connor L, Dixit V M 2000 Apoptosis signaling. Annu Rev Biochem 69: 217–245 (*Detailed review emphasising caspases, adaptor proteins, the death receptor family and the Bcl-2 family. Outlines the pathophysiological role of apoptosis*)
Zörnig M, Hueber A-O et al. 2001 Apoptosis regulators and their role in tumorigenesis. Biochem Biophys Acta 1551: F1–F37 (*Excellent comprehensive review*)

Growth factor signalling and the cell cycle

Assoian R K, Schwatz M A 2001 Coordinate signalling by integrins and receptor kinases in the regulation of G_1 phase cell-cycle progression. Curr Opin Genet Dev 11: 48–53 (*Discusses how cooperative signalling between integrins and receptor tryosine kinases regulates progression through G_1 phase. Annotated references*)
English J M, Cobb M H 2002 Pharmacological inhibitors of MAPK pathways. Trends Pharmacol Sci 23: 40–45 (*Lists mitogen-activated protein kinases (MAPKs) and discusses small molecule inhibitors under investigation*)
Blume-Jensen P, Hunter T 2001 Oncogenic kinase signalling. Nature 411: 355–365 (*Excellent article. Emphasises oncogenic receptor tyrosine kinases and cytoplasmic tyrosine kinases. Useful figures and tables. Note that there are eight other relevant articles in the same issue of Nature*)
Favoni R E, de Cupis A 2000 The role of polypeptide growth factors in human carcinomas: new targets for a novel pharmacological approach. Pharmacol Rev 52: 179–206 (*Thorough coverage. Outlines growth factor signalling; describes 14 growth factor families and their possible role in cancer; discusses possible drug action on signalling pathways*)
Funk J O 1999 Cancer cell cycle control. Anticancer Res 19: 4772–4780 (*Lucid article outlining the cell cycle, stressing the check points and the role of Rb and p53 proteins. Discusses the alterations of the cell cycle regulators in cancer, and DNA tumour virus oncoproteins. Has very useful tables*)
Johnson D G, Walker C L 1999 Cyclins and cell cycle checkpoints. Annu Rev Pharmacol Toxicol 39: 295–312 (*Admirably clear description of the cell cycle, detailing the progression from G_0 through the cycle, the inhibitors of cyclin-dependent kinases, the alterations seen in cancer and therapeutic targets*)
Knockaert M, Greengard P, Miejer L 2001 Pharmacological inhibitors of cyclin-dependent kinases. Trends Pharmacol Sci 23: 417–425 (*Brief review listing possible inhibitors, giving their structures and outlining possible therapeutic uses*)
Li J M, Brooks G 1999 Cell cycle regulatory molecules (cyclins, cyclin-dependent kinases and cyclin-dependent kinase inhibitors) and the cardiovascular system: potential targets for therapy. Eur Heart J 20: 406–420 (*Adroit overview of the cell cycle. Considers cycle control in vascular disease and potential therapeutic manipulation*)
Molinari M 2000 Cell cycle checkpoints and their inactivation in human cancer. Cell Prolif 33: 261–274 (*Clear well-written article describing the cell cycle engine, the G_0–G_1 transition, the G_2–M transition and the spindle check point*)
Senderowicz A M, Sausville E A 2000 Preclinical and clinical development of cyclin-dependent kinase modulators. J Natl Cancer Inst 92: 376–387 (*Outlines cell cycle control and targets for intervention and discusses preclinical pharmacology of agents in clinical trial*)
Talapatra S, Thompson C B 2001 Growth factor signaling in cell survival: implications for cancer treatment. J Pharmacol Exp Ther 298: 873–878 (*Succinct overview of death receptor-induced apoptosis, the role of growth factors in preventing it, and potential drugs*)
Zömig M, Hueber A-O, Baum W, Evans G 2001 Apoptosis regulators and their role in tumorigenesis. Biochim Biophys Acta 1551: F1–F37 (*Excellent review*)

Integrins, extracellular matrix, metalloproteinases, angiogenesis

Carmeliet P, Jain R K 2000 Angiogenesis in cancer and other diseases. Nature 407: 249–257 (*Gives details of mechanisms involved in angiogenesis, lists biological activators and inhibitors, and agents in clinical trials. Excellent figures*)
Chang C, Werb Z 2001 The many faces of metalloproteinases: cell growth, invasion, angiogenesis and metastasis. Trends Cell Biol 11: S37–S43 (*Covers the role of matrix metalloproteinases in cell proliferation, the release of growth regulators and angiogenesis*)
Dedhar S 2000 Cell–substrate interactions and signaling through ILK. Curr Opin Cell Biol 2000 12: 250–256 (*Discusses the role integrin-linked kinase in the cross-talk between integrin and growth factor signalling for cell cycle progression and cell growth*)
Eliceiri B P 2001 Integrin and growth factor receptor cross-talk. Circ Res 89: 1104–1110 (*Gives experimental evidence for cooperation between integrins and growth factors in cell growth and angiogenesis*)
Giancotti F G 1997 Integrin signalling: specificity and control of cell survival and cell cycle progression. Curr Opin Cell Biol 9: 691–700 (*Clear coverage of integrin signalling; useful diagrams*)
Griffioen A, Molema G 2000 Angiogenesis: potentials for pharmacologic intervention in the treatment of cancer, cardiovascular diseases and chronic inflammation. Pharmacol Rev 52: 237–268 (*Comprehensive review covering virtually all aspects of angiogenesis and the potential methods of modifying it*)
Haralson M A 1993 Extracellular matrix and growth factors: an integrated interplay controlling tissue repair and progression to disease. Lab Invest 69: 369–372 (*Editorial giving succinct overview*)
Hoekstra R, Eskens F A L M, Verveij J 2001 Matrix metalloproteinase inhibitors: current developments and future perspectives. Oncologist 6: 415–427 (*Reviews the results of preclinical and clinical trials and discusses future possibilities*)
Howe A, Aplin A E, Alahari S K, Juliano R L 1998 Integrin signaling and cell growth control. Curr Opin Cell Biol 10: 220–231 (*Discusses integrin involvement in cell adhesion, activation of the MAPK cascade, modulation of growth factor signalling and the cell cycle*)
Kresse H, Schönherr E 2001 Proteoglycans of the extracellular matrix and growth control. J Cell Physiol 189: 266–274 (*Describes how proteoglycans can affect cell growth directly and through modulation of growth factor activities*)
Marinissen M J, Gutkind, J S 2001 G-protein-coupled receptors and signaling networks: emerging paradigms. Trends Pharmacol Sci 22: 368–376 (*Discusses the participation of G-protein-coupled receptors in a range of intracellular signalling networks, including gene transcription for cell proliferation*)
McCawley L J, Matrisian L M 2001 Matrix metalloproteinases: they're not just for matrix anymore. Curr Opin Cell Biol 13: 534–540 (*Succinct coverage; discusses matrix and non-matrix metalloproteinase substrates involved in cell growth, apoptosis or tumour progression*)
Nelson A R, Fingleton B, Rothenberg M L, Matrisian LM 2000 Matrix metalloproteinase: biological activity and clinical implications. J Clin Oncol 18: 1135–1149 (*Gives classification of matrix metalloproteinases and their expression in cancers: lists inhibitors that are in phase I trials*)
Rosen L 2000 Antiangiogenic strategies and agents in clinical trial. Oncologist 5: 20–27 (*Succinct coverage; useful summary tables*)
Schwartz MA, Baron V 1999 Interactions between mitogenic stimuli, or a thousand and one cross-connections. Curr Opin Cell Biol 11: 197–202 (*Covers cross-talk between receptor kinase receptors, G-protein-coupled receptors and integrins*)
Sternlicht M D, Werb Z 2001 How matrix metalloproteinases regulate cell behaviour. Annu Rev Cell Dev Biol 17: 463–516 (*Comprehensive review of the regulation of metalloproteinases, their regulation of cell signalling and their role in development and disease*)
Stetler-Stevenson W G 1999 Matrix metalloproteinases in angiogenesis: a moving target for therapeutic intervention J Clin Invest 103: 1237–1241 (*Discussion of angiogenesis*)
Ulrich H, von Andrian U H, Englehardt B 2003 α4 Integrins as therapeutic targets in autoimmune disease. N Engl J Med 348: 68–70 (*Editorial commenting on two articles in the journal that describe the use of natalizumab, a recombinant monoclonal antibody, for the treatment of the inflammatory/immune diseases: multiple sclerosis and Crohn's disease. Natalizumab binds to α4 integrins on haemopoietic cells and prevents them from binding to their endothelial receptors.*)

6 Method and measurement in pharmacology

Overview 80

Bioassay 80
— General principles of bioassay 82
— Bioassays in humans 83

Animal models of disease 84

Clinical trials 86

Balancing benefit and risk 89

OVERVIEW

We emphasised in Chapters 2 and 3 that drugs, being molecules, produce their effects by interacting with other molecules. This interaction can lead to effects at all levels of biological organisation, from molecules to human populations* (Fig. 6.1).

In this chapter, we cover the principles of metrication at the various organisational levels, ranging from laboratory methods to clinical trials. Assessment of therapeutic drug action at the population level is the concern of *pharmacoepidemiology* and *pharmacoeconomics* (see Ch. 1), disciplines that are beyond the scope of this book.

We consider first the general principles of bioassay, and its extension to studies in human beings, and then the development of animal models to bridge the predictive gap between animal physiology and human disease. Clinical trials used to evaluate therapeutic efficacy in a clinical setting are discussed and, finally, we consider the principles of balancing benefit and risk.

BIOASSAY

Methods for measuring drug effects are needed in order that we may compare the properties of different substances, or the same substance under different circumstances, requirements that are met by the techniques of *bioassay,* defined as the estimation of the concentration or potency of a substance by measurement of the biological response that it produces. Nowadays, one of the main aims of bioassay is to provide information that will predict the effect of the drug in the clinical situation (where the aim is to improve function in patients suffering from the effects of disease). The choice of laboratory test systems (in vitro and in vivo 'models') that provide this predictive link is an important aspect of quantitative pharmacology. As our understanding of drug action at the molecular level advances (Ch. 3), this knowledge, and the technologies underlying it, have greatly extended the range of models that are available for measuring drug effects. By the 1960s, pharmacologists had become adept at using isolated organs and laboratory animals (usually under anaesthetic) for quantitative experiments and had developed the principles of bioassay to allow reliable measurements to be made with these sometimes difficult and unpredictable test systems. Such systems address drug action at the physiological level—roughly, the mid-range of the organisational heirarchy shown in Figure 6.1. Subsequent developments have extended the range of available models in both directions, towards the molecular and towards the clinical. The introduction of binding assays (Ch. 3) in the 1970s was a significant step towards analysis at the molecular level. More recently, the use of cell lines engineered to express specific human receptor subtypes has become widespread as a screening tool for drug discovery (see Ch. 54). Indeed, the range of techniques for analysing drug effects at the molecular and cellular levels is now very impressive. Bridging the gap between measuring effects at the physiological and the therapeutic levels has, however, proved much more difficult, because human illness cannot, in many cases, be accurately reproduced in experimental animals. The use of transgenic animals to model human disease represents a real advance, and this is discussed in more detail below.

USES OF BIOASSAY

The uses of bioassay** are:

- to measure the pharmacological activity of new or chemically undefined substances
- to investigate the function of endogenous mediators
- to measure drug toxicity and unwanted effects.

*Consider the effect of cocaine on organised crime, of organophosphate 'nerve gases' on the stability of dictatorships, or of anaesthetics on the feasibility of surgical procedures for examples of molecular interactions that affect the behaviour of populations and societies.

**In the past, bioassay was often used to measure the *concentration* of drugs and other active substances in the blood or other body fluids, an application now superseded by analytical chemistry techniques.

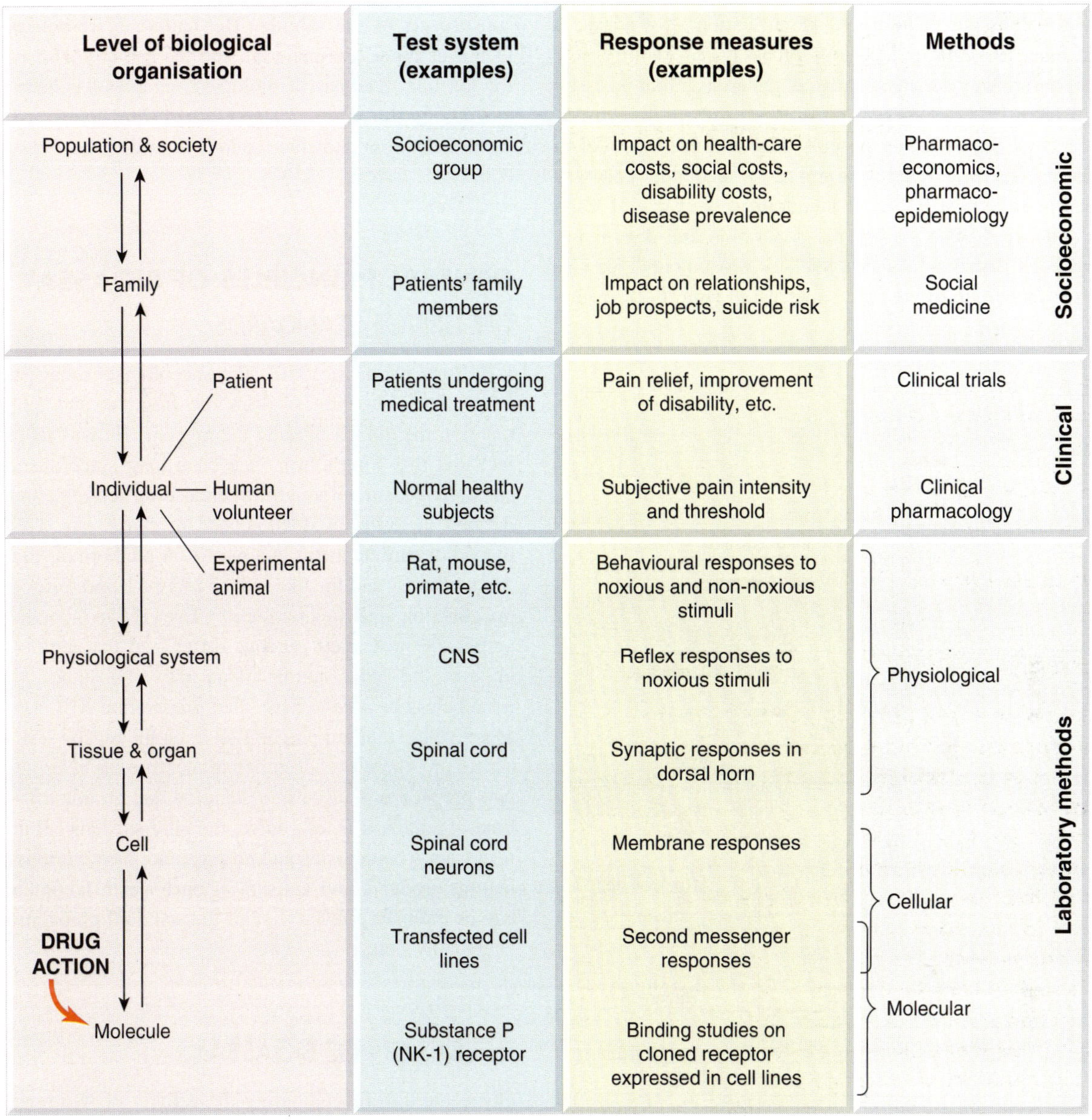

Fig. 6.1 Levels of biological organisation and types of pharmacological measurement.

Clinical trials, used to assess the effectiveness of drug treatments, embody the same principles as other types of bioassay, adapted to the situation. Increasingly, they are being extended to measure drug effects at the population level and to evaluate them in social and economic terms, moving into the realm of *pharmaco-epidemiology* and *pharmacoeconomics* (Ch. 1).

Bioassay plays a key role in the development of new drugs, discussed in Chapter 54.

At the scientific level, bioassay is useful in the study of new hormonal or other chemically mediated control systems. Mediators in such systems are often first recognised by the biological effects that they produce. The first clue may be the finding that a tissue extract or some other biological sample produces an effect on an assay system. For example, the ability of extracts of the posterior lobe of the pituitary to produce a rise in blood pressure and contraction of the uterus was observed at the beginning of the 20th century. These actions were developed as quantitative assay procedures and a standard preparation of the extract was established by international agreement in 1935. By use of these assays, it was shown that two distinct peptides—antidiuretic hormone (vasopressin) and oxytocin—were responsible, and they were eventually identified and synthesised in 1953. Biological assay had already revealed much about the synthesis, storage and release of the hormones, and it was essential for their purification and identification. Nowadays, it does not take 50 years of laborious bioassays to identify new hormones before they are chemically characterised,* but bioassay still plays a key role.

Bioassays on different test systems may be run in parallel to reveal the profile of activity of an unknown mediator. This was developed to an almost Baroque splendour in the work of Vane and his colleagues, who studied the generation and destruction of endogenous active substances, such as prostanoids (see Ch. 15), by the technique of cascade superfusion (Fig. 6.2). In this technique the sample is run sequentially over a series of test preparations chosen to differentiate between different active constituents of the sample. The pattern of responses produced identifies the active material, and the use of such assay systems for 'on line' analysis of biological samples has been invaluable in studying the production and fate of short-lived mediators such as prostanoids and the endothelium-derived relaxing factor (Ch. 14).

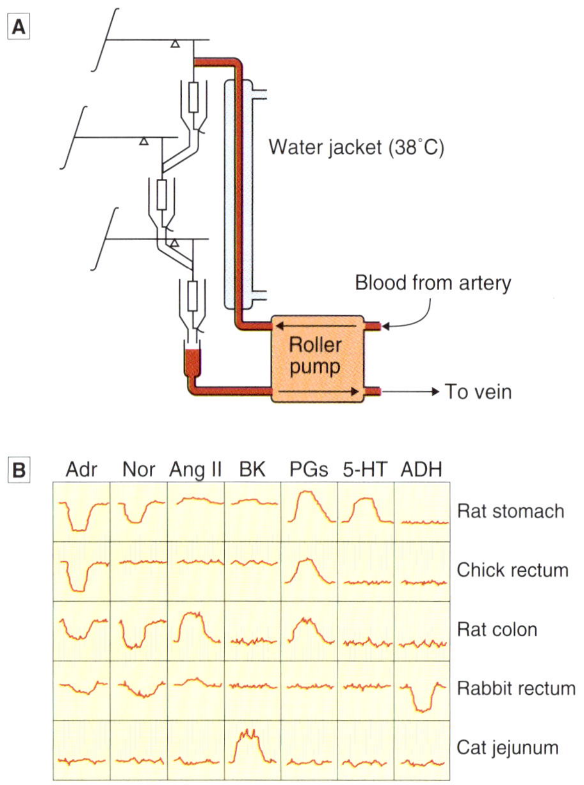

Fig. 6.2 Parallel assay by the cascade superfusion technique. A Blood is pumped continuously from the test animal over a succession of test organs, the responses of which are measured by a simple transducer system. B The response of these organs to a variety of test substances (at 0.1 ng/ml) is shown. Each active substance produces a distinct pattern of responses, enabling unknown materials present in the blood to be identified and assayed. (Adr, adrenaline; Nor, noradrenaline; Ang II, angiotensin II; BK, bradykinin; PG, prostaglandin; 5-HT, 5-hydroxytryptamine; ADH, antidiuretic hormone.) (From Vane J R 1969 Br J Pharmacol 35: 209-242.)

GENERAL PRINCIPLES OF BIOASSAY

THE USE OF STANDARDS

J H Burn wrote in 1950: 'Pharmacologists today strain at the king's arm, but they swallow the frog, rat and mouse, not to mention the guinea pig and the pigeon.' He was referring to the fact that the 'king's arm' had been long since abandoned as a standard measure of length, whereas drug activity continued to be defined in terms of dose needed to cause, say, vomiting in a pigeon or cardiac arrest in a mouse. A plethora of 'pigeon units', 'mouse units' and the like, which no two laboratories could agree on, contaminated the literature.** Even if two laboratories cannot agree—because their pigeons differ—on the activity in pigeon units of the same sample of an active substance, they should nonetheless be able to agree that preparation X is, say, 3.5 times as active as standard preparation Y on the pigeon test. Biological assays are, therefore, designed to measure the *relative* potency of two preparations, usually a standard and an unknown. The best kind of standard is, of course, the pure substance, but it is often necessary to establish standard preparations of various hormones, natural products and antisera against which laboratory samples can be calibrated, even though the standard preparations are not chemically pure.

THE DESIGN OF BIOASSAYS

Given the aim of comparing the activity of two preparations, a standard (S) and an unknown (U), on a particular preparation, a bioassay must provide an estimate of the dose or concentration of U that will produce the same biological effect as that of a known dose or concentration of S. As Figure 6.3 shows, provided that the $\log_{10}$-dose–effect curves for S and U are parallel, the *potency ratio*, *M*, of equiactive doses will not depend on the magnitude of response chosen. Thus, *M* provides an estimate of the potency ratio of the two preparations. A comparison of the magnitude of the effects produced by equal doses of S and U does not provide an estimate of *M* (see Fig. 6.3).

*In 1988, a Japanese group (Yanagisawa et al., 1988) described in a single remarkable paper the bioassay, purification, chemical analysis and synthesis, and DNA cloning of a new vascular peptide, endothelin (see Ch. 18).

**More picturesque examples of absolute units of the kind that Burn would have frowned upon are the PHI and the mHelen. PHI, cited by Colquhoun (1971), stands for 'purity in heart index' and measures the ability of a virgin pure-in-heart to transform, under appropriate conditions, a he-goat into a youth of surpassing beauty. The mHelen is a unit of beauty, 1 mHelen being sufficient to launch 1 ship.

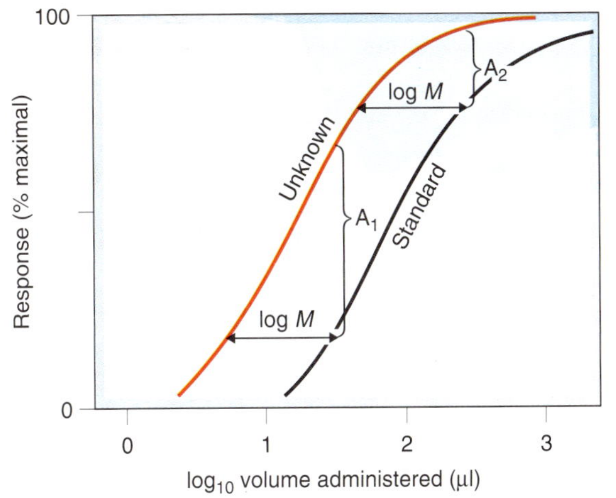

Fig. 6.3 Comparison of the potency of unknown and standard by bioassay. Note that comparing the magnitude of responses produced by the same dose (i.e. volume) of standard and unknown gives no quantitative estimate of their relative potency. (The differences, A1 and A2, depend on the dose chosen.) Comparison of equi-effective doses of standard and unknown gives a valid measure of their relative potencies. Since the lines are parallel, the magnitude of the effect chosen for the comparison is immaterial; i.e. $\log_{10} M$ is the same at all points on the curve.

The main problem with all types of bioassay is that of *biological variation*, and the design of bioassays is aimed at:

- minimising variation
- avoiding systematic errors resulting from variation
- estimation of the limits of error of the assay result.

Many different experimental designs have been proposed to maximise the efficiency and reliability of bioassays (see Laska & Meisner, 1987). Commonly, comparisons are based on analysis of dose–response curves, from which the matching doses of S and U are calculated. Such calculations become much simpler if the dose–response curves are linear. In many cases this can be achieved (see Ch. 2) by using a logarithmic ($\log_{10}$) dose scale and restricting observations to the middle region of the log-dose–effect curve, which is usually close to a straight line. The use of a logarithmic dose scale means that the curves for S and U will normally be parallel, and the potency ratio of U, relative to S, is determined by the horizontal distance between the two curves (Fig. 6.3). Assays of this type are known as parallel line assays, the minimal design being the 2+2 assay, in which two doses of standard (S_1 and S_2) and two of unknown (U_1 and U_2) are used. The doses are chosen to give responses lying on the linear part of the $\log_{10}$-dose–response curve, and are given repeatedly in randomised order, providing an inherent measure of the variability of the test system, which can be used, by means of straightforward statistical analysis, to estimate the confidence limits of the final result.

In practice, most bioassays will give results with 5% confidence limits lying within ±20% and many will do better than this.

The 2+2 assay also detects whether or not the two $\log_{10}$-dose–effect lines deviate significantly from parallelism. If the lines are not parallel, which may be the case if the assay is used to compare two drugs with differing mechanisms of action, it is not possible to define the relative potencies of S and U unambiguously in terms of a simple ratio. The experimenter must then face up to the fact that there are qualitative as well as quantitative differences between the two, so that comparison requires measurement of more than a single dimension of potency. An example of this kind of difficulty is met when diuretic drugs (Ch. 20) are compared. Some ('low ceiling') diuretics are capable of producing only a small diuretic effect, no matter how much is given; others ('high ceiling') can produce a very intense diuresis (described as 'torrential' by authors with vivid imaginations). A comparison of two such drugs requires not only a measure of the doses needed to produce an equal low-level diuretic effect, but also a measure of the relative heights of the ceilings.

QUANTAL AND GRADED RESPONSES

▼ An assay may be based on a *graded response* (e.g. change in blood glucose concentration, contraction of a strip of smooth muscle, change in the time taken for a rat to run a maze) or on *all-or-nothing responses* (e.g. death, loss of righting reflex, success in maze-running within a stipulated time). With the latter, sometimes known as a *discontinuous* or *quantal response*, the proportion of animals responding will increase with dose. The shape and slope of such a curve is governed by the individual variation between animals—the more uniform the population, the steeper the curve, and the more precise the assay. With graded responses, the steepness of the dose–response curve is a property of the test system and has nothing to do with biological variation. Quantal responses can be used in essentially the same way as graded responses for the purposes of bioassay, though the appropriate statistical procedures are slightly different.

BIOASSAYS IN HUMANS

Studies involving human subjects fall into two distinct categories: *human and clinical pharmacology* and *clinical trials*. The former focusses on using human subjects (either healthy volunteers or patients) essentially as experimental animals, for example to check whether mechanisms that operate in other species also apply to humans, or to take advantage of the much broader response capabilities of a person compared with a rat. The scientific principles underlying such measurements are the same, but the ethical and safety issues are paramount, and ethical committees associated with all medical research centres tightly control the type of experiment that can be done.

▼ An example of an experiment to compare two analgesic drugs (see Ch. 40) in humans is shown in Figure 6.4. Though many animal tests have been devised (for example, measuring the effect of an analgesic drug on the mean time taken for groups of mice to jump off a surface heated to a mildly painful temperature), they often fail to predict accurately the subjective relief of pain in humans. Figure 6.4 shows a comparison of morphine and codeine in humans, based on a modified 2 + 2 design. Each of the four doses was given on different occasions to each of the four subjects, the order being randomised and both subject and observer being unaware of the dose given. Subjective pain relief was assessed by a trained observer, and the results showed morphine to be 13 times as potent as codeine. This, of course, does not prove its superiority but merely shows that a smaller dose is needed to produce the same effect. Such a measurement is, however, an essential preliminary to assessing the relative therapeutic merits of the two drugs, for any comparison of other factors, such as side-effects, duration of action, tolerance or dependence, needs to be done on the basis of doses that are equiactive as analgesics.

Clinical trials aim to measure therapeutic effectiveness and constitute an important and highly specialised form of biological assay. The need to use patients for experimental purposes imposes many restrictions. Below, we discuss some of the basic principles involved in clinical trials; the role of such trials in the course of drug development is described in Chapter 54.

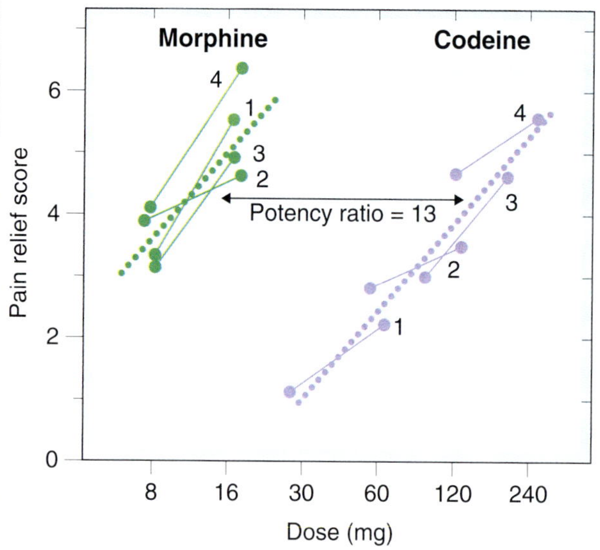

Fig. 6.4 Assay of morphine and codeine as analgesics in humans. Each of four patients (numbered 1–4) was given, on successive occasions in random order, four different treatments (high and low morphine, and high and low codeine) by intramuscular injection, and the subjective pain relief score calculated for each. The calculated regression lines gave a potency ratio estimate of 13 for the two drugs. (After: Houde R W et al. 1965 In: Analgesics. Academic Press, New York)

ANIMAL MODELS OF DISEASE

There are many examples where simple intuitive models predict with fair accuracy therapeutic efficacy in humans. Ferrets, when housed in swaying cages, respond by vomiting, and drugs that prevent this are also found to relieve motion sickness and other types of nausea in humans. Irritant chemicals injected into rats' paws cause them to become swollen and tender, and this test predicts very well the efficacy of drugs used for symptomatic relief in inflammatory conditions such as rheumatoid arthritis in humans. As discussed elsewhere in this book, animal models are available for many important disorders, such as epilepsy, diabetes, hypertension, gastric ulceration, etc., based on knowledge of the physiology of the condition. These models have been used successfully to produce new drugs, even though their success in predicting therapeutic efficacy is far from perfect.* Generalising, we can say that an animal model should ideally resemble the human disease in the following ways:

- similar phenotype
- common cause
- similar pathophysiology
- similar response to treatment.

In practice, there are many difficulties, and the shortcomings of animal models are one of the main road-blocks that bar the route from basic medical science to improvements in therapy. The difficulties encompass each of the criteria listed above.

Phenotype Many diseases, particularly in psychiatry, are defined by phenomena in humans that are difficult or impossible

Bioassay

- Bioassay is the measurement of potency of a drug or unknown mediator from the magnitude of the biological effect that it produces.
- Bioassay normally involves comparison of the unknown preparation with a standard. Estimates that are not based on comparison with standards are usually unreliable and will vary from laboratory to laboratory.
- Comparisons are best made on the basis of dose–response curves, which allow estimates of the equiactive concentrations of unknown and standard to be used as a basis for the potency comparison. Parallel line assays follow this principle.
- The biological response may be quantal (the proportion of tests in which a given all-or-nothing effect is produced) or graded. Different statistical procedures are appropriate in each case.
- Different approaches to metrication apply according to the level of biological organisation at which the drug effect needs to be measured. Approaches range through molecular and chemical techniques, in vitro and in vivo animal studies, clinical studies on volunteers and patients, to measurement of effects at the socioeconomic level.

*There have been many examples of drugs that were highly effective in experimental animals (e.g. in reducing brain damage following cerebral ischaemia) but ineffective in humans (stroke victims). How many errors in the opposite direction may have occurred, we shall never know, since such drugs will not have been tested in humans.

to observe in animals. As far as we know, mania or delusions have no counterpart in laboratory animals, nor can we recognise in them anything resembling a migraine attack or psychopathic behaviour.

Common cause The 'cause' of many human diseases is complex or unknown. For many degenerative diseases (e.g. Alzheimer's disease, osteoarthritis, Parkinson's disease) we need to model the upstream (causative) factors, rather than the downstream (symptomatic) features of the disease, though the latter are the basis of most of the simple physiological models used hitherto.

Similarity of pathophysiology This is also inapplicable to conditions such as depression or anxiety disorders, where no clear brain pathology has been defined.

Treatment response Relying on response to treatment as a test of validity carries the risk that drugs acting by novel mechanisms could be missed, since the model will have been selected on the basis of its responsiveness to known drugs. With schizophrenia (Ch. 37), for example, it is clear that dopamine antagonists are effective, and many of the models used are designed to reflect dopamine function in the brain, rather than other potential mechanisms that need to be identified if drug discovery is to move on.

GENETIC APPROACHES

Nowadays genetic approaches are increasingly used as an adjunct to conventional physiological and pharmacological approaches to disease modelling.

By selective breeding, it is possible to obtain pure animal strains with characteristics closely resembling certain human diseases. Genetic models of this kind include spontaneously hypertensive rats, genetically obese mice, epilepsy-prone dogs and mice, rats with deficient antidiuretic hormone secretion, and many other examples. In most cases, the genes responsible have not been identified.

More recently, deliberate genetic manipulation of the germline is increasingly used to generate *transgenic animals* with defined mutations, as a means of replicating human disease states in experimental animals and thereby providing animal models that are expected to be more predictive of therapeutic drug effects in humans (see reviews by Maerki & Hearri, 1996; Polites, 1996; Rudolph & Moehler, 1999). This technology, first reported in 1980, allows the inactivation of existing genes ('knock-outs') or the insertion of new genes ('knock-ins') in breeding colonies of animals. Examples of such models include transgenic mice that overexpress mutated forms of the amyloid precursor protein (APP) or presenilins (see Yamada & Nabeshima, 2000), which are important in the pathogenesis of Alzheimer's disease (see Ch. 34). When they are a few months old, these mice develop pathological lesions and cognitive changes resembling Alzheimer's disease, and this provides a very useful model with which to test possible new therapeutic approaches to the disease. Another neurodegenerative condition, Parkinson's disease (Ch. 34), has been modelled in transgenic mice which overexpress synuclein, a protein found in the brain inclusions that are characteristic of the disease (see Beal, 2001). Mice in which the gene for a particular adenosine receptor subtype has been inactivated show distinct behavioural and cardiovascular abnormalities, such as increased aggression, reduced response to noxious stimuli and raised blood pressure (Ledent et al., 1997). These findings serve to pinpoint the physiological role of this receptor, the function of which was hitherto unknown, and to suggest new ways in which agonists or antagonists for these receptors might be developed for therapeutic use (e.g. to reduce aggressive behaviour or to treat hypertension).

The use of transgenic animals in pharmacological research is increasing rapidly as the technology improves. Recent developments are reviewed by Rudolph & Moehler (1999). There are several limitations. One is that the gene switch may cause the animals to die during gestation, or shortly after birth. A second is that adaptive changes may compensate for the lack, or overexpression, of a particular gene and complicate interpretation of the phenotypic changes seen in the transgenic animals. Third, the incorporation of new genetic material may alter the control or function of other genes. To overcome these problems, ways of achieving *conditional mutagenesis* are being developed (Plueck, 1996; Rudolph & Moehler, 1999), whereby the introduced genes are engineered so that they are expressed only in particular cells (e.g. neurons), or so that they can be switched on or off by an external signal, such as administration of interferon, allowing the animal to develop normally up to this point. At present, the technology is mainly confined to the mouse, which breeds quickly but is inconveniently small for many experimental purposes.

Animal models

- Animal models of disease are important for the discovery of new therapeutic agents. Animal models generally reproduce imperfectly only certain aspects of human disease states. Models of psychiatric illness are particularly problematic.
- Transgenic animals are produced by introducing mutations into the germ cells of animals (usually mice) which allow new genes to be introduced ('knock-ins') or existing genes to be inactivated ('knock-outs') or mutated in the animals in a breeding colony.
- Insertion or deletion of certain genes sometimes results in phenotypic changes resembling human disease and is an increasingly used approach to developing disease models for drug testing. Many such models are now available.
- The induced mutation operates throughout the development and lifetime of the animal, and may be lethal. The new technique of conditional mutagenesis is an advance which should allow the abnormal gene to be switched on or off at a chosen time.

CLINICAL TRIALS

A clinical trial is a method for comparing objectively, by a prospective study, the results of two or more therapeutic procedures. For new drugs, this is carried out during phases II and III of clinical development (Ch. 54). It is important to realise that, until the 1970s, methods of treatment were chosen on the basis of clinical impression and personal experience rather than objective testing.* Though, on the one hand, many drugs, with undoubted effectiveness, remain in use without ever having been subjected to a controlled clinical trial; on the other hand, *digitalis* (see Ch. 17) was used for 200 years to treat cardiac failure before a controlled trial showed it to be of very limited value except in a particular type of patient. Any new drug is now required to have been tested in this way before being licensed for general clinical use.**

A good account of the principles and organisation of clinical trials is given by Friedman et al. (1996). A clinical trial aims to compare the response of a test group of patients receiving a new treatment (A) with that of a control group receiving an existing 'standard' treatment (B). Treatment A might be a new drug or a new combination of existing drugs, or any other kind of therapeutic intervention such as a surgical operation, diet, physiotherapy and so on. The standard against which it is judged (treatment B) might be a currently used drug treatment or (if there is no currently available effective treatment) a placebo or no treatment at all.

The use of controls is crucial in clinical trials. Claims of therapeutic efficacy based on reports that, for example, 16 out of 20 patients receiving drug X got better within 2 weeks are of no value without a knowledge of how 20 patients receiving no treatment, or a different treatment, would have fared. Usually, the controls are provided by a separate group of patients from those receiving the test treatment, but sometimes a cross-over design is possible in which the same patients are switched from test to control treatment or vice versa, and the results compared. Randomisation is essential to avoid bias in assigning individual patients to test or control groups. Hence, the *randomised controlled clinical trial* is now regarded as the essential tool for assessing clinical efficacy of new drugs.

Concern inevitably arises over the ethics of assigning patients at random to an untreated control group when the doctor in charge believes the test treatment to have advantages. However, the reason for setting up a trial is that doubt exists in the minds of many doctors that the treatment is efficacious, so for these doctors there is no ethical dilemma. If individual doctors are personally convinced that the treatment is beneficial, they should clearly avoid participating in a controlled trial. All would agree on the principle of informed consent,*** whereby each patient must be told the nature of the trial and agree to participate on the basis that he or she will be randomly and unknowingly assigned to either the test or the control group.

Unlike the kind of bioassay discussed earlier, the clinical trial does not normally give any information about potency or the form of the dose–response curve, it merely compares the response produced by two stipulated therapeutic regimens. Additional questions may be posed, such as the prevalence and severity of side-effects, or whether the treatment works better or worse in particular classes of patient, but only at the expense of added complexity and numbers of patients. Most trials are kept as simple as possible. The investigator must decide in advance what dose to use and how often to give it, and the trial will only reveal whether the chosen regimen performed better or worse than the control treatment. It will not say whether increasing or decreasing the dose would have improved the response; another trial would be needed to ascertain that. The basic question posed by a clinical trial is, therefore, simpler than that addressed by most conventional bioassays. However, the organisation of clinical trials, with the problem of avoiding bias, is immeasurably more complicated, time-consuming and expensive than that of any laboratory-based assay.

AVOIDANCE OF BIAS

There are two main strategies that aim to minimise bias in clinical trials:

- randomisation
- the double-blind technique.

If two treatments are being compared on a series of selected patients, the simplest form of randomisation is to allocate each patient to A or B by reference to a series of random numbers. One difficulty with simple randomisation, particularly if the groups are small, is that the two groups may turn out to be ill-matched with respect to characteristics such as age, sex or disease severity. *Stratified randomisation* is often used to avoid the difficulty. Thus the subjects might be divided into age categories, random allocation to A or B being used within each category. It is possible to treat two or more characteristics of the trial population in this way, but the number of strata can quickly become large, and the process is self-defeating when the number of subjects in each group becomes too small. As well as avoiding error resulting

*Not exclusively. James Lind conducted a controlled trial in 1753 on 12 mariners which showed that oranges and lemons offered protection against scurvy. However, 40 years passed before the British Navy acted on his advice, and a further century before the US Navy did.

**It is fashionable in some quarters to argue that to require evidence of efficacy of therapeutic procedures in the form of a controlled trial runs counter to the doctrines of 'holistic' medicine. This is a fundamentally antiscientific view, for science advances only by generating predictions from hypotheses and by subjecting the predictions to experimental test. Standing up for the scientific approach is the *evidence-based medicine* movement (see Sackett et al., 1996), which sets out strict criteria for assessing therapeutic efficacy based on randomised, controlled clinical trials, and urges scepticism about therapeutic doctrines where the efficacy has not been so demonstrated.

***Even this can be contentious, since patients who are unconscious, demented or mentally ill are unable to give such consent, yet no-one would want to preclude trials that might offer improved therapies to these needy patients.

from imbalance of groups assigned to A and B, stratification can also allow more sophisticated conclusions to be reached. B might, for example, prove to be better than A in a particular group of patients even if it is not significantly better overall.

The *double-blind technique*, which means that neither subject nor investigator is aware at the time of the assessment which treatment is being used, is intended to minimise subjective bias. It has been repeatedly shown that, with the best will in the world, subjects and investigators both contribute to bias if they know which treatment is which, so the use of a double-blind technique is an important safeguard. It is not always possible, however. A dietary regimen or a surgical operation, for example, can seldom be disguised, and even with drugs, pharmacological effects may reveal to the patient what is being taken and predispose the patient to report accordingly.* In general, however, the use of a double-blind procedure, with precautions if necessary to disguise such clues as the taste or appearance of the two drugs, is an important principle.

Maintaining the blind can be problematic. In an attempt to determine whether **melatonin** is effective in countering jet-lag, a pharmacologist selected a group of fellow pharmacologists attending a congress in Australia, providing them with unlabelled capsules of melatonin or placebo, with a jet-lag questionnaire to fill in when they arrived. Many of them (one of the authors included), with analytical resources easily to hand, opened the capsules and consigned them to the bin on finding that they contained placebo. Pharmacologists are only humans.

THE SIZE OF THE SAMPLE

Both ethical and financial considerations dictate that the trial should involve the minimum number of subjects, and much statistical thought has gone into the problem of deciding in advance how many subjects will be required to produce a useful result. The results of a trial cannot, by their nature, be absolutely conclusive. This is because it is based on a sample of patients and there is always a chance that the sample was atypical of the population from which it came. Two types of erroneous conclusion are possible, referred to as *type I* and *type II errors*.

A type I error occurs if a difference is found between A and B when none actually exists (false positive). A type II error occurs if no difference is found though A and B do actually differ (false negative). A major factor that determines the size of sample needed is the degree of certainty the investigator seeks in avoiding either type of error. The probability of incurring a type I error is expressed as the *significance* of the result. To say that A and B are different at the 0.05 level of significance means that the probability of obtaining a false-positive result (i.e. incurring a type I error), is less than 1 in 20. For most purposes, this level of significance is considered acceptable as a basis for drawing conclusions.

The probability of avoiding a type II error (i.e. failing to detect a real difference between A and B) is termed the *power* of the trial. We tend to regard type II errors more leniently than type I errors, and trials are often designed with a power of 0.8–0.9. To increase the significance and the power of a trial requires more patients. The second factor that determines the sample size required is the magnitude of difference between A and B that is regarded as clinically significant. For example, to detect that a given treatment reduces the mortality in a certain condition by at least 10 percentage points, say from 50% (in the control group) to 40% (in the treated group) would require 850 subjects, assuming that we wanted to achieve a 0.05 level of significance and a power of 0.9. If we were content only to reveal a reduction by 20 percentage points (and very likely miss a reduction by 10 points) only 210 subjects would be needed. In this example, missing a real 10-point reduction in mortality could result in abandonment of a treatment that would save 100 lives for every 1000 patients treated—an extremely serious mistake from society's point of view. This simple example emphasises the need to assess clinical benefit (which is often difficult to quantify) in parallel with statistical considerations (which are fairly straightforward) in planning trials.

▼ The use of *sequential trials*, introduced by Armitage in 1975, is intended to minimise the number of subjects used by computing the results continuously as the trial proceeds, and stopping it as soon as a result (at a predetermined level of significance) is achieved. In this type of trial, the subjects are usually paired, one subject receiving each treatment. The result of each individual comparison is scored as A better than B, B better than A, or no discernible difference; as soon as a result is reached that meets the necessary criteria with respect to significance and power, the trial is stopped. In practice, sequential trials based on individual pairwise comparisons are not often feasible. Patients do not generally present themselves in matched pairs, and assessment of the result of treatment may take a long time (e.g. where death rates are being compared) so that all the subjects will have been committed to the trial before any results are obtained.

Various 'hybrid' trial designs, which have the advantage of sequential trials in minimising the number of patients needed but do not require strict pairing of subjects, have been devised (see Friedman et al., 1996). Even with conventional trials, successive interim analyses of the accumulated data (by monitoring groups independent of the investigators) are generally made as the trial progresses, which allows the trial to be terminated as soon as a clear result is achieved. In a large-scale trial (Beta-blocker Heart Attack Trial Research Group, 1982) of the value of long-term treatment with the β-adrenoceptor blocking drug propranolol (Ch. 11) following heart attacks, the interim results showed a significant reduction in mortality, which led to the early termination of the trial.

CLINICAL OUTCOME MEASURES

The measurement of clinical outcome can be a complicated business, and it is becoming increasingly so as society becomes more preoccupied with assessing the efficacy of therapeutic procedures in terms of improved quality of life, societal and economic benefit, rather than in terms of objective clinical effects, such as lowering of blood pressure, improved airways conductance or increased life expectancy. Various scales for assessing 'health-related quality of life' have been devised and tested (see Drummond et al., 1997; Walley & Haycocks, 1997),

*The distinction between a true pharmacological response and a beneficial clinical effect produced by the knowledge (based on the pharmacological effects that the drug produces) that an active drug is being administered is not easy to draw, and we should not expect a mere clinical trial to resolve such a fine semantic issue.

and the tendency is to combine these with measures of life expectancy to arrive at the measure 'quality-adjusted life-years' (QALYs) as an overall measure of therapeutic efficacy. This attempts to combine both survival time and relief from suffering in assessing overall benefit.* In planning clinical trials, it is necessary to decide the purpose of the trial in advance and to define the outcome measures accordingly.

PLACEBOS

▼ A placebo is a dummy medicine containing no active ingredient (or alternatively, a dummy surgical procedure, diet or other kind of therapeutic intervention), which the patient believes is (or could be, in the context of a controlled trial) the real thing. The 'placebo response' is widely believed to be a powerful therapeutic effect, producing a significant beneficial effect in up to one third of patients. While many clinical trials include a placebo group that shows improvement, only a small minority have compared this group with untreated controls. A recent survey of these trial results (Hróbjartsson & Grøtsche, 2001) showed that the placebo effect was generally insignificant, except in the case of pain relief, where it was small but significant. They concluded that the popular belief in the strength of the placebo effect is misplaced and probably reflects, in part, the tendency of many symptoms to improve spontaneously and, in part, the reporting bias of patients who want to please their doctors. The ethical case for using placebos as therapy, which has been the subject of much public discussion, may, therefore, be weaker than has been argued. The risks of placebo therapies should not be underestimated. The use of active medicines may be delayed. The necessary element of deception risks undermining the confidence of patients in the integrity of doctors. A state of 'therapy-dependence' may be produced in people who are not ill, since there is no way of assessing whether a patient still 'needs' the placebo.

META-ANALYSIS

▼ It is possible, by the use of statistical techniques, to combine the data obtained in several individual trials (provided each has been conducted according to a randomised design) in order to gain greater power and significance. This procedure, known as *meta-analysis* or *overview analysis*, can be very useful in arriving at a conclusion on the basis of several published trials, of which some claimed superiority of the test treatment over the control while others did not. As an objective procedure, it is certainly preferable to the 'take-your-pick' approach to conclusion-forming adopted by most humans beings when confronted with contradictory data. It has several drawbacks, however (see Naylor 1997), the main one being 'publication bias', since negative studies are generally considered less interesting and are, therefore, less likely to be published than positive studies. Double counting, caused by the same data being incorporated into more than one trial report, is another problem.

*As may be imagined, trading off duration and quality of life involves issues about which many of us feel decidedly squeamish. Not so economists, however. They approach the problem by asking such questions as: 'How many years of life would you be prepared to sacrifice in order to live the rest of your life free of the disability you are currently experiencing?' Or, even more disturbingly: 'If you could gamble on surviving free of disability for your normal lifespan, or (if you lose the gamble) dying immediately, what odds would you accept?' Imagine being asked this by your doctor. 'But I only wanted something for my sore throat' you protest weakly.

THE ORGANISATION OF CLINICAL TRIALS

The organisation of large-scale clinical trials involving hundreds or thousands of patients at many different centres is a massive and expensive undertaking. It makes up one of the major costs of developing a new drug, and it can easily go wrong.

One large trial (Anturane Reinfarction Trial Research Group 1978) involved 1620 patients at 26 research centres in the USA and Canada, 98 collaborating researchers, and a formidable list of organising committees, including two independent audit committees to check that the work was being carried out in conformity with the strict protocols established. The conclusion was that the drug under test (**sulfinpyrazone**) reduced by almost one half the mortality from repeat heart attacks in the 8-month

Clinical trials

- A clinical trial is a special type of a bioassay done to compare the clinical efficacy of a new drug or procedure with that of a known drug or procedure (or a placebo).
- Generally the aim is a straight comparison of unknown (A) with standard (B) at a single dose level. The result may be: 'B better than A', 'B worse than A', or 'no difference detected'. Efficacy, not potency, is compared.
- To avoid bias, clinical trials should be:
  —controlled (comparison of A with B, rather than study of A alone)
  —randomised (assignment of subjects to A or B on a random basis)
  —double-blind (neither subject nor assessor knows whether A or B is being used).
- Type I errors (concluding that A is better than B when the difference is actually the result of chance) and type II errors (concluding that A is no better than B because a real difference has escaped detection) can occur; the likelihood of either kind of error gets less as the sample size and number of end-point events is increased.
- Sequential trials are appropriate in some cases and provide a way of limiting the number of subjects studied.
- Clinical trials require very careful planning and execution and are inevitably expensive.
- Clinical outcome measures may comprise
  —physiological measures (e.g. blood pressure, liver function tests)
  —long-term outcome (e.g. survival)
  —subjective assessments (e.g. pain relief)
  —overall 'quality-of-life' measures
  —'quality-adjusted life years' (QUALYs), which combines survival with quality of life.
- Meta-analysis is a statistical technique used to pool the data from several independent trials.

period after a first attack, and could save many lives. The US Food and Drug Administration, however, refused to grant a licence for the use of the drug, criticising the trial as unreliable and biased in several respects. Their independent analysis of the data showed the beneficial effect of the drug to be slight and insignificant. Further analysis and further trials, however, supported the original conclusion, but by then the efficacy of aspirin in this condition had been established, so the use of sulfinpyrazone never found favour.

BALANCING BENEFIT AND RISK

THERAPEUTIC INDEX

Ehrlich recognised that a drug must be judged not only by its useful properties but also by its toxic effects, and he expressed the *therapeutic index* of a drug in terms of the ratio between the average minimum effective dose and the average maximum tolerated dose in group of subjects:

$$\text{Therapeutic index} = \frac{\text{Maximum non-toxic dose}}{\text{Minimum effective dose}}$$

Unfortunately, the variability between individuals is not taken into account in this definition. Even if for a particular subject there is a large margin between the maximum tolerated dose and minimum effective dose, individuals may vary widely in their sensitivity, so it is quite possible that the effective dose in some individuals will be toxic to others.

An often-quoted definition, which aims to take into account individual variation is:

$$\text{Therapeutic index} = LD_{50}/ED_{50}$$

where LD_{50} is the dose that is lethal in 50% of the population, and ED_{50} is the dose that is 'effective' in 50%.

Thus defined, therapeutic index is intended to indicate the margin of safety in use of a drug, by drawing attention to the relationship between the effective and toxic doses, but it has obvious limitations and is, therefore, very rarely quoted as a number. For many reasons, it is not a useful guide to the safety of a drug in clinical use.

- LD_{50} does not reflect toxicity in the therapeutic setting, where unwanted effects are common, but rarely death.
- ED_{50} is often not definable, since it depends on what measure of effectiveness is used. For example, the ED_{50} for aspirin used for a mild headache is much lower than for aspirin as an antirheumatic drug.
- Some very important forms of toxicity are *idiosyncratic* (i.e. only a small proportion of individuals are susceptible; see Ch. 51). In other cases, toxicity depends greatly on the clinical state of the patient. For example, **propranolol** is dangerous to an asthmatic patient in doses that are harmless to a normal individual. More generally, we can say that wide individual variation (see Ch. 51) in either the effective dose or the toxic dose of a drug makes it inherently less predictable, and therefore less safe, though this is not reflected in the therapeutic index.

In conclusion, therapeutic index is of little value as a measure of the clinical usefulness of a drug, It may have some relevance as a measure of the impunity with which an overdose may be given. For example, one reason why the **benzodiazepines** replaced **barbiturates** as hypnotic drugs (see Ch. 36) is that their therapeutic index is much greater, and they are much less likely to kill when taken in accidental or deliberate overdose. Ironically, though, **thalidomide**—probably the most harmful drug ever marketed—was promoted specifically on the basis of its exceptionally high therapeutic index.

Though therapeutic index expresses a valid general concept by emphasising the balance between risk and benefit, its pseudo-quantitative precision is misleading, and it provides no measure of the usefulness of a drug.

OTHER MEASURES OF BENEFIT AND RISK

Alternative ways of quantifying the benefits and risks of drugs in clinical use have received much attention. One useful approach is to estimate from clinical trial data the proportion of test and control patients who will experience (a) a defined level of clinical benefit (for example, survival beyond 2 years, pain relief to a certain predetermined level, slowing of cognitive decline by a given amount), and (b) adverse effects of defined degree. These estimates of proportions of patients showing beneficial or harmful reactions can be expressed as *'number needed to treat'* (NNT, i.e. the number of patients who need to be treated in order for one to show the given effect, whether beneficial or adverse). For example, in a recent study of pain relief by antidepressant drugs compared with placebo, the findings were: for benefit (a defined level of pain relief), NNT = 3; for minor unwanted effects, NNT = 3; for major adverse effects, NNT = 22. Therefore, of 100 patients treated with the drug, on average 33 will experience pain relief, 33 will experience

Determination of risk and benefit

- Therapeutic index (lethal dose for 50% of the population divided by effective dose for 50%) provides a very crude measure of the safety of any drug as used in practice. Its main limitations are:
  - —it is based on animal toxicity data, which may not reflect forms of toxicity that are important clinically
  - —it takes no account of idiosyncratic toxic reactions.
- More sophisticated measures of risk–benefit analysis for drugs in clinical use are coming into use and include the 'number-needed-to-treat' (NNT) principle.

minor unwanted effects, and 4 or 5 will experience major adverse effects, information that is helpful in guiding therapeutic choices. One advantage of this type of analysis is that it can take into account the underlying disease severity in quantifying benefit. For example, if drug A halves the mortality of an often-fatal disease (reducing it from 50% to 25%, say), the NNT to save one life is 4; if drug B halves the mortality of a rarely fatal disease (reducing it from 5% to 2.5%, say), the NNT to save one life is 40. Notwithstanding other considerations, drug A is judged to be more valuable than drug B, even though both reduce mortality by a half. Furthermore, the clinician must realise that to save one life with drug B, 40 patients must be exposed to a risk of adverse effects, whereas only 4 are exposed for each life saved with drug A.

REFERENCES AND FURTHER READING

Anturane Reinfarction Trial Research Group 1978 Sulfinpyrazone in the prevention of cardiac death after myocardial infarction. N Engl J Med 298: 289–295 (*Example of a large-scale clinical trial*)

Beal M F 2001 Experimental models of Parkinson's disease. Nat Rev Neurosci 2: 325–332 (*Review of the various approaches to producing valid models for PD, including transgenics. Though focus is on one disorder, the principles apply generally*)

Beta-blocker Heart Attack Trial Research Group 1982 A randomised trial of propranolol in patients with acute myocardial infarction. 1. Mortality results. JAMA 247: 1707–1714 (*A trial that was terminated early when clear evidence of benefit emerged*)

Colquhoun D 1971 Lectures on biostatistics. Oxford University Press, Oxford (*Standard textbook*)

Drummond M F, O'Brien B, Stoddart G I, Torrance G W 1997 Methods for the economic evaluation of health care programmes. Oxford University Press, Oxford (*Includes good explanation of the principles of pharmacoeconomics*)

Friedman L M, Furberg C D, de Mets D L 1996 Fundamentals of clinical trials, 3rd edn. Mosby, St Louis, MO (*Standard textbook*)

Hróbjartsson A, Grøtsche P C 2001 Is the placebo powerless? An analysis of clinical trials comparing placebo with no treatment. New Engl J Med 344: 1594–1601 (*An important survey of clinical trial data, which shows, contrary to common belief, that placebos in general have no significant effect on clinical outcome, except—to a small degree—in pain relief trials*)

Laska E M, Meisner M J 1987 Statistical methods and the applications of bioassay. Annu Rev Pharmacol 27: 385–397 (*Useful references for those concerned with statistical principles of assay design and analysis*)

Ledent C, Veaugois J-M, Schiffmann S N et al. 1997 Aggressiveness, hypoalgesia and high blood pressure in mice lacking the adenosine A_{2A} receptor. Nature 388: 674–676 (*Examples of the use of a transgenic model to study receptor function*)

Maerki U, Haerri A 1996 Transgenic technology: principles. Int J Exp Pathol 77: 247–250 (*Short review article*)

Naylor C D 1997 Meta-analysis and the meta-epidemiology of clinical research. Br Med J 315: 617–619 (*Thoughtful review on strengths and weaknesses of meta-analysis*)

Plueck A 1996 Conditional mutagenesis in mice: the *cre/loxP* recombination system. Int J Exp Pathol 77: 269–278 (*An emerging technology for allowing genes to be switched on or off during the lifetime of an animal*)

Polites H G 1996 Transgenic model applications to drug discovery. Int J Exp Pathol 77: 257–262 (*Useful general review*)

Rudolph U, Moehler H 1999 Genetically modified animals in pharmacological research: future trends. Eur J Pharmacol 375: 327–337 (*Good review of uses of transgenic animals in pharmacological research, including application to disease models*)

Sackett D L, Rosenburg W M C, Muir-Gray J A, Haynes R B, Richardson W S 1996 Evidence-based medicine: what it is and what it isn't. Br Med J 312: 71–72 (*Balanced account of the value of 'evidence-based medicine'—an important recent trend in medical thinking*)

Walley T, Haycocks A 1997 Pharmacoeconomics: basic concepts and terminology. Br J Clin Pharmacol 43: 343–348 (*Useful introduction to analytical principles that are becoming increasingly important for therapeutic policy-makers*)

Yamada K, Nabeshima T 2000 Animal models of Alzheimer's disease and evaluation of anti-dementia drugs. Pharmacol Ther 88: 93–113 (*Good review of models of Alzheimer's disease, including transgenics*)

Yanagisawa M, Kurihara H, Kimura S et al. 1988 A novel potent vasoconstrictor peptide produced by vascular endothelial cells. Nature 332: 411–415 (*The first paper describing endothelin—a remarkably full characterisation of an important new mediator*)

Vane J R 1969 Br J Pharmacol 35: 209–242 (*The technique of cascade perfusion to study endogenous active substances*)

Absorption and distribution of drugs

7

Overview 91

Translocation of drug molecules 91
- The movement of drug molecules across cell barriers 91
- Binding of drugs to plasma proteins 96
- Partition into body fat and other tissues 96

Drug disposition 97

Drug absorption 98
- Routes of administration 98
- Distribution of drugs in the body 101

Special drug delivery systems 104

OVERVIEW

In order to work, drugs need to achieve an adequate concentration in their target tissues. The two fundamental processes that determine the concentration of a drug at any moment and in any region of the body are:

- **translocation of drug molecules**
- **chemical transformation.**

In this chapter, we discuss drug translocation and the factors that determine absorption and distribution. These are critically important for choosing appropriate routes of administration, and this aspect is emphasised. Chemical transformation by drug metabolism, and other processes involved in drug elimination, are described in Chapter 8.

TRANSLOCATION OF DRUG MOLECULES

Drug molecules move around the body in two ways:

- bulk flow transfer (i.e. in the bloodstream)
- diffusional transfer (i.e. molecule by molecule, over short distances).

The chemical nature of a drug makes no difference to its transfer by bulk flow. The cardiovascular system provides a very fast long-distance bulk flow distribution system. In contrast, diffusional characteristics differ markedly between different drugs. In particular, ability to cross hydrophobic diffusion barriers is strongly influenced by lipid solubility. Aqueous diffusion is also part of the overall mechanism of drug transport, since it is this process that delivers drug molecules to and from the non-aqueous barriers. The rate of diffusion of a substance depends mainly on its molecular size, the diffusion coefficient for small molecules being inversely proportional to the square root of molecular weight. Consequently, while large molecules diffuse more slowly than small ones, the variation with molecular weight is modest. Many drugs fall within the molecular weight range 200–1000, and variations in aqueous diffusion rate have only a small effect on their overall pharmacokinetic behaviour. For most purposes, we can regard the body as a series of interconnected well-stirred compartments within each of which the drug concentration is uniform. It is movement between compartments, generally involving penetration of non-aqueous diffusion barriers, that determines where, and for how long, a drug will be present in the body after it has been administered. The analysis of drug movements with the help of a simple compartmental model is discussed in Chapter 8.

THE MOVEMENT OF DRUG MOLECULES ACROSS CELL BARRIERS

Cell membranes form the barriers between aqueous compartments in the body. A single layer of membrane separates the intracellular from the extracellular compartments. An epithelial barrier, such as the gastrointestinal mucosa or renal tubule, consists of a layer of cells tightly connected to each other so that molecules must traverse at least two cell membranes (inner and outer) to pass from one side to the other. Vascular endothelium is more complicated, its anatomical disposition and permeability varying from one tissue to another. Gaps between endothelial cells are packed with a loose matrix of proteins that act as filters, retaining large molecules and letting smaller ones through. The cut off of molecular size is not exact: water transfers rapidly whereas molecules of 80 000–100 000 Da transfer very slowly. In some organs, especially the central nervous system (CNS) and the placenta, there are tight junctions between the cells and the endothelium is encased in an impermeable layer of periendothelial cells (*pericytes*). These features prevent potentially harmful molecules from leaking from the blood into these organs and have major pharmacokinetic consequences for drug distribution. In other organs (e.g. the liver and spleen)

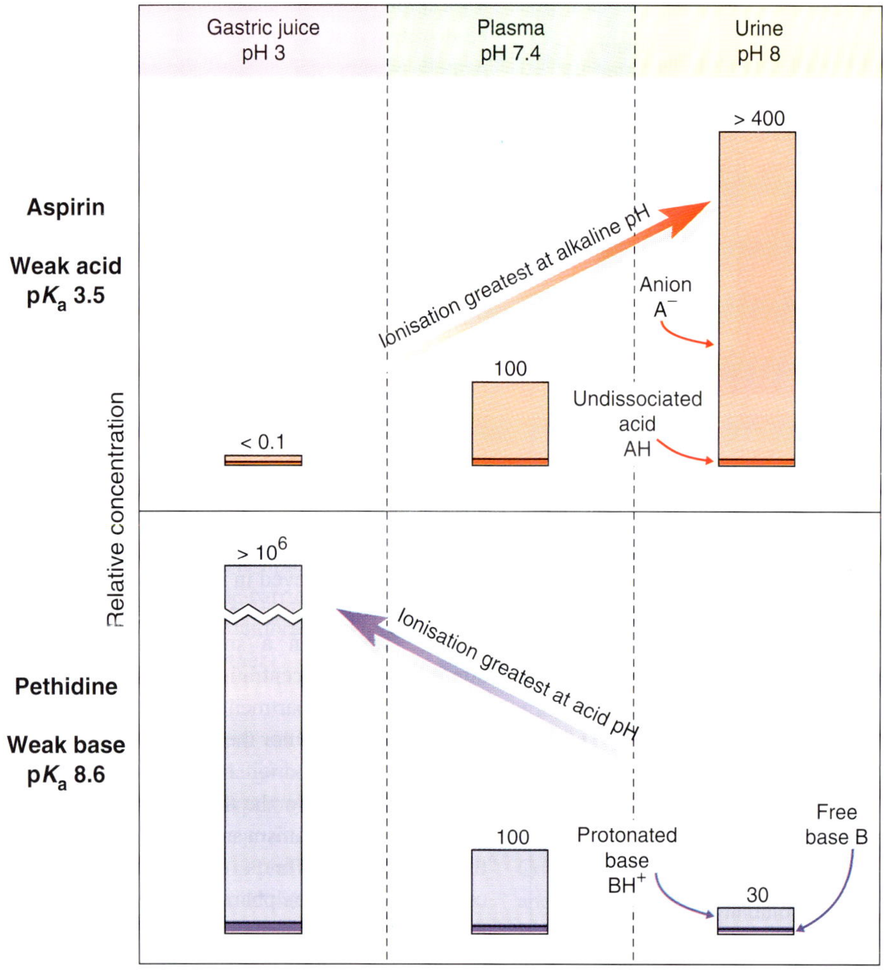

Fig. 7.3 Theoretical partition of a weak acid (aspirin) and a weak base (pethidine) between aqueous compartments (urine, plasma and gastric juice) according to the pH difference between them. Numbers represent relative concentrations (total plasma concentration = 100). It is assumed that the uncharged species in each case can permeate the cellular barrier separating the compartments and, therefore, reaches the same concentration in all three. Variations in the fractional ionisation as a function of pH give rise to the large total concentration differences with respect to plasma.

means to alkalinise urine in treating aspirin overdose (see p. 365): bicarbonate and acetazolamide each increase urine pH and hence increase salicylate elimination, but bicarbonate reduces whereas acetazolamide increases distribution of salicylate to the CNS.

CARRIER-MEDIATED TRANSPORT

Many cell membranes possess specialised transport mechanisms that regulate entry and exit of physiologically important molecules, such as sugars, amino acids, neurotransmitters and metal ions. Generally, such transport systems involve a carrier molecule, i.e. a transmembrane protein which binds one or more molecules or ions, changes conformation and releases them on the other side of the membrane. Such systems may operate purely passively, without any energy source; in this case they merely facilitate the process of transmembrane equilibration of the transported species in the direction of its electrochemical gradient and the mechanism is called *facilitated diffusion*. Alternatively, they may be coupled to the electrochemical gradient of Na^+; in this case transport can occur against an electrochemical gradient and is called *active transport*. Carrier-mediated transport, because it involves a binding step, shows the characteristic of saturation. With simple diffusion, the rate of transport increases directly in proportion to the concentration gradient, whereas with carrier-mediated transport the carrier sites become saturated at high ligand concentrations and the rate of transport does not increase beyond this point. Furthermore, competitive inhibition of transport can occur in the presence of a second ligand that binds the carrier.

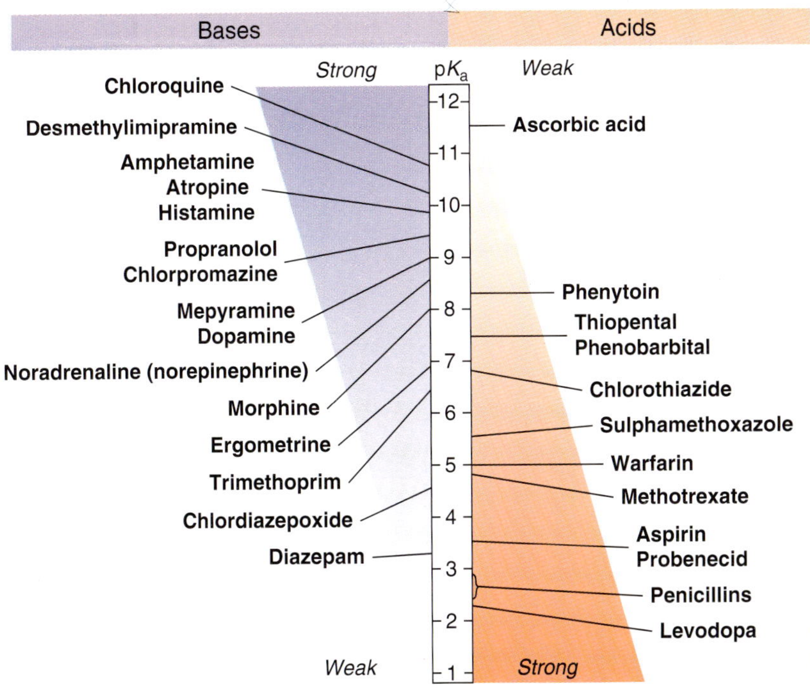

Fig. 7.4 pK_a **values for some acidic and basic drugs.**

Carriers of this type are ubiquitous and many pharmacological effects are the result of interference with them. Thus, nerve terminals have transport mechanisms for accumulating specific neurotransmitters, and there are many examples of drugs that act by inhibiting these transport mechanisms (see Chs 10, 11 and 31). From a pharmacokinetic point of view, though, there are only a few sites in the body where carrier-mediated drug transport is important, the main ones being:

- the renal tubule
- the biliary tract
- the blood–brain barrier
- the gastrointestinal tract.

P-glycoprotein (the drug transporter responsible for multidrug resistance in neoplastic cells, pp. 706–707) is present in renal tubular brush border membranes, in bile canaliculi, in astrocyte foot processes in brain microvessels and in the gastrointestinal tract. It plays an important part in absorption, distribution and elimination of many drugs. The characteristics of transport systems are discussed later when patterns of distribution and elimination in the body as a whole are considered more fully.

In addition to the processes so far described, which govern the transport of drug molecules across the barriers between different aqueous compartments, two additional factors have a major influence on drug distribution and elimination. These are:

- binding to plasma proteins
- partition into body fat and other tissues.

Movement of drugs across cellular barriers

- To traverse cellular barriers (e.g. gastrointestinal mucosa, renal tubule, blood–brain barrier, placenta), drugs have to cross lipid membranes.
- Drugs cross lipid membranes mainly (a) by passive diffusional transfer and (b) by carrier-mediated transfer.
- The main factor that determines the rate of passive diffusional transfer across membranes is a drug's lipid solubility. Molecular weight is a less important factor.
- Many drugs are weak acids or weak bases; their state of ionisation varies with pH according to the Henderson–Hasselbalch equation.
- With weak acids or bases, only the uncharged species (the protonated form for a weak acid; the unprotonated form for a weak base) can diffuse across lipid membranes; this gives rise to pH partition.
- pH partition means that weak acids tend to accumulate in compartments of relatively high pH, whereas weak bases do the reverse.
- Carrier-mediated transport (e.g. in the renal tubule, blood–brain barrier, gastrointestinal epithelium) is important for some drugs that are chemically related to endogenous substances.

BINDING OF DRUGS TO PLASMA PROTEINS

At therapeutic concentrations in plasma, many drugs exist mainly in bound form. The fraction of drug that is free in aqueous solution can be as low as 1%, the remainder being associated with plasma protein. It is the unbound drug that is pharmacologically active. The most important plasma protein in relation to drug binding is *albumin*, which binds many acidic drugs (for example **warfarin**, non-steroidal anti-inflammatory drugs, sulfonamides) and a smaller number of basic drugs (for example tricyclic antidepressants, **chlorpromazine**). Other plasma proteins, including β-globulin and an acid glycoprotein that increases in inflammatory disease, have also been implicated in the binding of certain basic drugs, such as **quinine**.

The amount of a drug that is bound to protein depends on three factors:

- the concentration of free drug
- its affinity for the binding sites
- the concentration of protein.

As a first approximation, the binding reaction can be regarded as a simple association of the drug molecules with a finite population of binding sites, exactly analogous to drug–receptor binding (see Ch. 2).

$$\underset{\text{free drug}}{D} + \underset{\text{binding site}}{S} \rightleftharpoons \underset{\text{complex}}{DS}$$

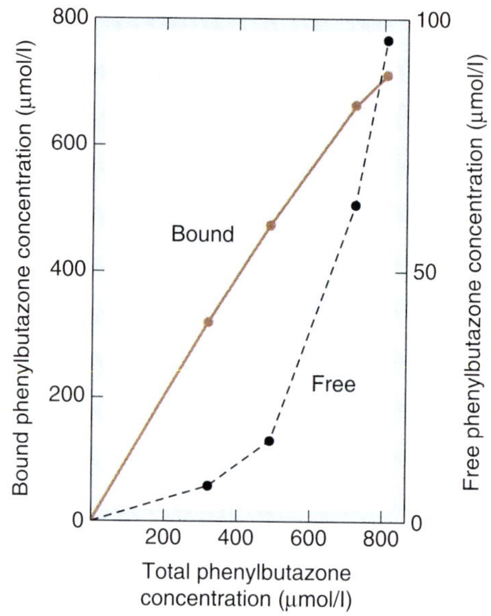

Fig. 7.5 Binding of phenylbutazone to plasma albumin. The graph shows the disproportionate increase in free concentration as the total concentration increases, owing to the binding sites approaching saturation. (Data from: Brodie B, Hogben C A M 1957 J Pharm Pharmacol 9: 345.)

The usual concentration of albumin in plasma is about 0.6 mmol/l (4 g/100 ml). With two sites per albumin molecule, the drug-binding capacity of plasma albumin would, therefore, be about 1.2 mmol/l. For most drugs, the total plasma concentration required for a clinical effect is much less than 1.2 mmol/l, so with usual therapeutic doses the binding sites are far from saturated, and the concentration bound [DS] varies nearly in direct proportion to the free concentration [D]. Under these conditions the fraction bound, [DS]/([D] + [DS]), is independent of the drug concentration. However, some drugs, for example **tolbutamide** (Ch. 25) and some **sulfonamides** (Ch. 44), work at plasma concentrations at which the binding to protein is approaching saturation (i.e. on the flat part of the binding curve). This means that addition of more drug to the plasma will increase the free concentration disproportionately. Doubling the dose of such a drug can, therefore, more than double the free (pharmacologically active) concentration. This is illustrated in Figure 7.5.

Binding sites on plasma albumin bind many different drugs, so competition can occur between them. Administration of drug B can thereby reduce the protein binding, and hence increase the free plasma concentration, of drug A. To do this, drug B needs to occupy an appreciable fraction of the binding sites. Few therapeutic drugs affect the binding of other drugs because they occupy, at therapeutic plasma concentrations, only a tiny fraction of the available sites. Sulfonamides (Ch. 45) are an exception because they occupy about 50% of the binding sites at therapeutic concentrations and so can cause unexpected effects by displacing other drugs or, in premature babies, bilirubin (Ch. 50). Much has been made of binding interactions of this kind as a source of untoward drug interactions in clinical medicine, but this type of competition is less important than was once thought (see Ch. 51).

PARTITION INTO BODY FAT AND OTHER TISSUES

Fat represents a large, non-polar compartment. In practice, this is important for only a few drugs, mainly because the effective fat:water partition coefficient is relatively low for most drugs. **Morphine**, for example, though quite lipid soluble enough to cross the blood–brain barrier, has a lipid:water partition coefficient of only 0.4, so sequestration of the drug by body fat is of little importance. **Thiopental**, by comparison (fat:water partition coefficient approximately 10), accumulates substantially in body fat. This has important consequences that limit its usefulness as an intravenous anaesthetic to short-term initiation ('induction') of anaesthesia (Ch. 35).

The second factor that limits the accumulation of drugs in body fat is its low blood supply—less than 2% of the cardiac output. Consequently, drugs are delivered to body fat rather slowly and the theoretical equilibrium distribution between fat and body water is approached slowly. For practical purposes, therefore, partition into body fat when drugs are given acutely is important only for a few highly lipid-soluble drugs (e.g. general anaesthetics; Ch. 35). When lipid-soluble drugs are given chronically, however, accumulation in body fat is often significant (e.g. benzodiazepines; Ch. 36). Furthermore, there are

Binding of drugs to plasma proteins

- Plasma albumin is most important; β-globulin and acid glycoprotein also bind some drugs.
- Plasma albumin binds mainly acidic drugs (approximately two molecules per albumin molecule). Basic drugs may be bound by β-globulin and acid glycoprotein.
- Saturable binding sometimes leads to a non-linear relation between dose and free (active) drug concentration.
- Extensive protein binding slows drug elimination (metabolism and/or excretion by glomerular filtration).
- Competition between drugs for protein binding can lead, rarely, to clinically important drug interactions.

some environmental contaminants ('xenobiotics'), such as insecticides, that are poorly metabolised. If ingested regularly, such xenobiotics accumulate slowly but progressively in body fat.

Body fat is not the only tissue in which drugs can accumulate. **Chloroquine**—an antimalarial drug (Ch. 47) used additionally to treat rheumatoid arthritis (Ch. 16)—has a high affinity for melanin and is taken up by tissues such as retina that are rich in melanin granules, which may account for the retinopathy that can occur during prolonged treatment of patients with rheumatoid disease. Tetracyclines (Ch. 45) accumulate slowly in bones and teeth, because they have a high affinity for calcium, and should not be used in children for this reason. Very high concentrations of **amiodarone** (an antidysrhythmic drug; Ch. 17) accumulate in liver and lung as well as fat.

DRUG DISPOSITION

We will now consider how the physical processes described above—diffusion, penetration of membranes, binding to plasma protein and partition into fat and other tissues—influence the overall disposition of drug molecules in the body. Drug disposition is divided into four stages:

- absorption from the site of administration
- distribution within the body
- metabolism
- excretion.

Absorption and distribution are considered here, metabolism and excretion in Chapter 8. The main routes of drug administration and elimination are shown schematically in Figure 7.6.

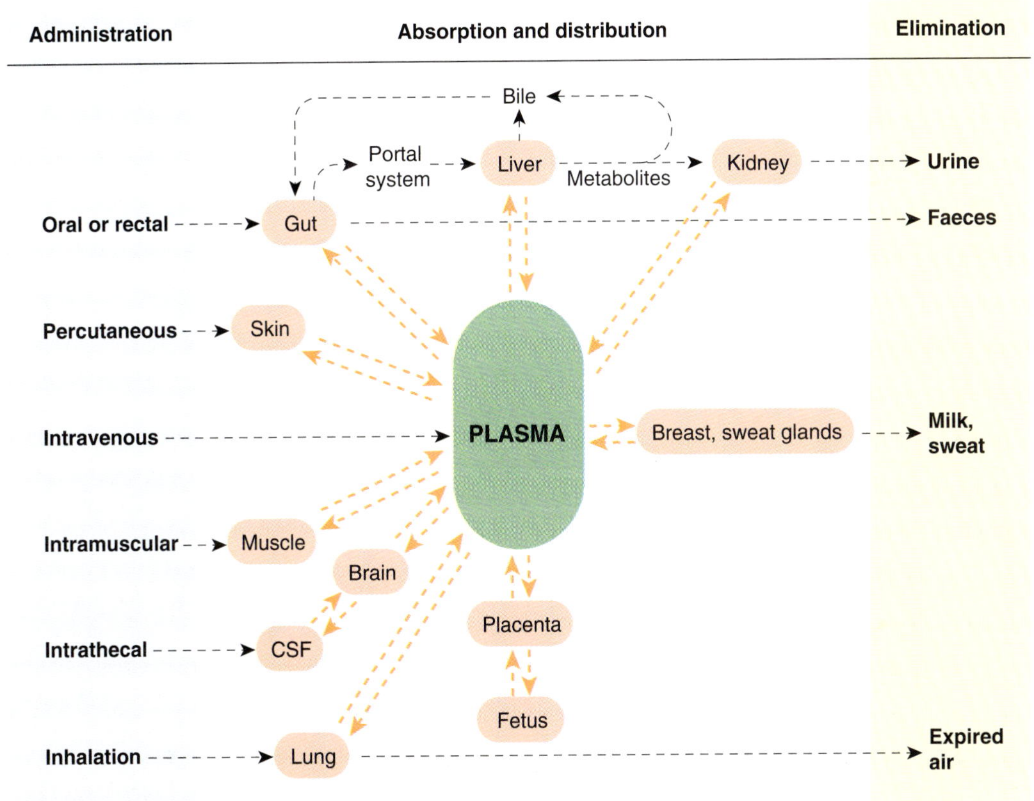

Fig. 7.6 **The main routes of drug administration and elimination.**

DRUG ABSORPTION

ROUTES OF ADMINISTRATION

Absorption is defined as the passage of a drug from its site of administration into the plasma. It is, therefore, important for all routes of administration, except intravenous injection. There are instances, such as inhalation of a bronchodilator aerosol to treat asthma (Ch. 22), where absorption as just defined is not required for the drug to act, but in most cases the drug must enter plasma before reaching its site of action.

The main routes of administration are:

- oral
- sublingual
- rectal
- application to other epithelial surfaces (e.g. skin, cornea, vagina and nasal mucosa)
- inhalation
- injection
  —subcutaneous
  —intramuscular
  —intravenous
  —intrathecal.

ORAL ADMINISTRATION

Most drugs are taken by mouth and swallowed. Little absorption occurs until the drug enters the small intestine.

Drug absorption from the intestine

The mechanism of drug absorption is the same as for other epithelial barriers, namely passive transfer at a rate determined by the ionisation and lipid solubility of the drug molecules. Figure 7.7 shows the absorption of a series of weak acids and bases as a function of pK_a. As expected, strong bases of pK_a 10 or higher are poorly absorbed, as are strong acids of pK_a less than 3, because they are fully ionised. The arrow poison curare used by South American Indians contained quaternary ammonium compounds that block neuromuscular transmission (Ch 10). These strong bases are poorly absorbed from the gastrointestinal tract, so the meat from animals killed in this way was safe to eat.

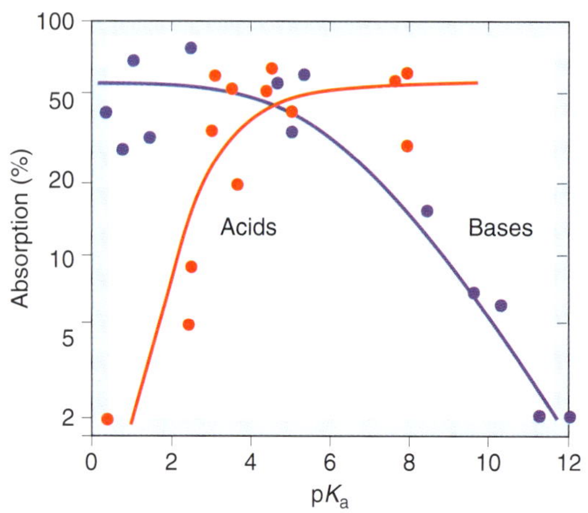

Fig. 7.7 Absorption of drugs from the intestine as a function of pK_a, for acids and bases. Weak acids and bases are well absorbed; strong acids and bases are poorly absorbed. (Redrawn from: Schanker L S et al. 1957 J Pharmacol 120: 528.)

There are a few instances where intestinal absorption depends on carrier-mediated transport rather than simple lipid diffusion. Examples include **levodopa**, used in treating Parkinson's disease (see Ch. 34), which is taken up by the carrier that normally transports phenylalanine, and **fluorouracil** (Ch. 49), a cytotoxic drug that is transported by the system that carries natural pyrimidines (thymine and uracil). Iron is absorbed via specific carriers in the surface membranes of jejunal mucosa, and calcium is absorbed by means of a vitamin D-dependent carrier system.

Factors affecting gastrointestinal absorption

Typically, about 75% of a drug given orally is absorbed in 1–3 hours, but numerous factors alter this, some physiological and some to do with the formulation of the drug. The main factors are:

- gastrointestinal motility
- splanchnic blood flow
- particle size and formulation
- physicochemical factors.

Gastrointestinal motility has a large effect. Many disorders (e.g. migraine, diabetic neuropathy) cause gastric stasis and slow drug absorption. Drug treatment can also affect motility, either reducing (e.g. drugs that block muscarinic receptors; see Ch. 10) or increasing it (e.g. **metoclopramide**, which is used in migraine to facilitate absorption of analgesic). Excessively rapid movement of gut contents can impair absorption. A drug taken after a meal is often more slowly absorbed because its progress to the small intestine is delayed. There are exceptions, however, and several drugs (e.g. **propranolol**) reach a higher plasma concentration if they are taken after a meal, probably because food increases splanchnic blood flow. Conversely, splanchnic blood flow is greatly reduced in hypovolaemic states, with a resultant slowing of drug absorption.

Particle size and formulation have major effects on absorption. In 1971, patients in a New York hospital were found to require unusually large maintenance doses of **digoxin** (Ch. 17). In a study on normal volunteers, it was found that standard digoxin tablets from different manufacturers resulted in grossly different plasma concentrations (Fig.7.8) even though the digoxin content of the tablets was the same, because of differences in particle size. Because digoxin is rather poorly absorbed, small differences in the pharmaceutical formulation can make a large difference to the extent of absorption.

Therapeutic drugs are formulated pharmaceutically to produce desired absorption characteristics. Capsules may be designed to remain intact for some hours after ingestion in order to delay absorption, or tablets may have a resistant coating to give the same effect. In some cases, a mixture of slow- and fast-release

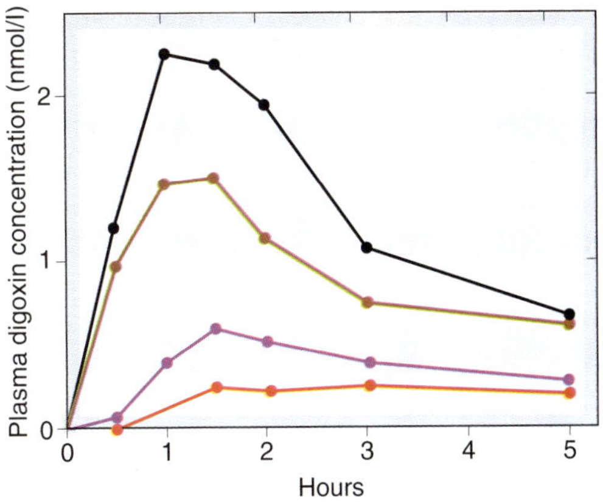

Fig. 7.8 Variation in oral absorption among different formulations of digoxin. The four curves show the mean plasma concentrations attained for the four preparations, each of which was given on separate occasions to four subjects. The large variation has caused the formulation of digoxin tablets to be standardised since this study was published. (From: Lindenbaum J et al. 1971 N Engl J Med 285: 1344.)

particles is included in a capsule to produce rapid but sustained absorption. More elaborate pharmaceutical systems include various modified-release preparations (e.g. a long-acting form of **nifedipine** that permits once daily use). Such preparations not only increase the dose interval but also reduce adverse effects related to high peak plasma concentrations following administration of a conventional formulation (e.g. flushing following regular nifedipine). Osmotically driven 'mini-pumps' can be implanted experimentally, and some oral extended-release preparations that are used clinically use the same principle, the tablet containing an osmotically active core and being bounded by an impermeable membrane with a precisely engineered pore to allow drug to exit in solution, delivering drug at an approximately constant rate into the bowel lumen. Such preparations may, however, cause problems related to high local concentrations of drug in the intestine (an osmotically released preparation of the anti-inflammatory drug **indometacin** had to be withdrawn because it caused small bowel perforation) and are subject to variations in small bowel transit time that occur during ageing and with disease.

Physicochemical factors (including some drug interactions; Ch. 50) affect drug absorption. **Tetracycline** binds strongly to Ca^{2+}, and calcium-rich foods (especially milk) prevent its absorption (Ch. 44). Bile acid-binding resins such as **colestyramine** (used to treat certain forms of hypercholesterolaemia; Ch. 19) bind several drugs, for example **warfarin** (Ch. 20) and **thyroxine** (Ch. 28).

When drugs are administered by mouth, the intention is usually that they should be absorbed and cause a systemic effect, but there are exceptions. **Vancomycin** is very poorly absorbed and is administered orally to eradicate toxin-forming *Clostridium difficile* from the gut lumen in patients with pseudomembranous colitis (an adverse effect of broad-spectrum antibiotics caused by appearance of this organism in the bowel). **Mesalazine** is a formulation of 5-aminosalicylic acid in a pH-dependent acrylic coat that degrades in the terminal ileum and proximal colon and is used to treat inflammatory bowel disease affecting this part of the gut. **Olsalazine** is a pro-drug consisting of a dimer of two molecules of 5-aminosalicylic acid that is cleaved by colonic bacteria in the distal bowel and is used to treat patients with distal colitis.

Bioavailability

To get from the lumen of the small intestine into the systemic circulation, a drug must not only penetrate the intestinal mucosa, it must also run the gauntlet of enzymes that may inactivate it in gut wall and liver. The term *bioavailability* is used to indicate the proportion of drug that passes into the systemic circulation after oral administration, taking into account both absorption and local metabolic degradation. It is a convenient term for making bland generalisations, but the concept creaks badly if attempts are made to use it with quantitative precision, or even to define it.* One problem is that it is not a characteristic solely of the drug preparation: variations in enzyme activity of gut wall or liver, in gastric pH or intestinal motility all affect it. Because of this, one cannot speak strictly of the bioavailability of a particular preparation, but only of that preparation in a given individual on a particular occasion. Even with these caveats, the concept is of limited use because it relates only to the total proportion of the drug that reaches the systemic circulation and neglects the *rate* of absorption. If a drug is completely absorbed in 30 minutes, it will reach a much higher peak plasma concentration (and have a more dramatic effect) than if it were absorbed more slowly. One rarely sees a numerical value assigned to 'bioavailability', and it is well to be wary of ostensibly measurable quantities that are used impressionistically, but not actually given values. For these reasons, regulatory authorities—which have to make decisions about the licensing of products that are 'generic equivalents' of patented products—lay importance on evidence of *bioequivalence*, i.e. evidence that the new product behaves sufficiently similarly to the existing one to be substituted for it without causing clinical problems.

SUBLINGUAL ADMINISTRATION

Absorption directly from the oral cavity is sometimes useful (provided the drug does not taste too horrible) when a rapid response is required, particularly when the drug is either unstable at gastric pH or rapidly metabolised by the liver. **Glyceryl**

*The definition of bioavailability offered by the US Food and Drug Administration is: 'The rate and extent to which the therapeutic moiety is absorbed and becomes available to the site of drug action'. You may be forgiven for finding this confusing. The double use of 'and' gives the definition four possible meanings, two of which are obfuscated by the uncertain meaning of the phrase 'becomes available to the site of drug action'.

trinitrate is an example of a drug that is often given sublingually (Ch. 17). Drugs absorbed from the mouth pass straight into the systemic circulation without entering the portal system and so escape first-pass metabolism.

RECTAL ADMINISTRATION

Rectal administration is used for drugs that are required either to produce a local effect (e.g. anti-inflammatory drugs for use in ulcerative colitis) or to produce systemic effects. Absorption following rectal administration is often unreliable, but this route can be useful in patients who are vomiting or are unable to take medication by mouth (e.g. postoperatively). It is used to administer **diazepam** to children who are in status epilepticus (Ch. 39) in whom it is difficult to establish intravenous access.

APPLICATION TO EPITHELIAL SURFACES

Cutaneous administration

Cutaneous administration is used when a local effect on the skin is required (e.g. topically applied steroids). Appreciable absorption may nonetheless occur and lead to systemic effects.

Most drugs are absorbed very poorly through unbroken skin. However, a number of organophosphate insecticides (see Ch. 10), which need to penetrate an insect's cuticle in order to work, are absorbed through skin, and accidental poisoning occurs in farm workers.

▼ A case is recounted of a 35-year-old florist in 1932. 'While engaged in doing a light electrical repair job at a work bench he sat down in a chair on the seat of which some "Nico-Fume liquid" (a 40% solution of free nicotine) had been spilled. He felt the solution wet through his clothes to the skin over the left buttock, an area about the size of the palm of his hand. He thought nothing further of it and continued at his work for about 15 minutes, when he was suddenly seized with nausea and faintness...and found himself in a drenching sweat. On the way to hospital he lost consciousness.' He survived, just, and then 4 days later: 'On discharge from the hospital he was given the same clothes that he had worn when he was brought in. The clothes had been kept in a paper bag and were still damp where they had been wet with the nicotine solution.' The sequel was predictable. He survived again but felt thereafter 'unable to enter a greenhouse where nicotine was being sprayed'. Transdermal dosage forms of nicotine are now used to reduce the withdrawal symptoms that accompany stopping smoking (Ch. 52).

Transdermal dosage forms, in which the drug is incorporated in a stick-on patch applied to an area of thin skin, are used increasingly, and several drugs—for example **estrogen** for hormone replacement (Ch. 29)—are available in this form. Such patches produce a steady rate of drug delivery and avoid presystemic metabolism. However, the method is suitable only for lipid-soluble drugs and is relatively expensive.

Nasal sprays

Some peptide hormone analogues, for example antidiuretic hormone (Ch. 23), gonadotrophin-releasing hormone (see Ch. 29) and calcitonin, are given as nasal sprays. These peptides are inactive when given orally as they are quickly destroyed in the gastrointestinal tract, but enough is absorbed through the nasal mucosa to provide a therapeutic effect. Such absorption is believed to take place through mucosa overlying nasal-associated lymphoid tissue. This is similar to mucosa overlying Peyer's patches in the small intestine, which is also unusually permeable.

Eye drops

Many drugs are applied as eye drops, relying on absorption through the epithelium of the conjunctival sac to produce their effects. Desirable local effects within the eye can be achieved without causing systemic side effects; for example, **dorzolamide** is a carbonic anhydrase inhibitor that is given as eye drops to lower ocular pressure in patients with glaucoma. It achieves this without affecting the kidney (see Ch. 23), thus avoiding the acidosis that is caused by oral administration of **acetazolamide**. Some systemic absorption from the eye occurs, however, and can result in unwanted effects (e.g. bronchospasm in asthmatic patients using **timolol** eye drops for glaucoma).

Administration by inhalation

Inhalation is the route used for volatile and gaseous anaesthetics (see Ch. 35), the lung serving as the route both of administration and elimination. The rapid exchange resulting from the large surface area and blood flow makes it possible to achieve rapid adjustments of plasma concentration. The pharmacokinetic behaviour of inhalation anaesthetics is discussed more fully in Chapter 35. Recently, the potential of the lung as a site of absorption of peptides and proteins has been appreciated, and inhaled human insulin is being investigated for use in diabetes mellitus (see Ch 25).

Drugs used for their effects on the lung are also given by inhalation, usually as an aerosol. Glucocorticoids (e.g. **beclometasone dipropionate**) and bronchodilators (e.g. **salbutamol**; Ch. 22) are given in this way to achieve high local concentrations in the lung while minimising systemic side-effects. However, drugs given by inhalation in this way are usually partly absorbed into the circulation, and systemic side-effects (e.g. tremor following salbutamol) can occur. Chemical modification of a drug may minimise such absorption. For example, **ipratropium**, a muscarinic receptor antagonist (Chs 10 and 22), is a quaternary ammonium ion analogue of **atropine**. It is used as an inhaled bronchodilator because its poor absorption minimises systemic adverse effects.

ADMINISTRATION BY INJECTION

Intravenous injection is the fastest and most certain route of drug administration. Bolus injection produces a very high concentration of drug, first in the right heart and lungs and then in the systemic circulation. The peak concentration reaching the tissues depends critically on the rate of injection. Administration by steady intravenous infusion avoids the uncertainties of absorption from other sites, while avoiding high peak plasma concentrations caused by bolus injection. Drugs given intravenously include several antibiotics, anaesthetics such as **propofol** (Ch. 35), and **diazepam** for patients with status epilepticus (Ch. 39).

Subcutaneous or intramuscular injection of drugs usually produces a faster effect than oral administration, but the rate of absorption depends greatly on the site of injection and on local blood flow. The rate-limiting factors in absorption from the injection site are:

- diffusion through the tissue
- removal by local blood flow.

Absorption from a site of injection is increased by increased blood flow. Hyaluronidase (an enzyme that breaks down the intercellular matrix thereby increasing diffusion) also increases drug absorption from the site of injection. Conversely, absorption is reduced in patients with circulatory failure ('shock') in whom tissue perfusion is reduced (Ch 18).

Methods for delaying absorption

It may be desirable to delay absorption, either to reduce the systemic actions of drugs that are being used, to produce a local effect, or to prolong systemic action. For example, addition of **adrenaline (epinephrine)** to a local anaesthetic reduces absorption of the anaesthetic into the general circulation. This usefully prolongs the anaesthetic effect, as well as reducing systemic toxicity.

Another method of delaying absorption from intramuscular or subcutaneous sites is to use a relatively insoluble 'slow-release' form, for example a poorly soluble salt, ester or complex, injected either as an aqueous suspension or an oily solution. **Procaine penicillin** (Ch. 45) is a poorly soluble salt of penicillin; when injected as an aqueous suspension it is slowly absorbed and exerts a prolonged action. Esterification of steroid hormones (e.g. **medroxyprogesterone acetate**, **testosterone propionate**; see Ch. 29) and antipsychotic drugs (e.g. **fluphenazine decanoate**; Ch. 37) increases their solubility in oil and slows their rate of absorption when they are injected in an oily solution.

The physical characteristics of a preparation may also be changed so as to influence the rate of absorption. Examples of this are the insulin zinc suspensions (see Ch. 25); insulin forms a complex with zinc, the physical form of which can be altered by varying the pH. One form consists of a fine amorphous suspension from which insulin is absorbed rapidly, and another consists of a suspension of crystals from which insulin absorption is slow. These can be mixed to produce an immediate, but sustained, effect.

Another method used to achieve slow and continuous absorption of certain steroid hormones (e.g. estradiol; Ch. 29) is the subcutaneous implantation of solid pellets. The rate of absorption is proportional to the surface area of the implant.

Intrathecal injection

Injection of a drug into the subarachnoid space via a lumbar puncture needle is used for some specialised purposes. **Methotrexate** (Ch. 50) is administered in this way in the treatment of certain childhood leukaemias to prevent relapse in the CNS. Regional anaesthesia can be produced by intrathecal administration of a local anaesthetic such as **bupivacaine** (see Ch. 43); opiate analgesics can also be used in this way (Ch. 40).

Drug absorption and bioavailability

- Drugs of very low lipid solubility, including those that are strong acids or bases, are generally poorly absorbed from the gut.
- A few drugs (e.g. levodopa) are absorbed by carrier-mediated transfer.
- Absorption from the gut depends on many factors, including:
  - —gastrointestinal motility
  - —gastrointestinal pH
  - —particle size
  - —physicochemical interaction with gut contents (e.g. chemical interaction between calcium and tetracycline antibiotics).
- Bioavailability is the fraction of an ingested dose of a drug that gains access to the systemic circulation. It may be low because absorption is incomplete, or because the drug is metabolised in the gut wall or liver before reaching the systemic circulation.
- Bioequivalence implies that if one formulation of a drug is substituted for another no clinically untoward consequences will ensue.

Baclofen (a gamma-aminobutyric acid (GABA) analogue, Ch. 32) is used to treat disabling muscle spasms. It has been administered intrathecally to minimise its adverse effects. Some antibiotics (e.g. aminoglycosides) cross the blood–brain barrier very slowly, and in rare clinical situations where they are essential (e.g. nervous system infections with bacteria resistant to other antibiotics) can be given intrathecally or directly into the cerebral ventricles via a reservoir.

DISTRIBUTION OF DRUGS IN THE BODY

BODY FLUID COMPARTMENTS

Body water is distributed into four main compartments as shown in Figure 7.9. The total body water as a percentage of body weight varies from 50 to 70%, being rather less in women than in men.

Extracellular fluid comprises the blood plasma (about 4.5% of body weight), interstitial fluid (16%) and lymph (1.2%). Intracellular fluid (30–40%) is the sum of the fluid contents of all cells in the body. Transcellular fluid (2.5%) includes the cerebrospinal, intraocular, peritoneal, pleural and synovial fluids and digestive secretions. The fetus may also be regarded as a special type of transcellular compartment. Within each of these aqueous compartments, drug molecules usually exist both in free solution and in bound form; furthermore, drugs that are weak acids or bases will exist as an equilibrium mixture of the charged and uncharged forms, the position of the equilibrium depending on the pH (see p. 92).

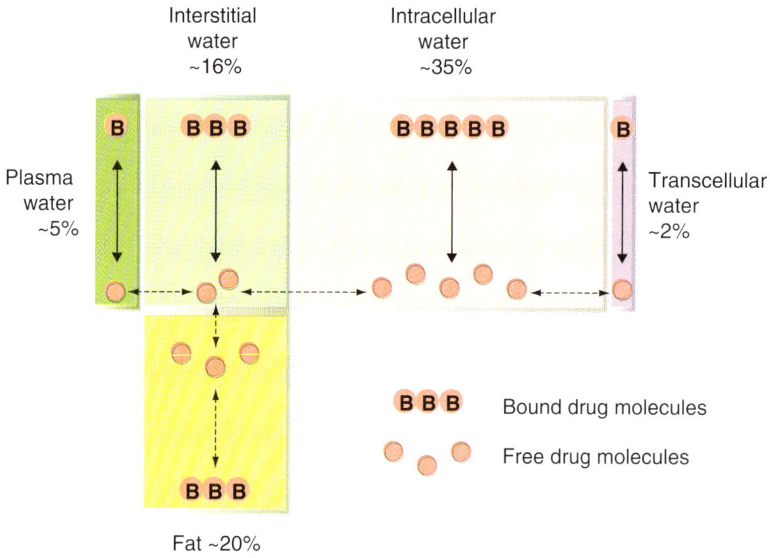

Fig. 7.9 The main body fluid compartments, expressed as a percentage of body weight. Drug molecules exist in bound or free form in each compartment, but only the free drug is able to move between the compartments.

The equilibrium pattern of distribution between the various compartments will, therefore, depend on:

- permeability across tissue barriers
- binding within compartments
- pH partition
- fat:water partition.

To enter the transcellular compartments from the extracellular compartment, a drug must cross a cellular barrier, a particularly important example in the context of pharmacokinetics being the blood–brain barrier.

THE BLOOD–BRAIN BARRIER

The concept of the blood–brain barrier was introduced by Paul Ehrlich to explain his observation that intravenously injected dye stained most tissues yet the brain remained unstained. The barrier consists of a continuous layer of endothelial cells joined by tight junctions. The brain is consequently inaccessible to many drugs, including many anticancer drugs and some antibiotics such as the aminoglycosides, with a lipid solubility that is insufficient to allow penetration of the blood–brain barrier. However, inflammation can disrupt the integrity of the blood–brain barrier, allowing normally impermeant substances to enter the brain (Fig. 7.10); consequently, penicillin (Ch. 45) can be given intravenously (rather than intrathecally) to treat bacterial meningitis (which is accompanied by intense inflammation).

Furthermore, in some parts of the CNS, including the chemoreceptor trigger zone, the barrier is leaky. This enables **domperidone**, a dopamine receptor antagonist (Ch. 24) that does not penetrate the blood–brain barrier but does access the chemoreceptor trigger zone, to be used to prevent the nausea caused by dopamine agonists such as **apomorphine** when these are used to treat advanced Parkinson's disease. This is achieved

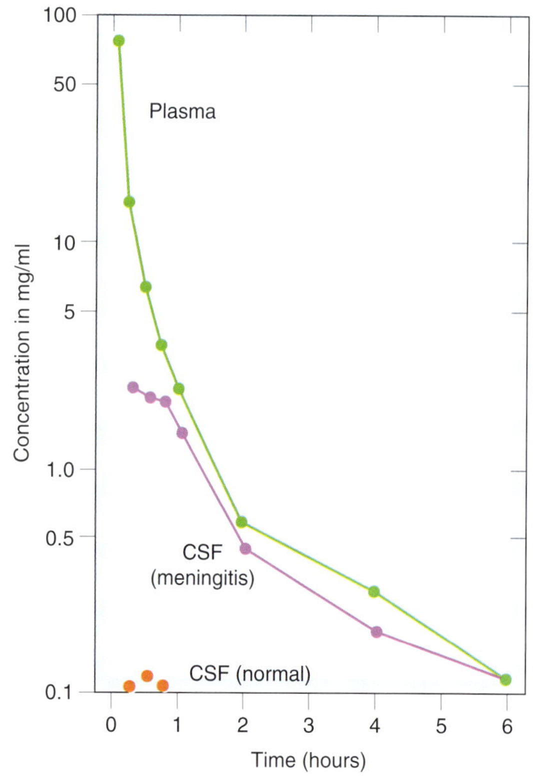

Fig. 7.10 Plasma and cerebrospinal fluid (CSF) concentrations of an antibiotic (thienamycin) following an intravenous dose (25 mg/kg). In normal rabbits, no drug reaches the CSF, but in animals with experimental *Escherichia coli* meningitis, the concentration of drug in CSF approaches that in the plasma. (From: Patamasucon & McCracken 1973 Antimicrob Agents Chemother 3: 270.)

without loss of efficacy because dopamine receptors in the basal ganglia are only accessible to drugs that have traversed the blood–brain barrier.

An opioid antagonist (ADL 8-2698) with extremely limited gastrointestinal absorption has been developed to prevent ileus, the transient reduction in bowel motility that often complicates abdominal surgery. It does not cross the blood–brain barrier. When given by mouth postoperatively it speeds recovery of bowel function without impairing the pain relief provided by opioid analgesics.

Several peptides, including bradykinin and enkephalins, increase blood–brain barrier permeability. There is interest in exploiting this to improve penetration of chemotherapy during treatment of brain tumours. In addition, extreme stress renders the blood–brain barrier permeable to drugs such as pyridostigmine (Ch. 10), which normally act peripherally.*

VOLUME OF DISTRIBUTION

The apparent volume of distribution, V_d, is defined as the volume of fluid required to contain the total amount, Q, of drug in the body at the same concentration as that present in the plasma, C_p.

$$V_d = \frac{Q}{C_p}$$

Values of V_d** have been measured for many drugs (Table 7.1). Some general patterns can be distinguished, but it is important to avoid identifying a given range of V_d too closely with a particular anatomical compartment. For example, insulin has a measured V_d similar to the volume of plasma water but exerts its effects on muscle, fat and liver via receptors that are exposed to interstitial fluid but not to plasma (Ch. 25).

Drugs confined to the plasma compartment

The plasma volume is about 0.05 l/kg body weight. A few drugs, such as heparin (Ch. 20), are confined to plasma because the molecule is too large to cross the capillary wall easily. More often, retention of a drug in the plasma following a single dose reflects strong binding to plasma protein. It is, nevertheless, the free drug in the interstitial fluid that exerts a pharmacological effect. Following repeated dosing, equilibration occurs and measured V_d increases. Some dyes, such as Evans blue, bind so strongly to plasma albumin that its V_d is used experimentally to measure plasma volume.

Table 7.1 Distribution volumes for some drugs compared with volume of body fluid compartments

Volume (l/kg body weight)	Compartment	Volume of distribution (V_d; l/kg body weight)	
0.05	Plasma	0.05–0.1	Heparin Insulin
		0.1–0.2	Warfarin Sulfamethoxazole Glibenclamide Atenolol
0.2	Extracellular fluid	0.2–0.4	Tubocurarine
		0.4–0.7	Theophylline
0.55	Total body water		Ethanol Neostigmine Phenytoin
		1–2	Methotrexate Indometacin Paracetamol Diazepam Lidocaine
		2–5	Glyceryl trinitrate Morphine Propranolol Digoxin Chlorpromazine
		> 10	Nortriptyline Imipramine

*This has been invoked to explain the central symptoms of cholinesterase inhibition experienced by some soldiers during the Gulf War. These soldiers may have been exposed to cholinesterase inhibitors (developed as chemical weapons and also, somewhat bizarrely, used externally during the conflict to prevent insect infestation) in the context of the stress of warfare.

**The experimental measurement of V_d is complicated by the fact that Q does not stay constant (because of metabolism and excretion of the drug) during the time that it takes for it to be distributed among the various body compartments that contribute to the overall V_d. It, therefore, has to be calculated indirectly from a series of measurements of plasma concentrations as a function of time (see p. 117).

Drug distribution

- The major compartments are:
  - —plasma (5% of body weight)
  - —interstitial fluid (16%)
  - —intracellular fluid (35%)
  - —transcellular fluid (2%)
  - —fat (20%).
- Volume of distribution (V_d) is defined as the volume of plasma that would contain the total body content of the drug at a concentration equal to that in the plasma.
- Lipid-insoluble drugs are mainly confined to plasma and interstitial fluids; most do not enter the brain following acute dosing.
- Lipid-soluble drugs reach all compartments, and may accumulate in fat.
- For drugs that accumulate outside the plasma compartment (e.g. in fat, or by being bound to tissues) V_d may exceed total body volume.

Drugs distributed in the extracellular compartment

The total extracellular volume is about 0.2 l/kg, and this is the approximate V_d for many polar compounds, such as **vecuronium** (Ch. 10), **gentamicin** and **carbenicillin** (Ch. 45). These drugs cannot easily enter cells because of their low lipid solubility, and they do not traverse the blood–brain or placental barriers freely.

Distribution throughout the body water

Total body water represents about 0.55 l/kg. This approximates the distribution of relatively lipid-soluble drugs that readily cross cell membranes, such as **phenytoin** (Ch. 39) and **ethanol** (Ch. 52). Binding of drug outside the plasma compartment, or partitioning into body fat, increases V_d beyond total body water. Consequently, there are many drugs with V_d greater than the total body volume, such as **morphine** (Ch. 40), tricyclic antidepressants (Ch. 38) and **haloperidol** (Ch. 37). Such drugs are not efficiently removed from the body by haemodialysis, which is, therefore, unhelpful in managing overdose with such agents.

SPECIAL DRUG DELIVERY SYSTEMS

Several approaches are being explored in an attempt to improve drug delivery. They include:

- biologically erodable microspheres
- pro-drugs
- antibody–drug conjugates
- packaging in liposomes.
- coating implantable devices

Biologically erodable microspheres

Microspheres of biologically erodable polymers can be engineered to adhere to mucosal epithelium in the gut. Such microspheres can be loaded with drugs, including high-molecular-weight substances, as a means of improving absorption, which occurs both through mucosal absorptive epithelium and also through epithelium overlying Peyer's patches. This approach has yet to be used clinically, but microspheres made from polyanhydride copolymers of fumaric and sebacic acids by a technique known as phase inversion nanoencapsulation have been used to produce systemic absorption of insulin and of plasmid DNA following oral administration in rats. Since drug delivery is a critical problem in gene therapy (Ch. 53), this is potentially momentous!

Pro-drugs

Pro-drugs are inactive precursors that are metabolised to active metabolites; they are described in Chapter 8. Some of the examples in clinical use confer no obvious benefits and have been found to be pro-drugs only retrospectively, not having been designed with this in mind. However, some do have advantages. For example, the cytotoxic drug **cyclophosphamide** (see Ch. 50) becomes active only after it has been metabolised in the liver; it can, therefore, be taken orally without causing serious damage to the gastrointestinal epithelium. **Levodopa** is absorbed from the gastrointestinal tract and crosses the blood–brain barrier via an amino acid transport mechanism before conversion to active dopamine in nerve terminals in the basal ganglia (Ch. 34). **Zidovudine** is phosphorylated to its active trisphosphate metabolite only in cells containing appropriate reverse transcriptase, hence conferring selective toxicity toward cells infected with the human immunodeficiency virus (Ch. 46). **Valaciclovir** and **famciclovir** are each ester pro-drugs of pro-drugs: respectively, of **aciclovir** and of **penciclovir**. Their bioavailability is greater than that of aciclovir and penciclovir, each of which is converted into active metabolites in virally infected cells (Ch. 46).

Other problems could theoretically be overcome by the use of suitable pro-drugs; for example instability of drugs at gastric pH, direct gastric irritation (**aspirin** was synthesised in the 19th century in a deliberate attempt to produce a pro-drug of salicylic acid that would be tolerable when taken by mouth), failure of drug to cross the blood–brain barrier and so on. Progress with this approach remains slow, however, and the optimistic pro-drug designer was warned as long ago as 1965: 'he will have to bear in mind that an organism's normal reaction to a foreign substance is to burn it up for food'.

Antibody–drug conjugates

One of the aims of cancer chemotherapy is to improve the selectivity of cytotoxic drugs (see Ch. 50). One interesting possibility is to attach the drug to an antibody directed against a tumour-specific antigen, which will bind selectively to tumour cells. Such approaches look promising in experimental animals, but it is still too early to say whether they will succeed in humans.

Packaging in liposomes

Liposomes are minute vesicles produced by sonication of an aqueous suspension of phospholipids. They can be filled with non-lipid-soluble drugs or nucleic acids (Ch. 53), which are retained until the liposome is disrupted. Liposomes are taken up by reticuloendothelial cells, especially in the liver. They are also concentrated in malignant tumours and there is a possibility of achieving selective delivery of drugs in this way. **Amphotericin**, an antifungal drug used to treat systemic mycoses (Ch. 47), is available in a liposomal formulation that is less nephrotoxic and better tolerated than the conventional form, albeit considerably more expensive. In the future, it may be possible to direct drugs or genes selectively to a specific target by incorporating antibody molecules into liposomal membrane surfaces.

Coated implantable devices

Impregnated coatings have been developed that permit localised drug delivery from implants. Examples include hormonal delivery to the endometrium from intrauterine devices and delivery of antithrombotic and antiproliferative agents (drugs or radiopharmaceuticals) to the coronary arteries from stents (devices inserted via a catheter after a diseased coronary artery has been dilated with a balloon). Stents reduce the occurrence of restenosis, but this can still occur at the margin of the device. Recent results from studies of stents coated with drugs such as **sirolimus** (a potent immunosuppressant) embedded in a surface polymer suggest that these can prevent this important clinical problem.

REFERENCES AND FURTHER READING

Abbott N J, Romero I A 1996 Transporting therapeutics across the blood–brain barrier. Mol Med Today 2: 106–113 (*Strategies for overcoming/bypassing the blood–brain barrier*)

Audus K L, Chikhale P J, Miller D W, Thompson S E, Borchadt R T 1992 Brain uptake of drugs: chemical and biological factors. Adv Drug Res 23: 1–64 (*Highlights chemical and biological factors regulating permeability of the blood–brain barrier to drugs as a basis for drug delivery to the CNS*)

Brogden R N, McTavish D 1995 Nifedipine gastrointestinal therapeutic system (GITS). A review of its pharmacodynamic and pharmacokinetic properties and therapeutic efficacy in hypertension and angina pectoris. Drugs 50: 495–512 (*Novel formulation permitting once daily dosing and reduced adverse effects*)

Chonn A, Cullis P R 1995 Recent advances in liposomal drug-delivery systems. Curr Opin Biotechnol 6: 698–708 (*Discusses delivery of recombinant proteins, antisense oligonucleotides and cloned genes*)

Cooper G J, Boron W F 1998 Effect of pCMBS on the CO_2 permeability of Xenopus oocytes expressing aquaporin 1 or its C189S mutant. Am J Physiol 275: C1481–C1486 (*Carbon dioxide acidification depends on transfer via a channel called aquaporin 1, rather than free diffusion as thought previously*)

Fix J A 1996 Strategies for delivery of peptides utilizing absorption-enhancing agents. J Pharmacol Sci 85: 1282–1285 (*Brief review emphasising unresolved difficulties*)

Friedman A, Kaufer D, Shemer J, Hendler I, Soreq H, Tur-Kaspa I 1996 Pyridostigmine brain penetration under stress enhances neuronal excitability and induces early immediate transcriptional response. Nat Med 2: 1382–1385 (*Peripherally acting drugs administered during severe stress may unexpectedly penetrate the blood–brain barrier. See also accompanying comment: Hanin I The Gulf War, stress and a leaky blood brain barrier, pp. 1307–1308*)

Keppler D, Arias I M 1996 Hepatic canalicular membrane. Introduction: transport across the hepatocyte cannalicular membrane FASEB J 11: 15–18 (*Succinct review*)

Koch-Weser J, Sellers E M 1976 Binding of drugs to serum albumin (2 parts). N Engl J Med 294: 311–316, 526–531 (*Classic review*)

Kremer J M H, Wilting J, Janssen L M H 1988 Drug binding to human α_1-acid glycoprotein in health and disease. Pharmacol Rev 40: 1–47

Langer R 1995 1994 Whittacker lecture: polymers for drug delivery and tissue engineering. Annu Biomed Eng 23: 101–111

Le Couter J et al. 2001 Identification of an angiogenic mitogen selective for endocrine gland endothelium. Nature 412: 877–884 (*See also accompanying editorial comment: Carmeliet P Creating unique blood vessels pp. 868–869*)

Leveque D, Jehl F 1995 P-glycoprotein and pharmacokinetics. Anticancer Res 15: 331–336 (*Update on impact of P-glycoprotein on drug disposition*)

Mathiovitz E, Jacob J S, Jong Y S et al. 1997 Biologically erodable microspheres as potential oral drug delivery systems. Nature 386: 410–414 (*Oral delivery of three model substances of different molecular size: dicoumarol, insulin and plasmid DNA*)

Oliyai R, Stella V J 1993 Prodrugs of peptides and proteins for improved formulation and delivery. Annu Rev Pharmacol Toxicol 33: 521–544 (*Review of pro-drug strategy for peptide absorption/delivery*)

Partridge W M, Golden P L, Kang Y S, Bickel U 1997 Brain microvascular and astrocyte localization of P-glycoprotein. J Neurochem 68: 1278–1285 (*Immunoreactive P-glycoprotein in brain microvasculature is localised to astrocyte foot processes and the role of P-glycoprotein in the blood–brain barrier*)

Sayani A P, Chien Y W 1996 Systemic delivery of peptides and proteins across absorptive mucosae. Crit Rev Ther Drug Carrier Syst 13: 85–184 (*Discusses insulin, enkephalin and calcitonin in particular*)

Skyler J S, Cefalu W T, Kourides I A et al. 2001 Efficacy of inhaled human insulin in type 1 diabetes mellitus: a randomized proof-of-concept study. Lancet 357: 324–325 (*Pre-prandial inhaled insulin is a less invasive alternative to injection*)

Somogyi A 1996 Renal transport of drugs: specificity and molecular mechanisms. Clin Exp Pharmacol Physiol 23: 986–989 (*Short review of selective organic anion and cation transporters in the proximal tubule*)

Taguchi A, Sharma N, Saleem R M 2001 Selective postoperative inhibition of gastrointestinal opioid receptors. N Engl J Med 345: 935–940 (*Speeds recovery of bowel function and shortens hospitalisation: notionally 'poor' absorption is used to advantage by providing a selective action on the gut*)

8 Drug elimination and pharmacokinetics

Overview 106

Introduction 106

Drug metabolism 106
- Phase I reactions 107
- Phase II reactions 109
- Induction of microsomal enzymes 109
- First-pass (presystemic) metabolism 110
- Pharmacologically active drug metabolites 111

Renal excretion of drugs and drug metabolites 111
- Glomerular filtration 111
- Tubular secretion 112
- Diffusion across the renal tubule 112
- Drug elimination expressed as clearance 113

Biliary excretion and enterohepatic circulation 113

Pharmacokinetics 114
- Single-compartment model 114
- More complicated kinetic models 116

OVERVIEW

In the first part of this chapter, we describe the main pathways of drug metabolism, factors that influence drug elimination by the kidney, and biliary excretion and enterohepatic recirculation of drugs. The second part presents a simple pharmacokinetic model that describes how the characteristics of absorption, distribution, metabolism and excretion determine the time course of the drug concentration in the blood with different dosing regimens.

INTRODUCTION

Drug elimination is the irreversible loss of drug from the body; it occurs by two processes, metabolism and excretion. Metabolism involves enzymic conversion of one chemical entity to another, whereas excretion consists of elimination from the body of chemically unchanged drug or its metabolites. The main routes by which drugs and their metabolites leave the body are:

- the kidneys
- the hepatobiliary system
- the lungs (important for volatile/gaseous anaesthetics).

Most drugs leave the body in the urine, either unchanged or as polar metabolites. Some drugs are secreted into bile via the liver, but most of these are then reabsorbed from the intestine. There are, however, instances (e.g. **rifampicin**) where faecal loss accounts for the elimination of a substantial fraction of unchanged drug in healthy individuals, and faecal elimination of drugs such as digoxin that are normally excreted in urine becomes progressively more important in patients with advancing renal failure. Excretion via the lungs occurs only with highly volatile or gaseous agents (e.g. general anaesthetics). Small amounts of some drugs are also excreted in secretions such as milk or sweat. Elimination by these routes is quantitatively negligible compared with renal excretion, although excretion into milk can sometimes be important because of effects on the baby.

Lipophilic substances are not eliminated efficiently by the kidney. Consequently, most lipophilic drugs are metabolised to more polar products, which are then excreted in urine. Drug metabolism occurs predominantly in the liver, especially by the *cytochrome P450* (*CYP*) system. Some P450 enzymes are extrahepatic and play an important part in several synthetic pathways including steroid biosynthesis in the adrenal gland, the biosynthesis of prostaglandin I_2 (PGI_2, prostacyclin) and thromboxanes (Ch. 15), and possibly of endothelium-derived hyperpolarising factor ('EDHF'; Ch. 18), but here we shall be concerned with catabolism of drugs by the hepatic P450 system.

DRUG METABOLISM

Animals have evolved complex systems that detoxify foreign chemicals, including carcinogens and toxins present in poisonous plants. Drugs are a special case of such foreign chemicals and, like plant alkaloids, they often exhibit distinct chirality (i.e. there is more than one stereoisomer), which affects their overall metabolism. Drug metabolism involves two kinds of biochemical reaction known as *phase I* and *phase II* reactions. These often, though not invariably, occur sequentially.

Phase I reactions are catabolic (e.g. oxidation, reduction or hydrolysis), and the products are often more chemically reactive and hence, paradoxically, sometimes more toxic or carcinogenic than the parent drug. Phase II reactions are synthetic (anabolic) and involve conjugation, which usually results in inactive products (although there are exceptions, for example the active sulfate metabolite of **minoxidil**, a potassium channel activator used to treat severe hypertension; Ch. 18). Phase I reactions often introduce a relatively reactive group, such as hydroxyl, into the molecule (a process known as 'functionalisation'). This functional group then serves as the point of attack for the conjugating system to attach a substituent such as glucuronide (Fig. 8.1). Both stages usually decrease lipid solubility, thus increasing renal elimination.

Phase I and phase II reactions take place mainly in the liver, though some drugs are metabolised in plasma (e.g. hydrolysis of **suxamethonium** by plasma cholinesterase; see Ch. 10), lung (e.g. various prostanoids; see Ch. 15) or gut (e.g. **tyramine**, **salbutamol**; Chs 9, 22). Many hepatic drug-metabolising enzymes, including cytochrome P450, are embedded in the smooth endoplasmic reticulum. They are often called 'microsomal' enzymes because, on homogenisation and differential centrifugation, the endoplasmic reticulum is broken into very small fragments that sediment only after prolonged high-speed centrifugation in the 'microsomal' fraction. To reach these metabolising enzymes in life, a drug must cross the plasma membrane. Polar molecules do this less readily than non-polar molecules except where there are specific transport mechanisms (Ch. 7), so intracellular metabolism is in general less important for polar drugs than for lipid-soluble drugs, and the former tend to be excreted unchanged in the urine. Conversely, non-polar drugs can readily access intracellular enzymes but are eliminated very inefficiently by the kidneys because of passive tubular reabsorption (see p. 112 below).

Stereoselectivity

Many clinically important drugs, such as **sotalol** (Ch. 17), **warfarin** (Ch. 20) and **cyclophosphamide** (Ch. 50), are mixtures of stereoisomers, the components of which differ not only in their pharmacodynamic activity but also in their metabolism, which may follow completely distinct pathways. Several clinically important drug interactions involve stereospecific inhibition of metabolism of one drug by another (Ch. 50). In some cases, drug toxicity appears to be mainly linked to one of the stereoisomers, not necessarily the pharmacologically active one. Where practicable, regulatory authorities now urge that new drugs should consist of pure stereoisomers to avoid these complications.

PHASE I REACTIONS

THE P450 MONOOXYGENASE SYSTEM

Nature, classification and mechanism of P450 enzymes

Cytochrome P450 enzymes are haem proteins, comprising a large family ('superfamily') of related but distinct enzymes (each referred to as CYP followed by a defining set of numbers and letter). These enzymes differ from one another in amino acid sequence, in regulation by inhibitors and inducing agents, and in the specificity of the reactions that they catalyse (see Nelson et al., 1996 for a review). Different members of the family have distinct, but often overlapping, substrate specificities, with some enzymes acting on the same substrates as each other but at

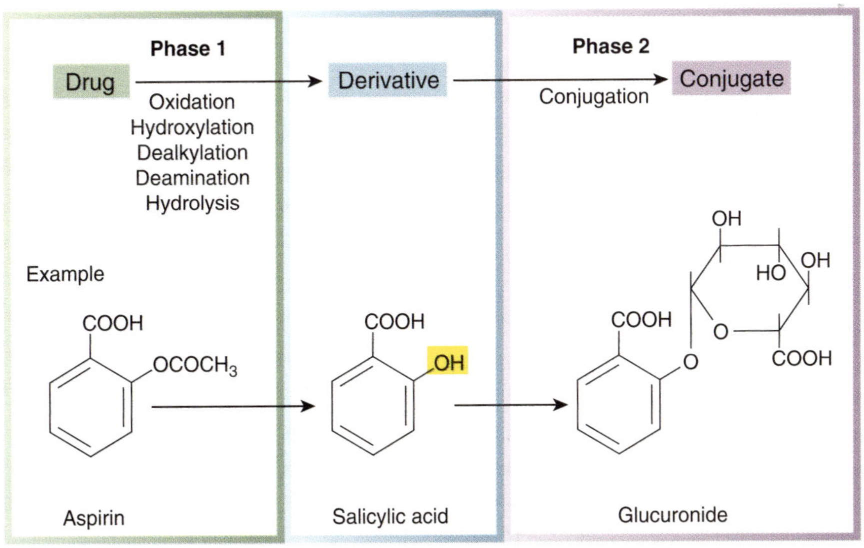

Fig. 8.1 The two phases of drug metabolism.

different rates. Purification of P450 enzymes and cDNA (complementary DNA) cloning form the basis of the current classification system, which is based on amino acid sequence similarities. So far, 74 CYP gene families have been described, of which three main ones (CYP1, CYP2 and CYP3) are involved in drug metabolism in human liver. CYP1A2 is one of the main enzymes. Examples of therapeutic drugs that are substrates for CYP1A2, and other important P450 enzymes and their substrates, are shown in Table 8.1. Drug oxidation by the monooxygenase P450 system requires drug (substrate, 'DH'), P450 enzyme and, in addition, molecular oxygen, NADPH and a flavoprotein (NADPH-P450 reductase). The mechanism involves a complex cycle (Fig. 8.2), but the overall net effect of the reaction is quite simple, namely the addition of one atom of oxygen (from molecular oxygen) to the drug to form a hydroxyl group (product, 'DOH'), the other atom of oxygen being converted to water.

▼ The P450 enzymes have unique spectral properties and the reduced forms combine with carbon monoxide to form a pink compound (hence 'P') with absorption peaks near 450 nm (range 447–452 nm). The first evidence that there is more than one form of cytochrome P450 came from the observation that treatment of rats with 3-methylcholanthrene, an inducing agent (see below), causes a shift in the absorption maximum from 450 to 448 nm.

Table 8.1 Examples of common drugs that are substrates for P450 isoenzymes

Isoenzyme P450	Drug
CYP1A1	Theophylline
CYP1A2	Caffeine, paracetamol, tacrine, theophylline
CYP2A6	Methoxyflurane
CYP2C8	Taxol
CYP2C9	Ibuprofen, phenytoin, tolbutamide, warfarin
CYP2C19	Omeprazole
CYP2D6	Clozapine, codeine, debrisoquine, metoprolol
CYP2E1	Alcohol, enflurane, halothane
CYP3A4/5	Ciclosporin, losartan, nifedipine, terfenadine

From: Pichard et al. (1995) Predictability of drug metabolism from in vitro studies. In: Alvan G et al. (eds) COST B1 conference on variability and specificity in drug metabolism. European Commission, Luxembourg, pp. 45–56.

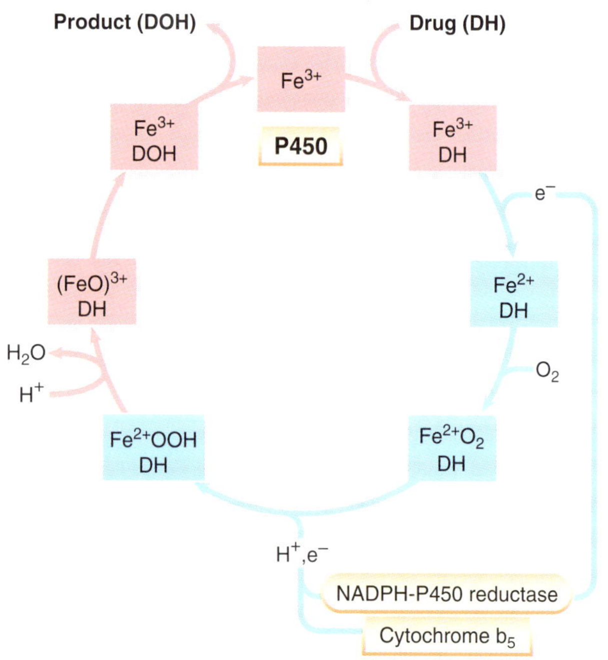

Fig. 8.2 The monooxygenase P450 cycle. P450 containing ferric iron (Fe^{3+}) combines with a molecule of drug (DH), receives an electron from NADPH-P450 reductase, which reduces the iron to Fe^{2+}, combines with molecular oxygen, a proton and a second electron (either from NADPH-P450 reductase or from cytochrome b_5) to form an $Fe^{2+}OOH{\cdot}DH$ complex. This combines with another proton to yield water and a ferric oxene $(FeO)^{3+}{\cdot}DH$ complex. $(FeO)^{3+}$ extracts a hydrogen atom from DH with the formation of a pair of short-lived free radicals (see text), liberation from the complex of oxidised drug (DOH) and regeneration of P450 enzyme.

CYP enzymes have unique redox properties that are fundamental to their diverse functions. These relate to the variable spin state (high/low) of the haem iron, which lies in an octahedral complex with six ligands and within which it can adopt either a penta- or hexa-coordinate configuration. NADPH-P450 reductase supplies one or both electrons needed for the oxidation and restores the redox state of the P450. Cyclic oxidation/reduction of haem iron occurs in conjunction with substrate binding and oxygen activation. The ferric iron (Fe^{3+}) in free P450 is mainly in a low spin form. After binding DH, a conformational change converts the ferric Fe^{3+} iron to the high spin state, making it easier to reduce. Reduction from Fe^{3+} to Fe^{2+} is achieved by a single electron, which is relayed from NADPH (electron donor) to P450 via the flavoprotein NADPH-P450 reductase. Molecular oxygen binds the reduced $Fe^{2+}{\cdot}DH$ complex to form a $Fe^{2+}O_2{\cdot}DH$ complex. This then accepts a second electron from NADPH-P450 reductase (or alternatively from cytochrome b_5) and a proton, to yield a peroxide complex: $Fe^{2+}OOH{\cdot}DH$. Addition of a second proton cleaves the $Fe^{2+}OOH{\cdot}DH$ complex to yield water and a ferric oxene $(FeO)^{3+}$ drug complex: $(FeO)^{3+}{\cdot}DH$. $(FeO)^{3+}$ extracts a hydrogen atom from DH to form a pair of transient free radicals $D^{\bullet}$ and $Fe^{2+}OH^{\bullet}{\cdot}D^{\bullet}$ acquires the bound $OH^{\bullet}$ radical to form hydroxylated drug (DOH), which is released from the complex with regeneration of P450 in its initial state.

P450 and biological variation

There are important variations in the expression and regulation of P450 enzymes between species. For instance, the activation pathways of certain dietary heterocyclic amines (formed when meat is cooked) to genotoxic products involves one member of the P450 superfamily (CYP1A2) that is constitutively present in humans and rats (which develop colon tumours after treatment with such amines) but not in cynomolgus monkeys (which do not). Such species differences have crucial implications for the choice of species to be used for toxicity and carcinogenicity testing during the development of new drugs for use in humans.

Within human populations there are major sources of interindividual variation in P450 enzymes that are of great importance in therapeutics. These include genetic polymorphisms: for example, one variant of the gene *CYP2D6* leads to poor or extensive hydroxylation of **debrisoquine**. Environmental factors (Ch. 51) are also important. Enzyme inhibitors and inducers are present in the diet and environment. For example, grapefruit juice and St John's wort (used to treat depression in 'alternative' medicine) inhibit drug metabolism (leading to potentially disastrous consequences, including cardiac dysrhythmias; Ch. 51) whereas Brussels sprouts and cigarette smoke induce P450 enzymes.

Inhibition of P450

Inhibitors of P450 differ in their selectivity toward different isoforms of the enzyme and are classified by their mechanism of action. Some drugs compete for the active site but are not themselves substrates (e.g. **quinidine** is a potent competitive inhibitor of CYP2D6 but is not a substrate for it). Non-competitive inhibitors include drugs such as **ketoconazole**, which forms a tight complex with the Fe^{3+} form of the haem iron of CYP3A4 causing reversible non-competitive inhibition. So-called mechanism-based inhibitors require oxidation by a P450 enzyme. Examples include **gestodene** (CYP3A4), **diethylcarbamate** (CYP2E1) and **furafylline** (CYP1A2). An oxidation product (e.g. a postulated epoxide intermediate of gestodene) binds covalently to the enzyme, the result of which then destroys itself ('suicide inhibition'). Many clinically important interactions between drugs are the result of inhibition of P450 enzymes (see Ch. 51).

OTHER PHASE I REACTIONS

Not all drug oxidation reactions exclusively involve the P450 system. For example, **ethanol** is metabolised by a soluble cytoplasmic enzyme, alcohol dehydrogenase, in addition to CYP2E1. Other exceptions include xanthine oxidase, which inactivates 6-mercaptopurine (Ch. 49) and monoamine oxidase, which inactivates many biologically active amines (e.g. *noradrenaline, tyramine, 5-hydroxytryptamine*; see Chs 11 and 12).

Reductive reactions are much less common than oxidations, but some are important. For example, **warfarin** (Ch. 20) is inactivated by conversion of a ketone to a hydroxyl group by CYP2A6.

Hydrolytic reactions do not involve hepatic microsomal enzymes but occur in plasma and in many tissues. Both ester and (less readily) amide bonds are susceptible to hydrolysis.

PHASE II REACTIONS

If a drug molecule has a suitable 'handle' (e.g. a hydroxyl, thiol or amino group), either in the parent molecule or in a product resulting from phase I metabolism, it is susceptible to conjugation, i.e. attachment of a substituent group. This synthetic step is called a phase II reaction. The resulting conjugate is almost always pharmacologically inactive and less lipid soluble than its precursor and is excreted in urine or bile.

The groups most often involved in conjugate formation are glucuronyl (Fig. 8.3), sulfate, methyl, acetyl, glycyl and glutathione. Glucuronide formation involves the formation of a high-energy phosphate compound, uridine diphosphate (UDP) glucuronic acid (UDPGA), from which glucuronic acid is transferred to an electron-rich atom (N, O or S) on the substrate, forming an amide, ester or thiol bond. UDP glucuronyl transferase, which catalyses these reactions, has very broad substrate specificity embracing many drugs and other foreign molecules. Several important endogenous substances, such as bilirubin and adrenal corticosteroids, are also conjugated by the same system.

Acetylation and methylation reactions occur with acetyl-CoA and *S*-adenosyl methionine, respectively, acting as the donor compounds. Many of these conjugation reactions occur in the liver, but other tissues, such as lung and kidney, are also involved.

INDUCTION OF MICROSOMAL ENZYMES

A number of drugs such as **rifampicin** (Ch. 45), **ethanol** (Ch. 52), **carbamazepine** (Ch. 39) increase the activity of microsomal oxidase and conjugating systems when administered repeatedly. Many carcinogenic chemicals (e.g. benzpyrene, 3-methylcholanthrene) also have this effect, which can be substantial; Figure 8.4 shows a nearly 10-fold increase in the rate of benzpyrene metabolism 2 days after a single dose. The effect is referred to as induction and is the result of increased synthesis of microsomal enzymes.

Enzyme induction can increase as well as decrease drug toxicity. There are drugs, for example **paracetamol**, where the

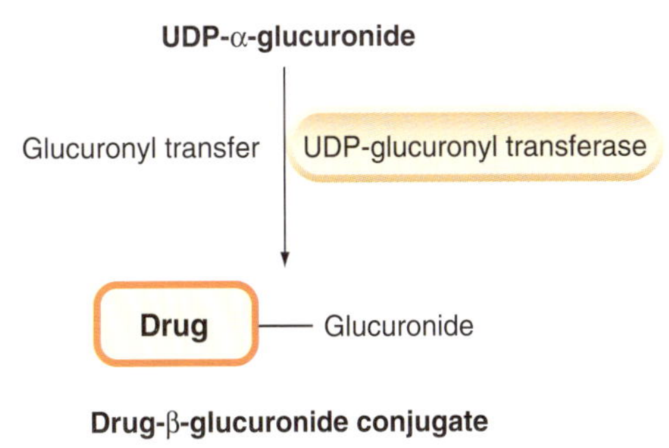

Fig. 8.3 The glucuronide conjugation reaction.

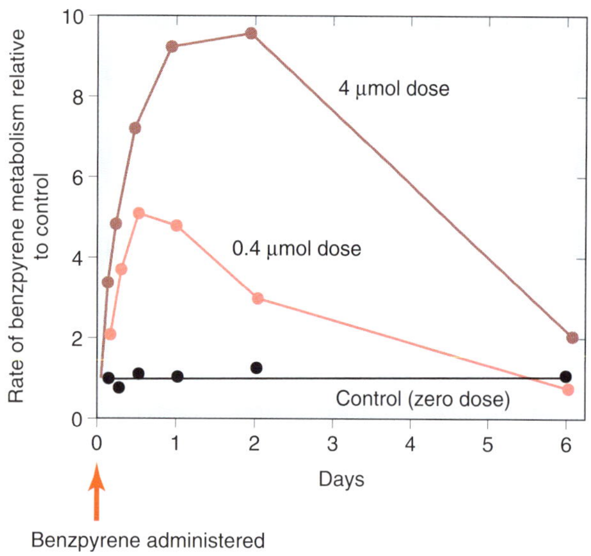

Fig. 8.4 Stimulation of hepatic metabolism of benzpyrene. Young rats were given benzpyrene (intraperitoneally) in the doses shown, and the benzpyrene metabolising activity of liver homogenates was measured at times up to 6 days. (From: Conney A H et al. 1957 J Biol Chem 228: 753.)

phase I metabolites are mainly responsible for their toxicity (see Ch. 52); consequently toxicity is increased following enzyme induction. The carcinogenic action of some polycyclic hydrocarbons is associated with increased hepatic formation of highly reactive oxidative products (e.g. epoxides) that can damage DNA.

The mechanism of induction is incompletely understood but is similar to that involved in the action of steroid and other hormones that bind to nuclear receptors (see Ch. 3). The most thoroughly studied inducing agents are polycyclic aromatic hydrocarbons. These bind to the ligand-binding domain of a soluble protein, termed the aromatic hydrocarbon (Ah-) receptor. This complex is transported to the nucleus by an Ah-receptor nuclear translocator and binds Ah-receptor response elements in the DNA, thereby promoting transcription of the gene *CYP1A1*. In addition to enhanced transcription, some inducing agents (e.g. ethanol which induces CYP2E1 in humans) also stabilise mRNA or P450 protein.

FIRST-PASS (PRESYSTEMIC) METABOLISM

The liver (or sometimes the gut wall) extracts and metabolises some drugs so efficiently that the amount reaching the systemic circulation is considerably less than the amount absorbed. This is known as *first-pass* or *presystemic* metabolism, which causes low bioavailability even when a drug is well absorbed from the gut. It is important for many clinically important drugs (Table 8.2).

Table 8.2 Examples of drugs that undergo substantial first-pass elimination

Aspirin
Glyceryl trinitrate
Isosorbide dinitrate
Levodopa
Lidocaine
Metoprolol
Morphine
Propranolol
Salbutamol
Verapamil

First-pass metabolism is generally a nuisance in practice, because:

- a much larger dose of the drug is needed when it is given orally than when it is given by other routes
- marked individual variations occur in the extent of first-pass metabolism of a given drug (see Ch. 51), resulting in unpredictability when such drugs are taken orally.

Drug metabolism

- Phase I reactions involve oxidation, reduction and hydrolysis:
  - —usually form more chemically reactive products, sometimes pharmacologically active, toxic or carcinogenic
  - —often involve monooxygenase system in which cytochrome P450 plays a key role.
- Phase II reactions are conjugation (e.g. glucuronidation) of a reactive group (often inserted during phase I reaction) and usually form inactive and readily excretable products.
- Some conjugated products are excreted via bile, are reactivated in the intestine and then reabsorbed.
- Induction of enzymes by other drugs and chemicals can greatly accelerate hepatic drug metabolism.
- Some drugs show rapid 'first-pass' hepatic metabolism, and thus poor oral bioavailability.

PHARMACOLOGICALLY ACTIVE DRUG METABOLITES

In some cases (see Table 8.3) a drug becomes pharmacologically active only after it has been metabolised. For example, **azathioprine**, an immunosuppressant drug (Ch. 16), is metabolised to **mercaptopurine**; and **enalapril**, an angiotensin-converting enzyme inhibitor (Ch.18), is hydrolysed to its active form **enalaprilat**. Such drugs, in which the parent compound lacks activity of its own, are known as *pro-drugs*. These are sometimes designed deliberately to overcome problems of drug delivery (Ch. 7). Metabolism can alter the pharmacological actions of a drug qualitatively. **Aspirin** inhibits some platelet functions and has anti-inflammatory activity (Chs 16 and 20). It is hydrolysed to salicylic acid (Fig. 8.1), which has anti-inflammatory but not antiplatelet activity. In other instances, metabolites have pharmacological actions similar to the parent compound (e.g. benzodiazepines, many of which form long-lived active metabolites that cause sedation to persist after the parent drug has disappeared). There are also cases in which metabolites are responsible for toxicity. Hepatotoxicity of **paracetamol** is one example (see Ch. 52), and bladder toxicity of **cyclophosphamide**, which is caused by its toxic metabolite acrolein, is another. Methanol and ethylene glycol both exert their toxic effects via metabolites formed by alcohol dehydrogenase. Poisoning with these agents is treated with ethanol (or with a more potent inhibitor), which competes for the active site of the enzyme. **Terfenadine**, a non-sedating antihistamine, can, rarely, cause serious cardiac dysrhythmias by blocking cardiac potassium channels. Its pharmacologically active metabolite (fexofenadine) blocks histamine H_1-receptors but not cardiac potassium channels, and it has now largely replaced terfenadine in therapeutic use for this reason. Hepatic necrosis is a rare but sometimes fatal complication of halothane anaesthesia. It is caused by immune sensitisation to new antigens formed by trifluoroacetylation of liver protein (Ch. 52). **Disulfiram** inhibits CYP2E1 and reduces substantially the formation of trifluoroacetic acid during halothane anaesthesia, raising the intriguing possibility that it could prevent halothane hepatitis.

RENAL EXCRETION OF DRUGS AND DRUG METABOLITES

Drugs differ greatly in the rate at which they are excreted by the kidney, ranging from **penicillin** (Ch. 45), which is cleared from the blood almost completely on a single transit through the kidney, to **diazepam** (Ch. 36), which is cleared extremely slowly. Most drugs fall somewhere inbetween, and metabolites are nearly always cleared more quickly than the parent drug. Three fundamental renal processes account for renal drug excretion:

- glomerular filtration
- active tubular secretion
- passive diffusion across tubular epithelium.

GLOMERULAR FILTRATION

Glomerular capillaries allow drug molecules of molecular weight below about 20 000 to diffuse into the glomerular filtrate. Plasma albumin (68 000) is almost completely impermeable, but most

Table 8.3 Some drugs that produce active or toxic metabolites

Inactive (pro-drugs)	Active drug	Active metabolite		Toxic metabolite	See Ch.
Azathioprine →		Mercaptopurine			16
Cortisone →		Hydrocortisone			27
Prednisone →		Prednisolone			27
Enalapril →		Enalaprilat			18
Zidovudine →		Zidovudine trisphosphate			46
Cyclophosphamide →		Phosphoramide mustard →		Acrolein	50
	Diazepam →	Nordiazepam →	Oxazepam		36
	Morphine →	Morphine 6-glucuronide			40
	Halothane →			Trifluoroacetic acid	35
	Methoxyflurane →			Fluoride	35
	Paracetamol →			*N*-Acetyl-*p*-benzoquinone imine	16, 52

drugs—with the exception of macromolecules such as **heparin** (Ch. 20)—cross the barrier freely. If a drug binds appreciably to plasma albumin, its concentration in the filtrate will be less than the total plasma concentration. If, like **warfarin** (Ch. 20), a drug is approximately 98% bound to albumin, the concentration in the filtrate is only 2% of that in plasma and clearance by filtration is correspondingly reduced.

TUBULAR SECRETION

Up to 20% of renal plasma flow is filtered through the glomerulus, leaving at least 80% of delivered drug to pass on to the peritubular capillaries of the proximal tubule. Here drug molecules are transferred to the tubular lumen by two independent and relatively non-selective carrier systems. One of these transports acidic drugs (as well as various endogenous acids, such as uric acid), while the other handles organic bases. Some of the more important drugs that are transported by these two carrier systems are shown in Table 8.4. The carriers can transport drug molecules against an electrochemical gradient and can, therefore, reduce the plasma concentration nearly to zero. Since at least 80% of the drug delivered to the kidney is presented to the carrier, tubular secretion is potentially the most effective mechanism of renal drug elimination. Unlike glomerular filtration, carrier-mediated transport can achieve maximal drug clearance even when most of the drug is bound to plasma protein.* **Penicillin** (Ch. 44), for example, though about 80% protein bound and therefore cleared only slowly by filtration, is almost completely removed by proximal tubular secretion, and its overall rate of elimination is very high.

Many drugs compete for the same transport system (Table 8.4), leading to drug interactions. For example, **probenecid** was developed to prolong the action of **penicillin** by retarding its tubular secretion.

Table 8.4 Important drugs and related substances actively secreted into the proximal renal tubule

Acids	Bases
p-Aminohippuric acid (PAH)	Amiloride
Furosemide (frusemide)	Dopamine
Glucuronic acid conjugates	Histamine
Glycine conjugates	Mepacrine
Indometacin	Morphine
Methotrexate	Pethidine
Penicillin	Quaternary ammonium compounds
Probenecid	Quinine
Sulphate conjugates	5-Hydroxytryptamine (serotonin)
Thiazide diuretics	Triamterene
Uric acid	

DIFFUSION ACROSS THE RENAL TUBULE

As glomerular filtrate traverses the tubule, water is reabsorbed, the volume of urine emerging being only about 1% of that of the filtrate. If the tubule is freely permeable to drug molecules, the drug concentration in the filtrate will remain close to that in the plasma, and some 99% of the filtered drug will be reabsorbed passively. Drugs with high lipid solubility, and hence high tubular permeability, are, therefore, excreted slowly. If the drug is highly polar, and, therefore, of low tubular permeability, filtered drug remains in the tubule, and its concentration rises until it is about 100 times as high in the urine as in the plasma. Drugs handled in this way include **digoxin**, and aminoglycoside antibiotics. Many drugs, being weak acids or weak bases, change their ionisation with pH (see pp. 92–93), and this can markedly affect renal excretion. The ion-trapping effect means that a basic drug is more rapidly excreted in an acid urine, because the low pH within the tubule favours ionisation and thus inhibits reabsorption. Conversely, acidic drugs are most rapidly excreted if the urine is alkaline (Fig. 8.5). Urinary alkalinisation is used to accelerate the excretion of aspirin in treating selected cases of overdose.

Elimination of drugs by the kidney

- Most drugs, unless highly bound to plasma protein, cross the glomerular filter freely.
- Many drugs, especially weak acids and weak bases, are actively secreted into the renal tubule, and thus more rapidly excreted.
- Lipid-soluble drugs are passively reabsorbed by diffusion across the tubule so are not efficiently excreted in the urine.
- Because of pH partition, weak acids are more rapidly excreted in alkaline urine, and vice versa.
- Several important drugs are removed predominantly by renal excretion and are liable to cause toxicity in elderly persons and patients with renal disease.

*Because filtration involves isosmotic movement of both water and solutes, it does not affect the free concentration of drug in the plasma. Thus the equilibrium between free and bound drug is not disturbed, and there is no tendency for bound drug to dissociate as blood traverses the glomerular capillary. The rate of clearance of a drug by filtration is, therefore, reduced directly in proportion to the fraction that is bound. In the case of active tubular secretion, this is not so; secretion may be retarded very little even though the drug is mostly bound. This is because the carrier transports drug molecules unaccompanied by water. As free drug molecules are taken from the plasma, therefore, the free plasma concentration falls, causing dissociation of bound drug from plasma albumin. Consequently, effectively 100% of the drug, bound and free, is available to the carrier.

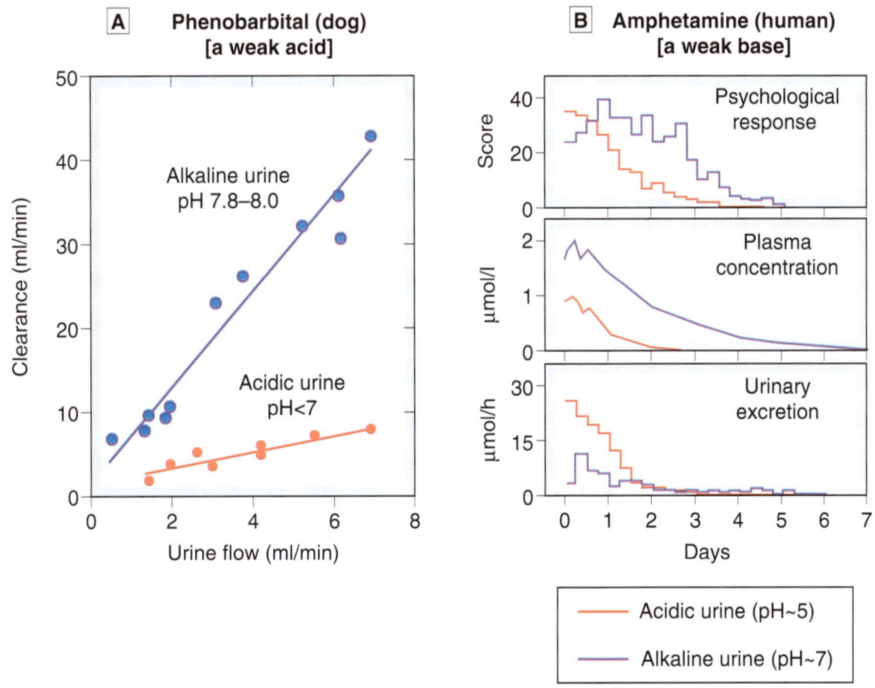

Fig. 8.5 The effect of urinary pH on drug excretion. A Phenobarbital clearance in the dog as a function of urine flow. Because phenobarbital is acidic, alkalinising the urine increases clearance about five fold. B Amphetamine excretion in humans. Acidifying the urine increases the rate of renal elimination of amphetamine, reducing its plasma concentration and its effect on the subject's mental state. (Data from: Gunne & Anggard 1974 In: Torrell T et al. (eds) Pharmacology and pharmacokinetics. Plenum, New York.)

DRUG ELIMINATION EXPRESSED AS CLEARANCE

Renal clearance, CL_r, is defined as the volume of plasma containing the amount of substance that is removed by the kidney in unit time. It is calculated from the plasma concentration, C_p, the urinary concentration, C_u, and the rate of flow of urine, V_u, by the equation:

$$CL_r = \frac{C_u V_u}{C_p} \qquad (8.1)$$

CL_r varies greatly for different drugs, from less than 1 ml/min to the theoretical maximum set by the renal plasma flow (about 700 ml/min, measured by *p*-aminohippuric acid (PAH) clearance; renal extraction of PAH is nearly 100%). The main determinants, as explained above, are the rate of active tubular secretion and the rate of passive reabsorption. For a small but important group of drugs that are not inactivated by metabolism, the rate of renal elimination is the main factor that determines their duration of action (Table 8.5). These drugs have to be used with special care in individuals whose renal function may be impaired, including the elderly and patients with renal disease or any severe acute illness.

The clearance concept is also useful in quantifying the metabolism of drugs. This can be expressed in terms of the volume of plasma containing the amount of drug that is metabolised in unit time. In this case CL_{met} denotes the rate of metabolism.

BILIARY EXCRETION AND ENTEROHEPATIC CIRCULATION

Liver cells transfer various substances, including drugs, from plasma to bile by means of transport systems similar to those of

Table 8.5 Drugs that are excreted largely unchanged in the urine

Percentage excreted	Drugs
100–75	Furosemide (frusemide), gentamicin, methotrexate, atenolol, digoxin
75–50	Benzylpenicillin, cimetidine, oxytetracycline, neostigmine
~50	Propantheline, tubocurarine

the renal tubule and which involve P-glycoprotein (see Ch. 7). Various hydrophilic drug conjugates (particularly glucuronides) are concentrated in bile and delivered to the intestine where the glucuronide is usually hydrolysed, releasing active drug once more; free drug can then be reabsorbed and the cycle repeated (enterohepatic circulation). The effect of this is to create a 'reservoir' of recirculating drug that can amount to about 20% of total drug in the body and prolongs drug action. Examples where this is important include **morphine** (Ch. 40) and **ethinylestradiol** (Ch. 29). Several drugs are excreted to an appreciable extent in bile. **Vecuronium** (a non-depolarising muscle relaxant; Ch. 10) is an example of a drug that is excreted mainly unchanged in bile. **Rifampicin** (Ch. 45) is absorbed from the gut and slowly deacetylated, retaining its biological activity. Both forms are secreted in the bile, but the deacetylated form is not reabsorbed, so eventually most of the drug leaves the body in this form in the faeces.

PHARMACOKINETICS

The relationship between the time course of drug concentrations attained in different regions of the body during and after dosing is termed pharmacokinetics ('what the body does to the drug'), to distinguish it from pharmacodynamics ('what the drug does to the body' i.e. events consequent on interaction of the drug with its receptor or other primary site of action). The distinction is useful, though the words cause dismay to etymological purists. In this section, a simple quantitative model is presented that synthesises the effects on drug concentration of the simultaneous operation of absorption, distribution, metabolism and excretion. This enables us to predict the time course of drug action, which is extremely important from a clinical viewpoint, since it underpins selection of an appropriate dosing regimen.

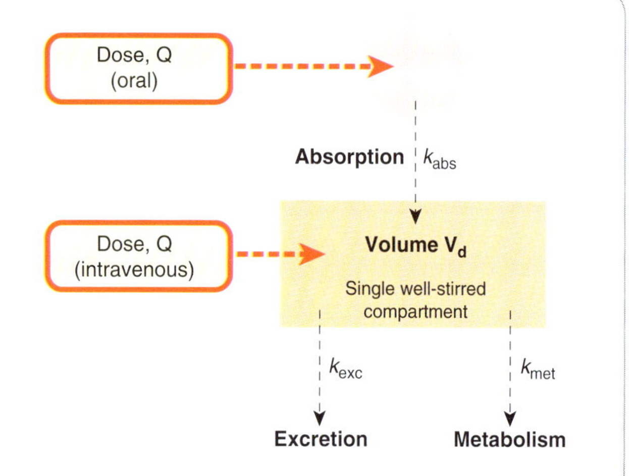

Fig. 8.6 Single-compartment pharmacokinetic model.

SINGLE-COMPARTMENT MODEL

Consider first a highly simplified model of a human being, which consists of a single well-stirred compartment (of volume V_d (distribution volume)) into which a quantity of drug Q is introduced rapidly by intravenous injection, and from which it can escape either by being metabolised or by being excreted (Fig. 8.6). The initial concentration, $C(0)$, will be Q/V_d. The concentration $C(t)$ at a later time t will depend on the rate of elimination of the drug (i.e. its total clearance CL_s, which is equal to the sum of the clearance by metabolism and by renal excretion.

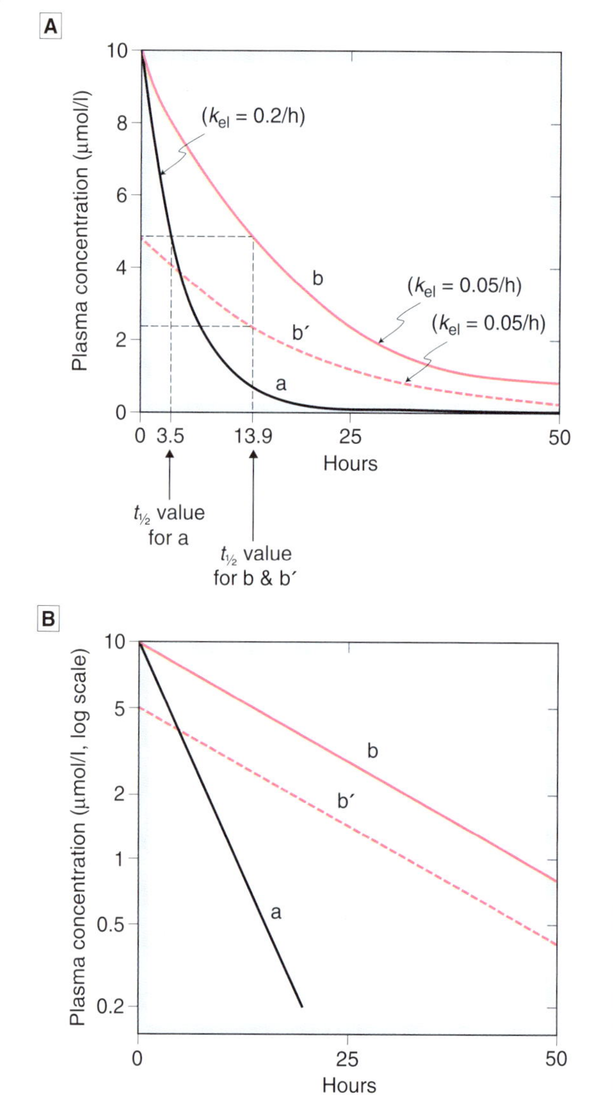

Fig. 8.7 Predicted behaviour of single-compartment model following intravenous drug administration at time 0. Drugs a and b differ only in their elimination rate constant, k_{el}. Curve b shows the plasma concentration time course for a smaller dose of B. Note that the half-life ($t_{1/2}$) (indicated by broken lines) does not depend on the dose. **A** Linear concentration scale. **B** Logarithmic concentration scale.

▼ Most drugs exhibit first-order kinetics where the rate of elimination is directly proportional to drug concentration. Drug concentration then decays exponentially (Fig. 8.7), being described by the equation:

$$C(t) = C(0)\exp\frac{-CL_s}{V_d}t \qquad (8.2)$$

Taking logarithms:

$$\ln C(t) = \ln C(0) - \frac{CL_s}{V_d}t \qquad (8.3)$$

Plotting $C(t)$ logarithmically against t yields a straight line with slope $-CL_s/V_d$. The inverse of this slope (CL_s/V_d) is the elimination rate constant, k_{el}. The half-life, $t_{1/2}$, is an easily conceptualised parameter inversely related to k_{el}. It is the time taken for $C(t)$ to decrease by 50% and is equal to $\ln 2/k_{el}$ ($0.693/k_{el}$). The plasma half-life is, therefore, determined by V_d and CL_s.

EFFECT OF REPEATED DOSAGE

Drugs are usually given as repeated doses rather than single injections. A continuous infusion can be regarded as the extreme of a repeated dose schedule. In this case, the plasma concentration increases until a steady-state concentration, C(steady state), is reached where the rate of infusion, X, equals the rate of elimination. The rate of elimination is equal to $CL_s \times C$(steady state), so that:

$$C(\text{steady state}) = \frac{X}{CL_s} \qquad (8.4)$$

The drug concentration approaches this steady-state value exponentially (Fig. 8.8). Repeated injections (each of dose Q) give a more complicated pattern, but the principle is the same. The concentration will rise to a mean steady-state concentration with an approximately exponential time course but will oscillate (through a range Q/V_d). The smaller and more frequent the doses, the more closely the situation approaches that of a continuous infusion and the smaller the swings in concentration. The exact dosage schedule, however, does not affect the mean steady-state concentration, nor the rate at which it is approached. In practice, a steady state is effectively achieved after three to five half-lives. Speedier attainment of the steady state can be achieved by starting with a larger dose. Such a *loading dose* is sometimes useful when starting treatment with a drug with a half-life that is long compared with the urgency of the clinical situation, as may be the case when treating cardiac dysrhythmias with drugs such as **amiodarone** or **digoxin** (Ch. 17). It must again be emphasised that the simple behaviour predicted by the single-compartment model only roughly corresponds to real life. Inclusion of other body compartments, particularly slowly equilibrating ones such as body fat, results in additional exponential components in the overall kinetic behaviour and, in practice, two or three compartments are often necessary to produce a realistic simulation (see below).

EFFECT OF VARIATION IN RATE OF ABSORPTION

If a drug is absorbed slowly from the gut or from an injection site into the plasma, it is (in terms of a compartmental model) as though it were being injected slowly into the bloodstream. For the purpose of kinetic modelling, the transfer of drug from the site of administration to the central compartment can be represented approximately by a rate constant, k_{abs} (see Fig. 8.6). This assumes that the rate of absorption is directly proportional, at any moment,

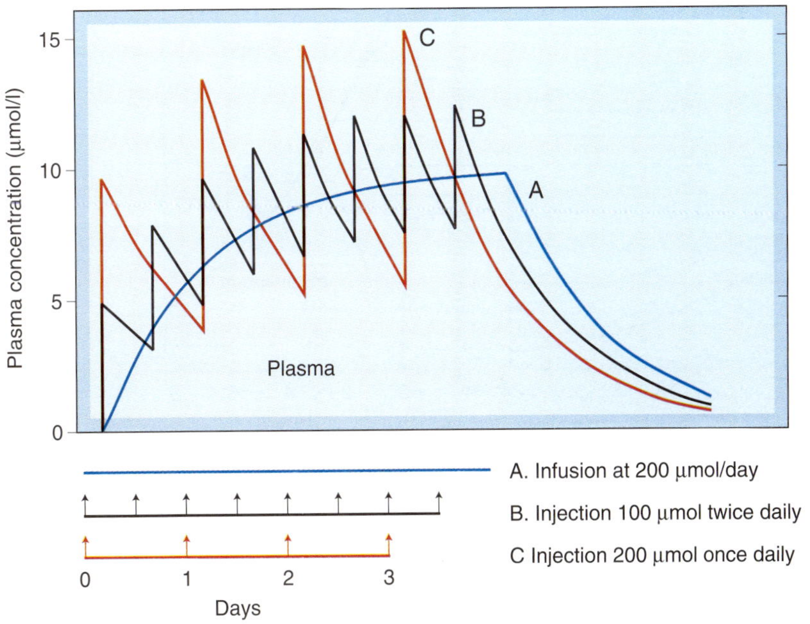

Fig. 8.8 Predicted behaviour of single-compartment model with continuous or intermittent drug administration. Smooth curve A shows the effect of continuous infusion for 4 days; curve B the same total amount of drug given in eight equal doses; and curve C the same total amount of drug given in four equal doses. The drug has a half life of 17 hours and a volume of distribution of 20 litres. Note that in each case a steady state is effectively reached after about 2 days (about three half-lives), and that the mean concentration reached in the steady state is the same for all three schedules.

to the amount of drug still unabsorbed, which is at best a rough approximation to reality. The effect of slow absorption on the time course of the rise and fall of the plasma concentration is shown in Figure 8.9. The curves show the effect of spreading out the absorption of the same total amount of drug over different times. In each case, the drug is absorbed completely, but the peak concentration appears later and is lower and less sharp if absorption is slow. Once absorption is complete, the plasma concentration declines with the same half-time, irrespective of the rate of absorption.

▼ For the kind of pharmacokinetic model discussed here, the area under the plasma concentration–time curve (often abbreviated to AUC, for area under the curve) is directly proportional to the total amount of drug introduced into the plasma compartment, irrespective of the rate at which it enters. Comparison of the AUC following oral and intravenous administration can, therefore, be used to determine the fraction of the oral dose that enters the bloodstream, and thus to measure bioavailability (see p. 99). If unmetabolised drug is absorbed completely after oral administration, the AUC will be the same as after intravenous administration, so bioavailability is 100%. Incomplete absorption, or destruction by first-pass metabolism before the drug reaches the plasma compartment, reduces AUC after oral administration. Changes in the *rate* of absorption, however, do not affect AUC. Again it is worth noting that provided absorption is complete the relation between the rate of administration and the steady-state plasma concentration (equation 8.4) is unaffected by k_{abs}, though the size of the oscillation of plasma concentration with each dose will be reduced if absorption is slow.

MORE COMPLICATED KINETIC MODELS

So far we have considered a single-compartment pharmacokinetic model in which the rates of absorption, metabolism and excretion are all assumed to be directly proportional to the concentration of drug in the compartment from which transfer is occurring. This is a useful way to illustrate some basic principles but is clearly a physiological oversimplification. The characteristics of different parts of the body, such as brain, body fat and muscle, are quite different in terms of their blood supply, partition coefficient for drugs and the permeability of their capillaries to drugs. These differences, which the single-compartment model ignores, can considerably affect the time course of drug distribution and drug action, and much theoretical work has gone into the mathematical analysis of more complex models (see Rowland & Tozer, 1995). They are beyond the scope of this book, and perhaps also beyond the limit of what is actually useful, for the experimental data on pharmacokinetic properties of drugs are seldom accurate or reproducible enough to enable complex models to be tested critically.

The two-compartment model, which introduces a separate 'peripheral' compartment to represent the tissues, in communication with the 'central' plasma compartment, more closely resembles the real situation without involving excessive complications.

TWO-COMPARTMENT MODEL

The two-compartment model is a widely used approximation in which the tissues are lumped together as a peripheral compartment. Drug molecules can enter and leave the peripheral compartment only via the central compartment (Fig. 8.10), which usually represents the plasma (or plasma plus some extravascular space in the case of a few drugs that distribute especially rapidly).

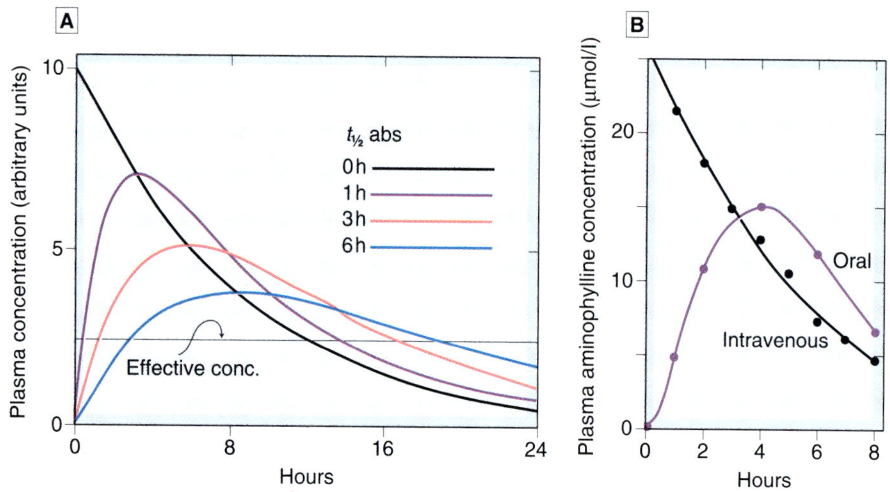

Fig. 8.9 The effect of slow drug absorption on plasma drug concentration. A Predicted behaviour of single-compartment model with drug absorbed at different rates from the gut or an injection site. The elimination half-time is 6 hours. The absorption half-times ($t_{1/2}$ abs) are marked on the diagram. (Zero indicates instantaneous absorption, corresponding to intravenous administration.) Note that the peak plasma concentration is reduced and delayed by slow absorption, and the duration of action is somewhat increased. B Measurements of plasma aminophylline concentration in humans following equal oral and intravenous doses. (Data from: Swintowsky J V 1956 J Am Pharm Assoc 49: 395.)

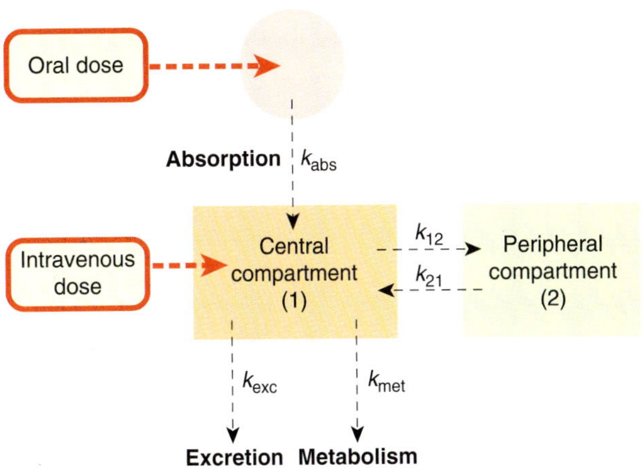

Fig. 8.10 Two-compartment pharmacokinetic model.

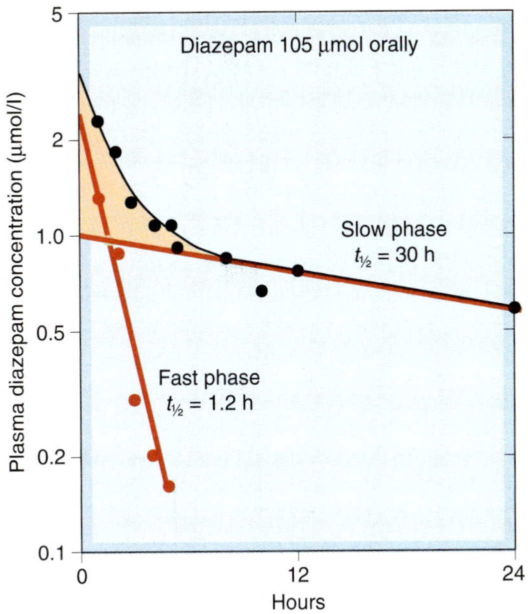

Fig. 8.11 Kinetics of diazepam elimination in humans following a single oral dose. The graph shows a semilogarithmic plot of plasma concentration versus time. The experimental data (black symbols) follow a curve that becomes linear after about 8 hours (slow phase). Plotting the deviation of the early points (pink shaded area) from this line on the same coordinates (red symbols) reveals the fast phase. This type of two-component decay is consistent with the two-compartment model (Fig. 8.10) and is obtained with many drugs. (Data from: Curry S H 1980 Drug disposition and pharmacokinetics. Blackwell, Oxford)

The effect of adding a second compartment to the model is to introduce a second exponential component into the predicted time course of the plasma concentration, so that it comprises a fast and a slow phase. This pattern is often found experimentally and is most clearly revealed when the concentration data are plotted semilogarithmically (Fig. 8.11). If, as is often the case, the transfer of drug between the central and peripheral compartments is relatively fast compared with the rate of elimination, then the fast phase (often called the α-phase) can be taken to represent the redistribution of the drug (i.e. drug molecules passing from plasma to tissues thereby rapidly lowering the plasma concentration). The plasma concentration reached when the fast phase is complete, but before any elimination has occurred, allows a measure of the combined distribution volumes of the two compartments; the half-time for the slow phase (the β-phase) provides an estimate of k_{el}. If a drug is rapidly metabolised, the α- and β-phases are not well separated and the calculation of V_d and k_{el} is not straightforward. Problems also arise with drugs (e.g. very fat-soluble drugs) for which it is unrealistic to lump all the peripheral tissues together.

It is important to realise that the addition of extra compartments to the basic model affects only the predicted time course of drug action, and not the steady state. Thus the relation between plasma concentration and dose derived for the single-compartment model (equation 8.4) still applies.

SATURATION KINETICS

In a few cases, such as **ethanol**, **phenytoin** and **salicylate**, the time course of disappearance of drug from the plasma does not follow the exponential or biexponential patterns shown in Figures 8.7 and 8.11 but is initially linear (i.e. drug is removed at a constant rate that is independent of plasma concentration). This is often called *zero-order kinetics* to distinguish it from the usual *first-order kinetics* that we have considered so far (these terms

Pharmacokinetics

- For many drugs, disappearance from the plasma follows an exponential time course characterised by the plasma half-life.
- Plasma half-life, in the simple case, is directly proportional to the volume of distribution, and inversely proportional to the overall rate of clearance.
- With repeated dosage or sustained delivery of a drug, the plasma concentration approaches a steady value within 3–5 plasma half-lives.
- A two-compartment model is often needed. In this case the kinetics are biexponential. The two components roughly represent the processes of transfer between plasma and tissues (α-phase) and elimination from the plasma (β-phase).
- Some drugs show non-exponential 'saturation' kinetics, with important clinical consequences, especially a disproportionate increase in steady-state plasma concentration when daily dose is increased.

have their origin in chemical kinetic theory). *Saturation kinetics* is a better term. Figure 8.12 shows the example of ethanol. It can be seen that the rate of disappearance of ethanol from the plasma is constant at about 4 mmol/l per hour irrespective of its plasma concentration. The explanation for this is that the rate of oxidation by the enzyme alcohol dehydrogenase reaches a maximum at low ethanol concentrations because of limited availability of the cofactor NAD^+ (see Ch. 52).

Saturation kinetics has several important consequences (see Fig. 8.13). One is that the duration of action is more strongly dependent on dose than is the case with drugs that do not show metabolic saturation. Another consequence is that the relationship between dose and steady-state plasma concentration is steep and unpredictable, and it does not obey the proportionality rule implicit in equation 8.4 for non-saturating drugs. The maximum rate of metabolism sets a limit to the rate at which the drug can be administered; if this rate is exceeded, the amount of drug in the body will, in principle, increase indefinitely and never reach a steady state (Fig. 8.13). This does not actually happen because there is always some dependence of the rate of elimination on the plasma concentration (usually because other, non-saturating metabolic pathways or renal excretion contribute significantly at high concentrations). Nevertheless, steady-state plasma concentrations of drugs of this kind vary widely and unpredictably with dose. Similarly, variations in the rate of metabolism (e.g. through enzyme induction) cause disproportionately large changes in the plasma concentration.

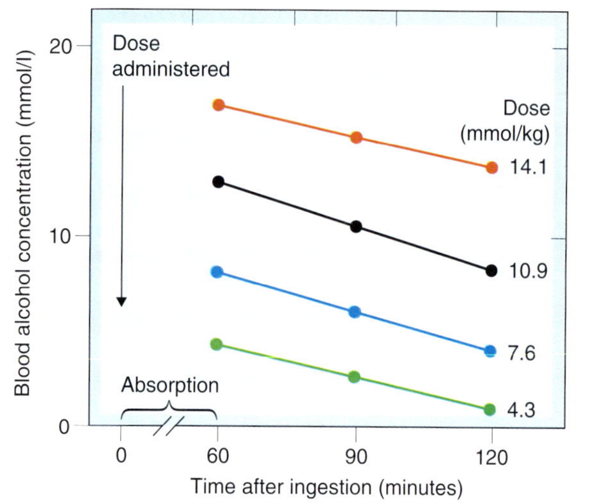

Fig. 8.12 Saturating kinetics of alcohol elimination in humans. The blood alcohol concentration falls linearly rather than exponentially, and the rate of fall does not vary with dose. (From: Drew G C et al. 1958 Br Med J 2: 5103.)

These problems are well recognised for drugs such as **phenytoin**, an anticonvulsant for which plasma concentration needs to be closely controlled to achieve an optimal clinical effect (see Ch. 39).

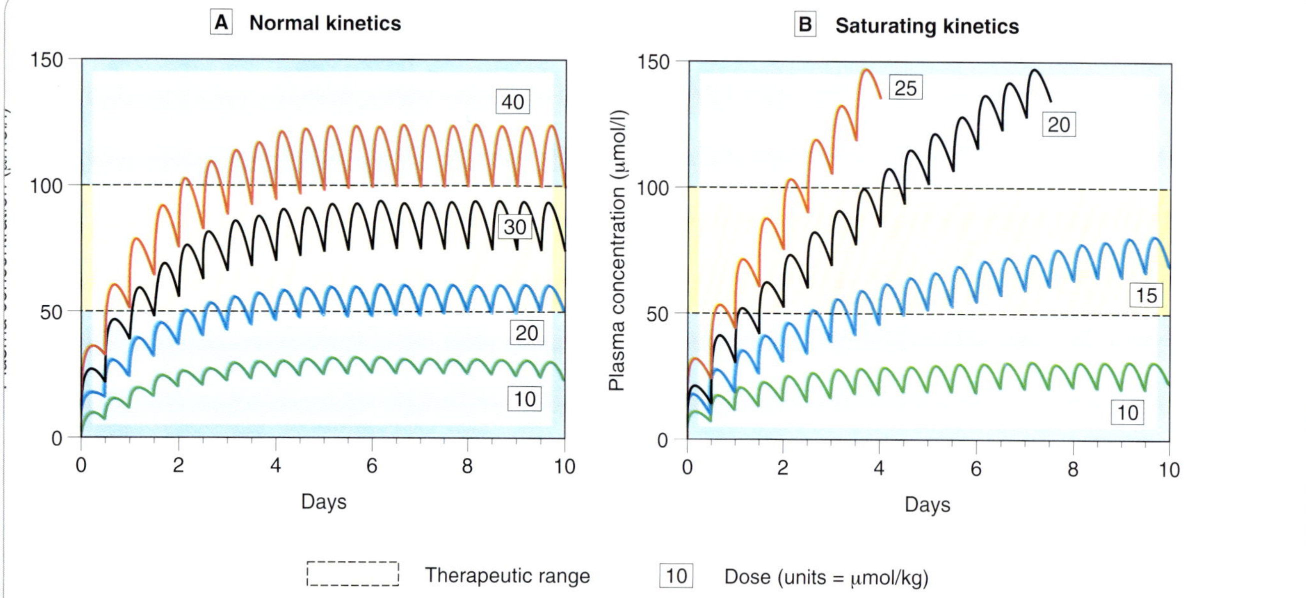

Fig. 8.13 Comparison of non-saturating and saturating kinetics for drugs given orally every 12 hours. A The curves show an imaginary drug, similar to the antiepileptic drug phenytoin at the lowest dose, but with linear kinetics. B The curves for saturating kinetics are calculated from the known pharmacokinetic parameters of phenytoin (see Ch. 39). Note (i) that no steady state is reached with higher doses of phenytoin and (ii) that a small increment in dose results after a time in a disproportionately large effect on plasma concentration. With linear kinetics, the steady-state plasma concentration is directly proportional to dose. (Curves were calculated with the 'Sympak' pharmacokinetic modelling program written by Dr J G Blackman, University of Otago.)

REFERENCES AND FURTHER READING

Benton R E, Honig P K, Zamani K, Cantilena L R, Woosley R L 1996 Grapefruit juice alters terfenadine pharmacokinetics, resulting in prolongation of repolarization on the electrocardiogram. Clin Pharmacol Ther 59: 383–388 (*Grapefruit juice sets the stage for a potentially fatal, albeit very uncommon, interaction*)

Boobis A R, Edwards R J, Adams D A, Davies D S 1996 Dissecting the function of P450. Br J Clin Pharmacol 42: 81–89 (*Use of antipeptide antibodies directed against defined regions of human P450 enzymes*)

Gonzalez F J, Korzekwa K R 1995 Cytochromes P450 expression systems. Annu Rev Pharmacol Toxicol 35: 369–390 (*Catalytically active P450 enzymes can be expressed in bacterial, yeast or mammalian cells*)

Gooderham N J, Murray S, Lynch A M et al. 1996 Heterocyclic amines: evaluation of their role in diet associated human cancer. Br J Clin Pharmacol 42: 91–98 (*Heterocyclic amines are formed during cooking. They are absorbed after eating meat and converted into genotoxic hydroxylamines by CYP1A2 in human liver; they are both mutagenic and carcinogenic in bioassays. More nightmares!*)

Halpert J R 1995 Structural basis of selective cytochrome P450 inhibition. Annu Rev Pharmacol Toxicol 35: 29–53 (*Complementary properties of isoform-selective P450 inhibitors and their target enzymes determine inhibitor selectivity*)

Henderson L et al. 2002 St John's wort (*Hypericum perforatum*): drug interactions and clinical outcomes. Br J Clin Pharmacol 54: 349–356 (*Reviews the induction of CYP450 isoenzymes and of P-glycoprotein by constituents in this herbal 'remedy'*)

Hutt A J, Tan S C 1996 Drug chirality and its clinical significance. Drugs 52: 1–12 (*Short review*)

Kane G C, Lipsky J J 2000 Drug–grapefruit juice interactions. Mayo Clinic Proc 75: 933–942

Kharasch E D, Hankins D, Mautz D, Thummel K E 1996 Identification of the enzyme responsible for oxidative halothane metabolism: implications for prevention of halothane hepatitis. Lancet 347: 1367–1371 (*Evidence that CYP2E1 is important in human oxidative halothane metabolism: 'single dose disulfiram may prove effective prophylaxis against halothane hepatitis'*)

Lin J H, Lu A Y 2001 Interindividual variability in inhibition and induction of cytochrome P450 enzymes. Annu Rev Pharmacol Toxicol 41: 535–567

Nelson D R, Koymans L, Kamataki T et al. 1996 P450 superfamily: update on new sequences, gene mapping, accession numbers and nomenclature. Pharmacogenetics 6: 1–42 (*Classification of the superfamily of P450 enzymes*)

Park B K, Kitteringham N R, Pirmohamed M, Tucker G T 1996 Relevance of induction of human drug-metabolizing enzymes: pharmacological and toxicological implications. Br J Clin Pharmacol 41: 477–491 (*Reviews the mechanism and biological importance of enzyme induction, including implications for toxicity/carcinogenicity testing of new drugs*)

Raunio H, Pasanen M, Maenpaa J, Hakkola J, Pelkonen O 1995 Expression of extrahepatic cytochrome P450 in humans. In: Pacifici G M, Fracchia G M (ed) Advances in drug metabolism in man. European Commission, Luxembourg pp. 233–287 (*Reviews anabolic functions of P450 enzymes in humans*)

Rowland M, Tozer T N 1995 Clinical pharmacokinetics: concepts and applications, 3rd edn. Williams & Wilkins, Baltimore, MD (*Excellent text, overmodestly described by its authors as a 'primer'. Emphasises clinical applications*)

Sueyoshi T, Negishi M 2001 Phenobarbital response elements of cytochrome P450 genes and nuclear receptors. Annu Rev Pharmacol Toxicol 41: 123–143

SECTION 2

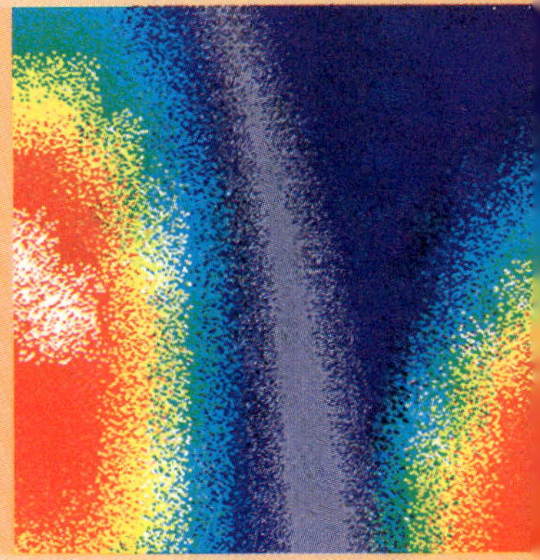

CHEMICAL MEDIATORS

9 Chemical mediators and the autonomic nervous system

Overview 122

Historical aspects 122

The peripheral nervous system 123
- Basic anatomy and physiology of the autonomic nervous system 123
- Transmitters in the autonomic nervous system 126

Some general principles of chemical transmission 126
- Dale's principle 126
- Denervation supersensitivity 126
- Presynaptic modulation 128
- Postsynaptic modulation 130
- Transmitters other than acetylcholine and noradrenaline 130
- Co-transmission 130
- Termination of transmitter action 131

Basic steps in neurochemical transmission: sites of drug action 133

OVERVIEW

The network of chemical signals and associated receptors by which cells in the body communicate with one another provides many targets for drug action, and this has always been a focus of attention for pharmacologists. Chemical transmission in the peripheral nervous system, and the various ways in which the process can be pharmacologically subverted, are discussed in this chapter. In addition to neurotransmission, we also consider briefly the less clearly defined processes, collectively termed *neuromodulation*, by which many mediators and drugs exert control over the function of the nervous system. The relative anatomical and physiological simplicity of the peripheral nervous system has made it the proving ground for most of the important discoveries about chemical transmission, and the same general principles apply to the central nervous system (CNS; see Ch. 31). For more detail than is given here, see Broadley (1996), Cooper et al. (1996), Brading (1999) and Nestler et al. (2001).

HISTORICAL ASPECTS

▼ Studies initiated on the peripheral nervous system have been central to the understanding and classification of many major types of drug action, so it is worth recounting a little history. An excellent account is given by Bacq (1975).

Experimental physiology became established as an approach to the understanding of the function of living organisms in the middle of the 19th century. The peripheral nervous system, and particularly the autonomic nervous system, received a great deal of attention. The fact that electrical stimulation of nerves could elicit a whole variety of physiological effects—from blanching of the skin to arrest of the heart—presented a real challenge to comprehension, particularly of the way in which the signal was passed from the nerve to the effector tissue. In 1877 Du Bois-Reymond was the first to put the alternatives clearly: 'Of known natural processes that might pass on excitation, only two are, in my opinion, worth talking about—either there exists at the boundary of the contractile substance a stimulatory secretion...; or the phenomenon is electrical in nature.' The latter view was generally favoured. In 1869 it had been shown that an exogenous substance, **muscarine**, could mimic the effects of stimulating the vagus nerve, and that **atropine** could inhibit the actions both of muscarine and of nerve stimulation. In 1905, Langley showed the same for **nicotine** and **curare** acting at the neuromuscular junction. Most physiologists interpreted these phenomena as stimulation and inhibition of the nerve endings, respectively, rather than as evidence for chemical transmission. Hence, the suggestion of T. R. Elliott, in 1904, that **adrenaline** might act as a chemical transmitter mediating the actions of the sympathetic nervous system was coolly received, until Langley, the Professor of Physiology at Cambridge and a powerful figure at that time, suggested, a year later, that transmission to skeletal muscle involved the secretion by the nerve terminals of a substance related to nicotine.

One of the key observations for Elliott was that degeneration of sympathetic nerve terminals did not abolish the sensitivity of smooth muscle preparations to adrenaline (which the electrical theory predicted) but actually enhanced it. The hypothesis of chemical transmission was put to direct test by Dixon in 1907, who tried to show that vagus nerve stimulation released from a dog's heart into the blood a substance capable of inhibiting another heart. The experiment failed, and the atmosphere of scepticism prevailed.

It was not until 1921, in Germany, that Loewi showed that stimulation of the vagosympathetic trunk to an isolated and cannulated frog's heart could cause the release into the cannula of a substance ('Vagusstoff') that, if the cannula fluid was transferred from the first heart to a second, would inhibit the second heart. This is a classic and much-quoted experiment that proved extremely difficult for even Loewi to perform reproducibly. In an autobiographical sketch, Loewi tells us that the idea of chemical transmission arose in a discussion that he had in 1903 but no way of testing it experimentally occurred to him until he dreamed of the appropriate experiment one night in 1920. He wrote some notes of this very important dream in the middle of the night, but in the morning could not read them. The dream obligingly returned the next night, and, taking no chances, he went to the laboratory at 3 a.m. and carried out the experiment successfully. Loewi's experiment may be, and was, criticised on numerous grounds (it could, for example, have been potassium rather than a neurotransmitter that was acting on the recipient heart), but a series of further experiments proved him to be right. His findings can be summarised as follows.

- Stimulation of the vagus caused the appearance in the perfusate of the frog heart of a substance capable of producing, in a second heart, an inhibitory effect resembling vagus stimulation.
- Stimulation of the sympathetic nervous system caused the appearance of a substance capable of accelerating a second heart. By fluorescence measurements, Loewi concluded later that this substance was adrenaline.
- Atropine prevented the inhibitory action of the vagus on the heart but did not prevent release of Vagusstoff. Atropine thus prevented the effects, rather than the release, of the transmitter.
- When 'Vagusstoff' was incubated with ground-up frog heart muscle it became inactivated. This effect is now known to be the result of enzymic destruction of acetylcholine by cholinesterase.
- **Physostigmine** (**eserine**), which potentiated the effect of vagus stimulation on the heart, prevented destruction of 'Vagusstoff' by heart muscle, providing evidence that the potentiation is the result of inhibition of cholinesterase, which normally destroys the transmitter substance acetylcholine.

A few years later, in the early 1930s, Dale showed convincingly that acetylcholine was also the transmitter substance at the neuromuscular junction of striated muscle and at autonomic ganglia. One of the keys to Dale's success lay in the use of very highly sensitive bioassays, especially the leech dorsal muscle, for measuring acetylcholine release (see Ch. 6). Chemical transmission at sympathetic nerve terminals was demonstrated at about the same time as cholinergic transmission and by very similar methods. Cannon and his colleagues at Harvard first showed unequivocally the phenomenon of chemical transmission at sympathetic nerve endings, by experiments in vivo in which tissues made supersensitive to adrenaline by prior sympathetic denervation were shown to respond, after a delay, to the transmitter released by stimulation of the sympathetic nerves to other parts of the body. The chemical identity of the transmitter, tantalisingly like adrenaline but not identical to it, caused confusion for many years, until in 1946 von Euler showed it to be the non-methylated derivative **noradrenaline**.

THE PERIPHERAL NERVOUS SYSTEM

The peripheral nervous system consists of the following principal elements:

- autonomic nervous system, which includes the enteric nervous system
- somatic efferent nerves, innervating skeletal muscle
- somatic and visceral afferent nerves.

In this chapter, we focus on the autonomic nervous system, which for a long time occupied centre stage in the pharmacology of chemical transmission. Aspects of the somatic efferent system are considered in Chapter 10. Afferent nerves (particularly the non-myelinated nerves subserving nociceptive and other functions; see Ch. 40) also have important effector functions in the periphery, mediated mainly by neuropeptides (Ch. 13). Many afferent fibres are present in autonomic nerves and are anatomically part of the autonomic nervous system, but it is the efferent pathways that are the main concern of this chapter.

BASIC ANATOMY AND PHYSIOLOGY OF THE AUTONOMIC NERVOUS SYSTEM

The autonomic nervous system (see Appenzeller & Oribe, 1997; Brading, 1999) consists of three main anatomical divisions, sympathetic and parasympathetic (see Fig. 9.1), and the enteric nervous system. The latter consists of the intrinsic nerve plexuses of the gastrointestinal tract, which are closely interconnected with the sympathetic and parasympathetic systems.

The autonomic nervous system conveys all of the outputs from the central nervous system (CNS) to the rest of the body except for the motor innervation of skeletal muscle. The enteric nervous system has sufficient integrative capabilities to allow it to function independently of the CNS, but the sympathetic and parasympathetic systems are agents of the CNS, and cannot function without it. The autonomic nervous system is largely outside the influence of voluntary control. The main processes that it regulates are:

- contraction and relaxation of smooth muscle
- all exocrine and certain endocrine secretions
- the heartbeat
- energy metabolism, particularly in liver and skeletal muscle.

A degree of autonomic control also affects many other systems, including the kidney, immune system and somatosensory system, though its physiological importance is not yet clear.

The main difference between the autonomic and the somatic efferent pathways is that the former consists of two neurons arranged in series, whereas in the latter a single motoneuron connects the CNS to the skeletal muscle fibre (Fig. 9.2). The two neurons in the autonomic pathway are known, respectively, as *preganglionic* and *postganglionic*. In the sympathetic nervous system, the intervening synapses lie in *autonomic ganglia*, which are outside the CNS and contain the nerve endings of preganglionic fibres and the cell bodies of postganglionic fibres. In parasympathetic pathways, the postganglionic cells are mainly found in the target organs, discrete parasympathetic ganglia being found only in the head and neck.

The sympathetic preganglionic neurons have their cell bodies in the lateral horn of the grey matter of the thoracic and lumbar segments of the spinal cord, and the fibres leave the spinal cord in the spinal nerves as the *thoracolumbar sympathetic outflow*. The preganglionic fibres synapse in the *paravertebral chain* of sympathetic ganglia, lying bilaterally on either side of the spinal column. These ganglia contain the cell bodies of the postganglionic sympathetic neurons, the axons of which rejoin the spinal nerves. Many of the postganglionic sympathetic fibres reach their peripheral destinations via the branches of the spinal nerves. Others, destined for abdominal and pelvic viscera, have their cell bodies in a group of unpaired *prevertebral ganglia* in

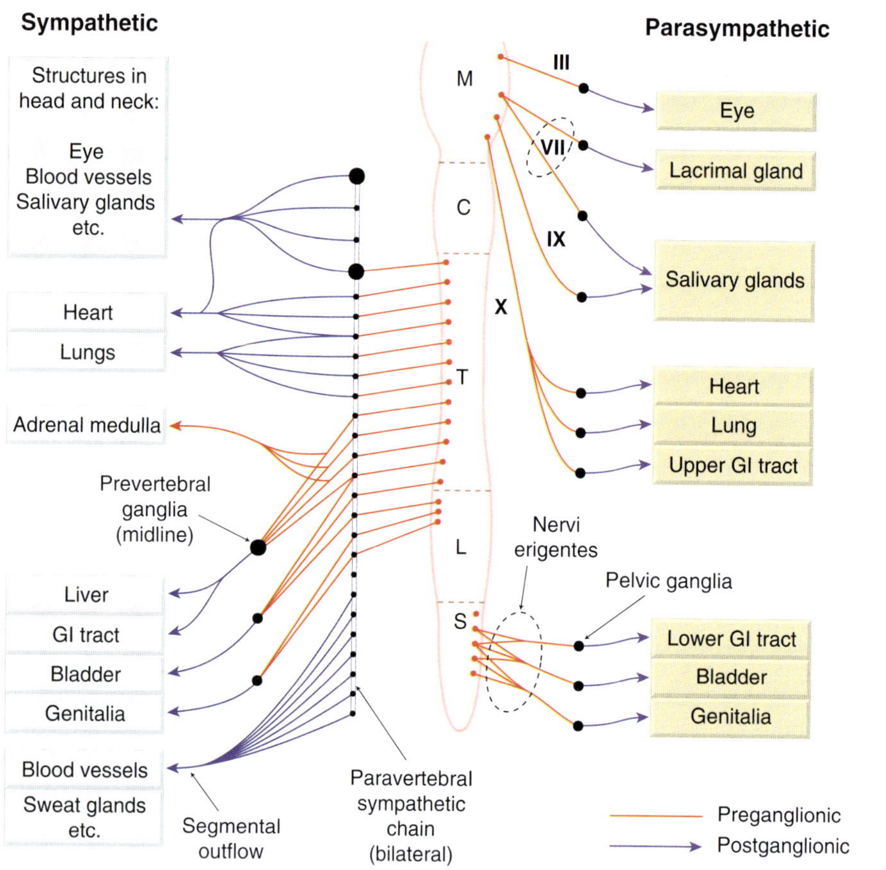

Fig. 9.1 Basic plan of the mammalian autonomic nervous system. (M, medullary; C, cervical; T, thoracic; L, lumbar, S, sacral; GI, gastrointestinal.)

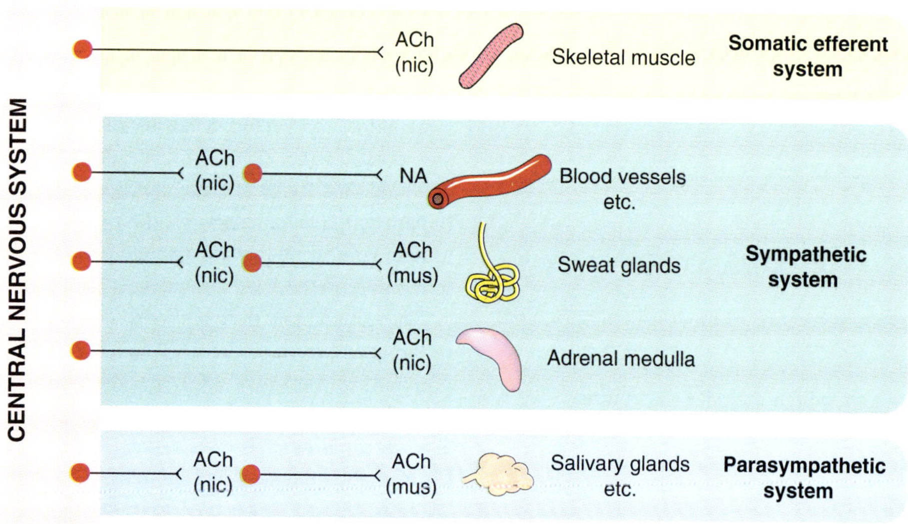

Fig. 9.2 Acetylcholine (ACh) and noradrenaline (NA) as transmitters in the peripheral nervous system. The main two types of acetylcholine receptor, nicotinic (nic) and muscarinic (mus) (see Ch.10), are indicated.

the abdominal cavity. The only exception to the two-neuron arrangement is the innervation of the adrenal medulla. The catecholamine-secreting cells of the adrenal medulla are, in effect, modified postganglionic sympathetic neurons, and the nerves supplying the gland are equivalent to preganglionic fibres.

The parasympathetic nerves emerge from two separate regions of the CNS. The *cranial outflow* consists of preganglionic fibres in certain cranial nerves, namely the oculomotor nerve (carrying parasympathetic fibres destined for the eye), the facial and glossopharyngeal nerves (carrying fibres to the salivary glands and the nasopharynx) and the vagus nerve (carrying fibres to the thoracic and abdominal viscera). The ganglia lie scattered in close relation to the target organs; the postganglionic neurons are very short compared with those of the sympathetic system. Parasympathetic fibres destined for the pelvic and abdominal viscera emerge as the *sacral outflow* from the spinal cord in a bundle of nerves known as the *nervi erigentes* (since stimulation of these nerves evokes genital erection—a fact of some importance to those responsible for artificial insemination of livestock). These fibres synapse in a group of scattered pelvic ganglia, whence the short postganglionic fibres run to target tissues such as the bladder, rectum and genitalia. The pelvic ganglia carry both sympathetic and parasympathetic fibres, and the two divisions are not anatomically distinct in this region.

The *enteric nervous system* (reviewed by Furness & Costa, 1987; Goyal & Hirano, 1996) consists of the neurons from cell bodies that lie in the intramural plexuses in the wall of the intestine. It is estimated that there are more cells in this system than in the spinal cord, and functionally they do not fit simply into the sympathetic/parasympathetic classification. Incoming nerves from both the sympathetic and the parasympathetic systems terminate on enteric neurons, as well as running directly to smooth muscle, glands and blood vessels. Some enteric neurons function as mechanoreceptors or chemoreceptors, providing local reflex pathways that can control gastrointestinal function without external inputs. The enteric nervous system is pharmacologically more complex than the sympathetic or parasympathetic systems, involving many neuropeptide and other transmitters (such as 5-hydroxytryptamine, (5-HT, serotonin) nitric oxide and ATP) and is often described as a collection of 'little brains' outside the CNS, rather like those of many invertebrates.

In some places (e.g. in the visceral smooth muscle of the gut and bladder and in the heart) the sympathetic and the parasympathetic systems produce opposite effects, but there are others where only one division of the autonomic system operates. The sweat glands and most blood vessels, for example, have only a sympathetic innervation, whereas the ciliary muscle of the eye has only a parasympathetic innervation. Bronchial smooth muscle has only a parasympathetic (constrictor) innervation (though its tone is highly sensitive to circulating adrenaline—acting probably to inhibit the constrictor innervation rather than on the smooth muscle directly). Resistance arteries (see Ch. 18) have a sympathetic vasoconstrictor innervation, but no parasympathetic innervation; instead, the constrictor tone is opposed by a background release of nitric oxide from the endothelial cells (see Ch. 14). There are other examples, such as the salivary glands, where the two systems produce similar, rather than opposing, effects.

It is, therefore, a mistake to think of the sympathetic and parasympathetic systems as physiological opponents. Each serves its own physiological function and can be more or less active in a

Basic anatomy of the autonomic nervous system

- The autonomic nervous system comprises three divisions: sympathetic, parasympathetic and enteric.
- Basic (two-neuron) pattern of the sympathetic and parasympathetic systems consists of preganglionic neurons with cell bodies in the CNS and postganglionic neurons with cell bodies in the autonomic ganglion.
- Parasympathetic system is connected to the CNS via:
  - cranial nerve outflow (III, VII, IX, X)
  - sacral outflow.
- Parasympathetic ganglia usually lie close to or within the target organ.
- Sympathetic outflow leaves the CNS in thoracic and lumbar spinal roots. Sympathetic ganglia form two paravertebral chains, plus some midline ganglia.
- The enteric nervous system consists of neurons lying in the intramural plexuses of the gastrointestinal tract. It receives inputs from sympathetic and parasympathetic systems but can act on its own to control the motor and secretory functions of the intestine.

Physiology of the autonomic nervous system

- The autonomic system controls smooth muscle (visceral and vascular), exocrine (and some endocrine) secretions, rate and force of the heart and certain metabolic processes (e.g. glucose utilisation).
- Sympathetic and parasympathetic systems have opposing actions in some situations (e.g. control of heart rate, gastrointestinal smooth muscle) but not in others (e.g. salivary glands, ciliary muscle).
- Sympathetic activity increases in stress (fight-or-flight response) whereas parasympathetic activity predominates during satiation and repose. Both systems exert a continuous physiological control of specific organs under normal conditions, when the body is at neither extreme.

particular organ or tissue according to the need of the moment. Cannon rightly emphasised the general role of the sympathetic system in evoking 'fight-or-flight' reactions in an emergency, but emergencies are rare for most animals. In everyday life, the autonomic nervous system functions continuously to control specific local functions, such as adjustments to postural changes or exercise (see Jänig & MacLachlan 1992); the popular concept of a continuum from the extreme 'rest-and-digest' state (parasympathetic active, sympathetic quiescent) to the extreme emergency 'fight-or-flight' state (sympathetic active, parasympathetic quiescent) is a misleading oversimplification.

Table 9.1 lists some of the more important autonomic responses in humans.

TRANSMITTERS IN THE AUTONOMIC NERVOUS SYSTEM

The two main neurotransmitters that operate in the autonomic system are **acetylcholine** and **noradrenaline**; their sites of action are shown diagrammatically in Figure 9.2. This diagram also shows the type of postsynaptic receptor with which the transmitters interact at the different sites. (Discussed more fully in Chs 10 and 11.) Some general rules apply.

- All motor nerve fibres leaving the CNS release acetylcholine, which acts on nicotinic receptors (although in autonomic ganglia a minor component of excitation is the result of activation of muscarinic receptors (see Ch. 10).
- All postganglionic parasympathetic fibres release acetylcholine, which acts on muscarinic receptors.
- All postganglionic sympathetic fibres (with one important exception) release noradrenaline, which may act on either α- or β-adrenoceptors (see Ch. 11). The exception is the sympathetic innervation of sweat glands, where transmission is caused by acetylcholine acting on muscarinic receptors. In some species, but not humans, vasodilatation in skeletal muscle is produced by cholinergic sympathetic nerve fibres.

Acetylcholine and noradrenaline are the grandees among autonomic transmitters and are central to understanding autonomic pharmacology. However, many other chemical mediators are also released by autonomic neurons (see below), and their functional significance is gradually becoming clearer.

SOME GENERAL PRINCIPLES OF CHEMICAL TRANSMISSION

The essential processes in chemical transmission—the release of mediators and their interaction with receptors on target cells—are described in Chapters 4 and 3, respectively. Here we consider some general characteristics of chemical transmission of particular relevance to pharmacology. Many of these principles apply also to the CNS and are taken up again in Chapter 31.

DALE'S PRINCIPLE

Dale's principle, advanced in 1934, states, in its modern form: 'A mature neurone releases the same transmitter (or transmitters) at all of its synapses'.

▼ Dale considered it unlikely that a single neuron could store and release different transmitters at different nerve terminals, and his view has been substantiated by physiological and neurochemical evidence. It is known, for example, that the axons of motor neurons have branches that synapse on interneurons in the spinal cord, in addition to the main branch that innervates skeletal muscle fibres in the periphery. The transmitter at both the central and the peripheral nerve endings is acetylcholine, in accordance with Dale's principle.

Recent work, however (see Marder, 1999), suggests that there are situations where different transmitters are released from different terminals of the same neuron. Further, we now know that most neurons release more than one transmitter (see Co-transmission, below) and may change their transmitter repertoire, for example during development or in response to injury. Moreover (see below), the balance of the cocktail of mediators released by a nerve terminal can vary with stimulus conditions, and in response to presynaptic modulators. Dale's principle was, of course, framed long before these complexities were discovered, and it has probably now outlived its usefulness, though purists seem curiously reluctant to let it go.

DENERVATION SUPERSENSITIVITY

It is known, mainly from the work of Cannon on the sympathetic system, that if a nerve is cut and its terminals allowed to degenerate, the structure supplied by it becomes supersensitive to the transmitter substance released by the terminals. For example, skeletal muscle, which normally responds to injected acetylcholine only if a large dose is given directly into the arterial blood supply, will, after denervation, respond by contracture to much smaller amounts. Other organs, such as salivary glands and blood vessels, show similar supersensitivity to acetylcholine and noradrenaline when the postganglionic nerves degenerate, and there is evidence that pathways in the CNS show the same phenomenon.

▼ Several mechanisms are known to contribute to denervation supersensitivity, and the extent and mechanism of the phenomenon varies from organ to organ.

- *Proliferation of receptors* This is particularly marked in skeletal muscle, in which the number of acetylcholine receptors increases 20-fold or more after denervation; the receptors, normally localised to the endplate region of the fibres, spread over the whole surface. Elsewhere, much smaller increases in receptor number (about twofold) have often been reported, but there are examples where no change occurs.
- *Loss of mechanisms for transmitter removal* At noradrenergic synapses, the loss of neuronal uptake of noradrenaline (see Ch. 11) contributes substantially to denervation supersensitivity. At cholinergic synapses, a partial loss of cholinesterase occurs (see Ch. 10).
- *Increased postjunctional responsiveness* In some cases, the postsynaptic cells become supersensitive without a corresponding increase in the number of receptors. For example, smooth muscle cells become partly depolarised and hyperexcitable, and this phenomenon contributes appreciably to their supersensitivity. The mechanism of this change and its importance for other synapses is not known.

Table 9.1 The main effects of the autonomic nervous system

Organ	Sympathetic effect	Adrenergic receptor type	Parasympathetic effect	Cholinergic receptor type
Heart				
Sinoatrial node	Rate ↑	β_1	Rate ↓	M_2
Atrial muscle	Force ↑	β_1	Force ↓	M_2
Atrioventricular node	Automaticity ↑	β_1	Conduction velocity ↓	M_2
			Atrioventricluar block	M_2
Ventricular muscle	Automaticity ↑ Force ↑	β_1	No effect	
Blood vessels				
Arterioles				
Coronary	Constriction	α		
Muscle	Dilatation	β_2	No effect	
Viscera	Constriction	α	No effect	
Skin	Constriction	α	No effect	
Brain	Constriction	α	No effect	
Erectile tissue	Constriction	α	Dilatation	? M_3
Salivary gland	Constriction	α	Dilatation	? M_3
Veins	Constriction	α	No effect	
	Dilatation	β_2	No effect	
Viscera				
Bronchi				
Smooth muscle	No sympathetic innervation, but dilated by circulating adrenaline	β_2	Constriction	M_3
Glands	No effect		Secretion	M_3
Gastrointestinal tract				
Smooth muscle	Motility ↓	α_1, α_2, β_2	Motility ↑	M_3
Sphincters	Constriction	α_2, β_2	Dilatation	M_3
Glands	No effect		Secretion	M_3
			Gastric acid secretion	M_1
Uterus				
Pregnant	Contraction	α	Variable	
Non-pregnant	Relaxation	β_2		
Male sex organs	Ejaculation	α	Erection	? M_3
Eye				
Pupil	Dilatation	α	Constriction	M_3
Ciliary muscle	Relaxation (slight)	β	Contraction	M_3
Skin				
Sweat glands	Secretion (mainly cholinergic)	α	No effect	
Pilomotor	Piloerection	α	No effect	
Salivary glands	Secretion	α, β	Secretion	M_3
Lacrimal glands	No effect		Secretion	M_3
Kidney	Renin secretion	β_2	No effect	
Liver	Glycogenolysis Gluconeogenesis	α, β_2	No effect	

The adrenergic and cholinergic receptor types shown are described more fully in Chapters 10 and 11. Transmitters other than acetylcholine and noradrenaline contribute to many of these responses (see Table 9.2).

Supersensitivity can occur, but is less marked, when transmission is interrupted by processes other than nerve section. For example, if pharmacological block of ganglionic transmission is sustained for a few days, it causes some degree of supersensitivity of the target organs; long-term blockade of postsynaptic receptors also causes receptors to proliferate, leaving the cell supersensitive when the blocking agent is removed. Phenomena such as this are of importance in the CNS, where such supersensitivity can cause 'rebound' effects when drugs that impair synaptic transmission are given for some time and then stopped.

PRESYNAPTIC MODULATION

The presynaptic terminals that synthesise and release transmitter in response to electrical activity in the nerve fibre are often themselves sensitive to transmitter substances and to other substances that may be produced locally in tissues (for reviews see Starke et al., 1989; Fuder & Muscholl, 1995). Such presynaptic effects most commonly act to inhibit transmitter release, but they may enhance it. Figure 9.3 shows the inhibitory effect of adrenaline on the release of acetylcholine (evoked by electrical stimulation) from the postganglionic parasympathetic nerve terminals of the intestine. The release of noradrenaline from nearby sympathetic nerve terminals can also inhibit release of acetylcholine. Noradrenergic and cholinergic nerve terminals often lie close together in the myenteric plexus; consequently, the opposing effects of the sympathetic and parasympathetic systems result not only from the opposite effects of the two transmitters on the smooth muscle cells but also from the inhibition of acetylcholine release by noradrenaline acting on the parasympathetic nerve terminals. A similar situation exists in the heart, where a mutual presynaptic inhibition has been demonstrated; noradrenaline inhibits acetylcholine release, as in the myenteric plexus, and acetylcholine also inhibits noradrenaline release. These are examples of *heterotropic* interactions, where one neurotransmitter affects the release of another. *Homotropic* interactions also occur, where the transmitter, by binding to presynaptic autoreceptors, affects the nerve terminals from which it is being released. This type of autoinhibitory feedback acts powerfully at noradrenergic nerve terminals (Starke et al., 1989). One of the strongest pieces of evidence is that the amount of noradrenaline released from tissues in response to repetitive stimulation of sympathetic nerves is increased 10-fold or more in the presence of an antagonist that blocks the presynaptic noradrenaline receptors (Ch. 11). This suggests that the released noradrenaline can inhibit further release by at least 90%.

A similar state of affairs probably exists also at cholinergic nerve terminals, where release of transmitter can also be increased by antagonists that block the autoinhibitory action of acetylcholine on the terminal. In both the noradrenergic and cholinergic systems, the presynaptic autoreceptors are pharmacologically distinct from the postsynaptic receptors (see Chs 10 and 11), and there are drugs that act selectively, as agonists or antagonists, on the pre- or postsynaptic receptors.

Cholinergic and noradrenergic nerve terminals respond not only to acetylcholine and noradrenaline, as described above, but also to other substances that are released as co-transmitters, such as *ATP* and *neuropeptide Y*, or derived from other sources, including *nitric oxide, prostaglandins, adenosine, dopamine, 5-HT, gamma-aminobutyric acid (GABA), opioid peptides* and many other substances. The physiological role and pharmacological significance of these various interactions is still unclear (see review by Vizi, 2001), but the description of the autonomic nervous system represented in Figure 9.1 is undoubtedly oversimplified. Figure 9.4 shows some of the main presynaptic interactions between autonomic neurons and summarises the many chemical influences that regulate transmitter release from noradrenergic neurons.

Presynaptic receptors regulate transmitter release mainly by affecting Ca^{2+} entry into the nerve terminal (see Ch. 4). Most presynaptic receptors are of the G-protein-coupled type (see Ch. 3), which control the function of calcium and potassium channels, either through second messengers that regulate the state of phosphorylation of the channel proteins or by a direct interaction of G-proteins with the channels. Transmitter release is inhibited when calcium channel opening is inhibited, or when potassium channel opening is increased (see Ch. 4); in many cases, both mechanisms operate simultaneously. Presynaptic regulation by receptors linked directly to ion channels (ionotropic receptors, see Ch. 3), rather than to G-proteins also occurs (see MacDermott et al., 1999). Nicotinic acetylcholine receptors are particularly important in this respect. They facilitate the release of other transmitters, such as glutamate (see Ch. 32), and it is believed that most of the nicotine receptors expressed in the CNS are located presynaptically. Another example is the $GABA_A$ receptor, which acts to inhibit transmitter release (see Chs 4 and 32). It is likely

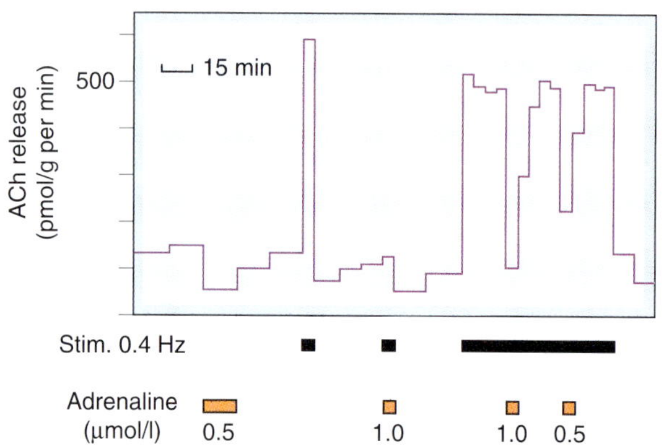

Fig. 9.3 Inhibitory effect of adrenaline on acetylcholine (ACh) release from postganglionic parasympathetic nerves in the guinea-pig ileum. The intramural nerves were stimulated electrically where indicated, and the acetylcholine released into the bathing fluid determined by bioassay. Adrenaline strongly inhibits acetylcholine release. (From: Vizi E S 1979 Prog Neurobiol 12: 181.)

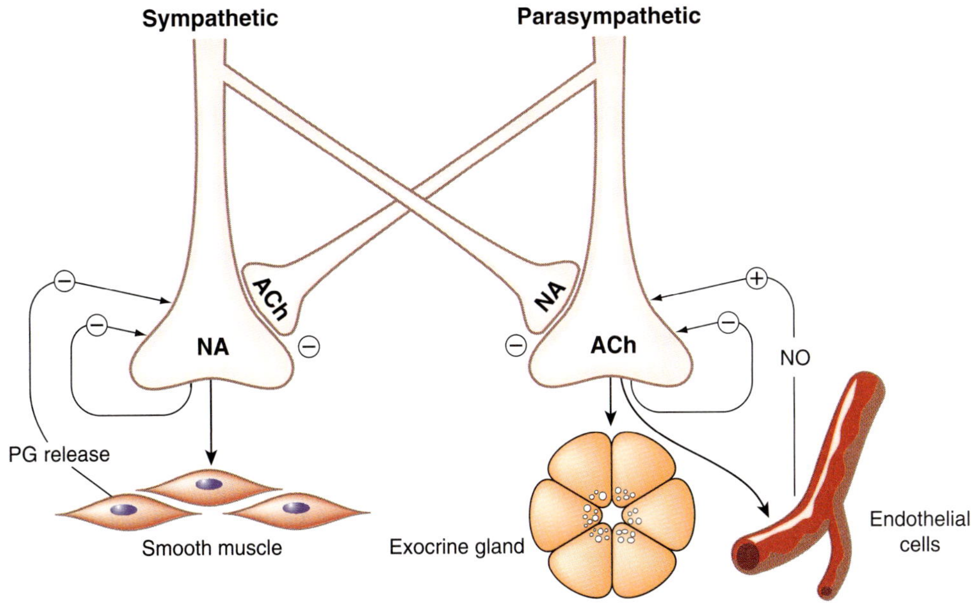

B

Mediator	Receptor type
ACh	Musc.
NA/A	α_2
5-HT	5-HT_1
Adenosine	P_1
PGE	EP
Histamine	H_2
Enkephalin	δ
Dopamine	D_2
ATP	P_2

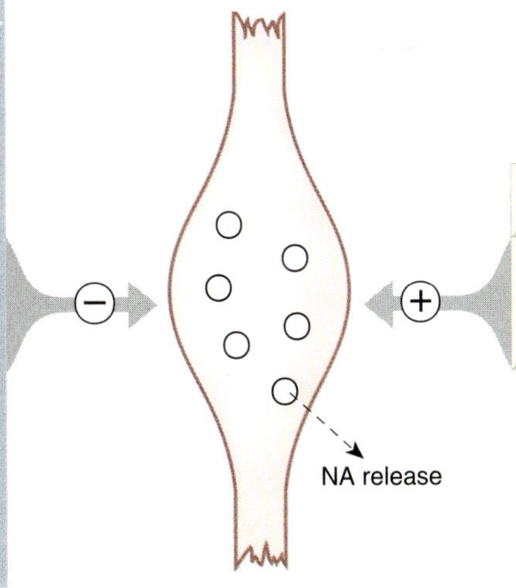

Receptor type	Mediator
β_2	A
AT_1	Angiotensin II

Fig. 9.4 Presynaptic regulation of transmitter release from noradrenergic and cholinergic nerve terminals. A Postulated homotropic and heterotropic interactions between sympathetic and parasympathetic nerves. B Some of the known inhibitory and facilitatory influences on noradrenaline release from sympathetic nerve endings. (ACh, acetylcholine; A, adrenaline; NA, noradrenaline; NO, nitric oxide; NPY, neuropeptide Y; PG, prostaglandin; PGE, prostaglandin E; 5-HT, 5-hydroxytryptamine.)

that other ionotropic receptors, such as those activated by ATP and 5-HT (Ch. 12), also affect transmitter release, but the evidence is less conclusive than that for acetylcholine and GABA.

POSTSYNAPTIC MODULATION

Chemical mediators often act on postsynaptic structures, including neurons, smooth muscle cells, cardiac muscle cells, etc., in such a way that their excitability or spontaneous firing pattern is altered. In many cases, as with presynaptic modulation, the mechanisms appear to involve changes in calcium and/or potassium channel function mediated by a second messenger. We give only a few examples here.

- The slow excitatory effect produced by various mediators, including acetylcholine and peptides such as substance P (see Ch. 40), on many peripheral and central neurons results mainly from a decrease in K^+ permeability. By comparison, the inhibitory effect of various opiates is mainly a result of increased K^+ permeability.
- **Benzodiazepine** tranquillisers (Ch. 36) act directly on receptors for GABA (Ch. 32) to facilitate their inhibitory effect. There is some evidence that drugs such as **galantamine** act similarly on nicotinic acetylcholine receptors to facilitate the excitatory effect of acetylcholine in the brain, which may have relevance for the use of such drugs to treat dementia (see Ch. 34).
- Neuropeptide Y, which is released as a co-transmitter with noradrenaline at many sympathetic nerve endings, enhances the vasoconstrictor effect of noradrenaline, thus greatly facilitating transmission (Fig. 9.5); the mechanism is not known.

The pre- and postsynaptic effects described above are often described as *neuromodulation* since the mediator acts to increase or decrease the efficacy of synaptic transmission without participating directly as a transmitter. Many neuropeptides, for example, affect membrane ion channels in such a way as to increase or decrease excitability, and thus control the firing pattern of the cell. Neuromodulation is a loosely defined term, and we cannot distinguish unequivocally, on functional, anatomical or biochemical grounds, exactly how a neurotransmitter differs from a neuromodulator. In general, though, neuromodulation involves slower processes (taking seconds to days) than neurotransmission (which occurs in milliseconds); furthermore, neuromodulation operates through cascades of intracellular messengers (Ch. 3), rather than directly on ligand-gated ion channels. Some aspects of this problem of terminology are discussed in Chapter 15.

TRANSMITTERS OTHER THAN ACETYLCHOLINE AND NORADRENALINE

As mentioned above, acetylcholine or noradrenaline are not the only autonomic transmitters. The rather grudging realisation that this was so dawned many years ago when it was noticed that autonomic transmission in many organs could not be completely blocked by drugs that abolish responses to these transmitters. The dismal but tenacious term *non-noradrenergic non-cholinergic* (*NANC*) transmission was coined. Later, fluorescence and immunocytochemical methods showed that neurons, including autonomic neurons, contain many potential transmitters, often several in the same cell. Compounds believed to function as NANC transmitters include ATP, vasoactive intestinal peptide, neuropeptide Y and nitric oxide (see Fig. 9.6 and Table 9.2), which function at postganglionic nerve terminals, as well as substance P, 5-HT, GABA and dopamine, which play a role in ganglionic transmission (see Lundberg (1996) for a comprehensive review).

CO-TRANSMISSION

It is probably the rule rather than the exception that neurons release more than one transmitter or modulator (Lundberg, 1996), each of which interacts with specific receptors and produces effects, often both pre- and postsynaptically. We are only just beginning to understand the functional implications of this

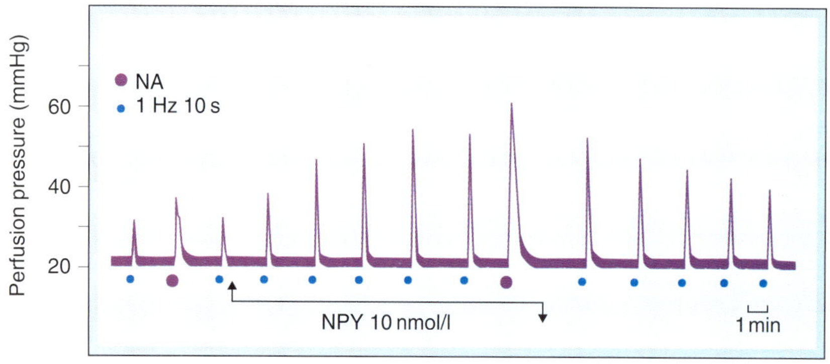

Fig. 9.5 Effect of neuropeptide Y (NPY) on noradrenergic transmission. Vasoconstriction (upward deflection) of the rabbit ear artery occurs in response to injections of noradrenaline (NA) or to a brief period of sympathetic nerve stimulation. Infusion of a low concentration of NPY greatly increases the response to both. (From: Rand M J et al. 1987 Cardiovasc Pharmacol 10(suppl 12): S33–S44.)

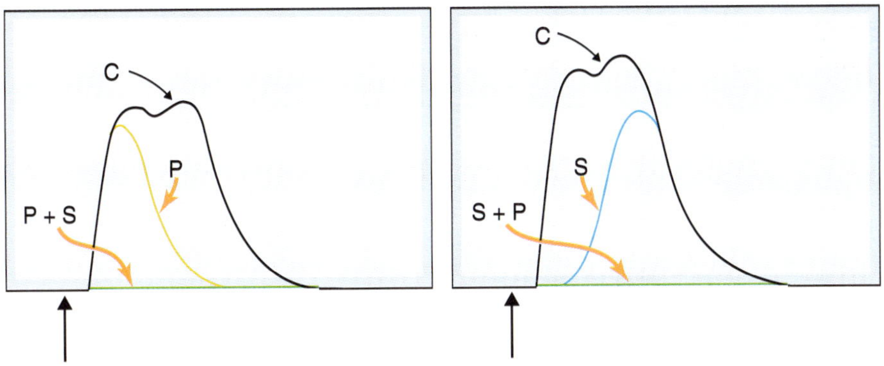

Fig. 9.6 Noradrenaline/ATP cotransmission in the guinea-pig vas deferens. Contractions of the tissue are shown in response to a single electrical stimulus causing excitation of sympathetic nerve endings. With no blocking drugs present, a twin-peaked response is produced (C). The early peak is selectively abolished by the ATP antagonist suramin (S), while the late peak is blocked by the α_1-adrenoceptor antagonist prazosin (P). The response is completely eliminated when both drugs are present. (Reproduced with permission from: von Kugelglen & Starke 1991 Trends Pharmacol Sci 12: 319–324.)

(Kupfermann, 1991). The example of noradrenaline/ATP co-transmission at the sympathetic nerve endings is shown in Figure 9.6, and the best-studied examples and mechanisms are summarised in Table 9.2 and Figures 9.7 and 9.8.

What, one might well ask, could be the functional advantage of co-transmission, compared with a single transmitter acting on various different receptors? There are at least two possible advantages.

- One constituent of the cocktail (e.g. a peptide) may be removed or inactivated more slowly than the other (e.g. a monoamine) and, therefore, reach targets further from the site of release and produce longer-lasting effects. This appears to be the case, for example, with acetylcholine and gonadotrophin-releasing hormone in sympathetic ganglia (Jan & Jan, 1983).
- The balance of the transmitters released may vary under different conditions. At sympathetic nerve terminals, for example, where noradrenaline and neuropeptide Y are stored in separate vesicles, the latter is preferentially released at high stimulation frequencies (Stjarne, 1989), so differential release of one or other mediator may result from varying impulse patterns. Differential effects of presynaptic modulators are also possible; for example, activation of β-adrenoceptors inhibits ATP release, while enhancing noradrenaline release from sympathetic nerve terminals (Gonçalves et al., 1996).

Transmitters of the autonomic nervous system

- The principal transmitters are acetylcholine and noradrenaline.
- Preganglionic neurons are cholinergic; ganglionic transmission occurs via nicotinic acetylcholine receptors (though excitatory muscarinic acetylcholine receptors are also present on postganglionic cells).
- Postganglionic parasympathetic neurons are cholinergic, acting on muscarinic receptors in target organs.
- Postganglionic sympathetic neurons are mainly noradrenergic, though a few are cholinergic (e.g. sweat glands).
- Transmitters other than noradrenaline and acetylcholine (NANC transmitters) are also used extensively in the autonomic nervous system. The main ones are nitric oxide and vasoactive intestinal peptide (parasympathetic), ATP and neuropeptide Y (sympathetic). Others, such as 5-hydroxytryptamine (5-HT), gamma-aminobutyric acid (GABA) and dopamine, also play a role.
- Cotransmission is a general phenomenon.

TERMINATION OF TRANSMITTER ACTION

Chemically transmitting synapses other than the peptidergic variety (Ch. 13) invariably incorporate a mechanism for rapidly disposing of the released transmitter, so that its action remains brief and localised. At cholinergic synapses (Ch. 10), the released acetylcholine is inactivated very rapidly in the synaptic cleft by acetylcholinesterase, but in most cases (see Fig. 9.9), transmitter action is terminated by active reuptake into the presynaptic nerve, or into supporting cells such as glia. Such reuptake depends on transporter proteins, each being specific for a particular transmitter (Borowsky & Hoffmann, 1995; Nelson, 1998). These

Table 9.2 Examples of NANC (non-noradrenergic, non-cholinergic) transmitters and cotransmitters in the peripheral nervous system

Transmitter	Location	Function
Non-peptides		
ATP	Postganglionic sympathetic neurons (e.g. blood vessels, vas deferens)	Fast depolarisation/contraction of smooth muscle cells
GABA, 5-HT	Enteric neurons	Peristaltic reflex
Dopamine	Some sympathetic neurons (e.g. kidney)	Vasodilatation
NO	Pelvic nerves	Erection
NO	Gastric nerves	Gastric emptying
Peptides		
Neuropeptide Y	Postganglionic sympathetic neurons (e.g. blood vessels)	Facilitates constrictor action of NA; inhibits NA release
VIP	Parasympathetic nerves to salivary glands NANC innervation of airways smooth muscle	Vasodilatation; cotransmitter with ACh Bronchodilatation
GnRH	Sympathetic ganglia	Slow depolarisation; cotransmitter with ACh
Substance P	Sympathetic ganglia	Slow depolarisation
	Enteric neurons	Cotransmitter with ACh
CGRP Substance P	Non-myelinated sensory neurons	Vasodilatation; vascular leakage; neurogenic inflammation

GABA, gamma-aminobutyric acid; 5-HT, 5-hydroxytryptamine; NO, nitric oxide; NA, noradrenaline; ACh, acetylcholine; GnRH, gonadotrophin-releasing hormone; CGRP, calcitonin gene-related peptide; VIP, vasoactive intestinal peptide.

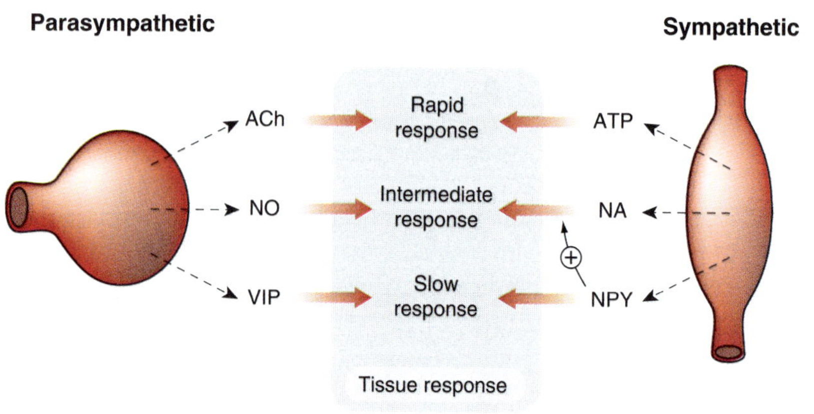

Fig. 9.7 The main cotransmitters at postganglionic parasympathetic and sympathetic neurons. The different mediators generally give rise to fast, intermediate and slow responses of the target organ. (ACh, acetylcholine; NO, nitric oxide; VIP, vasoactive intestinal peptide; NA, noradrenaline; NPY, neuropeptide Y.)

proteins belong to a distinct family of membrane proteins, each possessing 12 transmembrane helices. Different members of the family show selectivity for each of the main monoamine transmitters (e.g. the *norepinephrine transporter, NET*, which transports noradrenaline, the *serotonin transporter, SERT*, which transports 5-HT); transporters for glutamate and GABA show greater diversity, several subtypes of each having been described (Seal & Amara, 1999; Nestler et al., 2001). *Vesicular transporters* (Ch. 4), which load synaptic vesicles with transmitter molecules, are closely related to the membrane transporters. Membrane transporters usually act as co-transporters of Na^+, Cl^- and transmitter molecules, and it is the inwardly directed 'downhill' gradient for Na^+ that provides the energy for the inward 'uphill' movement of the transmitter. The simultaneous transport of ions along with the transmitter means that the process generates a net current across the membrane,

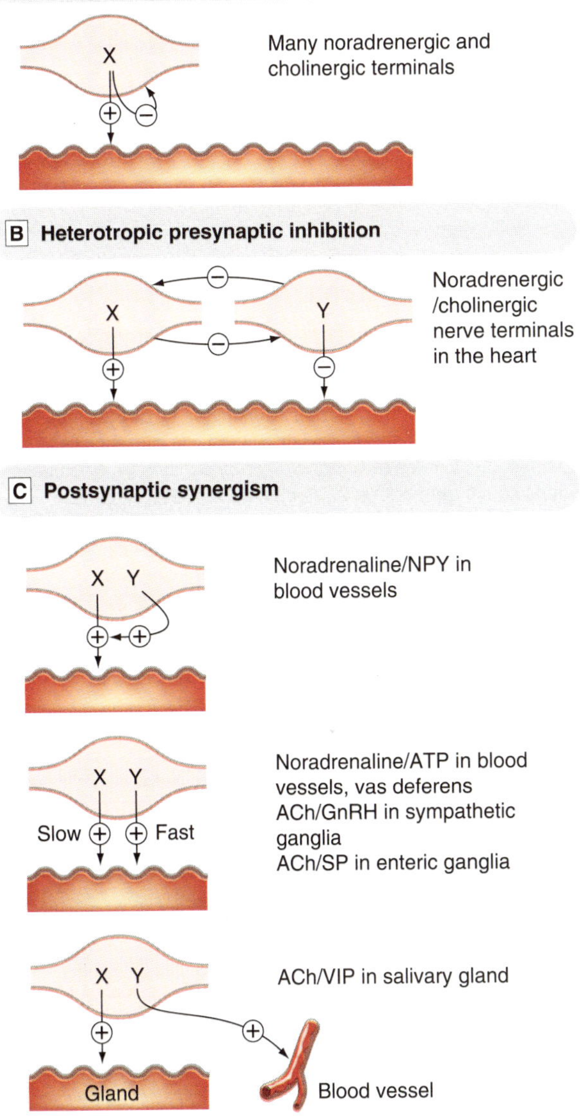

Fig. 9.8 Co-transmission and neuromodulation—some examples. A Presynaptic inhibition. B Heterotropic presynaptic inhibition. C Postsynaptic synergism. (ACh, acetylcholine; NPY, neuropeptide Y; GnRH, gonadotrophin-releasing hormone (luteinising hormone-releasing hormone); SP, substance P; VIP, vasoactive intestinal peptide.)

which can be measured directly and used to monitor the transport process (Brew & Attwell, 1988). Very similar mechanisms are responsible for other physiological transport processes, such as glucose uptake (Ch. 25) and renal tubular transport of amino acids. Since it is the electrochemical gradient for Na^+ that drives the inward transport of transmitter molecules, a reduction of this gradient can reduce or even reverse the flow of transmitter. This is probably not important under normal conditions, but when the nerve terminals are depolarised or abnormally loaded with Na^+ (e.g. in ischaemic conditions; see Attwell et al. 1993) the resulting non-vesicular release of transmitter (and inhibition of the normal synaptic reuptake mechanism) may play a significant role in the effects of ischaemia on tissues such as heart and brain (see Chs 17 and 34).

As we shall see in subsequent chapters, both membrane and vesicular transporters are the target for various drug effects, and defining the physiological role and pharmacological properties of these molecules is the focus of much current research.

BASIC STEPS IN NEUROCHEMICAL TRANSMISSION: SITES OF DRUG ACTION

Figure 9.9 summarises the main processes that occur in a classical chemically transmitting synapse and provides a useful basis for understanding the actions of the many different classes of drug, discussed in later chapters, which act by facilitating or blocking neurochemical transmission.

All of the steps shown in Figure 9.9 (except for transmitter diffusion, step 8) can be influenced by drugs. For example, the enzymes involved in synthesis or inactivation of the transmitter can be inhibited by drugs, as can the transport systems responsible for the neuronal and vesicular uptake of the transmitter or its precursor. The actions of the great majority of drugs that act on the peripheral nervous system (Chs 10 and 11) and the CNS fit into this general scheme.

Neuromodulation and presynaptic interactions

- As well as functioning directly as neurotransmitters, chemical mediators may regulate:
  —presynaptic transmitter release
  —neuronal excitability.
- Both are examples of neuromodulation, and generally involve second messenger regulation of membrane ion channels.
- Presynaptic receptors may inhibit or increase transmitter release, the former being more important.
- Inhibitory presynaptic autoreceptors occur on noradrenergic and cholinergic neurons, causing each transmitter to inhibit its own release (autoinhibitory feedback).
- Many endogenous mediators (e.g. gamma-aminobutyric acid (GABA), prostaglandins, opioid and other peptides) as well as the transmitters themselves exert presynaptic control (mainly inhibitory) over autonomic transmitter release.

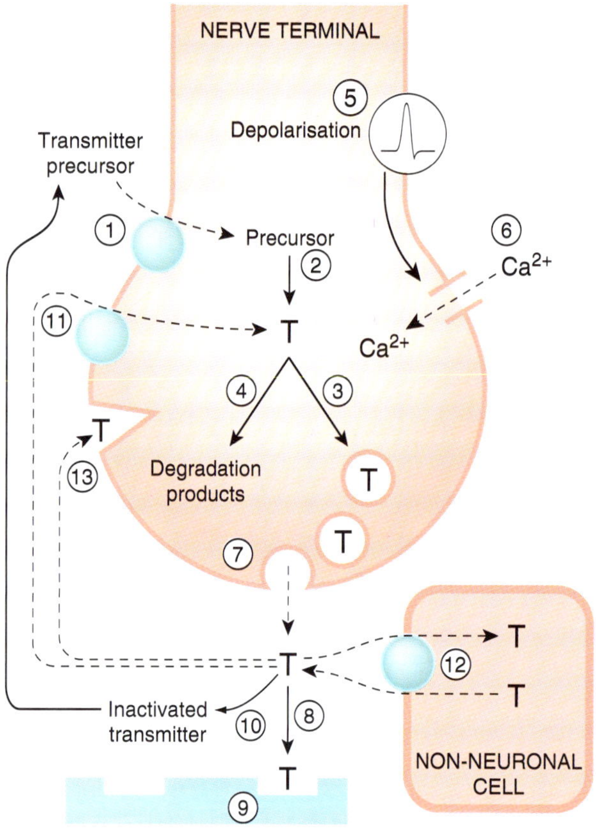

Fig. 9.9 The main processes involved in synthesis, storage and release of amine and amino acid transmitters. 1, uptake of precursors; 2, synthesis of transmitter; 3, storage of transmitter in vesicles; 4, degradation of surplus transmitter; 5, depolarisation by propagated action potential; 6, influx of Ca^{2+} in response to depolarisation; 7, release of transmitter by exocytosis; 8, diffusion to postsynaptic membrane; 9, interaction with postsynaptic receptors; 10, inactivation of transmitter; 11, reuptake of transmitter or degradation products by nerve terminals; 12, uptake of transmitter by non-neuronal cells; 13, interaction with presynaptic receptors. The transporters (11 and 12) can release transmitter under certain conditions by working in reverse. These processes are well characterised for many transmitters (e.g. acetylcholine, monoamines, amino acids, ATP). Peptide mediators (see Ch.13) differ in that they may be synthesised and packaged in the cell body rather than the terminals.

REFERENCES AND FURTHER READING

Appenzeller O, Oribe E 1997 The autonomic nervous system: an introduction to basic and clinical concepts, 5th edn. Elsevier, New York (*Comprehensive textbook*)

Attwell D, Barbour B, Szatkowski M 1993 Non-vesicular release of neurotransmitter. Neuron 11: 401–407 (*Summarises evidence for, and potential significance of, non-vesicular release*)

Bacq Z M 1975 Chemical transmission of nerve impulses: a historical sketch. Pergamon Press, Oxford (*Lively account of the history of the discovery of chemical transmission*)

Borowsky B, Hoffmann B J 1995 Neurotransmitter transporters: molecular biology, function and regulation. Int Rev Neurobiol 38: 139–199 (*Detailed review article*)

Brading A F 1999 The autonomic nervous system and its effectors. Blackwell, Oxford

Brew H, Attwell D I 1988 Electrogenic glutamate uptake is a major current carrier in the membrane of axolotl retinal ganglion cells. Nature 327: 707–709 (*Elegant physiological analysis of glutamate transport by neurons*)

Broadley K J 1996 Autonomic Pharmacology. Taylor & Francis, London (*Comprehensive textbook*)

Cooper J C, Bloom F E, Roth R H 1996 The biochemical basis of neuropharmacology, 7th edn. Oxford University Press, New York (*Excellent general account, covering a broad area of neuropharmacology*)

Fuder H, Muscholl E 1995 Heteroreceptor-mediated modulation of noradrenaline and acetylcholine release from peripheral nerves. Rev Physiol Biochem Pharmacol 126: 263–412 (*Comprehensive review of presynaptic modulation*)

Furness J B, Costa M 1987 The enteric nervous system. Churchill Livingstone, Edinburgh

Gonçalves J, Bueltmann R, Driessen B 1996 Opposite modulation of cotransmitter release in guinea-pig vas deferens: increase of noradrenaline and decrease of ATP release by activation of prejunctional β-receptors. Naunyn-Schmiedebergs Arch Pharmacol 353: 184–192 (*Shows that presynaptic regulation can affect specific transmitters in different ways*)

Goyal R K, Hirano I 1996 The enteric nervous system. N Engl J Med 334: 1106–1115 (*Excellent review article*)

Jan Y N, Jan L Y 1983 A LHRH-like peptidergic neurotransmitter capable of 'action at a distance' in autonomic ganglia. Trends Neurosci 6: 320–325 (*Electrophysiological analysis of cotransmission*)

Jänig W, McLachlan E M 1992 Characteristics of function-specific pathways in the sympathetic nervous system. Trends Neurosci 15: 475–481 (*Short article emphasising that the sympathetic system is far from being an all-or-none alarm system*)

Kupfermann I 1991 Functional studies of cotransmission. Physiol Rev 71: 683–732 (*Good review article*)

Lundberg J M 1996 Pharmacology of co-transmission in the autonomic nervous system: integrative aspects on amines, neuropeptides, adenosine triphosphate, amino acids and nitric oxide. Pharmacol Rev 48: 114–192 (*Detailed and informative review article*)

MacDermott A B, Role L W, Siegelbaum S A 1999 Presynaptic ionotropic receptors and the control of transmitter release. Annu Rev Pharmacol 22: 442–485 (*Detailed review of presynaptic ionotropic receptor mechanisms—as distinct from the more familiar G-protein-coupled receptors—controlling transmitter release*)

Marder E 1999 Neural signalling: does colocalization imply cotransmission? Curr Biol 9: R809–R811 (*Short commentary on a paper showing that a particular neuron in the crab nervous system releases different transmitters at different terminals: a rare example which directly contradicts Dale's principle*)

Nelson N 1998 The family of Na^+/Cl^- neurotransmitter transporters. J Neurochem 71: 1785–1803 (*Review article describing the molecular characteristsics of the different familes of neurotransporters*)

Nestler E J , Hyman S E, Malenka R C 2001 Molecular neuropharmacology. McGraw-Hill, New York (*A very good advanced textbook covering the actions of mediators and neuroactive drugs at the molecular and cellular level*)

Seal R P, Amara S G 1999 Excitatory amino acid transporters: a family in

flux. Annu Rev Pharmacol Toxicol 39: 431–456 (*Review article describing the molecular properties of glutamate transporters and their possible role in brain disorders*)
Starke K, Gothert M, Kilbinger H 1989 Modulation of neurotransmitter release by presynaptic autoreceptors. Physiol Rev 69: 864–989 (*Comprehensive review article*)
Stjarne L 1989 Basic mechanisms and local modulation of nerve impulse-induced secretion of neurotransmitters from individual sympathetic nerve varicosities. Rev Physiol Biochem Pharmacol 112: 4–137 (*Excellent review on presynaptic regulation*)
Vizi E S 2001 Role of high-affinity receptors and membrane transporters in non-synaptic communication and drug action in the central nervous system. Pharmacol Rev 52: 63–89 (*Comprehensive review on pharmacological relevance of presynaptic receptors and transporters. Useful for reference*)

10 Cholinergic transmission

Overview 136

Muscarinic and nicotinic actions of acetylcholine 136

Acetylcholine receptors 137
- Nicotinic receptors 137
- Muscarinic receptors 137

Physiology of cholinergic transmission 139
- Acetylcholine synthesis and release 139
- Electrical events in transmission at cholinergic synapses 141

Effects of drugs on cholinergic transmission 143
- Drugs affecting muscarinic receptors 143
- Drugs affecting autonomic ganglia 147
- Neuromuscular-blocking drugs 149
- Drugs acting presynaptically 154
- Drugs that enhance cholinergic transmission 155

OVERVIEW

This chapter is concerned mainly with cholinergic transmission in the periphery, and the ways in which drugs affect it. Cholinergic mechanisms in the central nervous system (CNS) and their relevance to dementia are discussed in Chapters 31 and 34.

MUSCARINIC AND NICOTINIC ACTIONS OF ACETYLCHOLINE

The discovery of the pharmacological action of acetylcholine arose from work on adrenal glands. Adrenal extracts were known to produce a rise in blood pressure owing to their content of adrenaline. In 1900, Reid Hunt found that after adrenaline had been removed from such extracts, they produced a fall in blood pressure instead of a rise. He attributed the fall to their content of choline but later concluded that a more potent derivative of choline must be responsible. With Taveau he tested a number of choline derivatives and discovered that acetylcholine was some 100 000 times more active than choline in lowering the rabbit's blood pressure. Although Hunt's studies suggested that acetylcholine was present in tissues, its physiological function was not apparent at that time and it remained a pharmacological curiosity until Dale and his colleagues discovered its transmitter role in the 1930s.

In a study of the pharmacological actions of acetylcholine carried out in 1914, Dale distinguished two types of activity, which he designated as *muscarinic* and *nicotinic*. The muscarinic actions of acetylcholine are those that can be reproduced by the injection of **muscarine**, the active principle of the poisonous mushroom *Amanita muscaria*, and can be abolished by small doses of **atropine** (the poisonous constituent of deadly nightshade). On the whole, muscarinic actions correspond to those of parasympathetic stimulation, as shown in Table 9.1. After the muscarinic effects have been blocked by atropine, larger doses of acetylcholine produce another set of effects, closely similar to those of **nicotine**. They include:

- stimulation of all autonomic ganglia
- stimulation of voluntary muscle
- secretion of adrenaline from the adrenal medulla.

The muscarinic and nicotinic actions of acetylcholine are demonstrated in Figure 10.1 in an experiment on the blood pressure of an anaesthetised cat. Small and medium doses of acetylcholine produce a transient fall in blood pressure owing to arteriolar vasodilatation and slowing of the heart—muscarinic effects that are abolished by atropine. A large dose of acetylcholine given after atropine produces nicotinic effects: an initial rise in blood pressure owing to a stimulation of sympathetic ganglia and consequent vasoconstriction, and a secondary rise resulting from secretion of adrenaline.

Dale's classification was originally made on pharmacological grounds, but it corresponds closely to the main physiological functions of acetylcholine in the body. The muscarinic actions correspond to those of acetylcholine released at postganglionic parasympathetic nerve endings, with two significant exceptions:

- Acetylcholine causes generalised vasodilatation, even though most blood vessels have no parasympathetic innervation. This is an indirect effect: acetylcholine (like many other

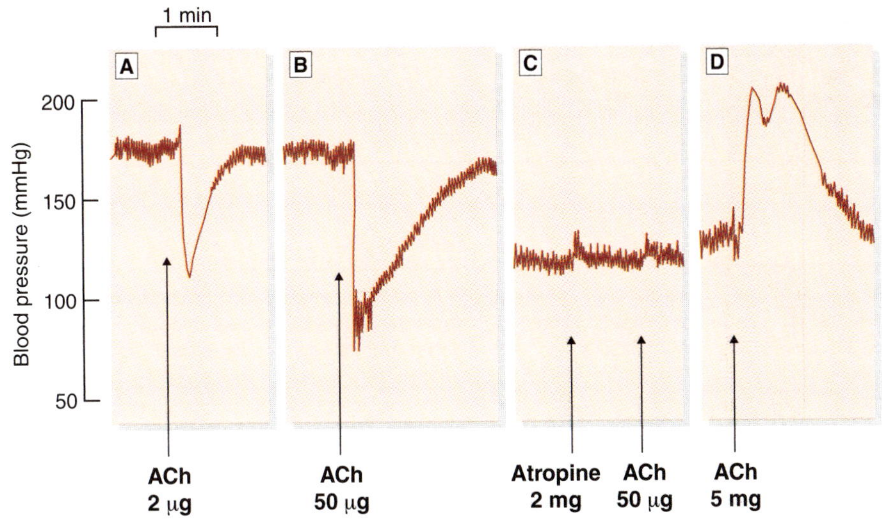

Fig. 10.1 Dale's experiment showing that acetylcholine (ACh) produces two kinds of effect on the cat's blood pressure. Arterial pressure was recorded with a mercury manometer from a spinal cat. [A] ACh causes a fall in blood pressure owing to vasodilatation. [B] A larger dose also produces bradycardia. Both A and B are muscarinic effects. [C] After atropine (muscarinic antagonist), the same dose of ACh has no effect. [D] Still under the influence of atropine, a much larger dose of ACh causes a rise in blood pressure (by stimulation of sympathetic ganglia), accompanied by tachycardia, followed by a secondary rise (owing to release of adrenaline from the adrenal gland). These effects result from its action on nicotinic receptors. (From: Burn J H 1963 Autonomic pharmacology. Blackwell, Oxford.)

mediators) acts on vascular endothelial cells to release nitric oxide; see Ch. 14) which relaxes smooth muscle. The physiological function of this is uncertain, since acetylcholine is not normally present in circulating blood.

- Acetylcholine evokes secretion from sweat glands, which are innervated by cholinergic fibres of the sympathetic nervous system (see Table 9.1).

The nicotinic actions correspond to those of acetylcholine acting on autonomic ganglia of the sympathetic and parasympathetic systems, the motor endplate of voluntary muscle and the secretory cells of the adrenal medulla.

ACETYLCHOLINE RECEPTORS

Though Dale himself dismissed the concept of receptors as sophistry rather than science, his classification provided the basis for distinguishing the two major classes of acetylcholine receptor (see Ch. 3): nicotinic and muscarinic.

NICOTINIC RECEPTORS

Nicotinic receptors fall into three main classes, the muscle, ganglionic and CNS types; they are typical of ligand-gated ion channels (Fig. 3.4, p. 30) and their subunit composition is summarised in Table 10.1. Muscle receptors are confined to the skeletal neuromuscular junction; ganglionic receptors are responsible for transmission at sympathetic and parasympathetic ganglia; CNS-type receptors are widespread in the brain and are heterogeneous with respect to their molecular composition and location (see Ch. 34).

▼ All nicotinic receptors are pentameric structures which function as ligand-gated ion channels (see Ch. 3). The five subunits that form the receptor–channel complex are similar in structure, and so far 16 different members of the family have been identified and cloned, designated α (nine types), β (four types), γ, δ and ε (one of each). The five subunits each possess four membrane-spanning helical domains, and one of these helices (M_2) from each subunit defines the central pore (see Ch. 3). All but one of the various nicotine receptor subtypes contain α- and β-subunits, the exception being the $(\alpha7)_5$ subtype found mainly in the brain (Ch. 34). The adult muscle receptor has the composition $(\alpha1)_2\beta1\gamma\varepsilon$ while the main ganglionic subtype is $(\alpha3)_2(\beta4)_3$. The two binding sites for acetylcholine (both of which need to be occupied to cause the channel to open) reside at the interface between the extracellular domain of each of the α-subunits and its neighbour. The diversity of the nicotine receptor family (see Trends in Neuroscience Supplement, 2000, for details) which emerged from cloning studies in the 1980s, took pharmacologists somewhat by surprise. Though they knew that the neuromuscular and ganglionic synapses differed pharmacologically, and suspected that cholinergic synapses in the CNS might be different again, the actual extent of the diversity goes far beyond this, and the functional significance of what has been revealed remains largely unknown (for reviews, see McGehee & Role (1995) and Cordero-Erauskin et al. (2000)).

The different action of agonists and antagonists on ganglionic and neuromuscular synapses is of practical importance and mainly reflects the differences between the muscle and neuronal nicotinic receptors (Table 10.1).

MUSCARINIC RECEPTORS

Gene cloning has revealed five distinct types of muscarinic receptor (see Wess, 1996), but only four have been distinguished

Table 10.1 Nicotinic acetylcholine receptor subtypes

Characteristic	Muscle type: $(\alpha1)_2\beta1\delta\varepsilon$ (adult form)	Ganglion type: $(\alpha3)_2(\beta4)_3$	CNS type		Comment
			$(\alpha4)_2(\beta2)_3$	$(\alpha7)_5$	
Main synaptic location	Skeletal neuromuscular junction: mainly postsynaptic	Autonomic ganglia: mainly postsynaptic	Many brain regions: pre- and postsynaptic	Many brain regions: pre- and postsynaptic	
Membrane response	Excitatory Increased cation permeability (mainly Na^+, K^+)	Excitatory Increased cation permeability (mainly Na^+, K^+)	Pre- and postsynaptic excitation Increased cation permeability (mainly Na^+, K^+)	Pre- and postsynaptic excitation Increased Ca^{2+} permeability	$(\alpha7)_5$ receptor produces large Ca^{2+} entry, evoking transmitter release
Agonists	ACh CCh Suxamethonium	ACh CCh Nicotine Epibatidine, DMPP	Nicotine Epibatidine ACh Cytosine	Epibatidine DMPP	$(\alpha4)_2(\beta2)_3$ is responsible for CNS effects of nicotine $(\alpha7)$ is brain bungarotoxin-binding site (Ch. 33)
Antagonists Atracurium Vecuronium α-Bungarotoxin α-Conotoxin	Tubocurarine Pancuronium Hexamethonium α-Conotoxin	Mecamylamine Trimetaphan	Mecamylamine Methylaconitine α-Conotoxin	Methylaconitine α-Bungarotoxin	

Ach, acetylcholine; CCh, carbachol; DMPP, dimethylphenylpiperazinium
Note: This table shows only the main subtypes expressed in mammalian tissues. Several other subtypes are expressed in selected brain regions, and also in the peripheral nervous system and in non-neuronal tissues. For further details, see Chapter 33, and reviews by indstrom (2000), Jones et al. (1999), Cordero-Erausquin et al (2000).

functionally and pharmacologically (see Goyal, 1989). Three of these (M_1, M_2, M_3) are well characterised (Table 10.2). M_1-receptors ('neural') are found mainly on CNS and peripheral neurons and gastric parietal cells. They mediate excitatory effects, for example the slow muscarinic excitation mediated by acetylcholine in sympathetic ganglia (Ch. 9) and central neurons. This excitation is produced by a decrease in K^+ conductance, which causes membrane depolarisation. Deficiency of this kind of acetylcholine-mediated effect in the brain is possibly associated with dementia (see Ch. 34). M_1-receptors are also involved in the increase of gastric acid secretion following vagal stimulation (see Ch. 24).

M_2-receptors ('cardiac') occur in the heart, and also on the presynaptic terminals of peripheral and central neurons. They exert inhibitory effects, mainly by increasing K^+ conductance and by inhibiting calcium channels (see Ch. 4). M_2-receptor activation is responsible for the vagal inhibition of the heart, as well as presynaptic inhibition in the CNS and periphery (Ch. 9).

M_3-receptors ('glandular/smooth muscle') produce mainly excitatory effects, i.e. stimulation of glandular secretions (salivary, bronchial, sweat, etc.) and contraction of visceral smooth muscle. M_3-receptors also mediate relaxation (mainly vascular) of smooth muscle, which results from the release of nitric oxide from neighbouring endothelial cells (Ch. 14). M_1-, M_2- and M_3-receptors occur also in specific locations in the CNS (see Ch. 27). M_4- and M_5-receptors are largely confined to the CNS, and their functional role is not well understood.

The pharmacological classification of these receptor types relies on the limited selectivity of certain agonists and antagonists that can distinguish between them. Most agonists are non-selective, but two experimental compounds, **McNA343** and **oxotremorine**, are selective for M_1-receptors; **carbachol** is relatively inactive on these receptors. There is more selectivity amongst antagonists. Though most of the classical muscarinic antagonists (e.g. **atropine**, **hyoscine**) are non-selective, **pirenzepine** is selective for M_1-receptors. **Gallamine**, better known as a neuromuscular-blocking drug (see p. 150), is also a selective M_2-receptor antagonist. Recently, toxins from the venom of the green mamba have been discovered to be highly selective muscarinic receptor antagonists (see Table 10.2), and there are also various synthetic compounds with some degree of selectivity (see Eglen et al. (1999) for more details). Compounds that have recently been approved for clinical use are described below (p. 145)

Muscarinic receptors all belong to the family of G-protein-coupled receptors (Ch. 3). The odd-numbered members of the

Table 10.2 Muscarinic acetylcholine receptor subtypes

Characteristic	M_1 ('neural')	M_2 ('cardiac')	M_3 ('glandular/smooth muscle')	M_4	M_5
Main locations	CNS: cortex, hippocampus Glands: gastric, salivary, etc	Heart: atria Smooth muscle: GI tract CNS: widely distributed	Exocrine glands: gastric, salivary, etc. Smooth muscle: GI tract, eye Blood vessels: endothelium	?Lung CNS: cortex, striatum	CNS: very localised expression in substantia nigra Salivary glands Iris/ciliary muscle
Cellular response	↑ IP_3, DAG Depolarisation Excitation (slow epsp) ↑ K^+ conductance	↓ cAMP Inhibition ↓ Ca^{2+} conductance ↑ K^+ conductance	↑ IP_3 Stimulation ↑ $[Ca^{2+}]_i$	As M_2	As M_3
Functional response	CNS excitation (?memory) Gastric secretion	Cardiac inhibition Neural inhibition Central muscarinic effects, e.g. tremor, hypothermia	Gastric, salivary secretion GI smooth muscle contraction Ocular accommodation Vasodilatation	Enhanced locomotion	Not known
Agonists (non-selective, except those in italics)	ACh Carbachol Oxotremorine *McNA343*	As M_1	As M_1	As M_1	As M_1
Antagonists (non-selective, except those in italics)	Atropine Dicycloverine* (dicyclomine) Tolterodine Oxybutynin Ipratropium *Pirenzepine* *Mamba toxin MT7*	Atropine Dicycloverine Tolterodine Oxybutynin Ipratropium *Gallamine*	Atropine Dicycloverine Tolterodine Oxybutynin Ipratropium	Atropine Dicycloverine Tolterodine Oxybutynin Ipratropium *Mamba toxin MT3*	Atropine Dicycloverine Tolterodine Oxybutynin Ipratropium

IP_3, inositol trisphosphate; DAG, diacylglycerol; GI, gastrointestinal.
Note: This table shows only the predominant subtypes expressed in mammalian tissues. All subtypes are expressed in selected brain regions, and also in the peripheral nervous system and in non-neuronal tissues. For further details, see Chapter 33, and reviews by Lindstrom (2000), Jones et al. (1999), Cordero-Erausquin et al (2000).
*Previously known as dicyclomine.

group (M_1, M_3, M_5) act through the inositol phosphate pathway (p. 36), while the even-numbered receptors (M_2, M_4) act by inhibiting adenylate cyclase and thus reducing intracellular cAMP (see Goyal, 1989).

PHYSIOLOGY OF CHOLINERGIC TRANSMISSION

The physiology of cholinergic transmission is described in detail by Ginsborg & Jenkinson (1976) and Nicholls et al. (2001). The main ways in which drugs can affect cholinergic transmission are shown in Figure 10.2.

▼ Acetylcholine is synthesised and stored in many tissues that lack cholinergic innervation, such as the placenta and cornea. Despite speculation about possible regulatory and trophic functions, (see review by Wessle et al., 1998), the role of non-neuronal acetycholine is uncertain.

ACETYLCHOLINE SYNTHESIS AND RELEASE

Acetylcholine metabolism is well reviewed by Parsons et al. (1993). Acetylcholine is synthesised within the nerve terminal from choline, which is taken up into the nerve terminal by a specific carrier (Ch. 9), similar to that which operates for many transmitters. The difference is that it transports the precursor choline, not acetylcholine, so it is not important in terminating the action of the transmitter. The concentration of choline in the blood and body fluids is normally about 10 μmol/l, but it increases in the immediate vicinity of cholinergic nerve terminals, probably to about 1 mmol/l, when the released

Acetylcholine receptors

- Main subdivision is into nicotinic (nAChR) and muscarinic (mAChR) subtypes.
- nAChRs are directly coupled to cation channels and mediate fast excitatory synaptic transmission at the neuromuscular junction, autonomic ganglia and at various sites in the CNS. Muscle and neuronal nAChR differ in their molecular structure and pharmacology.
- Both mAChR and nAChR occur presynaptically as well as postsynaptically and function to regulate transmitter release.
- mAChRs are G-protein-coupled receptors, causing:
  - —activation of phospholipase C (hence formation of inositol trisphosphate and diacylglycerol as second messengers)
  - —inhibition of adenylate cyclase
  - —activation of potassium channels or inhibition of calcium channels.
- mAChR mediate acetylcholine effects at postganglionic parasympathetic synapses (mainly heart, smooth muscle, glands), and contribute to ganglionic excitation. They occur in many parts of the CNS.
- Three main types of mAChR occur:
  - —M_1-receptors ('neural'), producing slow excitation of ganglia; they are selectively blocked by pirenzepine
  - —M_2-receptors ('cardiac'), causing decrease in cardiac rate and force of contraction (mainly of atria) and also mediate presynaptic inhibition: they are selectively blocked by gallamine
  - —M_3-receptors ('glandular'), causing secretion, contraction of visceral smooth muscle, vascular relaxation.
- All mAChR are activated by ACh and blocked by atropine. There are also subtype-selective agonists and antagonists.

acetylcholine is hydrolysed. More than 50% of this choline is normally recaptured by the nerve terminals. Free choline within the nerve terminal is acetylated by a cytosolic enzyme, *choline acetyltransferase*, which transfers the acetyl group from acetyl-CoA. The rate-limiting process in acetylcholine synthesis appears to be choline transport, the activity of which is regulated according to the rate at which acetylcholine is being released. *Cholinesterase* is present in the presynaptic nerve terminals and acetylcholine is continually being hydrolysed and resynthesised. Inhibition of the nerve terminal cholinesterase causes the accumulation of 'surplus' acetylcholine in the cytosol, which is not available for release by nerve impulses (though it is able to leak out via the choline carrier). Most of the acetylcholine synthesised, however, is packaged into synaptic vesicles, in which its concentration is very high (about 100 mmol/l), from where release occurs by exocytosis, triggered by Ca^{2+} entry into the nerve terminal (see Ch. 9).

Cholinergic vesicles accumulate acetylcholine actively, by means of a specific transporter (Usdin et al., 1995; Liu & Edwards, 1997) belonging to the family of amine transporters described in Chapter 9. Accumulation of acetylcholine is coupled to the large electrochemical gradient for H^+ that exists between intracellular organelles and the cytosol; it is blocked selectively by the experimental drug **vesamicol** (Parsons et al., 1993). Following its release, the acetylcholine diffuses across the synaptic cleft* to combine with receptors on the postsynaptic cell. Some of it succumbs on the way to hydrolysis by acetylcholinesterase (AChE), an enzyme which is bound to the basement membrane that lies between the pre- and postsynaptic membranes. At fast cholinergic synapses (e.g. the neuromuscular and ganglionic synapses), but not at slow ones (smooth muscle, gland cells, heart, etc.), the released acetylcholine is hydrolysed very rapidly (within 1 ms), so that it acts only very briefly.

At the neuromuscular junction, which is a highly specialised synapse, a single nerve impulse releases about 300 synaptic vesicles (altogether about three million acetylcholine molecules) from the nerve terminals supplying a single muscle fibre, which contain altogether about three million synaptic vesicles. Approximately two million acetylcholine molecules combine with receptors, of which there are about 30 million on each muscle fibre, the rest being hydrolysed without reaching a receptor. The acetylcholine molecules remain bound to receptors for, on average, about 2 ms, and are quickly hydrolysed after dissociating so that they cannot combine with a second receptor. The result is that transmitter action is very rapid and very brief, which is important for a synapse that has to initiate speedy muscular responses, and which may have to transmit signals faithfully at high frequency. Muscle cells are much larger than neurons and require much more synaptic current to generate an action potential. Consequently, all of the chemical events happen on a larger scale than at a neuronal synapse: the number of transmitter molecules in a quantum, the number of quanta released and the number of receptors activated by each quantum are all 10–100 times greater. Our brains would be huge, but not very clever, if their synapses were built on the industrial scale of the neuromuscular junction.

PRESYNAPTIC MODULATION

Acetylcholine release is regulated by mediators, including acetylcholine itself, acting on presynaptic receptors, as discussed in Chapter 9. At postganglionic parasympathetic nerve endings, inhibitory M_2-receptors participate in autoinhibition of acetylcholine release (see Kilbinger, 1984); other mediators, such as noradrenaline, also inhibit the release of acetylcholine (see Ch. 9). At the neuromuscular junction, in contrast, presynaptic

*At postsynaptic parasympathetic nerve terminals (e.g. those supplying intestinal smooth muscle) there is often no clearly defined 'synaptic cleft', such as exists at the neuromuscular or ganglionic synapse, and the transmitter may have to diffuse tens of micrometres to its site of actions.

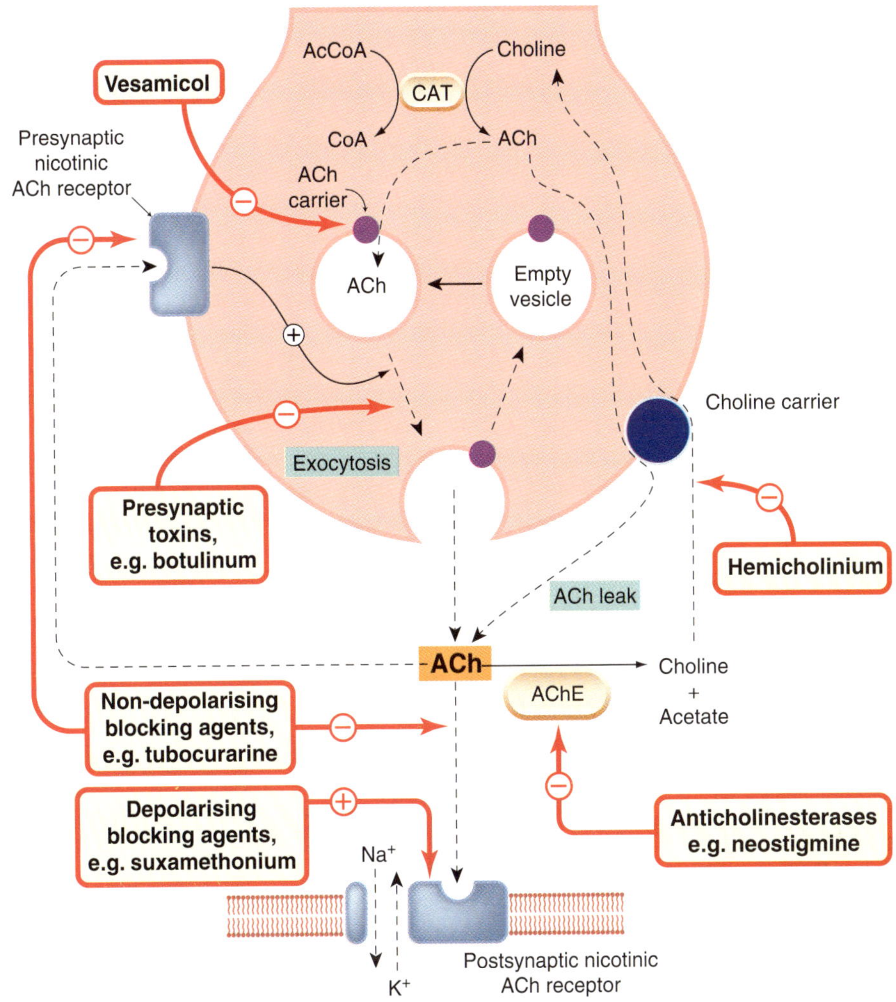

Fig. 10.2 Events and sites of drug action at a nicotinic cholinergic synapse. Acetycholine (ACh) is shown acting postsynaptically on a nicotinic receptor controlling a cation channel (e.g. at the neuromuscular or ganglionic synapse), and also on a presynaptic nicotine receptor, which acts to facilitate ACh release during sustained synaptic activity. The nerve terminal also contains acetylcholinesterase (not shown); when this is inhibited, the amount of free ACh, and the rate of leakage of ACh via the choline carrier, are increased. Under normal conditions, this leakage of ACh is insignificant. At muscarinic cholinergic junctions (e.g. heart, smooth muscle, exocrine glands), both postsynaptic and presynaptic (inhibitory) receptors are of the muscarinic type. (AcCoA, acetyl coenzyme A; CoA, coenzyme A; CAT, choline acetyltransferase; AChE, acetylcholinesterase.)

nicotinic receptors are believed to facilitate acetylcholine release (see Prior et al., 1995), a mechanism that may allow the synapse to function reliably during prolonged high-frequency activity. In the brain (see review by Wonnacott, 1997) most of the nicotinic receptors are located presynaptically and serve to facilitate transmission by other mediators, such as glutamate and dopamine.

ELECTRICAL EVENTS IN TRANSMISSION AT CHOLINERGIC SYNAPSES

Acetylcholine, acting on the postsynaptic membrane of a nicotinic (neuromuscular or ganglionic) synapse, causes a large increase in its permeability to cations, particularly to Na^+ and K^+, and to a lesser extent, Ca^{2+}. Because of the large inwardly directed electrochemical gradient for Na^+ across the cell membrane, an inflow of Na^+ occurs, causing depolarisation of the postsynaptic membrane. This transmitter-mediated depolarisation is called an *endplate potential* (epp) in a skeletal muscle fibre (Ginsborg & Jenkinson, 1976), or a *fast excitatory postsynaptic potential* (fast epsp) at the ganglionic synapse (Skok, 1980). In a muscle fibre, the localised epp spreads to adjacent, electrically excitable parts of the muscle fibre; if its amplitude reaches the threshold for excitation, an action potential is initiated, which propagates to the rest of the fibre and evokes a contraction (Ch. 4).

In a nerve cell, depolarisation of the soma or a dendrite by the fast epsp causes a local current to flow. This depolarises the axon hillock region of the cell, where, if the epsp is large enough, an action potential is initiated. Figure 10.3 shows that **tubocurarine**, a drug that blocks postsynaptic acetylcholine receptors (see p. 150), reduces the amplitude of the fast epsp until it no longer initiates an action potential, though the cell is still capable of responding when it is stimulated antidromically. Most ganglion cells are supplied by several presynaptic axons, and it requires simultaneous activity in more than one to make the postganglionic cell fire. At the neuromuscular junction, only one nerve fibre supplies each muscle fibre. Nevertheless, the amplitude of the epp is normally more than enough to initiate an action potential—indeed transmission still occurs when the epp is

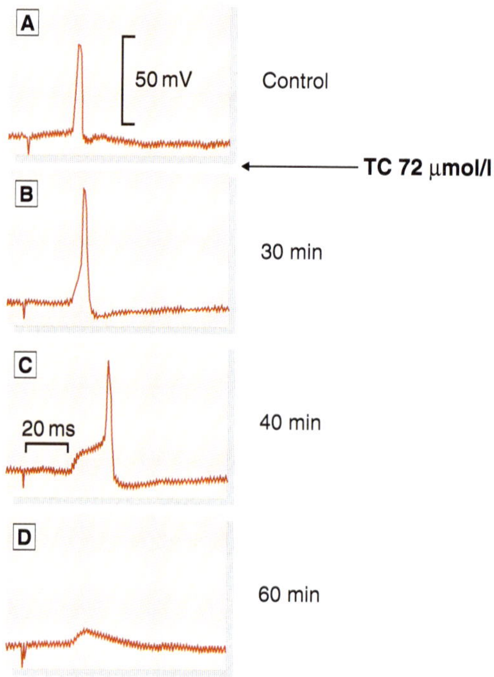

Fig. 10.3 Cholinergic transmission in an autonomic ganglion cell. Records were obtained with an intracellular microelectrode from a guinea-pig parasympathetic ganglion cell. The artefact at the beginning of each trace shows the moment of stimulation of the preganglionic nerve. Tubocurarine (TC), an acetylcholine antagonist, causes the exitatory postsynaptic potential (epsp) to become smaller. In record C it only just succeeds in triggering the action potential, and in D it has fallen below the threshold. Following complete block, antidromic stimulation (not shown) will still produce an action potential (cf. depolarisation block, Fig.10.4). (From: Blackman J G et al. 1969 J Physiol 201: 723.)

reduced by 70–80% and is said to show a large *margin of safety* so that fluctuations in transmitter release (e.g. during repetitive stimulation) do not affect transmission.

Transmission at the ganglionic synapse is more complex than at the neuromuscular junction. Though the primary event at both is the epp or fast epsp produced by acetylcholine acting on nicotinic receptors, this is followed in the ganglion by a succession of much slower postsynaptic responses, comprising:

- a slow inhibitory (hyperpolarising) potential (slow ipsp) lasting 2–5 seconds: this mainly reflects a M_2-receptor-mediated increase in conductance of K^+, but other transmitters, such as dopamine and adenosine, also contribute
- a slow epsp, which lasts for about 10 seconds; this is produced by acetylcholine acting on M_1-receptors, which close potassium channels
- a late slow epsp, lasting for 1–2 minutes: this is thought to be mediated by a peptide cotransmitter, which may be substance P in some ganglia and a gonadotrophin-releasing hormone-like peptide in others (see Ch. 9); like the slow epsp, it is produced by a decrease in K^+ conductance.

DEPOLARISATION BLOCK

Depolarisation block occurs at cholinergic synapses when the excitatory nicotinic receptors are persistently activated by nicotinic agonists, and it results from a decrease in the electrical excitability of the postsynaptic cell. This is shown in Figure 10.4. Application of **nicotine** to a sympathetic ganglion causes a depolarisation of the cell, which at first initiates action potential discharge. After a few seconds, this discharge ceases, and transmission is blocked. The loss of electrical excitability at this time is shown by the fact that antidromic stimuli also fail to produce an action potential. The main reason for the loss of electrical excitability during a period of maintained depolarisation is that the voltage-sensitive sodium channels (see Ch. 4) become inactivated (i.e. refractory) and no longer able to open in response to a brief depolarising stimulus.

▼ A second type of effect is also seen in the experiment shown in Figure 10.4. After nicotine has acted for several minutes, the cell partially repolarises, and its electrical excitability returns; in spite of this,

Cholinergic transmission

- Acetylcholine (ACh) synthesis:
  - —requires choline, which enters the neuron via carrier-mediated transport
  - —requires acetylation of choline, utilising acetyl-CoA as source of acetyl groups, which requires choline acetyltransferase, a cytosolic enzyme found only in cholinergic neurons.
- ACh is packaged into synaptic vesicles at high concentration by carrier-mediated transport.
- ACh release occurs by Ca^{2+}-mediated exocytosis. At the neuromuscular junction (NMJ), one presynaptic nerve impulse releases 100–500 vesicles.
- At the NMJ, ACh acts on nicotinic receptors to open cation channels, producing a rapid depolarisation (endplate potential), which normally initiates an action potential in the muscle fibre. Transmission at other 'fast' cholinergic synapses (e.g. ganglionic) is similar.
- At 'fast' cholinergic synapses, ACh is hydrolysed within about 1 ms by acetylcholinesterase, so a presynaptic action potential produces only one postsynaptic action potential.
- Transmission mediated by mucarinic receptors is much slower in its time course, and synaptic structures are less clearly defined. In most cases, ACh functions as a modulator rather than as a direct transmitter.
- Main mechanisms of pharmacological block: inhibition of choline uptake, inhibition of ACh release, block of postsynaptic receptors or ion channels, persistent postsynaptic depolarisation.

transmission remains blocked. This type of secondary, non-depolarising block occurs also at the neuromuscular junction if repeated doses of the depolarising drug **suxamethonium** (see below) are used. The main factor responsible for the secondary block (known clinically as phase II block) appears to be receptor desensitisation (see Ch. 2). This causes the depolarising action of the blocking drug to subside, but transmission remains blocked because the receptors are desensitised to acetylcholine.

EFFECTS OF DRUGS ON CHOLINERGIC TRANSMISSION

As shown in Figure 10.2, drugs can influence cholinergic transmission either by acting on postsynaptic acetylcholine receptors as agonists or antagonists (Tables 10.1 and 10.2), or by affecting the release or destruction of endogenous acetylcholine.

In the rest of this chapter we describe the following groups of drugs, subdivided according to their physiological site of action:

- drugs affecting muscarinic receptors
  —muscarinic agonists
  —muscarinic antagonists
- drugs affecting ganglia
  —ganglion-stimulating drugs
  —ganglion-blocking drugs
- drugs blocking neuromuscular transmission
  —non-depolarising drugs
  —depolarising drugs
  —inhibitors of acetylcholine synthesis or release
- drugs that enhance cholinergic transmission
  —inhibitors of cholinesterase
  —stimulants of acetylcholine release.

DRUGS AFFECTING MUSCARINIC RECEPTORS

MUSCARINIC AGONISTS

Structure–activity relationships

Muscarinic agonists, as a group, are often referred to as *parasympathomimetic* because the main effects that they produce in the whole animal resemble those of parasympathetic stimulation. The structures of the most important compounds are given in Table 10.3. Acetylcholine itself and related choline esters are agonists at both muscarinic and nicotinic receptors but act more potently on the former (see Fig. 10.1). Only **bethanechol** and **pilocarpine** are now used clinically.

The key features of the acetylcholine molecule that are important for its activity are the quaternary ammonium group, which bears a positive charge, and the ester group, which bears a partial negative charge and is susceptible to rapid hydrolysis by cholinesterase. Variants of the choline ester structure (Table 10.3) have the effect of reducing the susceptibility of the compound to hydrolysis by cholinesterase, and altering the relative activity on muscarinic and nicotinic receptors.

Carbachol and **methacholine** are used as experimental tools. Bethanechol, which is a hybrid of these two molecules, is stable to hydrolysis and selective for muscarinic receptors; it is occasionally used clinically. **Pilocarpine** is a partial agonist and shows some selectivity in stimulating secretion from sweat, salivary, lacrimal and bronchial glands, and contracting iris smooth muscle (see below), with weak effects on gastrointestinal smooth muscle and the heart.

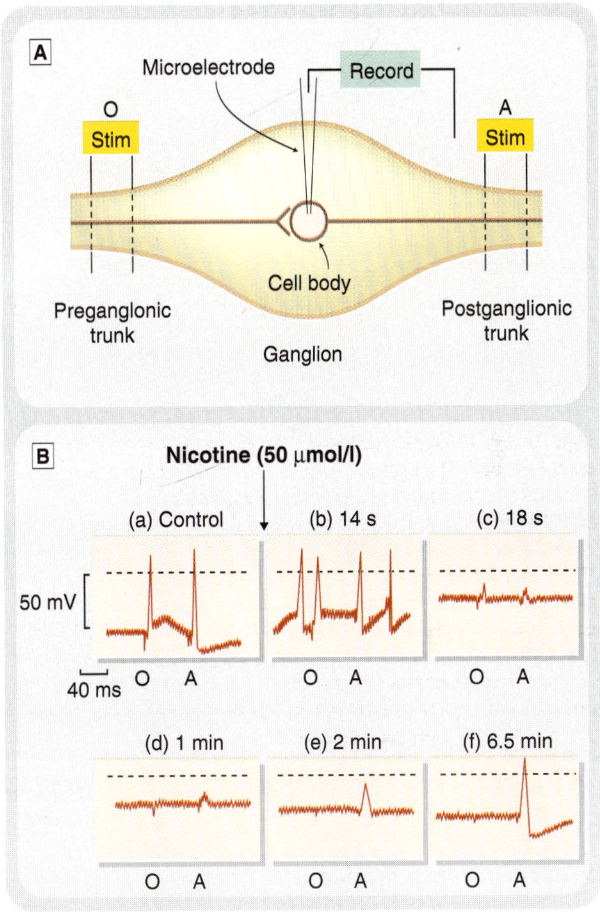

Fig. 10.4 Depolarisation block of ganglionic transmission by nicotine. A System used for intracellular recording from sympathetic ganglion cells of the frog, showing the location of orthodromic (O) and antidromic (A) stimulating (stim) electrodes. Stimulation at O excites the cell via the cholinergic synapse, whereas stimulation at A excites it by electrical propagation of the action potential. B The effect of nicotine: (a) Control records. The membrane potential is –55 mV (dotted line = 0 mV) and the cell responds to both O and A. (b) Shortly after adding nicotine the cell is slightly depolarised and spontaneously active, but still responsive to O and A. (c,d) The cell is further depolarised, to –25 mV and produces only a vestigial action potential. The fact that it does not respond to A shows that it is electrically inexcitable. (e,f) In the continued presence of nicotine, the cell repolarises and regains its responsiveness to A, but it is still unresponsive to O because the acetylcholine receptors are desensitised by nicotine. (From: Ginsborg B L, Guerrero S 1964 J Physiol 172: 189.)

Table 10.3 Muscarinic agonists

Drug	Structure	Receptor specificity		Hydrolysis by AChE	Clinical uses
		Musc	*Nic*		
Acetylcholine	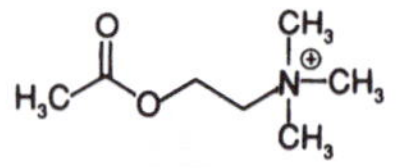	+++	+++	+++	None
Carbachol	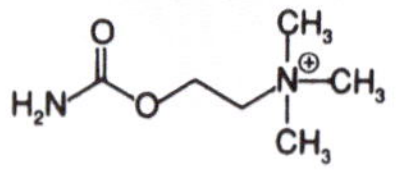	++	+++	—	None
Methacholine	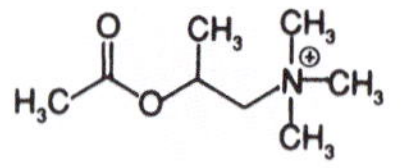	+++	+	++	None
Bethanechol	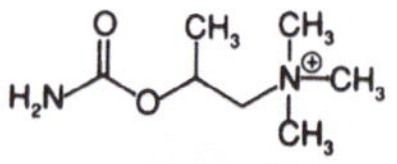	+++	—	—	Bladder* and GI hypotonia
Muscarine	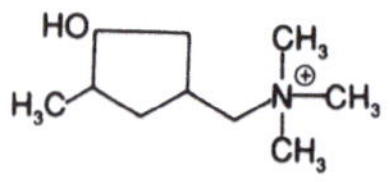	+++	—	—	None†
Pilocarpine	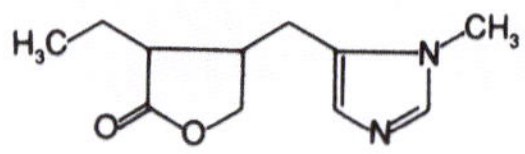	++	—	—	Glaucoma
Oxotremorine	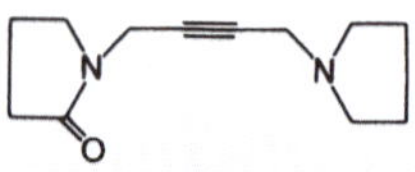	++	—	—	None

Musc, muscarinic; Nic, nicotinic.
*Necessary first to ensure that bladder neck is not obstructed.
†Cause of mushroom poisoning.

Effects of muscarinic agonists

The main actions of muscarinic agonists are readily understood in terms of the functions of the parasympathetic nervous system.

Cardiovascular effects These include cardiac slowing and a decrease in cardiac output. The latter action results mainly from a decreased force of contraction of the atria, since the ventricles have only a sparse parasympathetic innervation and a low sensitivity to muscarinic agonists. Generalised vasodilatation also occurs (a nitric oxide-mediated effect; see Ch. 14) and these two effects combine to produce a sharp fall in arterial pressure (Fig. 10.1). The mechanism of action of muscarinic agonists on the heart is discussed in Chapter 17.

Smooth muscle Smooth muscle other than vascular smooth muscle contracts in response to muscarinic agonists. Peristaltic activity of the gastrointestinal tract is increased, which can cause colicky pain, and the bladder and bronchial smooth muscle also contract.

Sweating, lacrimation, salivation and bronchial secretion These result from stimulation of exocrine glands. The combined effect of bronchial secretion and constriction can interfere with breathing.

Effects on the eye Such effects are of some importance. The parasympathetic nerves to the eye supply the *constrictor pupillae* muscle, which runs circumferentially in the iris, and the *ciliary muscle*, which adjusts the curvature of the lens (Fig. 10.5). Contraction of the ciliary muscle in response to activation of muscarinic receptors pulls the ciliary body forwards and inwards, thus relaxing the tension on the suspensory ligament of the lens, allowing the lens to bulge more and reducing its focal length. This parasympathetic reflex is, therefore, necessary to

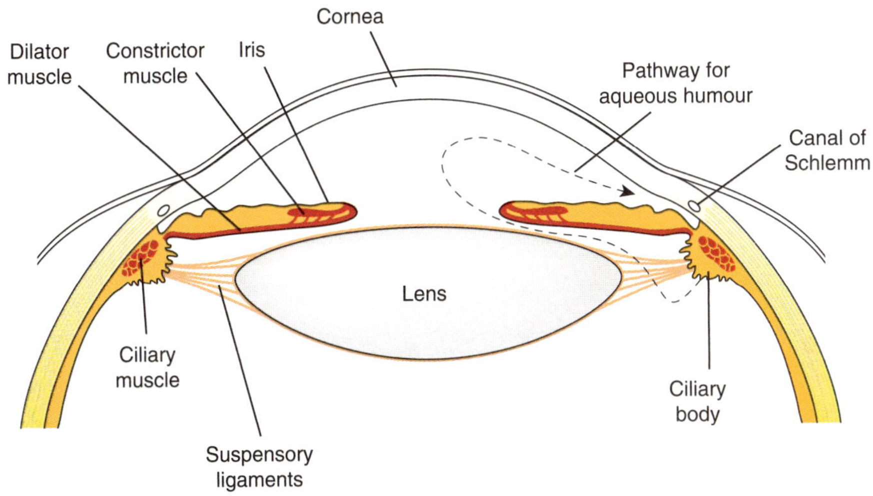

Fig. 10.5 **The anterior chamber of the eye, showing the pathway for secretion and drainage of the aqueous humour.**

accommodate the eye for near vision. The constrictor pupillae is important not only for adjusting the pupil in response to changes in light intensity but also in regulating the intraocular pressure. Aqueous humour is secreted slowly and continuously by the cells of the epithelium covering the ciliary body, and it drains into the canal of Schlemm (Fig. 10.5), which runs around the eye close to the outer margin of the iris. The intraocular pressure is normally 10–15 mmHg above atmospheric, which keeps the eye slightly distended. Abnormally raised intraocular pressure (associated with glaucoma) damages the eye and is one of the commonest preventable causes of blindness. In acute glaucoma, drainage of aqueous humour becomes impeded when the pupil is dilated because folding of the iris tissue occludes the drainage angle, causing the intraocular pressure to rise. Activation of the constrictor pupillae muscle by muscarinic agonists in these circumstances lowers the int raocular pressure, though in a normal individual it has little effect. The increased tension in the ciliary muscle produced by these drugs may also play a part in improving drainage by realigning the connective tissue trabeculae through which the canal of Schlemm passes.

Central effects In addition to these peripheral effects, muscarinic agonists that are able to penetrate the blood–brain barrier produce marked central effects, owing to activation mainly of M_1-receptors in the brain. These include tremor, hypothermia and increased locomotor activity, as well as improved cognition (see Ch. 33). M_1-selective agonists are being developed for possible use in treating dementia (see Eglen et al., 1999; Ch. 34), but are not yet in general use.

Clinical use

The main use of muscarinic agonists is in treating glaucoma, by local instillation in the form of eye drops. Pilocarpine is the most effective as, being a tertiary amine, it can cross the conjunctival membrane. It is a stable compound with an action that lasts for about 1 day.

A variety of drugs with different mechanisms of action are now available for the treatment of glaucoma and are summarised in Table 10.4.

Bethanechol is very occasionally used to assist bladder emptying or to stimulate gastrointestinal motility (Table 10.3). It acts mainly on M_3-receptors and has little effect on the heart. In principle, a selective M_2-agonist would be useful for treating cardiac dysrhythmias but such drugs remain to be discovered.

MUSCARINIC ANTAGONISTS

Muscarinic receptor antagonists (Table 10.5) are often referred to as *parasympatholytic* because they selectively block the effects of parasympathetic nerve activity. All of them are competitive antagonists, and their chemical structures usually contain ester and basic groups in the same relationship as acetylcholine, but they have a bulky aromatic group in place of the acetyl group. The two naturally occurring compounds, **atropine** and **hyoscine**, are alkaloids found in solanaceous plants. The deadly nightshade (*Atropa belladonna*) contains mainly atropine, whereas the thorn apple (*Datura stramonium*) contains mainly hyoscine. These are tertiary ammonium compounds that are sufficiently lipid soluble to be readily absorbed from the gut or conjunctival sac and, importantly, to penetrate the blood–brain barrier. The quaternary derivative of atropine, **atropine methonitrate**, has peripheral actions very similar to those of atropine but, because of its exclusion from the brain, lacks central actions. **Ipratropium**, another quaternary ammonium compound, is used by inhalation as a bronchodilator. **Cyclopentolate** and **tropicamide** are tertiary amines developed for ophthalmic use and administered as eye drops. **Pirenzepine** is a relatively selective M_1-receptor

Table 10.4 Drugs that lower intraocular pressure

Drug	Mechanism	Notes	Reference
Pilocarpine	Muscarinic agonist	Widely used as eye drops	This chapter
Ecothiopate	Anticholinesterase	Widely used as eye drops. Can cause muscle spasm and systemic effects	This chapter
Timolol, carteolol	β-Adrenoceptor antagonist	Given as eye drops but may still cause systemic side-effects: bradycardia, bronchoconstriction	Ch. 11
Acetazolamide, dorzolamide	Carbonic anhydrase inhibitor	Acetazolamide is given systemically. Side-effects include diuresis, loss of appetite, tingling, neutropenia. Dorzolamide is used as eye drops. Side-effects include bitter taste and burning sensation	Ch. 23
Clonidine, apraclonidine	α_2-Adrenoceptor agonist	Used as eye drops	Ch. 11
Latanoprost	Prostaglandin analogue	Can cause ocular pigmentation	Ch. 15

The most important drugs are shown in bold type.

antagonist. **Oxybutynin** and **tolterodine** are new drugs developed for treating urinary incontinence. Though lacking receptor selectivity, they appear to act preferentially on the bladder to inhibit micturition. Both produce unwanted effects typical of muscrinic antagonists, such as dry mouth, constipation and blurred vision.

Effects of muscarinic antagonists

All of the muscarinic antagonists produce basically similar peripheral effects, though some show a degree of selectivity (e.g. for the heart or the gastrointestinal tract), reflecting heterogeneity among muscarinic receptors (see p. 138).

The main uses of muscarinic antagonists are shown in Table 10.5 and the clinical box (p. 148). The main effects of atropine are as follows.

Atropine

Inhibition of secretions Salivary, lacrimal, bronchial and sweat glands are inhibited by very low doses of atropine, producing an uncomfortably dry mouth and skin. Gastric secretion is only slightly reduced. Mucociliary clearance in the bronchi is inhibited; as a result residual secretions tend to accumulate in the lungs. Ipratropium lacks this effect.

Effects on heart rate Atropine causes tachycardia through block of cardiac muscarinic receptors. The tachycardia is modest, up to 80–90 beats/min in humans. This is because there is no effect on the sympathetic system but only inhibition of the existing parasympathetic tone. At very low doses, atropine causes a paradoxical bradycardia, which results from a central action, increasing vagal activity. The response of the heart to exercise is unaffected. Arterial blood pressure is unaffected, since most resistance vessels have no cholinergic innervation.

Effects on the eye The pupil is dilated (*mydriasis*) by atropine administration and becomes unresponsive to light. Relaxation of the ciliary muscle causes paralysis of accommodation (*cycloplegia*); as a result, near vision is impaired. Intraocular pressure may rise; though this is unimportant in normal individuals, it can be dangerous in patients suffering from narrow-angle glaucoma.

Effects on the gastrointestinal tract Gastrointestinal motility is inhibited by atropine, though this requires larger doses than the other effects listed and the inhibition is not complete. This is because excitatory transmitters other than acetylcholine are important in normal function of the myenteric plexus (see Ch. 9). Atropine is used in pathological conditions in which there is increased gastrointestinal motility; agents selective for M_3-receptors, which are being developed, may be preferable. **Pirenzepine**, owing to its selectivity for M_1-receptors, inhibits gastric acid secretion in doses that do not affect other systems.

Effects on other smooth muscle Bronchial, biliary and urinary tract smooth muscle are all relaxed by atropine. Reflex bronchoconstriction (e.g. during anaesthesia) is prevented by atropine, whereas bronchoconstriction caused by local mediators, such as *histamine* and *leukotrienes* (e.g. in asthma; Ch. 22) is unaffected. Biliary and urinary tract smooth muscle are only slightly affected, probably because transmitters other than acetylcholine (see Ch. 6) are important in these organs; nevertheless, atropine and similar drugs commonly precipitate urinary retention in elderly men with prostatic enlargement.

Effects on the CNS Atropine produces mainly excitatory effects on the CNS. At low doses, this causes mild restlessness; higher doses cause agitation and disorientation. In atropine poisoning, which occurs mainly in young children who eat deadly nightshade berries, marked excitement and irritability result in

Table 10.5 Muscarinic antagonists

Compound	Pharmacological properties	Clinical uses	Notes
Atropine	Non-selective antagonist Well absorbed orally CNS stimulant	• Adjunct for anaesthesia (reduced secretions, bronchodilatation) • Anticholinesterase poisoning • Bradycardia • GI hypermotility (antispasmodic)	Belladonna alkaloid Main side-effects: • urinary retention • dry mouth • blurred vision Dicycloverine (dicyclomine) is similar and used mainly as antispasmodic agent
Hyoscine (scopolamine)	Similar to atropine CNS depressant	As atropine • Motion sickness	Belladonna alkaloid Causes sedation; other side-effects as atropine
Atropine methonitrate	Similar to atropine, but poorly absorbed and lacks CNS effects Significant ganglion-blocking activity	Mainly for GI hypermotility	Quaternary ammonium derivative. Similar drugs include hyoscine butylbromide, propantheline
Ipratropium	Similar to atropine methonitrate Does not inhibit mucociliary clearance from bronchi	By inhalation for asthma, bronchitis	Quaternary ammonium compound
Tropicamide	Similar to atropine May raise intraocular pressure	Ophthalmic use to produce mydriasis and cycloplegia (as eye drops) Short acting	
Cyclopentolate	Similar to tropicamide	As tropicamide (long acting)	
Pirenzepine	Selective for M_1-receptors Inhibits gastric secretion by action on ganglion cells Little effect on smooth muscle or in CNS	Peptic ulcer	Fewer side-effects than other muscarinic antagonists Largely superseded by other anti-ulcer drugs (see Ch. 24)

For chemical structures, see Hardman et al. (2001).

hyperactivity and a considerable rise in body temperature, which is accentuated by the loss of sweating. These central effects are the result of blocking muscarinic receptors in the brain, and they are opposed by anticholinesterase drugs such as **physostigmine**, which is an effective antidote to atropine poisoning. **Hyoscine** in low doses causes marked sedation but has similar effects in high dosage. Hyoscine also has a useful antiemetic effect and is used in treating motion sickness. Muscarinic antagonists also affect the extrapyramidal system, reducing the involuntary movement and rigidity of patients with Parkinson's disease (Ch. 34) and counteracting the extrapyramidal side-effects of many antipsychotic drugs (Ch. 37).

DRUGS AFFECTING AUTONOMIC GANGLIA

GANGLION STIMULANTS

Most nicotinic receptor agonists affect both ganglionic and motor endplate receptors, but **nicotine**, **lobeline** and **dimethylphenylpiperazinium** (DMPP) affect ganglia preferentially (Table 10.6).

Nicotine and lobeline are tertiary amines found in the leaves of tobacco and lobelia plants, respectively. Nicotine belongs in pharmacological folklore as it was the substance on the tip of Langley's paintbrush causing stimulation of muscle fibres when applied to the endplate region, leading him to postulate in 1905 the existence of a 'receptive substance' on the surface of the fibres (Ch. 9). DMPP is a synthetic compound that is selective for ganglionic receptors.

These substances are not used clinically, but only as experimental tools. Nicotine is discussed in Chapter 42. They cause complex peripheral responses associated with generalised stimulation of autonomic ganglia. The effects of nicotine on the gastrointestinal tract and sweat glands are familiar to neophyte smokers (see Ch. 42), though usually insufficient to act as an effective deterrent.

GANGLION-BLOCKING DRUGS

Ganglion block is often used in experimental studies on the autonomic nervous system but is of little clinical importance. It can occur by several mechanisms.

Clinical uses of muscarinic antagonists

Cardiovascular
- Treatment of sinus bradycardia (e.g. after myocardial infarction; see Ch. 17): atropine.

Ophthalmic
- To dilate the pupil: e.g. tropicamide eye drops or cyclopentolate eye drops (longer acting).

Neurological
- Prevention of motion sickness: e.g. hyoscine (orally or transdermally).
- Parkinsonism (see Ch. 34), especially to counteract movement disorders caused by antipsychotic drugs (see Ch. 37): e.g. benzhexol, benztropine.

Respiratory
- Asthma (see Ch. 22): ipratopium by inhalation.

Anaesthetic premedication
- To dry secretions: e.g. atropine, hyoscine. (Current anaesthetics are relatively non-irritant, see Ch. 35, so this use is now less important.)

Gastrointestinal
- To facilitate endoscopy and gastrointestinal radiology by relaxing gastrointestinal smooth muscle (antispasmodic action; see Ch. 24), e.g. hyoscine.
- As an antispasmodic in irritable bowel syndrome or colonic diverticular disease, e.g. dicycloverine (dicyclomine).
- To treat peptic ulcer disease by suppressing gastric acid secretion (see Ch. 24), e.g. pirenzepine (M_1-selective antagonist). This is used less since the introduction of histamine H_2-antagonists and proton pump inhibitors.

- By interference with acetylcholine release, as at the neuromuscular junction (see p. 000 and Ch. 9). **Botulinum toxin** and **hemicholinium** work in this way.
- By prolonged depolarisation. Nicotine (see Fig. 10.4) can block ganglia, after initial stimulation, in this way, as can acetylcholine itself if cholinesterase is inhibited so that it can exert a continuing action on the postsynaptic membrane.
- By interference with the postsynaptic action of acetylcholine. The few ganglion-blocking drugs of practical importance act by blocking neuronal nicotinic receptors or the associated ion channels.

▼ Paton & Zaimis, 50 years ago, investigated a series of linear bisquaternary compounds. Compounds with five or six carbon atoms (**hexamethonium**; Table 10.6) in the methylene chain linking the two quaternary groups produced ganglionic block, whereas compounds with nine or ten carbon atoms (**decamethonium**) produced neuromuscular block.*

Hexamethonium, though no longer used, deserves recognition as the first effective antihypertensive agent (see Ch. 18). The only ganglion-blocking drug currently in clinical use is **trimetaphan** (Table 10.6; see below).

At autonomic ganglia, hexamethonium and tubocurarine (see below) act exclusively on the ion channel, whereas at the neuromuscular junction, tubcurarine acts mainly on the receptor with only a small component of channel block.

Drugs acting on muscarinic receptors

Muscarinic agonists
- Important compounds include acetylcholine, carbachol, methacholine, muscarine and pilocarpine. They vary in muscarinic/nicotinic selectivity, and in susceptibility to cholinesterase.
- Main effects are bradycardia and vasodilatation (endothelium dependent), leading to fall in blood pressure; contraction of visceral smooth muscle (gut, bladder, bronchi, etc.); exocrine secretions; pupillary constriction and ciliary muscle contraction, leading to decrease of intraocular pressure.
- Main use is in treatment of glaucoma (especially pilocarpine).

Muscarinic antagonists
- Most important compounds are atropine, hyoscine, ipratropium and pirenzepine.
- Main effects are inhibition of secretions; tachycardia; pupillary dilatation and paralysis of accommodation; relaxation of smooth muscle (gut, bronchi, biliary tract, bladder); inhibition of gastric acid secretion (especially pirenzepine); CNS effects (mainly excitatory with atropine; depressant, including amnesia, with hyoscine), including antiemetic effect and antiparkinsonian effect.

Effects of ganglion-blocking drugs

The effects of ganglion-blocking drugs are numerous and complex, as would be expected, since both divisions of the autonomic nervous system are blocked indiscriminately. The description by Paton of 'hexamethonium man' cannot be bettered:

▼ He is a pink-complexioned person, except when he has stood in a queue for a long time, when he may get pale and faint. His handshake is warm and dry. He is a placid and relaxed companion; for instance he may laugh but he can't cry because the tears cannot come. Your rudest story

*Based on their structural similarity to acetylcholine, these compounds were originally believed to act as competitive antagonists. However, they are now known to act mainly by blocking the ion channel, rather than the receptor site itself.

Table 10.6 Nicotine receptor agonists and antagonists

Drugs	Main site	Type of action	Notes
Agonists			
Nicotine	Autonomic ganglia CNS	Stimulation then block Stimulation	No clinical uses For CNS effects, see Ch. 42
Lobeline	Autonomic ganglia Sensory nerve terminals	Stimulation Stimulation	
Epibatidine	Autonomic ganglia, CNS	Stimulation	Isolated from frog skin. Highly potent. No clinical uses
Suxamethonium	Neuromuscular junction	Depolarisation block	Used clinically as muscle relaxant
Decamethonium	Neuromuscular junction	Depolarisation block	No clinical use
Antagonists			
Hexamethonium	Autonomic ganglia	Transmission block	No clinical use
Trimetaphan	Autonomic ganglia	Transmission block	Blood pressure lowering in surgery (rarely used)
Tubocurarine	Neuromuscular junction	Transmission block	Now rarely used
Pancuronium Atracurium Vecuronium	Neuromuscular junction	Transmission block	Widely used as muscle relaxants in anaesthesia

will not make him blush, and the most unpleasant circumstances will fail to make him turn pale. His collars and socks stay very clean and sweet. He wears corsets and may, if you meet him out, be rather fidgety (corsets to compress his splanchnic vascular pool, fidgety to keep the venous return going from his legs). He dislikes speaking much unless helped with something to moisten his dry mouth and throat. He is long-sighted and easily blinded by bright light. The redness of his eyeballs may suggest irregular habits and in fact his head is rather weak. But he always behaves like a gentleman and never belches or hiccups. He tends to get cold and keeps well wrapped up. But his health is good; he does not have chilblains and those diseases of modern civilization, hypertension and peptic ulcer, pass him by. He gets thin because his appetite is modest; he never feels hunger pains and his stomach never rumbles. He gets rather constipated so that his intake of liquid paraffin is high. As old age comes on, he will suffer from retention of urine and impotence, but frequency, precipitancy and strangury will not worry him. One is uncertain how he will end, but perhaps if he is not careful, by eating less and less and getting colder and colder, he will sink into a symptomless, hypoglycaemic coma and die, as was proposed for the universe, a sort of entropy death.

In practice, the important effects are on the cardiovascular system. A marked fall in arterial blood pressure results mainly from block of sympathetic ganglia, which causes arteriolar vasodilatation. Most cardiovascular reflexes are blocked. In particular, the venoconstriction, that occurs normally when a subject stands up, and which is necessary to prevent the central venous pressure from falling sharply, is reduced. Standing, therefore causes a sudden fall in cardiac output and arterial pressure (postural hypotension), which can cause fainting. Similarly, the vasodilatation of vessels supplying skeletal muscle during exercise is normally accompanied by vasoconstriction elsewhere (e.g. splanchnic area) produced by sympathetic activity. If this adjustment is prevented, the overall peripheral resistance falls and the blood pressure also falls (postexercise hypotension).

Clinical use

Ganglion-blocking drugs, because of their many side-effects, are now clinically obsolete, with the exception of **trimetaphan**, a very short-acting drug that can be administered as an intravenous infusion for certain types of anaesthetic procedure. Tilting of the operating table results in controlled hypotension and is used to minimise bleeding during certain kinds of surgery. Trimetaphan can also be used to lower blood pressure as an emergency procedure.

NEUROMUSCULAR-BLOCKING DRUGS

The pharmacology of neuromuscular function is well reviewed by Bowman (1990). Drugs can block neuromuscular transmission either by acting presynaptically, to inhibit acetylcholine synthesis or release, or by acting postsynaptically, the latter being the site of action of all of the clinically important drugs (except for botulinum toxin; see below).

Clinically, neuromuscular block is used only as an adjunct to anaesthesia, when artificial ventilation is available; it is not a therapeutic intervention. The drugs that are used all work by interfering with the postsynaptic action of acetylcholine. They fall into two categories:

- non-depolarising blocking agents (the majority), which act by blocking acetylcholine receptors (and, in some cases, also by blocking ion channels)

- depolarising blocking agents, which are agonists at acetylcholine receptors.

NON-DEPOLARISING BLOCKING AGENTS

In 1856 Claude Bernard, in a famous experiment, showed that 'curare' causes paralysis by blocking neuromuscular transmission, rather than by abolishing nerve conduction or muscle contractility. Curare is a mixture of naturally occurring alkaloids found in various South American plants and used as arrow poisons by South American Indians. Many of these substances have neuromuscular-blocking activity, but the most important is **tubocurarine**, the structure of which was elucidated in 1935. Tubocurarine is now rarely used in clinical medicine, but a number of synthetic drugs with very similar actions have been developed, the most important ones being **pancuronium**, **vecuronium** and **atracurium** (Table 10.7), which differ mainly in their duration of action. **Gallamine** was the first useful synthetic successor to tubocurarine but has been superseded by compounds with fewer side-effects. These substances are all quaternary ammonium compounds, which means that they are poorly absorbed and generally rapidly excreted. They also fail to cross the placenta, which is important in relation to their use in obstetric anaesthaesia. The low oral absorption of tubocurarine allowed it to be used safely in the hunting of animals for food.

Drugs acting on autonomic ganglia

Ganglion-stimulating drugs

- Compounds include nicotine dimethylphenylpiperazinium (DMPP).
- Both sympathetic and parasympathetic ganglia are stimulated, so effects are complex, including tachycardia and increase of blood pressure, variable effects on gastrointestinal motility and secretions, increased bronchial, salivary and sweat secretions. Additional effects result from stimulation of other neuronal structures, including sensory and noradrenergic nerve terminals.
- Ganglion stimulation may be followed by depolarisation block.
- Nicotine also has important CNS effects.
- No therapeutic uses.

Ganglion-blocking drugs

- Compounds include hexamethonium, trimetaphan, tubocurarine (also nicotine; see above).
- Block all autonomic ganglia and enteric ganglia. Main effects are hypotension and loss of cardiovascular reflexes, inhibition of secretions, gastrointestinal paralysis, impaired micturition.
- Clinically obsolete, except for occasional use of trimetaphan to produce controlled hypotension in anaesthesia.

Mechanism of action

Non-depolarising blocking agents all act as competitive antagonists (see Ch. 2) at the acetylcholine receptors of the endplate, and this largely accounts for their actions. The amount of acetylcholine released by a nerve impulse normally exceeds by several fold what is needed to elicit an action potential in the muscle fibre. It is, therefore, necessary to block 70–80% of the receptor sites before transmission actually fails. When this happens, it is still possible to record a small epp in the muscle fibre though its amplitude fails to reach threshold (Fig. 10.6). In any individual muscle fibre, transmission is all-or-nothing, so graded degrees of block represent a varying proportion of muscle fibres failing to respond. In this situation, where the amplitude of epp in all of the fibres is close to threshold (just above in some, just below in others), small variations in the amount of transmitter released, or in the rate at which it is destroyed, will have a large effect on the proportion of fibres contracting; consequently, the degree of block is liable to vary according to various physiological circumstances (e.g. stimulation frequency, temperature, cholinesterase inhibition, etc.) that normally have relatively little effect on the efficiency of transmission.

In addition to blocking receptors, some of these drugs also block ion channels in a manner similar to the ganglion-blocking drugs, though this is probably of little importance in practice. Furthermore (see Prior et al., 1995), some non-depolarising blocking agents also appear to block presynaptic autoreceptors and thus inhibit the release of acetylcholine during repetitive stimulation of the motor nerve. This may play a part in causing the 'tetanic fade' seen with these drugs (see p. 153).

Effects of non-depolarising blocking drugs

The effects of non-depolarising neuromuscular-blocking agents are mainly a result of motor paralysis, though some of the drugs also produce clinically significant autonomic effects. The first muscles to be affected are the extrinsic eye muscles (causing double vision) and the small muscles of the face, limbs and pharynx (causing difficulty in swallowing). Respiratory muscles are the last to be affected and the first to recover. An experiment in 1947 in which a heroic volunteer was fully curarised under artificial ventilation established this orderly paralytic march and showed that consciousness and awareness of pain were quite normal even when paralysis was complete. The special characteristics of non-depolarising block, and the ways in which it differs from depolarisation block, are described on page 153.

Unwanted effects

The main side-effect of tubocurarine is a fall in arterial pressure, chiefly a result of ganglion block. An additional cause is the release of histamine from mast cells (see Ch. 15), which can also give rise to bronchospasm in sensitive individuals. This is unrelated to nicotinic receptors and is an effect common to many strongly basic drugs. The other non-depolarising blocking drugs, especially vecuronium, lack these side-effects and hence cause less hypotension. Gallamine, and to a lesser extent pancuronium, block muscarinic receptors, particularly in the heart, which results in tachycardia.

Table 10.7 Characteristics of neuromuscular-blocking drugs

Drug	Speed of onset	Duration of action	Main side-effects	Notes
Tubocurarine	Slow (>5 min)	Long (1–2 h)	Hypotension (ganglion block plus histamine release) Bronchoconstriction (histamine release)	Plant alkaloid, now rarely used **Alcuronium** is a semisynthetic derivative with similar properties but fewer side-effects
Gallamine	Slow	Long	Tachycardia (muscarinic antagonist)	100% renal excretion; therefore, to be avoided in patients with poor renal function The first synthetic alternative to tubocurarine, now rarely used
Pancuronium	Intermediate (2–3 min)	Long	Slight tachycardia. No hypotension	The first steroid-based compound. Better side-effect profile than tubocurarine. Widely used **Pipecuronium** is similar
Vecuronium	Intermediate	Intermediate (30–40 min)	Few side-effects	Widely used. Occasionally causes prolonged paralysis, probably owing to active metabolite **Rocuronium** is similar, with faster onset
Atracurium	Intermediate	Intermediate (<30 min)	Transient hypotension (histamine release)	Unusual mechanism of elimination (spontaneous non-enzymic chemical degradation in plasma). Degradation slowed by acidosis Widely used **Doxacurium** is chemically similar but stable in plasma, giving it long duration of action **Cisatracurium** is the pure isomeric constituent of atracurium, similar but with less histamine release
Mivacurium	Fast (~2 min)	Short (~15 min)	Transient hypotension (histamine release)	New drug, chemically similar to atracurium but rapidly inactivated by plasma cholinesterase (therefore, longer acting in patients with liver disease or with genetic cholinesterase deficiency (see p. 153)
Suxamethonium	Fast	Short (~10 min)	Bradycardia (muscarinic agonist effect) Cardiac dysrhythmias (increased plasma K^+ concentration—avoid in patients with burns or severe trauma) Raised intraocular pressure (nicotinic agonist effect on extraocular muscles) Postoperative muscle pain	Acts by depolarisation of endplate (nicotinic agonist effect)—the only drug of this type still in use Paralysis is preceded by transient muscle fasciculations Short duration of action owing to hydrolysis by plasma cholinesterase (prolonged action in patients with liver disease or genetic deficiency of plasma cholinesterase) Used for brief procedures (e.g. tracheal intubation, electroconvulsive shock therapy). Rocuronium has similar speed of onset and recovery with fewer unwanted effects

For chemical structures, see Hardman et al. (2001).

Pharmacokinetic aspects

Neuromuscular-blocking agents are used mainly in anaesthesia to produce muscle relaxation. They are given intravenously but differ in their rates of onset and recovery (Table 10.7, Fig. 10.7).

Most of the non-depolarising blocking agents are metabolised by the liver or excreted unchanged in the urine, exceptions being **atracurium**, which hydrolyses spontaneously in plasma, and **mivacurium**, which, like **suxamethonium**, is hydrolysed by plasma cholinesterase. Their duration of action varies between about 15 minutes and 1–2 hours (Table 10.7), by which time the patient regains enough strength to cough and breathe properly, though residual weakness may persist for much longer. The route of elimination is important, since many patients undergoing

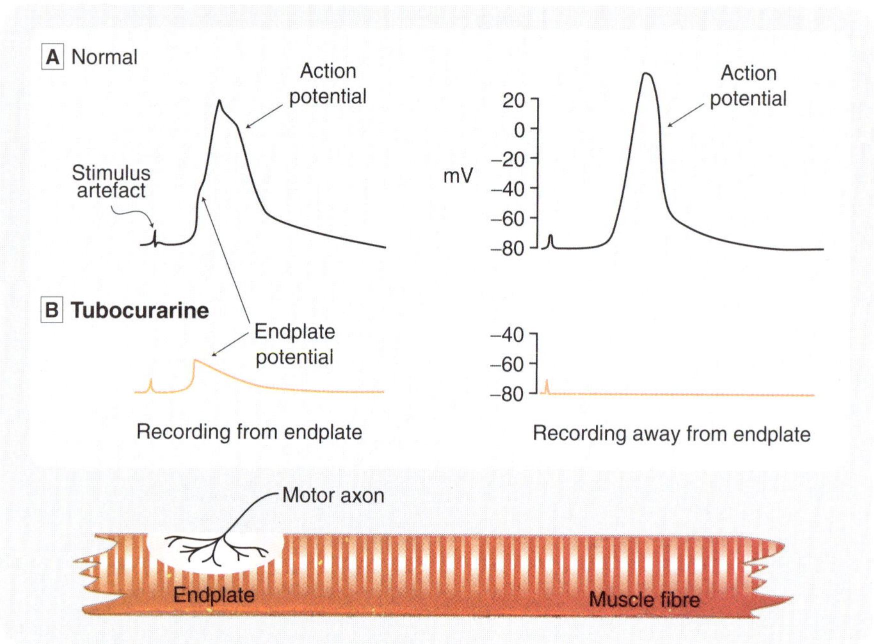

Fig. 10.6 The effect of tubocurarine on neuromuscular transmission. A Microelectrode recording at the endplate (left) normally shows a complex response to nerve stimulation, consisting of an endplate potential (epp), from the peak of which the action potential is initiated. The action potential is distorted by the local increase in conductance produced by the transmitter. Away from the endplate; a simple propagated action potential is recorded. B Tubocurarine reduces the epp amplitude, so that no action potential is generated.

anaesthesia have impaired renal or hepatic function, which, depending on the drug used, can enhance or prolong the paralysis to an important degree. The action of gallamine, for example, may be dangerously prolonged in patients with renal failure.

Atracurium was designed to be chemically unstable at physiological pH (splitting into two inactive fragments by cleavage at one of the quaternary nitrogen atoms), though indefinitely stable when stored at an acid pH. It has a short duration of action, which is unaffected by renal or hepatic function. Because of the marked pH dependence of its degradation, however, its action becomes considerably briefer during respiratory alkalosis caused by hyperventilation.

DEPOLARISING BLOCKING AGENTS

The depolarising action of neuromuscular-blocking drugs were discovered by Paton & Zaimis in their study of the effects of symmetrical bisquaternary ammonium compounds (see Paton, 1954). One of these, **decamethonium**, was found to cause paralysis without appreciable ganglion-blocking activity. Several features of its action showed it to be different from competitive blocking drugs such as tubocurarine.

In particular, decamethonium was found to produce a transient twitching of skeletal muscle (fasciculation) before causing block, and when it was injected into chicks it caused a powerful extensor spasm,* whereas tubocurarine simply caused flaccid paralysis. In 1951, Burns & Paton showed that its action was to cause a maintained depolarisation at the endplate region of the muscle fibre, which led to a loss of electrical excitability (see p. 142), and they coined the term 'depolarisation block'. Fasciculation occurs because the developing endplate depolarisation initially causes a discharge of action potentials in the muscle fibre. This subsides after a few seconds as the electrical excitability of the endplate region of the fibre is lost.

Decamethonium itself was used clinically but has the disadvantage of too long a duration of action. Suxamethonium (Table 10.7) is closely related in structure to both decamethonium and acetylcholine (consisting of two acetylcholine molecules linked by their acetyl groups). Its action is shorter than that of decamethonium because it is quickly hydrolysed by plasma cholinesterase. Suxamethonium and decamethonium act—like acetylcholine—as agonists on the receptors of the motor endplate. However, when given as drugs, they diffuse relatively slowly to the endplate and remain there for long enough that the depolarisation causes loss of electrical excitability. Acetylcholine, in contrast, when released from the nerve, reaches the endplate in very brief spurts and is rapidly hydrolysed in situ, so it never causes sufficiently prolonged depolarisation to result in block. If cholinesterase is inhibited, however (see p. 158), it is possible for the circulating acetylcholine concentration to reach a level sufficient to cause depolarisation block.

*Birds possess a special type of skeletal muscle, rare in mammals, that has many endplates scattered over the surface of each muscle fibre. A drug that causes endplate depolarisation produces a widespread depolarisation in such muscles, resulting in a maintained contracture. In normal skeletal muscle, with only one endplate per fibre, endplate depolarisation is too localised to cause contracture on its own.

Two potent neurotoxins, namely **botulinum toxin** and **β-bungarotoxin**, act specifically to inhibit acetylcholine release. Botulinum toxin is a protein produced by the anaerobic bacillus *Clostridium botulinum*, an organism that can multiply in preserved food and can cause botulism, an extremely serious type of food poisoning. The potency of botulinum toxin is extraordinary, the minimum lethal dose in a mouse being less than 10^{-12} g: only a few million molecules. It belongs to the group of potent bacterial exotoxins that includes tetanus and diphtheria toxins. They possess two subunits, one of which binds to a membrane receptor and is responsible for cellular specificity. By this means the toxin enters the cell, where the other subunit produces the toxic effect (Montecucco & Schiavo, 1995). Botulinum toxin contains several components (A to G). They are peptidases that cleave specific proteins involved in exocytosis (*synaptobrevins, syntaxins*, etc.—see Ch. 9), thereby producing a long-lasting block of synaptic function. Each toxin component inactivates a different functional protein—a remarkably coordinated attack by a humble bacterium on a vital component of mammalian physiology.

Botulinum poisoning causes progressive parasympathetic and motor paralysis, with dry mouth, blurred vision and difficulty in swallowing, followed by progressive respiratory paralysis. Treatment with antitoxin is effective only if given before symptoms appear, for once the toxin is bound its action cannot be reversed. Mortality is high, and recovery takes several weeks. Anticholinesterases and drugs that increase transmitter release (see p. 156) are ineffective in restoring transmission. Among the more spectacular outbreaks of botulinum poisoning was an incident on Loch Maree in Scotland in 1922 when all eight members of a fishing party died after eating duck pâté for their lunch. Their ghillies, consuming humbler fare no doubt, survived. The inn-keeper committed suicide.

Botulinum toxin, injected locally into muscles, is used to treat a form of persistent and disabling eyelid spasm (blepharospasm) as well as other types of local muscle spasm, for example in spasticity (Tsui, 1996).*

Beta-bungarotoxin is a protein contained in the venom of various snakes of the cobra family and has a similar action to botulinum toxin, though its active component is a phospholipase rather than a peptidase. The same venoms also contain **α-bungarotoxin**, which blocks postsynaptic acetylcholine receptors—so these snakes evidently cover all eventualities as far as causing paralysis of their victims is concerned.

DRUGS THAT ENHANCE CHOLINERGIC TRANSMISSION

Drugs that enhance cholinergic transmission act either by inhibiting cholinesterase (the main group) or by increasing acetylcholine release. In this chapter, we focus on the peripheral actions of such drugs; drugs affecting cholinergic transmission in the CNS, used to treat senile dementia, are discussed in Chapter 34.

DISTRIBUTION AND FUNCTION OF CHOLINESTERASE

There are two distinct types of cholinesterase, namely *acetylcholinesterase* (AChE) and *butyrylcholinesterase* (BChE), closely related in molecular structure but differing in their distribution, substrate specificity and functions (see Chatonnet & Lockridge 1989). Both consist of globular catalytic subunits, which constitute the soluble forms found in plasma (BChE) and cerebrospinal fluid (AChE). Elsewhere, the catalytic units are linked to collagen-like proteins or to glycolipids, through which they are tethered, like a bunch of balloons, to the cell membrane or the basement membrane at various sites, such as the erythrocyte and the motor endplate.

AChE is bound to the basement membrane in the synaptic cleft at cholinergic synapses, where its function is to hydrolyse the released transmitter. The soluble form of AChE is also present in cholinergic nerve terminals, where it seems to have a role in regulating the free acetylcholine concentration, and from which it may be secreted; the function of the secreted enzyme is so far unclear. The membrane-bound form also occurs in unexpected places such as the erythrocyte, where its function is unknown. AChE is quite specific for acetylcholine and closely related esters such as methacholine. Certain neuropeptides, such as substance P (Ch. 13), are inactivated by AChE, but it is not known whether this is of physiological significance. Overall, there is poor correspondence between the distibution of cholinergic synapses and that of AChE, both in the brain and in the periphery, and AChE most probably has functions other than disposal of acetylcholine, though the details remain unclear (see review by Soreq & Sediman 2001).

BChE (or pseudocholinesterase) has a widespread distribution, being found in tissues such as liver, skin, brain and gastrointestinal smooth muscle, as well as in soluble form in the plasma. It is not particularly associated with cholinergic synapses and has a broader substrate specificity than AChE. It hydrolyses butyrylcholine more rapidly than acetylcholine, as well as other esters such as **procaine**, **suxamethonium** and **propanidid** (a short-acting anaesthetic agent; see Ch. 35). The function of this enzyme is not known, but the plasma enzyme is important in relation to the inactivation of the drugs listed above. Genetic variants of BChE occur (see Ch. 52), and these partly account for the variability in the duration of action of these drugs.

The very short duration of action of acetylcholine given intravenously (see Fig. 10.1) results from its rapid hydrolysis in the plasma. Normally AChE and BChE between them keep the plasma acetylcholine at an undetectably low level, so acetylcholine (unlike noradrenaline) is strictly a neurotransmitter and not a hormone.

AChE and BChE belong to the class of serine hydrolases that includes many proteases, such as trypsin. The active site of AChE

*'Botox' is also fashionable as a wrinkle-remover, removing frown-lines by paralysing the superficial muscles that pucker the skin. For the same agent to figure in popular beauty magazines as well as in manuals of biological warfare reflects strangely on the modern world.

(Fig. 10.9) comprises two distinct regions, an *anionic site* (glutamate residue), which binds the basic (choline) moiety of acetylcholine, and an *esteratic site* (histidine + serine). As with other serine hydrolases, the acidic (acetyl) group of the substrate is transferred to the serine hydroxyl group, leaving (transiently) an acetylated enzyme molecule and a molecule of free choline. Spontaneous hydrolysis of the serine acetyl group occurs rapidly, and the overall turnover number of AChE is extremely high (over 10 000 molecules of acetylcholine hydrolysed per second by a single active site).

DRUGS THAT INHIBIT CHOLINESTERASE

Peripherally acting anticholinesterase drugs fall into three main groups according to the nature of their interaction with the active site, which determines their duration of action. Most of them inhibit AChE and BChE about equally. Centrally acting anticholinesterases, developed for the treatment of dementia, are discussed in Chapter 34.

Short-acting anticholinesterases

The only important drug among the short-acting anticholinesterases is **edrophonium** (Table 10.8), a quaternary ammonium compound that binds to the anionic site of the enzyme only. The ionic bond formed is readily reversible and the action of the drug is very brief. It is used mainly for diagnostic purposes, since improvement of muscle strength by an anticholinesterase is characteristic of myasthenia gravis (see p. 159) but does not occur when muscle weakness is from other causes.

Table 10.8 Anticholinesterase drugs

Drug	Structure	Duration of action (long/medium/short)	Main site of action	Notes
Edrophonium	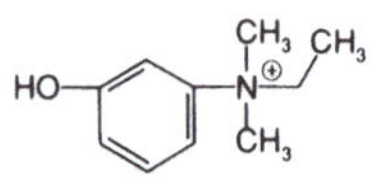	S	NMJ	Used mainly in diagnosis of myasthenia gravis Too short acting for therapeutic use
Neostigmine	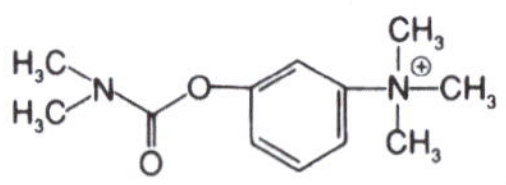	M	NMJ	Used i.v. to reverse competitive neuromuscular block Used orally in treatment of myasthenia gravis Visceral side-effects
Physostigmine	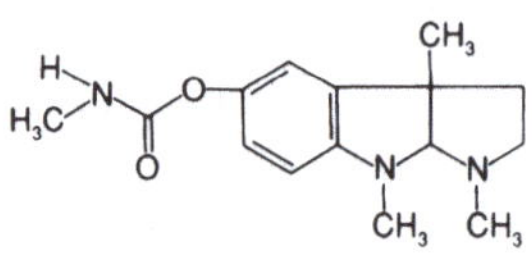	M	P	Used as eye drops in treatment of glaucoma
Pyridostigmine	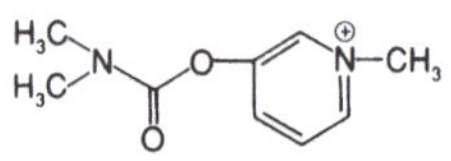	M	NMJ	Used orally in treatment of myasthenia gravis Better absorbed than neostigmine and has longer duration of action
Dyflos	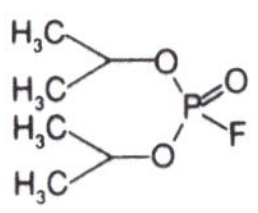	L	P	Highly toxic organophosphate, with very prolonged action Has been used as eye drops for glaucoma
Ecothiopate	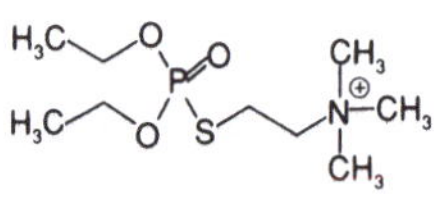	L	P	Used as eye drops in treatment of glaucoma Prolonged action; may cause systemic effects
Parathion	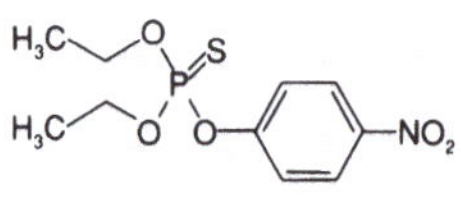	L	—	Converted to active metabolite by replacement of sulfur by oxygen Used as insecticide but commonly causes poisoning in humans

NMJ, neuromuscular junction; P, postganglionic parasympathetic junction; i.v., intravenous.

Medium-duration anticholinesterases

The medium-duration anticholinesterases (Table 10.8) include **neostigmine** and **pyridostigmine**, which are quaternary ammonium compounds of clinical importance, and **physostigmine** (eserine), a tertiary amine, which occurs naturally in the Calabar bean.*

These drugs are all carbamyl, as opposed to acetyl, esters and all possess basic groups that bind to the anionic site. Transfer of the carbamyl group to the serine hydroxyl group of the esteratic site occurs as with acetylcholine, but the carbamylated enzyme is very much slower to hydrolyse (Fig. 10.9), taking minutes rather than microseconds. The anticholinesterase drug is, therefore, hydrolysed, but at a negligible rate compared with acetylcholine, and the slow recovery of the carbamylated enzyme means that the action of these drugs is quite long lasting.

*Otherwise known as the ordeal bean. Extracts of these poisonous beans were once used to assess the guilt or innocence of suspected criminals and heretics; death implied guilt.

Irreversible anticholinesterases

Irreversible anticholinesterases (Table 10.8) are pentavalent phosphorus compounds containing a labile group such as fluoride (in **dyflos**) or an organic group (in **parathion** and **ecothiopate**). This group is released, leaving the serine hydroxyl group of the enzyme phosphorylated (Fig. 10.9). Most of these organophosphate compounds, of which there are many, were developed as war gases and pesticides as well as for clinical use.

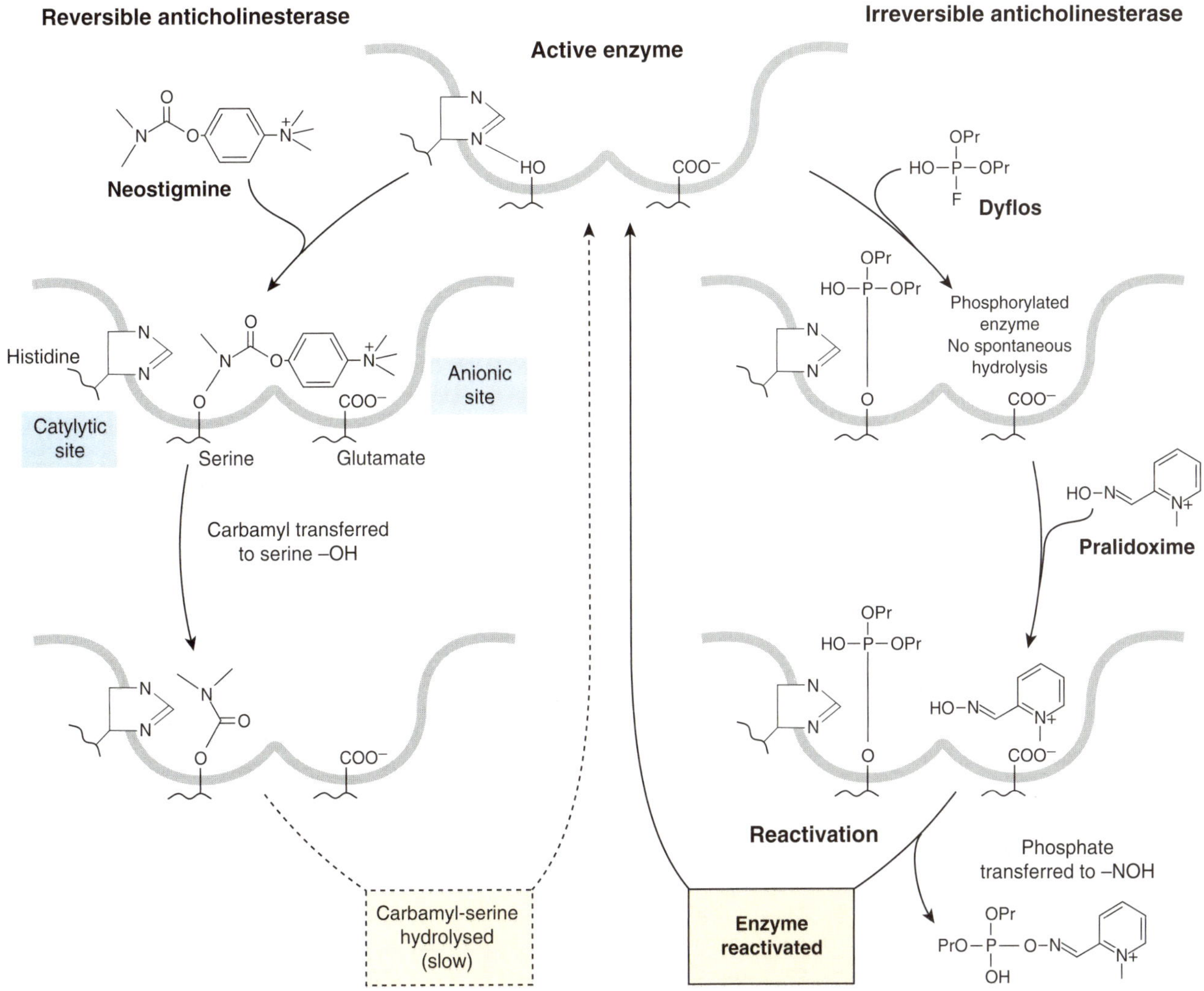

Fig. 10.9 Action of anticholinesterase drugs. With a reversible anticholinesterase (neostigmine), recovery of activity by hydrolysis of the carbamylated enzyme takes many minutes. An irreversible anticholinesterase (dyflos) gives a form (phosphorylated) that cannot be spontaneously regenerated. The addition of pralidoxime allows reactivation of the cholinesterase by transfer of the phosphate group.

They interact only with the esteratic site of the enzyme and have no cationic group. Ecothiopate is an exception in having a quaternary nitrogen group designed to bind also to the anionic site.

The inactive phosphorylated enzyme is usually very stable. With drugs such as dyflos, no appreciable hydrolysis occurs, and recovery of enzymic activity depends on the synthesis of new enzyme molecules, a process that may take weeks. With other drugs, such as ecothiopate, slow hydrolysis occurs over the course of a few days, so that their action is not strictly irreversible. Dyflos and parathion are volatile non-polar substances of very high lipid solubility and are rapidly absorbed through mucous membranes and even through unbroken skin and insect cuticles; the use of these agents as war gases or insecticides relies on this property. The lack of a specificity-conferring quaternary group means that most of these drugs block other serine hydrolases (e.g. trypsin, thrombin), though their pharmacological effects result mainly from cholinesterase inhibition.

Effects of anticholinesterase drugs

Cholinesterase inhibitors affect peripheral as well as central cholinergic synapses.

Some organophosphate compounds can produce, in addition, a form of neurotoxicity not associated with cholinesterase inhibition.

Effects on autonomic cholinergic synapses These mainly reflect enhancement of acetylcholine activity at parasympathetic postganglionic synapses (i.e. increased secretions from salivary, lacrimal, bronchial and gastrointestinal glands, increased peristaltic activity, bronchoconstriction, bradycardia and hypotension, pupillary constriction, fixation of accommodation for near vision, fall in intraocular pressure). Large doses can stimulate, and later block, autonomic ganglia, producing complex autonomic effects. The block, if it occurs, is a depolarisation block and is associated with a build-up of acetylcholine in the plasma and body fluids. Neostigmine and pyridostigmine tend to affect neuromuscular transmission more than the autonomic system, whereas physostigmine and organophosphates show the reverse pattern. The reason is not clear, but therapeutic usage takes advantage of this partial selectivity.

Anticholinesterase poisoning (e.g. from contact with insecticides or war gases) causes severe bradycardia, hypotension and difficulty in breathing. Combined with a depolarising neuromuscular block, and central effects (see below), the result may be fatal.

Effects on the neuromuscular junction The twitch tension of a muscle stimulated via its motor nerve is increased by anticholinesterases, owing to repetitive firing in the muscle fibre, and is associated with prolongation of the epp. Normally, the acetylcholine is hydrolysed so quickly that each stimulus initiates only one action potential in the muscle fibre, but when AChE is inhibited, this is converted to a short train of action potentials in the muscle fibre, and hence greater tension. Much more important is the effect produced when transmission has been blocked by a competitive blocking agent, such as tubocurarine. In this case, addition of an anticholinesterase can dramatically restore transmission. If a large proportion of the receptors are blocked, the majority of acetylcholine molecules will normally encounter, and be destroyed by, an AChE molecule before reaching a vacant receptor; inhibiting AChE will increase the number of acetylcholine molecules that will find a vacant receptor, and thus increase the epp so that it reaches threshold. In myasthenia gravis (see below), transmission fails because there are too few acetylcholine receptors, and cholinesterase inhibition improves transmission just as it does in curarised muscle. In large doses, such as can occur in poisoning, anticholinesterases initially cause twitching of muscles. This is because spontaneous acetylcholine release can give rise to epp that reach the firing threshold. Anticholinesterases may later cause a paralysis through a depolarisation block, which is associated with the build-up of acetylcholine in the plasma and tissue fluids.

Effects on the CNS Tertiary compounds, such as physostigmine, and the non-polar organophosphates penetrate the blood–brain barrier freely and affect the brain. The result is an initial excitation, which can result in convulsions, followed by depression, which can cause unconsciousness and respiratory failure. These central effects result mainly from the activation of muscarinic receptors and are antagonised by atropine. The potential use of brain-selective anticholinesterases to treat senile dementia is discussed in Chapter 34.

Neurotoxicity of organophosphates Many organophosphates can cause a severe type of peripheral nerve demyelination, leading to slowly developing weakness and sensory loss. This is not a problem with clinically used anticholinesterases but occasionally occurs with accidental poisoning. In 1931, an estimated 20 000 Americans were affected, some fatally, by contamination of fruit juice with an organophosphate insecticide, and other similar outbreaks have been recorded. The mechanism of this reaction is only partly understood, but it seems to result from inhibition of an esterase (not cholinesterase itself) specific to myelin.

The main uses of anticholinesterases are summarised in the clinical box.

CHOLINESTERASE REACTIVATION

Spontaneous hydrolysis of phosphorylated cholinesterase is extremely slow, a fact that makes poisoning with organophosphates very dangerous. **Pralidoxime** (Figs 10.9 and 10.10) reactivates the enzyme by bringing an oxime group into close proximity with the phosphorylated esteratic site. This group is a strong nucleophile and attracts the phosphate group from the serine hydroxyl group of the enzyme. The effectiveness of pralidoxime in reactivating plasma cholinesterase activity in a poisoned subject is shown in Figure 10.10. The main drawback to its use as an antidote to organophosphate poisoning is that within a few hours the phosphorylated enzyme undergoes a change ('ageing') that renders it no longer susceptible to reactivation, so pralidoxime must be given early in order to work. Pralidoxime does not enter the brain, but related compounds have been developed to treat the central effects of organophosphate poisoning.

Myasthenia gravis

▼ The neuromuscular junction is a robust structure that very rarely fails, myasthenia gravis being one of the very few disorders that specifically affects it (see Graus & de Baets 1993; Lindstrom 2000). This disease affects about 1 in 2000 individuals, who show muscle weakness and increased fatiguability resulting from a failure of neuromuscular transmission. The tendency for transmission to fail during repetitive activity can be seen in Figure 10.11. Functionally, it results in the inability of muscles to produce sustained contractions, of which the characteristic drooping eyelids of myasthenic patients are a sign. The effectiveness of anticholinesterase drugs in improving muscle strength in myasthenia was discovered in 1931, long before the cause of the disease was known.

The cause of the transmission failure is an autoimmune response that causes a loss of nicotinic acetylcholine receptors from the neuromuscular junction, first revealed in studies showing that the number of bungarotoxin-binding sites at the endplates of myasthenic patients was reduced by about 70% compared with normal. It had been suspected that myasthenia had an immunological basis, since removal of the thymus gland was frequently of benefit. Immunisation of rabbits with purified acetylcholine receptor causes, after a delay, symptoms very similar to those of human myasthenia gravis. The presence of antibody directed

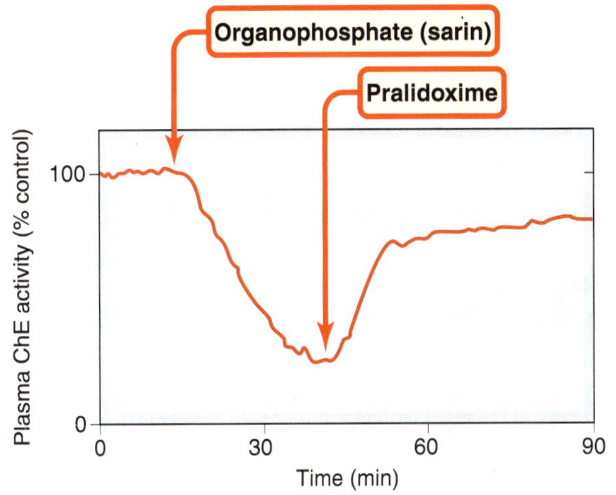

Fig. 10.10 Reactivation of plasma cholinesterase (ChE) in a volunteer subject by intravenous injection of pralidoxime. (Redrawn from: Sim V M 1965 J Am Med Assoc 192: 404.)

Cholinesterase and anticholinesterase drugs

- There are two main forms of cholinesterase both enzymes belong to the family of serine hydrolases:
  —acetylcholinesterase (AChE), which is mainly membrane bound, relatively specific for ACh and responsible for rapid ACh hydrolysis at cholinergic synapses
  —butyrylcholinesterase (BuChE) or pseudocholinesterase, which is relatively non-selective and occurs in plasma and many tissues.
- Anticholinesterase drugs are of three main types: short-acting (edrophonium), medium-acting (neostigmine, physostigmine), irreversible (organophosphates, dyflos, ecothiopate). They differ in the nature of their chemical interaction with the active site of cholinesterase.
- Effects of anticholinesterase drugs are mainly a result of enhancement of cholinergic transmission at cholinergic autonomic synapses and at the neuromuscular junction.
- Anticholinesterase drugs that cross the blood–brain barrier (e.g. physostigmine, organophosphates) also have marked CNS effects.
- Autonomic effects include bradycardia, hypotension, excessive secretions, bronchoconstriction, gastrointestinal hypermotility, decrease of intraocular pressure.
- Neuromuscular action causes muscle fasciculation and increased twitch tension and can produce depolarisation block.
- Anticholinesterase poisoning may occur from exposure to insecticides or nerve gases.

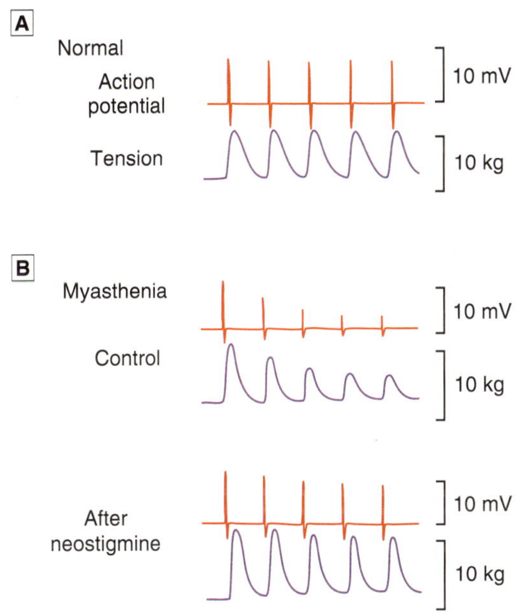

Fig. 10.11 Neuromuscular transmission in a normal and a myasthenic human subject. Electrical activity was recorded with a needle electrode in the adductor pollicis muscle, in response to ulnar nerve stimulation (3 Hz) at the wrist. [A] In a normal subject, the electrical and mechanical response is well sustained. [B] In a myasthenic patient, transmission fails rapidly when the nerve is stimulated. Treatment with neostigmine improves transmission. (From: Desmedt J E 1962 Bull Acad Roy Med Belg VII 2: 213.)

Clinical uses of anticholinesterase drugs

- Neostigmine is admistered by anaesthetists to reverse the action of non-depolarising neuromuscular-blocking drugs at the end of an operation.
- Neostigmine (2–4 hour duration) or pyridostigmine (3–6 hour duration) is used to treat myasthenia gravis.
- Edrophonium (a short-acting drug) is given intravenously as a test for myasthenia gravis; it is also used to distinguish between weakness caused by anticholinesterase overdosage ('cholinergic crisis') and the weakness of myasthenia itself ('myasthenic crisis').
- Ecothiopate eye drops are used to treat glaucoma.

against the acetylcholine receptor protein can be detected in the serum of myasthenic patients, but the reason for the development of the autoimmune response in humans is still unknown (Lindstrom, 2000).

The improvement of neuromuscular function by anticholinesterase treatment (shown in Fig. 10.11) can be dramatic, but if the disease progresses too far, the number of receptors remaining may become too few to produce an adequate epp, and anticholinesterase drugs will then cease to be effective.

Alternative approaches to the treatment of myasthenia are to remove circulating antibody by plasma exchange, which is transiently effective, or, for a more prolonged effect, to inhibit antibody production with steroids (e.g. **prednisolone**) or immunosuppressant drugs (e.g. **azathioprine**; see Ch. 16).

OTHER DRUGS THAT ENHANCE CHOLINERGIC TRANSMISSION

It was observed many years ago that **tetraethylammonium**, better known as a ganglion-blocking drug, could reverse the neuromuscular-blocking action of tubocurarine, and this was shown to be because it increases the release of transmitter evoked by nerve stimulation. Subsequently, **aminopyridines** (see Ch. 3), which block potassium channels and thus prolong the action potential in the presynaptic nerve terminal, were found to act similarly and to be considerably more potent and selective in their actions than tetraethylammonium. These drugs are not selective for cholinergic nerves but increase the evoked release of many different transmitters; consequently, they have too many unwanted effects to be useful in treating neuromuscular disorders.

REFERENCES AND FURTHER READING

Bowman W C 1990 Pharmacology of neuromuscular function. Wright, Bristol, England (*Detailed textbook*)

Chatonnet A, Lockridge O 1989 Comparison of butyrylcholinesterase and acetylcholinesterase. Biochem J 260: 625–634 (*Short review on nature and functions of cholinesterases*)

Cordero-Erauskin M, Marubio L M, Clink R, Changeux J-P 2000 Nicotinic receptor function: new perspectives from knockout mice. Trends Pharmacol Sci 21: 211–217

Drachman D B 1981 The biology of myasthenia gravis. Annu Rev Neurobiol 4: 195–225 (*Autoimmune nature of myasthenia*)

Eglen R M, Choppin A, Dillon M P, Hedge S 1999 Muscarinic receptor ligands and their therapeutic potential. Curr Opin Chem Biol 3: 426–432 (*Review of future development of muscarinic agonists and antagonists for different indications*)

Ginsborg B L, Jenkinson D H 1976 Transmission of impulses from nerve to muscle. In: Zaimis E J (ed) Neuromuscular junction. Handbook of experimental pharmacology. Springer-Verlag, Berlin, vol. 42, pp. 229–364 (*Excellent general account of neuromuscular physiology and pharmacology*)

Goyal R K 1989 Muscarinic receptor subtypes: physiology and clinical implications. N Engl J Med 321: 1022–1029 (*Good general review*)

Graus Y M, de Baets M H 1993 Myasthenia gravis: an autoimmune response against the acetylcholine receptor. Immunol Res 12: 78–100

Hardman J G, Limbird L E, Gilman A G, Goodman-Gilman A 2001 Goodman and Gilman's pharmacological basis of therapeutics, 10th edn. McGraw-Hill, New York (*Comprehensive and authorative textbook*)

Kilbinger H 1984 Presynaptic muscarinic receptors modulating acetylcholine release. Trends Pharmacol Sci 5: 103–105 (*Short review article*)

Lindstrom J M 2000 Acetylcholine receptors and myasthenia. Muscle Nerve 23: 453–477 (*Good review article on nicotinic acetylcholine receptor subtypes and current views on the pathophysiology of myasthenia gravis and related neuromuscular disorders*)

Liu Y, Edwards R H 1997 The role of vesicular transport proteins in synaptic transmission and neural degeneration. Annu Rev Neurosci 20: 125–156 (*Review of recent ideas about functional role of transporters*)

McGehee D S, Role L W 1995 Physiological diversity of nicotinic acetylcholine receptors expressed by vertebrate neurons. Annu Rev Physiol 57: 521–546 (*Summarises molecular and physiological diversity among neuronal receptors in CNS and periphery*)

Montecucco C, Schiavo G 1995 Structure and function of botulinum neurotoxins. Q Rev Biophys 28: 423–472 (*Discusses the mode of action of an important group of presynaptic neurotoxins*)

Nicholls J G, Martin A R, Wallace B G, Fuchs P 2001 From neuron to brain. Sinauer, Sunderland, MA (*Excellent general textbook*)

Parsons S M, Prior C, Marshall I G 1993 Acetylcholine transport, storage and release. Int Rev Neurobiol 35: 279–390 (*Useful review of the local metabolism of acetylcholine*)

Paton W D M 1954 The principles of ganglion block. Lectures on the scientific basis of medicine, vol. 2. Athlone Press, London

Prior C, Tian L, Dempster J, Marshall I G 1995 Prejunctional actions of muscle relaxants: synaptic vesicles and transmitter mobilization as sites of action. Gen Pharmacol 26: 659–666 (*Emphasises the role of presynaptic inhibition in the action of neuromuscular-blocking drugs*)

Skok V I 1980 Ganglionic transmission: morphology and physiology. In: Kharkevich D A (ed) Pharmacology of ganglionic transmission. Handbook of experimental pharmacology. Springer-Verlag, Berlin, vol. 53, pp. 9–39 (*Comprehensive account of ganglion-blocking drugs*)

Soreq H, Sediman S 2001 Acetycholinesterase—new roles for an old actor. Nature Rev Neurosci 2: 294–302 (*Speculative review of evidence suggesting functions for AChE other than acetylcholine hydrolysis*)

Tsui J K C 1996 Botulinum toxin as a therapeutic agent. Pharmacol Ther 72: 13–24 (*A lethal toxin can be useful in therapeutics*)

Usdin T B, Eiden L E, Bonner T I, Erickson J D 1995 Molecular biology of the vesicular acetylcholine transporter. Trends Neurosci 18: 218–224

Wess J 1996 Molecular biology of muscarinic acetylcholine receptors. Crit Rev Neurobiol 10: 69–99 (*Describes receptor subtypes in detail*)

Wessle I, Kilpatrick C J, Racke K 1998 Non-neuronal acetylcholine, a locally-acting molecule, widely distributed in biological systems: expression and function in humans. Pharmacol Ther 77: 59–79 (*Speculation of possible roles for non-neuronal acetylcholine*)

Wonnacott S 1997 Presynaptic nicotinic ACh receptors. Trends Neurosci 20: 92–98 (*Summarises evidence for a role of nicotinic acetylcholine receptors as presynaptic regulators; most authors having postulated a postsynaptic excitatory role, which has proved elusive to pin down*)

Noradrenergic transmission

11

Overview 161

Classification of adrenoceptors 161

Physiology of noradrenergic transmission 164
– The noradrenergic neuron 164

Drugs acting on adrenoceptors 168
– Structure–activity relationships 168
– Adrenoceptor agonsists 169
– Adrenoceptor antagonists 172

Drugs that affect noradrenergic neurons 176
– Drugs that affect noradrenaline synthesis 176
– Drugs that affect noradrenaline storage 176
– Drugs that affect noradrenaline release 176
– Inhibitors of noradrenaline uptake 178

OVERVIEW

The noradrenergic neuron is an important target for drug action, both as an object for investigation in its own right and as a point of attack for many clinically useful drugs. In this chapter, we describe the physiology and function of noradrenergic neurons and the properties of adrenoceptors, and we discuss the various classes of drug that affect them. For convenience, much of the pharmacological information is summarised in Table 11.3 at the end of the chapter.

CLASSIFICATION OF ADRENOCEPTORS

In 1896, Oliver & Schafer demonstrated that injection of extracts of adrenal gland caused a rise in arterial pressure. Following the subsequent isolation of **adrenaline** as the active principle, it was shown by Dale in 1913 that adrenaline causes two distinct kinds of effect, namely vasoconstriction in certain vascular beds (which normally predominates and causes the rise in arterial pressure) and vasodilatation in others. Dale showed that the vasoconstrictor component disappeared if the animal was first injected with an ergot derivative* (see p. 188) and noticed that adrenaline then caused a fall, instead of a rise, in arterial pressure. This result paralleled Dale's demonstration of the separate muscarinic and nicotinic components of the action of acetylcholine (see Ch. 10). He avoided interpreting it in terms of different types of receptor, but later pharmacological work, beginning with that of Ahlquist in 1948, showed clearly the existence of several subclasses of adrenoceptor. Ahlquist found that the rank order of the potencies of various

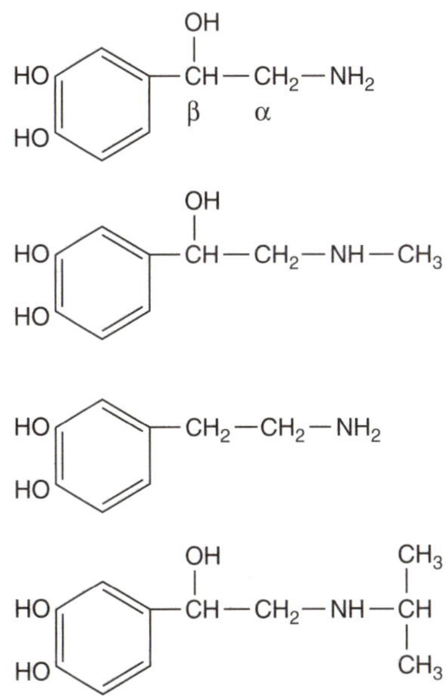

Fig. 11.1 Structures of the major catecholamines.

*Dale was a new recruit in the laboratories of the Wellcome pharmaceutical company, given the job of checking the potency of batches of adrenaline coming from the factory. He tested one batch at the end of a day's experimentation on a cat, which he had earlier injected with an ergot preparation. Because it produced a fall in blood pressure rather than the expected rise, he advised that the whole expensive consignment should be rejected. Unknown to him, he was given the same sample to test a few days later and reported it to be normal (based on its effect in a cat that had not received ergot). How he explained this to Wellcome's management is not recorded.

catecholamines,* including **adrenaline**, **noradrenaline** and **isoprenaline** (a synthetic catecholamine; see Fig. 11.1), fell into two distinct patterns, depending on what response was being measured. He postulated the existence of two kinds of receptor, α and β, defined in terms of agonist potencies as follows:

α: noradrenaline > adrenaline > isoprenaline
β: isoprenaline > adrenaline > noradrenaline.

It was then recognised that certain ergot alkaloids, which Dale had studied, act as selective α-adrenoceptor antagonists, and that Dale's adrenaline reversal experiment reflected the unmasking of the β effects of adrenaline by α-adrenoceptor blockade. Selective β-adrenoceptor antagonists were not developed until 1955, when their effects fully confirmed Ahlquist's original classification, and also suggested the existence of further subdivisions of both α- and β-adrenoceptors. Subsequent studies with agonists and antagonists have confirmed the existence of two main α-adrenoceptor subtypes (α_1 and α_2) and three β-adrenoceptor subtypes (β_1, β_2 and β_3; Table 11.1).

All adrenoceptors are typical G-protein-coupled receptors, and cloning has revealed that α_1- and α_2-adrenoceptors each comprise three further subclasses, which are expressed in different locations but have functions that are, for the most part, still unclear (Bylund, 1994; Insel, 1996).

Each of these receptor classes is associated with a specific second messenger system (Table 11.1; see Summers & McMartin, 1993). For example, α_1-adrenoceptors are coupled to phospholipase C and produce their effects mainly by the release of intracellular Ca^{2+}; α_2-adrenoceptors are negatively coupled to adenylate cyclase and reduce cAMP formation, as well as inhibiting calcium channels. All three types of β-adrenoceptor act by stimulation of adenylate cyclase. The major effects that are produced by these receptors, and the main drugs that act on them, are shown in Table 11.1.

The distinction between β_1- and β_2-adrenoceptors is an important one, for β_1-adrenoceptors are found mainly in the heart, where they are responsible for the positive inotropic and chronotropic effects of catecholamines (see Ch. 17). The β_2-adrenoceptors, in contrast, are responsible for causing smooth muscle relaxation in many organs. The latter is often a useful therapeutic effect, while the former is more often harmful; consequently, considerable efforts have been made to find selective β_2-agonists, which would relax smooth muscle without affecting the heart, and selective β_1-antagonists, which would exert a useful blocking effect on the heart without at the same time blocking β_2-adrenoceptors in bronchial smooth muscle (see Table 11.1). It is important to realise that the selectivity of these drugs is relative rather than absolute. Thus, compounds used as selective β_1-antagonists invariably have some action on β_2-adrenoceptors as well, which can cause unwanted effects such as bronchoconstriction. Furthermore, the high degree of receptor specificity found for some compounds in laboratory animals is not invariably found in humans. Also, it appears that both types of β-adrenoceptor contribute to some effects, such as the chronotropic action, with the relative contribution of each varying from species to species. In relation to vascular control, it is broadly true that α_1- and β_2-adrenoceptors act mainly on the smooth muscle cells themselves, while α_2-adrenoceptors act on presynaptic terminals, but different vascular beds deviate from this general rule. Both α- and β-adrenoceptor subtypes are expressed in smooth muscle cells, nerve terminals and endothelial cells, and their role in physiological regulation and pharmacological responses of the cardiovascular system is only partly understood (see Guimaraes & Moura, 2001)

Classification of adrenoceptors

- Main pharmacological classification into α- and β-subtypes, based originally on order of potency among agonists, later on selective antagonists.
- There are two main α-adrenoceptor subtypes (α_1 and α_2, each divided into three further suptypes) and three β-adrenoceptor subtypes (β_1, β_2, β_3). All belong to the superfamily of G-protein-coupled receptors.
- Second messengers:
  - —α_1-adrenoceptors activate phospholipase C, thus producing inositol trisphosphate and diacylglycerol as second messengers
  - —α_2-adrenoceptors inhibit adenylate cyclase and thus decrease cAMP formation
  - —all types of β-adrenoceptor stimulate adenylate cyclase.
- The main effects of receptor activation are:
  - —α_1-adrenoceptors: vasoconstriction, relaxation of gastrointestinal smooth muscle, salivary secretion and hepatic glycogenolysis
  - —α_2-adrenoceptors: inhibition of transmitter release (including noradrenaline and acetylcholine release from autonomic nerves), platelet aggregation, contraction of vascular smooth muscle, inhibition of insulin release
  - —β_1-adrenoceptors: increased cardiac rate and force
  - —β_2-adrenoceptors: bronchodilatation, vasodilatation, relaxation of visceral smooth muscle, hepatic glycogenolysis and muscle tremor
  - —β_3-adrenoceptors: lipolysis.

---

*Catecholamines are compounds containing a catechol moiety (a benzene ring with two adjacent hydroxyl groups) and an amine side-chain. Pharmacologically, the most important ones are:

- **noradrenaline** (now officially **norepinephrine**), a transmitter released by sympathetic nerve terminals
- **adrenaline (epinephrine)**, a hormone secreted by the adrenal medulla
- **dopamine**, the metabobolic precursor of noradrenaline and adrenaline, also a transmitter/neuromodulator in the central nervous system
- **isoprenaline** (US: **isoproterenol**), a synthetic derivative of noradrenaline, not present in the body.

We use the conventional (UK) nomenclature, with which most students will be familiar; for the naturally occurring forms but follow the EC Directive and give both the British Approved Name (BAN) and the Recommended Internation Non-proprietary Name (r INN) for the drug forms.

Table 11.1 Characteristics of adrenoceptors

	α_1	α_2	β_1	β_2	β_3
Tissues and effects					
Smooth muscle:					
Blood vessels	Constrict	Constrict/dilate		Dilate	
Bronchi	Constrict			Dilate	
GI tract	Relax	Relax (presynaptic effect)		Relax	
GI sphincters	Contract				
Uterus	Contract			Relax	
Bladder detrusor				Relax	
Bladder sphincter	Contract				
Seminal tract	Contract			Relax	
Iris (radial muscle)	Contract				
Ciliary muscle				Relax	
Heart					
Rate			Increase		
Force of contraction			Increase		
Skeletal muscle				Tremor Increased muscle mass and speed of contraction Glycogenolysis	Thermogenesis
Liver	Glycogenolysis			Glycogenolysis	
Fat					Lipolysis Thermogenesis
Pancreatic islets		Decrease insulin secretion			
Nerve terminals					
Adrenergic		Decrease release		Increase release	
Cholinergic		Decrease release			
Salivary gland	K^+ release		Amylase secretion		
Platelets		Aggregation			
Mast cells				Inhibition of histamine release	
Brainstem		Inhibits sympathetic outflow			
Second messengers and effectors	PLC activation ↑ IP_3 ↑ DAG ↑ Ca^{2+}	↓ cAMP ↓ Calcium channels ↑ Potassium channels	↑ cAMP	↑ cAMP	↑ cAMP
Agonist potency order	NA ≥ A ≫ ISO	A > NA ≫ ISO	ISO > NA > A	ISO > A > NA	ISO > NA = A
Selective agonists	Phenylephrine, methoxamine	Clonidine, clenbuterol	Dobutamine, xamoterol	Salbutamol, terbutaline, salmeterol, formoterol	BRL 37344
Selective antagonists	Prazosin, doxazocin	Yohimbine, idazoxan	Atenolol, metoprolol	Butoxamine	

A, adrenaline; cAMP, cyclic 3′,5′-adenosine monophosphate; DAG, diacylglycerol; ISO, isoprenaline; IP_3, inositol trisphosphate; NA, noradrenaline; PLC, phospholipase C.

Partial agonist effects

▼ Several drugs that act on adrenoceptors have the characteristics of partial agonists (see Ch. 2), i.e. they block receptors and thus antagonise the actions of full agonists, but also have a weak agonist effect of their own. Examples include **ergotamine** (α_1-adrenoceptors) and **clonidine** (α_2-adrenoceptors). Some β-adrenoceptor-blocking drugs (β-blockers, e.g. **alprenolol**, **oxprenolol**) cause, under resting conditions, an increase of heart rate, while at the same time opposing the tachycardia produced by sympathetic stimulation. This has been interpreted as a partial agonist effect, though there is evidence that mechanisms other than β-adrenoceptor activation may contribute to the tachycardia.

The possible clinical significance of partial agonists is discussed under the headings of individual drugs later in this chapter. The pharmacology of ergot derivatives is discussed in Chapter 12.

PHYSIOLOGY OF NORADRENERGIC TRANSMISSION

THE NORADRENERGIC NEURON

Noradrenergic neurons in the periphery are postganglionic sympathetic neurons; their cell bodies lie in sympathetic ganglia. They generally have long axons that end in a series of varicosities strung along the branching terminal network. These varicosities contain numerous synaptic vesicles, which are the sites of synthesis and release of noradrenaline and of coreleased mediators such as ATP and neuropeptide Y (see Ch. 12). Fluorescence histochemistry, in which formaldehyde treatment is used to convert catecholamines to fluorescent quinone derivatives, shows that noradrenaline is present at high concentration in these varicosities, where it is stored in large dense-core vesicles, and is released by exocytosis. In most peripheral tissues, and also in the brain, the tissue content of noradrenaline closely parallels the density of the sympathetic innervation. With the exception of the adrenal medulla, sympathetic nerve terminals account for all of the noradrenaline content of peripheral tissues. Organs such as the heart, spleen, vas deferens and some blood vessels are particularly rich in noradrenaline (5–50 nmol/g tissue) and have been widely used for studies of noradrenergic transmission. For detailed information on noradrenergic neurons, see Cooper et al. (1996), Fillenz (1990) and Trendelenburg & Weiner (1988).

NORADRENALINE SYNTHESIS

The biosynthetic pathway for noradrenaline synthesis is shown in Figure 11.2. The metabolic precursor for noradrenaline is L-tyrosine, an aromatic amino acid present in the body fluids, which is taken up by adrenergic neurons. *Tyrosine hydroxylase*, a cytosolic enzyme that catalyses the conversion of tyrosine to dihydroxyphenylalanine (dopa), is found only in catecholamine-containing cells. It is a rather selective enzyme; unlike other enzymes involved in catecholamine metabolism, it does not accept indole derivatives as substrates and so is not involved in 5-hydroxytryptamine (5-HT) metabolism. This first hydroxylation step is the main control point for noradrenaline synthesis. Tyrosine hydroxylase is inhibited by the end-product of the biosynthetic pathway, noradrenaline, and this provides the mechanism for the moment-to-moment regulation of the rate of synthesis; much slower regulation, taking hours or days, occurs by changes in the rate of production of the enzyme.

The tyrosine analogue **α-methyltyrosine** strongly inhibits tyrosine hydroxylase; it is used clinically in patients with the rare problem of inoperable phaeochromocytoma (see below) and may be used experimentally to block noradrenaline synthesis.

The next step, conversion of dopa to dopamine, is catalysed by *dopa decarboxylase*, a cytosolic enzyme that is by no means confined to catecholamine-synthesising cells. It is a relatively non-specific enzyme and catalyses the decarboxylation of various other L-aromatic amino acids, such as L-histidine and L-tryptophan, which are precursors in the synthesis of histamine and 5-HT, respectively. Activity of dopa decarboxylase is not rate limiting for noradrenaline synthesis. Though various factors,

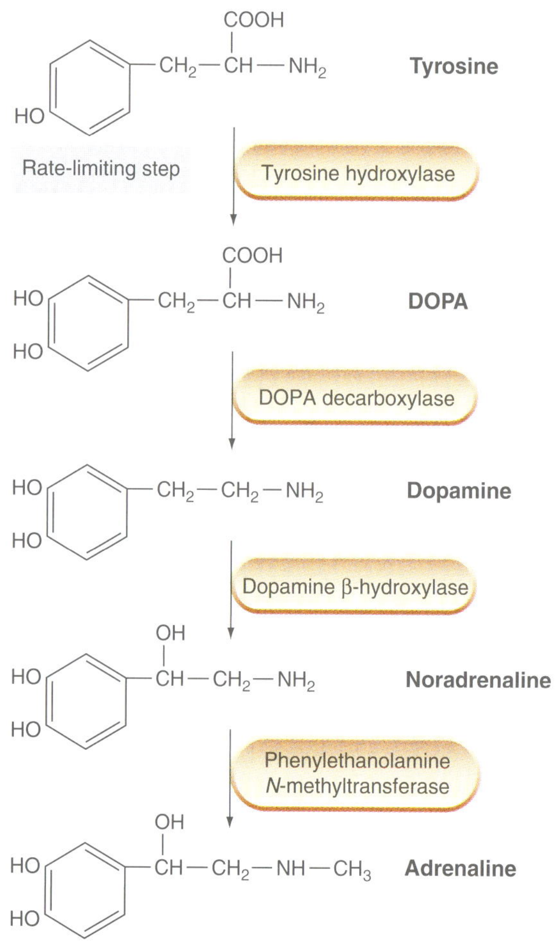

Fig. 11.2 Biosynthesis of catecholamines (dopa, dihydroxyphenylalanine.)

including certain drugs, affect the enzyme, it is not an effective means of regulating noradrenaline synthesis.

Dopamine-β-hydroxylase (DBH) is also a relatively non-specific enzyme but is restricted to catecholamine-synthesising cells. It is located in synaptic vesicles, mainly in membrane-bound form. A small amount of the enzyme is released from adrenergic nerve terminals with noradrenaline; representing the small proportion in a soluble form within the vesicle. Unlike noradrenaline, the released DBH is not subject to rapid degradation or uptake, so its concentration in plasma and body fluids can be used as an index of overall sympathetic nerve activity.

Many drugs inhibit DBH, including copper-chelating agents and **disulfiram** (a drug used mainly for its effect on ethanol metabolism; see Chs 8 and 52). Such drugs can cause a partial depletion of noradrenaline stores and interference with sympathetic transmission.

Phenylethanolamine N-*methyltransferase* (PNMT) catalyses the N-methylation of noradrenaline to adrenaline. The main location of this enzyme is in the adrenal medulla, which contains a population of adrenaline-releasing (A) cells separate from the smaller proportion of noradrenaline-releasing (N) cells. The A cells, which appear only after birth, lie adjacent to the adrenal cortex, and the production of PNMT is induced by the steroid hormones secreted by the adrenal cortex (see Ch. 27). PNMT is also found in certain parts of the brain, where adrenaline may function as a transmitter, but little is known about its role.

Noradrenaline turnover can be measured under steady-state conditions as accumulation of labelled noradrenaline from a labelled precursor, such as tyrosine or dopa. The turnover time is the time taken for an amount of noradrenaline equal to the total tissue content to be degraded and resynthesised. In peripheral tissues, the turnover time is generally about 5–15 hours, but it becomes much shorter if sympathetic nerve activity is increased. Under normal circumstances, the rate of synthesis closely matches the rate of release, so that the noradrenaline content of tissues is constant regardless of how fast it is being released.

NORADRENALINE STORAGE

Most of the noradrenaline in nerve terminals or chromaffin cells is contained in vesicles; only a little is free in the cytoplasm under normal circumstances. The concentration in the vesicles is very high (0.3–1.0 mol/l) and is maintained by a transport mechanism similar to the amine transporter responsible for noradrenaline uptake into the nerve terminal, but using the transvesicular proton gradient as its driving force (see Liu & Edwards, 1997). Certain drugs, such as **reserpine** (see below, Table 11.2), block this transport and cause nerve terminals to become depleted of their noradrenaline stores. The vesicles contain two major constituents besides noradrenaline, namely ATP (about four molecules per molecule of noradrenaline) and a protein called *chromogranin A*. These substances are released along with noradrenaline, and it is generally assumed that a reversible complex, depending partly on the opposite charges on the molecules of noradrenaline and ATP, is formed within the vesicle. This would serve both to reduce the osmolarity of the vesicle contents and to reduce the tendency of noradrenaline to leak out of the vesicles within the nerve terminal.

ATP itself has a transmitter function at adrenergic synapses (see Lundberg, 1996; Ch. 12) being responsible for the fast excitatory synaptic potential and the rapid phase of contraction produced by sympathetic nerve activity in many smooth muscle tissues. Noradrenergic neurons also store and release, from separate vesicle pods, various neuropetides (pp. 131, 133).

NORADRENALINE RELEASE

The processes linking the arrival of a nerve impulse at a noradrenergic nerve terminal to the release of noradrenaline are basically the same as those at other chemically transmitting synapses (see Ch. 4). Depolarisation of the nerve terminal membrane opens calcium channels in the nerve terminal membrane, and the resulting entry of Ca^{2+} promotes the fusion and discharge of synaptic vesicles. A surprising feature of the release mechanism at the varicosities of noradrenergic nerves is that the probability of release, even of a single vesicle, when a nerve impulse arrives at a varicosity is very low (less than 1 in 50; see Cunnane, 1984). A single neuron possesses many thousand varicosities, so one impulse leads to the discharge of a few hundred vesicles, scattered over a wide area. This contrasts sharply with the cholinergic synapse, where the release probability at a single bouton is high, but the boutons are few in number; the total release is similar, but it is sharply localised. Noradrenaline release can be produced without exocytosis, by drugs that displace it from vesicles (p. 177).

Regulation of noradrenaline release

Noradrenaline release is affected by a variety of substances that act on presynaptic receptors (see Fig. 9.4, p. 129). Many different types of nerve terminal (cholinergic, noradrenergic, dopaminergic, 5-HT-ergic, etc.) are subject to this type of control, and many different mediators (e.g. acetylcholine, acting through muscarinic receptors; catecholamines acting through α- and β-adrenoceptors; angiotensin II; prostaglandins; purine nucleotides; neuropeptides; etc.) can act on presynaptic terminals. Presynaptic modulation represents an important physiological control mechanism throughout the nervous system.

Furthermore, noradrenaline, by acting on presynaptic receptors, can regulate its own release and that of coreleased ATP (see Ch. 9). This is believed to occur physiologically, so that released noradrenaline exerts a local inhibitory effect on the terminals from which it came—the so-called *autoinhibitory feedback* mechanism (Fig. 11.3; see Starke et al., 1989). Agonists or antagonists affecting these presynaptic receptors can have large effects on sympathetic transmission. The physiological significance of presynaptic autoinhibition in the sympathetic nervous system is contentious, and there is evidence that, in most tissues, it is less influential than biochemical measurements of transmitter overflow would imply. For example, although large changes in noradrenaline overflow occur when the autoreceptors

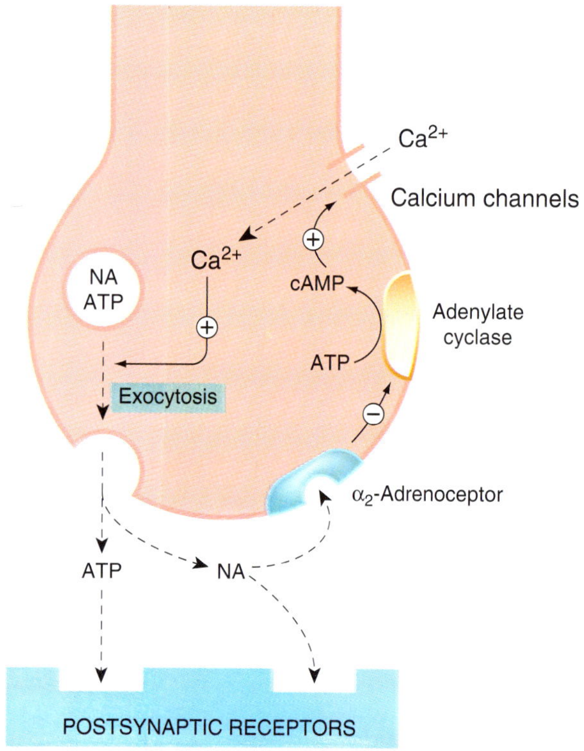

Fig. 11.3 Feedback control of noradrenaline release. The presynaptic α_2-adrenoceptor inhibits adenylate cyclase, thereby reducing intracellular cAMP. cAMP acts to promote Ca^{2+} influx in response to membrane depolarisation and hence to promote the release of noradrenaline and ATP.

are blocked, the associated changes in the tissue response to sympathetic nerve activity are often small. This suggests that what is measured in overflow experiments may not be the physiologically important component of transmitter release.

The inhibitory feedback mechanism operates through α_2-adrenoceptors, which inhibit adenylate cyclase and prevent the opening of calcium channels. Sympathetic nerve terminals also possess β_2-adrenoceptors, coupled to activation of adenylate cyclase, which cause an increased noradrenaline release. Whether they have any physiological function is not yet clear.

UPTAKE AND DEGRADATION OF CATECHOLAMINES

The action of released noradrenaline is terminated mainly by reuptake of the transmitter into noradrenergic nerve terminals. Some is also sequestered by other cells in the vicinity. Circulating adrenaline and noradrenaline are degraded enzymically, but much more slowly than acetylcholine (see Ch. 10), where synaptically located acetylcholinesterase inactivates the transmitter in milliseconds. The two main catecholamine-metabolising enzymes are located intracellularly; consequently, uptake into cells necessarily precedes metabolic degradation.

Uptake of catecholamines

Indirect evidence that sympathetic nerves can take up amines from the circulation and release them again as transmitter came originally from the work of Burn and his colleagues. In 1932, Burn found that the pressor effect of indirectly acting sympathomimetics (e.g. **tyramine**; see below) in whole animals was increased if the injection was preceded by injection of adrenaline, and he showed that this was because adrenaline was able to replenish the releasable amine stores of the nerve terminals. Later, it was demonstrated that tritiated noradrenaline was rapidly taken up from the circulation into tissues. Part of this

Noradrenergic transmission

- Transmitter synthesis involves the following steps:
  - —L-tyrosine is converted to dopa by tyrosine hydroxylase (rate-limiting step). Tyrosine hydroxylase occurs only in catecholaminergic neurons.
  - —dopa is converted to dopamine by dopa decarboxylase.
  - —dopamine is converted to noradrenaline by dopamine β-hydroxylase (DBH), located in synaptic vesicles
  - —in the adrenal medulla, noradrenaline is converted to adrenaline by phenylethanolamine *N*-methyltransferase.
- Transmitter storage: noradrenaline is stored at high concentration in synaptic vesicles, together with ATP, chromogranin and DBH, all of which are released by exocytosis. Transport of noradrenaline into vesicles occurs by a reserpine-sensitive carrier. Noradrenaline content of cytosol is normally low, owing to monoamine oxidase in nerve terminals.
- Transmitter release occurs normally by Ca^{2+}-mediated exocytosis from varicosities on the terminal network. Non-exocytotic release occurs in response to indirectly acting sympathomimetic drugs (e.g. amphetamine), which displace noradrenaline from vesicles. Noradrenaline escapes via uptake 1 (reverse transport).
- Transmitter action is terminated mainly by reuptake of noradrenaline into nerve terminals. This uptake (uptake 1) is blocked by tricyclic antidepressant drugs and cocaine.
- Noradrenaline release is controlled by autoinhibitory feedback, mediated by α_2-adrenoceptors.
- Cotransmission occurs at many noradrenergic nerve terminals, ATP and neuropeptide Y being frequently coreleased with noradrenaline. ATP mediates the early phase of smooth muscle contraction in response to sympathetic nerve activity.

uptake was by sympathetic neurons (for it disappeared when sympathetic nerves were allowed to degenerate), and the amine could be released again by sympathetic nerve stimulation. In a study of noradrenaline uptake by isolated rat hearts, Iversen identified two distinct uptake mechanisms, each having the characteristics of a saturable active transport system capable of accumulating catecholamines against a large concentration gradient. These two mechanisms, called *uptake 1* and *uptake 2*, correspond to neuronal and extraneuronal uptake, respectively. They have different kinetic properties as well as different substrate and inhibitor specificity, as summarised in Table 11.2.

Uptake 1 is a high-affinity system, relatively selective for noradrenaline and with a low maximum rate of uptake, whereas uptake 2 has low affinity and transports adrenaline and isoprenaline as well as noradrenaline, but at a much higher maximum rate. The effects of several important drugs that act on noradrenergic neurons depend on their ability either to inhibit uptake 1 or to enter the nerve terminal with its help (see Table 11.2).

Noradrenaline transporters belong to the family of neurotransmitter transporter proteins (NET, DAT, SERT, etc.) specific for different amine transmitters, described in Chapter 9; these act as cotransporters of Na^+ and Cl^- with the amine in question, using the electrochemical gradient for Na^+ as a driving force. Changes in this gradient can alter, or even reverse, the operation of uptake 1, with marked effects on the availability of the released transmitter at postsynaptic receptors.

Metabolic degradation of catecholamines

Endogenous and exogenous catecholamines are metabolised mainly by two enzymes, *monoamine oxidase* (MAO) and *catechol-O-methyl transferase* (COMT). MAO occurs within cells bound to the surface membrane of mitochondria. It is abundant in noradrenergic nerve terminals but is also present in many other places, such as liver and intestinal epithelium. MAO converts catecholamines to their corresponding aldehydes, which, in the periphery, are rapidly metabolised by aldehyde dehydrogenase to the corresponding carboxylic acid (Fig. 11.4). In the case of noradrenaline, this yields *dihydroxymandelic acid* (DOMA). MAO can also oxidise other monoamines, important ones being dopamine and 5-HT. It is inhibited by various drugs (see Table 11.3, below), which are used mainly for their effects on the central nervous system where these three amines all have transmitter functions (see Ch. 31). These drugs have important side-effects that are related to disturbances of peripheral adrenergic transmission. Within sympathetic neurons, MAO controls the content of dopamine and noradrenaline, and the releasable store of noradrenaline increases if the enzyme is inhibited. MAO and its inhibitors are discussed in more detail in Chapter 38.

The second major pathway for catecholamine metabolism involves methylation of one of the catechol hydroxyl groups to give a methoxy derivative. COMT is a widespread enzyme that occurs in both neuronal and non-neuronal tissues. It acts on both

Table 11.2 Characteristics noradrenaline transport systems

	Uptake 1[a]	Uptake 2	Vesicular transporter[a]
Transport of noradrenaline (rat heart)			
V_{max} (nmol/g per min)	1.2	100	
K_m (μmol/l	0.3	250	~0.2
Specificity	NA > A > ISO	A > NA > ISO	NA = A = ISO
Location	Neuronal membrane	Non-neuronal cell membrane (smooth muscle, cardiac muscle, endothelium)	Synaptic vesicle membrane
Other substrates	Methylnoradrenaline Tyramine Adrenergic neuron-blocking drugs (e.g. guanethidine)	(+)-Noradrenaline Dopamine 5-HT Histamine	Dopamine 5-HT Guanethidine MPP+ (see Ch. 34)
Inhibitors	Cocaine Tricyclic antidepressants (e.g. desipramine) Phenoxybenzamine Amphetamine	Normetanephrine Steroid hormones (e.g. corticosterone) Phenoxybenzamine	Reserpine Tetrabenazine

NA, noradrenaline; A, adrenaline; ISO, isoprenaline; 5-HT, 5-hydroxytryptamine; MPP^+, methylphenylpyridinium.
[a]Transporters corresponding to uptake 1 and vesicular transporter have been cloned and termed norepinephrine transporter (NET) and vesicular monoamine transporter (VMAT), respectively (see review by Nelson, 1998). The uptake 2 transporter has not yet been identified.

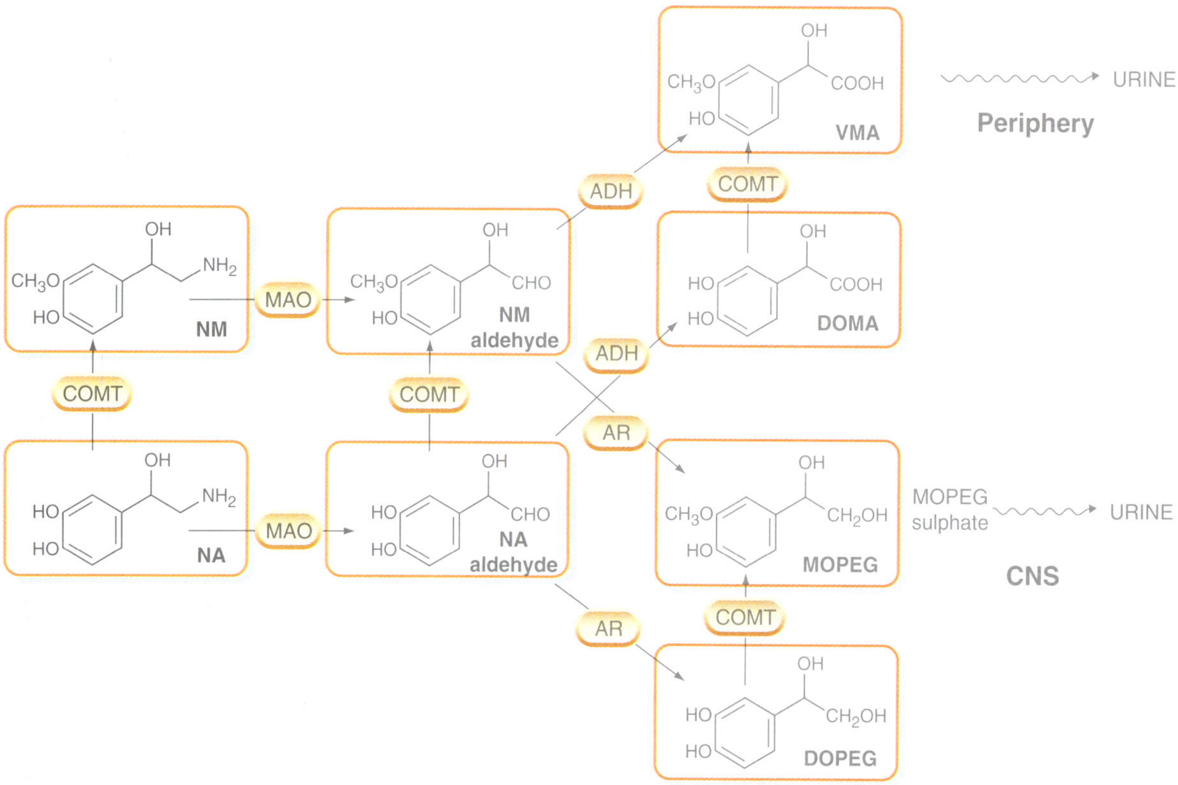

Fig. 11.4 The main pathways of noradrenaline metabolism in the brain and in the periphery. In the periphery, the oxidative branch (catalysed by ADH) predominates, giving VMA as the main urinary metabolite. In the brain, the reductive branch (catalysed by AR) predominates, producing MOPEG, which is conjugated to give MOPEG sulfate before being excreted. (NA, noradrenaline; NM, normetanephrine; VMA, vanillylmandelic acid; DOMA, 3,2-dihydroxymandelic acid; MOPEG, 3-methoxy-4-hydroxyphenylglycol; DOPEG, 3,4-dihydroxyphenylglycol; MAO, monoamine oxidase; COMT, catechol-*O*-methyltransferase; ADH, aldehyde dehydrogenase; AR, aldehyde reductase.)

the catecholamines themselves and the deaminated products, such as DOMA, that are produced by the action of MAO. The main final metabolite of adrenaline and noradrenaline is *3-methoxy-4-hydroxymandelic acid* (VMA). In patients with tumours of chromaffin tissue that secrete these amines (a rare cause of high blood pressure), the urinary excretion of VMA is markedly increased, this being used as a diagnostic test for this condition.

In the periphery, neither MAO nor COMT is primarily responsible for the termination of transmitter action, most of the released noradrenaline being quickly recaptured by uptake 1. Circulating catecholamines are usually removed by a combination of uptake 1, uptake 2 and COMT, the relative importance of these processes varying according to the agent concerned. Thus, circulating noradrenaline is removed mainly by uptake 1, whereas adrenaline is more dependent on uptake 2. Isoprenaline is not a substrate for uptake 1 and is removed by a combination of uptake 2 and COMT.

The metabolism of noradrenaline in the central nervous system (CNS) follows a different course (see Ch. 31 and Fig. 11.4). MAO is more important as a means of terminating transmitter action than it is in the periphery, and the resulting aldehydes are mainly reduced to the corresponding alcohols. The main excretory product of noradrenaline released in the brain is an ethyleneglycol derivative (MOPEG). Thus measurement of urinary VMA and MOPEG enables the central and peripheral release of noradrenaline to be quantified.

DRUGS ACTING ON ADRENOCEPTORS

STRUCTURE–ACTIVITY RELATIONSHIPS

The overall potency and receptor specificity of drugs that exert their effects by combining with adrenoceptors depends on several factors:

- affinity for, and efficacy on, adrenoceptors
- interaction with neuronal uptake systems
- interaction with MAO and COMT.

The relationship of these different factors with chemical structure is, not surprisingly, complex, but there are certain useful generalisations that can be made. The noradrenaline molecule can be modified in several different ways to yield compounds that interact with adrenoceptors (Fig. 11.5).

- Increasing the bulkiness of substituents on the N-atom produces compounds (**adrenaline, isoprenaline** and **salbutamol**) of relatively greater potency as β-agonists and that are less susceptible to uptake 1 and MAO.
- Addition of an α-methyl group (**α-methylnoradrenaline, metaraminol**) increases α_2-adrenoceptor selectivity and also renders compounds resistant to MAO, though they remain susceptible to uptake 1.
- Removal of the side-chain –OH group (**dopamine**) greatly reduces interaction with α- and β-adrenoceptors.
- Modification of the catechol –OH groups renders compounds resistant to COMT and uptake 1 (**salbutamol** and many β-adrenoceptor antagonists), but retains receptor activity.
- Removal of one or both –OH groups (**tyramine, amphetamine, ephedrine**) abolishes affinity for receptors, though these compounds are still indirectly acting sympathomimetic amines as they are substrates for uptake 1.
- Extension of the alkyl side-chain, with isopropyl substitution on the N-atom, and modification of catechol –OH groups (**propranolol, oxprenolol**, etc.) produce potent β-adrenoceptor antagonists.

These general rules account fairly well for the properties of many directly and indirectly acting sympathomimetic drugs and for β-adrenoceptor antagonists. The α-adrenoceptor antagonists are much more heterogeneous, however, and defy such generalisations.

ADRENOCEPTOR AGONISTS

Examples of the main types of adrenoceptor agonist are given in Table 11.1 and the characteristics of individual drugs are summarised in Table 11.3, below.

Actions

The major physiological effects mediated by different types of adrenoceptor are summarised in Table 11.1.

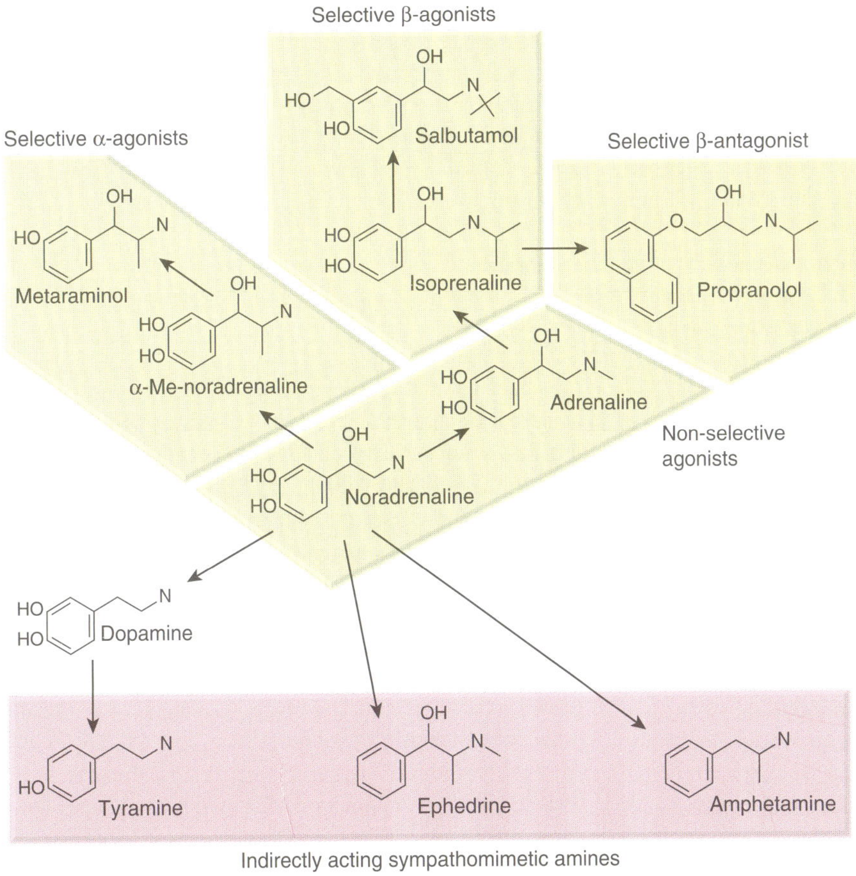

Fig. 11.5 Structure–activity relationships among catecholamines and related compounds.

Smooth muscle

All types of smooth muscle, except that of the gastrointestinal tract, contract in response to stimulation of α_1-adrenoceptors, through activation of the signal transduction mechanism described in Chapter 4.

When α-agonists are given systemically to experimental animals or humans, the most important action is on vascular smooth muscle, particularly in the skin and splanchnic vascular beds, which are strongly constricted. Large arteries and veins, as well as arterioles, are also constricted, resulting in decreased vascular compliance, increased central venous pressure and increased peripheral resistance. All of these contribute to an increase in systolic and diastolic arterial pressure. Some vascular beds (e.g. cerebral, coronary and pulmonary) are relatively little affected.

In the whole animal, baroreceptor reflexes are activated by the rise in arterial pressure produced by α-agonists, causing reflex bradycardia and inhibition of respiration.

Smooth muscle in the vas deferens, spleen capsule and eyelid retractor muscles (or nictitating membrane, in some species) is also stimulated by α-agonists and these organs are often used for pharmacological studies.

The α-adrenoceptors involved in smooth muscle contraction are mainly α_1 in type, though vascular smooth muscle possesses both α_1- and α_2-adrenoceptors. It appears that α_1-adrenoceptors lie close to the sites of release (and are mainly responsible for neurally mediated vasoconstriction), while α_2-adrenoceptors lie elsewhere on the muscle fibre surface, and are activated by circulating catecholamines (see McGrath & Wilson, 1988; Broadley, 1996).

Stimulation of β-adrenoceptors causes relaxation of most kinds of smooth muscle by increasing cAMP formation (see Ch. 4). Additionally, β-adrenoceptor activation enhances Ca^{2+} extrusion and intracellular Ca^{2+} binding, both effects acting to reduce free intracellular Ca^{2+} concentrations.

Relaxation is usually produced by β_2-adrenoceptors, though the receptor that is responsible for this effect in gastrointestinal smooth muscle is not clearly β_1 or β_2. In the vascular system, β_2-mediated vasodilatation is (particularly in humans) mainly endothelium-dependent and mediated by nitric oxide release (see Ch. 14). It occurs in many vascular beds and is especially marked in skeletal muscle.

The powerful inhibitory effect of the sympathetic system on gastrointestinal smooth muscle is produced by both α- and β-adrenoceptors, the gastrointestinal tract being unusual in that α-adrenoceptors cause relaxation in most regions. Part of the effect is the result of stimulation of presynaptic α_2-adrenoceptors (see below), which inhibit the release of excitatory transmitters (e.g. acetylcholine) from intramural nerves, but there are also α-adrenoceptors on the muscle cells, stimulation of which hyperpolarises the cell (by increasing the membrane permeability to K^+) and inhibits action potential discharge. The sphincters of the gastrointestinal tract are contracted by α-adrenoceptor activation.

Bronchial smooth muscle is strongly dilated by activation of β_2-adrenoceptors, and selective β_2-agonists are important in the treatment of asthma (see Ch. 22). Uterine smooth muscle responds similarly, and these drugs are also used to delay premature labour.

Alpha-adrenoceptors also mediate a long-lasting trophic response, stimulating smooth muscle proliferation in various tissues, for example in blood vessels and in the prostate gland, which is of clinical importance. Benign prostatic hyperplasia (see Ch. 29) is commonly treated with α-adrenoceptor antagonists (see the clinical box on p. 173). 'Cross-talk' between the α_1-adrenoceptor and the growth factor signalling pathways (see Ch. 3) probably accounts for this effect.

Nerve terminals

Presynaptic adrenoceptors are present on both cholinergic and adrenergic nerve terminals (see Chs 4 and 9). The main effect (α_2-mediated) is inhibitory, but a weaker facilitatory action of β-adrenoceptors on adrenergic nerve terminals has also been described.

Heart

Catecholamines, acting on β_1-adrenoceptors, exert a powerful stimulant effect on the heart (see Ch. 17). Both the heart rate (chronotropic effect) and the force of contraction (inotropic effect) are increased, resulting in a markedly increased cardiac output and cardiac oxygen consumption. The cardiac efficiency (see Ch. 17) is reduced. Catecholamines can also cause disturbance of the cardiac rhythm, culminating in ventricular fibrillation. In normal hearts, the dose required to cause marked dysrhythmia is greater than that which produces the chronotropic and inotropic effects, but in ischaemic conditions dysrhythmias are produced much more readily. Figure 11.6 shows the overall pattern of cardiovascular responses to catecholamine infusions in humans, reflecting their actions on both the heart and vascular system.

Cardiac hypertrophy occurs in response to activation of α_1-adrenoceptors, probably by a mechanism similar to the hypertrophy of vascular and prostatic smooth muscle. This may be important in the pathophysiology of hypertension and cardiac failure (see Ch. 17).

Metabolism

Catecholamines encourage the conversion of energy stores (glycogen and fat) to freely available fuels (glucose and free fatty acids), and cause an increase in the plasma concentration of the latter substances. The detailed biochemical mechanisms (see review by Nonogaki, 2000) vary from species to species, but in most cases the effects on carbohydrate metabolism in liver and muscle (Fig. 11.7) are mediated through β_1-adrenoceptors (though hepatic glucose release can also be produced by α-agonists), and the stimulation of lipolysis is produced by β_3-adrenoceptors (see Table 11.1). Insulin secretion is also affected, the main influence being inhibitory, through α_2-adrenoceptors, an effect which further contributes to the hyperglycaemia. Additionally, the production of **leptin** by adipose tissue (see Ch. 26) is inhibited. Adrenaline-induced hyperglycaemia in humans is blocked completely by a combination of α- and β-antagonists but not by either on its own. Selective β_3-adrenoceptor agonists (e.g. BRL 37344) have been developed and may prove useful in the treatment of obesity, but they are not yet approved for clinical use.

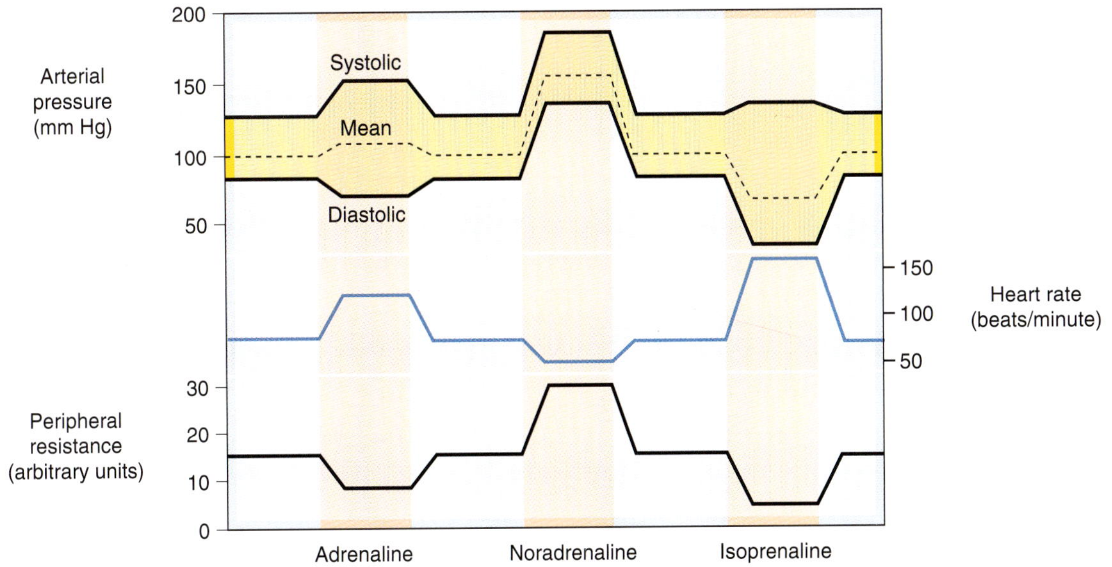

Fig. 11.6 Schematic representation of the cardiovascular effects of intravenous infusions of adrenaline, noradrenaline and isoprenaline in humans. Noradrenaline (predominantly α-agonist) causes vasoconstriction and increased systolic and diastolic pressure, with a reflex bradycardia. Isoprenaline (β-agonist) is a vasodilator, but strongly increases cardiac force and rate. Mean arterial pressure falls. Adrenaline combines both actions.

Other effects

Skeletal muscle is affected by adrenaline, acting on β_2-adrenoceptors, though the effect is far less dramatic than that on the heart. The twitch tension of fast-contracting fibres (white muscle) is increased by adrenaline, particularly if the muscle is fatigued, whereas the twitch of slow (red) muscle is reduced. These effects depend on an action on the contractile proteins, rather than on the membrane, and the mechanism is poorly understood. In humans, adrenaline and other β_2-agonists cause a marked tremor: the shakiness that accompanies fear, excitement or the excessive use of β_2-agonists (e.g. salbutamol) in the treatment of asthma are examples of this. It probably results from an increase in muscle spindle discharge, coupled with an effect on the contraction kinetics of the fibres, these effects combining to produce an instability in the reflex control of muscle length. Beta-adrenoceptor antagonists are sometimes used to control pathological tremor. The β_2-agonists also cause long-term changes in the expression of the sarcoplasmic reticular proteins that control contraction kinetics and thereby increase the rate and force of contraction of skeletal muscle (see Zhang et al., 1996). **Clenbuterol**, an 'anabolic' drug used illicitly by sportsmen to improve performance, is a β_2-agonist that acts in this way.

Histamine release by human and guinea-pig lung tissue in response to anaphylactic challenge (see Ch. 15) is inhibited by catecholamines, acting apparently on β_2-adrenoceptors.

Lymphocytes and other cells of the immune system also express adrenoceptors (mainly β-adrenoceptors). Lymphocyte proliferation, lymphocyte-mediated cell killing and production of many cytokines are inhibited by β-adrenoceptor agonists. The physiological and clinical importance of these effects has not yet been established. For a review of the effects of the sympathetic nervous system on immune function, see Elenkov et al. (2000).

Adrenoceptor agonists

- Noradrenaline and adrenaline show relatively little receptor selectivity.
- Selective α_1-agonists include phenylephrine and oxymetazoline.
- Selective α_2-agonists include clonidine, α-methylnoradrenaline. They cause a fall in blood pressure, partly by inhibition of noradrenaline release, and partly by a central action. Methylnoradrenaline is formed as a false transmitter from methyldopa, developed as a hypotensive drug (now largely obsolete).
- Selective β_1-agonists include dobutamine. Increased cardiac contractility may be useful clinically, but all β_1-agonists can cause cardiac dysrhythmias.
- Selective β_2-agonists include salbutamol, terbutaline and salmeterol, used mainly for their bronchodilator action in asthma.
- Selective β_3-agonists are being developed for the control of obesity.

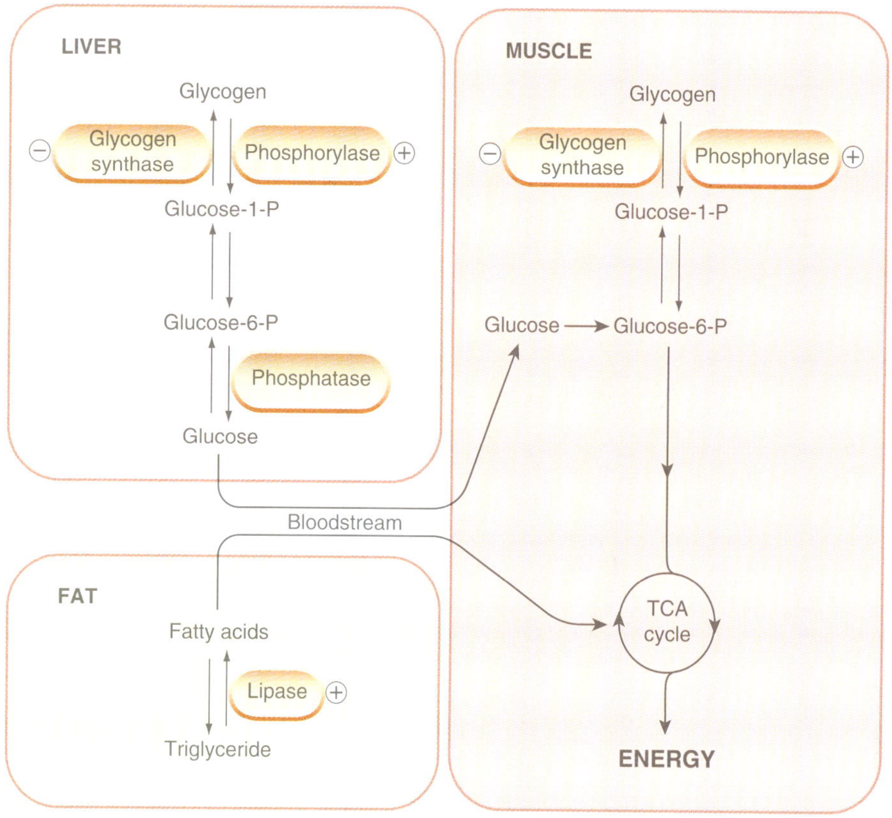

Fig. 11.7 Regulation of energy metabolism by catecholamines. The main enzymic steps that are affected by β-adrenoceptor activation are indicated by + and – signs, denoting stimulation and inhibition, respectively. The overall effect is to mobilise glycogen and fat stores to meet energy demands.

Clinical uses of adrenoceptor agonists

- Cardiovascular system
  - —cardiac arrest: **adrenaline**
  - —cardiogenic shock (see Ch.18): **dobutamine** (β_1-agonist)
  - —heart block: β-agonists (e.g. **isoprenaline**) can be used temporarily while electrical pacing is being arranged.
- Anaphylactic shock (acute hypersensitivity, see Ch. 15)
  - —**adrenaline** is the first-line treatment
- Respiratory system
  - —asthma (see Ch. 22): selective β_2-receptor agonists (**salbutamol, terbutaline, salmeterol, formoterol**)
  - —nasal decongestion:drops containing **oxymetazoline** or **ephedrine** for short-term use.
- Miscellaneous indications
  - —**adrenaline** can be used to prolong local anaesthetic action (see Ch. 42)
  - —inhibition of premature labour (**salbutamol**; see Ch. 29)
  - —miscellaneous indication for α_2-agonists (e.g. **clonidine**) include hypertension (Ch.18), menopausal flushing, lowering intraocular pressure and migraine prophylaxis (Ch. 12).

Clinical use

The main clinical uses of adrenoceptor agonists are summarised in the clinical box.

ADRENOCEPTOR ANTAGONISTS

The main adrenoceptor antagonists are listed in Table 11.1, and further information is given in Table 11.3, below. In contrast to the situation with agonists, most adrenoceptor antagonists are selective for α- or β-adrenoceptors, and many are also subtype selective.

ALPHA-ADRENOCEPTOR ANTAGONISTS

The main groups of α-adrenoceptor antagonists are:

- non-selective α-adrenoceptor antagonists (e.g. **phenoxybenzamine, phentolamine**)
- α_1-selective antagonists (e.g. **prazosin, doxazosin, terazosin**)
- α_2-selective antagonists (e.g. **yohimbine, idazoxan**)
- ergot derivatives (e.g. **ergotamine, dihydroergotamine**). This group of compounds has many actions in addition to α-adrenoceptor block and is discussed in Chapter 12. Their action on α-adrenoceptors is of pharmacological interest (see p. 161) but they are not used therapeutically.

Non-selective α-adrenoceptor antagonists

Phenoxybenzamine is not specific for α-adrenoceptors and also antagonises the actions of acetylcholine, histamine and 5-HT. It is long lasting because it binds covalently to the receptor. **Phentolamine** is more selective, but it binds reversibly and its action is short lasting. In humans, these drugs cause a fall in arterial pressure (because of block of α-adrenoceptor-mediated vasoconstriction) and postural hypotension. The cardiac output and heart rate are increased. This is a reflex response to the fall in arterial pressure, mediated through β-adrenoceptors. The concomitant block of α_2-adrenoceptors tends to increase noradrenaline release, which has the effect of enhancing the reflex tachycardia that occurs with any blood-pressure-lowering agent.

Labetalol and **carvedilol** are mixed α- and β-adrenoceptor-blocking drugs, though clinically they act predominantly on β-adrenoceptors. Much has been made of the fact that they combine both activities in one molecule. To a pharmacologist, accustomed to putting specificity of action high on the list of pharmacological saintly virtues, they may seem like a step backwards rather than forwards. Carvedilol is used mainly to treat hypertension and heart failure (see Chs 17 and 18); labetalol is used occasionally to treat hypertension in pregnancy.

Selective α_1-antagonists

Prazosin was the first α_1-selective antagonist. Similar drugs with longer half-lives (e.g. **doxazosin**, **terazosin**), which have the advantage of allowing once-daily dosing, are now available. They are highly selective and cause vasodilatation and fall in arterial pressure, but less tachycardia than occurs with non-selective α-adrenoceptor antagonists, presumably because they do not increase noradrenaline release from sympathetic nerve terminals. Some postural hypotension may occur.

The α_1-adrenoceptor antagonists cause relaxation of the smooth muscle of the bladder neck and prostate capsule, which may be useful in patients with urinary retention associated with benign prostatic hypertrophy. **Tamsulosin**, an α_{1A}-adrenoceptor antagonist, shows some selectivity for the bladder and causes less hypotension than drugs such as prazosin.

There is also evidence that particular α_1-adrenoceptor subtypes play a part in the pathological hypertrophy of prostatic and vascular smooth muscle, and also in the cardiac hypertrophy that occurs in hypertension. The use of subtype-selective α_1-adrenoceptor antagonists to treat these chronic conditions is under investigation.

Clinical uses of α-adrenoceptor antagonists

- Hypertension(see Ch.15): α_1-selective antagonists. **Prazosin** is short-acting. Preferred drugs are longer-acting (e.g. **doxazosin**, **terazosin**), used either alone in mild hypertension, or in combination with other drugs.
- Benign prostatic hypertrophy (especially **tamsulosin**, a selective α_1A-receptor antagonist).
- Phaeochromocytoma: **phenoxybenzamine** used in conjunction with α_1-receptor antagonist in preparation for surgery.

Selective α_2-antagonists

Yohimbine is a naturally occurring alkaloid; various synthetic analogues have been made, such as idazoxan. These drugs are used experimentally to analyse α-adrenoceptor subtypes, and yohimbine, probably by virtue of its vasodilator effect, enjoys a certain notoriety as an aphrodisiac, but they are not used therapeutically.

General clinical uses and unwanted effects of α-adrenoceptor antagonists

The main uses of α-adrenoceptor antagonists are related to their cardiovascular actions and are summarised in the clinical box. They have been tried for many purposes but have only limited therapeutic applications. In hypertension, non-selective α-blocking drugs are unsatisfactory, because of their tendency to produce tachycardia, cardiac dysrhythmias and increased gastrointestinal activity. Selective α_1-adrenoceptor antagonists (especially the longer-acting compounds **doxazosin** and **terazosin**) are, however, useful. They do not affect cardiac function appreciably, and postural hypotension is less troublesome than with prazosin or non-selective α-adrenoceptor antagonists. There has been a recent resurgence in the use of these drugs to treat hypertension (see Ch. 18). Unlike other antihypertensive drugs, they cause a modest decrease in low density lipoproteins and an increase in high density lipoprotein cholesterol (see Ch. 19), though the clinical importance of these ostensibly beneficial effects is uncertain. They are used to control urinary retention in benign prostatic hypertrophy.

A common side-effect of α-adrenceptor antagonists is impotence.

Phaeochromocytoma is a catecholamine-secreting tumour of chromaffin tissue, and one of its effects is to cause episodes of severe hypertension. A combination of α- and β-adrenoceptor antagonists is the most effective way of controlling blood pressure. The tumour may be surgically removable, and it is essential to block α- and β-adrenoceptors before surgery is begun to avoid the effects of a sudden release of catecholamines when the tumour is disturbed. A combination of phenoxybenzamine and atenolol is effective for this purpose.

BETA-ADRENOCEPTOR ANTAGONISTS

The β-adrenoceptor antagonists are an important group of drugs. They were first discovered in 1958, 10 years after Ahlquist had postulated the existence of β-adrenoceptors. The first compound, **dichloroisoprenaline**, had fairly low potency, and was a partial agonist. Further development led to **propranolol**, which is much more potent and a pure antagonist that blocks β_1- and β_2-adrenoceptors equally. The potential clinical advantages of drugs with some partial agonist activity, and/or with selectivity for β_1-adrenoceptors, led to the development of **practolol** (selective for

β_1-adrenoceptors but no longer used clinically because of its toxicity), **oxprenolol** and **alprenolol** (non-selective with considerable partial agonist activity), and **atenolol** (β_1-selective with no agonist activity). Many very similar drugs have been developed, and the characteristics of the most important compounds are set out in Tables 11.1 and 11.3. Most β-adrenoceptor antagonists are inactive on β_3-adrenoceptors so do not affect lipolysis.

Actions

The pharmacological actions of β-adrenoceptor antagonists can be deduced from Table 11.1. The effects produced in humans depend on the degree of sympathetic activity and are slight in subjects at rest. The most important effects are on the cardiovascular system and on bronchial smooth muscle (see Chs 17, 18 and 22).

In a subject at rest, propranolol causes little change in heart rate, cardiac output or arterial pressure, but it reduces the effect of exercise or excitement on these variables (Fig. 11.8). Drugs with partial agonist activity, such as oxprenolol, increase the heart rate at rest but reduce it during exercise. Maximum exercise tolerance is considerably reduced in normal subjects, partly because of the limitation of the cardiac response and partly because the β-mediated vasodilatation in skeletal muscle is reduced. Coronary flow is reduced, but relatively less than the myocardial oxygen consumption, so oxygenation of the myocardium is improved, an effect of importance in the treatment of angina pectoris (see Ch. 17).

In normal subjects, the reduction of the force of contraction of the heart is of no importance, but it may have serious consequences for patients with heart disease (see below).

An important, and somewhat unexpected, effect of β-adrenoceptor antagonists is their antihypertensive action (see Ch. 18). Patients with hypertension (though not normotensive subjects) show a gradual fall in arterial pressure that takes several days to develop fully. The mechanism is complex and involves:

- reduction in cardiac output
- reduction of renin release from the juxtaglomerular cells of the kidney
- a central action, reducing sympathetic activity.

Blockade of the facilitatory effect of presynaptic β-adrenoceptors on noradrenaline release may also contribute to the antihypertensive effect. The antihypertensive effect of β-adrenoceptor antagonists is clinically very useful. Because reflex vasoconstriction is preserved, postural and exercise-induced hypotension (see Ch. 18) are less troublesome than with many other antihypertensive drugs.

Many β-adrenoceptor antagonists have an antidysrhythmic effect on the heart, which is of clinical importance (see Ch. 17).

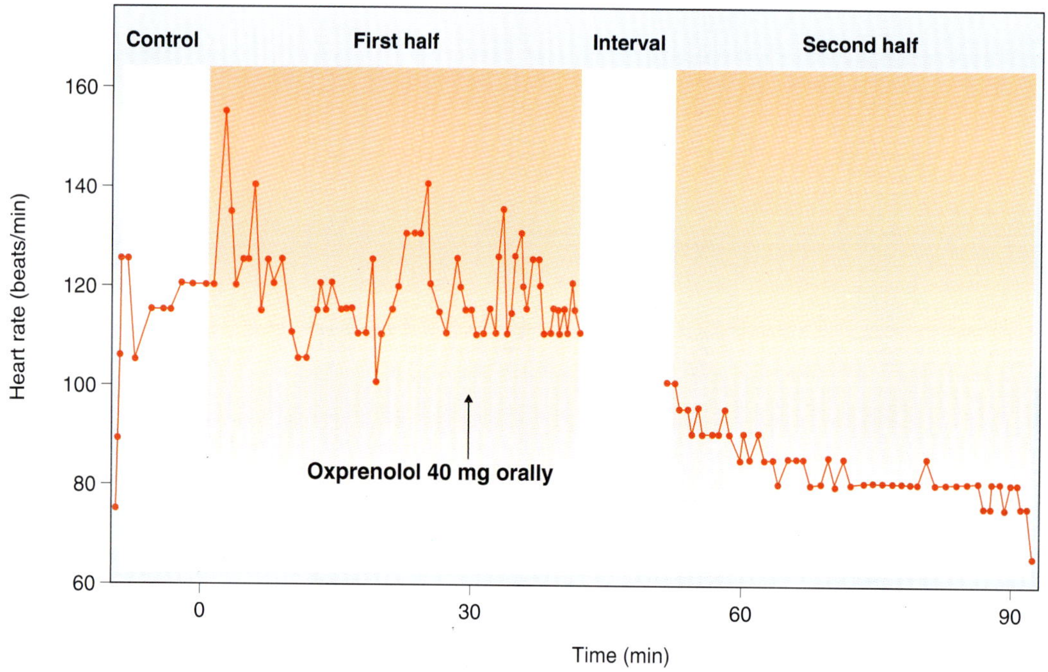

Fig. 11.8 Heart rate recorded continuously in a spectator watching a live football match, showing the effect of the β-adrenoceptor antagonist oxprenol. (From: Taylor S H, Meeran M K 1973 In Burley et al. (eds) New perspectives in beta-blockade. CIBA Laboratories, Horsham)

Airways resistance in normal subjects is only slightly increased by β-adrenoceptor antagonists, and this is of no consequence. In asthmatic subjects, however, non-selective β-adrenoceptor antagonists (such as propranolol) can cause severe bronchoconstriction, which does not, of course, respond to the usual doses of drugs such as salbutamol or adrenaline. This danger is less with β_1-selective antagonists, but none is so selective that this danger can be ignored.

In spite of the involvement of β-adrenoceptors in the hyperglycaemic actions of adrenaline, β-adrenoceptor antagonists cause only minor metabolic changes in normal subjects. They do not affect the onset of hypoglycaemia following an injection of insulin, but somewhat delay the recovery of blood glucose concentration. In diabetic patients, the use of β-adrenoceptor antagonists increases the likelihood of exercise-induced hypoglycaemia because the normal adrenaline-induced release of glucose from the liver is diminished.

Clinical use

The main uses of β-adrenoceptor antagonists are connected with their effects on the cardiovascular system and are discussed in Chapters 17 and 18. They are as summarised in the clinical box.

Unwanted effects

The main side-effects of β-adrenoceptor antagonists result from their receptor-blocking action.

Adrenoceptor antagonists

- Compounds are either α- or β-adrenoceptor selective, and some show further subtype selectivity.
- Drugs that block α_1- and α_2-adrenoceptors (e.g. phenoxybenzamine, phentolamine) were once used to produce vasodilatation in treatment of peripheral vascular disease, now largely obsolete.
- Selective α_1-antagonists (e.g. prazosin, doxazosin, terazosin) are used in treating hypertension. Postural hypotension and impotence are unwanted effects.
- Yohimbine is a selective α_2-antagonist. It is not used clinically.
- Tamsulosin is α_{1A}-selective and acts mainly on urogenital tract.
- α-Adrenoceptor antagonists include propranolol, alprenolol, oxprenolol (non-selective between α_1 and α_2), atenolol (α_1-selective). Some (alprenolol, oxprenolol) have partial agonist activity. Used mainly to treat hypertension, cardiac dysrhythmias, angina and myocardial infarction. They are also used to treat anxiety. Important hazards are bronchoconstriction, bradycardia and cardiac failure (possibly less with partial agonists). Side-effects include cold extremities, insomnia, depression. Some show rapid first-pass metabolism, hence poor bioavailability.

Clinical uses of β-adrenoceptor antagonists

- Cardiovascular system (see Chs 17 and 18)
  - —hypertension
  - —angina pectoris
  - —following myocardial infarction (protection against dysrhythmias and repeated infarction)
  - —cardiac dysrhythmias
- Clinically stable cardiac failure (prolong survival).
- Other uses
  - —glaucoma, e.g. **timolol** eye drops
  - —thyrotoxicosis (see Ch. 28), as adjunct to definitive treatment (e.g. properatively)
  - —anxiety states (see Ch. 36), to control somatic symptoms associated with sympathetic overactivity, such as palpitations and tremor
  - —migraine prophylaxis (see Ch. 12)
  - —benign essential tremor (a familial disorder).

Bronchoconstriction.

Bronchoconstiction is of little importance in the absence of airways disease, but in asthmatic patients, this effect can be dramatic and life threatening. It is also of clinical importance in patients with other forms of obstructive lung disease (e.g. chronic bronchitis, emphysema).

Cardiac failure

Patients with heart disease may rely on a degree of sympathetic drive to the heart to maintain an adequate cardiac output, and removal of this by blocking β-adrenoceptors will produce a degree of cardiac failure.* In theory, drugs with partial agonist activity (e.g. oxprenolol, alprenolol) offer an advantage since they can, by their own action, maintain a degree of β_1-adrenoceptor activation, while at the same time blunting the cardiac response to increased sympathetic nerve activity or to circulating adrenaline. Clinical trials so far, however, have not shown a clear advantage of these drugs measurable as a reduced incidence of cardiac failure.

Bradycardia

Bradycardia can progress to life-threatening heart block. It can occur in patients with coronary disease, particularly if they are being treated with antidysrhythmic drugs that impair cardiac conduction (see Ch. 18).

Hypoglycaemia

Glucose release in response to adrenaline is a safety device that may be important to diabetic patients and to other individuals

*Paradoxically, β-adrenoceptor antagonists are increasingly being used in low doses to *treat* cardiac failure, though at the outset there is a danger of exacerbating the problem. Several mechanisms may contribute, including inhibition of central sympathetic outflow and direct vasodilator effects (see review by Pfeffer & Stevenson, 1996). **Carvedilol** is often used for this purpose.

prone to hypoglycaemic attacks. The sympathetic response to hypoglycaemia produces symptoms (especially tachycardia) that warn patients of the urgent need for carbohydrate (usually in the form of a sugary drink). The use of β-adrenoceptor antagonists reduces these symptoms, so incipient hypoglycaemia is more likely to go unnoticed by the patient. The use of β-adrenoceptor antagonists is generally to be avoided in patients with poorly controlled diabetes. There is a theoretical advantage in using β_1-selective agents, since glucose release from the liver is controlled by β_2-adrenoceptors.

Fatigue

Patients taking β-adrenoceptor-blocking drugs often complain of fatigue, which is probably a result of reduced cardiac output and reduced muscle perfusion in exercise.

Cold extremities

Cold at the extremities results presumably from a loss of β-adrenoceptor-mediated vasodilatation in cutaneous vessels and is a common side-effect. Again, β_1-selective drugs ought to be less likely to produce this effect, but it is not clear that this is so in practice.

Other effects

Other side-effects associated with β-adrenoceptor antagonists are not obviously the result of β-adrenoceptor blockade. One is the occurrence of bad dreams, which occur mainly with highly lipid-soluble drugs such as propranolol, which enter the brain easily. Practolol was withdrawn from clinical use because it produced a serious *oculomucocutaneous syndrome*, as a rare idiosyncratic reaction (see Ch. 51).

DRUGS THAT AFFECT NORADRENERGIC NEURONS

Emphasis in this chapter is placed on peripheral sympathetic transmission. The same principles, however, are applicable to the CNS (see Ch. 33), where many of the drugs mentioned here also act.

DRUGS THAT AFFECT NORADRENALINE SYNTHESIS

Only a few clinically important drugs affect noradrenaline synthesis directly. Examples are **α-methyltyrosine**, which inhibits tyrosine hydroxylase and has been used in the treatment of phaeochromocytoma, and **carbidopa**, a hydrazine derivative of dopa, which inhibits dopa decarboxylase and is used in the treatment of parkinsonism (see Ch. 34).

Methyldopa, a drug still occasionally used in the treatment of hypertension during pregnancy (see Ch. 18), is taken up by noradrenergic neurons, where it is converted to the false transmitter α-methylnoradrenaline. This substance is not deaminated within the neuron by MAO, so it accumulates and displaces noradrenaline from the synaptic vesicles. Alpha-methylnoradrenaline is released in the same way as noradrenaline but is less active than noradrenaline on α_1-adrenoceptors and thus is less effective in causing vasoconstriction. However, it is more active on presynaptic (α_2) adrenoceptors; consequently, the autoinhibitory feedback mechanism operates more strongly than normal, thus reducing transmitter release below the normal levels. Both of these effects (as well as a central effect, probably caused by the same cellular mechanism) contribute to the hypotensive action. It produces side-effects typical of centrally acting antiadrenergic drugs (e.g. sedation) as well carrying a risk of immune haemolytic reactions and liver toxicity, so it is now little used, except for hypertension in late pregnancy.

6-Hydroxydopamine (identical with dopamine except that it possesses an extra ring –OH group) is a neurotoxin of the Trojan horse kind. It is taken up selectively by noradrenergic nerve terminals, where it is converted to a reactive quinone, which destroys the nerve terminal, producing a 'chemical sympathectomy'. The cell bodies survive and eventually the sympathetic innervation recovers. The drug is useful for experimental purposes but has no clinical uses. If injected directly into the brain, it selectively destroys those nerve terminals (i.e. dopaminergic, noradrenergic and adrenergic) that take it up, but it does not reach the brain if given systemically. **MPTP** (1-methyl-4-phenyl-1,2,3,5-tetrahydropyridine; see Ch. 34) is a rather similar selective neurotoxin acting selectively on dopaminergic neurons.

DRUGS THAT AFFECT NORADRENALINE STORAGE

Reserpine is an alkaloid from the shrub *Rauwolfia* that has been used in India for centuries for the treatment of mental disorders. Reserpine, at very low concentration, blocks the transport of noradrenaline and other amines into synaptic vesicles by binding to the transport protein (see Liu & Edwards, 1997). Noradrenaline accumulates instead in the cytoplasm, where it is degraded by MAO. The noradrenaline content of tissues drops to a low level, and sympathetic transmission is blocked. Reserpine also causes depletion of 5-HT and dopamine from neurons in the brain in which these amines are transmitters (see Ch. 33). Reserpine is now only used experimentally, but was at one time used as an antihypertensive drug (see Ch. 18); its central effects, especially depression, which probably result from impairment of noradrenergic and 5-HT-mediated transmission in the brain (see Ch. 38), are a serious disadvantage.

DRUGS THAT AFFECT NORADRENALINE RELEASE

Drugs can affect noradrenaline release in four main ways:

- by directly blocking release (noradrenergic neuron-blocking drugs)
- by evoking noradrenaline release in the absence of nerve terminal depolarisation (indirectly acting sympathomimetic drugs)
- by interacting with presynaptic receptors that indirectly inhibit or enhance depolarisation-evoked release (e.g. α_2-

agonists, angiotensin II, dopamine, prostaglandins, etc.): effects mediated through α_2-adrenoceptors are discussed elsewhere in this chapter; the other mechanisms are probably more important in the central than in the peripheral nervous system
- by increasing or decreasing available stores of noradrenaline (e.g. reserpine, see above; MAO inhibitors). These drugs are discussed elsewhere in this chapter, and in Chapter 38, and are not considered further in this section.

NORADRENERGIC NEURON-BLOCKING DRUGS

Noradrenergic neuron-blocking drugs (e.g. **guanethidine**) were first discovered in the mid-1950s when alternatives to ganglion-blocking drugs, for use in the treatment of hypertension, were being sought. The main effect of guanethidine is to inhibit the release of noradrenaline from sympathetic nerve terminals. It has little effect on the adrenal medulla, and none on nerve terminals that release transmitters other than noradrenaline. Drugs very similar to it include **bretylium**, **betanidine** and **debrisoquin** (which is of interest mainly as a tool for studying drug metabolism; see Ch. 8).

Actions

Drugs of this class reduce or abolish the response of tissues to sympathetic nerve stimulation but do not affect (or may potentiate) the effects of circulating noradrenaline. Their ability to block noradrenaline release can be demonstrated by measurement, for example, of the release of radioactivity from organs such as the spleen or vas deferens in response to stimulation of the sympathetic nerves after the transmitter stores have been labelled by infusion of radioactive noradrenaline.

The action of guanethidine on noradrenergic transmission is complex (see Broadley, 1996). It is selectively accumulated by noradrenergic nerve terminals, being a substrate for uptake 1. Its initial blocking activity depends on impairment of impulse conduction in the nerve terminals through this selective accumulation (Brock & Cunnane, 1988). Its action is prevented by drugs, such as amphetamine (see below), which block uptake 1.

Guanethidine is also concentrated in synaptic vesicles by means of the vesicular transporter, possibly interfering with their ability to undergo exocytosis and also displacing noradrenaline. In this way, it causes a gradual and long-lasting depletion of noradrenaline in sympathetic nerve endings, similar to the effect of reserpine.

Given in large doses, guanethidine causes structural damage to noradrenergic neurons, which is probably because of the accumulation of the drug in high concentration in the terminals. It can, therefore, be used as a selective neurotoxin.

Guanethidine is no longer used clinically. Though extremely effective in lowering blood pressure, it produces severe side-effects associated with the loss of sympathetic reflexes. The most troublesome are postural hypotension, diarrhoea, nasal congestion and failure of ejaculation. Bretylium is sometimes used to treat ventricular dysrhythmias resistant to other agents during cardiac resuscitation (see Ch. 17); its mechanism of action in this setting is unknown.

INDIRECTLY ACTING SYMPATHOMIMETIC AMINES

Mechanism of action and structure–activity relationships

The most important drugs in the indirectly acting sympathomimetic amine category are **tyramine**, **amphetamine** and **ephedrine**, which are structurally related to noradrenaline (Fig. 11.5), and **methylphenidate,** which is used for its central effects (Ch. 41). They have only weak actions on adrenoceptors but sufficiently resemble noradrenaline to be transported into nerve terminals by uptake 1.

Once inside the nerve terminals, they are taken up into the vesicles by the vesicular monoamine transporter, in exchange for noradrenaline, which escapes into the cytosol. Some of the cytosolic noradrenaline is degraded by MAO, while the rest escapes via uptake 1, in exchange for the foreign monoamine, to act on postsynaptic receptors (Fig. 11.9). Exocytosis is not

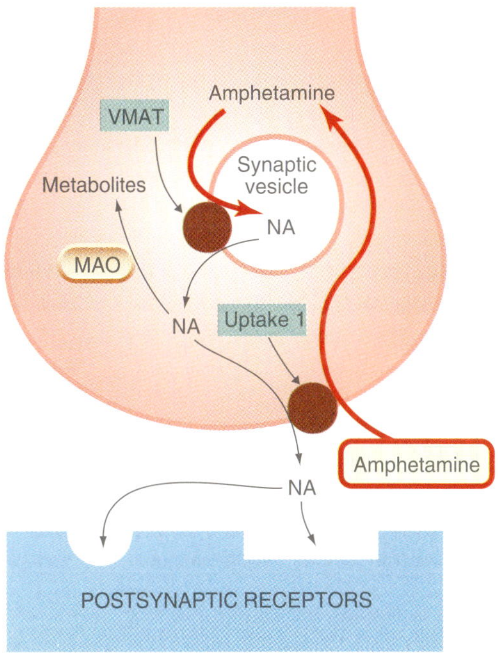

Fig. 11.9 The mode of action of amphetamine, an indirectly acting sympathomimetic amine. Amphetamine enters the nerve terminal via the NA transporter (uptake 1) and enters synaptic vesicles via the vesicular monoamine transporter (VMAT), in exchange for noradrenaline (NA), which accumulates in the cytosol. Some of the NA is degraded by monoamine oxidase (MAO) within the nerve terminal and some escapes, in exchange for amphetamine via the NA transporter, to act on postsynaptic receptors. Amphetamine also reduces NA reuptake via the transporter, so enhancing the action of the released NA.

involved in the release process, so these actions do not require the presence of Ca^{2+}. These drugs are not completely specific in their actions and act partly by a direct effect on adrenoceptors, partly by inhibiting uptake 1 (thereby enhancing the effect of the released noradrenaline) and partly by inhibiting MAO.

As would be expected, the effects of these drugs are strongly influenced by other drugs that modify noradrenergic transmission. Thus, reserpine and 6-hydroxydopamine, abolish their effects by depleting the terminals of noradrenaline. MAO inhibitors, however, strongly potentiate their effects by preventing inactivation, within the terminals, of the transmitter displaced from the vesicles. MAO inhibition particularly enhances the action of **tyramine** because this substance is itself a substrate for MAO. Normally, dietary tyramine is destroyed by MAO in the gut wall and liver before reaching the systemic circulation. When MAO is inhibited, this is prevented, and ingestion of tyramine-rich foods, such as fermented cheese (e.g. ripe Brie), can then provoke a sudden and dangerous rise in blood pressure (see Ch. 38). Inhibitors of uptake 1, such as **imipramine** (see below), interfere with the effects of indirectly acting sympathomimetic amines by preventing their uptake into the nerve terminals.

Indirectly acting sympathomimetic drugs, especially amphetamine, have important effects on the CNS (see Ch. 38) that depend on their ability to release not only noradrenaline but also 5-HT and dopamine from nerve terminals in the brain. An important characteristic of the effects of indirectly acting sympathomimetic amines is that marked tolerance develops. Repeated doses of amphetamine or tyramine, for example, produce progressively smaller pressor responses. This is probably caused by a depletion of the releasable store of noradrenaline, since the response can be restored, in experimental animals by infusion of noradrenaline, which has the effect of replenishing the releasable store. A similar tolerance to the central effects also develops with repeated administration, which partly accounts for the liability of amphetamine and related drugs to cause dependence.

Actions

The peripheral actions of the indirectly acting sympathomimetic amines include bronchodilatation, raised arterial pressure, peripheral vasoconstriction, increased heart rate and force of myocardial contraction, and inhibition of gut motility. They have important central actions, which account for their significant abuse potential and for their limited therapeutic applications (see Chs 41 and 52). Apart from ephedrine, which is still sometimes used as a nasal decongestant since it has much less central action, these drugs are no longer used for their peripheral sympathomimetic effects.

INHIBITORS OF NORADRENALINE UPTAKE

Neuronal reuptake of released noradrenaline (uptake 1) is the most important mechanism by which its action is brought to an end. Many drugs inhibit this transport and thereby enhance the effects of both sympathetic nerve activity and circulating noradrenaline. Uptake 1 is not responsible for clearing circulating adrenaline so these drugs do not affect responses to this amine.

Drugs acting on noradrenergic nerve terminals

- Drugs that inhibit noradrenaline (NA) synthesis include:
  - —**α-methyltyrosine**: blocks tyrosine hydroxylase, not used clinically
  - —**carbidopa**: blocks dopa decarboxylase and is used in treatment of parkinsonism (see Ch. 34); little effect on NA synthesis.
- **Methyldopa** gives rise to false transmitter (methylnoradrenaline) which is a potent α_2-agonist, thus causing powerful presynaptic inhibitory feedback (also central actions). Occasionally used as antihypertensive agent.
- **Reserpine** blocks carrier-mediated NA accumulation in vesicles, thus depleting NA stores and blocking transmission. Effective in hypertension but may cause severe depression.
- Noradrenergic neuron-blocking drugs (e.g. **guanethidine, betanidine**) are selectively concentrated in terminals (uptake 1) and in vesicles (vesicular transporter). They block transmitter release, partly by local anaesthetic action. Effective in hypertension but cause severe side-effects (postural hypotension, diarrhoea, nasal congestion, etc.) so now little used.
- **6-Hydroxydopamine** is selectively neurotoxic for noradrenergic neurons because it is taken up and converted to a toxic metabolite. Used experimentally to eliminate noradrenergic neurons, not clinically.
- Indirectly acting sympathomimetic amines (e.g. **amphetamine, ephedrine, tyramine**) are accumulated by uptake 1 and displace NA from vesicles, allowing it to escape. Effect is much enhanced by monoamine oxidase (MAO) inhibition, which can lead to severe hypertension following ingestion of tyramine-rich foods by patients treated with MAO inhibitors.
- Drugs that inhibit uptake 1 include **cocaine** and **tricyclic antidepressant drugs**. Sympathetic effects are enhanced by such drugs.

The main class of drug with a primary action to inhibit uptake 1 is the **tricyclic antidepressants** (see Ch. 38), for example **desipramine**. These drugs have their major effect on the CNS but also cause tachycardia and cardiac dysrhythmias, reflecting their peripheral effect on sympathetic transmission. **Cocaine**, known mainly for its abuse liability (Ch. 42) and local anaesthetic activity (Ch. 43), enhances sympathetic transmission, causing tachycardia and increased arterial pressure. Its central effects of euphoria and excitement (Ch. 41) are probably a manifestation of the same mechanism acting in the brain. It strongly potentiates the actions of noradrenaline in experimental animals or in isolated tissues provided the sympathetic nerve terminals are intact.

Table 11.3 Summary of drugs that affect noradrenergic transmission

Type	Drug[a]	Main action	Uses/function	Unwanted effects	Pharmacokinetic aspects	Notes
Sympathomimetic (directly acting)	Norepinephrine[b]	α/β-Agonist	Not used clinically. Transmitter at postganglionic sympathetic neurons, and in CNS. Hormone of adrenal medulla	Hypertension, vasoconstriction, tachycardia (or reflex bradycardia), ventricular dysrhythmias	Poorly absorbed by mouth. Rapid removal by tissues. Metabolised by MAO and COMT. Plasma $t_{1/2}$ ~ 2 min	
	Epinephrine[b]	α/β-Agonist	Asthma (emergency treatment), anaphylactic shock, cardiac arrest. Added to local anaesthetic solutions. Main hormone of adrenal medulla	As norepinephrine	Given i.m. or s.c. As norepinephrine	See Chapter 22
	Isoprenaline	β-Agonist (non-selective)	Asthma (obsolete). Not an endogenous substance	Tachycardia, dysrhythmias	Some tissue uptake, followed by inactivation (COMT) Plasma $t_{1/2}$ ~ 2 h	Now replaced by salbutamol in treatment of asthma (see Ch. 22)
	Dobutamine	$β_1$-Agonist (non-selective)	Cardiogenic shock	Dysrhythmias	Plasma $t_{1/2}$ ~ 2 min Given i.v.	Ch. 17
	Salbutamol	$β_2$-Agonist	Asthma, premature labour	Tachycardia, dysrhythmias, tremor, peripheral vasodilatation	Given orally or by aerosol Mainly excreted unchanged. Plasma $t_{1/2}$ ~ 4 h	Ch. 22
	Salmeterol	$β_2$-Agonist	Asthma	As salbutamol	Given by aerosol. Long acting	Formoterol is similar
	Terbutaline	$β_2$-Agonist	Asthma	As salbutamol	Poorly absorbed orally. Given by aerosol. Mainly excreted unchanged. Plasma $t_{1/2}$ ~ 4 h	Ch. 22
	Clenbuterol	$β_2$-Agonist	'Anabolic' action to increase muscle strength	As salbutamol	Active orally. Long acting	Illicit use in sport
	Phenylephrine	$α_1$-Agonist	Nasal decongestion	Hypertension, reflex bradycardia	Given intranasally. Metabolised by MAO Short plasma $t_{1/2}$	
	Methoxamine	α-Agonist (non-selective)	Nasal decongestion	As phenylephrine	Given intranasally. Plasma $t_{1/2}$ ~ 1 h	
	Clonidine	$α_2$-Partial agonist	Hypertension, migraine	Drowsiness, orthostatic hypotension, oedema and weight gain, rebound hypertension	Well absorbed orally. Excreted unchanged and as conjugate. Plasma $t_{1/2}$ ~ 12 h	See Chapter 18

Table 11.3 (continued)

Type	Drug[a]	Main action	Uses/function	Unwanted effects	Pharmacokinetic aspects	Notes
Sympathomimetic (indirectly acting)	Tyramine	NA release	No clinical uses. Present in various foods	As norepinephrine	Normally destroyed by MAO in gut. Does not enter brain	Ch. 38
	Amphetamine	NA release, MAO inhibitor, uptake 1 inhibitor, CNS stimulant	Used as CNS stimulant in narcolepsy, also (paradoxically) in hyperactive children. Appetite suppressant. Drug of abuse	Hypertension, tachycardia, insomnia. Acute psychosis with overdose. Dependence	Well absorbed orally Penetrates freely into brain. Excreted unchanged in urine. Plasma $t_{1/2}$ ~ 12 h, depending on urine flow and pH	Ch. 41 Methylphenidate is similar
	Ephedrine	NA release, β-agonist, weak CNS stimulant	Nasal decongestion	As amphetamine, but less pronounced	Similar to amphetamine	Contraindicated if MAO inhibitors are given
Adrenoceptor antagonists	Phenoxybenzamine	α-Antagonist (non-selective, irreversible), Uptake 1 inhibitor	Phaeochromocytoma	Hypotension, flushing, tachycardia, nasal congestion, impotence	Absorbed orally. Plasma $t_{1/2}$ ~ 12 h	Action outlasts presence of drug in plasma, because of covalent binding to receptor
	Phentolamine	α-Antagonist (non-selective), vasodilator	Rarely used	As phenoxybenzamine	Usually given i.v. Metabolised by liver. Plasma $t_{1/2}$ ~ 2 h	Tolazoline is similar
	Prazosin	α_1-Antagonist	Hypertension	As phenoxybenzamine	Absorbed orally. Metabolised by liver, Plasma $t_{1/2}$ ~ 4 h	Doxazosin, terazosin are similar but longer-acting. See Ch. 18
	Tamsulosin	α_1-Antagonist ('uroselective')	Prostatic hyperplasia	Failure of ejaculation	Absorbed orally Plasma $t_{1/2}$ ~ 5h	Selective for α_{1A}-adrenoceptor
	Yohimbine	α_2-Antagonist	Not used clinically. Claimed to be aphrodisiac	Excitement, hypertension	Absorbed orally. Metabolised by liver. Plasma $t_{1/2}$ ~ 4 h	Idazoxan is similar
	Propranolol	β-Antagonist (non-selective)	Angina, hypertension, cardiac dysrhythmias, anxiety tremor, glaucoma	Bronchoconstriction, cardiac failure, cold extremities, fatigue and depression, hypoglycaemia	Absorbed orally. Extensive first-pass metabolism. About 90% bound to plasma protein. Plasma $t_{1/2}$ ~ 4 h	Timolol is similar, and used mainly to treat glaucoma. See Ch. 17
	Alprenolol	β-Antagonist (non-selective) (partial agonist)	As propranolol	As propranolol	Absorbed orally Metabolised by liver. Plasma $t_{1/2}$ ~ 4 h	Oxprenolol and pindolol are similar. See Ch. 17
	Practolol	β_1-Antagonist	Hypertension, angina, dysrhythmias	As propranolol, also oculomucocutaneous syndrome	Absorbed orally. Excreted unchanged in urine Plasma $t_{1/2}$ ~ 4 h	Withdrawn from clinical use
	Metoprolol	β_1-Antagonist	Angina, hypertension, dysrhythmias	As propranolol, less risk of bronchoconstriction	Absorbed orally. Mainly metabolised in liver Plasma $t_{1/2}$ ~ 3 h	Atenolol is similar with a longer half-life See Ch. 17

Table 11.3 (continued)

Type	Drug[a]	Main action	Uses/function	Unwanted effects	Pharmacokinetic aspects	Notes
Adrenoceptor antagonists (continued)	Butoxamine	β_2-Antagonist, weak α-agonist	No clinical uses			
	Labetalol	α/β-Antagonist	Hypertension in pregnancy	Postural hypotension, bronchoconstriction	Absorbed orally. Conjugated in liver. Plasma $t_{1/2}$ ~ 4 h	Chs 17 and 18
	Carvedilol	α/β-Antagonist	Heart failure	As for other β-blockers Exacerbation of heart failure Renal failure	Absorbed orally $t_{1/2}$ ~ 10 h	Additional actions may contribute to clinical benefit (Ch. 17)
Drugs affecting noradrenaline synthesis	α-Methyl-*p*-tyrosine	Inhibits tyrosine hydroxylase	Occasionally used in phaeochromocytoma	Hypotension, sedation		
	Carbidopa	Inhibits DOPA decarboxylase	Used as adjunct to levodopa to prevent peripheral effects		Absorbed orally. Does not enter brain	Ch. 34
	Methyldopa	False transmitter precursor	Hypertension in pregnancy	Hypotension, drowsiness, diarrhoea, impotence, hypersensitivity reactions	Absorbed slowly by mouth. Excreted unchanged or as conjugate. Plasma $t_{1/2}$ ~ 6 h	Ch. 18
	Reserpine	Depletes NA stores by inhibiting vesicular uptake of NA	Hypertension (obsolete)	As methyldopa. Also depression, parkinsonism, gynaecomastia	Poorly absorbed orally. Slowly metabolised.. Plasma $t_{1/2}$ ~ 100 h Excreted in milk	Antihypertensive effect develops slowly, and persists when drug is stopped
Drugs affecting noradrenaline release	Guanethidine	Inhibits NA release. Also causes NA depletion, and can damage NA neurons irreversibly	Hypertension (obsolete)	As methyldopa. Hypertension on first administration	Poorly absorbed orally. Mainly excreted unchanged in urine. Plasma $t_{1/2}$ ~ 100 h	Action prevented by uptake 1 inhibitors. Bethanidine and debrisoquin are similar
Drugs affecting noradrenaline uptake	Imipramine	Blocks uptake 1. Also has atropine-like action	Depression	Atropine-like side-effects. Cardiac dysrhythmias in overdose	Well absorbed orally. 95% bound to plasma protein. Converted to active metabolite (desmethylimipramine). Plasma $t_{1/2}$ ~ 4h	Desipramine and amitriptyline are similar. See Ch. 38
	Cocaine	Local anaesthetic; blocks uptake 1, CNS stimulant	Rarely used local anaesthetic. Major drug of abuse	Hypertension, excitement, convulsions, dependence	Well absorbed orally	See Chs 41 and 52

NA, noradrenaline; MAO, monoamine oxidase; COMT, catechol-*O*-methyltransferase; i.m.. intramuscular; s.c., subcutaneous; i.v., intravenous; $t_{1/2}$, half-life.
[a]For chemical structures, see Hardman et al (2001).
[b]Note that norepinephrine and epinephrine are the recommended drug names for noradrenaline and adrenaline respectively.

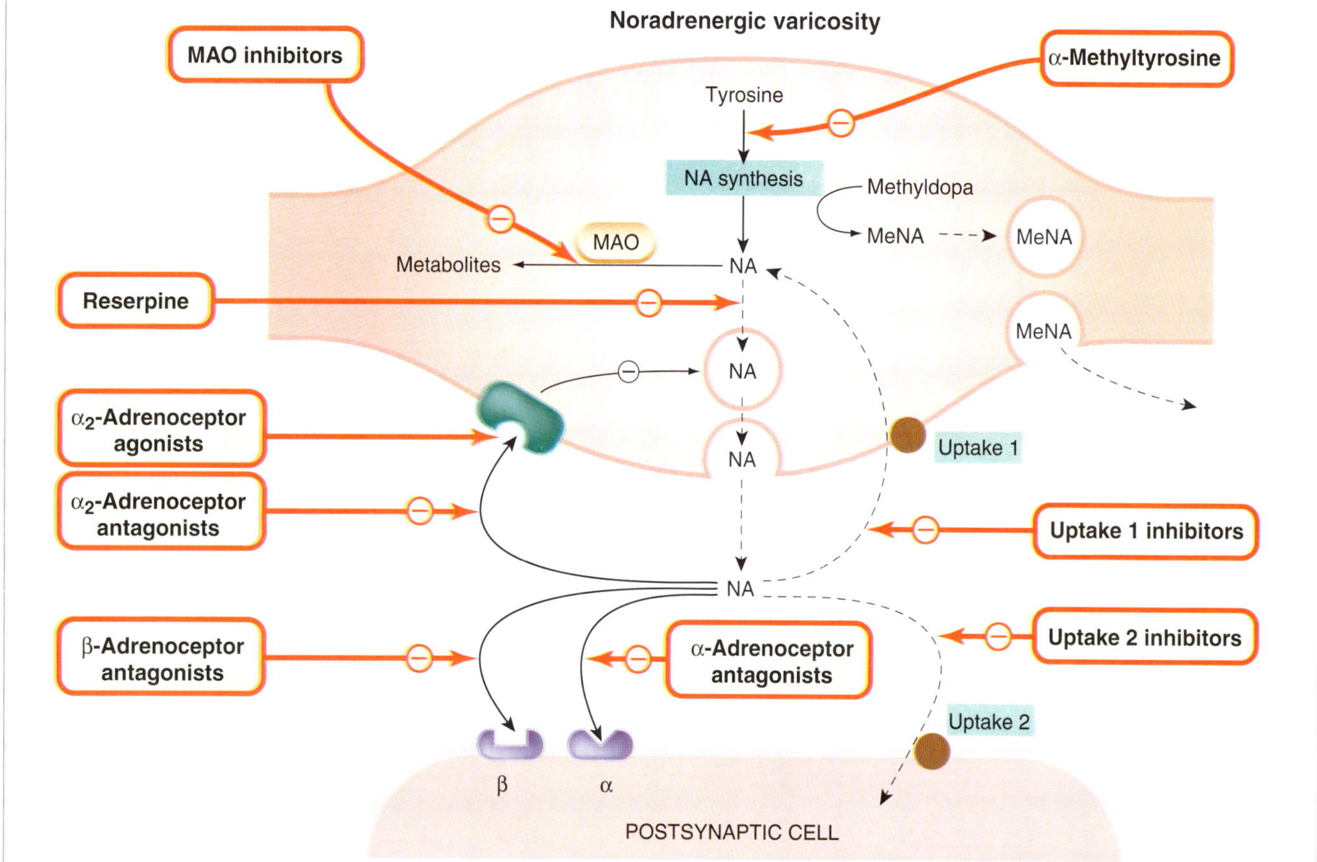

Fig. 11.10 Generalised diagram of a noradrenergic nerve terminal showing sites of drug action. Action of indirectly acting sympathomimetic drugs not shown (see Fig. 11.9). (NA, noradrenaline; MAO, monoamine oxidase; MeNA, methylnoradrenaline.)

Many drugs that act mainly on other steps in sympathetic transmission also inhibit uptake 1 to some extent, presumably because the carrier molecule bears a steric relationship to other noradrenaline recognition sites, such as receptors and degradative enzymes. Examples include **amphetamine**, **phenoxybenzamine** and **guanethidine**.

Extraneuronal uptake (uptake 2), which is important in clearing circulating adrenaline from the bloodstream, is not affected by most of the drugs that block uptake 1. It is inhibited by phenoxybenzamine, however, and also by various **corticosteroids** (see Ch. 17). This action of corticosteroids may have some relevance to their therapeutic effect in conditions such as asthma but is probably of minor importance.

The main sites of action of drugs that affect adrenergic transmission are summarised in Figures 11.9 and 11.10.

REFERENCES AND FURTHER READING

Broadley K J 1996 Autonomic pharmacology. Taylor & Francis, London (*Detailed textbook*)

Brock J A, Cunnane T C 1988 Studies on the mode of action of bretylium and guanethidine in post-ganglionic sympathetic nerve fibres. Naunyn-Schmiedebergs Arch Pharmacol 338: 504–509 (*Elegant electrophysiological analysis of action of sympathetic neuron-blocking drugs*)

Bylund D B 1994 Nomenclature of adrenoceptors. Pharmacol Rev 46: 121–136 (*Rationalisation of the taxonomy of adrenoceptors*)

Cooper J R, Bloom F E, Roth R H 1996 The biochemical basis of neuropharmacology. Oxford University Press, New York (*Excellent standard textbook*)

Cunnane T C 1984 The mechanism of neurotransmitter release from sympathetic nerves. Trends Neurosci 7: 248–253 (*Points out important differences between adrenergic and cholinergic neurons*)

Elenkov I J, Wilder R L, Chrousos G P, Vizi E S 2000. The sympathetic nerve—an integrative interface between two supersystems: the brain and the immune system. Pharmacol Rev 52: 595–638 (*Detailed catalogue of effects of catecholamines and the sympathetic nervous system on the immune system*)

Fillenz M 1990 Noradrenergic neurons. Cambridge University Press, Cambridge (*Comprehensive monograph*)

Insel P A 1996 Adrenergic receptors—evolving concepts and clinical implications. N Engl J Med 334: 580–585 (*Excellent review, focussing on applications*)

Guimaraes S, Moura D 2001 Vascular adrenoceptors: an update. Pharmacol

Rev 53: 319–356 (*Review describing the complex roles of different adrenoceptors in blood vessels*)

Hardman J G, Limbird L E, Gilman A G, Goodman-Gilman A 2001 Goodman and Gilman's pharmacological basis of therapeutics, 10th edn. McGraw-Hill, New York (*Comprehensive and authorative textbook*)

Liu Y, Edwards R H 1997 The role of vesicular transport proteins in synaptic transmission and neural degeneration. Annu Rev Neurosci 20: 125–156 (*Review of recent ideas about functional role of transporters*)

Lundberg J M 1996 Pharmacology of co-transmission in the autonomic nervous system: integrative aspects on amines, neuropeptides, adenosine triphosphate, amino acids and nitric oxide. Pharmacol Rev 48: 114–192 (*Comprehensive and informative review*)

McGrath J C, Wilson V 1988 α-Adrenoceptor subclassification by classical and response-related methods: same question, different answers. Trends Pharmacol Sci 9: 162–165 (*Discusses problems of adrenoceptor taxonomy*)

Nelson N 1998 The family of Na^+/Cl^- neurotransmitter transporters. J Neurochem 71: 1785–1803 (*General review article*)

Nonogaki K 2000 New insights into sympathetic regulation of glucose and fat metabolism. Diabetologia 43: 533–549 (*Review of the complex adrenoceptor-mediated effects on the metabolism of liver, muscle and adipose tissue. Up-to-date, but not a particularly easy read*)

Pfeffer M A, Stevenson L W 1996 β-Adrenergic blockers and survival in heart failure. N Engl J Med 334: 1396–1397 (*Shows that β-adrenergic blockers in low doses can be beneficial in heart failure*)

Starke K, Göthert M, Kilbinger H 1989 Modulation of transmitter release by presynaptic autoreceptors. Physiol Rev 69: 864–989 (*Comprehensive review*)

Summers R J, McMartin L R 1993 Adrenoceptors and their second messenger systems. J Neurochem 60: 10–23 (*Short review article*)

Trendelenburg U, Weiner N 1988 Catecholamines. Handbook of experimental pharmacology. Springer-Verlag, Berlin, vol. 90, part 1,2 (*Massive compilation of knowledge to date*)

Zhang K-M, Hu P, Wang S-W et al. 1996 Salbutamol changes the molecular and mechanical properties of canine skeletal muscle. J Physiol 496: 211–220 (*Surprising finding that salbutamol affects muscle function by non-receptor mechanisms*)

12 Other peripheral mediators: 5-hydroxytryptamine and purines

Overview 184

5-Hydroxytryptamine 184
- Distibution, biosynthesis and degradation 184
- Pharmacological effects 185
- Classification of 5-HT receptors 186
- Drugs acting on 5-HT receptors 188
- Clinical conditions in which 5-HT plays a role 190

Purines 192
- ATP as a neurotransmitter 192
- ADP and platelets 194
- Adenosine as a mediator 194
- Purine receptors 194

OVERVIEW

In this chapter we discuss two types of mediator, both of which play a role as neurotransmitters in the brain and periphery and also probably function as local hormones. 5-Hydroxytryptamine (5-HT) has a longer pharmacological history than purines (*nucleosides* and *nucleotides*), and numerous drugs in current use act wholly or partly on 5-HT receptors, of which no fewer than 14 subtypes have been identified; purine pharmacology is much sparser. In both cases, the physiological significance—and hence therapeutic relevance—of the various receptor subtypes is still being unravelled; in our discussion, we will focus on the more secure hypotheses, recognising that the picture is far from complete. The pharmaceutical industry has seized on the opportunity offered by these potential new drug targets and is producing a profusion of specific agonists and antagonists, which are, in turn, being used to clarify the physiological role of the various receptor systems. There is expectation of therapeutic advances on the horizon, but the student may be forgiven for finding the taxonomic niceties somewhat unrewarding at this stage. Useful reviews for the insatiable include Hoyer et al. (1994), Fredholm et al. (1994) and North & Barnard (1997).

5-HYDROXYTRYPTAMINE

Serotonin was the name given to an unknown vasoconstrictor substance found in the serum after blood has clotted. It was identified chemically as 5-hydroxytryptamine (5-HT) in 1948 and shown to originate from the platelets. It was subsequently found in the gastrointestinal tract and central nervous system (CNS) and shown to function both as a neurotransmitter and as a local hormone in the peripheral vascular system. As knowledge advances, we get the picture of a mediator that has a subsidiary role in many functions. In the words of one pundit, 5-HT seems to be 'involved in everything, but responsible for nothing', a kind of mediator-without-portfolio. This chapter deals with the metabolism, distribution and possible physiological roles of 5-HT in the periphery, and with the different types of 5-HT receptor and the drugs that act on them. Further information on the role of 5-HT in the brain, and its relationship to psychiatric disorders and the actions of psychotropic drugs, is presented in Chapters 31, 37 and 38. More detailed information on 5-HT in the CNS and in the periphery can be found in Fozard (1989) and Cooper et al. (1996).

DISTRIBUTION, BIOSYNTHESIS AND DEGRADATION

5-HT occurs in the highest concentrations in three situations in the body.

- *In the wall of the intestine* About 90% of the total amount in the body is present in *enterochromaffin cells*, which are cells derived from the neural crest, similar to those of the adrenal medulla, that are interspersed with mucosal cells, mainly in the stomach and small intestine. Some 5-HT also occurs in nerve cells of the myenteric plexus, where it functions as an excitatory neurotransmitter (see Chs 9 and 24).
- *In blood* 5-HT is present in high concentration in platelets, which accumulate it from the plasma by an active transport system and release it when they aggregate at sites of tissue damage (see Ch. 20).
- *In the CNS* 5-HT is a transmitter in the CNS (see Ch. 33) and is present in high concentrations in localised regions of the midbrain. Its functional role is discussed in Chapter 33.

Though 5-HT is present in the diet, most of this is metabolised before entering the bloodstream. Endogenous 5-HT arises by biosynthesis, which follows a pathway similar to that of noradrenaline (see Ch. 11), except that the precursor amino acid is tryptophan instead of tyrosine (Fig. 12.1). Tryptophan is converted to 5-hydroxytryptophan (in chromaffin cells and neurons, but not in platelets) by the action of *tryptophan hydroxylase* (an enzyme confined to 5-HT-producing cells). The 5-hydroxytryptophan is then decarboxylated to 5-HT, by a ubiquitous *amino-acid decarboxylase* that also participates in the synthesis of catecholamines (Ch. 11) and histamine (Ch. 15). Platelets (and neurons) possess a high affinity 5-HT uptake mechanism, and platelets become loaded with 5-HT as they pass through the intestinal circulation, where the local concentration is relatively high. The mechanisms of synthesis, storage, release and reuptake of 5-HT are very similar to those of noradrenaline, and many drugs affect both processes indiscriminately (see Chs 11 and 38). 5-HT is often stored in neurons and chromaffin cells as a co-transmitter together with various peptide hormones, such as **somatostatin, substance P** or **vasoactive intestinal polypeptide** (VIP).

Degradation of 5-HT (Fig. 12.1) occurs mainly through oxidative deamination, catalysed by *monoamine oxidase,* followed by oxidation to *5-hydroxyindoleacetic acid* (5-HIAA), the pathway being the same as that of noradrenaline catabolism. 5-HIAA is excreted in the urine and serves as an indicator of 5-HT production in the body. This is used, for example, in the diagnosis of *carcinoid syndrome* (see below).

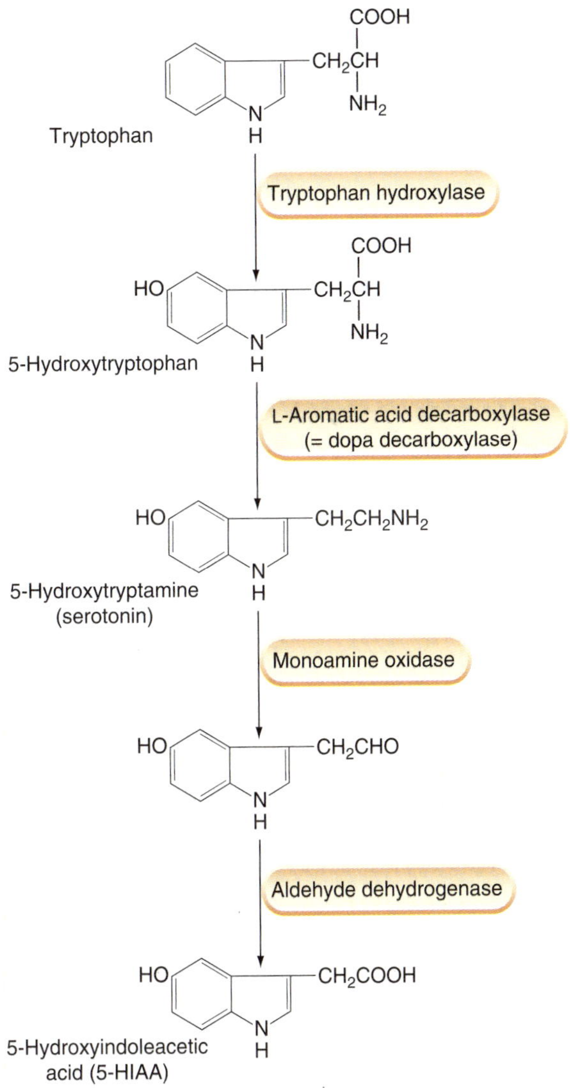

Fig. 12.1 Biosynthesis and metabolism of 5-hydroxytryptamine.

Distribution, biosynthesis and degradation of 5-hydroxytryptamine (5-HT)

- Structures rich in 5-HT are:
  —gastrointestinal tract (chromaffin cells and enteric neurons)
  —platelets
  —central nervous system.
- Metabolism closely parallels that of noradrenaline.
- 5-HT is formed from dietary tryptophan, which is converted to 5-hydroxytryptophan by tryptophan hydroxylase, then to 5-HT by a non-specific decarboxylase.
- 5-HT is transported into 5-HT-containing cells by a specific transport system.
- Degradation occurs mainly by monoamine oxidase, forming 5-HIAA (5-hydroxyindoleacetic acid), which is excreted in urine.

PHARMACOLOGICAL EFFECTS

The actions of 5-HT are numerous and complex, and there is considerable species variation. This complexity reflects a profusion of 5-HT receptor subtypes, which has been revealed in recent years (see below). The main sites of action are as follows.

Gastrointestinal tract 5-HT stimulates gastrointestinal motility (see Taniyama et al., 2000), this being partly through a direct effect on the smooth muscle cells (5-HT_2-receptors) and partly as a result of an indirect excitatory effect on enteric neurons (5-HT_3- and 5-HT_4-receptors). 5-HT also stimulates fluid secretion and elicits nausea and vomiting by stimulating smooth muscle and sensory nerves in the stomach (5-HT_3- and 5-HT_4-receptors). The peristaltic reflex, evoked by increasing the pressure within a segment of intestine, is mediated, partly at least, by the release of 5-HT from chromaffin cells in response to the mechanical stimulus. Chromaffin cells also respond to vagal stimulation by releasing 5-HT.

Smooth muscle Elsewhere in the body (e.g. *uterus and bronchial tree)* smooth muscle is also contracted by 5-HT in many species, but only to a minor extent in humans.

Blood vessels The effect of 5-HT on blood vessels depends on various factors, including the size of the vessel, the species and the prevailing sympathetic activity. Large vessels, both arteries and veins, are usually constricted by 5-HT, though the sensitivity varies greatly. This is a direct action on vascular smooth muscle cells, mediated through 5-HT_{2A}-receptors (see below). Activation of 5-HT_1-receptors causes constriction of large intracranial vessels, dilation of which contributes to headache (see below). 5-HT can also cause vasodilatation, partly by acting on endothelial cells to release nitric oxide (see Ch. 14) and partly by inhibiting noradrenaline release from sympathetic nerve terminals. If 5-HT is injected intravenously, the blood pressure usually first rises, owing to the constriction of large vessels, and then falls, owing to arteriolar dilatation.

Platelets 5-HT causes platelet aggregation (see Ch. 19), via 5-HT_{2A}-receptors, and the platelets that collect in the vessel release more 5-HT. If the endothelium is intact, 5-HT release from adherent platelets causes vasodilatation, which helps to sustain blood flow; if it is damaged (e.g. by atherosclerosis), 5-HT causes constriction and impairs blood flow further. These effects of platelet-derived 5-HT are thought to be important in vascular disease.

Actions and functions of 5-hydroxytryptamine (5-HT)

- Important actions are:
  - —increased gastrointestinal motility (direct excitation of smooth muscle and indirect action via enteric neurons)
  - —contraction of other smooth muscle (bronchi, uterus)
  - —mixture of vascular constriction (direct and via sympathetic innervation) and dilatation (endothelium dependent)
  - —platelet aggregation
  - —stimulation of peripheral nociceptive nerve endings
  - —excitation/inhibition of CNS neurons.
- Postulated physiological and pathophysiological roles include:
  - —in periphery: peristalsis, vomiting, platelet aggregation and haemostasis, inflammatory mediator, sensitisation of nociceptors and microvascular control
  - —in CNS: many postulated functions, including control of appetite, sleep, mood, hallucinations, stereotyped behaviour, pain perception and vomiting.
- Clinical conditions associated with disturbed 5-HT function include migraine, carcinoid syndrome, mood disorders and anxiety (see Chs 36 and 38).

Nerve endings 5-HT stimulates nociceptive (pain-mediating) sensory nerve endings, an effect mediated mainly by 5-HT_3-receptors. If injected into the skin, 5-HT causes pain; given systemically, it elicits a variety of autonomic reflexes through stimulation of afferent fibres in the heart and lungs, which further complicate the cardiovascular response. Nettle stings contain 5-HT, amongst other things. 5-HT also inhibits transmitter release from adrenergic neurons in the periphery, as mentioned above.

Central nervous system 5-HT excites some neurons and inhibits others; it also acts presynaptically to inhibit transmitter release from nerve terminals. Different receptor types and different membrane mechanisms mediate these effects (see Table 12.1; Barnes & Sharp, 1999; Branchek & Blackburn, 2000). The role of 5-HT in the CNS is discussed in Chapter 33.

CLASSIFICATION OF 5-HT RECEPTORS

It was long ago realised that the actions of 5-HT are not all mediated by receptors of the same type, and various pharmacological classifications have come and gone. The current classification (Hoyer et al., 1994) was agreed after long deliberation at a summit meeting of 5-HT aficionados and delivered, with puffs of white smoke and much celebration, in 1992. It is summarised in Table 12.1. This classification takes into account sequence data derived from cloning, signal transduction mechanisms and pharmacological specificity. Currently, there are seven main receptor types, 5-HT_{1-7}, of which types 1 and 2 (also 5, about which we know little) are further subdivided.*

Recently, transgenic mice lacking functional 5-HT_1- or 5-HT_2-receptors have been produced (see Bonasera & Tecott, 2000). The functional deficits in such animals are generally quite subtle, suggesting that these receptors may serve to tune, rather than to enable, physiological responses.

▼ *5-HT_1-receptors* occur mainly in the brain, the subtypes being distinguished on the basis of their regional distribution and their pharmacological specificity. They function mainly as inhibitory presynaptic receptors and are linked to inhibition of adenylate cyclase. The 5-HT_{1A} subtype is particularly important in the brain, in relation to mood and behaviour (see Chs 24, 27, and 29). The 5-HT_{1D} subtype, which is expressed in cerebral blood vessels, is believed to be important in migraine (see below) and is the target for **sumatriptan,** an agonist at 5-HT_{1D}-receptors that is used to treat acute attacks. The cerebral vessels are unusual in that vasoconstriction is mediated by 5-HT_1-receptors; in most vessels, 5-HT_2-receptors are responsible. The hapless '5-HT_{1C}-receptor'—actually the first to be cloned—has been officially declared non-existent, having been ignominiously reclassified as the 5-HT_{2C}-receptor when it was found to be linked, not to adenylate cyclase, but to inositol trisphosphate (IP_3) production.

5-HT_2-receptors are particularly important in the periphery. The effects of 5-HT on smooth muscle and platelets, which have been known for many

*With a total of 14 subtypes—13 G-protein-coupled receptors (GPCRs) plus one ionotropic receptor identified so far, 5-HT receptors hold the record for diversity (even if we ignore splice variants, about which we know little except that they occur). ATP-receptors, with four GPCRs and seven ionotropic subtypes (see p. 194), come close.

Table 12.1 The main 5-HT receptor subtypes

Receptor	Location	Main effects	Second messenger	Agonists	Antagonists
1A	CNS	Neuronal inhibition Behavioural effects: sleep, feeding, thermoregulation, anxiety	↓ cAMP	5-CT 8-OH-DPAT Buspirone (PA)	Spiperone Methiothepin Ergotamine (PA)
1B	CNS Vascular smooth muscle	Presynaptic inhibition Behavioural effects Pulmonary vasoconstriction	↓ cAMP	5-CT Ergotamine (PA)	Methiothepin
1D	CNS Blood vessels	Cerebral vasoconstriction Behavioural effects: locomotion	↓ cAMP	5-CT Sumatriptan	Methiothepin Ergotamine (PA)
2A	CNS PNS Smooth muscle Platelets	Neuronal excitation Behavioural effects Smooth muscle contraction (gut, bronchi, etc.) Platelet aggregation Vasoconstriction/vasodilatation	↑ IP_3/DAG	α-Me-5-HT LSD (CNS) LSD (periphery)	Ketanserin Cyproheptadine Pizotifen (non-selective) Methysergide
2B	Gastric fundus	Contraction	↑ IP_3/DAG	α-Me-5-HT	
2C	CNS Choroid plexus	CSF secretion	↑ IP_3/DAG	α-Me 5-HT LSD	Methysergide
3	PNS CNS	Neuronal excitation (autonomic, nociceptive neurons) Emesis Behavioural effects: anxiety	None—ligand-gated cation channel	2-Me-5-HT Chlorophenyl-biguanide	Ondansetron Tropisetron Granisetron
4	PNS (GI tract) CNS	Neuronal excitation GI motility	↑ cAMP	5-Methoxy-tryptamine Metoclopramide	Various experimental compounds (e.g GR113808, SB207266)
5	CNS	Not known	Not known	Not known	Not known
6	CNS	Not known	Not known	Not known	Not known
7	CNS GI tract Blood vessels	Not known	↑ cAMP	5-CT, LSD No selective agonists	Various 5-HT_2-antagonists No selective antagonists

PNS, peripheral nervous system; GI, gastrointestinal tract; CSF, cerebrospinal fluid; IP_3, inositol trisphosphate; DAG, diacylglycerol; 5-HT, 5-hydroxytrypamine; 5-CT, 5-carboxamidotryptamine; 8-OH-DPAT, 8-hydroxy-2-(di-n-propylamino)tetraline; α-Me-5-HT, α-methyl 5-HT; LSD, lysergic acid diethylamide; 2-Me-5-HT, 2-methyl-5-HT; PA, partial agonist. For further details, see Hoyer et al. (1994).
The list of agonists and antagonists includes only the better-known compounds. Many new selective 5-HT receptor ligands, known only by code numbers, are being developed.

years, are mediated by the 5-HT_{2A}-*receptor*, as are some of the behavioural effects of agents such as **lysergic acid diethylamide (LSD**; see Table 12.1 and Ch. 41). 5-HT_2-*receptor*s are linked to phospholipase C and thus stimulate IP_3 formation. The 5-HT_{2A} subtype is functionally the most important, the others having a much more limited distribution and functional role. The role of 5-HT_2-*receptor*s in normal physiological processes is probably a minor one, but it becomes more prominent in pathological conditions such as asthma and vascular thrombosis (see Chs 19, 20 and 22).

5-HT_3-receptors occur mainly in the peripheral nervous system, particularly on nociceptive sensory neurons (see Ch. 40) and on autonomic and enteric neurons, on which 5-HT exerts a strong excitatory effect. 5-HT itself evokes pain when injected locally; when given intravenously it elicits a fine display of autonomic reflexes, which result from excitation of many types of vascular, pulmonary and cardiac sensory nerve fibres. 5-HT_3-receptors also occur in the brain, particularly in the *area postrema,* a region of the medulla involved in the vomiting reflex, and selective 5-HT_3 antagonists are used as antiemetic drugs (see Ch. 21). 5-HT_3-receptors are exceptional in being directly linked to membrane ion channels (Ch. 3); they cause excitation directly, without involvement of any second messenger step.

5-HT_4-receptors occur in the brain, as well as in peripheral organs, such as the gastrointestinal tract, bladder and heart. Their main physiological role appears to be in the gastrointestinal tract, where they produce neuronal excitation and mediate the effect of 5-HT in stimulating peristalsis.

Little is so far known about the functions of the remaining types: 5, 6 and 7.

DRUGS ACTING ON 5-HT RECEPTORS

Table 12.1 lists some of the agonists and antagonists for the different receptor types. Most are only partly selective, though more selective compounds have been synthesised and may be developed for clinical use. The improved understanding of the location and function of the different receptor subtypes has, however, caused an upsurge of interest in developing compounds with improved receptor selectivity, and useful new drugs are likely to appear in the near future.

Important drugs that act on 5-HT receptors in the periphery include:

- 5-HT_{1D}-receptor agonists (e.g. **sumatriptan**) used for treating migraine (see below). Selective 5-HT_{1A} agonists, such as 8-OH-DPAT (8-hydroxy-2-(di-n-propylamino) tetralin; Table 12.1), are potent hypotensive agents, acting by a central mechanism, but are not used clinically.
- 5-HT_3-receptor antagonists (e.g. **ondansetron, granisetron, tropisetron**) are used as antiemetic drugs (see Ch. 24) particularly for controlling the severe nausea and vomiting that occurs with many forms of cancer chemotherapy: a major advance, since this side-effect is one of the main factors limiting the effective use of chemotherapy (Ch. 50).
- 5-HT_2-receptor antagonists (e.g. **dihydroergotamine, methysergide, cyproheptadine, ketanserin, ketotifen, pizotifen**) act mainly on 5-HT_2-receptors but also block other 5-HT receptors, as well as α-adrenoceptors and histamine receptors. Dihydroergotamine and methysergide belong to the ergot family (see below) and are used mainly for migraine prophylaxis. Ketotifen is sometimes used to treat asthma (Ch. 22) but the role of 5-HT receptors in this condition is unclear. Other 5-HT_2 antagonists are used to control the symptoms of carcinoid tumours.
- 5-HT_4-receptor agonists, which stimulate coordinated peristaltic activity (known as a 'prokinetic action'), are used for treating gastrointestinal disorders (see Ch. 24). **Metoclopramide** acts in this way, though it also affects dopamine receptors. The new drug **tegaserod** is more selective and is used to treat irritable bowel syndrome.

5-HT receptors

- There are seven types (5-HT_{1-7}), with further subtypes (A–D) of 5-HT_1 and 5-HT_2. All are G-protein-coupled receptors, except 5-HT_3, which is a ligand-gated cation channel.
- 5-HT_1-receptors occur mainly in CNS (all subtypes) and some blood vessels (5-HT_{1D} subtype). Effects are neural inhibition and vasoconstriction. Act by inhibiting adenylate cyclase. Specific agonists include **sumatriptan** (used in migraine therapy) and buspirone (used in anxiety). **Ergotamine** is a partial agonist. Specific antagonists include **spiperone** and **methiothepin**.
- 5-HT_2-receptors occur in CNS and many peripheral sites (especially blood vessels, platelets, autonomic neurons). Neuronal and smooth muscle effects are excitatory. Some blood vessels dilated as a result of nitric oxide release from endothelial cells. 5-HT_2-receptors acts through phospholipase C/inositol trisphosphate pathway. Specific ligands include LSD (lysergic acid diethylamide; agonist in CNS, antagonist in periphery). Specific antagonists are **ketanserin**, **methysergide** and **cyproheptadine**.
- 5-HT_3-receptors occur in peripheral nervous system, especially nociceptive afferent neurons and enteric neurons, and in CNS. Effects are excitatory, mediated via direct receptor-coupled ion channels. Specific agonist is 2-methyl-5-HT. Specific antagonists are **ondansetron** and **tropisetron**. Antagonists are used mainly as antiemetic drugs but may also be anxiolytic.
- 5-HT_4-receptors occur mainly in the enteric nervous system (also in CNS). Effects are excitatory, causing increased gastrointestinal motility. Act by stimulating adenylate cyclase. Specific agonists include **metoclopramide** (used to stimulate gastric emptying).
- Little is known so far about the function and pharmacology of 5-HT_{5-7}-receptors.
- Many new receptor-selective agonists and antagonists are being developed

5-HT is also important as a transmitter in the CNS, and several important antipsychotic and antidepressant drugs owe their actions to effects on these pathways (see Chs 33, 37 and 38). **LSD** is a relatively non-selective 5-HT receptor agonist or partial agonist, which acts centrally as a potent hallucinogen (see Ch. 41)

ERGOT ALKALOIDS

Ergot alkaloids constitute a hard-to-classify group of drugs that have preoccupied pharmacologists for more than a century. Many of them act on 5-HT receptors, but not selectively, and their actions are complex and diverse. Ergot alkaloids occur naturally in a fungus *(Claviceps purpurea)* that infests cereal crops. Epidemics of ergot poisoning have occurred, and still occur, when contaminated grain is used for food. The symptoms produced include mental disturbances and intensely painful peripheral vasoconstriction, leading to gangrene, which came to be known in the Middle Ages as *St Anthony's fire,* because it could be cured by a visit to the Shrine of St Anthony (which happened to be in an ergot-free region of France). Ergot contains many active substances, and it was the study of their pharmacological properties that led Dale to many important discoveries concerning acetylcholine, histamine and catecholamines.

Ergot alkaloids are complex molecules based on **lysergic acid** (a naturally occurring tetracyclic alkaloid). The important members of the group (Table 12.2) are various naturally occurring and synthetic derivatives containing different substituent groups attached to the basic nucleus. These compounds display many different types of pharmacological action, and it is difficult to discern any clear relationship between chemical structure and pharmacological properties.

Actions

Most of the effects of ergot alkaloids appear to be mediated through 5-HT receptors, adrenoceptors or dopamine receptors (Table 12.2), though some effects may be produced through other mechanisms. They all cause stimulation of smooth muscle, some being relatively selective for vascular smooth muscle, and others acting mainly on the uterus. **Ergotamine** and **dihydroergotamine** are, respectively, a partial agonist and an antagonist at α-adrenoceptors; **bromocriptine** is an agonist on dopamine receptors, particularly in the CNS; **methysergide** is an antagonist at 5-HT_2-receptors.

The main pharmacological actions and uses of these drugs are summarised in Table 12.2. As one would expect of drugs with so many actions, their physiological effects are complex and rather poorly understood. Ergotamine, dihydroergotamine and methysergide are discussed here; further information on ergometrine and bromocriptine is given in Chapters 29 and 34.

Vascular effects When injected into an anaesthetised animal, **ergotamine** causes a sustained rise in blood pressure, caused by activation of α-adrenoceptors leading to vasoconstriction. At the same time, ergotamine reverses the pressor effect of adrenaline (epinepthrine; see Ch. 9). The vasoconstrictor effect of ergotamine is responsible for the peripheral gangrene of St Anthony's fire, and probably also for some of the effects of ergot on the CNS. Methysergide and dihydroergotamine have much less vasoconstrictor effect.

Actions on 5-HT receptors Methysergide is a potent 5-HT_2-receptor antagonist, whereas ergotamine and dihydroergotamine act selectively on 5-HT_1-receptors. Though generally classified as antagonists, they show partial agonist activity in some tissues,

Table 12.2 Properties of ergot alkaloids

Drug	5-HT receptor	α-Adrenoceptor	Dopamine receptor	Uterine contraction	Main uses	Side-effects etc.
Ergotamine	Antagonist/partial agonist (5-HT_1)	Partial agonist (blood vessels) Antagonist (other sites)	Inactive	++	Migraine	Emesis Vasoconstriction (avoid in peripheral vascular disease) Avoid in pregnancy
Dihydro-ergotamine	Antagonist/partial agonist (5-HT_1)	Antagonist	Inactive	+	Migraine (largely obsolete)	Less emesis than ergotamine
Ergometrine	Antagonist/partial agonist (5-HT_1) (weak)	Weak antagonist/ partial agonist	Weak	+++	Prevention of postpartum haemorrhage	
Bromocriptine	Inactive	Weak antagonist	Agonist/partial agonist	–	Parkinson's disease (Ch. 34) Endocrine disorders (Ch. 27)	Emesis
Methysergide	Antagonist/partial agonist (5-HT_2)	–	–	–	Carcinoid syndrome Migraine (prophylaxis)	Retroperitoneal and mediastinal fibrosis Emesis

5-HT, 5-hydroxytryamine.

Ergot alkaloids

- These active substances are produced by a fungus that infects cereal crops; it is responsible for occasional poisoning incidents.
- The most important compounds are:
  —ergotamine, dihydroergotamine, used in migraine
  —ergometrine, used in obstetrics to prevent postpartum haemorrhage
  —methysergide, used to treat carcinoid syndrome, and occasionally for migraine prophylaxis
  —bromocriptine, used in parkinsonism and endocrine disorders.
- Main sites of action are 5-HT receptors, dopamine receptors and adrenoceptors (mixed agonist, antagonist and partial agonist effects).
- Unwanted effects include nausea and vomiting, vasoconstriction (ergot alkaloids are contraindicated in patients with peripheral vascular disease).

and this may account for their activity in treating migraine attacks (see below).

Clinical use

The only use of ergotamine is in the treatment of attacks of migraine unresponsive to simple analgesics (see below). Methysergide is occasionally used for migraine prophylaxis, but its main use is in treating the symptoms of carcinoid tumours (see below). All of these drugs can be used orally or by injection.

Unwanted effects

Ergotamine often causes nausea and vomiting, and it must be avoided in patients with peripheral vascular disease because of its vasoconstrictor action. Methysergide also causes nausea and vomiting, but its most serious side-effect, which restricts its clinical usefulness considerably, is retroperitoneal and mediastinal fibrosis, which can impair the functioning of the gastrointestinal tract, kidneys, heart and lungs. The mechanism of this is unknown, but it is noteworthy that similar fibrotic reactions also occur in carcinoid syndrome (see below) in which there is a high circulating level of 5-HT.

CLINICAL CONDITIONS IN WHICH 5-HT PLAYS A ROLE

In this section, we discuss two situations in which the peripheral actions of 5-HT are believed to be important, namely *migraine* and *carcinoid syndrome*. Further information is reviewed by Houston & Vanhoutte (1986). The possible role of 5-HT in vomiting, and the usefulness of 5-HT_3 antagonists in treating drug-induced emesis are discussed in Chapter 24. Interference with 5-HT-mediated transmission in the CNS is probably a factor in the actions of antidepressant and antipsychotic drugs (see Chs 33, 37 and 38).

MIGRAINE AND ANTI-MIGRAINE DRUGS

Migraine is a common and debilitating condition, affecting 10–15% of people, the causation of which is not well understood (see Moskowitz, 1992; Edvinsson, 1999). The classical pattern of events in a migraine attack consists of an initial visual disturbance (the *aura),* in which a flickering pattern, followed by a blind spot, progresses gradually across an area of the visual field. This visual disturbance is followed, about 30 minutes later, by a severe throbbing headache, starting unilaterally, often with photophobia, nausea, vomiting and prostration, which lasts for several hours. In fact, the classical visual aura occurs only in about 20% of migraine sufferers, though many experience other kinds of premonitory sensation. Sometimes attacks are precipitated by particular foods or by visual stimuli, but more often they occur without obvious cause.

Pathophysiology

Though controversy abounds, and religious wars continue, there are three fundamental views of the physiological mechanisms underlying migraine, linking it to primary events in *blood vessels*, the *brain* or *sensory nerves*.

The classical 'vascular' theory, proposed around 50 years ago by Wolff, implicated an initial humorally mediated intracerebral vasoconstriction causing the aura, and an ensuing extracerebral vasodilatation phase causing the headache. This hypothesis has not, however, been generally supported by more recent blood flow studies involving non-invasive monitoring techniques in patients with migraine (see review by Friberg, 1999). In episodes of migraine with aura, there is indeed a biphasic change in cerebral blood flow (Fig. 12.2), with a reduction of 20–30% preceding the premonitory aura, followed by a highly variable increase of similar magnitude. However, the headache usually begins during the initial vasoconstrictor phase, and blood flow changes of similar magnitude caused by other factors do not produce symptoms. The vasoconstriction starts posteriorly and gradually spreads forwards over the rest of the hemisphere,

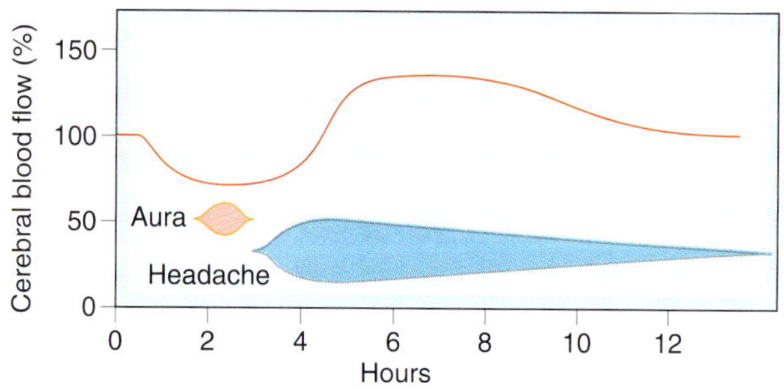

Fig. 12.2 Cerebral blood flow changes during migraine. (After Olesen et al. 1990.)

implying a neural rather than a humoral cause. It only occurs in association with the aura, and not in the remaining 80% of migraine sufferers; no consistent blood flow changes are associated with the headache phase.

Headache originates not in the brain itself but in extracerebral structures lying within the cranial cavity, such as the meninges or large arteries, which are innervated by nociceptive sensory nerve fibres belonging to the trigeminal pathway. The vascular theory attributes the headache to dilatation in these large arteries. While some studies have shown a unilateral widening of the middle cerebral artery on the side of the headache, others have shown no clear change; overall the evidence for arterial dilatation as the cause of the headache is controversial (see Thomsen, 1997).

The 'brain' hypothesis (see Lauritzen, 1987) links migraine to the phenomenon of cortical *spreading depression*. This is a dramatic, though poorly understood, phenomenon, thought to occur in concussion and triggered in experimental animals by local application of K^+ to the cortex. This causes an advancing wave of profound neural inhibition, which progresses slowly over the cortical surface at a rate of about 2 mm/min. In the depressed area, the ionic balance is grossly disturbed, with an extremely high extracellular K^+ concentration, and the blood flow is reduced. There is strong evidence to suggest that the aura phase of a migraine attack is associated with a wave of spreading depression, though what initiates it remains unknown. However, in animal models, spreading depression does not lead to activation or sensitisation of trigeminal afferents (Ebersberger et al., 2001). It is believed that the aura is associated with spreading depression, but that this is not a necessary step in the pathogenesis of the migraine attack.

The 'sensory nerve' hypothesis (see Moskowitz, 1992) suggests that activation of trigeminal nerve terminals in the meninges and extracranial vessels is the primary event in a migraine attack. This will cause pain directly and will also induce inflammatory changes through the release of neuropeptides from the sensory nerve terminals (neurogenic inflammation; see Chs 15 and 40). This theory is supported by experiments showing that one such peptide (calcitonin gene-related peptide; see Ch. 13) is released into the meningeal circulation during a migraine attack.

The main theories are summarised in Figure 12.3. Many variants of these mechanisms have been proposed, but it is noteworthy that none can explain at the biochemical level what initiates a migraine attack or define the underlying abnormality that predisposes particular individuals to suffer such attacks,

Whether one inclines to the view that migraine is a vascular disorder, kind of spontaneous concussion, an inflammatory disease or just a bad headache, there is strong evidence to implicate 5-HT in its pathogenesis.

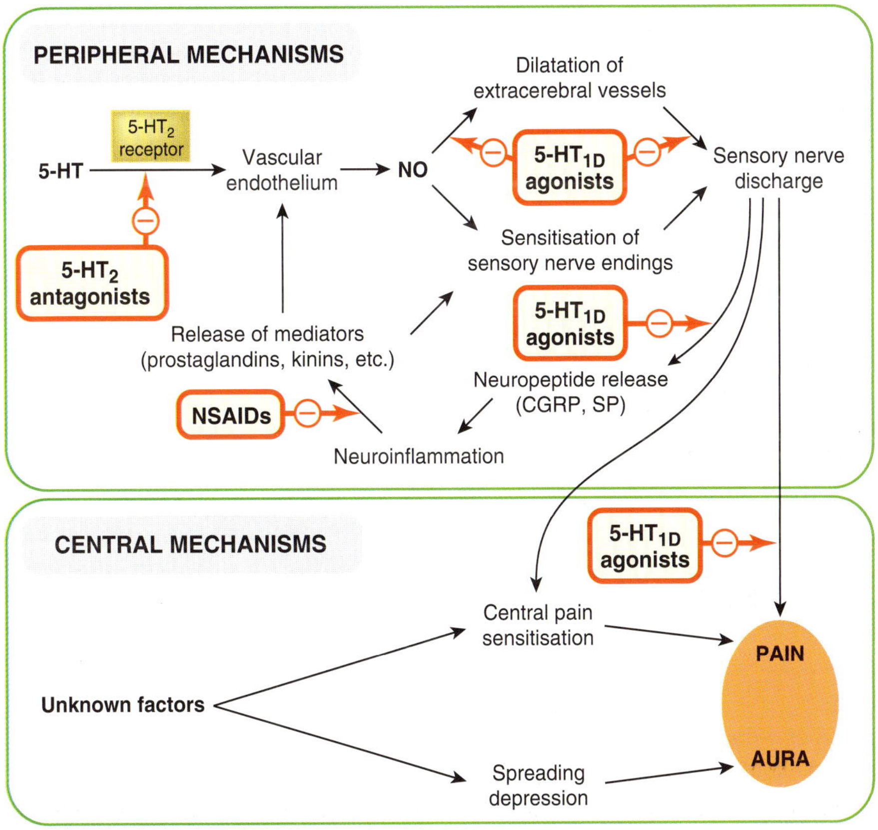

Fig. 12.3 Postulated pathogenesis of migraine. The initiating event is uncertain but in some cases may be an abnormal neuronal discharge, set off by emotional or biochemical disturbances This leads to localised 'spreading depression' which causes the aura and may also lead to sensitisation of central pain pathways. In migraine without aura, the primary event is excitation (cause unknown) of nociceptive nerve terminals in the meningeal vessels, leading to the cycle of neurogenic inflammation shown in the upper part of the diagram. (SP, substance P; CGRP, calcitonin gene-related peptide; 5-HT, 5-hydroxytryptamine; NO, nitric oxide; NSAIDs, non-steroidal anti-inflammatory drugs.)

- There is a sharp increase in the urinary excretion of the main 5-HT metabolite, 5-HIAA, during the attack. The blood concentration of 5-HT falls, probably because of depletion of platelet 5-HT.
- Many of the drugs that are effective in treating migraine are 5-HT receptor agonists or antagonists. See Figure 12.3 and the clinical box for further information.

Antimigraine drugs

The main drugs used to treat migraine are summarised in Table 12.3, and their postulated sites of action are shown in Figure 12.3. It is important to distinguish between drugs used to treat acute attacks of migraine (appropriate when the attacks are fairly infrequent, and prophylaxis is not justified) and drugs used for prophylaxis. Apart from 5-HT_2-receptor antagonists, the drugs used prophylactically are a mixed bag, and their mechanism of action is poorly understood.

CARCINOID SYNDROME

▼ Carcinoid syndrome (see Creutzfeld & Stockmann, 1987) is a rare disorder associated with malignant tumours of enterochromaffin cells, usually arising in the small intestine and metastasising to the liver. These tumours secrete a variety of hormones. 5-HT is the most important, but neuropeptides, such as substance P (Ch. 13), and other agents, such as prostaglandins and bradykinin (Ch. 15), are also produced. The release of these substances into the bloodstream results in various unpleasant symptoms, including flushing, diarrhoea and bronchoconstriction, as well as hypotension, which may cause dizziness or fainting. Stenosis of heart valves also occurs, which can result in cardiac failure. The relationship of this to hormone secretion is not understood.

The syndrome is readily diagnosed by measuring the excretion of 5-HIAA, the main metabolite of 5-HT, in the urine, the level of which may increase 20-fold. 5-HIAA is raised even during periods when the tumour is asymptomatic.

5-HT_2 antagonists, such as **cyproheptadine,** are effective in controlling some of the symptoms of carcinoid syndrome. **Methysergide** is also effective but is liable to cause retroperitoneal and mediastinal fibrosis, a potentially serious side-effect.

A complementary therapeutic approach is to use a long-acting analogue of somatostatin, namely **octreotide,** which suppresses hormone secretion from various neuroendocrine cells, including carcinoid cells (see Ch. 27).

Drugs used for migraine

Acute attack
- Simple analgesics (e.g. aspirin, paracetamol) can be given with metoclopramide to speed up absorption.
- Ergotamine (5-HT_{1D}-receptor partial agonist).
- Sumatriptan (5-HT_{1D} agonist) is effective but short acting (half-life about 2 hours). Newer compounds (e.g. zolmitriptan) are claimed to be faster acting and not to cause chest pain.

Prophylaxis (considered for patients with more than one severe attack per month)
- Beta-adrenoceptor antagonists (e.g. propranolol, metoprolol; see Ch. 11).
- Pizotifen (5-HT_2-receptor antagonist). Adverse effects include weight gain, antimuscarinic effects.
- Other 5-HT_2-receptor antagonists
  —cyproheptadine: also has antihistamine and calcium antagonist actions
  —methysergide: rarely used because of risk of retroperitoneal fibrosis and renal failure.
- Tricyclic antidepressants (e.g. amitriptyline; see Ch. 38). May be effective even though patients are not depressed.
- Clonidime, an α_2-adrenoceptor agonist (see Ch. 11). Has been used, but efficacy is doubtful.
- Calcium antagonists (e.g. dihydropyridines, verapamil; see Ch. 17): headache is a side-effect of these drugs but, paradoxically, may reduce frequency of migraine attacks. Their mechanism of action is unknown.

PURINES*

Nucleosides, especially *adenosine,* and nucleotides, especially *ADP* and *ATP,* produce a wide range of pharmacological effects that are unrelated to their role in energy metabolism. It was shown in 1929 that adenosine injected into anaesthetised animals causes cardiac slowing, a fall in blood pressure, vasodilatation and inhibition of intestinal movements, and purines are now known to participate in many physiological control mechanisms, such as the regulation of coronary flow and myocardial function (Chs 17 and 18), platelet aggregation and immune responses (Chs 15 and 20) and neurotransmission, in both the central and peripheral nervous system (Chs 9 and 33). (For reviews, see Illes et al., 2000; Cunha, 2001.) Figure 12.4 summarises the mechanisms by which purines are released and interconverted, and the main receptor types on which they act.

The full complexity of purinergic control systems, and their importance in many pathophysiological mechanisms, is only now emerging, and there is no doubt that therapeutic agents affecting these systems will assume growing significance.

ATP AS A NEUROTRANSMITTER

The idea that such a work-a-day metabolite as ATP might be a member of the neurotransmitter elite was resisted for a long time, but it is now firmly established. ATP is a transmitter in the periphery, both as a primary mediator and as a co-transmitter in noradrenergic nerve terminals (see Burnstock, 1985; Lundberg, 1996; Khakh, 2001). ATP is contained in synaptic vesicles of both adrenergic and cholinergic neurons, and it accounts for

*The important mediators are actually *nucleosides* and *nucleotides*, not purines at all, but 'purines' and 'purinergic' are now widely used as a convenient, though strictly incorrect, shorthand.

Table 12.3 Antimigraine drugs

Use	Drug	Mode of action	Side effects	Pharmacokinetic aspects	Notes
Acute	Sumatriptan	5-HT_{1D}-receptor agonist. Constricts large arteries, inhibits trigeminal nerve transmission	Coronary vasoconstriction, dysrhythmias	Poorly absorbed by mouth, hence delayed response Can be given subcutaneously Does not cross blood–brain barrier Plasma half-life ~1.5 h	Effective in ~70% of migraine attacks, but short duration of action is a drawback Contraindicated in patients with coronary disease
	Naratriptan Zolmitriptan Rizatriptan Alnitidan	As sumatriptan, with additional actions on CNS	Side-effects less than sumatriptan	Improved bioavailability and duration of action compared with sumatriptan Able to cross blood–brain barrier	Basically sumatriptan look-alikes, with improved pharmacokinetics and reduced cardiac side-effects
Acute	Ergotamine	5-HT_1-receptor partial agonist. Also affects α-adrenoceptors Vasoconstrictor Blocks trigeminal nerve transmission	Peripheral vasoconstriction, including coronary vessels Nausea, vomiting Contracts uterus and may cause fetal damage	Poorly absorbed. Sometimes given by suppository, inhalation, etc. Duration of action 12–24 h	Effective, but use limited by side-effects
Prophylaxis	Methysergide	$5HT_2$-receptor antagonist/partial agonist	Nausea, vomiting, diarrhoea Rarely, but seriously, retroperitoneal or mediastinal fibrosis	Used orally	Effective but rarely used, owing to side-effects and insidious toxicty
Prophylaxis	Pizotifen	$5HT_2$-receptor antagonist Also muscarinic acetylcholine antagonist	Weight gain Antimuscarinc side-effects	Used orally	
Prophylaxis	Cyproheptadine	$5HT_2$-receptor antagonist Also blocks histamine receptors and calcium channels.	Sedation, weight gain	Used orally	Rarely used
Prophylaxis	Propranolol and similar drugs (e.g. metoprolol)	β-Adrenoceptor antagonists Mechanism of antimigraine effect not clear	Fatigue Bronchoconstriction (Ch. 11)	Used orally	Effective and widely used for migraine

Notes:
1. Aspirin-like or opiate analgesic drugs (see Ch. 40) are often used to treat acute migraine attacks.
2. Other drugs used for migraine prohylaxis include calcium channel blockers (e.g. nifedipine, see Ch. 18), antidepressants (e.g. amitriptyline, see Ch. 38), valproate (see Ch. 39) and clonidine (Ch. 11). Their efficacy is limited..

many of the actions produced by stimulation of autonomic nerves that are not caused by acetylcholine or noradrenaline (see Ch. 9). These include effects such as relaxation of intestinal smooth muscle evoked by sympathetic stimulation, and contraction of the bladder produced by parasympathetic nerves. Burnstock and his colleagues have shown that ATP is released, in a Ca^{2+}-dependent fashion, on nerve stimulation, and that exogenous ATP in general mimics the effects of nerve stimulation in various preparations. Furthermore, **suramin**, a drug recently shown to block ATP-receptors (developed many years ago for treating trypanosome infections), blocks these synaptic responses. Recent work has also shown ATP to function as a conventional 'fast' transmitter in

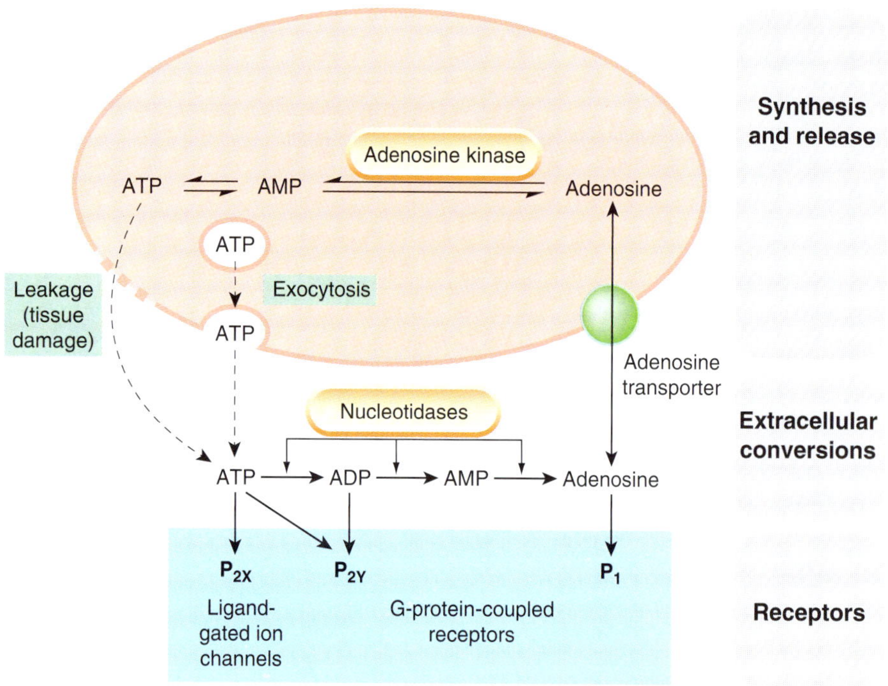

Fig. 12.4 Purines as mediators. ATP (and in platelets, ADP) is stored in vesicles and released by exocytosis. It is also present in the cytosol of all cells, from which large quantities may be released by cellular damage. Adenosine is present in the cytosol of all cells and is taken up and released via a specific membrane transporter. Released ATP and ADP are rapidly converted to adenosine by the action of tissue nucleotidases.

the CNS and in autonomic ganglia (see Khakh, 2001). ATP is present in all cells at millimolar concentrations and is released, independently of exocytosis, if the cells are damaged (e.g. by ischaemia). ATP released from cells is rapidly dephosphorylated by a range of tissue-specific *nucleotidases*, producing ADP and adenosine (Fig. 12.4), both of which produce a wide variety of receptor-mediated effects.

The role of *intracellular* ATP in controlling membrane potassium channels, which is important in the control of vascular smooth muscle (Ch. 17) and of insulin secretion (Ch. 25), is quite distinct from its transmitter function.

ADP AND PLATELETS

The secretory vesicles of blood platelets store both ATP and ADP in high concentrations, and release them when the platelets are activated (see Ch. 20). One of the many effects of ADP is to promote platelet aggregation, so this system provides positive feedback—an important mechanism, though one of many, for controlling this process.

ADENOSINE AS A MEDIATOR

Adenosine differs from ATP in that it is not stored by and released from secretory vesicles. Rather, it exists free in the cytosol of all cells and is transported in and out of cells mainly via a membrane transporter. Not much is known about the way in which this is controlled. Adenosine in tissues comes partly from this source and partly from released ATP or ADP (Fig. 12.4).

Adenosine produces many pharmacological effects, both in the periphery and in the CNS (see Brundege & Dunwiddie, 1997; Cunha, 2001). One of its functions appears to be as a protective agent when tissues are threatened (e.g. by coronary or cerebral ischaemia; see Chs 17 and 34), based on its ability to inhibit cell function and thus minimise the metabolic requirements of cells. Under less-extreme conditions, variations in adenosine release may play a role in controlling blood flow, matching it to the metabolic needs of the tissues.

Adenosine is destroyed or taken up within a few seconds when given intravenously (as in the treatment of supraventricular tachycardias; see Ch. 17), but longer-lasting analogues have been discovered that also show greater receptor selectivity. Adenosine uptake is blocked by **dipyridamole**, a vasodilator and antiplatelet drug (see Ch. 17).

PURINE RECEPTORS

Purine receptors, like those of other mediators, have undergone classification, reclassification, naming and renaming worthy of politics in the Balkans, and similarly acrimonious; order has now been achieved. There are two main types (see Fredholm et al., 1994), namely:

- *P_1-receptors* (subtypes A_1, A_2 and A_3): these respond to adenosine, and are G-protein-coupled receptors (GPCRs) linked to stimulation or inhibition of adenylate cyclase; they are present in many different tissues
- *P_2-receptors* (subtypes P_{2X} and P_{2Y}, each with several further subdivisions): these respond to ATP and/or ADP. P_{2X}-

receptors are multimeric ionotropic receptors (see Ch. 3), whereas P_{2Y}-receptors are GPCRs, coupled to adenylate cyclase or phosphoinositide metabolism.

These subtypes are distinguished on the basis of their agonist and antagonist selectivity, and their molecular structure (for recent reviews, see von Kügelglen & Wetter (2000), Fredholm et al. (2001) and Khakh (2001)). Though there are many experimental compounds with varying degrees of receptor selectivity, there are so far few therapeutic agents that act on these receptors, and we will confine this account to some functional aspects which may give rise to therapeutic drugs in the future.

FUNCTIONAL ASPECTS

Adenosine receptors

The main effects of adenosine, and the receptors involved are:

- vasodilatation, including coronary vessels (A_2), except in the kidney, where A_1-receptors produce vasoconstriction; adenosine infusion causes a fall in blood pressure
- inhibition of platelet aggregation (A_2)
- block of cardiac atrioventricular conduction (A_1) and reduction of force of contraction
- bronchoconstriction, especially in asthmatic subjects (A_1); the anti-asthmatic effect of methylxanthines may partly reflect A_1-receptor antagonism
- release of mediators from mast cells (A_3): this contributes to bronchoconstriction
- stimulation of nociceptive afferent neurons, especially in the heart (A_2): adenosine release in response to ischaemia has been suggested as a mechanism of anginal pain (Ch. 17); carotid body afferents are also stimulated, causing reflex hyperventilation
- inhibition of transmitter release at many peripheral and central synapses (A_1): in the CNS adenosine generally exerts a pre- and postsynaptic depressant action. reducing motor activity, depressing respiration, inducing sleep, and reducing anxiety, all of which effects are the opposite of those produced by methylxanthines (Ch. 41)
- neuroprotection, in cerebral ischaemia, probably through inhibition of glutamate release through A_1-receptors (see Rudolphi et al., 1992; Ch. 34).

In general, the A_1-receptor has been characterised as a 'homeostatic' receptor with protective functions in many tissues, whereas the A_2-receptor has more specific regulatory functions, especially in the brain, where it is widely expressed.

P_2-receptors and actions

P_2-receptors respond to various adenine nucleotides, generally preferring ATP to ADP or AMP. The role of ATP as a fast transmitter (see above) involves P_{2X}-receptors, of which seven subtypes have been identified. These occur as a variety of mixed (heteromeric) assemblies (see Khakh, 2001). Their functions are still unclear, apart from the following pointers.

- P_{2x1}-receptors are expressed on various smooth muscle cells. ATP is a co-transmitter released by sympathetic nerves (Ch. 11), and P_{2x1}-receptors are responsible for the initial contraction.
- P_{2x2}-receptors are expressed in many brain regions and mediate 'fast' transmission by ATP in the brain.
- P_{2x3}-receptors occur in nociceptive afferent neurons and may participate in pain associated with ATP released through tissue injury.

Purines as mediators

- ATP functions as a neurotransmitter (or co-transmitter) at peripheral neuroeffector junctions and central synapses.
- ATP is stored in vesicles and released by exocytosis. Cytoplasmic ATP may be released when cells are damaged. It also functions as an intracellular mediator, inhibiting the opening of membrane potassium channels.
- ATP acts on two types of purinoceptor (P_2), one of which (P_{2X}) is a ligand-gated ion channel responsible for fast synaptic responses. The other (P_{2Y}) is coupled to various second messengers. Suramin blocks the P_{2X}-receptor.
- Released ATP is rapidly converted to ADP and adenosine.
- ADP acts on platelets, causing aggregation. This is important in thrombosis. It also acts on vascular and other types of smooth muscle, as well as having effects in the CNS.
- Adenosine affects many cells and tissues, including smooth muscle and nerve cells. It is not a conventional transmitter but may be important as local hormone and 'homeostatic modulator'.
- Adenosine acts through A_1-, A_2- and A_3-receptors, coupled to inhibition or stimulation of adenylate cyclase. A_1- and A_2-receptors are blocked by xanthines, such as theophylline.
- The main effects of adenosine are:
  —hypotension (A_2) and cardiac depression (A_1)
  —inhibition of atrioventricular conduction (antidysrhythmic effect, A_1)
  —inhibition of platelet aggregation (A_2)
  —bronchoconstriction (probably secondary to mast cell activation, A_3)
  —presynaptic inhibition in CNS (responsible for neuroprotective effect, A_1).
- Adenosine is very short acting and is sometimes used for its antidysrhythmic effect.
- New adenosine agonists and antagonists are in development, mainly for treatment of ischaemic heart disease and stroke.

- P_{2X7}-receptors are unusual in that activation causes a large and non-selective increase in membrane permeability. They are expressed mainly by cells of the immune system, and they control the release of certain cytokines.

The other actions of ATP are mediated through P_{2Y}-receptors, of which five subtypes occur in mammals. They are GPCRs and are linked to various second messenger systems They occur in many tissues, and the lack of selective antagonists makes it difficult to define their functions individually, though the actions of ADP on platelets and vascular endothelial cells are ascribed to the P_{2Y1}-subtype.

Drugs acting selectively on P_2-receptors have not yet been developed for clinical purposes.

PHARMACOLOGICAL ASPECTS

Uses of adenosine

Because of its inhibitory effect on cardiac conduction, adenosine may be used as an intravenous bolus injection to terminate supraventricular tachycardia (Ch. 17). It is safer than alternative drugs such as β-adrenoceptor antagonists or verapamil, because of its short duration of action.

Otherwise adenosine is not used therapeutically, though longer lasting A_1-receptor agonists could prove useful in various conditions (e.g. hypertension, ischaemic heart disease, stroke, etc.). Selective adenosine receptor antagonists could also have advantages over theophylline in the treatment of asthma (see Ch. 22).

Drugs acting on purine receptors

Methylxanthines, especially analogues of **theophylline** (Ch. 22), are A_1/A_2-receptor antagonists; however, they also increase cAMP by inhibiting phosphodiesterase, which contributes to their pharmacological actions independently of adenosine receptor antagonism. CNS stimulation by methylxanthines such as **caffeine** (see Ch. 41) is partly a result of block of inhibitory A_1/A_2-receptors. Certain derivatives of theophylline are claimed to show greater selectivity for adenosine receptors over phosphodiesterase.

P_2-receptors are blocked by **suramin** and the experimental compound PPADS.

Intensive effort are under way to develop drugs with improved receptor selectivity for therapeutic purposes. There are many potential applications for such compounds in different indications, including heart disease, stroke, pain and immunological disorders. Probably, their time will come.

REFERENCES AND FURTHER READING

Barnes N M, Sharp T 1999 A review of central 5-HT receptors and their function. Neuropharmacology 38: 1083–1152 (*Useful general review, focusing on CNS*)

Bonasera S J, Tecott L H 2000 Mouse models of serotonin receptor function: towards a genetic dissection of serotonin systems. Pharmacol Ther 88: 133–142 (*Review of studies on transgenic mice lacking 5-HT$_1$- or 5-HT$_2$-receptors. Shows how difficult it can be to interpret such experiments*)

Branchek T A, Blackburn T P 2000 5-HT$_6$ receptors as emerging targets for drug discovery. Annu Rev Pharmacol Toxicol 40: 319–334 (*Summary of what is known about 5-HT$_6$-receptors, with emphasis on future therapeutic opportunities*)

Brundege J M, Dunwiddie T V 1997 Role of adenosine as a modulator of synaptic activity in the central nervous system. Adv Pharmacol 39: 353–391 (*Good review article*)

Burnstock G 1985 Purinergic mechanisms broaden their sphere of influence. Trends Neurosci 8: 5–6 (*Ideas about the functional role of purinergic transmission*)

Cooper J R, Bloom F E, Roth R H 1996 The biochemical basis of neuropharmacology. Oxford University Press, New York (*Excellent general textbook*)

Creutzfeld W, Stockmann F 1987 Carcinoids and carcinoid syndrome. Am J Med 82(Suppl 58): 4–16

Cunha R A 2001 Adenosine as a neuromodulator and as a homeostatic regulator in the nervous system: different roles, different sources and different receptors. Neurochem Int 38: 107–125 (*Speculative review on the functions of adenosine in the nervous system*)

Ebersberger A, Schaible H-G, Averbeck B, Richter F 2001 Is there a correlation between spreading depression, neurogenic inflammation, and nociception that might cause migraine pain? Ann Neurol 49: 7–13 (*Their conclusion is there is no connection—spreading depression does not produce inflammation or affect sensory neurons*)

Edvinsson L (ed) 1999 Migraine and headache pathophysiology. Martin Dunitz, London (*Collected articles summarising current, and often conflicting, views on the mechanism of migraine*)

Fozard J R (ed) 1989 The peripheral actions of 5-hydroxytryptamine. Oxford University Press, Oxford

Fredholm B B, Abbrachio M B, Burnstock G et al. 1994 Nomenclature and classification of purinoceptors. Pharmacol Rev 46: 143–156 (*Useful review*)

Fredholm B B, Arslan G, Halldner L, Kull B, Schulte G, Wasserman W 2001 Structure and function of adenosine receptors and their genes. Naunyn-Schmiedeberg Arch Pharmacol 362: 364–374 (*General review article*)

Friberg L 1999 Migraine pathophysiology, its relation to cerebral haemodynamic changes. In: Edvinsson L (ed) Migraine and headache pathophysiology. Martin Dunitz: London (*Useful summary of findings in a controversial area*)

Green A R (ed) 1985 Neuropharmacology of serotonin. Oxford University Press, Oxford (*Useful compilation of articles on 5-HT pharmacology*)

Houston D S, Vanhoutte P M 1986 Serotonin and the vascular system: role in health and disease, and implications for therapy. Drugs 31: 149–163

Hoyer D, Clarke D E, Fozard J R et al. 1994 VII International Union of Pharmacology classification of receptors for 5-hydroxytryptamine. Pharmacol Rev 46: 157–203 (*The official view on 5-HT receptor classification*)

Illes P, Klotz K-N, Lohse M J 2000 Signalling by extracellular nucleotides and nucleosides. Naunyn-Schmiedeberg Arch Pharmacology 362: 295–298 (*Introductory article in a series of useful reviews on purinergic mechanisms in the same issue*)

Khakh B S 2001 Molecular physiology of P_{2X} receptors and signalling at synapses. Nat Rev Neurosci 2: 165–174 (*Summarises data on ATP-mediated synaptic transmission*)

Klotz K-N 2000 Adenosine receptors and their ligands. Naunyn-Schmiedeberg Arch Pharmacol 362: 382–391 (*Account of known agonists and antagonists at adenosine receptors*)

von Kügelglen I, Wetter A 2000 Molecular pharmacology of P_{2Y} receptors. Naunyn-Schmiedeberg Arch Pharmacol 362: 310–323

Lauritzen M 1987 Cerebral blood flow in migraine and cortical spreading depression. Acta Neurol Scand Suppl 113: 140 (*Review of clinical measurements of cerebral blood flow in migraine, which overturn earlier hypotheses*)

Lundberg J M 1996 Pharmacology of co-transmission in the autonomic nervous system: integrative aspects on amines, neuropeptides, adenosine triphosphate, amino acids and nitric oxide. Pharmacol Rev 48: 114–192 (*Comprehensive and informative review*)

Moskowitz M A 1992 Neurogenic versus vascular mechanisms of sumatriptan and ergot alkaloids in migraine. Trends Pharmacol Sci 13: 307–311 (*Discussion of controversies about pathophysiology of migraine*)

North R A, Barnard E A 1997 Nucleotide receptors. Curr Opin Neurobiol 7: 346–357 (*Update on purinergic receptors*)

Rudolphi K A, Schubert P, Parkinson F E, Fredholm B B 1992 Neuroprotective role of adenosine in cerebral ischaemia. Trends Pharmacol Sci 13: 439–445 (*Argues that adenosine protects neurons against ischaemic damage—important therapeutic implications*)

Taniyama K et al. 2000 Functions of peripheral 5-hydroxytryptamine receptors, especially 5-HT_4 receptor, in gastrointestinal motility. J Gastroenterol 35: 575–582 (*Review describing the role of various 5-HT receptors in the gastrointestinal tract*)

Thomsen L L 1997 Investigations into the role of nitric oxide and the large intracranial arteries in migraine headache. Cephahalgia 17: 873–895 (*Revisits the old vascular theory of migraine in the light of evidence from blood flow studies in humans, and effects of nitric oxide*)

13 Peptides and proteins as mediators

Overview 198

General principles of peptide pharmacology 198
- Structure of peptides 198
- Types of peptide mediator 199

Biosynthesis and regulation of peptides 202
- Peptide precursors 202
- Diversity within peptide families 203
- Peptide trafficking and secretion 204

Peptide antagonists 204

Proteins and peptides as drugs 205

Concluding remarks 206

OVERVIEW

Much of today's pharmacology is based on signalling molecules that are of low molecular weight and non-peptide in nature. Since the 1970s, it has emerged that peptides and proteins are at least as important, maybe more so, as signalling molecules. Yet, the pharmacological manipulation of peptide signalling is still far less advanced than that of, say, the cholinergic, adrenergic or 5-hydroxytryptamine (5-HT) systems (Chs 10–12). Pharmacology, one could say, has some catching up to do. In this chapter, we give an overview of the main characteristics of peptides and proteins as mediators and as drugs, bringing out the contrasts between these and non-peptides, and we evaluate the present and possible future use of peptides as therapeutic agents. For reviews, with more detail than can be provided here, see Buckel (1996), Cooper et al. (1996), Hökfelt (1991), Hökfelt et al., (2000) and Nestler et al. (2001).

Historical aspects

▼ Historically, there are two main reasons why pharmacology has a strong bias towards non-peptides. One is that the subject began with the analysis of the actions of natural (mainly plant) products thought to have medicinal properties. Very few of these were peptides, and they did not, for the most part, interact with peptide signalling systems. The second reason is that the methodology required to study peptides is of more recent origin. Key technological advances were the introduction of solid phase peptide synthesis, the use of antibodies, both for radioimmunoassay and for immunocytochemical localisation of peptides, and the use of molecular biology approaches for studying the expression of peptides and their precursors. Solid phase synthesis developed in the 1960s was particularly important; prior to this, very few scientists were dogged enough to tackle peptide chemistry by classical methods.

In 1953, du Vigneaud made history, and earned a Nobel Prize, by determining the structure and carrying out the synthesis of oxytocin—the first peptide mediator to be characterised and the first to be synthesised commercially for use in medicine. There were many other examples of mediators, for example substance P, bradykinin (Ch. 15) and angiotensin (Ch. 18), which had been identified as peptides in the 1930s, but which had structures that remained unknown for many years. All are small peptides of 11 residues or fewer, but determination of their structure, and their chemical synthesis, was a major task; the structure of bradykinin was not known until 1960, while that of substance P was published in 1970. By contrast, the use of the newer, now routine, methods enabled endothelin (a much larger peptide; see Ch. 18 and below) to be fully characterised, synthesised and its gene cloned within about a year, the complete information being published in a single paper (Yanagisawa et al., 1988). Protein mediators, such as cytokines (Ch. 15) and growth factors (Chs 15 and 21), containing 50 or more residues are still very difficult to synthesise chemically, and the major advances since the early 1980s have relied very largely on molecular biological approaches. The use of recombinant proteins as therapeutic agents—a development driven mainly by the emergent biotechnology industry—is rapidly gaining ground.*

Whereas the discovery of new 'small molecule' mediators has virtually dried up, the discovery of new peptide mediators continues apace. Hökfelt et al. (2000) list 13 neuropeptides that have been discovered since 1990.

GENERAL PRINCIPLES OF PEPTIDE PHARMACOLOGY

STRUCTURE OF PEPTIDES

Peptide and protein mediators vary from 3 to about 200 amino acid residues in size (Fig. 13.1), the arbitrary dividing line between peptides and proteins being about 50 residues. For

*In 1990, one new 'biopharmaceutical' product and 36 'conventional' drugs were registered for therapeutic use; in 1998 the figures were 9 and 26, respectively.

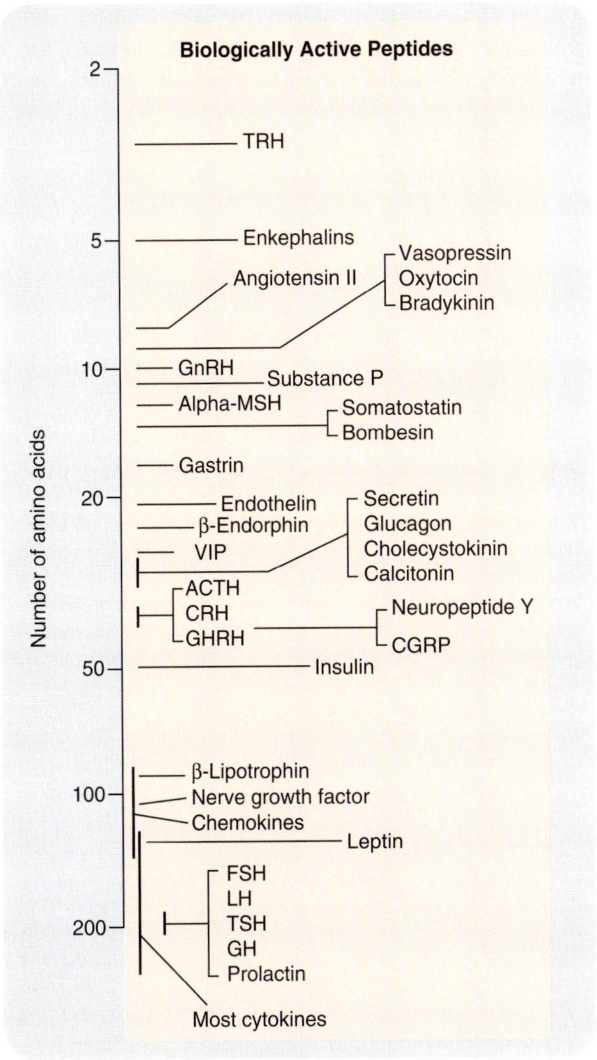

Fig. 13.1 Some typical peptide mediators. (TRH, thyrotrophin-releasing hormone; GHRH, growth hormone-releasing hormone; Alpha-MSH, α-melanocyte-stimulating hormone; VIP, vasoactive intestinal peptide; ACTH, adrenocorticotrophic hormone; CGRP, calcitonin gene-related peptide; CRH, corticotrophin-releasing hormone; GnRH, gonadotrophin-releasing hormone; FSH, follicle-stimulating hormone; LH, luteinising hormone; TSH, thyroid-stimulating hormone; GH, growth hormone.)

convenience, in this chapter, we use the term peptide to cover both classes. Peptides generally undergo post-translational modifications, such as C-terminal amidation, glycosylation, acetylation, carboxylation, sulfation or phosphorylation of specific residues. They often contain intramolecular disulfide bonds, so the molecule adopts a partially cyclic conformation, and they may comprise two or more separate chains linked by disulfide bonds. The conformation of peptides in solution is generally ill defined because they are so flexible, and peptides of less than about 40 residues have proved impossible to crystallise, which precludes the use of X-ray diffraction methods to study their conformation. To envisage them fitting into a receptor site in a precise 'lock-and-key' mode is to imagine that you can unlock your front door with a length of cooked spaghetti. Larger proteins adopt more restricted conformations, but because of their size, they generally interact with multiple sites on the receptor. These facts have greatly impeded the rational design of non-peptide analogues ('peptidomimetics') that mimic the structure of peptides and interact with peptide receptors. The use of random screening methods (somewhat to the chagrin of the rationalists) has nevertheless led in recent years to the discovery of many non-peptide antagonists—very few agonists—for peptide receptors (see below; Betancur et al., 1997).

TYPES OF PEPTIDE MEDIATOR

The soluble peptide mediators in the body, which are secreted by cells and act on surface receptors of other cells, can be very broadly divided into four groups:

- *neurotransmitters and neuroendocrine mediators*: (discussed further in this chapter)
- *hormones from non-neural sources*: plasma-derived peptides, notably angiotensin (Ch. 18) and bradykinin (Ch. 15), and substances such as insulin (Ch. 25) endothelin (Ch. 18), atrial natriuretic peptide (Ch. 18) and leptin (Ch. 26)
- *growth factors*: produced by many different cells and tissues and control cell growth and differentiation (see Chs 15 and 21)
- *mediators of the immune system*: (*cytokines* and *chemokines*; see Ch. 15).

Some important examples of peptide and protein mediators are shown in Figure 13.1.

Role of molecular biology

▼ Because peptide structures are represented directly in the genome, molecular biology has been the key to most of the recent advances in knowledge. It is used in many ways.

- Cloning of the genes encoding peptide precursors (see below) has shown how various active peptides can arise from a single precursor protein. Calcitonin gene-related peptide (CGRP) was discovered in this way.
- Cloning of the genes encoding peptide receptors has proved very informative. Nearly all peptide receptors belong either to the class of G-protein-coupled receptors or that of tyrosine kinase-linked receptors (see Ch. 3); very few peptides act on ligand-gated channels. Several new peptide mediators have been discovered by screening for ligands of 'orphan receptors'* (see Civelli et al., 2001).

*Recently, an orphan receptor (called ORL_1), closely resembling known opioid receptors, was identified by homology screening of brain complementary DNA (cDNA) libraries. Searching in an extract of brain peptides for possible ligands led to the identification of a hitherto unknown neuropeptide, christened *nociceptin* (Meunier et al., 1995). Its function remains unknown. Then, when the gene encoding nociceptin was cloned, it was found also to encode another peptide *nocistatin*, which has effects on pain transmission opposite to those of nociceptin, and seems to work on yet another receptor…(see Okuda-Ashitaka & Ito, 2000). The discovery of *orexins* (peptides involved in appetite and obesity; see Ch. 26) came through similar molecular orienteering.

- The control of precursor synthesis can be studied by measuring mRNA, for which highly sensitive and specific assays have been developed. The technique of *in situ hybridisation* enables the location and abundance of the mRNA to be mapped at microscopic resolution.
- Transgenic animals with peptide or receptor genes knocked out or overexpressed provide valuable clues to the functions of novel peptides. Antisense oligonucleotides can also be used to silence such genes.

PEPTIDES IN THE NERVOUS SYSTEM: COMPARISON WITH CONVENTIONAL TRANSMITTERS

The abundance of neuropeptides in the brain and elsewhere became evident in the 1970s and 1980s, and, as mentioned above, the tide of discovery of new members of this class of mediators continues to run strongly. In most respects, neuropeptide-mediated transmission resembles transmission by 'conventional' non-peptide mediators. The mechanisms for the storage and release (summarised in Fig. 13.2), and the receptor mechanisms through which their effects are produced (Ch. 3), are essentially the same for peptide and non-peptide transmitters, the main difference being that the vesicles are loaded with peptide precursors in the cell body, the active peptides being generated within the vesicles as they move to the nerve terminals. Having undergone exocytosis, the vesicles cannot be reloaded in situ but must be replaced with new pre-loaded vesicles. Transmitter turnover is, therefore, less rapid than with conventional mediators. Furthermore, recapture of the released mediators does not occur as it does with amine and amino acid mediators. As with other chemical mediators, the effects of peptides may be excitatory or inhibitory, pre- or postsynaptic, and exerted over short or long distances from the site of release. There are, however, certain monopolies of function between peptide and non-peptide mediators. For example, peptides do not activate ligand-gated ion channels and, therefore, do not function as fast neurotransmitters in the manner of non-peptides, such as acetylcholine, glutamate, glycine or gamma-aminobutyric acid (see Chs 10 and 31). Instead, they serve (as do many non-peptides) mainly as neuromodulators (Ch. 9), by activating G-protein-coupled receptors. In contrast, the ligands for tyrosine-kinase-linked receptors (see Ch. 3) are all peptides or proteins.

In summary, the similarities in function between peptide and non-peptide mediators are more striking than the differences. The main difference is constitutional rather than functional and stems from the fact that peptides, being gene products, represent variations on a single theme—a linear string of amino acids. Such sequences are much more susceptible to evolutionary change than are the structures of non-peptide mediators, and the number of known peptide mediators now greatly exceeds that of non-peptides. As Iversen pointed out in 1983: 'almost overnight, the number of putative transmitters in the mammalian nervous system has jumped from the ten or so monoamine and amino acid candidates to more than 40'. Since then, no new monoamine transmitters have appeared, but there are at least another 60 peptides.

Peptides as co-transmitters are discussed in Chapter 9. Two well-documented examples (reviewed by Lundberg, 1996) are the parasympathetic nerves supplying salivary glands (where the secretory response is produced by acetylcholine and the vasodilatation partly by *vasoactive intestinal peptide*) and the sympathetic innervation to various tissues, which involves release of the vasoconstrictor *neuropeptide Y* in addition to noradrenaline.

The distinction between neuropeptides and peripherally acting hormones is useful, but not absolute. Thus, *insulin*, *angiotensin*, *atrial natriuretic peptide* and *oxytocin* are best known as hormones that are formed, released and act in the periphery. They are, however, also found in the brain, though their role there is uncertain. Similarly, *endothelin* was first discovered in blood vessels but is now know to occur extensively in the brain as well.

MULTIPLE PHYSIOLOGICAL ROLES OF PEPTIDES

▼ In common with many non-peptide mediators, such as noradrenaline, dopamine, 5-HT or acetylcholine, the same peptides are often found, and presumably function as mediators, in several different parts of the body. Intriguingly, there often appears to be some connection between the effects of a peptide at different sites, in terms of coordinated physiological functions. For example, angiotensin acts on the cells of the hypothalamus to release antidiuretic hormone (vasopressin), which in turn causes water retention. Angiotensin also acts elsewhere in the brain to promote drinking behaviour and to increase blood pressure by activation of the sympathetic system; in addition, it releases aldosterone, which causes salt

Structure and function of peptide mediators

- Size varies from three to several hundred amino acid residues; conventionally, molecules of fewer than 50 residues are called peptides, larger molecules being proteins.
- Neural and endocrine mediators range in size from 3 to over 200 residues. Cytokines, chemokines and growth factors are generally larger than 100 residues.
- Most known peptide mediators come from the nervous system and endocrine organs. However, some are formed in the plasma, and many occur at other sites (e.g. vascular endothelium, heart, cells of the immune system, etc.). The same peptide may occur in several places and serve different functions.
- Small peptides and chemokines act mainly on G-protein-coupled receptors and act through the same second messenger systems as those used by other mediators. Cytokines and growth factors generally act through tyrosine-kinase-linked membrane receptors.
- Peptides frequently function in the nervous system as co-transmitters with other peptides or with non-peptide transmitters.
- The number of known peptide mediators now greatly exceeds that of non-peptides.

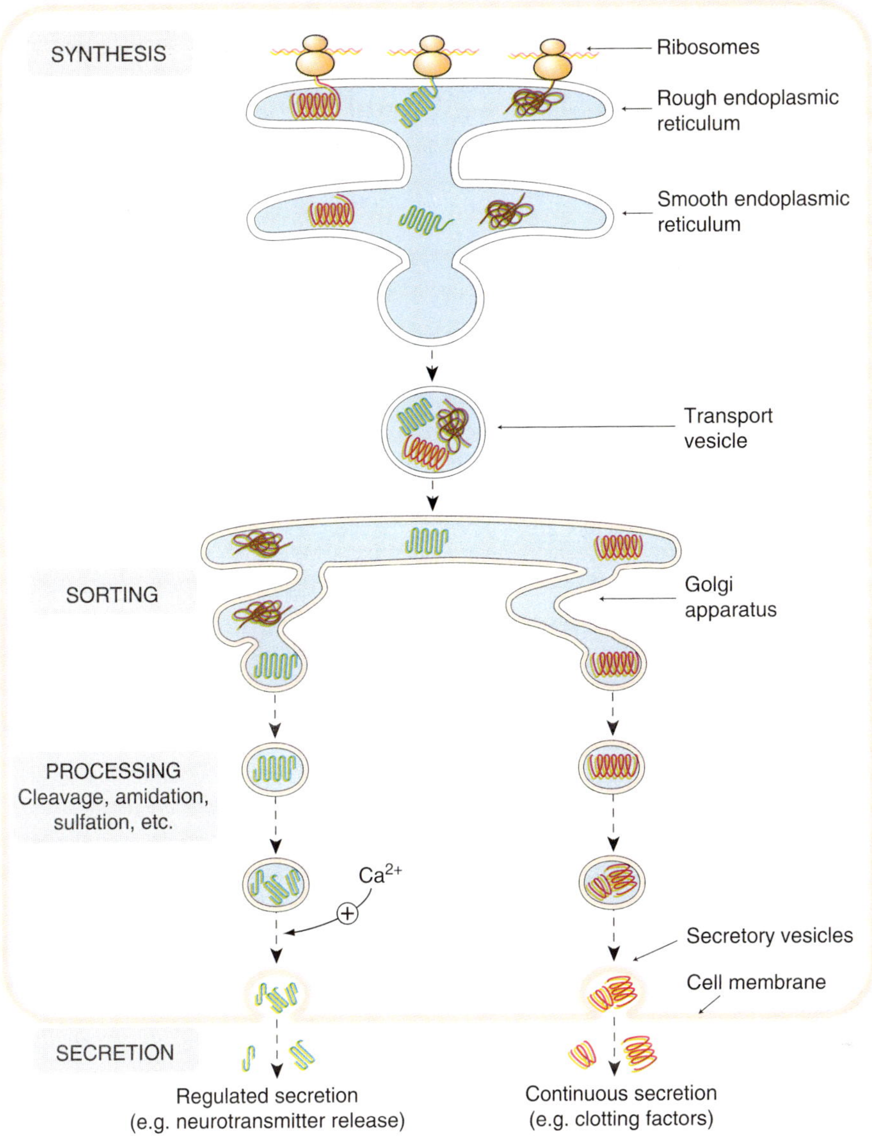

Fig. 13.2 Cellular mechanisms for peptide synthesis and release. Proteins synthesised by ribosomes are threaded through the membrane of the rough endoplasmic reticulum, from where they are conveyed via transport vesicles to the Golgi apparatus. Here they are sorted and packaged into secretory vesicles. Processing (cleavage, glycosylation, amidation, sulfation, etc.) occurs within the transport and secretory vesicles, and the products are released from the cell by exocytosis. Constitutive secretion (e.g. secretion of plasma proteins, clotting factors, etc. by liver cells) occurs continuously, and little material is stored in secretory vesicles. Regulated secretion, (e.g. neurosecretion or cytokine secretion) occurs in response to increased intracellular Ca^{2+} levels or other intracellular signals, and material is typically stored in significant amounts in an accumulation of secretory vesicles.

and water retention, and it acts directly to constrict blood vessels. Each of these effects plays a part in the overall response of the body to water deprivation and reduced circulating volume. There are other examples of what appears to be an orchestrated functional response produced by the various actions of a single mediator, but there are many more examples where the multiple effects just seem to be multiple effects.

So far, the stream of new information about neuropeptides since the 1970s has led to few useful generalisations about their functional role, and surprisingly few new drugs—with the exception of antihypertensive drugs acting on the renin–angiotensin system (see Ch. 18). For whatever reason, peptide pharmacology has proved to be something of a graveyard for drug discovery projects.*

*Substance P antagonists were confidently expected to be effective analgesic drugs, based on copious data from animal studies. When first tested in humans, non-peptide substance P antagonists proved to have no analgesic activity. Some face, but not much credibility, was saved when they were found instead to have unexpected anxiolytic properties.

BIOSYNTHESIS AND REGULATION OF PEPTIDES

Peptide structure is directly coded in the genome, in a manner that the structure of, say, acetylcholine is not. It is in some ways simpler for a cell to produce a peptide than a conventional neurotransmitter. To do the latter, it must produce a series of carrier molecules (to collect the necessary precursors and store the product) and enzymes to perform the synthesis. Peptide synthesis (Fig. 13.3) begins with the manufacture of a precursor protein in which the peptide sequence is embedded, along with specific proteolytic enzymes that excise the active peptide, a process of sculpture rather than synthesis. The precursor protein is packaged into vesicles at the point of synthesis, and the active peptide is formed in situ ready for release (Fig. 13.2). Thus there is no need for special uptake mechanisms for procuring the starting materials, and there are in general no mechanisms for recapturing released mediators, such as are important for non-peptides.

PEPTIDE PRECURSORS

The precursor protein, or *preprohormone* (Fig. 13.3), usually 100–250 residues in length, consists of an N-terminal *signal sequence* (*peptide*), followed by a variable stretch of unknown function, followed by a peptide-containing region in which several copies of active peptide fragments are contained. Often, several different peptides are found in one precursor, but sometimes there is only one in multiple copies. An extreme example occurs in the invertebrate *Aplysia*, in which the precursor contains 28 copies of the same short peptide. The signal peptide is strongly hydrophobic, which is important for insertion of the protein into the endoplasmic reticulum; it is cleaved off at an early stage, to form the *prohormone*. The active peptides are usually demarcated within the prohormone sequence by pairs of basic amino acids (Lys–Lys or Lys–Arg), which are cleavage points for the various trypsin-like proteases that act to release the peptides. This endoproteolytic cleavage generally occurs in the Golgi apparatus, or in the secretory vesicles. The enzymes responsible are known as *prohormone convertases*, of which two subtypes (PC1 and PC2) have been studied in detail (see Cullinan et al., 1991). Inspection of the prohormone sequence has often revealed likely cleavage points that demarcate unknown peptides. In some cases (e.g. CGRP; see below) new peptide mediators have been discovered in this way, but there are many examples where no function has yet been assigned. Whether they are, like strangers at a funeral, peptides waiting to declare their purpose or merely functionless relics remains a secret. There are also large stretches of the prohormone sequence lying between the active peptide fragments for which no function is known.

The levels of mRNA coding for different preprohormones, which reflect the level of gene expression, are very sensitive to physiological conditions, and this type of transcriptional control is one of the main mechanisms by which peptide expression and release are regulated over the medium-to-long term. Inflammation, for example, increases the expression, and hence the release, of various cytokines by immune cells (see Ch. 15). Sensory neurons respond to peripheral inflammation by increased expression of tachykinins, which is important in the genesis of inflammatory pain (see Ch. 40).

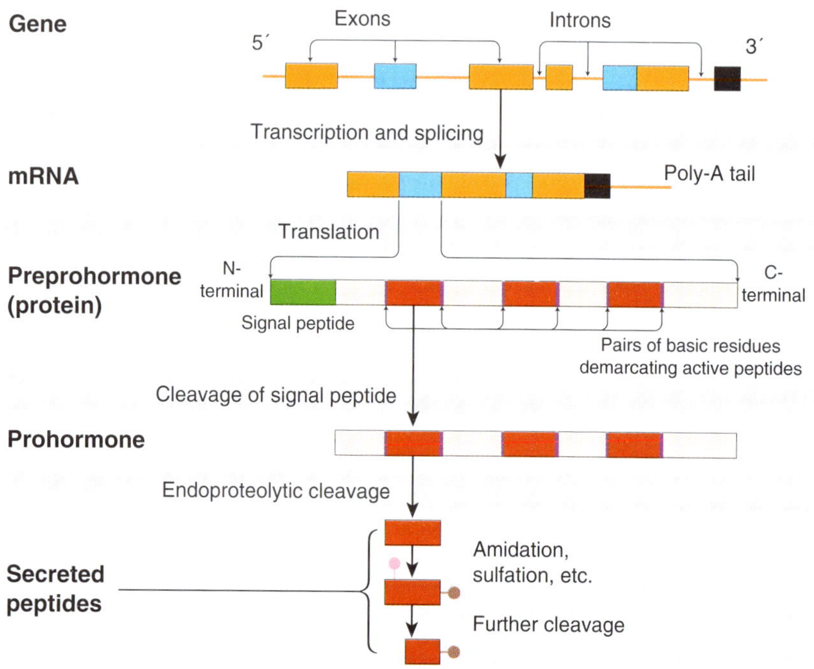

Fig. 13.3 Synthesis of a peptide mediator. The coding regions of the gene (exons) are transcribed and spliced to give rise to mRNA, segments of which (blue) are translated to produce preprohormones. Cleavage of the N-terminal signal peptide produces the prohormone, from which endopeptidases excise peptide fragments. These may be active as such or they may undergo further post-translational processing (amidation etc.).

DIVERSITY WITHIN PEPTIDE FAMILIES

▼ Peptides commonly occur in families, with sequences and actions that are basically similar. Opioid peptides (see Ch. 40) provide a good example of the representation of such a family at the genomic level. Opioid peptides, defined as peptides with opiate-like pharmacological effects, are coded by three distinct genes, whose products are, respectively, *preproopiomelanocortin* (POMC), *preproenkephalin* and *preprodynorphin*. Each of these precursors contains the sequences of a number of opioid peptides (Fig. 13.4). Hughes & Kosterlitz, who discovered the enkephalins in 1972, noticed that the sequence of metenkephalin is contained within that of a pituitary hormone, β-lipotrophin. About this time, three other peptides with morphine-like actions were discovered, α-, β- and γ-endorphin, which also were contained within stretches of the β-lipotrophin molecule. It was then found that the enkephalins actually come from the other gene products, proenkephalin and prodynorphin, POMC itself serving as a source of adrenocorticotrophic hormone (ACTH), melanocyte-stimulating hormones and β-endorphin, but not of enkephalins. The expression of the precursor proteins varies greatly in different tissues and brain areas. For example, POMC and its derived peptides are found mainly in the pituitary and hypothalamus, whereas enkephalins and their precursors are found throughout the central and peripheral nervous systems, and also in other organs such as the adrenal medulla. These peptides and precursors are restricted to individual cells, and distinct patterns of processing, leading to production of different peptides from the same precursor in different tissues and brain areas. In the brain, β-endorphin occurs mainly in neurons that project from the hypothalamus to the thalamus and brainstem, while the enkephalins are found mainly in short interneurons, in many brain areas.

In many cases, as with opioid peptides, the members of a peptide family are represented independently in the genome, but diversity can also arise by gene splicing or during post-translational processing of the prohormone.

Gene splicing as a source of peptide diversity

▼ Genes contain coding regions (*exons*) interspersed with non-coding regions (*introns*). The DNA forming the gene is initially totally transcribed to form RNA (hnRNA), which is then spliced to remove the introns, and some of the exons, forming the mRNA that is translated. Control of the splicing process allows a measure of cellular control over the peptides that are produced. The best examples of this are calcitonin/CGRP and substance P/substance K.

The calcitonin gene codes for calcitonin itself (Ch. 30) and also for a completely dissimilar peptide, CGRP. Alternative splicing allows cells to produce either procalcitonin (expressed in thyroid cells) or pro-CGRP (expressed in many neurons) from the same gene.

Substance P and neurokinin A are two closely related tachykinins belonging to the same family and are encoded on the same gene. Alternative splicing results in the production of two precursor proteins: one of these includes both peptides, the other includes only substance P. The ratio of the two varies widely between tissues, which correspondingly produce either one or both peptides. The control of the splicing process is not well understood.

Post-translational modifications as a source of peptide diversity

▼ Many peptides, such as tachykinins and peptides related to ACTH (see Ch. 27) are converted enzymically to amides, by amidation at the C-terminus, and this is important for their biological activity. Tissues may also generate peptides of varying length from the same primary sequence by the action of specific peptidases that cut the chain at different points. For example, procholecystokinin (pro-CCK) contains the sequences of at least five CCK-like peptides ranging in length from 4 to 58 amino acid residues, all with the same C-terminal sequence. CCK itself (33 residues) is the main peptide produced by the intestine, whereas the brain produces mainly CCK-8. The opioid precursor, prodynorphin, similarly gives rise to several peptides with a common terminal sequence, the proportions of which vary in different tissues and in different neurons in the brain. In some cases (e.g. the inflammatory mediator bradykinin; Ch. 15) peptide cleavage occurring after release gives rise to a new active peptide (des-Arg⁹-bradykinin), which acts on a different receptor, both peptides contributing to the inflammatory response.

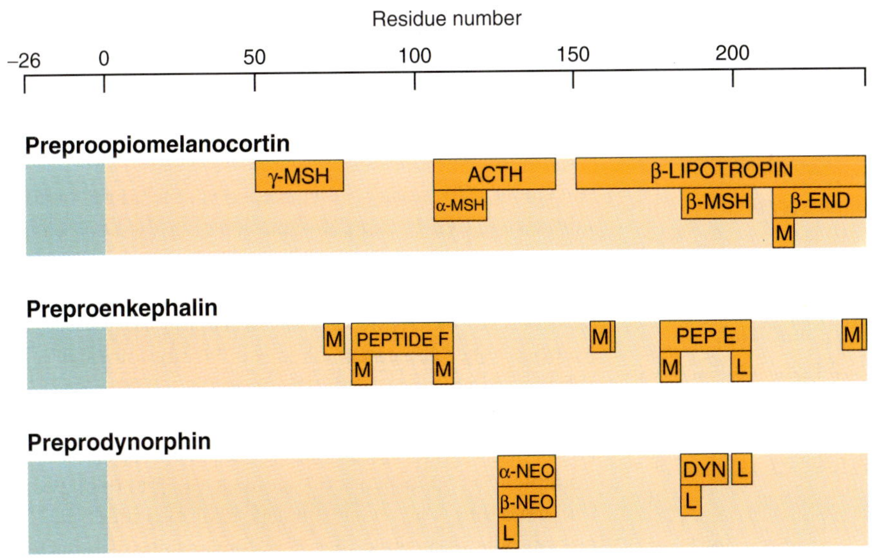

Fig. 13.4 Opioid precursors. Structures of the three opioid precursor proteins, showing the location of opioid and other peptides within the sequence. These contained peptides are bounded by pairs of basic amino acids, which form points of attack for enzymic cleavage. The signal peptide sequence is shown in green. (MSH, melanocyte-stimulating hormone; ACTH, adrenocorticotrophic hormone; β-END, β-endorphin; M, methionine enkephalin; L, leucine enkephalin; DYN, dynorphin; NEO, neoendorphin.)

PEPTIDE TRAFFICKING AND SECRETION

The basic mechanisms by which peptides are synthesised, packaged into vesicles, processed and secreted are summarised in Figure 13.2 (see review by Perone et al., 1997). Two secretory pathways exist, for constitutive and regulated secretion, respectively. Constitutively secreted proteins (e.g. plasma proteins, clotting factors*) are not stored in appreciable amounts, and secretion is controlled by the rate of synthesis. Regulated secretion is controlled mainly by intracellular calcium, as described for amine transmitters in Chapter 9, and the releasable peptides are stored in cytoplasmic vesicles. Specific protein–protein interactions appear to be responsible for the sorting of different proteins into different vesicles, and for their selective release. Though the details are not fully understood, it seems clear that peptide and protein secretion by cells utilises essentially the same mechanisms as the release of conventional neurotransmitters and hormones. Identification of the specific 'trafficking' proteins involved in particular secretory pathways should yield novel drug targets for the selective control of secretion, but the prospect is still some way off, and conventional receptor-based pharmacology will be the basis for shorter-term therapeutic developments.

Biosynthesis and release of peptides

- The genetically coded *preprohormone* is a large protein comprising a signal sequence (involved in transfer of the protein across the membrane) plus the *prohormone*, which contains the embedded sequences of one or more active peptides.
- The active peptides are produced intracellularly by selective enzymic cleavage, centred on pairs of adjacent Arg or Lys residues; in most cases the active peptides are stored (often in vesicles) in a releasable form.
- A single precursor gene may give rise to several peptides, by selective DNA splicing before transcription, by selective cleavage of the prohormone or by post-translational modification.
- There are many examples of closely related peptides, presumably produced by divergent evolution from a single gene, with different locations and physiological functions.
- Peptides and proteins are located in intracellular vesicles, which are budded off from the endoplasmic reticulum and Golgi apparatus.
- After sorting and post-translational processing of the peptide products, the vesicles differentiate into secretory vesicles, which discharge their contents by exocytosis.
- With *constitutive release* (e.g. plasma proteins, clotting factors), secretory vesicles are discharged as soon as they are formed, and secretion is continuous. With *regulated release* (neuropeptides and endocrine peptides), exocytosis is controlled by intracellular Ca^{2+}, as with release of conventional transmitters.

*Some clotting factors (e.g. factor Va, fibrinogen; see Ch. 20) are also stored in platelets and undergo regulated secretion.

PEPTIDE ANTAGONISTS

Selective antagonists are known for the great majority of non-peptide receptors. The first ones came from nature (e.g. tubocurarine, atropine, strychnine, ergot derivatives); subsequently, synthetic chemistry has succeeded in producing them in abundance. For many years, peptide antagonists (apart from opiate antagonists; Ch. 40) remained elusive, and only a few are so far in clinical use, though their therapeutic potential is considerable (see Betancur et al., 1997). Recently, though, progress has been made in what had seemed to be a rather sterile area. Substitution of unnatural amino acids, particularly D-amino acids, into the sequence of endogenous peptides sometimes produces antagonists; this was successful for substance P, angiotensin and bradykinin. For reasons discussed below, however, such peptide antagonists are of little use therapeutically, so effort has gone into discovering non-peptides that bind to peptide receptors. In a few cases, 'peptoids' have been produced by modifying the peptide backbone, while retaining as far as possible the disposition of the side-chain groups that are responsible for binding to the receptor. Such compounds have been developed as antagonists for several peptide receptors (e.g. CCK and neuropeptide Y). In other cases, random screening of large compound libraries has succeeded where rational approaches failed, resulting in highly potent and selective antagonists, some of which are in use, or under development, as therapeutic agents. The most important peptide receptor antagonists in clinical use—all of them non-peptides—are:

- **naloxone**, **naltrexone** (μ-opioid receptors): used to antagonise opiate effects (see Ch. 40)
- **losartan, valsartan, ibresartan**, etc. (angiotensin AT_1-receptors): used as antihypertensive drugs (see Ch. 18).
- **bosentan** (endothelin ET_1/ET_2-receptors).

Antagonists for many other peptides, including bradykinin, substance P, CGRP, corticotrophin-releasing factor, neuropeptide Y, neurotensin, oxytocin, antidiuretic hormone and somatostatin, have been discovered but not yet developed for clinical use. Details can be found in the Receptor and Ion Channel Nomenclature Supplement (Trends in Pharmacological Sciences, 2000), and in the review by Betancur et al. (1997).

Few, if any, agonists have been discovered by random screening, and morphine-like compounds remain the only examples of non-peptide agonists at peptide receptors. Understanding of what makes non-peptides chemically recognisable by peptide receptors remains elusive, much to the frustration of medicinal chemists who would dearly like to be able to design such compounds de novo. There remain many peptide mediators for which no antagonists are known, but strenuous efforts are being made to fill this gap in the hope of developing new therapeutic agents.

Not surprisingly, it has proved easier to find synthetic compounds that block receptors for small peptides (e.g. most neuropeptides), which have only a few points of attachment, than for large peptides and proteins (e.g. cytokines and growth factors), which interact with the receptor at many points. These receptors are not easily fooled by small molecules, and efforts to target them therapeutically rely on protein-based approaches (see below).

PROTEINS AND PEPTIDES AS DRUGS

Many proteins (about 70 in 1999), including antibodies, cytokines, enzymes, clotting factors, are registered for use as therapeutic agents in specific conditions; they are mainly given by injection but occasionally by other routes (see Table 13.1 for some examples; Bristow (1991), Buckel (1996) for further information). Many of the proteins currently in therapeutic use are functional human proteins prepared by recombinant technology,* which are used to supplement the action of endogenous mediators. Though their preparation requires advanced technology, such proteins are relatively straightforward to develop as drugs, since they rarely cause toxicity and have a more predictable therapeutic effect than synthetic drugs. The next stage will be to develop 'designer proteins'—genetically

*The use of recombinant material avoids the risk of transmitting viruses (e.g. hepatitis viruses or human immunodeficiency virus) or prion infections (particularly Creutzfeld–Jakob disease; see Ch. 34) with human-derived material. Human blood products are widely used, nonetheless.

Table 13.1 Peptides and protein as drugs

Drug	Use	Route
Peptides		
Captopril/enalapril (peptide-related)	Hypertension Heart failure (Ch. 18)	Oral
Antidiuretic hormone Desmopressin Lypressin	Diabetes insipidus (Ch. 27)	Intranasal, injection
Oxytocin	Induction of labour (Ch. 29)	Injection
GnRH analogues (e.g. buserelin)	Infertility, suppression of ovulation (Ch. 29) Prostate and breast tumours	Intranasal, injection
ACTH	Diagnosis of adrenal insufficiency (Ch. 27)	Injection
TSH/TRH	Diagnosis of thyroid disease (Ch. 28)	Injection
Calcitonin	Paget's disease of bone (Ch. 30)	Intranasal, injection
Insulin	Diabetes (Ch. 25)	Injection
Somatostatin, octreotide	Acromegaly, gastrointestinal tract tumours (Ch. 27)	Intranasal, injection
Growth hormone	Dwarfism (Ch. 27)	Injection
Ciclosporin	Immunosuppression (Ch. 16)	Oral
F(ab) fragment	Digoxin overdose	Injection
Proteins		
Streptokinase, tissue plasminogen activator	Thromboembolism (Ch. 20)	Injection
Asparaginase	Tumour chemotherapy (Ch. 15)	Injection
DNAase	Cystic fibrosis (Ch. 22)	Inhalation
Glucocerobrosidase	Gaucher's disease	Injection
Interferons	Tumour chemotherapy (Chs 16, 49) Multiple sclerosis (Ch. 34)	Injection
Erythropoietin, G-CSF, etc.	Anaemia (Ch. 21)	Injection
Clotting factors	Clotting disorders (Ch. 22)	Injection
Monoclonal antibodies, e.g. anti-TNF-α	Inflammatory diseases (Ch. 19)	Injection
Antibodies, vaccines, etc.	Infectious diseases	Injection or oral

GHRH, growth hormone-releasing hormone; TSH, thyroid-stimulating hormone; TRH, thyrotrophin-releasing hormone; ACTH, adrenocorticotrophic hormone; G-CSF, granulocyte colony-stimulating factor; TNF, tumour necrosis factor.

engineered variants of natural proteins—for specific purposes. One example is the production of fusion proteins consisting of an antibody (targeted, for example, at a tumour antigen) or a peptide (for example bombesin or somatostatin, which bind to receptors on tumour cells) linked to a toxin (such as ricin or diphtheria toxin) to kill the cells (see Ch. 50). Another example is the soluble extracellular domain of the human immunoglobulin receptor, intended to control allergic diseases by acting as a decoy to capture circulating immunoglobulins in order to prevent them from attaching to cellular receptors. Many ingenious ideas are being explored, and some prophets anticipate the dawn of a new era of therapeutics, as the dominion of small-molecule therapeutics begins to fade. Pharmacologists, needless to say, are somewhat sceptical, but nobody can afford to ignore the potential of biotechnology-based therapeutics in the future.

Smaller peptides are used therapeutically but, in general, peptides make bad drugs; there are several reasons for this.

- They cannot be given orally, either because they are hydrolysed in the gut or because they are not absorbed. Most are given by injection, some by nasal spray. (An important exception is ciclosporin, discussed in Ch. 16, which contains so many unnatural amino acids that no peptidase will touch it.)
- They are expensive to manufacture.
- They are usually quickly hydrolysed by plasma and tissue peptidases and so have a short biological half-life, though there are exceptions to this.
- They do not penetrate the blood–brain barrier.

A list of some important therapeutic proteins and peptides is given in Table 13.1 (see also Bristow, 1991; Buckel, 1996).

Peptides and proteins as drugs

- In spite of the large number of known peptide mediators, only a few peptides are, as yet, useful as drugs, most of these being close analogues of endogenous peptide mediators.
- In most cases, peptides make poor drugs, because:
  - —they are poorly absorbed when given orally
  - —they have a short duration of action because of rapid degradation in vivo
  - —they fail to cross the blood–brain barrier
  - —they are expensive to manufacture.
- Peptide antagonists were slow to be discovered, but many are now available for experimental purposes, and in development as therapeutic agents.
- Important peptide antagonists used clinically include **naloxone**, **losartan** and **bosentan**.
- Protein-based therapeutic agents are limited in number and include hormones (e.g. **insulin**, **growth hormone**), clotting factors, cytokines, antibodies and enzymes. In many cases, recombinant technology is used to produce them.
- 'Designer proteins' prepared by recombinant methods are expected to play an increasing therapeutic role in the future.

CONCLUDING REMARKS

The physiology and pharmacology of peptides—particularly neuropeptides—has stimulated a large amount of research since the early 1980s, and the flow of data continues unabated. With more than a dozen major families of peptides, and a host of minor players, it is beyond the scope of this book to cover them individually or in detail. Instead, we will introduce information on peptide pharmacology wherever it has relevance to the physiology and pharmacology under discussion (e.g. bradykinin in inflammation (Ch. 15), endothelins and angiotensin in cardiovascular regulation (Ch. 18), tachykinins in asthma (Ch. 22), tachykinins and opioid peptides in nociception (Ch. 40), leptin, neuropeptide Y and orexins in obesity (Ch. 26)). Useful general accounts of peptide pharmacology include Sherman et al. (1989), Hökfelt et al. (1991, 2000), Cooper et al. (1996) and Nestler et al., 2001).

REFERENCES AND FURTHER READING

Betancur C, Azzi M, Rostene W 1997 Nonpeptide antagonists of neuropeptide receptors. Trends Pharmacol Sci 18: 372–386 (*Describes success in finding non-peptide antagonists—for long elusive—and their possible therapeutic uses*)

Bristow A F 1991 The current status of therapeutic peptides and proteins. In: Hider R C, Barlow D (eds) Polypeptide and protein drugs. Ellis Horwood, Chichester (*Review article*)

Buckel P 1996 Recombinant proteins for therapy. Trends Pharmacol Sci 17: 450–456 (*Good account of therapeutic proteins*)

Civelli O, Nothacker H-P, Saito Y, Wang Z, Lin S H S, Reinsceid R K 2001 Novel neurotransmitters as natural ligands of orphan G-protein-coupled receptors. Trends Neurosci 24: 230–237 (*Describes how new peptide mediators have been discovered by screening orphan receptors*)

Cooper J R, Bloom F E, Roth R H 1996 Biochemical basis of neuropharmacology. Oxford University Press, New York (*Excellent standard textbook*)

Cullinan W E, Day N C, Schafer M K et al. 1991 Neuroanatomical and functional studies of peptide precursor-processing enzymes. Enzyme 45: 285–300 (*Review of enzyme mechanisms involved in neuropeptide processing*)

Hökfelt T 1991 Neuropeptides in perspective: the last ten years. Neuron 7: 867–879 (*Excellent overview by a neuropeptide pioneer*)

Hökfelt T Broberger C, Xu Z-Q D, Sergeyev V, Ubink R, Diez M 2000 Neuropeptides—an overview. Neuropharmacology 39: 1337–1356 (*Excellent summary of recent developments*)

Lundberg J M 1996 Pharmacology of co-transmission in the autonomic nervous system: integrative aspects on amines, neuropeptides, adenosine triphosphate, amino acids and nitric oxide. Pharmacol Rev 48: 114–192

Meunier J-C, Mollereau C, Toll L et al. 1995 Isolation and structure of the endogenous agonist of opioid receptor-like ORL_1 receptor. Nature 377: 532–535 (*Describes a new opioid-like peptide—a ligand for a hitherto 'orphan' receptor*)

Nestler E J, Hyman S E, Malenka R C 2001 Molecular neuropharmacology. McGraw-Hill, New York (*Good modern textbook*)
Okuda-Ashitaka E, Ito S 2000 Nocistatin: a novel neuropeptide encoded by the gene for the nociceptin/orphanin FQ precursos. Peptides 21: 1101–1109
Perone M J, Windeatt S, Castro M G 1997 Intracellular trafficking of prohormones and proneuropeptides: cell type-specific sorting and targeting. Exp Physiol 82: 609–628 (*Excellent review of mechanisms by which cells manage to avoid getting their many neuropeptides mixed up*)
Receptor and ion channel nomenclature supplement. Trend Pharmcol Sci 2000
Sherman T G, Akil H, Watson S J 1989 The molecular biology of neuropeptides. Disc Neurosci 6: 1–58 (*General review*)
Yanagisawa M, Kurihara H, Kimura S et al. 1988 A novel potent vasoconstrictor peptide produced by vascular endothelial cells. Nature 332: 411–415 (*The discovery of endothelin—a remarkable tour de force*)

14 Nitric oxide

Overview 208

Introduction 208

Biosynthesis of nitric oxide and its control 209

Degradation and carriage of nitric oxide 210

Effects of nitric oxide 212

Therapeutic approaches 213
- Nitric oxide 213
- Nitric oxide donors 213
- Inhibition of nitric oxide synthesis 213
- Potentiation of nitric oxide 214

Clinical conditions in which nitric oxide may play a part 214

OVERVIEW

The physiological role of nitric oxide (NO) is a relatively recent and rapidly expanding field. NO is a powerful modulator of many aspects of bodily function. It is generated by action of an enzyme, nitric oxide synthase, that occurs in an endothelial, a neuronal and an inducible isoform. In this chapter, we concentrate on general aspects of NO, especially its biosynthesis and its pharmacological control. We also touch on clinical conditions where disordered biosynthesis of NO is believed to play a part as a basis for a brief consideration of possible therapeutic uses of drugs that potentiate or donate NO, and of inhibitors of NO synthesis.

INTRODUCTION

Nitric oxide (NO), a free radical gas, is formed in the atmosphere during lightning storms. Less dramatically, but with far-reaching biological consequences, it is also formed in an enzyme-catalysed reaction between molecular oxygen and L-arginine. The convergence of several lines of research led to the realisation that NO is a key signalling molecule in the cardiovascular and nervous systems, and that it has a role in host defence.

A physiological function of NO was discovered in the vasculature when it was shown that the endothelium-derived relaxing factor described by Furchgott & Zawadzki in 1980 (Fig. 14.1) is accounted for by the formation of NO by endothelial cells (Fig 14.2). NO is the endogenous activator of soluble guanylate cyclase, leading to the formation of cyclic GMP (cGMP), which functions as a second messenger in many cells including nerves, smooth muscle, monocytes and platelets (Ch. 3). Nitrogen and oxygen are neighbours in the periodic table, and NO shares several properties with O_2, in particular a high affinity for haem and other iron–sulfur groups. This is important for activation of guanylate cyclase, which contains a haem group, and for the inactivation of NO by haemoglobin.

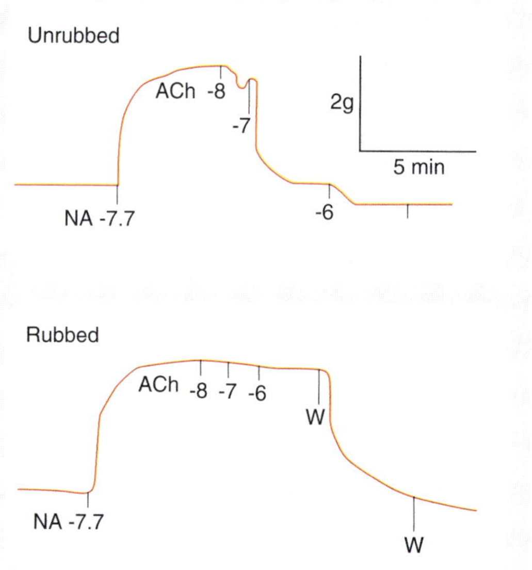

Fig. 14.1 Endothelium-derived relaxing factor (EDRF). Acetylcholine (ACh) relaxes a strip of rabbit aorta precontracted with noradrenaline (NA) if the endothelium is intact ('unrubbed': upper panel), but not if it has been removed by gentle rubbing ('rubbed': lower panel). The numbers are logarithms of molar concentrations of drugs. (From: Furchgott R F, Zawadzki J V 1980.)

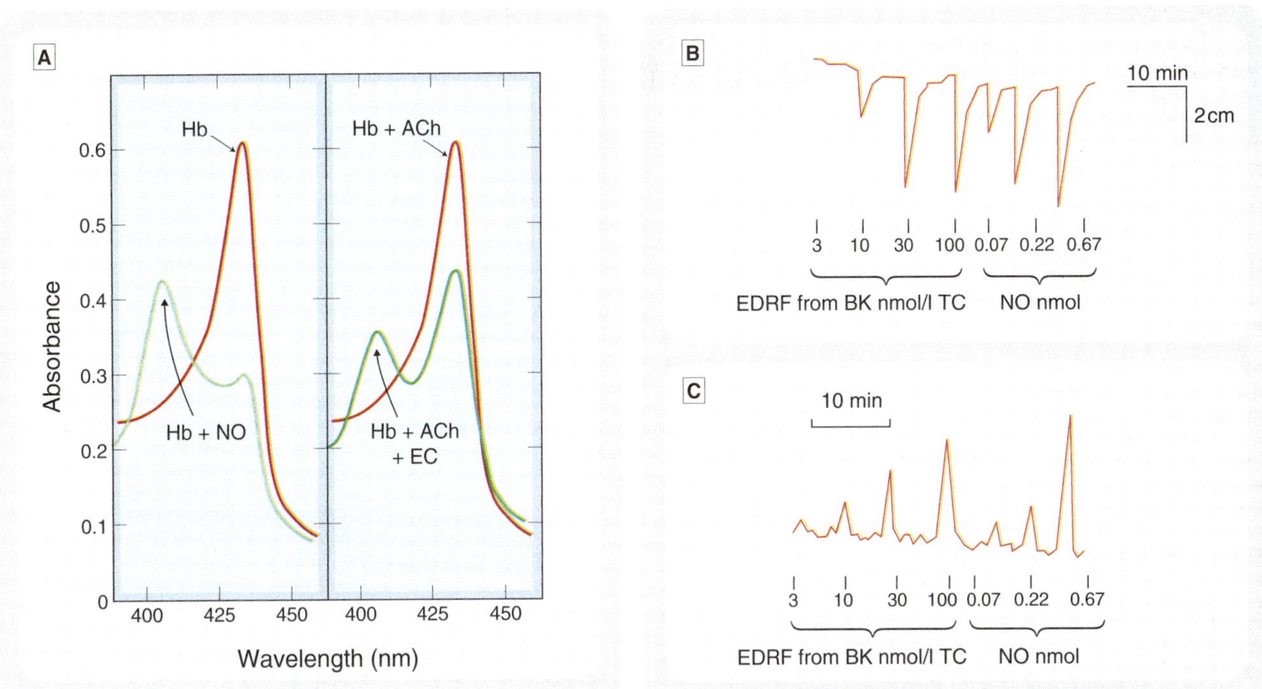

Fig. 14.2 Endothelium-derived relaxing factor (EDRF) is closely related to nitric oxide (NO). A EDRF released from aortic endothelial cells (EC) by acetylcholine (ACh) (right hand panel) has the same effect on the absorption spectrum of deoxyhaemoglobin (Hb) as does authentic NO (left panel). B EDRF is released from a column of cultured endothelial cells by bradykinin (BK 3–100 nmol) applied through the column of cells (TC) and relaxes a de-endothelialised precontracted bioassay strip, as does authentic NO (upper trace). C A chemical assay of NO based on chemiluminescence shows that similar concentrations of NO are present in the EDRF released from the column of cells as in equiactive authentic NO solutions. (From: (A) Ignarro et al. 1987 Circ Res 61: 866–879; (B,C) Palmer et al. 1987 Nature 327: 524–526.)

The role of NO in specific settings is described in other chapters: the endothelium in Chapter 18, the autonomic nervous system in Chapter 9, as a chemical transmitter and mediator of excitotoxicity in the central nervous system (CNS) in Chapters 31–34, and in the innate mediator-derived reactions of acute inflammation and the immune response in Chapter 15. Therapeutic uses of organic nitrates and of nitroprusside (NO donors) are described in Chapters 17 and 18.

BIOSYNTHESIS OF NITRIC OXIDE AND ITS CONTROL

NO synthase (NOS) enzymes are central to the control of NO biosynthesis. There are three known isoforms of NOS: an inducible form (iNOS or NOS-II: expressed in macrophages and Kupffer cells, neutrophils, fibroblasts, vascular smooth muscle and endothelial cells in response to pathological stimuli such as invading microorganisms) and two so-called 'constitutive' forms, which are present under physiological conditions in endothelium (eNOS or NOS-III) and in neurons (nNOS or NOS-I). eNOS is not restricted to endothelium. It is also present in cardiac myocytes, renal mesangial cells, osteoblasts and osteoclasts and, in small amounts, in platelets. The constitutive enzymes generate small amounts of NO, whereas the activity of iNOS is approximately a thousand times greater.

All three NOS isoenzymes are dimers. They are structurally and functionally complex, bearing similarities to the cytochrome P450 enzymes (described in Ch. 8) that are so important in drug metabolism. Each isoform contains iron protoporphyrin IX (haem), flavin adenine dinucleotide (FAD), flavin mononucleotide (FMN) and tetrahydrobiopterin as bound prosthetic groups. They also contain binding sites for L-arginine, reduced nicotinamide adenine dinucleotide phosphate (NADPH) and calcium–calmodulin. These prosthetic groups and ligands control the assembly of the enzyme into the active dimer. eNOS is dually acylated by N-myristoylation and cysteine palmitoylation, post-translational modifications that lead to its association with membranes in the Golgi apparatus and in **caveolae**: specialised microdomains in the plasma membrane derived from the Golgi apparatus. In the caveolae, eNOS is associated with *caveolin*, a transmembrane protein involved in signal transduction. Association of eNOS with caveolin is reversible, dissociation from caveolin activating the enzyme.

nNOS and iNOS are soluble rather than membrane-associated enzymes.

The nitrogen atom in NO is derived from the terminal guanidino group of L-arginine. Details of the reaction mechanism are controversial, but it is known that NOS enzymes are functionally 'bimodal' in that they combine oxygenase and reductase activities associated with distinct structural domains. The oxygenase domain contains haem, while the reductase domain binds calcium–calmodulin, FMN, FAD and NADPH. By analogy with cytochrome P450, it is believed that the flavins accept electrons from NADPH and transfer them to the haem iron, which binds oxygen and catalyses the stepwise oxidation of L-arginine to NO and citrulline. In pathological states, electron transfer between substrates, enzyme cofactors and products can become 'uncoupled', associated with structural change in the enzyme; electron transfer to molecular oxygen leads to the synthesis of superoxide anion rather than NO.

L-Arginine is usually present in excess in endothelial cell cytoplasm, so the rate of production of NO is determined by the activity of the enzyme rather than by substrate availability. Nevertheless, very high doses of L-arginine can restore endothelial NO biosynthesis in some pathological states (e.g. hypercholesterolaemia; see below) in which endothelial function is impaired. Possible explanations for this paradox include:

- compartmentation: i.e. existence of a distinct pool of substrate in a cell compartment with access to the synthase enzyme, which can become depleted despite apparently plentiful total cytoplasmic arginine concentrations
- competition with endogenous inhibitors of NOS such as asymmetric dimethylarginine (ADMA; see below), which might be increased in hypercholesterolaemia
- reassembly/reactivation of enzyme in which transfer of electrons has become uncoupled from L-arginine.

The activity of constitutive isoforms of NOS is controlled by intracellular calcium–calmodulin (Fig. 14.3). Control is exerted in two ways:

- many endothelium-dependent agonists (e.g. acetylcholine, bradykinin, substance P) increase the cytoplasmic concentration of calcium ions, $[Ca^{2+}]_i$; the consequent increase in calcium–calmodulin activates eNOS or nNOS
- phosphorylation of specific residues on eNOS renders it more active at a given concentration of calcium–calmodulin. This can increase NO synthesis in the absence of any change in $[Ca^{2+}]_i$.

The main physiological stimulus controlling endothelial NO synthesis in resistance vessels is probably *shear stress*. This is sensed by endothelial mechanoreceptors and transduced via a serine–threonine protein kinase called *Akt* or *protein kinase B*. Agonists that increase cAMP in endothelial cells (e.g. β_2-agonists) also influence the phosphorylation of eNOS,* as does insulin (via tyrosine kinase activation).

*The β_2-agonists, which have endothelium-dependent as well as endothelium-independent relaxing effects, probably work partly in this way.

In contrast to constitutive NOS isoforms, the activity of iNOS is independent of $[Ca^{2+}]_i$. Though iNOS contains a binding site for calcium–calmodulin, the very high affinity of this site for its ligand means that iNOS is activated even at the low values of $[Ca^{2+}]_i$ present under resting conditions. The enzyme is induced by bacterial lipopolysaccharide (LPS) and/or cytokines synthesised in response to LPS, notably interferon γ the antiviral effect of which can be explained by this action. Tumour necrosis factor-α and interleukin-1 are not effective in inducing iNOS in their own right, but they each synergise with interferon γ in this regard (see Ch. 15). Induction of iNOS is inhibited by glucocorticoids and by several cytokines, including transforming growth factor-β. There are important species differences in the inducibility of iNOS, which, despite the importance of iNOS in humans, is less readily induced in humans than in mouse cells.

DEGRADATION AND CARRIAGE OF NITRIC OXIDE

NO reacts with oxygen to form N_2O_4, which combines with water to produce a mixture of nitric and nitrous acids. Nitrite ions are oxidised to nitrate by oxyhaemoglobin. These reactions are summarised:

$$2NO + O_2 \rightarrow N_2O_4 \quad (14.1)$$
$$N_2O_4 + H_2O \rightarrow NO_3^- + NO_2^- + 2H^+ \quad (14.2)$$
$$NO_2^- + HbO \rightarrow NO_3^- + Hb \quad (14.3)$$

Nitric oxide: synthesis, inactivation and carriage

- NO is synthesised from L-arginine and molecular O_2 by NO synthase (NOS).
- NOS exists in three isoforms: inducible, and constitutive endothelial and neuronal forms (respectively iNOS, eNOS and nNOS). NOSs are dimeric flavoproteins, contain tetrahydrobiopterin and have homology with cytochrome P450. The constitutive enzymes are activated by Ca^{2+}–calmodulin. Sensitivity to Ca^{2+}–calmodulin is controlled by phosphorylation of specific sites on the enzymes.
- iNOS is induced in macrophages and other cells by interferon-γ.
- nNOS is present in the CNS (see Chs 31–34) and in NANC nerves (see Ch. 9).
- eNOS is present in platelets and other cells in addition to endothelium.
- NO is unstable but can form more stable nitrosothiols, particularly with a cysteine residue in globin; as a result red cells can act as a kind of NO buffer. NO is inactivated by combination with the haem of haemoglobin or by oxidation to nitrite and nitrate, which are excreted in urine.

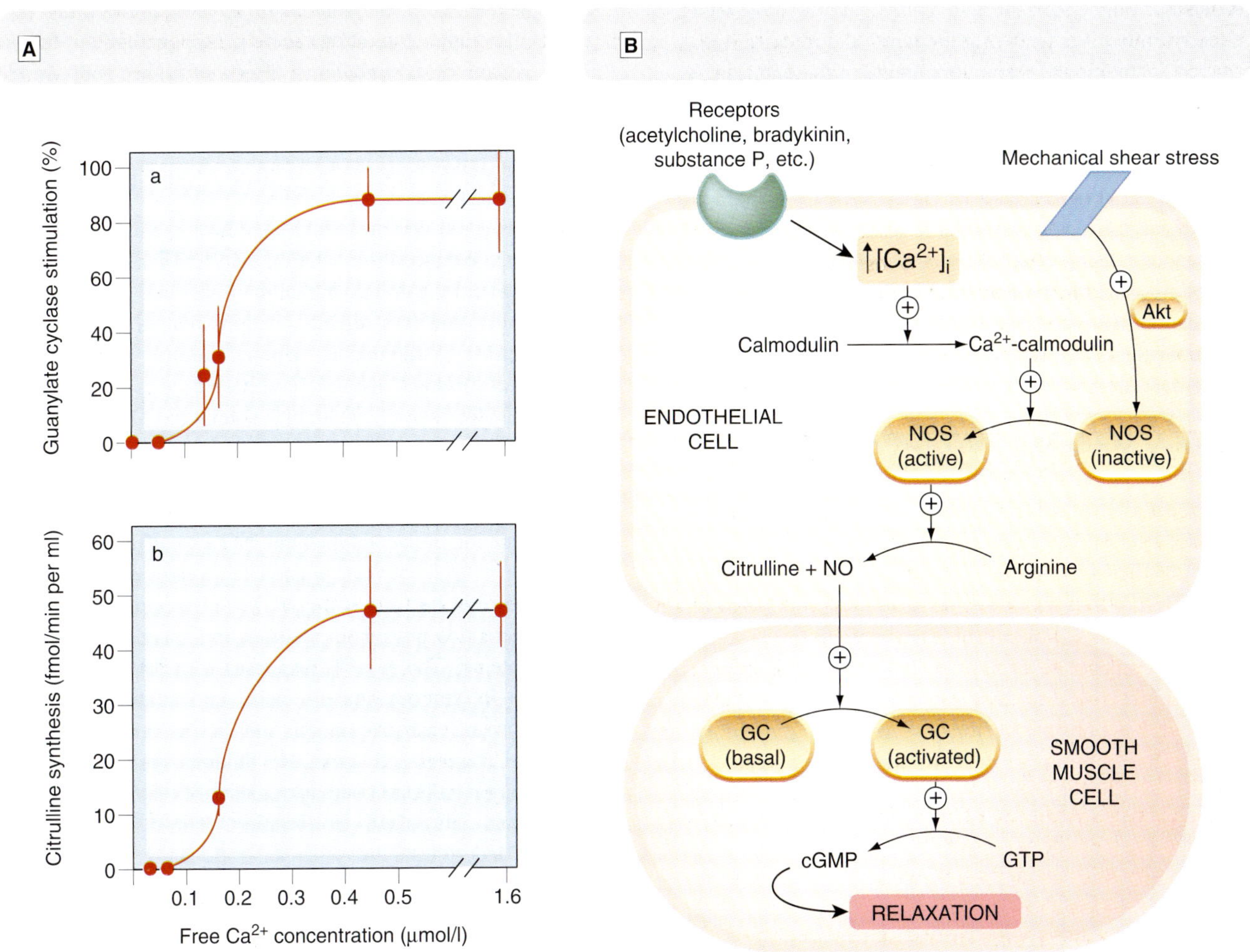

Fig. 14.3 Control of constitutive nitric oxide synthase (NOS) by Ca^{2+}–calmodulin. A Dependence on Ca^{2+} of nitric oxide (NO) and citrulline synthesis from L-arginine by rat brain synaptosomal cytosol. Rates of synthesis of NO from L-arginine were determined by stimulation of guanylate cyclase (GC) (a) or by synthesis of [^{3}H]-citrulline from L-[^{3}H]-arginine (b). B Regulation of GC in smooth muscle by NO formed in adjacent endothelium. Akt is a protein kinase that phosphorylates NOS, making it more sensitive to Ca^{2+}–calmodulin. (From: (A) Knowles R G et al. 1989 Proc Natl Acad Sci USA 86: 5159–5162.)

Low concentrations of NO are relatively stable in air because equation 14.1 is a second-order reaction. Consequently, small amounts of NO produced in the lung escape degradation and can be detected in exhaled air. In contrast, NO reacts very rapidly with even low concentrations of superoxide anion (O_2^-) to produce peroxynitrite anion ($ONOO^-$), which is responsible for some of its toxic effects.

Endothelium-derived NO acts locally on underlying vascular smooth muscle or on adherent monocytes or platelets. The potential for action at a distance is neatly demonstrated by *Rhodnius prolixus*, a blood-sucking insect that produces a salivary vasodilator/platelet inhibitor with the properties of a nitrovasodilator. This consists of a mixture of nitrosylated haemoproteins, which bind NO in the salivary glands of the insect but release it in the tissues of its prey. The consequent vasodilatation and inhibition of platelet activation presumably facilitates extraction of the bug's meal in liquid form.

Haem has an affinity for NO > 10 000 times greater than for oxygen. In the absence of oxygen, NO bound to haem is relatively stable but in the presence of oxygen, NO is converted to nitrate and the haem iron oxidised to methaemoglobin. Distinct from this inactivation reaction, evidence is accumulating that the globin part of haemoglobin carries NO under normal physiological conditions, optimising oxygen delivery in the periphery and contributing to the control of respiration. NO binds *reversibly* to a specific cysteine residue in globin. The resulting S-nitrosylated haemoglobin is believed to be involved in various NO-related activities including the control of vascular resistance, blood pressure and respiration. This is still controversial, particularly as regards quantitative aspects, but key features include:

- nitrosylation of haemoglobin is reversible
- it depends on the state (R or T) of the haemoglobin, which consequently takes up NO in the lungs and releases it in tissues, including the respiratory centre in the brain, in concert with release of oxygen
- NO is released not into the cytoplasm of erythrocytes (where it would be promptly hoovered up by haem) but is transported out of the red cells via cysteine residues in the haemoglobin-binding cytoplasmic domain of an anion exchanger called AE1. (AE1 is responsible for the exchange of chloride and bicarbonate ions across the cell membrane, the 'Hamburger shift' beloved of red cell physiologists. It is the most abundant protein in red cell membranes.)

EFFECTS OF NITRIC OXIDE

Some physiological and pathological effects of NO are shown in Table 14.1. NO activates guanylate cyclase by combining with its haem group, and the physiological effects of low concentrations of NO produced under normal conditions by the constitutive enzymes are mediated by cGMP. These effects are prevented by inhibitors of guanylate cyclase (e.g. **ODQ**), which are useful investigational tools in this regard. Effects of cGMP are terminated by phosphodiesterase enzymes. **Zaprinast** and **sildenafil** are inhibitors of phosphodiesterase type V, and sildenafil is used to treat erectile dysfunction because it potentiates NO actions in the corpora cavernosa by this mechanism (see Ch. 29). NO also combines with haem groups in other biologically important proteins (e.g. cytochrome *c* oxidase, where it may compete with oxygen, thus contributing to the control of cellular respiration), thereby influencing their function. Cytotoxic and/or cytoprotective effects of higher concentrations of NO relate to its chemistry as a free radical (see Ch. 34).

BIOCHEMICAL AND CELLULAR ASPECTS

Pharmacological effects of NO have been studied with NO gas dissolved in balanced salt solution that has first been thoroughly deoxygenated by gassing with an inert gas such as helium. More conveniently, but less directly, various donors of NO such as **nitroprusside**, ***S*-nitroso-acetylpenicillamine** ('SNAP') or ***S*-nitrosoglutathione** ('SNOG') have been used as surrogates. This has pitfalls: for example, vitamin C potentiates SNAP but inhibits responses to authentic NO.*

NO can activate guanylate cyclase in the same cells that produce it, giving rise to *autocrine* effects, for example on the barrier function of the endothelium. NO also diffuses from its site of synthesis and activates guanylate cyclase in neighbouring cells. The resulting increase in cGMP affects protein kinase G, cyclic nucleotide phosphodiesterases, ion channels and possibly other proteins. The $[Ca^{2+}]_i$ responses to various agonists are inhibited in smooth muscle cells and platelets. NO also hyperpolarises vascular smooth muscle, as a consequence of potassium channel activation. NO inhibits monocyte adhesion and migration, adhesion and aggregation of platelets and smooth muscle and fibroblast proliferation. These cellular effects probably underlie the anti-atherosclerotic action of NO (see Ch. 19).

Large amounts of NO (released following induction of NOS or excessive stimulation of NMDA (*N*-methyl-D-aspartate) receptors in the brain) cause cytotoxic effects (either directly or

*Vitamin C increases the rate of NO release from SNAP but accelerates NO degradation in solution, which could explain this divergence.

Table 14.1 Postulated roles of endogenous nitric oxide

System	Physiological role	Pathological role: Excess production	Pathological role: Inadequate production or action
Cardiovascular			
Endothelium/vascular smooth muscle	Control of blood pressure and regional blood flow	Hypotension (septic shock)	Atherogenesis, thrombosis, (e.g. in hypercholesterolaemia, diabetes mellitus)
Platelets	Limitation of adhesion/aggregation		
Host defence			
Macrophages, neutrophils, leucocytes	Defence against viruses, bacteria, fungi, protozoa, parasites		
Nervous system			
Central	Neurotransmission; long-term potentiation; plasticity (memory, appetite, nociception)	Excitotoxicity (Ch. 34) (e.g. ischaemic stroke, Huntington's disease, AIDS dementia)	
Peripheral	Neurotransmission (e.g. gastric empyting, penile erection)	–	Hypertrophic pyloric stenosis, erectile dysfunction

via peroxynitrite anions). These contribute to host defence, but also to the neuronal destruction that occurs when there is overstimulation of NMDA receptors by glutamate (see Chs 31 and 34). Paradoxically, NO is also cytoprotective under some circumstances (see Ch. 34).

VASCULAR EFFECTS (see also Ch. 18)

The endothelial L-arginine/NO pathway is tonically active in resistance vessels, reducing peripheral vascular resistance and hence systemic blood pressure. Mutant mice that lack the gene coding for eNOS are hypertensive, consistent with a role for NO biosynthesis in the physiological control of blood pressure. Increased endothelial NO generation may contribute to the generalised vasodilatation that occurs during pregnancy.

NEURONAL EFFECTS (see Chs 9 and 33)

NO is a non-noradrenergic non-cholinergic (NANC) neurotransmitter in many tissues (Ch. 9) and is important in the upper airways, gastrointestinal tract and control of penile erection (Chs 22, 24 and 29). It is implicated in the control of neuronal development and of synaptic plasticity in the CNS (Chs 31 and 33). Mice carrying a mutation disrupting the gene coding nNOS have grossly distended stomachs similar to human hypertrophic pyloric stenosis (a disorder characterised by pyloric hypertrophy causing gastric outflow obstruction, which occurs in approximately 1 in 150 male infants and is corrected surgically). nNOS knockout mice resist stroke damage caused by middle cerebral artery ligation but are aggressive and oversexed (characteristics that may not be unambiguously disadvantageous, at least in the context of natural selection!).

Actions of nitric oxide

- NO acts by:
  - —combining with haem in guanylate cyclase, activating the enzyme , increasing cGMP and thereby lowering $[Ca^{2+}]_i$
  - —combining with haem groups in other proteins (e.g. cytochrome *c* oxidase)
  - —combining with superoxide anion to yield the cytotoxic peroxynitrite anion
  - —nitrosation of proteins, lipids and nucleic acids.
- Effects of NO include:
  - —vasodilatation; inhibition of platelet and monocyte adhesion and aggregation; inhibition of smooth muscle proliferation; protection against atherogenesis
  - —synaptic effects in the peripheral and CNS (see Chs 9 and 31–34)
  - —host defence and cytotoxic effects on pathogens (see Ch.15)
  - —cytoprotection.

HOST DEFENCE (see Ch. 15)

Cytotoxic and/or cytostatic effects of NO are implicated in primitive non-specific host defence mechanisms against numerous pathogens, including bacteria, fungi, protozoa and parasites, and against tumour cells. The importance of this is evidenced by susceptibility to *Leishmania major* (to which wild-type mice are highly resistant) of mice lacking iNOS. Mechanisms whereby NO damages invading pathogens include nitrosylation of nucleic acids and combination with haem-containing enzymes, such as the mitochondrial enzymes involved in cell respiration.

THERAPEUTIC APPROACHES

NITRIC OXIDE

Inhalation of high concentrations of NO (as occurred when cylinders of nitrous oxide, N_2O, for anaesthesia were accidentally contaminated) causes acute pulmonary oedema and methaemoglobinaemia, but concentrations below 50 ppm (parts per million) are not toxic. NO (5–300 ppm) inhibits bronchoconstriction (at least in guinea-pigs), but the main action of inhaled NO is pulmonary vasodilatation. Two distinctive features make this action potentially important therapeutically. First, effects are most marked in the pulmonary circulation. Second, since NO is administered in inspired air it acts preferentially on ventilated alveoli. Inhaled NO could, therefore, be therapeutically useful in respiratory distress syndrome. This has a high mortality and is caused by diverse insults, of which infection is the most common in adults. It is characterised by intrapulmonary 'shunting' (i.e. pulmonary arterial blood entering the pulmonary vein without passing through capillaries in contact with ventilated alveoli), resulting in arterial hypoxaemia, and by acute pulmonary arterial hypertension. Inhaled NO dilates blood vessels in ventilated alveoli (which are exposed to the inspired gas) and thus reduces shunting. NO is used in intensive care units to reduce pulmonary hypertension and to improve oxygen delivery in patients with respiratory distress syndrome, but it is not known whether this improves long-term survival in these severely ill patients.

NITRIC OXIDE DONORS

Nitrovasodilators have been used therapeutically for over a century. The common mode of action of these drugs is as a source of NO (Chs 17 and 18). There is interest in the potential for selectivity of nitrovasodilators: for instance, glyceryl trinitrate is more potent on vascular smooth muscle than on platelets whereas *S*-nitrosoglutathione selectively inhibits platelet function.

INHIBITION OF NITRIC OXIDE SYNTHESIS

Drugs can inhibit NO synthesis or action by several mechanisms. Currently, the most useful drugs are arginine analogues, which compete with arginine for NOS and in some cases also compete for the carrier that transports arginine into endothelial cells. Several such compounds, e.g. N^G-monomethyl-L-arginine (L-NMMA) and N^G-nitro-L-arginine methyl ester (L-NAME), have proved of great value as experimental tools. One such compound, ADMA, is present in human urine and its plasma concentration has recently been found to correlate strongly with vascular mortality in patients receiving haemodialysis for chronic renal failure. Consequently, it appears likely that ADMA can influence the L-arginine/NO pathway under pathological conditions in vivo and there is considerable interest in the hydrolase enzymes that metabolise endogenous ADMA.

Infusion of L-NMMA into the brachial artery causes vasoconstriction (Fig. 14.4), owing to inhibition of the basal production of NO, without influencing blood pressure or causing other systemic effects, whereas intravenous L-NMMA increases blood pressure and causes vasoconstriction in renal, mesenteric, cerebral and striated muscle resistance vessels.

There is interest in selective inhibitors of different isoforms of NOS, although high (>100-fold) selectivity has yet to be achieved. *N*-Iminoethyl-L-lysine is a selective inhibitor of iNOS. 7-Nitroindazole inhibits mouse cerebellar NOS and, following intraperitoneal administration, inhibits nociception without altering arterial blood pressure; this selectivity apparently results from an incompletely understood pharmacokinetic effect related to access of the drug to NOS in brain.

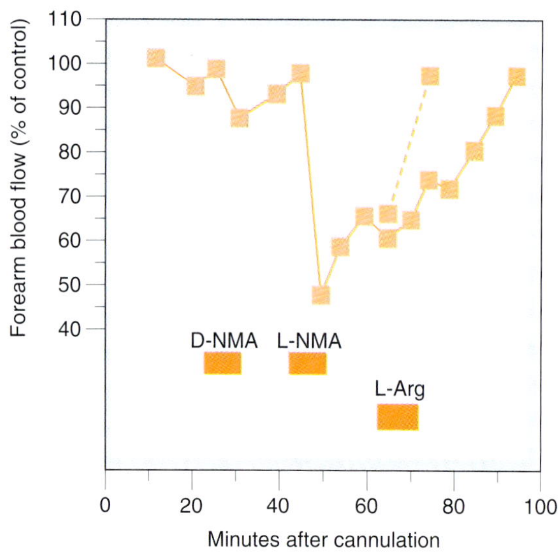

Fig. 14.4 Basal blood flow in the human forearm is influenced by nitric oxide (NO) biosynthesis. Forearm blood flow is expressed as a percentage of the flow in the non-cannulated control arm (which does not change). Brachial artery infusion of the D-isomer of the arginine analogue N^G-monomethyl-L-arginine (D-NMA) has no effect, while the L-isomer (L-NMA) causes vasoconstriction. L-Arginine (L-Arg) accelerates recovery from such vasoconstriction (dashed line). (From: Vallance et al. 1989 Lancet ii: 997–1000.)

Inhibition of the L-arginine/nitric oxide pathway

- Glucocorticoids inhibit biosynthesis of inducible (but not constitutive) nitric oxide synthase (NOS).
- Synthetic arginine analogues (e.g. L-NMMA, L-NAME; see text) compete with arginine and are useful experimental tools.
- Endogenous NOS inhibitors include ADMA (see text) and PIN (a protein which inhibits NOS dimerisation).
- Isoform selective inhibitors are being sought and have therapeutic potential.

An endogenous protein inhibitor of nNOS (termed 'PIN') works by an entirely different mechanism, namely destabilising the NOS dimer.

POTENTIATION OF NITRIC OXIDE

Several means whereby the L-arginine/NO pathway could be enhanced are under investigation. Some of these rely on existing drugs of proven value in other contexts. The hope (as yet unproven) is that by potentiating NO they will prevent atherosclerosis or its thrombotic complications or have other beneficial effects attributed to NO. Possibilities include:

- selective NO donors as 'replacement' therapy (see above)
- dietary supplementation with L-arginine (see above)
- antioxidants (to reduce superoxide anion formation and hence stabilise NO; Ch. 19)
- drugs that restore endothelial function in patients with metabolic risk factors for vascular disease (e.g. angiotensin-converting enzyme inhibitors, statins, insulin, oestrogens Chs 18, 19, 25 and 29)
- β_2-adrenoceptor agonists and related drugs (e.g. nebivolol, a β_1-adrenoceptor antagonist that is metabolised to an active metabolite that activates the L-arginine/NO pathway)
- sildenafil (see above and Ch. 29).

CLINICAL CONDITIONS IN WHICH NITRIC OXIDE MAY PLAY A PART

The wide distribution of NOS enzymes and diverse actions of NO suggest that abnormalities in the L-arginine/NO pathway could be involved in several clinical disorders. Either increased or reduced production could play a part in disease, and hypotheses abound. Evidence is harder to come by but has been sought using various indirect approaches including:

- analysing nitrate and/or cGMP in urine: these are bedeviled, respectively, by dietary nitrate and by membrane-bound guanylate cyclase (which is stimulated by natriuretic peptides, see Ch. 17)

- a considerable refinement is to administer [^{15}N]-arginine and use mass spectrometry to measure the enrichment of ^{15}N over naturally abundant [^{14}N]-nitrate in urine
- measuring effects of NOS inhibitors (e.g. L-NMMA)
- comparing responses to endothelium-dependent agonists (e.g. acetylcholine) and endothelium-independent agonists (e.g. nitroprusside)
- measuring responses to increased blood flow ('flow-mediated dilatation'), which are largely mediated by NO
- studying histochemical appearances and pharmacological responses in vitro of tissue obtained at operation (e.g. coronary artery surgery).

All these methods have limitations, and the dust is far from settled. Nevertheless, it seems clear that the L-arginine/NO pathway is indeed a player in the pathogenesis of several important diseases, opening the way to new therapeutic approaches. Some pathological roles of excessive or reduced NO production are summarised in Table 14.1. We touch only briefly on these clinical conditions and would caution the reader that not all of these exciting possibilities are likely to withstand the test of time!

Sepsis can cause multiple organ failure. Whereas NO benefits host defence by killing invading organisms, excessive NO production can cause harmful hypotension. Disappointingly, however, L-NMMA worsend survival in one controlled clinical trial. Chronic low-grade endotoxaemia occurs in patients with hepatic cirrhosis. Systemic vasodilatation is typical in such patients. Urinary excretion of cGMP is increased, and vasodilatation may be a consequence of induction of NOS leading to increased NO synthesis.

There is suggestive evidence that NO biosynthesis is reduced in patients with *hypercholesterolaemia* and some other disorders that predispose to atheromatous vascular disease, including cigarette smoking and *diabetes mellitus*. In hypercholesterolaemia, evidence of blunted NO release in forearm and coronary vascular beds is supported by evidence that this can be corrected by lowering plasma cholesterol (with a statin, see Ch. 19) or by supplementation with L-arginine.

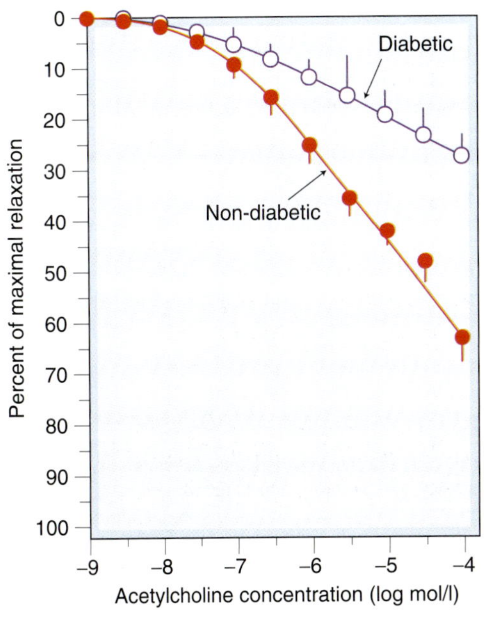

Fig. 14.5 Impaired endothelium-mediated relaxation of penile smooth muscle from diabetic men with erectile dysfunction. Mean (± SE) relaxation responses to acetylcholine in corpora cavernosa tissue (obtained at the time of performing surgical implants to treat impotence) from 16 diabetic men and 22 non-diabetics. (Data from: Saenz de Tejada et al. 1989 N Engl J Med 320: 1025–1030.)

Nitric oxide in pathophysiology

- NO is synthesised under physiological and pathological circumstances.
- Either reduced or increased NO production can contribute to disease processes.
- Underproduction of neuronal NO is reported in babies with hypertrophic pyloric stenosis. Endothelial NO production is reduced in patients with hypercholesterolaemia and some other risk factors for atherosclerosis, and this may contribute to atherogenesis.
- Overproduction of NO may be important in neurodegenerative diseases (see Ch. 34) and in septic shock.

Nitric oxide in therapeutics

- NO donors (e.g. **nitroprusside** and organic nitrovasodilators) are well established (see Chs 17 and 18).
- **Sildenafil** potentiates the action of NO on corpora cavernosa smooth muscle. It is used to treat erectile dysfunction (Ch. 29); other possible uses (e.g. in pulmonary hypertension, gastric stasis) are being investigated.
- Inhaled NO has therapeutic potential in respiratory distress syndrome but its effect on mortality is not known.
- Inhibition of NO biosynthesis (e.g. by L-NMMA; see text) is being investigated in disorders where there is overproduction of NO (e.g. inflammation and neurodegenerative disease). Disappointingly, LNMMA increases mortality in one such condition (sepsis).

Endothelial dysfunction in diabetic patients with erectile dysfunction occurs in tissue from the corpora cavernosum of penis, as evidenced by blunted relaxation to acetylcholine despite preserved responses to nitroprusside (Fig. 14.5). Vasoconstrictor responses to intra-arterial L-NMMA are reduced in forearm vasculature of insulin-dependent diabetics, especially in patients with traces of albumin in their urine (early evidence of glomerular endothelial dysfunction), suggesting that basal NO synthesis may be reduced throughout their circulation.

It is thought that failure to increase endogenous NO biosynthesis normally during pregnancy contributes to eclampsia. This is a hypertensive disorder that accounts for many maternal deaths and in which the normal vasodilatation seen in healthy pregnancy is lost.

Excessive NMDA receptor activation contributes to several forms of neurological damage (see Ch. 34). nNOS is absent in pyloric tissue from babies with ideopathic hypertrophic pyloric stenosis.*

Established clinical uses of drugs that influence the L-arginine/NO system are summarised in the clinical box.

*Are such individuals 'nNOS gene knockout humans'? What of their subsequent development?

REFERENCES AND FURTHER READING

Broeders M A W, Doevendans P A, Bekkers B C A M et al. 2000 Nebivolol: a third generation β-blocker that augments vascular nitric oxide release by endothelial β_2-adrenergic receptor-mediated nitric oxide production. Circulation 102: 677–684 (*This highly β_1-selective antagonist causes vasodilation through β_2-adrenergic receptor-mediated stimulation of the L-arginine/NO pathway*)

Davis K L, Martin E, Turko I V, Murad F 2001 Novel effects of nitric oxide. Annu Rev Pharmacol Toxicol 41: 203–236 (*Reviews non-cGMP mediated effects of NO including modifications of proteins, lipids and nucleic acids*)

Furchgott R F, Zawadzki J V 1980 The obligatory role of endothelial cells in the relaxation of arterial smooth muscle by acetylcholine. Nature 288: 373–376

Griffith O W, Stuehr D J 1995 Nitric oxide synthases: properties and catalytic mechanism. Annu Rev Physiol 57: 707–736 (*Mechanistic aspects of NOS catalysis*)

Gustafsson L E, Leone A M, Persson M G, Wiklund N P, Moncada S 1991 Endogenous nitric oxide is present in the exhaled air of rabbits, guinea-pigs and humans. Biochem Biophys Res Commun 181: 852–857

Hobbs A J 1997 Soluble guanylate cyclase: the forgotten sibling. Trends Pharmacol Sci 18: 484–491 (*'Forgotten' in comparison to its illustrious sibling adenylate cyclase*)

Hobbs A J, Higgs A, Moncada S 1999 Inhibition of nitric oxide synthase as a potential therapeutic target. Annu Rev Pharmacol Toxicol 39: 191–220 (*Overviews NOS inhibitors, concentrating on those that prevent binding of substrate*)

Huang P L, Huang Z, Mashimo H et al. 1995 Hypertension in mice lacking the gene for endothelial nitric oxide synthase. Nature 377: 239–242 (*Absent EDRF activity in aorta, and hypertension in the mutant mice*)

Jaffrey S R, Snyder S 1996 PIN: an associated protein inhibitor of neuronal nitric oxide synthase. Science 274: 774–777 (*Works by destabilising the nNOS dimer*)

Jia L, Bonaventura C, Bonaventura J, Stamler J S 1996 *S*-Nitroso-haemoglobin: a dynamic activity of blood involved in vascular control. Nature 380: 221–226 (*Challenges the previously orthodox view of NO as a paracrine mediator operating exclusively over a short range. See also accompanying editorial comment by Perutz M F pp. 205–206*)

Karupiah G, Xie Q, Buller M L, Nathan C, Duarte C, MacMicking J D 1993 Inhibition of viral replication by interferon-induced nitric oxide synthase. Science 261: 1445–1448

Liu J, Garcia-Cardena G, Sessa W C 1996 Palmitoylation of endothelial nitric oxide synthase is necessary for optimal stimulated release of nitric oxide: implications for caveolae localization. Biochemistry 35: 13277–13281 (*N-Myristoylation of eNOS is necessary for its association and targeting into the Golgi complex whereas palmitoylation influences its targeting to caveolae*)

Moncada S, Higgs A 1993 Mechanisms of disease: the L-arginine–nitric oxide pathway. N Engl J Med 329: 2002–2012 (*Excellent review of human/clinical aspects*)

Moore P K, Handy R C L 1997 Selective inhibitors of nitric oxide synthase—is no NOS really good NOS for the nervous system? Trends Pharmacol Sci 18: 204–211 (*Emphasis on compounds with selectivity for the neuronal isoform*)

Nelson R J, Demas G E, Huang P L et al. 1995 Behavioural abnormalities in male mice lacking neuronal nitric oxide synthase. Nature 378: 383–386 (*'A large increase in aggressive behaviour and excess, inappropriate sexual behaviour in nNOS knockout mice'*)

Pawlowski J R, Hess D T, Stamler J S 2001 Export by red cells of nitric oxide bioactivity Nature 409: 622–626 (*Movement of NO from red blood cells via anion echange protein AE1; see also editorial by SS Gross pp. 577–578*)

Ribiero J M C, Hazzard J M H, Nussenzveig R H, Champagne D E, Walker F A 1993 Reversible binding of nitric oxide by a salivary haem protein from a blood sucking insect. Science 260: 539–541 (*Action at a distance*)

Stuehr D J 1997 Structure–function aspects in the nitric oxide synthases. Annu Rev Pharmacol Toxicol 37: 339–359

Vallance P, Leone A, Calver A, Collier J, Moncada S 1992 Accumulation of endogenous inhibitor of nitric oxide synthesis in chronic renal failure. Lancet 339: 572–575 (*ADMA etc.; potential pathogenetic importance, and possible explanation of the 'arginine paradox'*)

Vanderwinden J-M, Mailleux P, Schiffmann S N, Vanderhaeghen J-J, de Laet M-H 1992 Nitric oxide synthase activity in infantile hypertrophic pyloric stenosis. N Engl J Med 327: 511–515

Wei X-Q, Charles I G, Smith A et al. 1995 Altered immune responses in mice lacking inducible nitric oxide synthase. Nature 375: 408–411 (*Homozygotes lacking iNOS were uniformly susceptible to infection by* Leishmania major)

Zoccali C et al. 2001 Plasma concentration of asymmetrical dimethylarginine and mortality in patients with end-stage renal disease: a prospective study. Lancet 358: 2113–2117 (*Accumulation of ADMA appears to be an important risk factor for cardiovascular disease in chronic renal failure*)

15

Local hormones, inflammation and immune reactions

Overview 217

Introduction 217

The components of the acute inflammatory reaction 217
- — The innate immune response 218
- — The adaptive immune response 222
- — Systemic responses in inflammation 227
- — Unwanted inflammatory and immune responses 228

The outcome of the inflammatory response 228

Mediators of inflammation and immune reactions 229
- — Histamine 229
- — Eicosanoids 231
- — Leukotrienes
- — Platelet-activating factor 237
- — Bradykinin 238
- — Nitric oxide 239
- — Neuropeptides 240
- — Cytokines 240

Current therapies based on manipulation of the immune response 241

Potential new therapies 242

OVERVIEW

This chapter deals with inflammatory/immune responses and the mediators (local hormones) that regulate them. We concentrate mainly on the acute inflammatory reaction—the response of the mammalian host to invading pathogen or noxious agent. It comprises both immune and non-immune elements.

We explain first the reason for emphasising this topic in a textbook of pharmacology. We follow this by an outline of the two components of the acute inflammatory reaction—the innate and the adaptive components—before giving a detailed description of the events that constitute them. We then describe the main chemical mediators that control the responses, emphasising their role in disease. Simple descriptions of the various topics covered will be found in Dale et al. (1994).

A glossary of some acronyms used in this chapter is given on p. 242.

INTRODUCTION

A mammalian organism facing an invasion by a disease-causing organism (pathogen) can call on a prodigious array of powerful defensive responses; the deployment of these constitutes the acute inflammatory/immune reaction. When these defences are lacking (as for example in the acquired immunodeficiency syndrome, AIDS) or are suppressed by drugs, organisms that are not normally pathogens can cause disease (opportunistic infections). However, in some circumstances, these defensive responses may be brought into play in response to other sorts of injury caused by chemicals, ultraviolet, heat, etc. In other circumstances they may be inappropriately deployed against innocuous substances from outside the body (e.g. pollen) or against the tissues of the body itself (in autoimmune conditions). When this happens, the responses themselves can produce damage and may indeed constitute part of the disease process—either acutely as, for example, in anaphylaxis, or chronically as, for example, in asthma (Ch. 22), rheumatoid arthritis (Ch. 16), or atherosclerosis (Ch. 19). It is for these sorts of conditions that anti-inflammatory or immunosuppressive drugs are used. An impressive variety of chemical mediators control or modulate these defensive responses of the host, and an understanding of the action, mechanism of action and clinical use of drugs that affect the inflammatory and the immune responses depends on an appreciation of the way in which the cells and the mediators interact with each other.

THE COMPONENTS OF THE ACUTE INFLAMMATORY REACTION

The acute inflammatory reaction has two components:

- an innate, non-adaptive response, thought to have been developed early in evolution and present in some form or other in most multicellular organisms
- the adaptive immune response.

The innate non-adaptive response

Some aspects of the innate response are non-immunological, for example the histamine-induced vascular changes to ultraviolet, some reactions of the neutrophil polymorphs, etc. Other aspects, particularly those which occur in response to an invading organism, are linked to, and are in essence part of, the overall immune response to infection and are referred to as the *innate immune response*. This is activated immediately after an infection, initiating the host response to the infecting organism and sending a wake-up signal to the adaptive immune response. It also has a role in preventing the adaptive response from targeting and damaging host cells.

The adaptive immune response

The adaptive immune response starts up only after a pathogen has been recognised by the innate immune response. It brings into play a whole panoply of reactions that are exquisitely specific for the invading organism as well as making the actions of the cells and mediators that participate in the innate response much more effective.

There are many 'back-up' systems so that a response to a pathogen can be produced in several ways, which is clearly important for a reaction with survival value.

Here we concentrate on the local manifestations of the reaction to an invading pathogen. The outline given will, of necessity, be a very general one. It may help if, in reading it, you keep in mind a picture of a boil, which is an acute inflammatory reaction caused by staphylococci, since most (but not all) of the events described will apply to it. At the macroscopic level, the inflamed area is reddened, swollen, hot and painful, and there is interference with, or alteration of, function. Examples of this last characteristic are the spasm of bronchiolar smooth muscle which occurs in asthma, or the restriction of movement in an inflamed joint.

In terms of what is happening locally within the tissues, the changes can be divided into cellular and vascular events. Mediators are generated both from plasma and from cells, and in turn they modify and regulate the vascular and cellular reactions.

The acute inflammatory reaction

- The term 'acute inflammatory reaction' refers to the events that occur in the tissues in response to an invading pathogen (disease-causing organism) or the presence of a noxious substance.
- It usually has two components: an innate non-adaptive response and an adaptive or specific immunological response.
- These reactions are protective, i.e. they have survival value, but if inappropriately deployed they are deleterious.
- The outcome can be healing with or without scarring or, if the pathogen or noxious substance persists, chronic inflammation.
- Many of the diseases that need drug treatment involve inflammatory processes. Understanding of the action and, therefore, the use of anti-inflammatory and immunosuppressive drugs necessitates an understanding of the inflammatory reaction.

THE INNATE IMMUNE RESPONSE

The innate immune response to infection with a microorganism has usually been rather airily dismissed by most immunologists as being an ancient throw-back that merely provides a temporary holding operation until the more effective specific adaptive immune response gets going. But it has recently become clear that the innate response has a much more important role in host defence, as mentioned above and described below.

An important initiating event in the innate immune response is the recognition by tissue macrophages of specific *pathogen-associated molecular patterns* (PAMPs) on the microorganism (see Medzhitov & Janeway, 2000; Brown, 2001). The PAMPs are highly conserved components that are shared between whole classes of pathogen (bacteria, viruses and fungi) and they are usually crucial parts of the pathogen's structure that are critical for its survival and pathogenicity.

Examples of bacterial PAMPs are:

- peptidoglycan: a constituent of the cell wall of virtually all bacteria (Ch. 44)
- bacterial lipopolysaccharide: a constituent of the outer membrane of all Gram-negative bacteria (Ch. 45).

The receptors that recognise PAMPs, (PAMP-recognition receptors)—some termed Toll receptors (TLRs)—are encoded in the host DNA* and are expressed on the surface of dendritic cells and macrophages, i.e. the professional antigen-presenting cells (APCs; see below).

The TLR–PAMP interaction triggers the dendritic cell or macrophage to respond immediately; proliferation is not required. The interaction triggers intracellular signal pathways that result in the production of the main pro-inflammatory cytokines:** tumour necrosis factor-α (TNF-α) and interleukin (IL-1). These act on vascular endothelial cells of the postcapillary venules causing:

- an increase in permeability, allowing the exudation of fluid (see Vascular events, below) that contains the components of enzyme cascades which give rise to more inflammatory mediators (e.g. the chemotaxin C5a, see Fig. 15.1)

*These receptors thus differ from the antigen receptors on T and B cells that are generated somatically as the T and B cells develop, endowing each lymphocyte clone with a structurally unique receptor. A new antiviral drug that works through the Toll receptor pathway to activate the immune system is under investigation.

**The term cytokine refers to a group of peptide cell regulators that includes lymphokines, chemokines, interleukins, interferons, etc.; see pp. 240–241.

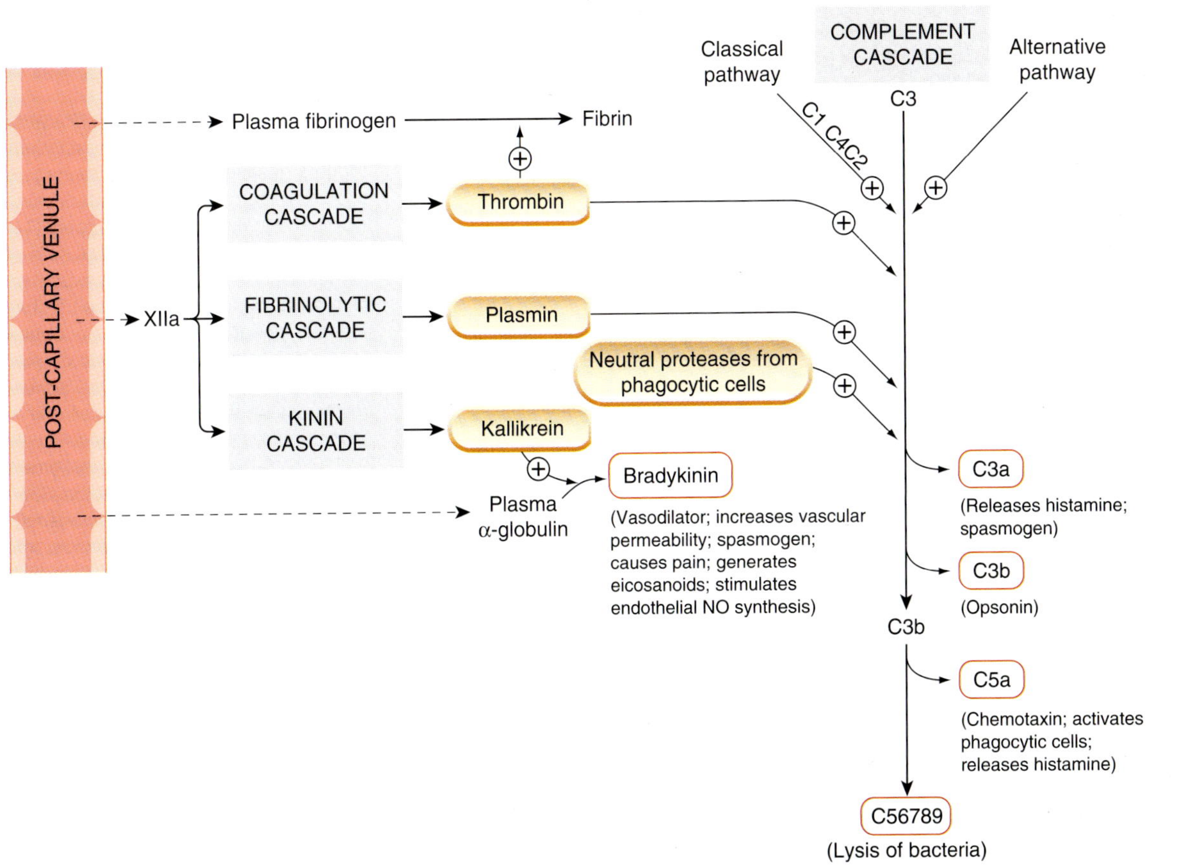

Fig. 15.1 Diagram showing the four enzyme cascades that are activated when plasma leaks out into the tissues as a result of the increased vascular permeability in an area of inflammation. Factors causing exudation are depicted in Figure 15.2. Mediators generated are shown in red-bordered boxes. Complement components are indicated by C1, C2, etc. When plasmin is formed it tends to increase kinin formation and decrease the coagulation cascade. (Adapted from: Dale et al. 1994.)

- the expression on the cells' intimal surface of adhesion molecules (see below).

▼ Both TNF-α and IL-1 induce signal pathways that lead to activation of transcription factor NF-κB. This transcription factor thus has a key role in the induction of inflammatory and immune responses.

In the unstimulated cell, NF-κB is inactive because complexed with an inhibitor, IkB. (Note that IkB is induced by glucocorticoids; see Ch. 27.) When a cell is stimulated, NF-κB is released, enters the nucleus and initiates transcription of genes for a variety of inflammatory and immune mediators.

White blood cells adhere to the endothelial cells through interactions between their cell surface integrins (see below) and the endothelial cells' adhesion molecules. This enables them to migrate out of the vessels, attracted to the site of the microorganisms by chemotaxins (see Fig. 15.2). Chemokines released by the TLR–PAMP interaction play an important part in this. (Cytokines and chemokines are considered on pp. 240–241.)

Numerous cells and mediators are involved in the innate response—constituting various back-up systems—and their interactions are very complex. A simplified outline is given in the box on page 222. More details of the vascular events and the role of individual cells and mediators are given below.

VASCULAR EVENTS AND THE MEDIATORS DERIVED FROM PLASMA

The vascular events are an initial dilatation of the small arterioles, resulting in increased blood flow, followed by slowing and then stasis of the blood and an increase in the permeability of the postcapillary venules, with exudation of fluid. The vasodilatation is brought about by various mediators (histamine, prostaglandins (PG) E_2 and I_2,* and so on) produced by the interaction of the microorganism with tissue. Some of these mediators (e.g. histamine, platelet-activating factor (PAF) and cytokines released

*Prostaglandin I_2 is also known as prostacyclin. It is referred to as PGI_2 in this book to accentuate its role as one of a series of prostaglandins.

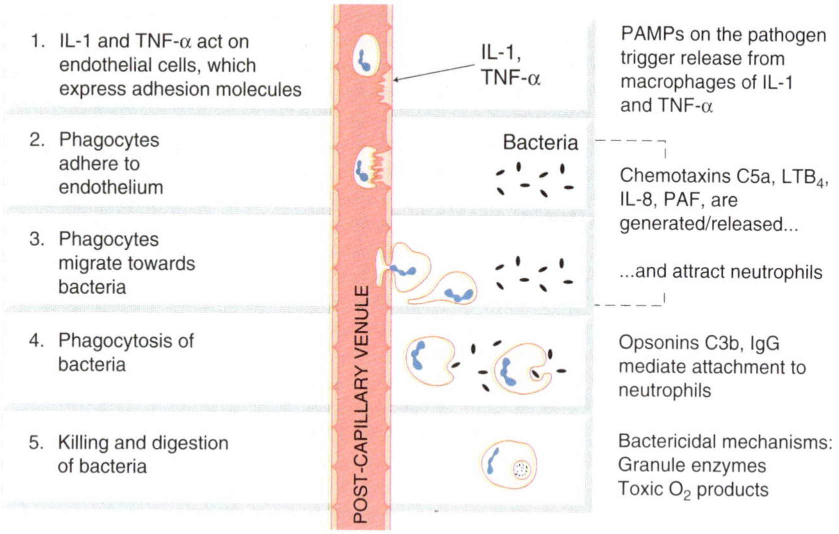

Fig. 15.2 Simplified diagram of some of the initial events in a local acute inflammatory reaction. Recognition by tissue macrophages of pathogen-associated molecular patterns (PAMPs) on the microorganism (e.g. a bacterium) triggers release from the macrophage of pro-inflammatory cytokines: interleukin-1 (IL-1) and tumour necrosis factor-α (TNF-α). These act on the endothelial cells of postcapillary venules causing exudation of fluid and expression of adhesion factors to which phagocytes (usually neutrophils in the initial stages) adhere. Adherence involves interaction between the adhesion molecules on the endothelial cell and those on the neutrophil. Subsequent steps are listed in the figure. (LTB_4, leukotriene B_4; PAF, platelet-activating factor; C5a and C3b are complement components; fMet.Leu.Phe is a bacterial peptide; IgG, immunoglobulin G; IL-8, interleukin-8.)

by TRL–PAMP interaction) are also responsible for the initial phase of increased vascular permeability.

The fluid exudate contains a variety of mediators, which influence the cells in the vicinity and the blood vessels themselves. These include the components for four proteolytic enzyme cascades: the *complement* system, the *coagulation* system, the *fibrinolytic* system, the *kinin* system (see Fig. 15.1). The components of these cascades are proteases that are inactive in their native form; they are activated by proteolytic cleavage, each activated component then activating the next.

The exudate is carried by lymphatics to local lymph glands or lymphoid tissue, where the products of the invading micro-organism can initiate an immune response.

▼ The complement system comprises nine major components, designated C1 to C9. Activation of the cascade can be initiated by substances derived from microorganisms, such as yeast cell walls, endotoxins, etc. This pathway of activation is termed 'the alternative pathway' (Fig. 15.1). (The 'classical pathway' involves antibody and is dealt with below.) One of the main events is the enzymic splitting of C3, which gives rise to various peptides. One of which, C3a (termed an *anaphylatoxin*), can stimulate mast cells to secrete chemical mediators and can also directly stimulate some smooth muscle, while another, C3b (termed an *opsonin*), can attach to the surface of a microorganism and facilitate its ingestion by white blood cells (see below). Enzymic action on a later component, C5, releases C5a which—in addition to causing release of mediators from mast cells—is powerfully chemotactic (i.e. acts as a chemical attractant) for white blood cells and also activates them. Some actions of these complement-derived mediators are considered below. Assembly of the last components in the sequence (C5 to C9) on the cell membranes of certain bacteria leads to the lysis of these organisms (see Ch. 44). Hence, complement can mediate the destruction of invading bacteria or damage multicellular parasites; however, it may sometimes cause injury to the host's own cells. The main event in the complement cascade—the splitting of C3—can also be brought about directly, by the principal enzymes of the coagulation and fibrinolytic cascades, thrombin and plasmin, and by enzymes released from white blood cells.

The coagulation system and the fibrinolytic system are described in Chapter 20. Factor XII is activated to XIIa (e.g. by collagen), and the end-product is *fibrin*, which when laid down in the tissues during a host–pathogen interaction can serve to limit the extension of the infection. The main enzyme of the coagulation system, *thrombin*, is involved in the activation of the complement and kinin systems (Fig. 15.1) and, indirectly, in fibrinolysis (see Ch. 20).

The kinin system is another enzyme cascade; it results in the production of several mediators of inflammation, in particular bradykinin (Fig. 15.1), which is dealt with in more detail below.

CELLULAR EVENTS

Of the cells involved in inflammation, some (vascular endothelial cells, mast cells and tissue macrophages) are normally present in tissues, while others (platelets and leucocytes) gain access to the area of inflammation from the blood. The *leucocytes* are actively motile cells and are of two classes:

- polymorphonuclear cells* (cells with many-lobed nuclei; also referred to as granulocytes), which are subdivided into neutrophils, eosinophils and basophils, according to the staining properties of the granules in their cytoplasm
- mononuclear cells (or cells with single-bodied nuclei), which are subdivided into monocytes and lymphocytes.

Mast cells

The mast cell membrane has receptors both for a special class of antibody, immunoglobulin E (IgE) see below), and for complement components C3a and C5a. The cell can be activated to secrete mediators through these receptors and also by direct physical damage.

*Some authors reserve the term 'polymorph' for neutrophils.

One of the main substances released by the mast cells is histamine (p. 229); others are heparin (see Ch. 20), leukotrienes (p. 235), PGD_2 (p. 234), PAF (p. 237), nerve growth factor and some interleukins (p. 240). For a simple overview of mast cells see Chapter 2 in Dale et al. (1994).

Polymorphonuclear leucocytes

Neutrophil polymorphs are the first of the blood leucocytes to enter the area of the inflammatory reaction (Fig. 15.2). They adhere to the vascular endothelial cells through interaction between adhesion molecules on the endothelial cell, e.g. the selectin and ICAM (intercellular adhesion molecule) families, with corresponding molecules on the neutrophil, e.g. the integrin family. The neutrophils then migrate out of the vessel to the site of the invading pathogen, attracted by chemicals termed *chemotaxins*: some released by the microorganism, such as formyl-Met–Leu–Phe, some produced locally, such as C5a (see above), leukotriene B_4 (LTB_4; p. 235) and various chemokines generated by macrophages (see above), in particular IL-8.

Neutrophils can engulf, kill and digest microorganisms. They, and the eosinophils, have surface receptors for the complement product C3b, which acts as an opsonin (see above), i.e. it forms a link between neutrophil and invading bacterium. (An even more effective link may be made by antibody; see below.) They kill by generating toxic oxygen products. Enzymic digestion of the microorganism then follows.

If the neutrophil is inappropriately activated, the toxic oxygen products and proteolytic enzymes can cause damage to the host's own tissues.

Eosinophils have similar capacities to neutrophils and, in addition, are armed with a number of potent granule constituents, which, when released extracellularly, can damage multicellular parasites (e.g. helminths). They include eosinophil cationic protein, a peroxidase, the eosinophil major basic protein and a neurotoxin. The eosinophil is now considered to be of primary importance in the pathogenesis of the late phase of asthma, in which its granule proteins cause damage to bronchiolar epithelium (see p. 343 and Fig. 22.3). Basophils are very similar in many respects to mast cells.

Monocytes/macrophages

The monocytes enter the area several hours after the polymorphs. Adhesion to endothelium and migration into the tissue follow a pattern similar to that of the neutrophils (see above), though chemotaxis of monocytes involves additional chemokines, for example MCP-1,* which, reasonably enough, stands for monocyte chemoattractant protein-1, and RANTES*, which (wait for it—immunological nomenclature has excelled itself here) stands for 'regulated upon activation, normal T cell expressed and secreted'.**

In the tissues, monocytes become transformed into macrophages (literally 'big eaters', compared with the neutrophil polymorphs, which were originally called microphages or 'little eaters'). Similar cells, all belonging to the mononuclear phagocyte system, are normally present in various tissues, probably all derived originally from blood-borne monocytes. The macrophage has a remarkable range of abilities, being not only a Jack-of-all-trades but also master of many (see below).

In innate reactions, macrophages bind lipopolysaccharide and other PAMPs by means of specific cell surface receptors. The binding stimulates generation and release of cytokines and chemokines (see above and p. 240) that act on vascular endothelial cells as described above, attract other leucocytes to the area and give rise to fever.

In areas of inflammation, macrophages engulf tissue debris and dead cells as well as microorganisms, and they are able to kill many (but not all) of the last (see below). When stimulated by **glucocorticoids**, they secrete lipocortin (a polypeptide that modulates the inflammatory response; see Ch. 27).

Vascular endothelial cells

The vascular endothelial cells (see also Chs 18 and 20)—originally considered as passive lining cells—are now known to play an active part in inflammation. The endothelial cells in the small arterioles secrete nitric oxide (NO)—which causes relaxation of the underlying smooth muscle (see Ch. 14)—and thus have a role in vasodilatation and in the delivery of plasma and blood cells to the area of inflammation; the cells of the postcapillary venules have a regulatory role in the flow of exudate and thus in the delivery of plasma-derived mediators (see Fig. 15.1).

On the luminal surface, vascular endothelial cells express several adhesion molecules (the ICAM and selectin families; see above, and Fig. 15.2) as well as a variety of receptors including those for histamine, acetylcholine, IL-1, etc.

In addition to NO, the cells can synthesise and release the vasodilator agent PGI_2 (p. 234), the vasoconstrictor agent endothelin (Ch. 18), plasminogen activator (Ch. 20), PAF (p. 237) and several cytokines. Endothelial cell function is also involved in angiogenesis (i.e. the growth of new blood vessels), which occurs in repair processes, chronic inflammation and cancer (see Chs 5 and 50).

Platelets

Platelets are involved primarily in coagulation and thrombotic phenomena (see Ch. 20) but may also play a part in inflammation. They have low-affinity receptors for IgE (see below) and are believed to contribute to the first phase of asthma (Fig. 22.3). In addition to generating thromboxane A_2 and PAF (Ch. 20), they can generate free radicals and pro-inflammatory cationic proteins. Platelet-derived growth factor contributes to the repair processes that follow inflammatory responses or damage to blood vessels (see below).

Neurons

Some sensory neurons, in addition to relaying impulses to the central nervous system (CNS), release inflammatory

*The human immunodeficiency virus 1 binds to the surface CD4 glycoprotein (see below) on monocyte/macrophages but is only able to penetrate the cell after also binding to the receptors for the chemokines MCP-1 and RANTES.

**RANTES is being renamed CCL5 and MCR1 will become CC13 and CCL4.

neuropeptides when appropriately stimulated. These neurons are fine afferents (capsaicin-sensitive C and Aδ fibres) with specific receptors at their peripheral terminals (Fig. 40.6, p. 568). Chemical mediators generated during injury and inflammation—kinins, 5-hydroxytryptamine (5-HT), etc. (discussed below)—act on the receptors, stimulating the release of neuropeptides, particularly two tachykinins (neurokinin A, substance P) and calcitonin gene-related peptide (CGRP). Neuropeptides are considered below and in Chapter 13.

Natural killer cells

Natural killer (NK) cells are specialised lymphocytes (see below) that, in an unusual version of a receptor-mediated reaction, kill target cells (virus-infected cells, tumour cells) which *lack* ligands for inhibitory receptors on the NK cells themselves. The ligands that are necessary are the major histocompatibility complex (MHC) molecules (described below). NK cells attack any cell unless it expresses these molecules—the mother turkey strategy.* If the inhibitory receptors recognise MHC molecules on the target cell, the NK cell does not kill the target cell. MHC molecules are proteins expressed on the surface of most host cells and, in simple terms, are specific for that individual, enabling the NK cells to avoid damaging host cells. The NK cells kill by antibody-mediated cytotoxicity.

NK cells have other functions in the immune response: they are equipped with Fc receptors and, in the presence of antibody against target cell components, they can kill the target cells (e.g. tumour cells) by antibody-dependent cellular cytotoxicity.

MEDIATORS DERIVED FROM CELLS

When inflammatory cells are stimulated or damaged, another major mediator system is called into play—the eicosanoids (see below, p. 231). Many of the current anti-inflammatory drugs act, at least in part, by interfering with synthesis of the eicosanoids. Other important inflammatory mediators derived from cells are histamine, PAF, NO, neuropeptides and the cytokines, details of which are given below (pp. 229, 237, 239, 240 and 240, respectively).

The innate non-adaptive response

- The innate response, which occurs soon after infection, has a component linked to the specific immunological response and also non-immunological vascular and cellular elements. Mediators are generated both from cells and from plasma and, in turn, modify and regulate the vascular and cellular events.
- Tissue macrophages recognise, by means of specific DNA-encoded receptors, specific *pathogen-associated molecular patterns* (PAMPs) on the microorganism; the interaction triggers release of cytokines, particularly interleukin-1 (IL-1) and tumour necrosis factor (TNF)-α and various chemokines.
- IL-1 and TNF-α act on local postcapillary venular endothelial cells causing:
  —vascular dilatation and exudation of fluid
  —expression of adhesion molecules on the cell surfaces.
- The fluid exudate contains the components of enzyme cascades that give rise to inflammatory mediators: bradykinin from the kinin system, C5a and C3a from the complement system; complement also gives rise to components that lyse bacteria.
- C5a and C3a stimulate mast cells to release histamine, which dilates local arterioles.
- Local tissue damage and the pro-inflammatory cytokines release eicosanoids: prostoglandins I_2 and E_2 (vasodilators), and leukotriene B_4 (chemotaxin).
- Cytokines stimulate synthesis of nitric oxide (vasodilator; increases vascular permeability).
- Leucocytes attach to the adhesion molecules then migrate out towards the pathogen site (attracted by chemokines, IL-8, C5a, leukotriene B_4) where phagocytosis and killing of bacteria takes place.

THE ADAPTIVE IMMUNE RESPONSE

The adaptive immunological response (the specific immunological response) to an invading organism makes the host's defensive response not only immeasurably more efficient but more specific for the invading pathogen. A simplified version will be given here, stressing only those aspects that are relevant for an understanding of current anti-inflammatory and immunosuppressant drugs and potential new therapeutic agents. (For more detailed coverage, see Janeway et al., 2001.)

The key cells are the *lymphocytes* of which there are three main groups:

- *B cells*, which are responsible for antibody production, i.e. the humoral immune response (Fig. 15.3)
- *T cells*, which are important in the induction phase of the immune response and are responsible for cell-mediated immune reactions (Fig. 15.3).
- *natural killer cells*, which are specialised non-T, non-B lymphoid cells that are active in the non-immunological, innate response (considered above).

It is a miraculous fact that we come equipped with the ability to *generate*, on T and B lymphocytes, antigen-specific receptors that can recognise and react with virtually all foreign proteins and polysaccharides (microbial products etc.) that we are likely to encounter during our lifetime.

*Richard Dawkins in River out of Eden, citing the zoologist Schliedt, explains that the 'rule of thumb a mother turkey uses to recognise nest robbers is a dismayingly brusque one; in the vicinity of the nest, attack anything that moves unless it makes a noise like a baby turkey' (quoted by Kärre & Welsh, 1997).

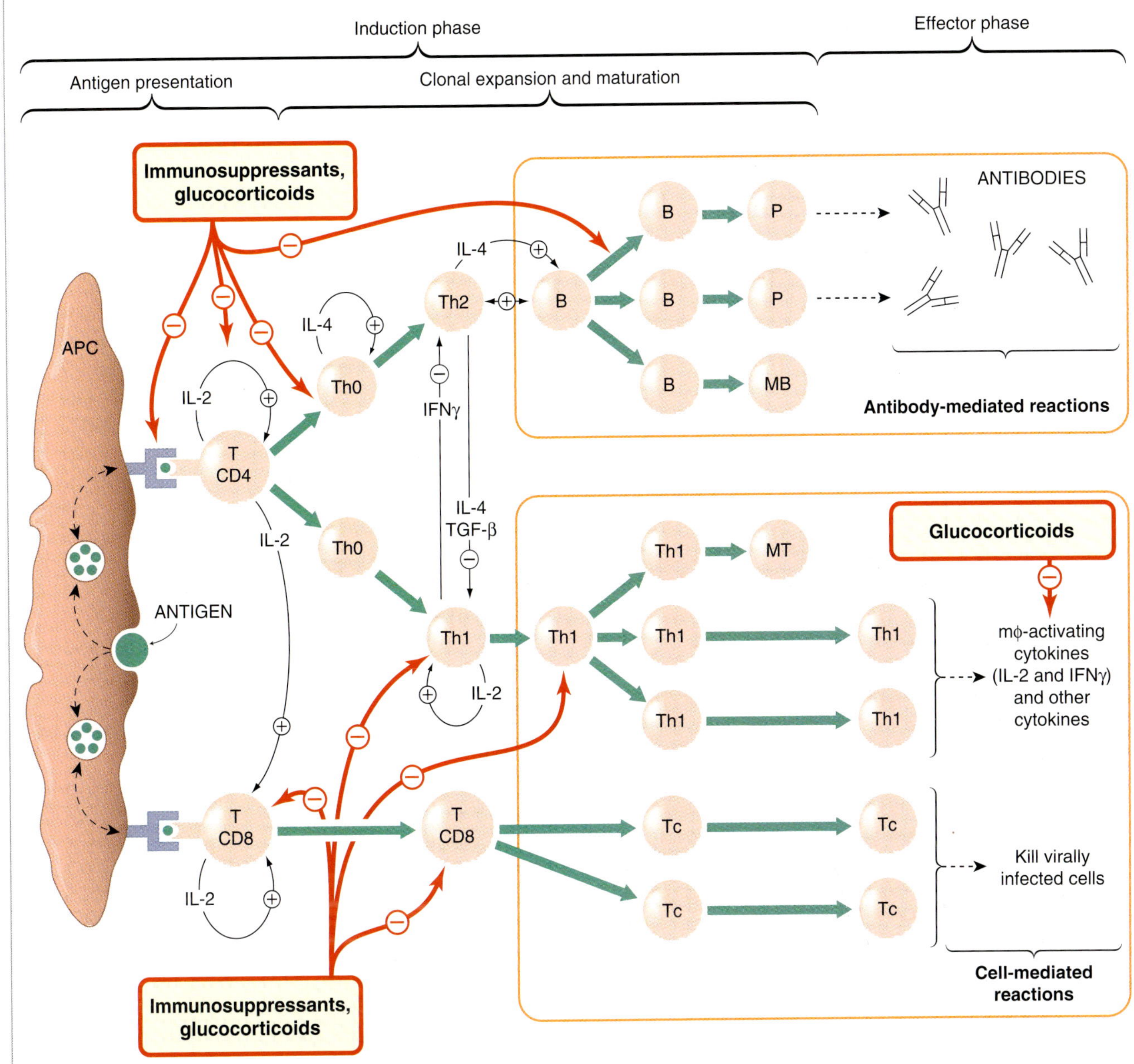

Fig. 15.3 Simplified diagram of the induction and effector phases of lymphocyte activation with the sites of action of immunosuppressants. Antigen-presenting cells (APC) ingest and process antigen (●) and present fragments of it (•) to naive, uncommitted CD4 T cells in conjunction with major histocompatibility complex (MHC) class II molecules and to naive CD8 T cells in conjunction with MCH class I molecules (-⊏), arming them. The armed CD4 T cells synthesise and express interleukin (IL)-2 receptors and release IL-2, which stimulates the cells by autocrine action, causing generation and proliferation of T-helper zero (Th0) cells. Autocrine cytokines (e.g. IL-4) cause proliferation of some Th0 cells to give Th2 cells, which are responsible for the development of antibody-mediated immune responses. These Th2 cells cooperate with and activate B cells to proliferate and give rise eventually to memory B cells (MB) and plasma cells (P), which secrete antibodies. Autocrine cytokines (e.g. IL-2) cause proliferation of some Th0 cells to give Th1 cells, which secrete cytokines that activate macrophages (responsible for some cell-mediated immune reactions).

The armed CD8 T cells also synthesise and express IL-2 receptors and release IL-2, which stimulates the cells by autocrine action to proliferate and give rise to cytotoxic T cells. These can kill virally infected cells. IL-2 secreted by $CD4^+$ cells also plays a part in stimulating $CD8^+$ cells to proliferate.

Note that the 'effector phase' depicted above relates to the 'protective' deployment of the immune response. When the response is inappropriately deployed—as in chronic inflammatory conditions such as rheumatoid arthritis—the Th1 wing of the immune response is dominant and the activated macrophages (mϕ) release IL-1 and TNF-α, which in turn trigger the release of the various chemokines and inflammatory cytokines that have a major role in the pathology of the disease (see Fig.16.5).

The involvement of lymphocytes in the specific immune response involves two phases: an induction phase and an effector phase, the latter consisting of two components—a humoral (antibody-mediated) component and a cell-mediated component. We give, first, a simple overview of the two phases:

1. During the *induction phase*, antigen is presented to T cells by large dendritic cells, APCs; this is followed by complex interactions of those T cells with B cells and other T cells. On first contact with an antigen (foreign protein or polysaccharide), the lymphocytes that have 'recognised' it (by means of surface receptors specific for that antigen) undergo a series of cell divisions, giving rise to a large clone of cells that all have the capacity to recognise and respond to that particular antigen. These latter cells are responsible eventually for the effector phase.
2. In the *effector phase*, these cells differentiate either into plasma cells or into memory cells. The plasma cells go on to produce antibodies (if they are B cells) or are involved in cell-mediated immune responses—activating macrophages or killing virus-infected host cells (if they are T cells). Other cells form an increased population of antigen-sensitive memory cells; a second exposure to the antigen to result in a much multiplied response.

The receptor repertoire on T and B cells is generated randomly and would recognise self proteins as well as foreign antigens. However, the body does not normally mount an immune response against its own tissues because tolerance to self antigens is produced during fetal life by apoptotic (Ch. 5) deletion of those clones of T cells that would have recognised and reacted against its own tissues. Dendritic cells and macrophages involved in the innate response also have a role in preventing damaging immune reactions against host's own cells (see below).

A simplified outline of the main interactions between cells and mediators is given in Figure 15.3.

THE INDUCTION PHASE

Antigenic molecules (e.g. bacterial products from the site of an infection or experimentally injected proteins) reach the local lymph nodes via the lymphatics. The antigen is presented to T lymphocytes on the surface of APCs. The APCs ingest and process the antigen and present it to:

- uncommitted (naive) $CD4^+$ T helper lymphocytes, termed Th cells, or T-helper precursor (Thp) cells, in association with class II MHC molecules (see Fig. 15.4)

and/or

- naive $CD8^+$ T lymphocytes in association with class 1 MHC molecules.*

*The main reason that it is difficult to transplant organs such as kidneys from one person to another is that their respective MHC molecules are different. Lymphocytes in the recipient of the transplant will react to non-self (allogeneic) MHC molecules in the transplanted tissue, which is thus likely to be rejected by a rapid and powerful immunological reaction.

CD4 and CD8** are coreceptors on T lymphocytes that cooperate with the main antigen-specific receptors in antigen recognition. Macrophages also carry surface CD4 proteins.

Activation of a T cell by an APC requires that several signals pass between the two cells (Fig. 15.4) (Medzhitov & Janeway, 2000). Research is underway on the elements involved in the interaction between the APC and the T cell shown in Figure 15.4 in the attempt to exploit them in the treatment of human immunodeficiency virus (HIV) infection and the therapy of immunologically mediated disease.

After activation, the T cells develop IL-2 receptors as well as generating IL-2, a cytokine that has autocrine*** action, causing proliferation of the cells that release it: giving rise to a clone of T cells termed Th0 cells, which in turn give rise to two different subsets of helper cells, Th1 cells and Th2 cells. (The proliferating T cells are said to develop into 'armed' effector T cells.) The action of specific interleukins determines whether Th1 or Th2 cells develop, IL-12 determining progress down the Th1 pathway, IL-4 determining progress down the Th2 pathway.

Each subset of Th cells then produces its own profile of cytokines, which control a unique set of immune responses: the Th1 pathway controlling mainly macrophage-initiated cell-mediated responses**** and the Th2 pathway antibody-mediated responses. The cytokines serve as autocrine growth factors for their own subset of T cells and have cross-regulatory actions on the development of the other subset (Abbas et al., 1996).

The relationship of Th1 and Th2 responses to disease

The T cell subsets are emphasised here because the balance between the functions of the two subsets clearly influences immunopathology. Diseases in which Th1 responses are dominant include insulin-dependent diabetes mellitus (Ch. 25), multiple sclerosis, *Helicobacter pylori*-induced peptic ulcer (Ch. 24), aplastic anaemia (Ch. 21) and rheumatoid arthritis***** (see Ch. 16). Th1 responses are implicated in allograft rejection (i.e. rejection of grafts between individuals of the same species); conversion of these Th1 responses to Th2 responses at the maternal/fetal interface prevents rejection of the fetal 'allograft'. Th2 responses are dominant in allergic conditions. AIDS progression is associated with loss of Th1 cells and is facilitated by Th2 responses. Progression of some diseases is associated with the Th1/Th2 balance; for example, in tuberculoid leprosy, Th1 responses predominate, in lepromatous leprosy Th2

**$CD4^+$ cells and NK cells recognise MHC class II molecules; $CD8^+$ cells recognise MHC class I molecules.

***Autocrine means 'acting on the cell that produces it' as opposed to paracrine, which means 'acting on nearby cells'.

****There is evidence that Th1 cytokines also have a role in some antibody-mediated responses, particularly in the production of opsonising antibodies (Abbas et al., 1996).

*****In rheumatoid arthritis and other chronic inflammatory diseases in which Th1 responses are dominant, macrophages release TNF-α and IL-1, which then, in turn, trigger the release of a host of other inflammatory cytokines (Fig. 16.5).

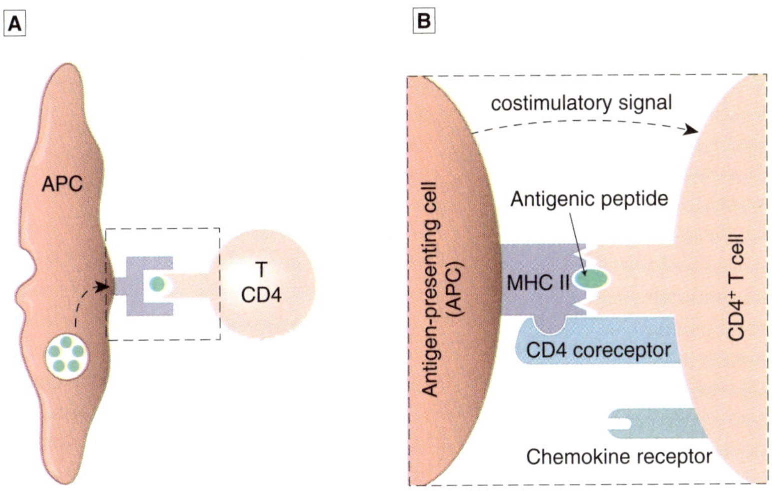

Fig. 15.4 The activation of a T cell by an antigen-presenting cell. A The activation process involves three stages. (i) Interaction between the complex of pathogen-derived antigen with peptide MHC class II and the antigen-specific receptor on the T cell. (ii) Interaction between the CD4 coreceptor on the T cell and an MHC molecule on the APC. (iii) A co-stimulatory signal from the APC to the T cell. The CD4 co-receptor is the main binding site for the HIV virus. A chemokine receptor (see Fig. 46.4) on the T cell is also involved in HIV binding.

predominate. (Th1/Th2 polarisation is summarised by Romagnani (1997).)

Understanding the relationship of the T cell subsets and their respective cytokine profiles with pathological conditions is expected to point the way to manipulation of immune responses for disease prevention and treatment. There are already many experimental models in which modulation of the Th1/Th2 balance with recombinant cytokines or cytokine antagonists alters the outcome of the disease.

Th1 cells and cell-mediated events

Th1 cells produce cytokines (IL-2, TNF-β and interferon-γ (IFNγ), which:

- activate macrophages; an important aspect of this effect is that activated macrophages can phagocytose and kill microbes (such as mycobacteria) that would otherwise survive and grow intracellularly
- stimulate $CD8^+$ lymphocytes to release IL-2; the IL-2 drives the $CD8^+$ lymphocytes' own proliferation and the subsequent maturation of the proliferated clone into cytotoxic cells that kill virally infected host cells (Fig. 15.3)
- inhibit Th2 cell functions (by IFNγ action).

Th2 cells and antibody-mediated events

Th2 cells produce cytokines (IL-4, TGF-β, IL-10*), which:

- stimulate B cells to proliferate; the clone so produced then matures into plasma cells that produce antibodies, particularly IgE—the antibody that fixes to mast cells and eosinophils
- stimulate differentiation and activation of eosinophils
- inhibit Th1 cell functions,* i.e. the activation of inflammatory cells and the cell-mediated reactions produced by Th1 cytokines.

*IL-4, TGF-β and IL-10 function as anti-inflammatory cytokines by virtue of inhibiting Th-1-induced activation of inflammatory cells.

The induction of antibody-mediated responses varies with the type of antigen. With most (but not all) antigens, a cooperative process between Th2 cells and B cells is necessary. B cells can also bind and present antigen to the T cell and the T cell then releases cytokines that act on the B cell.

The anti-inflammatory steroids (see Ch. 27) and the immunosuppressive drug **ciclosporin** (see Ch. 16) affect the events at the stage of induction. The cytotoxic immunosuppressive drugs (see Ch. 16) inhibit the proliferative phase of both B and T cells. Eicosanoids (see below) are believed to play a part in controlling these processes. For example, prostaglandins of the E series inhibit lymphocyte proliferation, probably by inhibiting the release of IL-2.

THE EFFECTOR PHASE

The reactions in the effector phase may be antibody mediated or cell mediated. The antibody-mediated (humoral) response is effective in the extracellular fluid (plasma and tissue fluid). However, antibodies cannot reach and deal with pathogens when these are within cells; cell-mediated immune mechanisms have evolved to deal with this.

The antibody-mediated (humoral) response

Antibodies are γ-globulins (immunoglobulins) that have two functions:

- to 'recognise' and interact specifically with particular antigens, i.e. proteins or polysaccharides foreign to the host
- to activate one or more of the host's defence systems.

The foreign substances may be part of an invading organism (the coat of a bacterium) or released by such an organism (a bacterial toxin), or they may be materials introduced experimentally in the laboratory in studies of the immune response (e.g. the injection of egg albumin into the guinea-pig).

An antibody is a Y-shaped protein molecule in which the arms of the Y (the 'Fab' portions) are the recognition sites for specific antigens, and the stem of the Y (the 'Fc' portion) activates host defence mechanisms. B lymphocytes, the cells that are responsible for antibody production, 'recognise' foreign molecules by means of receptors on their surfaces, the receptor being essentially the immunoglobulin which that B cell clone will eventually produce. The mammalian organism possesses a vast number of clones of B cells producing different antibodies with recognition sites for different antigens.

The ability to make antibodies has survival value; children born without this ability suffer repeated infections—pneumonia, skin infections, tonsillitis, etc. Before the days of antibiotics, they died in early childhood, and even today they require regular replacement therapy with immunoglobulin (see Ch. 16).

There are five classes of antibody—IgG, IgM, IgE, IgA and IgD—which differ from each other in certain structural respects (see Janeway & Travers, 2001).

Antibodies markedly improve the host's response to an invading pathogen. Apart from their ability to interact directly with invading pathogens such as viruses or with bacterial toxins, thus impairing their capacity for damage, antibodies can multiply manyfold the effectiveness and specificity of the host's defence reaction in several ways.

Antibodies and the complement sequence

When antibodies react with antigenic material on the pathogen, the antigen–antibody reaction leads to the exposure, on the Fc portion, of a binding site for complement. This results in activation of the complement sequence, with its biological repercussions (see p. 220 and Fig. 15.1). This route to C3 activation (the classical pathway) provides an especially selective way of activating complement in response to a particular pathogen, since the antigen–antibody reaction that initiates it is not only a highly specific recognition event but also occurs in close association with the pathogen. The lytic property of complement can be used therapeutically: monoclonal antibodies (mAbs) and complement together can be used to clean bone marrow of cancer cells as an adjunct to chemotherapy or radiotherapy (see Ch. 50). Complement lysis is also implicated in the action of antilymphocyte immunoglobulin (Ch. 16).

Antibodies and the phagocytosis of bacteria

Antibodies can attach to the particular antigens on the surface of microorganisms that have been 'recognised' by their Fab portions, leaving the Fc part of the molecule projecting. Phagocytic cells (neutrophils and macrophages) have receptors on their membranes for these projecting Fc portions of antibody. Antibody thus forms a very specific link between microorganism and phagocyte and is more effective than C3b as an opsonin in facilitating phagocytosis (see Fig. 15.2).

Antibodies and cellular cytotoxicity

In some cases, for example with parasitic worms, the invader may be too big to be ingested by phagocytes. Antibody molecules can form a link between parasite and the host's white cells (in this case, eosinophils), which are then able to damage or kill the parasite by surface or extracellular actions. NK cells with Fc receptors can also kill antibody-coated target cells (an example of antibody-dependent cell-mediated cytoxicity, mentioned above).

Antibodies and mast cells or basophils

Mast cells and basophils have receptors for a particular form of antibody—IgE—which can become attached to the cell membrane. When antigen reacts with this cell-fixed antibody, a whole panoply of pharmacologically active mediators is secreted. A complex reaction such as this, found widely throughout the animal kingdom, is unlikely to have been developed and retained during evolution unless it had survival value for the host. However, its precise biological significance in defence is not clear, though it may be of importance in association with eosinophil activity in reactions against parasitic worms. When inappropriately triggered by substances not inherently damaging to the host, it is implicated in certain types of allergic reaction (see below and Ch. 19) and contributes to illness in the modern world rather than survival.

The cell-mediated immune response

The lymphocytes involved in cell-mediated responses include both cytotoxic T cells (derived from $CD8^+$ cells) and inflammatory (cytokine-releasing) Th1 cells (see Fig. 15.3). They move into an area of inflammation by a process similar to that described for neutrophils and macrophages, namely interaction between adhesion molecules on both the endothelial cell and the lymphocyte and attraction to the inflammatory site by chemokines.

Cytotoxic T cells

Armed cytotoxic T cells are responsible for killing intracellular microorganisms such as viruses. When a virus infects a mammalian cell (which can be virtually any of the cells in the body), there are two aspects to the resulting immune response. The first step is the expression on the cell surface of peptides derived from the pathogen in association with MHC molecules. The second step is the recognition of the peptide–MHC complex by specific receptors on cytotoxic ($CD8^+$) T cells (Fig. 15.4 shows a similar process for a $CD4^+$ T cell; see also Fig. 46.2.). The cytotoxic T cells then destroy the virus-infected cell by programming them to undergo apoptosis (see Ch. 5). Cooperation with macrophages may be required for the kill.

Macrophage-activating $CD4^+$ Th1 cells

Some pathogens (e.g. mycobacteria, listeria) have evolved strategies for surviving and multiplying within macrophages after ingestion.

Armed $CD4^+$ Th1 cells release cytokines that activate macrophages to kill these intracellular pathogens. Th1 cells also recruit macrophages by releasing cytokines that act on vascular endothelial cells (e.g. TNF-α; see p. 218) and on chemokines (e.g. macrophage chemotactic factor-1 (MCF); see p. 221) that attract the macrophages to the sites of infection.

A complex of microorganism-derived peptide plus MHC molecule is expressed on the macrophage surface and is recognised by cytokine-releasing Th1 cells, which generate

The adaptive response

- The adaptive or specific immunological response vastly improves the effectiveness of the innate, non-immunological responses. It has two phases: the induction phase, and the effector phase, the latter consisting of (i) antibody-mediated and (ii) cell-mediated components.
- In the *induction phase*, naive T cells bearing either the CD4 coreceptor or the CD8 coreceptor are presented with antigen, which causes them to proliferate:
  - —CD8-bearing T cells proliferate further and develop into cytotoxic T cells, which can kill virally infected cells
  - —CD4-bearing Th cells are stimulated by cytokines to develop into Th1 or Th2 cells
  - —Th2 cells control mostly *antibody-mediated responses*; they interact with B cells, which proliferate giving rise to antibody-secreting plasma cells and memory cells
  - —Th1 cells proliferate, developing into cells that release macrophage-activating cytokines; these cells, along with cytotoxic T cells (above), control *cell-mediated responses*
  - —some develop into memory cells.
- The effector phase involves antibody- and cell-mediated responses.
- Antibodies provide:
  - —more selective activation of the complement cascade
  - —more effective ingestion of microorganisms
  - —more effective attachment to multicellular parasites, facilitating their killing
  - —neutralisation of some viruses and of some bacterial toxins.
- Cell-mediated reactions involve:
  - —CD8 cytotoxic T cells interacting with and killing virus-infected cells
  - —cytokine-releasing $CD4^+$ T cells; the cytokines enable macrophages to kill intracellular pathogens such as the tubercle bacillus.
  - —memory cells are cells primed to react rapidly to the antigen that gave rise to that clone of cells next time an organism bearing that antigen is encountered.
- Inappropriately deployed immune reactions are termed hypersensitivity reactions; these underlie the autoimmune diseases, i.e. diseases caused by immune reactions directed at the host's own tissues.
- Anti-inflammatory drugs and immunosuppressive agents are used when the normally protective inflammatory and/or immune responses are inappropriately deployed.

cytokines that enable the macrophage to deploy its killing mechanisms.

Activated macrophages (with or without intracellular pathogens) are factories for the production of chemical mediators and can generate and secrete not only many cytokines but also toxic oxygen metabolites and neutral proteases that can kill extracellular organisms (e.g. *Pneumocystis carinii** and various helminths), complement components, eicosanoids (see p. 231), NO (see below and Ch. 14), a fibroblast-stimulating factor, pyrogens and the 'tissue factor' that starts the extrinsic pathway of the coagulation cascade (Ch. 20), as well as various other coagulation factors. They are also important in repair processes. Among the cytokines secreted is IL-12, which has a positive feedback effect, driving the development of further Th1 cells.

It is primarily the cell-mediated reaction that is responsible for allograft rejection.

The specific immunological response, cell-mediated or humoral, is thus superimposed on the immunologically non-specific vascular and cellular reactions described previously, making them not only markedly more effective but much more specific for particular invading organisms. An important aspect of the specific immunological response is that the clone of lymphocytes that are programmed to respond to the antigens of the invading organism is greatly expanded after the first contact with the organism and now contains memory cells. Thus, subsequent exposure results in a greatly accelerated and more effective response. In some cases, the response becomes so prompt and so efficient that, after the first exposure which initiates the specific immune response, some microorganisms can virtually never gain a foothold in the host's tissues again. Immunisation procedures make use of this fact.

The general events of the inflammatory and hypersensitivity reactions specified above vary in some tissues. For example, in the inflammation that underlies asthma, eosinophils and neuropeptides have a particularly significant role (see Ch. 22). In inflammation in the CNS there is less infiltration of neutrophils, and monocyte infiltration is delayed—possibly owing to lack of adhesion molecule expression on CNS endothelium and deficient generation of chemotaxins. It has long been known that some tissues—the CNS parenchyma, the anterior chamber of the eye and the testis—are privileged sites in that a foreign antigen introduced directly does not provoke an immune reaction. However, introduction elsewhere of an antigen already in the CNS parenchyma allows development of immune/inflammatory responses in the CNS.

SYSTEMIC RESPONSES IN INFLAMMATION

In addition to the local changes in an inflammatory area, there are often various general responses such as a rise in temperature and an increase in blood leucocytes, termed 'leucocytosis' (or neutrophilia if the increase is in the neutrophils only). There is

*Patients with AIDS have a deficiency of $CD4^+$ T cells (see Ch. 44) and are, therefore, at risk from *P. carinii,* which can cause a fatal pneumonia.

also an increase in certain plasma proteins termed 'acute phase proteins' (see Gabay & Kushner, 1999). These include C-reactive protein, α_2-macroglobulin, fibrinogen (see Fig. 15.1), α_1-antitrypsin, and some complement components. C-reactive protein binds to certain microorganisms and the resulting complex activates complement

UNWANTED INFLAMMATORY REACTIONS AND IMMUNE RESPONSES

The responses described above can, in some circumstances, be inappropriately triggered by substances that are innocuous or even endogenous, as occurs in autoimmune* disease. It is when this happens that it becomes necessary to use anti-inflammatory or immunosuppressive drugs. Unwanted immune responses are termed allergic** or hypersensitivity reactions and have been classified into four types (Janeway et al., 2001).

Type I: immediate or anaphylactic hypersensitivity

Type I hypersensitivity (aka 'allergy') occurs in individuals who have a predominantly Th2 rather than a Th1 response to antigen. In these individuals, antigenic material that is not in itself noxious (such as grass pollen, products from dead house dust mites, certain foodstuffs or some drugs) evokes the production of antibodies of the IgE type, which fix to mast cells and, in the lung, to eosinophils. Subsequent contact with the material causes the release of histamine (p. 229), PAF (p. 237), eicosanoids (p. 231) and cytokines (p. 240) from mast cells. The effects may be localised to the nose (hay fever), the bronchial tree (the initial phase of asthma), the skin (urticaria) or the gastrointestinal tract. In some cases the reaction is more generalised and produces *anaphylactic shock*.

Roughly speaking, this type of hypersensitivity represents mainly inappropriate deployment of the processes outlined above in the discussion of antibodies and mast cells in the humoral immune response. Some important unwanted effects of drugs are anaphylactic hypersensitivity responses (see Ch. 52).

Type II: antibody-dependent cytotoxic hypersensitivity

Type II hypersensitivity occurs when the mechanisms outlined above are directed against cells within the host that are, or that appear to be, foreign; for example host's cells altered by drugs. The antigens form part of the surface of these cells and evoke antibodies. The antigen–antibody reaction initiates the complement sequence (with its repercussions) and can also provide a basis for the attack by killer cells.

Examples of this latter class are the alteration by drugs of neutrophil polymorphs, which may lead to agranulocytosis (see Ch. 51), and of platelets, which may lead to thrombocytopenic purpura (Ch. 20). Class II reactions are implicated in some types of autoimmune thyroiditis (e.g. Hashimoto's disease; see Ch. 28).

Type III: complex-mediated hypersensitivity

Type III hypersensitivity occurs when antibody reacts with soluble antigen. The antigen–antibody complexes can activate complement (see above) or attach to mast cells and stimulate the release of mediators (see above).

▼ An experimental example of type III hypersensitivity is a reaction termed the Arthus reaction, which occurs if a foreign protein is injected subcutaneously into a rabbit or guinea-pig that has a high concentration of circulating antibody against that protein. The area becomes red and swollen 3–8 hours later. This is because the antigen–antibody complexes settle in the small blood vessels, complement is activated, and neutrophils are attracted and activated (by C5a) to generate toxic oxygen products and to secrete enzymes. Mast cells are also stimulated by C3a to release mediators. Damage caused by this process is involved in serum sickness, in the reaction to mouldy hay (known as farmer's lung) and in certain types of autoimmune kidney and arterial disease. Type III hypersensitivity is also implicated in lupus erythematosus (a chronic, autoimmune inflammatory disease of connective tissue).

Type IV: cell-mediated hypersensitivity

The prototype of type IV hypersensitivity (also known as delayed hypersensitivity) is the tuberculin reaction—the reaction seen when proteins derived from cultures of the tubercle bacillus are injected into the skin of a person who has been sensitised to the bacillus by a previous infection or by immunisation.

▼ After 24 hours, the area becomes reddened and thickened. An 'inappropriate' cell-mediated immune response (p. 226) has been stimulated and there has been infiltration of mononuclear cells and the release of various cytokines. Cell-mediated hypersensitivity is the basis of the reaction seen with some rashes (e.g. in mumps and measles) and with mosquito and tick bites. It is also important in the skin reactions to drugs or industrial chemicals (see Ch. 52), and in these cases, the chemical combines with proteins in the skin to form the 'foreign' substance that evokes the cell-mediated immune response (Fig. 15.3). A substance acting in this way is called a *hapten*.

In essence, inappropriately deployed T cell activity underlies all types of hypersensitivity, being the initiating factor in types I, II and III and being involved in both the initiation and effector phase in type IV.

The hypersensitivity reactions given above are the basis of the clinically important group of autoimmune diseases. Some examples of autoimmune conditions have been given; other examples held to have a marked component of cell-mediated hypersensitivity are rheumatoid arthritis (Ch. 16), multiple sclerosis (p. 241)and type 1 (insulin-dependent) diabetes (Ch. 25).

Immunosuppressive drugs (Ch. 16) and/or **glucocorticoids** (Ch. 27) are employed as part of the treatment of some autoimmune diseases, and the use of cytokines and of antibodies to T cell surface antigens (e.g. the CD4 receptor) is being explored.

THE OUTCOME OF THE INFLAMMATORY RESPONSE

After this outline of the specific immune response, we need to return to a consideration of the host–pathogen interaction: the

*Autoimmune diseases are caused by the host's immune system attacking the host's own tissue, i.e. they result from inappropriately deployed immune responses.

**The term allergy is now generally restricted to type I hypersensitivity.

local acute inflammatory response. It should be clear that this may consist of the innate, immunologically non-specific vascular and cellular events described initially, together with a varying degree of participation of the specific immunological response (either humoral or cell mediated), the degree depending on several factors such as the nature of the pathogen and the organ or tissue involved.

What is the final result of the interaction? If the pathogen has been dealt with adequately, there may be complete healing and the tissue may be virtually normal thereafter. If there has been damage (death of cells, pus formation, ulceration), repair is usually necessary and may result in scarring. If the pathogen persists, the condition is likely to proceed to *chronic inflammation*, a slow smouldering reaction that continues for months or even years and involves destruction of tissue as well as local proliferation of cells and connective tissue. The principal cell types found in areas of chronic inflammation are *mononuclear cells* and abnormal cells derived from macrophages. In areas of healing and chronic inflammation, a variety of growth factors are active; there is *angiogenesis* (growth of new blood vessels) and also greatly increased activity of *fibroblasts*, which lay down fibrous tissue. The response to some microorganisms has the characteristic of chronicity from the start; examples are syphilis, tuberculosis and leprosy.

The cellular and mediator components of the chronic inflammatory response to microorganisms are also seen in many if not most chronic autoimmune and hypersensitivity diseases and are important targets for drug action in these conditions.

Mediators of importance in healing, repair processes and chronic inflammatory reactions are, amongst others, platelet-derived growth factor (p. 240), vascular endothelial growth factor, transforming growth factor, and various fibroblast growth factors. (See Fig. 5.3 for more information on growth factors.)

MEDIATORS OF INFLAMMATION AND IMMUNE REACTIONS

In the highly complex repertoire of reactions that constitutes the host response to invading pathogen (a repertoire which is inappropriately deployed in hypersensitivity and autoimmunity), the precise role of the various mediators has not been completely clarified. A putative mediator should fulfil certain criteria, modified from those outlined by Sir Henry Dale in 1933 for neurotransmitters. The modified criteria and the degree to which the known inflammatory mediators fulfil them is considered by Dale (1994).

The mediators of pharmacological significance will be described below. Drugs that affect the inflammatory and immune responses will be considered in the next chapter.

HISTAMINE

Most of the early studies on the biological actions of histamine were carried out by Sir Henry Dale and his colleagues.

▼ Dale had shown that a local anaphylactic reaction (a type I or 'immediate hypersensitivity reaction'; see above) was the result of an antigen–antibody reaction in sensitised tissue, and he subsequently demonstrated that histamine could largely mimic both the in vitro and in vivo anaphylactic responses. After the first generation of antihistamine drugs was produced, following the work of Bovet and his co-workers, it became clear (as a result of careful quantitative studies by Schild) that there were two types of histamine receptor in the body and that this first generation of antihistamine drugs affected only one type—the H_1-receptors. The second type, termed H_2-receptors and important particularly in gastric acid secretion, was unaffected. Black and his colleagues, following up the classification proposed by Schild, developed the second generation of antihistamine drugs—the H_2-receptor antagonists. Subsequently, Sir James Black was awarded the Nobel prize for his work on H_2-receptors (and β-adrenoceptors; Ch. 11). Later, evidence for the existence of a third type of histamine receptor—the H_3-receptor—was produced by Arrang et al. (1983).

Synthesis and storage of histamine

Histamine is a basic amine formed from histidine by histidine decarboxylase. It is found in most tissues of the body but is present in high concentrations in the lungs and the skin and in particularly high concentrations in the gastrointestinal tract. At the cellular level, it is found largely in mast cells and basophils, associated with heparin, but non-mast-cell histamine occurs in 'histaminocytes' in the stomach and in histaminergic neurons in the brain (see Ch. 33). The basophil content of the tissues is negligible—except in certain parasitic infections and hypersensitivity reactions (p. 735)—and basophils form only 0.5% of circulating white blood cells.

In mast cells and basophils, histamine is held in intracellular granules in a complex with an acidic protein and a heparin of high molecular weight, termed macroheparin. Together these comprise the matrix of the granule in which the basic molecule histamine is held by ionic forces, the histamine content being approximately 0.1–0.2 pmol per mast cell, and 0.01 pmol per basophil.

Histamine release

Histamine is released from mast cells by exocytosis during inflammatory or allergic reactions. As explained earlier in this chapter, stimuli include the interaction of complement components C3a and C5a with specific receptors on the cell surface, or the interaction of antigen with cell-fixed IgE antibodies. Secretion is initiated by a rise in cytosolic Ca^{2+}. Various basic drugs, such as **morphine** and **tubocurarine,** release histamine by non-receptor action.

Agents that increase cAMP formation (e.g. β-adrenoceptor agonists; see Ch. 11) inhibit histamine secretion. Replenishment of the histamine content of mast cell or basophil after secretion is a slow process, which may take days or weeks, whereas turnover of histamine in the gastric histaminocyte is very rapid.

Histamine is metabolised by histaminase and/or by the methylating enzyme imidazole *N*-methyltransferase.

Histamine receptors

Histamine produces its action by an effect on specific histamine receptors, which are of three* main types, H_1, H_2 and H_3,

*A fourth histamine receptor has recently been described, cloned and characterised. It is expressed in intestinal tissue, spleen, thymus and immune/inflammatory cells (T cells, neutrophils, eosinophils).

Table 15.1 Details of some agonist drugs used to define the three types of histamine receptors

Drug	Relative activity in vitro (histamine 100%)		
	H_1-receptors (ileum contraction)	H_2-receptors (stimulation of atrial rate)	H_3-receptors (histamine release from brain tissue)
Histamine	100	100	100
Dimaprit	<0.0001	71	0.0008
(*R*)-α-Methylhistamine	0.49	1.02	1550

Source: Data derived from Black J W et al. 1972 Nature 236: 385–390; Ganellin C R 1982 In: Ganellin C R, Parson M E (eds) Pharmacology of histamine receptor. Wright, Bristol, UK, pp. 11–102; Arrang J M et al. 1987 Nature 327: 117–123; van der Werf J F, Timmerman H 1989 Trends Pharmacol Sci 10: 159–162.

distinguished by means of selective antagonist drugs. Some details of the actions of antagonist and agonist drugs used to investigate and define the three types of histamine receptor are given in Tables 15.1 and 15.2. Selective antagonists at H_1-, H_2- and H_3-receptors are **mepyramine**, **cimetidine** and **thioperamide**, respectively. Selective agonists for H_2- and H_3-receptors are **dimaprit** and **(*R*)-methylhistamine**.

Histamine H_1 antagonists have clinical uses (see Chs 16 and 24), as do histamine H_2 antagonists (Ch. 24); H_3-receptor antagonists have been developed and may have a role in CNS pharmacology (see Ch. 33).

Table 15.2 Details of some antagonist drugs used to define the three types of histamine receptor

Drug	Binding constant (K_B; mol/l)		
	H_1	H_2	H_3
Mepyramine	0.4×10^{-9}	–	$> 3 \times 10^{-6}$
Cimetidine	4.5×10^{-4}	0.8×10^{-6}	3.3×10^{-5}
Thioperamide	$> 10^{-4}$	$> 10^{-5}$	4.3×10^{-9}

Source: Data derived from Black J W et al. 1972 Nature 236: 385–390; Ganellin C R 1982 In: Ganellin C R, Parson M E (eds) Pharmacology of histamine receptors. Wright, Bristol, UK, pp. 11–102; Arrang J M et al. 1987 Nature 327: 117–123; van der Werf J F, Timmerman H 1989 Trends Pharmacol Sci 10: 159–162.

Actions

Gastric secretion

Histamine stimulates the secretion of gastric acid by action on H_2-receptors. In clinical terms, this is the most important action of histamine, since it is implicated in the pathogenesis of peptic ulcer. It is considered in detail in Chapter 24.

Smooth muscle effects

Histamine, acting on H_1-receptors, causes contractions of the smooth muscle of the ileum, the bronchi and bronchioles, and the uterus.

The effect on the ileum is not as marked in humans as it is in the guinea-pig.* Histamine is one of the main mediators causing reduction of air flow in the first phase of bronchial asthma (see Ch. 22 and Fig. 22.3). Uterine muscle in most species is contracted.

Cardiovascular effects

Histamine dilates blood vessels in humans by an action on H_1-receptors, the effect being partly endothelium-dependent in some vascular beds. It increases the rate and the output of the heart by action on cardiac H_2-receptors.

Injected intradermally, histamine causes a reddening of the skin and a wheal with a surrounding flare—the 'triple response' described by Sir Thomas Lewis over 50 years ago. The reddening results from vasodilatation of the small arterioles and precapillary sphincters, and the wheal is caused by the increased permeability of the postcapillary venules. These effects are mainly mediated through activation of H_1-receptors. (Contrary to popular belief and the statements in some pathology textbooks, histamine does not increase capillary permeability; its locus of action in increasing permeability is on the postcapillary venules.) The flare is an 'axon reflex' that involves stimulation of sensory nerve fibres and the passage of antidromic impulses through neighbouring branches of the same nerve with release of a vasodilator mediator, probably CGRP (see Chs 13 and 15).

Itching

Itching occurs if histamine is injected into the skin or applied to a blister base; it is caused by stimulation of sensory nerve endings.

*The response of the guinea-pig ileum is the basis of the standard bioassay for histamine, familiar to students of experimental pharmacology.

Histamine

- Histamine is a basic amine, stored in granules within mast cells and basophils and secreted when complement components C3a and C5a interact with specific membrane receptors, or when antigen interacts with cell-fixed IgE.
- It produces effects by acting on H_1-, H_2- or H_3-receptors on target cells.
- The main actions in humans (with the receptors involved) are:
  —stimulation of gastric secretion (H_2)
  —contraction of most smooth muscle other than that of blood vessels (H_1)
  —cardiac stimulation (H_2)
  —vasodilatation (H_1)
  —increased vascular permeability (H_1).
- Injected intradermally, histamine causes the 'triple response': reddening from local vasodilatation, wheal by direct action on blood vessels and vasodilatation, and flare from an 'axon' reflex in sensory nerves releasing a peptide mediator.
- The main pathophysiological roles of histamine are:
  —as a stimulant of gastric acid secretion (treated with H_2-receptor antagonists)
  —as a mediator of type 1 hypersensitivity reactions such as urticaria and hay fever (treated with H_1-receptor antagonists).
- H_3-receptors occur at presynaptic sites and inhibit the release of a variety of neurotransmitters.

CNS effects

Histamine is a transmitter in the CNS (p. 485).

It will be clear from the above that histamine is released in inflammation and is capable of producing many of the effects of inflammation and hypersensitivity: vasodilatation, increased vascular permeability and the spasm of smooth muscle. However, histamine H_1 antagonists do not have much effect on the acute inflammatory response per se; other mediators are more important. Histamine has a significant role only in some sorts of type I hypersensitivity reaction, such as allergic rhinitis and urticaria. The use of H_1 antagonists in these and other conditions is dealt with in Chapter 16.

The main pathophysiological role of endogenous histamine is as a mediator of some types of vomiting by an action in the CNS (Ch. 24) and a stimulant of gastric acid secretion by an action on H_2-receptors (Ch. 24). It also has a physiological function as an inhibitor of neurotransmitter release, particularly in the CNS and the gastrointestinal tract.

EICOSANOIDS

Eicosanoids, unlike histamine, are not found preformed in the tissues; they are generated de novo from phospholipids. They are implicated in the control of many physiological processes and are among the most important mediators and modulators of the inflammatory reaction (Fig. 15.5).

Interest in eicosanoids arose in the 1930s after reports that semen contained a substance that contracted uterine smooth muscle. The substance was believed to originate in the prostate and was saddled with the misnomer prostaglandin. Later it became clear that prostaglandin was not just one substance but a whole family of compounds, that they were generated in many if not most tissues and derived from *arachidonic acid*.

Structure and biosynthesis

The main source of the eicosanoids is arachidonic acid (5,8,11,14-eicosatetraenoic acid), a 20-carbon unsaturated fatty acid containing four double bonds (hence 'eicosa' referring to the 20 carbon atoms, and 'tetraenoic' referring to the four double bonds). Arachidonic acid is found esterified in the phospholipids. The principal eicosanoids are the *prostaglandins*, the *thromboxanes* and the *leukotrienes*, though other derivatives of arachidonate, for example the *lipoxins*, are also produced. (The term *prostanoid* will be used here to encompass both prostaglandins and thromboxanes.)

The initial and rate-limiting step in eicosanoid synthesis is the liberation of arachidonate, either in a one-step process (Fig 15.6) or a two-step process (Fig. 15.7). The form of phospholipase A_2 (PLA_2) involved in the generation of arachidonic acid is mainly the intracellular form. Its action can give rise not only to arachidonic acid, and thus the eicosanoids, but also to lysoglyceryl-phosphorylcholine (lyso-PAF), which is the precursor of another mediator of inflammation—PAF (see Figs 15.5 and 15.10, below).

Many stimuli can liberate arachidonic acid, and they vary with the cell type, for example thrombin on platelets, C5a on neutrophils, bradykinin on fibroblasts and antigen–antibody reactions on mast cells. General cell damage also starts the process.

The free arachidonic acid is metabolised by several pathways:

- by fatty acid cyclooxygenase of which there are two forms, COX-1 and COX-2 (see below).* These enzymes initiate the biosynthesis of the prostaglandins and thromboxanes
- by various lipoxygenases (p. 235) which initiate the synthesis of the leukotrienes, the lipoxins and other compounds (Figs 15.5, 15.7 and 15.8).

The anti-inflammatory action of the *glucocorticoids* (Ch. 27) is largely the result of inhibition of induction of cyclooxygenase. These drugs may also stimulate production of the phospholipase A_2 inhibitor *lipocortin* (Fig. 15.5).

The anti-inflammatory action of the *non-steroidal anti-inflammatory drugs* (NSAIDs) results mainly from the fact that they inhibit the action of the fatty acid COXs (Fig. 15.5). Compounds that act selectively on COX-2, the form induced in inflammatory cells, are now available; and compounds that act at specific sites of eicosanoid synthesis (e.g. inhibitors of

*There is now evidence for a third form (Chandrasekharan et al, 2002).

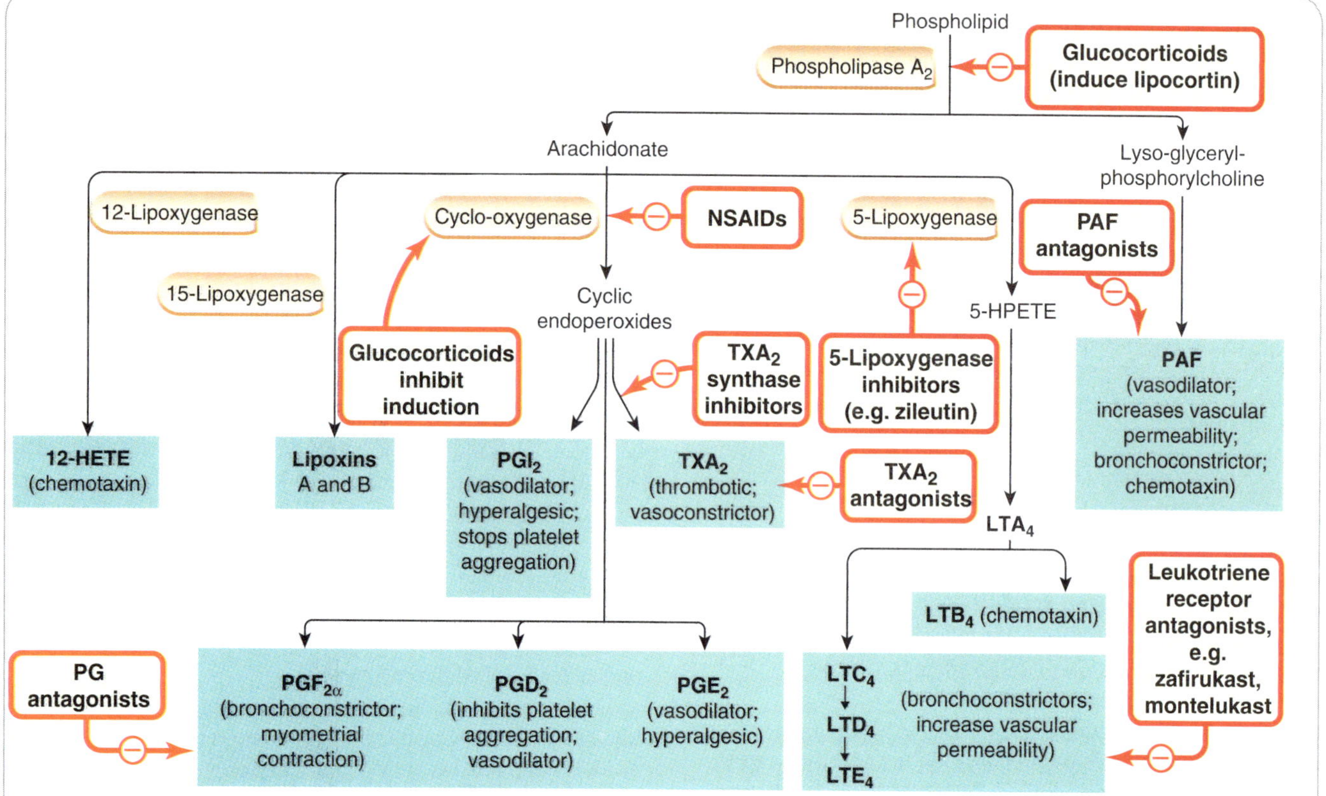

Fig. 15.5 Summary diagram of the inflammatory mediators derived from phospholipids with an outline of their actions, and the sites of action of anti-inflammatory drugs. The arachidonate metabolites are 'eicosanoids'. The glucocorticoids inhibit transcription of the gene for cyclooxygenase-2, which is induced in inflammatory cells by inflammatory mediators. The effects of PGE_2 depend on which of the three receptors for this prostanoid are activated; see text. (PG, prostaglandin; PGI_2, prostacyclin; TX, thromboxane; LT, leukotriene; HETE, hydroxyeicosatetraenoic acid; HPETE, hydroperoxyeicosatetraenoic acid; PAF, platelet-activating factor; NSAIDs, non-steroidal anti-inflammatory drugs; see Ch. 16.)

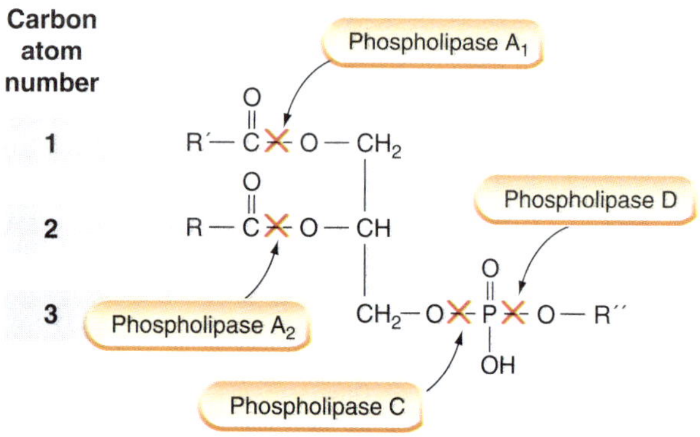

Fig. 15.6 Outline of the structure of phospholipids and the site of action of phospholipases—indicating how arachidonate can be released by a one-step process. The numbering of the carbon atoms in the glycerol 'backbone' is given on the left. Unsaturated fatty acids, such as arachidonic acid, are usually located at R on the second carbon. This figure shows O-acyl residues on carbon atoms 1 and 2, but O-alkyl residues can occur (see Fig. 15.10). (R′ = choline, ethanolamine, serine, inositol or hydrogen.)

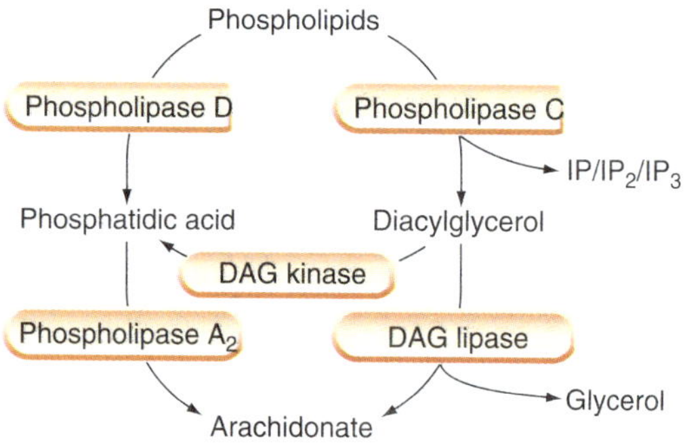

Fig. 15.7 Pathways of release of arachidonate from phospholipids by two-step processes. (IP, inositol phosphate; DAG, diacylglycerol.)

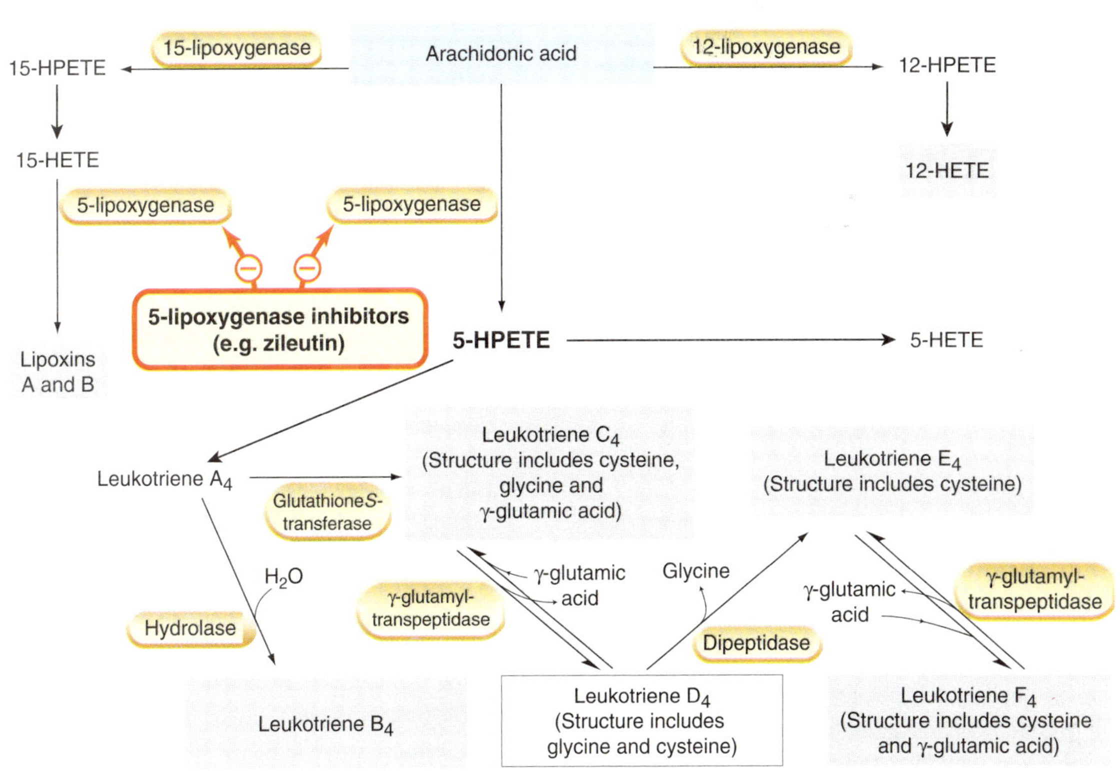

Fig. 15.8 The biosynthesis of leukotrienes from arachidonic acid. Compounds with biological action are shown in pink boxes. (HETE, hydroxyeicosatetraenoic acid; HPETE, hydroperoxyeicosatetraenoic acid.)

5-lipoxygenase and thromboxane synthetase) are being or have been developed, as have specific antagonists of the prostaglandins and leukotrienes (Figs 15.5 and 15.8).

PROSTANOIDS: PRODUCTS OF THE PATHWAY

COX exists in two forms—COX-1 and COX-2. COX-1 is found in most cells as a constitutive enzyme (i.e. it is always present) and it is thought that the prostanoids it produces are involved in normal homeostasis (e.g. regulating vascular responses). COX-2 is induced in inflammatory cells by an inflammatory stimulus. This division of labour, though not completely clear-cut, has relevance for the mechanism of action of present and future NSAIDs.

Subsequent steps in arachidonate metabolism differ in different cells. In platelets, the pathway leads to thromboxane A_2 synthesis, in vascular endothelium it leads to PGI_2 synthesis and in macrophages it leads mainly to synthesis of PGI_2. Mast cells synthesise PGI_2.

▼ The confusing nomenclature of the eicosanoids derives from the fact that the names of the first two prostaglandins were based on the separation procedure—PGE partitioned into ether, and PGF into the phosphate buffer (fosfat in Swedish). PGA and PGB (which are artefacts) were so-called because of their stability or otherwise in acids and bases. Thereafter other letters of the alphabet were filled in rather randomly. The subscripts refer to the number of double bonds; thus PGF_2 has two double bonds. The Greek letter subscript, the α in $PGE_{2\alpha}$, refers to the orientation of the hydroxyl above or below the plane of the ring.

PGE_2, PGI_2, PGD_2, $PGF_{2\alpha}$ and thromboxane A_2 are the most important products of the COX pathway. If the COX acts on eicosatrienoic acid instead of arachidonic acid, the resulting prostanoids have only a single double bond, for example PGE_1.

Catabolism of the prostanoids

Several intracellular enzymes are involved in inactivation of the prostaglandins. After carrier-mediated uptake, there is rapid inactivation by 'prostaglandin-specific' enzymes, then slow inactivation by general fatty-acid-oxidising enzymes. The prostaglandin-specific enzymes are present in high concentration in the lung, and 95% of infused PGE_2, PGE_1 or $PGF_{2\alpha}$ is inactivated on first passage. The half-life of most prostaglandins in the circulation is less than 1 minute.

PGI_2 is not taken up into cells by the transport system in the lung and thus survives passage through the lung. However, it is very short lived (half-life < 5 min).

Thromboxane A_2 is hydrolysed rapidly to the biologically inactive thromboxane B_2 (half-life 30 seconds).

Mediators derived from phospholipids

- The main phospholipid-derived mediators are the eicosanoids (prostanoids and leukotrienes) and platelet-activating factor (PAF).
- The eicosanoids are derivatives of arachidonate that can be released from phospholipid by phospholipase (PL) action, either in one step by PLA_2, or by two steps—PLC then diacylglycerol lipase. Arachidonate can be metabolised either by one of two cyclooxygenases to give rise to various prostanoids, or by 5-lipoxygenase to give rise to various leukotrienes.
- PAF is derived from phospholipid by PLA_2 giving rise to lyso-PAF, which is acetylated to give PAF.

Prostanoid receptors

There are five main classes of prostanoid receptors (Coleman et al., 1993), all of which are typical G-protein-coupled receptors. They are termed DP-, FP-, IP-, TP- and EP-receptors respectively, based on the five classes of natural prostanoids PGD_2, $PGF_{2\alpha}$, PGI_2, PGE_2 and thromboxane A_2; the EP-receptors are further subdivided into three subgroups.

Actions of the prostanoids

The prostanoids affect most tissues, having a bewildering variety of effects.

- PGD_2 causes vasodilatation, inhibition of platelet aggregation, relaxation of gastrointestinal muscle, uterine relaxation, modification of release of hypothalamic/pituitary hormones. (Its bronchoconstrictor effect is the result of an action on TP-receptors.)
- PGF_{2a} causes myometrial contraction in humans (see Ch. 29), luteolysis in some species (e.g. cattle) and bronchoconstriction in other species (cats and dogs).
- PGI_2 causes vasodilatation, inhibition of platelet aggregation (see Ch. 20), renin release and natriuresis via effects on tubular reabsorption of Na^+.
- Thromboxane A_2 causes vasoconstriction, platelet aggregation (see Ch. 20) and bronchoconstriction (the last more marked in guinea-pig than in humans).
- PGE_2 has the following actions:
  —on EP_1-receptors it causes contraction of bronchial and gastrointestinal smooth muscle
  —on EP_2-receptors it causes bronchodilatation, vasodilatation, stimulation of intestinal fluid secretion and relaxation of gastrointestinal smooth muscle
  —on EP_3-receptors it causes contraction of intestinal smooth muscle, inhibition of gastric acid secretion (see Ch. 24 and Fig. 24.2), increased gastric mucus secretion, inhibition of lipolysis, inhibition of autonomic neurotransmitter release and stimulation of contraction of the pregnant human uterus (Ch. 29).

Prostanoids

- The term 'prostanoids' encompasses the prostaglandins (PGs) and the thromboxanes (TXs).
- Cyclooxygenase acts on arachidonate to produce cyclic endoperoxides (PGG_2, PGH_2).
- There are two forms of cyclooxygenase: COX-1, a constitutive enzyme, and COX-2, which is induced in inflammatory cells by inflammatory stimuli.
- PGI_2 (prostacyclin) predominantly from vascular endothelium, acts on IP-receptors. Main effects are vasodilatation and inhibition of platelet aggregation.
- TXA_2 predominantly from platelets acts on TP-receptors. Main effects are platelet aggregation and vasoconstriction.
- PGE_2 is prominent in inflammatory responses and is a mediator of fever. Main effects are:
  —EP_1-receptors: contraction of bronchial and gastrointestinal tract (GIT) smooth muscle
  —EP_2-receptors: relaxation of bronchial, vascular and GIT smooth muscle
  —EP_3-receptors: inhibition of gastric acid secretion, increased gastric mucus secretion, contraction of pregnant uterus and of GIT smooth muscle, inhibition of lipolysis and of autonomic neurotransmitter release.
- $PGF_{2\alpha}$ acts on FP-receptors, which are found in smooth muscle and corpus luteum. Main effect in humans is contraction of the uterus.
- PGD_2 is derived particularly from mast cells and acts on DP-receptors. Its main effects are vasodilatation and inhibition of platelet aggregation.

The role of the prostanoids in inflammation

The inflammatory response is always accompanied by the release of prostanoids, the predominant product being PGE_2, though PGI_2 can also be found. In areas of acute inflammation, PGE_2 and PGI_2 are generated by the local tissues and blood vessels, and mast cells release PGD_2. In chronic inflammation, cells of the monocyte/macrophage series also release PGE_2 and thromboxane A_2.

The prostanoids have a sort of Yin-Yang action in inflammation—stimulating some responses and decreasing others, as follows.

PGE_2, PGI_2 and PGD_2 are powerful vasodilators in their own right and synergise with other inflammatory vasodilators such as histamine and bradykinin. It is this combined dilator action on precapillary arterioles that contributes to the redness and increased blood flow in areas of acute inflammation. These prostanoids do not directly increase the permeability of the postcapillary venules, but they potentiate this effect of histamine and bradykinin. Similarly, they do not themselves produce pain but potentiate the effect of bradykinin by sensitising afferent C

Clinical uses of prostanoids

- Gynaecological and obstetric (see Ch.29):
  - —for termination of pregnancy: **gemeprost** or **misoprostol** (a metabolically stable prostaglandin (PG) E analogue)
  - —for induction of labour: **dinoprostone** or misoprostol
  - —for postpartum haemorrhage: **carboprost** (if no response to other oxytocics).
- Gastrointestinal:
  - —to prevent peptic ulcers in patients taking non-steroidal anti-inflammatory agents: **misoprostol** (see Ch. 24).
- Cardiovascular:
  - —to maintain the patency of the ductus arteriosus until surgical correction of the defect in babies with certain congenital heart malformations: **alprostadil** (PGE_1).
  - —to inhibit platelet aggregation during haemodialysis: PGI_2 (**epoprostenol**) is given if heparin is contraindicated (see Ch. 20). PGI_2 is also used to treat primary pulmonary hypertension.
- Ophthalmic:
  - —open-angle glaucoma: **latanoprost** eyedrops.

fibres (see Ch. 40). The anti-inflammatory effects of the NSAIDs result largely from prevention of these actions of the prostaglandins.

Prostaglandins of the E series are also implicated in the production of fever. High concentrations are found in cerebrospinal fluid in infections, and there is evidence that the increase in temperature generated by endogenous fever-inducing cytokines is mediated by PGE_2. The antipyretic action of NSAIDs (Ch. 16) is the result partly of inhibition of the synthesis of PGE_2 in the hypothalamus.

In addition to the pro-inflammatory mediator function mentioned above, prostaglandins have been shown to have a significant anti-inflammatory modulator role on inflammatory cells, decreasing their activities. For example, PGE_2 decreases lysosomal enzyme release, the generation of toxic oxygen metabolites from neutrophils and histamine release from mast cells. Several prostanoids are available for clinical use (see the box).

LEUKOTRIENES

Leukotrienes are the products of the lipoxygenase pathways. The lipoxygenases, soluble enzymes located in the cytosol, are found in lung, platelets, mast cells and white blood cells.

▼ The main enzyme in this group is 5-lipoxygenase—the first enzyme in the biosynthesis of the leukotrienes ('leuko' because they are found in white cells and 'trienes' because they contain a conjugated triene system of double bonds). On cell activation, this enzyme translocates to the cell membrane where it becomes associated with a protein termed the 'five-lipoxygenase activating protein' (FLAP), which is necessary for leukotriene synthesis in intact cells. The 5-lipoxygenase adds a hydroperoxy group to C5 in arachidonic acid (Fig. 15.8). The next step in the pathway is the synthesis of LTA_4. This compound may be converted enzymically to LTB_4 and is also the precursor for an important class of cysteinyl-containing leukotrienes: LTC_4, LTD_4, LTE_4 and LTF_4 (also referred to as the sulfidopeptide leukotrienes). The first three of this latter group together constitute 'slow-reacting substance of anaphylaxis, (SRS-A), a substance shown many years ago to be generated in guinea-pig lung during anaphylaxis. LTB_4 is produced mainly by neutrophils, and the cysteinyl-leukotrienes mainly by eosinophils, mast cells, basophils and macrophages.

Lipoxins and other active products are also produced from arachidonate (Fig. 15.8).

Metabolism of the leukotrienes

▼ LTB_4 can be converted to 20-hydroxy-LTB_4 by a unique membrane-bound P450 enzyme that occurs in the neutrophil, and it is then further oxidised to 20-carboxy-LTB_4. LTC_4 and LTD_4 are metabolised to LTE_4, which is excreted in the urine.

Actions and receptors* of the leukotrienes

LTB_4 LTB_4 acts on specific LTB_4-receptors, defined by selective agonists and antagonists, the transduction mechanism being generation of inositol trisphosphate and increase of cytosolic Ca^{2+}. LTB_4 is a powerful chemotactic agent for both neutrophils and macrophages (see Fig. 15.2), acting in picogram amounts. On neutrophils, it also causes upregulation of the membrane adhesion molecules and increases the production of toxic oxygen products and the release of granule enzymes. On

*Receptors for the leukotrienes are termed LT-receptors: BLT for the class exemplified by LTB_4 and CysLT for the cysteinyl-leukotrienes LTC_4, LTD_4 and LTE_4, all of which act on the same CysLT-receptor.

Leukotrienes

- 5-Lipoxygenase acts on arachidonate to give 5-hydroperoxyeicosatetraenoic acid (5-HPETE), which is converted to leukotriene (LT) A_4. This, in turn, can be converted to either LTB_4 or to a series of cysteinyl-leukotrienes, LTC_4, LTD_4 and LTE_4, which have amino acids incorporated in their structure.
- LTB_4, acting on specific receptors, causes adherence, chemotaxis and activation of polymorphs and monocytes, and stimulates proliferation and cytokine production from macrophages and lymphocytes.
- The cysteinyl-leukotrienes cause:
  - —contraction of bronchial muscle
  - —vasodilatation in most vessels, but coronary vasoconstriction.
- LTB_4 is an important mediator in all types of inflammation; the cysteinyl-leukotrienes are of particular importance in asthma.

macrophages and lymphocytes, it stimulates proliferation and cytokine release.

Cysteinyl-leukotrienes Specific receptors for LTD_4 have been defined on the basis of numerous selective antagonists. Cysteinyl-leukotrienes have actions on the respiratory and cardiovascular systems.

- *The respiratory system* They are potent spasmogens, causing dose-related contraction of human bronchiolar muscle in vitro. LTE_4 is less potent than LTC_4 and LTD_4, but its effect is much longer lasting. All cause an increase in mucus secretion. Given by aerosol in vivo to human volunteers, they reduce specific airway conductance and maximum expiratory flow rate, the effect being more protracted than that produced by histamine (Fig. 15.9).
- *The cardiovascular system* Small amounts of LTC_4 or LTD_4 given intravenously cause a rapid, short-lived fall in blood pressure, and significant constriction of small coronary resistance vessels. Given subcutaneously they are equipotent with histamine in causing wheal and flare. Given topically in the nose, LTD_4 increases nasal blood flow and increases local vascular permeability.

The role of leukotrienes in inflammation

LTB_4 can be found in inflammatory exudates and is present in the tissues in many inflammatory conditions, including rheumatoid arthritis, psoriasis (a chronic skin disease) and ulcerative colitis. The cysteinyl-leukotrienes are present in the sputum of chronic bronchitis in amounts that are biologically active. On antigen challenge, they are released from samples of human asthmatic lung in vitro and into nasal lavage fluid in vivo in subjects with allergic rhinitis. There is evidence that they contribute to the underlying bronchial hyper-reactivity in asthmatics and it is thought that they are among the main mediators of both the early and late phases of asthma (p. 343 and Fig. 22.2). The CysLT-receptor antagonists **zarfirlukast** and **montelukast** are now in use in the treatment of asthma—the former as adjunct to other anti-asthma drugs, the latter in prevention of the acute attack (see Ch. 22). Iralukast is in the preclinical pipeline.

It is also possible that cysteinyl-leukotrienes have a role in the cardiovascular changes of acute anaphylaxis.

Agents that inhibit the enzymes that generate the leukotrienes—5-lipoxygenase inhibitors—are under development as anti-asthmatic agents (see Ch. 22) and anti-inflammatory agents. **Zileuton** is available but does not seem to have won a definite place in therapy yet.

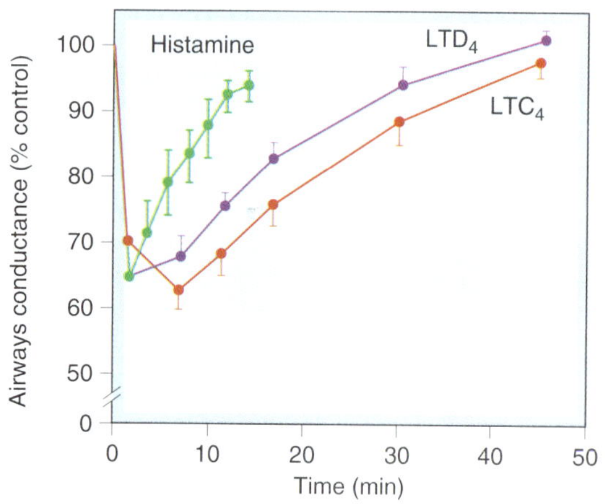

Fig. 15.9 The time course of action on specific airways conductance of the cysteinyl-leukotrienes and histamine, in six normal subjects. Specific airways conductance was measured in a constant volume whole body plethysmograph and the drugs were given by inhalation. (From: Barnes P J, Piper P J, Costello J K 1984 Thorax 39: 500.)

LIPOXINS

Recent work has indicated that lipoxins, products of 15-lipoxygenase (Fig. 15.8), act on specific receptors on polymorphs to oppose the action of LTB_4, giving what might be called 'stop signals' to some aspects of inflammation.

PLATELET-ACTIVATING FACTOR

PAF, which is also variously termed PAF-acether and AGEPC (acetyl-glyceryl-ether-phosphorylcholine), is a biologically active lipid that can produce effects at exceedingly low concentrations (less than 10^{-10} mol/l). The platelet-activating part of the name is misleading, since PAF has actions on a variety of different target cells and is believed to be an important mediator in both acute and persisting allergic and inflammatory phenomena.

PAF (Fig. 15.10) is derived from its precursor, acyl-PAF, by phospholipase A_2 activity, resulting in lyso-PAF, which is then acetylated to give PAF. This, in turn, can be deacetylated to lyso-PAF (Fig. 15.11).

Platelet-activating factor (PAF)

- PAF is released indirectly from many activated inflammatory cells by phopholipase A_2 activity and acts on specific receptors in many cell types.
- Pharmacological actions includes vasodilatation, increased vascular permeability, chemotactic for leucocytes (especially eosinophils), activation of leucocytes, activation and aggregation of platelets and spasmogenic for smooth muscle.
- It is a mediator in many types of inflammation and is implicated in bronchial hyper-responsiveness and in the delayed phase of asthma.

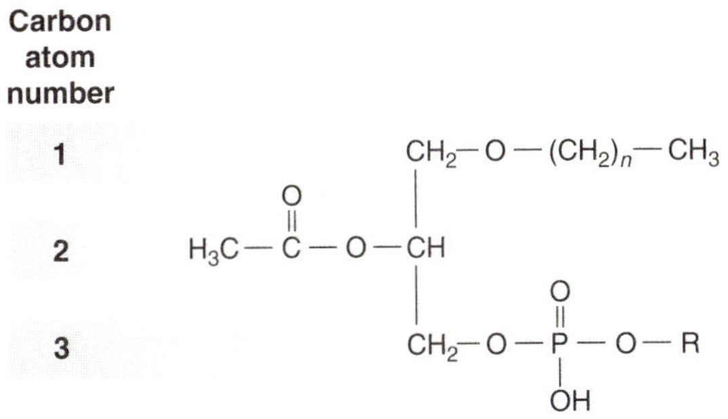

Fig. 15.10 The structure of platelet-activating factor (PAF). An O-alkyl residue is attached to carbon atom 1 (cf. Fig. 15.6). It may be hexadecyl or octadecyl; compounds containing either of these have PAF activity. (R = choline.)

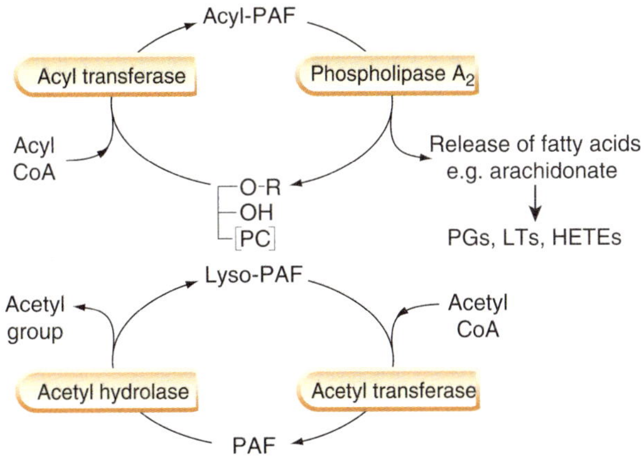

Fig. 15.11 The synthesis and breakdown of platelet-activating factor (PAF). (PC, phosphorylcholine; PG, prostaglandin; LT, leukotriene; HETE, hydroxyeicosatetraenoic acid.)

Sources of PAF

PAF is generated and released from most inflammatory cells when these are stimulated and from platelets on stimulation with thrombin.

Actions and role in inflammation

Acting on specific receptors, PAF has a wide range of pathophysiological actions and is capable of producing many of the phenomena of inflammation. Injected locally, it produces not only local vasodilatation, and thus erythema, but also increased vascular permeability and wheal formation. Higher doses produce hyperalgesia. It is a potent chemotaxin for neutrophils and monocytes and is important in recruiting eosinophils into the bronchial mucosa in the late phase of asthma (Fig. 22.3). It can activate phospholipase A_2 to generate eicosanoids.

On platelets, it causes shape change and the release of the granule contents. This effect is associated with metabolism of arachidonate and thromboxane A_2 generation and is important in haemostasis and thrombosis (see Ch. 20). PAF is also a spasmogen on both bronchial and ileal smooth muscle.

The anti-inflammatory actions of the glucocorticoids may be caused, at least in part, by inhibition of PAF synthesis (Fig. 15.5).

Competitive antagonists of PAF and/or specific inhibitors of lyso-PAF acetyltransferase could well be useful anti-inflammatory drugs and/or anti-asthmatic agents. The PAF antagonist lexipafant is in clinical trial in the treatment of acute pancreatitis. Several other antagonists are being examined in preclinical studies (e.g. apafant and numerous compounds known as yet only by numbers: Web 2086, SR-27417, etc.).

BRADYKININ

Bradykinin and the closely related peptide *kallidin* are vasoactive peptides formed by the action of enzymes on protein substrates termed kininogens (Fig. 15.1). The two peptides are virtually identical (see Fig. 15.13), kallidin possessing one additional amino acid residue.

Source and formation of bradykinin

An outline of the formation of bradykinin from high-molecular-weight kininogen in plasma by kallikrein is given in Figure 15.12.

▼ Prekallikrein is present in plasma as the inactive precursor of the proteolytic enzyme kallikrein. The substrate is kininogen, a plasma α-globulin. There are two forms of kininogen in plasma: high-molecular-weight kininogen (M_r 110 000) and low-molecular-weight kininogen (M_r 70 000). Prekallikrein can be converted to the active enzyme (which is a serine protease) in a variety of ways. One of the physiological activators, particularly in the context of inflammation, is Hageman factor (factor XII of the blood clotting sequence; see Ch. 20 and Fig. 15.1). Hageman factor is normally in an inactive form in the plasma and is activated by contact with surfaces having a negative charge, such as collagen, basement membrane, bacterial lipopolysaccharides, urate crystals and so on. As a

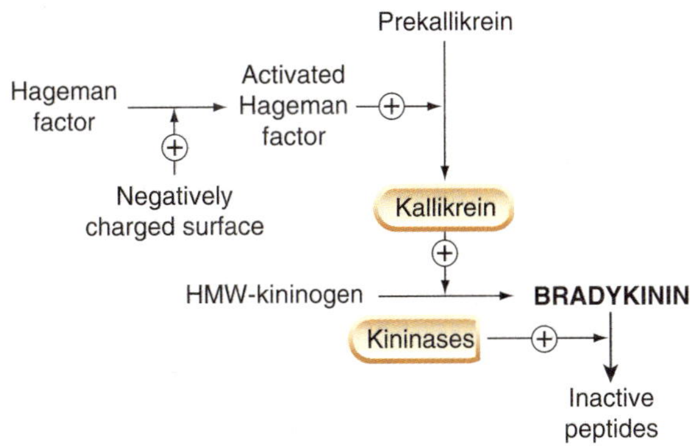

Fig. 15.12 The generation and breakdown of bradykinin. High-molecular-weight kininogen (HMW-kininogen) probably acts both as a substrate for kallikrein and as a cofactor in the activation of prekallikrein.

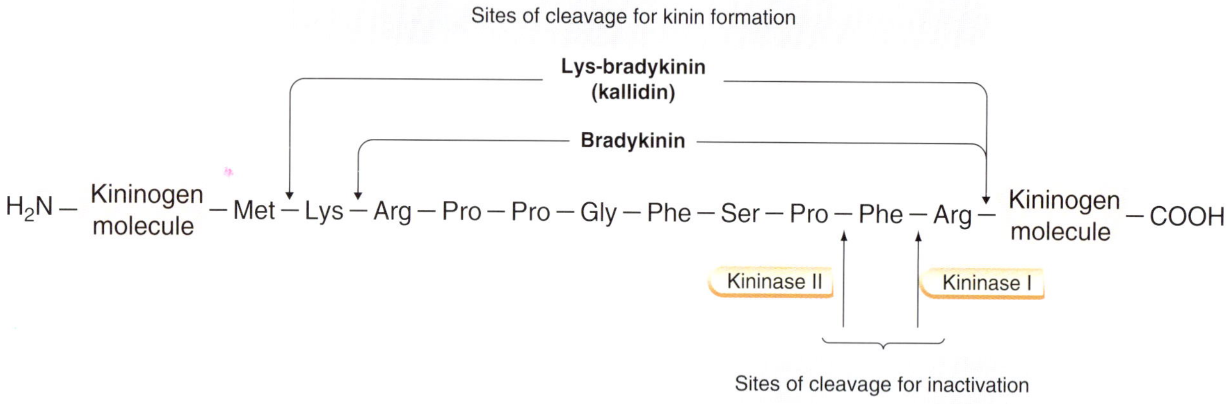

B_2- receptor antagonist, Hoe 140: D-Arg – Arg – Pro – Hyp – Gly – Thi – Ser – D-Tic – Oic – Arg

B_2- receptor antagonist, des-Arg Hoe 140: D-Arg – Arg – Pro – Hyp – Gly – Thi – Ser – D-Tic – Oic

Fig. 15.13 Structure of bradykinin and some bradykinin antagonists. The sites of proteolytic cleavage for formation of kallidin and bradykinin by kallikrein from high-molecular-weight kininogen are shown in the upper half of the figure; the sites of cleavage for bradykinin inactivation are shown in the lower half. The B_2-receptor antagonist icatibant (Hoe 140) has a pA_2 of 9, and the competitive B_1-receptor antagonist des-Arg Hoe 140 has a pA_2 of 8. The Hoe compounds contain unnatural amino acids: Thi, D-Tic and Oic, which are analogues of phenylalanine and proline.

result of the increased vascular permeability that occurs in inflammation, Hageman factor, prekallikrein and the kininogens leak out of the vessels with the plasma (see Fig. 15.1). Contact with the negatively charged surfaces promotes the interaction of prekallikrein and Hageman factor, and this leads to kinin generation, bradykinin being clipped out of the high-molecular-weight kininogen molecules by the enzyme, which acts at two sites to release the nonapeptide (Fig. 15.13). Kallikrein can also activate the complement system and can convert plasminogen to plasmin (see Fig. 15.1 and Ch. 20).

In addition to the plasma kallikrein described above, there are other kinin-generating kallikreins found in pancreas, salivary glands, colon and skin. Tissue kallikreins act on both high- and low-molecular-weight kininogens and generate mainly lysyl-bradykinin (or kallidin), a peptide with actions similar to those of bradykinin.

Inactivation of bradykinin

The main enzymes that inactivate bradykinin and related kinins are called kininases (Figs 15.12 and 15.13). One of these, kininase II, is the same as angiotensin-converting enzyme (see Ch. 18).

▼ Kininase II is a peptidyl dipeptidase that removes the two C-terminal amino acid residues from the kinin, thus inactivating it (Fig. 15.13). The enzyme is bound to the luminal surface of endothelial cells and is found mostly in the lung. It also cleaves the two C-terminal residues from the inactive peptide angiotensin I, converting it to the active vasoconstrictor peptide angiotensin II (see Chs 18 and 23). Thus, the enzyme inactivates a vasodilator and activates a vasoconstrictor.

Kinins are also inactivated by various less-specific kininases; one of these, a carboxypeptidase present in serum (Fig. 15.13), removes the C-terminal arginine from bradykinin, generating des-Arg^9-bradykinin, which is a specific agonist at one of the two main classes of bradykinin receptor (see below).

Actions and role of bradykinin in inflammation

Bradykinin (BK) causes vasodilatation and increased vascular permeability. Its vasodilator action is partly a result of generation of PGI_2 (Fig. 15.5) and the release of NO (Ch. 14). It is a potent pain-producing agent (Ch. 40), an effect that is potentiated by the prostaglandins (see Ch. 40, Fig. 40.6).

Bradykinin is spasmogenic for several types of smooth muscle including that of the intestine and the uterus; bronchial muscle is also contracted in some species. The contraction is slow and sustained in comparison with that produced by histamine (hence brady, which means 'slow').

▼ The pathophysiological function of bradykinin is still a matter of conjecture. The release of bradykinin by tissue kallikrein may be of importance in controlling blood flow to certain exocrine glands, and thus influencing the secretions of the glands. It is known to stimulate ion transport and fluid secretion by various epithelia, including that of the intestine, the airways and the gall bladder. Excessive bradykinin production is probably a factor in causing diarrhoea in many gastrointestinal disorders, and in stimulating nasopharyngeal secretion in allergic rhinitis. It also plays a part in pancreatitis.

On the basis of experimental observations, bradykinin is capable of producing many of the phenomena seen in the inflammatory reaction—pain, vasodilatation, increased vascular permeability and spasm of smooth muscle—but its role in inflammation and allergy has not been clearly defined, not least because its effects

Bradykinin (BK)

- Bradykinin is a nonapeptide. It is clipped out of kininogen, a plasma α-globulin, by a proteolytic enzyme, kallikrein.
- It is converted by kininase I to an octapeptide, BK_{1-8} (des-Arg-BK), which is inactivated by angiotensin-converting enzyme in the lung.
- Pharmacological actions:
  —vasodilatation (largely endothelial cell-dependent, caused both by generation of nitric oxide and by activation of phospholipase A_2, thus releasing prostaglandin I_2)
  —increased vascular permeability
  —stimulation of pain nerve endings
  —stimulation of epithelial ion transport and fluid secretion in airways and gastrointestinal tract
  —contraction of intestinal and uterine smooth muscle.
- There are two main subtypes of BK receptors: B_2, which is constitutively present, and B_1, which is induced in inflammation.
- There are selective competitive antagonists for both B_1-receptors (des-Arg Hoe 140; pA_2:8) and B_2-receptors (icatibant, pA_2:9).

are often part of a complex cascade of events that includes other mediators.

Bradykinin receptors

There are two types of bradykinin receptor, B_1 and B_2, which mediate very similar effects. Both are typical G-protein-coupled receptors.

B_1-receptors are absent in most normal tissues, but are strongly inducible within a few hours under conditions of inflammation and tissue damage; cytokines such as IL-1 are mainly responsible for this induction. B_1-receptors respond to the bradykinin metabolite (des-Arg^9-bradykinin), but not to bradykinin itself, and are selectively blocked by various peptide antagonists. It is likely that B_1-receptors play a significant role in inflammation and hyperalgesia.

B_2-receptors are constitutively present in many normal cells and tissues and are activated by bradykinin and kallidin, but not by the bradykinin metabolite (des-Arg^9-bradykinin). Peptide and non-peptide antagonists have been developed, the best known being icatibant (Hoe 140). None are yet available for clinical use.

NITRIC OXIDE

Chapter 14 discusses NO in detail; here we consider only its role in inflammation.

It is mainly the inducible form of NO synthase (iNOS) that is involved in inflammatory reactions. Virtually all inflammatory cells express the inducible form of the enzyme in response to cytokine stimulation. NOS is also present in the bronchial epithelium of asthmatic subjects, in the mucosa of the colon in patients with ulcerative colitis and in synoviocytes in inflammatory joint disease. NO has mainly pro-inflammatory actions: it is a potent vasodilator; it increases vascular permeability and it increases the production of pro-inflammatory prostaglandins. NO, or compounds derived from it, have cytotoxic action against bacteria, fungi, virus and metazoan parasites, and NO is thought to enhance local defence mechanisms. However, produced in excess, it can be harmful to host cells. Some of its actions are, however, anti-inflammatory since, released from endothelial cells, it inhibits adhesion of neutrophils and platelets and platelet aggregation.

Inhibitors of iNOS are under investigation for treatment of inflammatory conditions. Patients with septic shock have benefited from inhibitors of iNOS, and in experimental arthritis, iNOS inhibitors have significantly reduced disease activity.*

NEUROPEPTIDES

Neuropeptides released from sensory neurons contribute to inflammatory reactions—constituting the phenomenon known as 'neurogenic inflammation' (Maggi, 1996). The main peptides involved are substance P, neurokinin A and CGRP. Substance P and neurokinin A (members of the tachykinin family) act on mast cells, releasing histamine and other mediators, and produce smooth muscle contraction and mucus secretion; CGRP is a potent vasodilator (see Chs 13, 18, 22 and 40). Neurogenic inflammation is implicated in the pathogenesis of several inflammatory conditions including the delayed phase of asthma, allergic rhinitis, inflammatory bowel disease and some types of arthritis.

CYTOKINES

The term cytokine is an elastic one,** generally referring to protein or large peptide mediators released by cells of the immune system.

More than 100 cytokines have been identified, and the cytokine superfamily includes:

- interleukins
- chemokines
- interferons
- colony-stimulating factors (Ch. 21)
- growth factors and tumour necrosis factors.***

Cytokines generally act by autocrine and paracrine mechanisms. On the target cell they bind to and activate specific, high-affinity

*When it comes to the inhibition of the non-inducible form of NOS, it is not the case that no NOS is good NOS.

**Terms like cytokine (and neurotrophin) really belong—like a lot of scientific terms—to tribal dialects, reminding one of the umpteen different words for snow in Icelandic.

***For insulin-like growth factor (IGF-1) see Chapter 30 p. 447; for other growth factors see Chapters 5 and 50 and Figure 50.10.

receptors, which, in most cases, are upregulated in the cell when it is stimulated. Except for chemokines that act on G-protein-coupled receptors, most cytokines act on kinase-linked receptors, which regulate phosphorylation cascades and thereby affect gene expression (Ch. 3).

In addition to their own direct actions on cells, some cytokines induce formation of other cytokines (constituting an amplification cascade); some induce the receptors for other cytokines, and some have synergistic or antagonistic interactions with other cytokines. Cytokines have been likened to a complex signalling language, with the final response of a particular cell involved being determined by a number of different messages received concurrently at the cell surface.

Various classifications of the cytokines can be found in the literature as can a multitude of diagrams depicting complex networks of cytokines interacting with each other and with a range of target cells. The cytokine aficionado can find classification tables in Casciari et al. (1996) and Janeway et al. (2001).

A comprehensive coverage of this area is not possible here. For the purposes of this chapter, we will divide cytokines into two main groups:

- those involved in the induction of the immune response—described above and outlined in Figure 15.5
- those involved in the effector phase of the immune/inflammatory response, which we will consider now.

The effector phase cytokines include both pro-inflammatory and anti-inflammatory peptides.

Pro-inflammatory cytokines These are the cytokines that participate in acute and chronic inflammatory reactions and repair processes. The primary pro-inflammatory cytokines are TNF-α and IL-1* see above (p. 218 and Fig. 15.2). These are released from macrophages and many other cells and can start a cascade of secondary cytokines amongst which are the *chemokines* (see below). Various cytokine growth factors (e.g. platelet-derived growth factor, fibroblast growth factor, vascular endothelial growth factor) are important in repair processes and are implicated in chronic inflammation (see Ch. 5).

The anti-inflammatory cytokines These comprise those that inhibit aspects of the inflammatory reaction) include TGF-β, IL-4, IL-10 and IL-13. They can inhibit the production of chemokines and the last three can inhibit responses mediated by Th1 cells, i.e. those cells whose inappropriate activation is involved in several diseases (see above, p. 224).

CHEMOKINES

Chemokines are defined as chemoattractant cytokines that control the migration of leucocytes, functioning as traffic coordinators in immune and inflammatory reactions.

The nomenclature (and the classification) is a little confusing here since some non-cytokine mediators also control leucocyte movement (C5a, LTB_4, f-Met–Leu–Phe (a bacterial peptide; see p. 221 above and Fig. 15.2)) as do some interleukins (e.g. IL-8; see Fig. 15.2). Furthermore, many chemokines have actions other than as leucocyte attractants, causing mast cell degranulation or promoting angiogenesis.

More than 40 chemokines have been identified and for the simple purposes of those of us who are not professional chemokinologists they can be considered as falling into two main groups depending on chemical structure: the C-X-C group and the C-C group.**

The C-X-C chemokines (main example IL-8; see p. 241 and Fig. 15.2) act on neutrophils and are predominantly involved in acute inflammatory responses. The C-C chemokines (main examples MCP-1 and RANTES, see p. 221) act on monocytes, eosinophils and other cells, and are involved predominantly in chronic inflammatory responses. (RANTES is in the process of being rechristened as CCL5 and MCP-1 as CCL3 and CCL4.)

For most cytokines, the signal transduction mechanisms in the target cell involve the Jak/Stat pathway (see Fig. 50.1), but the chemokines act through G-protein-coupled receptors (Ch. 3).

Alteration or inappropriate expression of chemokine receptors is thought to be implicated in multiple sclerosis, some cancers, rheumatoid arthritis and some cardiovascular diseases (Gerard & Rollins, 2001). Alteration of the chemokine system is known to be involved in some viral infections in that several types of virus (herpesvirus, cytomegalovirus poxvirus and members of the retrovirus family) can exploit the system to subvert the host's response (Murphy, 2001). Numerous viral proteins have been shown to have this ability: some by mimicking host chemokines or chemokine receptors, some by acting as antagonists at chemokine receptors and some by posing as growth factors and angiogenic factors (see Ch. 46, p. 656).

The most audacious exploitation of the host chemokine system is that by the AIDS-causing HIV virus. This virus has a protein (gp120) in its envelope that recognises and binds to CD4 on T cells and also to a chemokine receptor on the T cell surface, which thus functions as a coreceptor for virus binding. This interaction allows viral penetration of the T cell (see Ch. 46, p. 657).

Interferons are considered in more detail below; the colony-stimulating factors are considered in Chapter 21.

INTERFERONS

There are three classes of interferon, termed IFNα, IFNβ and IFNγ. IFNα is not a single substance but a family of approximately 20 proteins with similar activities.

IFNα and IFNβ have antiviral activity and IFNα has some antitumour action. Both are released from virus-infected cells and activate antiviral mechanisms in neighbouring cells.

IFNγ has a role in induction of Th1 responses (p. 225 and Fig. 15.3; see also Abbas et al., 1996).

*IL-1 is really a family of three cytokines consisting of two agonists, IL-1a, IL-1b, and, surprisingly, an endogenous IL-1-receptor *antagonist* (IL-1ra).

**In the C-X-C cytokines, the first two cysteine residues are separated by an intervening amino acid, in the C-C group they are not (Adams & Lloyd, 1997).

Cytokines

- Cytokines are peptides that, in immune and inflammatory reactions, are released from and regulate the action of inflammatory and immune system cells.
- The cytokine superfamily includes the interferons, numerous interleukins, tumour necrosis factor (TNF), various growth factors, the chemokines and the colony-stimulating factors.
- They act in a complex interconnecting network on leucocytes, vascular endothelial cells, mast cells, fibroblasts, haemopoietic stem cells and osteoclasts, controlling proliferation, differentiation and/or activation through autocrine or paracrine mechanisms.
- Interleukin-1 and TNF-α are important primary inflammatory cytokines, inducing the formation of other cytokines.
- The interferons (IFNs) α and β have antiviral activity and IFNα is used as an adjunct in the treatment of viral infections. IFN-γ has significant immunoregulatory function and is used in the treatment of multiple sclerosis.

Clinical use of interferons

IFNα is used in the treatment of chronic hepatitis B and C, has some action against herpes zoster and in the prevention of the common cold. Antitumour action against some lymphomas and solid tumours had been reported. A variety of dose-related side-effects may occur.

IFNβ is used in some patients with multiple sclerosis.

IFNγ is used in chronic granulomatous disease in conjunction with antibacterial drugs.

CURRENT THERAPIES BASED ON MANIPULATION OF THE IMMUNE RESPONSE

IMMUNOGLOBULINS

Normal human immunoglobulin (IgG) derived from pooled human plasma can be used as a replacement therapy in antibody-deficiency states and to protect susceptible subjects against infections with hepatitis A virus, measles, mumps or rubella (German measles). IgG from individuals with high concentrations of antibody specific for certain serious conditions (hepatitis B, rabies, tetanus) is also available.

Monoclonal antibodies

The mAbs are genetically engineered immunoglobulins (IgGs) that react with specific molecular targets. They may be part mouse, part human (termed *humanised* or *chimeric*) or *fully human*. In chimeric mAbs, the antigen-recognising portion of a mouse antibody is joined to the framework of a human IgG molecule. Several are available to treat disease.

- **infliximab**, a chimeric mAb against the cytokine TFN-α used for rheumatoid arthritis (Ch. 16) and Crohn's disease
- **basiliximab**, a chimeric mAb against the receptor for the cytokine IL-2 on activated T cells; used in acute rejection of kidney transplants
- **abciximab**, a chimeric mAb against the clotting receptor GpIIb/IIIa on platelets; used to prevent clotting in patients undergoing coronary angioplasty (Ch. 21)
- **daclizumab**, a humanised mAb against the receptor for the cytokine IL-2 on activated T cells; used in acute rejection of kidney transplants
- **palivusamab**, a humanised mAb against a protein of respiratory syncytial virus (RSV); used to treat RSV infection in children
- **gemtuzumab**, a humanised mAb against an antigen on leukaemia cells, used to treat relapsed acute myeloid leukaemia
- **alemtuzumab**, a humanised mAb against an antigen on T and B lymphocytes used to treat B cell leukaemia
- **rituximab**, a humanised mAb against the cytokine CD20 receptor on B cells; used in non-Hodgkin's lymphoma

Etanercept is a TNF receptor joined to the Fc domain of a human IgG molecule; it is used in rheumatoid arthritis (Ch. 16).

Other mAbs are in the pipeline, notably some that carry radioactive chemicals or toxins directed at tumours.

POTENTIAL NEW THERAPIES

CYTOKINES

The new understanding of the cytokine system, particularly that of specific cytokine–receptor reactions, is expected to result in new therapies for inflammatory and immune-based disease. That this approach could be fruitful is shown by the currently available cytokine-system-based therapies specified above.

Chemokines and their receptors are particularly attractive targets for new drugs because of their selectivity, in that chemokines act on specific receptors on specific subsets of cells (Mackay et al., 1999).

A small non-peptide antagonist of the HIV CCR5 coreceptor on T cells has been shown to have potent and selective anti-HIV activity. It has low toxicity and is in phase I trial. Many more compounds that modify the cytokine system are in development.

IMMUNOTHERAPY

The possibility that peptide immunotherapy, DNA vaccination, immunostimulatory oligonucleotides and vaccination with bacterial products could be used to prevent atopic disease is being considered (see Walker & Zuany-Amorini, 2001).

GLOSSARY OF ACRONYMS

APCs	antigen-presenting cells
C	complement (as in C3a, C5a, C3b, etc.)
CD4 and CD8	co-receptors in T lymphocytes for MHC molecules classes II and I, respectively
COX-1 and COX-2	isoforms of cyclooxygenases
ICAM	intercellular adhesion molecule
IFN	interferon (as in IFN-α, IFN-β, IFN-γ)
IL	interleukin (as in IL-1, IL-2, etc.)
LT	leukotriene (as in LTB_4, LTC_4, LTD_4)
mAbs	monoclonal antibodies
MCP-1	monocyte chemoattractant protein-1
MHC	major histocompatibility complex
NK	natural killer lymphocyte
NSAID	non-steroidal anti-inflammatory drug
PAF	platelet-activating factor
PAMPs	pathogen-associated molecular patterns
PG	prostoglandin (as in PGE_2, PGI_2, etc.)
RANTES	regulated upon activation normal T cell expressed and secreted
Th	T helper lymphocyte (occurs as Th1 and Th2)
TLRs	Toll receptors
TNF-α	tumour necrosis factor-alpha

REFERENCES AND FURTHER READING

Abbas A K, Murphy K M, Sher A 1996 Functional diversity of helper lymphocytes. Nature 383: 787–793 (*Excellent review, helpful diagrams. Commendable coverage of Th1 and Th2 cells and their respective cytokine subsets*)

Adams D H, Lloyd A R 1997 Chemokines: leucocyte recruitment and activation cytokines. Lancet 349: 490-495 (*Commendable review*)

Akira S, Takeda K, Kaisho T 2001 Toll-like receptors: critical proteins linking innate and acquired immunity. Nat Immunol 2: 675–680 (*Article covering the receptors for pathogen-associated molecular patterns (PAMPs) shared by large groups of microorganisms. Stimulation of these receptors by components of microorganisms activates innate immunity, which can be a prerequisite for triggering acquired immunity. Useful diagrams*)

Arrang J M, Garbarg M, Schwartz J C 1983 Autoinhibition of brain histamine release mediated by a novel class (H_3) of histamine receptor. Nature 302: 832–834 (*Seminal article on the existence of H_3-receptors*)

Basan N G, Flower R J 2002 Lipid signals in pain control. Nature 420: 135–138 (*Succinct article describing the significance of the findings of Chandrasekharan et al. (2002) on COX-3*)

Beutler B 2000 The toll-like receptors as the primary sensors of the innate immune system. Immunologist 8: 123–130 (*Clear succinct coverage; good figures*)

Black J W, Duncan W A M, Durant G J et al. 1972 Definition and antagonism of histamine H_2-receptors. Nature 236: 385–390 (*Definitive, seminal article on H_2-receptors*)

Brown P 2001 Cinderella goes to the ball. Nature 410: 1018–1020 (*Pithy lucid review of the new understanding of innate immunity*)

Casciari J J, Sato H et al. 1996 Tabular lexicon of cytokine structure and function. In: Chabner B A, Longo D N (eds) Cancer chemotherapy and biotherapy, 2nd edn. Lippincott-Raven, Philadelphia, pp. 787–793 (*Useful classification bringing order to a confusing field*)

Chandrasekharan N V et al., 2002 COX-3, a cyclooxygenase-1 variant inhibited by acetaminophen and other analgesic/antipyretic drugs: cloning, structure, and expression. Proc Natl Acad Sci 2002 99: 13926–31 (*A new COX isozyme is described: COX-3. In humans, COX-3 mRNA is expressed most abundantly in cerebral cortex and heart. It is selectively inhibited by analgesic/antipyretic drugs such as paracetamol (acetaminophen) and is inhibited by some other NSAIDs. It is suggested that this could be how these drugs decrease pain and possibly fever.*)

Coleman R A, Humphrey P A et al. 1993 Prostanoid receptors: their function and classification. In: Vane J, O'Grady J (eds) Therapeutic applications of prostaglandins. Edward Arnold, London, ch. 2, pp. 15–36 (*Useful coverage; includes structures of prostanoids, their analogues and antagonists. A classification that brought order to chaos*)

Dale M M 1994 Summary of section on mediators. In: Dale M M, Foreman J C, Fan T-P (eds) Textbook of immunopharmacology, 3rd edn. Blackwell Scientific, Oxford, pp. 206–207 (*Considers which mediators meet defined criteria*)

Dale M M, Foreman J C, Fan T-P (eds) 1994 Textbook of immunopharmacology, 3rd edn. Blackwell Scientific, Oxford (*Simple textbook written with second and third year medical and science students in mind*)

Delves P J, Roitt I M 2000 The immune system. N Engl J Med 343: 37–49, 108–117 (*A good overview of the immune system—a mini-textbook of major areas in immunology. Colourful three-dimensional figures*)

Ezzell C 2001 Magic bullets fly again. Sci Am Oct: 28–35 (*Simple clear article on monoclonal antibodies; excellent figures*)

Foreman J C 1994 Mast cells and basophil leucocytes. In: Dale M M, Foreman J C, Fan T-P (eds) Textbook of immunopharmacology, 3rd edn. Blackwell Scientific, Oxford, ch. 2, pp. 21–34 (*Simple outline of the role of these cells in inflammation*)

Gabay C, Kushner I 1999 Acute phase proteins and other systemic responses to inflammation. N Engl J Med 340: 448–454 (*Lists the acute phase proteins and outlines the mechanisms controlling acute phase protein changes by cytokines and other chemical mediators*)

Gerard C, Rollins B 2001 Chemokines and disease. Nat Immunol 2: 108-115 (*Discusses various diseases that are associated with inappropriate activation of the chemokine network and discusses therapeutic implications. Describes mimicry of the chemokine system by viral proteins enabling viruses to evade the immune responses*)

Glennie M J, Johnson P W M 2000 Clinical trials of antibody therapy. Immunol Today 21:403–410 (*Proficient coverage of monoclonal antibodies (mAbs) and their potential in treatment. A table lists 70 currently in development for a variety of conditions, many in phase I, II or III trial*)

Horuk R 2001 Chemokine receptors. Cytokine Growth Factor Rev 12: 313–335 (*Comprehensive review focusing on recent findings in chemokine receptor research and discussing the molecular, physiological and biochemical properties of each chemokine receptor*)

Janeway C A, Travers P, Walport M, Shlomchik M 2001 Immunobiology: the immune system in health and disease, 2nd edn. Churchill Livingstone, Edinburgh (*Excellent textbook, good diagrams*)

Kärre K, Welsh R M 1997 Viral decoy vetoes killer cell. Nature 386: 446-447 (*Elegant short article*)

Kay A B 2001 Allergic diseases and their treatment. N Engl J Med 344: 30–37, 109–113 (*Covers atopy and Th2 cells; the role of Th2 cytokines in allergies, IgE, the main types of allergy and new therapeutic approaches*)

Luster A D 1998 Mechanisms of disease: chemokines—chemotactic cytokines that mediate inflammation. N Engl J Med 338: 436–445 (*Excellent review; outstanding diagrams*)

Mackay C R 2001 Chemokines: immunology's high impact factors. Nat Immunol 2: 95–101 (*Clear elegant coverage of the role of chemokines in leukocyte–endothelial interaction, control of primary immune responses and T/B cell interaction, T cells in inflammatory diseases and viral subversion of immune responses*)

Mackay C R, Lanzavecchia A, Sallusto F 1999 Chemoattractant receptors and immune responses. Immunologist 7: 112–118 (*Masterly short review covering the role of chemoattractants in orchestrating immune responses—both the innate reaction and Th1 and Th2 responses*)

Maggi C A 1996 Pharmacology of the efferent function of primary sensory neurones. In: Geppetti P, Holzer P (eds) Neurogenic inflammation. CRC Press, London (*Worthwhile. Covers neurogenic inflammation: the release of neuropeptides from sensory nerves by inflammatory mediators. Discusses agents that inhibit release and pharmacological modulation of the receptors mediating release*)

Mantovani A, Bussolino F, Introna M 1997 Cytokine regulation of endothelial cell function: from molecular level to the bedside. Immunol Today 5: 231–239 (*Pathophysiology of endothelial cell–cytokine interactions; detailed diagrams*)

Medzhitov R 2001 Toll-like receptors and innate immunity. Nat Rev Immunol 1: 135–145 (*Excellent review of the role of Toll-like receptors in (a) the detection of microbial infection and (b) the activation of innate non-adaptive responses, which in turn lead to antigen-specific adaptive responses*)

Medzhitov R, Janeway C 2000 Innate immunity. N Engl J Med 343: 338–344 (*Outstanding clear coverage of the mechanisms involved in innate immunity and its significance for the adaptive immune response*)

Murphy P M 2001 Viral exploitation and subversion of the immune system through chemokine mimicry. Nat Immunol 2: 116–122 (*Excellent description of viral/immune system interaction*)

Panes J, Perry M, Granger D N 1999 Leucocyte–endothelial cell adhesion: avenues for therapeutic intervention. Br J Pharmacol 126: 537–550 (*Brief coverage of main cell adhesion molecules and factors affecting leucocyte–endothelial adhesion precedes consideration of potential therapeutic targets*)

Parkin J, Cohen B 2001 An overview of the immune system. Lancet 357: 1777–1789 (*A competent straightforward review covering the role of the immune system in recognising, repelling and eradicating pathogens and reacting against molecules foreign to the body*)

Roitt I, Brostoff J, Male D 1998 Immunology, 9th edn. Blackwell Science, Oxford (*Excellent textbook; well illustrated*)

Romagnani S 1996 Short analytical review: Th1 and Th2 in human diseases. Clin Immunol Immunopathol 80: 225–235 (*Admirable coverage of the pathophysiology of Th1 and Th2 responses*)

Romagnani S 1997 The Th1/Th2 paradigm. Immunol Today 18: 263–265 (*Excellent succinct coverage of Th1/Th2 polarisation. Helpful diagrams*)

Roth J, LeRoith D et al. 1982 The evolutionary origins of hormones, neurotransmitters and other extracellular chemical messengers. N Engl J Med 306: 523–527 (*Details evidence that chemical mediators/neurotransmitters which we assume occur only in humans are in fact evolutionary ancient devices for inter- and intracellular communication*)

Samuelsson B 1983 Leukotrienes: mediators of immediate hypersensitivity reactions and inflammation. Science 220: 568–575 (*Seminal article on leukotrienes*)

Szolcsànyi J 1996 Neurogenic inflammation: reevaluation of the axon reflex theory. In: Geppetti P, Holzer P (eds) Neurogenic inflammation. CRC Press, London, ch. 3, pp. 33–42 (*Good coverage of the basis of neurogenic inflammation*)

Ulrich H, von Andrian U H, Englehardt B 2003 α4 Integrins as therapeutic targets in autoimmune disease. N Engl J Med 348: 68–70 (*Editorial commenting on two articles in the journal that describe the use of natalizumab, a recombinant monoclonal antibody, for the treatment of the inflammatory/immune diseases: multiple sclerosis and Crohn's disease. Natalizumab binds to α4 integrins on haemopoietic cells and prevents them from binding to their endothelial receptors.*)

Vane J R 1971 Inhibition of prostaglandin synthesis as a mechanism of action for aspirin-like drugs. Nat New Biol 231: 232–239 (*Definitive, seminal article on the mechanism of action of aspirin as inhibitor of prostanoid synthesis*)

Walker C, Zuany-Amorini C 2001 New trends in immunotherapy to prevent atopic disease. Trends Pharmacol Sci 22: 84–91 (*Discusses potential therapies based on recent advances in the understanding of the immune mechanisms of atopy*)

Wills-Karp M, Santeliz J, Karp C L 2001 the germless theory of allergic diseases. Nat Rev Immunol 1: 69–75 (*Discusses the hypothesis that early childhood infections inhibit the tendency to develop allergic disease*)

16 Anti-inflammatory and immunosuppressant drugs

Overview 244

Non-steroidal anti-inflammatory drugs 244
- Pharmacological actions 244
- Mechanism of action 247
- Common unwanted effects 247
- Some important NSAIDs 250
- Agents selective for cyclooxygenase 2 252

Antagonists of histamine 252

Drugs used in gout 254

Antirheumatoid drugs 255

Immunosuppressant drugs 257

Possible future developments 260

OVERVIEW

This chapter deals with the drugs used to treat inflammatory and immune disorders. Inappropriate inflammatory or immune reactions are involved in many if not most of the diseases that the clinician will meet, and the drugs used to treat these conditions are very extensively used in medical practice.

The main *anti-inflammatory agents* are the *glucocorticoids* and the *non-steroidal anti-inflammatory drugs* (NSAIDs). The glucocorticoids are dealt with in detail in Chapter 27 and their immunosuppressive actions are discussed briefly at the end of this chapter. The NSAIDs are dealt with below and, in dealing with them, we describe the pharmacological actions common to all of them, their mechanism of action and unwanted effects. Then we deal in a little more detail with aspirin, paracetamol and the new drugs that are selective for cyclooxygenase 2.

Other anti-inflammatory drugs considered in this chapter are the *antirheumatoid agents* and drugs used to treat gout. The *histamine H_1-receptor antagonists*, though not strictly anti-inflammatory agents, are also dealt with under this heading.

The main drugs affecting the immune response are the *immunosuppressants*.

NON-STEROIDAL ANTI-INFLAMMATORY DRUGS

Non-steroidal anti-inflammatory drugs (NSAIDs) are among the most widely used of all therapeutic agents worldwide. Some important examples are listed in Table 16.1. They are frequently prescribed for 'rheumatic' musculoskeletal complaints and are often taken without prescription for minor aches and pains. There are now more than 50 different NSAIDs on the market and none of these is ideal in controlling or modifying the signs and symptoms of inflammation, particularly those that occur in the common inflammatory joint diseases. Virtually all currently available NSAIDs, more particularly the 'classical' NSAIDs, can have significant unwanted effects, especially in the elderly. Newer agents have fewer and less serious adverse actions.

PHARMACOLOGICAL ACTIONS

NSAIDs include a variety of different agents of different chemical classes. Most of these drugs have three major types of effect:

- anti-inflammatory effects: modification of the inflammatory reaction
- analgesic effect: reduction of certain sorts of pain
- antipyretic effect: lowering of a raised temperature.

In general, all of these effects are related to the primary action of the drugs—inhibition of arachidonate cyclooxygenase and thus inhibition of the production of prostaglandins and thromboxanes—though some aspects of the action of individual drugs may occur by different mechanisms; in addition, some drugs have actions other than those on inflammation.

There are two types of cyclooxygenase enzyme,* namely COX-1 and COX-2. COX-1 is a constitutive enzyme expressed in most tissues, including blood platelets. It has a house-keeping role in the body being involved in tissue homeostasis. COX-2 is induced in inflammatory cells when they are activated, and the primary inflammatory cytokines—interleukin-1 (IL-1) and

*A third form, COX-3, has recently been described (Chandrasekharan et al, 2002).

Table 16.1 Comparison of some commonly used NSAIDs

Drug	Plasma half-life (hours)	Comments
Non-selective COX inhibitors		
Aspirin	3–5	See text, p. 250
Diflunisal	8–13	Less GIT irritation than aspirin; long acting (is related to aspirin)
Ibuprofen	2	First-choice drug; lowest incidence of unwanted effects
Fenbufen	10	A pro-drug, activated in the liver; less risk of GIT, reactions, more risk of skin reactions
Naproxen	14	The same chemical class as ibuprofen but rather more potent; reasonable efficacy, moderate risk of adverse reactions
Mefenamic acid	4	Only moderate anti-inflammatory action; diarrhoea likely; haemolytic anaemia has been reported; possible interaction with warfarin; skin reactions can occur
Nabumetone	24[a]	A pro-drug, activated in the liver; adverse effects less marked than with aspirin, antipyretic action more marked
Paracetamol	2–4	See text, p. 251
Diclofenac	1–2	Moderate potency; moderate risk of adverse GIT effects
Sulindac	7 (18)[a]	A pro-drug interconvertible with active sulfide metabolite; moderate risk of side-effects; chemically related to indometacin but less potent
Indometacin	2	Potent inhibitor of COX in vitro; high incidence of non-GIT side-effects;[b] headache, dizziness, etc.
Tolmetin	5	Efficacy as for ibuprofen; moderate risk of adverse effects
Piroxicam	45	GIT irritation in 20% of patients; tinnitus; rashes
Tenoxicam	72	Steady-state plasma concentration only after 2 weeks
Etodalac	7	Possibly fewer GIT effects than other non-selective NSAIDs
Meloxicam	20	Possibly fewer GIT effects than other non-selective NSAIDs
COX-2 inhibitors		
Celecoxib	11	New compound; markedly less GIT toxicity
Rofecoxib	17	New compound; markedly less GIT toxicity

GIT, gastrointestinal tract; COX, cyclooxygenase.
[a]Half-life of metabolite.
[b]See MacDonald et al., 1997.

tumour necrosis factor-α (TNF-α) (see Ch. 15)—are important in this regard. Thus COX-2 is responsible for the production of the prostanoid mediators of inflammation* (Vane & Botting, 2001). Most traditional NSAIDs in current use are inhibitors of both isoenzymes, though they vary in the degree of inhibition of each (Fig. 16.1).

It has become clear that the anti-inflammatory action of the NSAIDs is mainly related to their inhibition of COX-2 and that, when used as anti-inflammatory agents, their unwanted effects—particularly those affecting the gastrointestinal tract—are largely a result of their inhibition of COX-1. Compounds with a selective action on COX-2 are now in clinical use, and more are in development. It is expected that these COX-2 inhibitors could transform the approach to the treatment of inflammatory conditions. The relative selectivity for COX-2 of the currently available NSAIDs is given in Figure 16.1

There are no really significant differences in the main pharmacological actions cited above between the currently used NSAIDs, with the exception that paracetamol** is generally believed to have little or no anti-inflammatory action and both indometacin and piroxicam are more strongly anti-inflammatory than the others;** but there are marked differences in toxicity and some degree of difference in patient tolerance. Aspirin, however, has other qualitatively different pharmacological actions (see pp. 250–251).

The main pharmacological actions and the common side-effects of the NSAIDs are outlined below, followed by a more

*COX-2 has other roles, unrelated to inflammation. Constitutive COX-2 is found in the CNS; it is known to be important in renal haemodynamics and there is evidence that it is involved in the development of malignancy since there is increased expression of COX-2 in tumours such as breast cancer and colon cancer (see Ch. 50).

**There is a difference of opinion about this, see below.

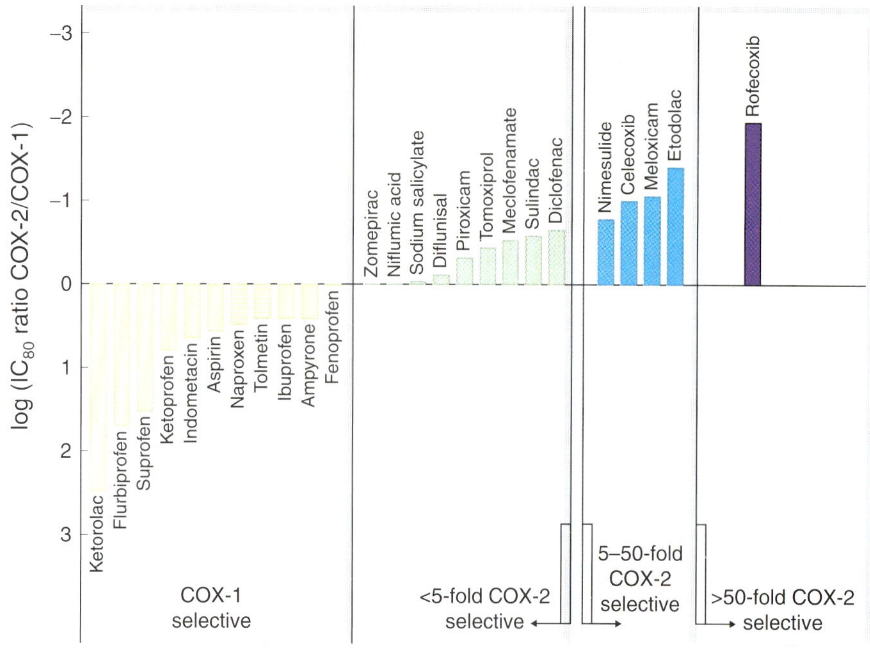

Fig. 16.1 A comparison of cyclooxygenase (COX) isozyme selectivity of non-steroidal anti-inflammatory drugs (NSAIDs). The graph shows the effect of various NSAIDs on COX-1 at a dose that gives an 80% inhibition of COX-2. The 0 line indicates equal potency. Those below the line have selectivity for COX-1. Some above the line have a less than fivefold selectivity to COX-2. The next group, containing meloxicam, etodolac, celecoxib and nimuselide, have a 50-fold selectivity towards COX-2; but note that all can produce full inhibition of COX-1. Only rofecoxib has a greater than 50-fold selectivity for COX-2. Activity measured in whole blood assay. (Modified from Warner et al. 1999 Proc Natl Acad USA 96: 7563–7568 as adapted by Vane 2000 Thorax 55: S3–S9.)

The cyclooxygenase (COX) enzymes

- There are two COX enzymes: COX-1 and COX-2.
- COX-1 is a constitutive, housekeeping enzyme involved in tissue homeostasis.
- COX-2 is induced in inflammatory cells and produces the prostanoid mediators of inflammation.
- Cox-3 has recently been described

detailed coverage of aspirin and paracetamol, an outline of the pharmacology of the selective COX-2 inhibitors and finally the clinical applications of the group as a whole.

ANTIPYRETIC EFFECT

Normal body temperature is regulated by a centre in the hypothalamus that ensures a balance between heat loss and heat production. Fever occurs when there is a disturbance of this hypothalamic 'thermostat', which leads to the set-point of body temperature being raised. NSAIDs reset the thermostat. Once there has been a return to the normal set-point, the temperature-regulating mechanisms (dilatation of superficial blood vessels, sweating, etc.) then operate to reduce temperature. Normal temperature is not affected by NSAIDs.

NSAIDs are thought to be antipyretic largely through inhibition of prostaglandin production in the hypothalamus. During an inflammatory reaction, bacterial endotoxins cause the release from macrophages of a pyrogen—IL-1 (Ch. 15)—which stimulates the generation, in the hypothalamus, of E-type prostaglandins (PGEs) and these, in turn, cause the elevation of the set-point for temperature. COX-2 may have a role here since it is induced by IL-1 in blood vessel endothelium in the hypothalamus. COX-3 may be implicated in fever.

There is some evidence that prostaglandins are not the only mediators of fever; hence NSAIDs may have an additional antipyretic effect by mechanisms as yet unknown.

ANALGESIC EFFECT

NSAIDs are mainly effective against pain associated with inflammation or tissue damage because they decrease production of the prostaglandins that sensitise nociceptors to inflammatory mediators such as bradykinin (see Chs 15 and 40). Therefore, they are effective in arthritis, bursitis, pain of muscular and vascular origin, toothache, dysmenorrhoea, the pain of postpartum states and the pain of cancer metastases in bone—all conditions that are associated with increased prostaglandin synthesis. In combination with opioids, they decrease postoperative pain and in some cases can reduce the requirement for opioids by as much as one third. Their ability to relieve headache may be related to the abrogation of the vasodilator effect of prostaglandins on the cerebral vasculature.

There is some evidence that they have a central effect by an action mainly in the spinal cord.

ANTI-INFLAMMATORY EFFECTS

As has been described in Chapter 15, there are many chemical mediators of the inflammatory and allergic response. Each facet of the response—vasodilatation, increased vascular permeability, cell accumulation, etc.—can be produced by several different mechanisms. Furthermore, different mediators may be of particular importance in different inflammatory and allergic conditions and some mediators have complex interactions with others; for example, small amounts of nitric oxide (NO) stimulate cyclooxygenase activity, while large amounts inhibit it.

Drugs such as the NSAIDs reduce mainly those components of the inflammatory and immune response in which the products of COX-2 action play a significant part, namely:

- vasodilatation
- oedema (by an indirect action: the vasodilatation facilitates and potentiates the action of mediators such as histamine that increase the permeability of postcapillary venules; see p. 230)
- pain (see above).

Cyclooxygenase inhibitors, per se, have no effect on those processes (lysosomal enzyme release, toxic oxygen radical production) that contribute to tissue damage in chronic inflammatory conditions such as rheumatoid arthritis, vasculitis and nephritis.

MECHANISM OF ACTION

The main action of NSAIDs is, as stated above, inhibition of arachidonic acid-metabolising activity of COX (see Figs 15.5 and 16.2), as described originally by Vane in 1971.

The cyclooxygenase enzymes are bifunctional, having two distinct activities: the main action, which gives PGG_2, and a peroxidase action, which converts PGG_2 to PGH_2. Both COX-1 and COX-2 inhibitors inhibit only the main cyclooxygenation reaction. Both COX-1 and COX-2 are associated with the membrane and each consists of a long channel with a bend at the end, the channel being wider in COX-2 (Fig. 16.2). The opening of the channel is largely hydrophobic. Arachidonic acid enters, is twisted round the bend and has two oxygens inserted and a free radical extracted, resulting in the 5-carbon ring characteristic of the prostaglandins (Hawkey, 1999).

▼ A simplified explanation of the effect of inhibitors of the COX enzymes is as follows. The traditional NSAIDs block both enzymes halfway down the channel by hydrogen bonding to a polar arginine at position 120. Most NSAIDs act reversibly, mainly by excluding arachidonate, but aspirin binds to and acetylates the serine at position 530, causing irreversible inactivation of the enzymes.

The crucial difference between the two COX enzymes is at position 523; here COX-1 has a bulky isoleucine while COX-2 has a valine—a smaller molecule that leaves a gap which gives access to a side-pocket (see Fig. 16.2). It is this side-pocket that is believed to be the binding site for COX-2-selective agents, which, in general, have a rigid side-extension that can reach across the channel and interact with the pocket. This aspect of their structure appears to be the basis of their selectivity for COX-2: they may be too bulky to fit into the COX-1 channel (Hawkey, 1999).

COX-1 inhibition, in general, is instantaneous and competitively reversible. (But note that aspirin action is qualitatively different; see above.) COX-2 inhibition is time dependent, i.e. its effect increases with time.

Other actions besides inhibition of COX may contribute to the anti-inflammatory effects of some NSAIDs. Reactive oxygen radicals produced by neutrophils and macrophages are implicated in tissue damage in some conditions, and NSAIDs that have particularly strong oxygen-radical-scavenging effects as well as COX-inhibitory activity (such as **sulindac**) may decrease tissue damage. Aspirin has been shown to inhibit expression of the transcription factor NF-κB, which has a key role in the transcription of the genes for inflammatory mediators (p. 219).

Non-steroidal anti-inflammatory drugs (NSAIDs)

NSAIDs have three major pharmacologically desirable actions, all of which result mainly from the inhibition of arachidonic acid cyclooxygenase in inflammatory cells (the COX-2 isoenzyme), and the resultant decrease in prostanoid synthesis. They are:

- An anti-inflammatory action: the decrease in vasodilator prostaglandins (PGE_2, prostacyclin) means less vasodilatation and, indirectly, less oedema. Accumulation of inflammatory cells is not reduced.
- An analgesic effect: decreased prostaglandin generation means less sensitisation of nociceptive nerve endings to inflammatory mediators such as bradykinin and 5-hydroxytryptamine. Relief of headache is probably a result of decreased prostaglandin-mediated vasodilatation.
- An antipyretic effect: this is partly owing to a decrease in the mediator prostaglandin (which is generated in response to the inflammatory pyrogen interleukin-1) that is responsible for elevating the hypothalamic set-point for temperature control, thus causing fever.

Some important examples are aspirin, ibuprofen, naproxen, indometacin, piroxicam, paracetamol. Newer agents with more selective inhibition of COX-2 (and thus fewer adverse effects on the gastrointesinal tract) are celecoxib and rofecoxib.

COMMON UNWANTED EFFECTS

NSAIDs are responsible for numerous adverse reactions worldwide, and they also feature in the reports of drug-related deaths. Although this may be partly because NSAIDs are used extensively in the elderly, the inherent toxicity of these drugs is clearly a contributory factor. When the classical NSAIDs are used in joint diseases (which usually necessitates fairly large doses and long-continued use), there is a high incidence of side-effects—more particularly in the gastrointestinal tract but also in liver,

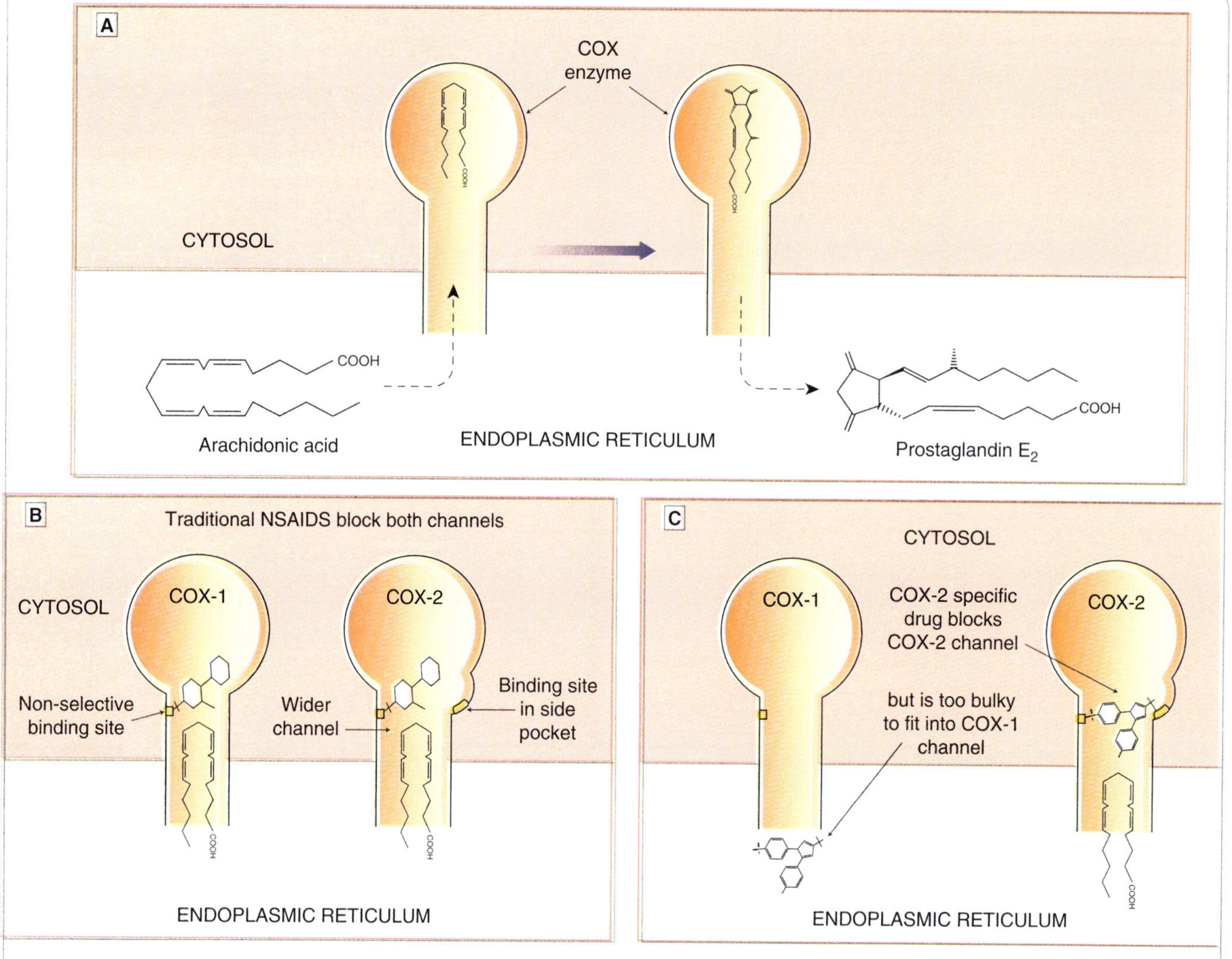

Fig. 16.2 Schematic diagram comparing the action of traditional non-steroidal anti-inflammatory drugs (NSAIDs) and NSAIDs that are selective for cyclooxygenase (COX) 1 or 2. A Arachidonic acid enters the COX enzyme channel and is converted first to prostaglandin G_2 then to prostaglandin H_2 (these steps not shown) then into a prostaglandin, the example shown here being prostaglandin E_2. B Flurbiprofen blocks both COX-1 and COX-2 channels. C The predicted basis of the specificity of the COX-2-selective agents; a COX-2-selective agent is effective in blocking the COX-2 channel but has little effect on COX-1. (Modified from Hawkey 1999.)

kidney, spleen, blood and bone marrow. The new COX-2-selective drugs have minimal gastrointestinal toxicity (see below).

GASTROINTESTINAL DISTURBANCES

Adverse gastrointestinal events are the commonest unwanted effects of the NSAIDs and result mainly from inhibition of COX-1. COX-1 action is responsible for the synthesis of the prostaglandins that normally inhibit acid secretion, as well as having a protective action on the mucosa (see p. 370 and Fig. 24.2).

Common gastrointestinal side-effects are dyspepsia, diarrhoea (but sometimes constipation), nausea and vomiting and, in some cases, gastric bleeding and ulceration. It has been estimated that one in five chronic users of non-selective NSAIDs will have gastric damage, which can be silent but which carries a small but definite risk of serious haemorrhage and/or perforation. Figure 16.3 gives the relative risks of gastrointestinal damage with some of the traditional NSAIDs. Oral administration of prostaglandin analogues such as **misoprostol** (Ch. 15, clinical box on p. 235) can diminish the gastric damage produced by these agents.

It had been predicted that the use of COX-2-selective agents (p. 231) would result in less gastric damage; and two large,

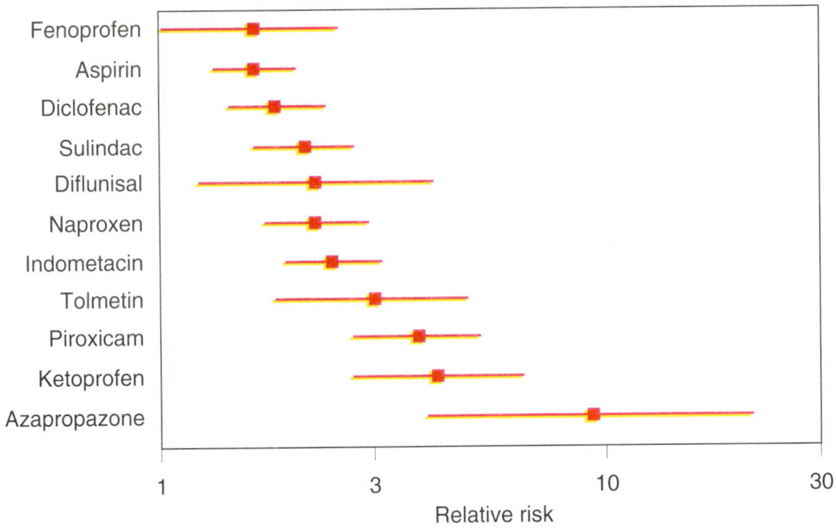

Fig. 16.3 The risk of gastrointestinal complications with various non-steroidal anti-inflammatory drugs (NSAIDs), relative to the risk with ibuprofen (relative risk = 1). Ibuprofen, given in a dose of 1200 mg daily, itself carries a risk double that of placebo. The lines represent 95% confidence intervals. (From a figure by Hawkey C J 2001. Data derived from a meta-analysis of 12 comparative studies in Henry et al. 1996.)

randomised, double-blind studies comparing a selective COX-2 inhibitor with a COX-1 inhibitor in patients with arthritis have proved this to be so. The COX-2 inhibitors caused significantly less damage, but they were associated with small but potentially clinically relevant cardiovascular changes in some patients (Boers, 2001; Fitzgerald & Partonto, 2001). Boers analyses the two trials cited and draws the conclusion that 'in patients who do not require platelet inhibition, selective COX-2 inhibitors seem to be a true advance and an attractive alternative to classic NSAIDs combined with gastroprotective strategies', but points out that cardiologists and rheumatologists should routinely consider gastroprotection alongside cardioprotection.

SKIN REACTIONS

Skin reactions are the second most common unwanted effects of NSAIDs, particularly with **mefenamic acid** (10–15% frequency) and **sulindac** (5–10% frequency). The type of skin condition seen varies from mild rashes, urticaria and photosensitivity reactions to more serious and potentially fatal diseases (which are fortunately rare).

ADVERSE RENAL EFFECTS

Therapeutic doses of NSAIDs in healthy individuals pose little threat to kidney function, but in susceptible patients they cause acute renal insufficiency, which is reversible on stopping the drug. This occurs through the inhibition of the biosynthesis of those prostanoids (PGE_2 and prostaglandin I_2 (PGI_2, prostacyclin)) involved in the maintenance of renal blood dynamics, and more particularly in the PGE_2-mediated compensatory vasodilatation that occurs in response to the action of noradrenaline or angiotensin II (see Ch. 23).

Chronic NSAID consumption can cause 'analgesic nephropathy': chronic nephritis and renal papillary necrosis. Phenacetin, now withdrawn, was the main culprit. It is rapidly metabolised to paracetamol and there is now a suggestion that paracetamol (and possibly some other NSAIDs) taken regularly in high doses over a long period could increase the risk of similar

General unwanted effects of NSAIDs

Unwanted effects, owing largely to inhibition of the constitutive housekeeping enzyme cyclooxygenase-1, are common, particularly in the elderly, and include:

- Dyspepsia, nausea and vomiting; also gastric damage in chronic users, with risk of haemorrhage, resulting from abrogation of the protective effect of prostaglandin (PG) on gastric mucosa.
- Skin reactions.
- Reversible renal insufficiency (in individuals who have noradrenergic- or angiotensin-mediated vasoconstriction) through lack of compensatory PGE_2-mediated vasodilatation.
- 'Analgesic-associated nephropathy'; this can occur following long-continued high doses of NSAIDs (e.g. paracetamol) and is often irreversible.
- Less commonly, liver disorders, bone marrow depression.
- Bronchospasm in 'aspirin-sensitive' asthmatics.

renal disease. However, the daily use of small doses of an NSAID, on its own, is not reported to be hazardous for the kidney.

More detail on the toxic effects of NSAIDs on the kidney is given in Chapter 52, pp. 728–729; see also de Broe & Elseviers (1998).

OTHER UNWANTED EFFECTS

Other, much less common, unwanted effects of NSAIDs include bone marrow disturbances and liver disorders, the latter more likely if there is already renal impairment. Overdose of paracetamol causes liver failure (see below). NSAIDs (in particular, aspirin) may precipitate asthma in NSAID-sensitive asthmatic patients (see Ch. 22).

SOME IMPORTANT NSAIDS

Table 16.1 lists commonly used NSAIDs and the clinical uses of the NSAIDs are summarised in the clinical box. Here we discuss aspirin and paracetamol.

ASPIRIN

Aspirin (acetylsalicylic acid) was amongst the earliest drugs synthesised and is now one of the most commonly consumed drugs, worldwide. It is relatively insoluble but its sodium and calcium salts are readily soluble. A newer member of this group is **diflunisal** (Table 16.1).

Aspirin in non-inflammatory conditions

It is becoming increasingly clear that aspirin—previously thought of as an old anti-inflammatory workhorse—is now approaching the status of wonder drug in that it is of benefit not only in inflammation but in an increasing number of other conditions:

- cardiovascular disorders:* through the antiplatelet action (the mechanism of which is detailed in Ch. 20) of low-dose aspirin
- colonic and rectal cancer: regular and sustained use of aspirin is reported to reduce (virtually halve) the risk of cancer of the colon and possibly also rectal cancer, which between them cause 25 000 deaths a year in the UK (but note that the selective COX-2 inhibitors may be more effective)
- Alzheimer's disease: there is preliminary evidence that aspirin reduces the risk and retards the onset of Alzheimer's disease (Ch. 34)
- radiation-induced diarrhoea.

*Clinicians increasingly now regard aspirin as a cardiovascular drug and query whether it should be classified as an NSAID. We include it here because, being primarily pharmacologists, our approach is to consider drugs in terms of their mechanisms of action. When you get into the clinic you can declassify aspirin.

Clinical uses of NSAIDs

- For analgesia in painful conditions (e.g. headache, dysmenorrhoea, backache, bony metastases of cancers, postoperative pain):
  - —the drugs of choice for short-term analgesia are aspirin, paracetamol and ibuprofen; more potent, longer-acting drugs (diflunisal, naproxen, piroxicam) are useful for chronic pain
  - —the requirement for narcotic analgesics can be markedly reduced by NSAIDs in some patients with bony metastases or postoperative pain
- For anti-inflammatory effects in chronic or acute inflammatory conditions (e.g. rheumatoid arthritis and related connective tissue disorders, gout and soft tissue diseases). With many NSAIDs, the dosage required for chronic inflammatory disorders is greater than for simple analgesia and treatment may be prolonged, so side-effects are common. Treatment can be started with a drug with a low incidence of side-effects, such as ibuprofen, more potent agents (see Table 16.1) being used only if necessary. For patients with a history of peptic ulcer or upper gastrointestinal bleeding a COX2-selective drug (e.g. celecoxib, rofecoxib) can be considered.
- To lower temperature. Paracetamol is preferred because it lacks gastrointestinal side-effects and, unlike aspirin, has not been associated with Reye's syndrome in children.
- There is substantial individual variation in clinical response to NSAIDs and considerable unpredictable patient preference for one drug rather than another.

Pharmacokinetic aspects

Aspirin, being a weak acid, is largely un-ionised in the acid environment of the stomach and its absorption is thus facilitated. Most absorption, however, occurs in the ileum because of the extensive surface area of the microvilli. Aspirin is hydrolysed by esterases in the plasma and the tissues—particularly the liver—yielding salicylate.

Approximately 25% of the salicylate is oxidised; some is conjugated to give the glucuronide or sulfate before excretion and about 25% is excreted unchanged, the rate of excretion being higher in alkaline urine (see Ch. 8).

The plasma half-life of aspirin will depend on the dose but the duration of action is not directly related to the plasma half-life because of the irreversible nature of the action of the drug.

Unwanted effects

Salicylates may produce local and systemic toxic effects.

Aspirin has many of the general unwanted effects of NSAIDs outlined above. In addition there are certain specific unwanted effects that occur with aspirin and other salicylates.

Salicylism

Salicylism can occur with repeated ingestion of fairly large doses of salicylate. It is a syndrome consisting of tinnitus (a high-pitched buzzing noise in the ears), vertigo, decreased hearing and sometimes also nausea and vomiting.

Other unwanted systemic effects

There is an association between aspirin intake and *Reye's syndrome*, which is a rare disorder in children. It is a combination of liver disorder and encephalopathy (central nervous system (CNS) disturbances) that can follow an acute viral illness and has a 20–40% mortality. It is not entirely clear to what extent aspirin is in fact implicated in its causation, but the drug is best avoided in children altogether.

Salicylate poisoning

Salicylates also cause various metabolic changes, the nature of which depends on the dose. Large therapeutic doses alter the acid–base balance and the electrolyte balance, and toxic doses have serious effects on these functions. The sequence of events with high doses is as follows. Salicylates uncouple oxidative phosphorylation (mainly in skeletal muscle) leading to increased oxygen consumption and thus increased production of carbon dioxide. This stimulates respiration, which is also stimulated by a direct action on the respiratory centre. The resulting hyperventilation causes a respiratory alkalosis that is normally compensated by renal mechanisms involving increased bicarbonate excretion. Larger doses can cause a depression of the respiratory centre, which leads eventually to retention of carbon dioxide and thus an increase in plasma carbon dioxide. Since this is superimposed on a reduction in plasma bicarbonate, an uncompensated respiratory acidosis will occur. This may be complicated by a metabolic acidosis, which results from the accumulation of metabolites of pyruvic, lactic and acetoacetic acids (an indirect consequence of interference with carbohydrate metabolism) and the acid load associated with the salicylate itself.

Hyperpyrexia is likely to be present owing to the increased metabolic rate, and dehydration may follow from repeated vomiting.

With toxic doses of salicylates, disturbance of haemostasis can also occur, mainly as a result of an action on platelet aggregation. The effect of these doses on the CNS is, initially, stimulation with excitement but eventually coma and respiratory depression.

Salicylate poisoning, with the signs and symptoms outlined above, occurs more commonly, and is more serious, in children than in adults. The acid–base disturbance seen in children is usually a metabolic acidosis whereas that in adults is a respiratory alkalosis. Salicylate poisoning constitutes a medical emergency.

Aspirin

- Aspirin (acetylsalicylic acid) causes irreversible inactivation of cyclooxygenase, acting on both COX-1 and COX-2.
- In addition to its anti-inflammatory actions, aspirin inhibits platelet aggregation (see Ch. 20) and its main clinical importance now is in the therapy of myocardial infarction (see Ch.17).
- It is given orally and is rapidly absorbed; 75% is metabolised in the liver.
- Elimination follows first-order kinetics with low doses (half-life 4 hours) and saturation kinetics with high doses (half-life over 15 hours).
- Unwanted effects:
  - —with therapeutic doses: some gastric bleeding, usually minimal, is common
  - —with large doses: dizziness, deafness and tinnitus ('salicylism'); compensated respiratory alkalosis may occur
  - —with toxic doses (e.g. from self-poisoning): uncompensated respiratory acidosis plus metabolic acidosis, the latter seen particularly in children
  - —aspirin is epidemiologically linked with an encephalitis (Reye's syndrome) if given to children with viral infections.
- If given concomitantly with warfarin, aspirin can cause a potentially hazardous increase in the risk of bleeding.

Some important interactions with other drugs

Aspirin causes a potentially hazardous increase in the effect of warfarin, partly by displacing it from plasma proteins (Ch. 51) and partly because its effect on platelets interferes with haemostatic mechanisms (see Ch. 20). Aspirin interferes with the effect of uricosuric agents such as **probenecid** and **sulfinpyrazone**, and since low doses of aspirin may, on their own, reduce urate excretion, aspirin should not be used in gout.

PARACETAMOL

Paracetamol (called acetaminophen in the USA) is one of the most commonly used non-narcotic analgesic–antipyretic agents. It has relatively weak anti-inflammatory activity.* Paracetamol is reported to be a selective inhibitor of COX-3 (see footnote p. 244).

Pharmacokinetic aspects

Paracetamol is given orally and is well absorbed; peak plasma concentrations are reached in 30–60 minutes and it is inactivated in the liver, being conjugated to give the glucuronide or sulfate. The plasma half-life of paracetamol with therapeutic doses is 2–4 hours but with toxic doses it may be extended to 4–8 hours.

Unwanted effects

With therapeutic doses, side-effects are few and uncommon, though allergic skin reactions sometimes occur. It is possible that regular intake of large doses over a long period may increase the risk of kidney damage (p. 728).

*There is some disagreement about this; Skjelbred et al. (1984) reported evidence of significant anti-inflammatory action.

Toxic doses* (i.e. two to three times the maximum therapeutic dose) cause a serious, potentially fatal hepatotoxicity. Renal toxicity can also occur. These toxic effects occur when the liver enzymes catalysing the normal conjugation reactions are saturated, causing the drug to be metabolised by the mixed function oxidases (reaction 3 in Fig. 16.1). The resulting toxic metabolite, *N*-acetyl-*p*-benzoquinone imine, is inactivated by conjugation with glutathione (reaction 4 in Fig. 16.1), but when glutathione is depleted the toxic intermediate accumulates and reacts with nucleophilic constituents in the cell. This causes necrosis in the liver and also in the kidney tubules (reaction 5 in Fig. 16.1).

The initial symptoms of acute paracetamol poisoning are nausea and vomiting, the hepatotoxicity being a delayed manifestation that occurs 24–48 hours later. Treatment entails gastric lavage followed by oral activated charcoal. Further details of the toxic effects of paracetamol are given in Chapter 52. If the patient is seen sufficiently soon after ingestion, the liver damage can be prevented by giving agents that increase glutathione formation in the liver (acetylcysteine intravenously, or methionine orally).

If more than 12 hours have passed since the ingestion of a large dose, the antidotes, which themselves can cause adverse effects (nausea, allergic reactions), are less likely to be useful.

AGENTS SELECTIVE FOR CYCLOOXYGENASE 2

Two agents selective for COX-2 are now available for clinical use: **celecoxib** and **rofecoxib**. Both are effective antiarthritic agents and have shown analgesic efficacy in pain such as occurs during dysmenorrhoea and after dental or orthopaedic surgery.

> **Paracetamol**
>
> - Paracetamol has potent analgesic and antipyretic actions but rather weaker anti-inflammatory effects.
> - It is given orally and metabolised in liver (half-life 2–4 hours).
> - Toxic doses cause nausea and vomiting, then, after 24–48 hours, potentially fatal liver damage by saturating normal conjugating enzymes, causing the drug to be converted by mixed function oxidases to *N*-acetyl-*p*-benzoquinone imine. This, if not inactivated by conjugation with glutathione, reacts with cell proteins and kills the cell.
> - Agents that increase glutathione (acetylcysteine intravenous or methionine orally) can prevent liver damage if given early.

*A large dose of paracetamol is fairly frequently used for attempted suicide.

The oral bioavailability of rofecoxib is over 92% and its elimination half-life is about 13 hours. The bioavailability of celecoxib is about 36% and its elimination half-life is about 11 hours. Both are metabolised in the liver.

Unwanted effects

The possibility of gastrointestinal disturbances with these agents is discussed above (p. 245). Both celecoxib and rofecoxib increase blood pressure if given with antihypertensive drugs. Since patients with rheumatoid arthritis may already have or be at risk from cardiovascular problems, use of the selective COX-2 agents may increase this risk (see Boers, 2001). Like the COX-1 inhibitors, these COX-2-selective agents also reduce glomerular filtration rates in elderly individuals.

Other COX-2 selective agents are in the pipeline.

ANTAGONISTS OF HISTAMINE

There are three classes of histamine antagonists: H_1-, H_2- and H_3-receptor antagonists. The first group was introduced first by Bovet and his colleagues in the 1930s, at a time when the classification of the histamine receptors had not been elucidated. (Indeed, the elucidation was possible only because these agents were available.) The term *antihistamine* conventionally refers to the H_1-receptor antagonists, which affect various inflammatory and allergic mechanisms. These drugs are discussed in this section. The more recently developed H_2-receptor antagonists, the main clinical effect of which is on gastric secretion, are discussed in Chapter 24. Several H_3-receptor agonists and antagonists are now available and the potential for their clinical use (mainly in CNS conditions) is being explored.

H_1-RECEPTOR ANTAGONISTS (H_1-ANTIHISTAMINES)

Details of some characteristic H_1-receptor antagonists are shown in Table 16.2.

Pharmacological actions

Many of the pharmacological actions of the H_1-receptor antagonists follow from the actions of histamine outlined in Chapter 15. For example, in vitro they decrease histamine-mediated contraction of the smooth muscle of the bronchi, the intestine and the uterus. They inhibit histamine-induced bronchospasm in the guinea-pig in vivo but are of little value in allergic bronchospasm in humans. They reduce the increased vascular permeability caused by histamine.

Some of the actions of these drugs do not appear to be related to blockade of H_1-receptors and may well be the result of antagonist effects at other receptors, such as 5-hydroxytryptamine (5-HT) receptors, α_1-adrenoceptors and acetylcholine muscarinic receptors, both peripherally and in the CNS.

Table 16.2 Comparison of some commonly used H_1-receptor antagonists

Drug	Plasma half-life (hours)	Sedative	Comments action
Diphenhydramine	7	++	Some local anaesthetic activity and marked muscarinic-receptor antagonism; used in motion sickness
Promethazine	12	++	Some local anaesthetic action and fairly marked muscarinic receptor antagonism; weak α_1-adrenoceptor antagonism; antiemetic; injection can be painful
Chlorpheniramine	23	+	Potent H_1-receptor antagonism; if injected it can cause transient CNS stimulation
Mequitazine	38	Nil	Potent H_1-receptor antagonism; has minimal muscarinic receptor antagonism; peak plasma concentration after 6 h; high doses can impair CNS function

Some H_1-receptor antagonists have pronounced effects in the CNS. These are usually listed as 'side-effects' but they may be more clinically useful than the peripheral H_1-antagonist effects and should be recognised as such. Some are fairly strong sedatives and may be used for this action (e.g. **promethazine**, a phenothiazine compound; see Table 16.2). Several are antiemetic and are used to prevent motion sickness (e.g. **cyclizine**, **dimenhydrinate**, **cinnarizine**; see Ch. 24, Fig. 24.5).

Many H_1-receptor antagonists (e.g. **diphenhydramine**) also show significant antimuscarinic effects, though their affinity is much lower for muscarinic than for histamine receptors. (As measured on the guinea-pig ileum, the pA_2 (see Ch. 2) of **mepyramine** (the prototype antihistamine) for the H_1-receptors is 9.2 and for the muscarinic receptors is 5.0). For circumstances in which selective H_1-receptor antagonism is desired, untrammelled by CNS effects, newer drugs have been developed, such as **mequitazine** (Table 16.2) and **terfenadine.** These non-sedating antihistamines, terfenadine in particular, can cause serious cardiac dysrhythmias (pp. 111 and 720). The risk is extremely low but is increased if grapefruit juice or agents that inhibit cytochrome P450 in the liver are taken concomitantly (see Ch. 6). Fexofenadine, the non-toxic, pharmacologically active metabolite of terfenadine, is now available.

Other, newer drugs that lack sedative action are **loratadine** and **cetirizine**.

Several H_1-receptor antagonists show weak blockade at α_1-adrenoceptors (an example is the phenothiazine promethazine). **Cyproheptadine** is a 5-HT antagonist as well as being an H_1-receptor antagonist.

The clinical uses of H_1-receptor antagonists are summarised in the clinical box.

Pharmacokinetic aspects

Most H_1-receptor antagonists are given orally, are well absorbed, reach their peak effect in 1–2 hours and are effective for 3–6 hours, though there are exceptions (see Table 16.2). Most appear to be widely distributed throughout the body, but some do not penetrate the blood–brain barrier, for example the non-sedative drugs (see Table 16.2). They are metabolised in the liver and excreted in the urine.

Unwanted effects

What is defined as 'unwanted' will depend to a certain extent on what the drugs are used for. When used for purely peripheral actions, all the CNS effects are unwanted, the main ones being sedation through the blockade of H_1-receptors. Occasionally these drugs are used for this CNS effect (e.g. in small children

Clinical use of histamine H_1-receptor antagonists

- For allergic reactions (see Ch.15) including allergic rhinitis (hay fever), urticaria, insect bites, drug hypersensitivities. Drugs that lack sedative or muscarinic receptor antagonist actions (e.g. fexofenadine or cetirizine) are preferred. Topical preparations (e.g. for eye, nose) are available. Injections are used as an adjunct to adrenaline (epinephrine) in the emergency treatment of anaphylaxis.
- As antiemetics for the prevention of motion sickness or other causes of nausea, especially those associated with vertigo (e.g. labyrinthine disorders). Muscarinic receptor antagonist actions of some antihistamines (e.g. cinnarizine, cyclizine) probably contribute to efficacy but also cause side-effects.
- For sedation: some H_1-receptor antagonists (e.g. promethazine; see Table 16.3) are fairly strong sedatives and may be used for this action.

approaching bedtime). When used for their sedative or antiemetic actions, some of the CNS effects such as dizziness, tinnitus and fatigue are unwanted. Excessive doses can cause excitation and may produce convulsions in children.

The peripheral antimuscarinic actions are always unwanted. The commonest of these is dryness of the mouth, but blurred vision, constipation and retention of urine can also occur.

Unwanted effects not related to the drugs' pharmacological actions are also seen; gastrointestinal disturbances are fairly common while allergic dermatitis can follow topical application.

DRUGS USED IN GOUT

Gout is a metabolic disease in which plasma urate concentration is raised because of overproduction or impaired excretion of purines. It is characterised by intermittent attacks of acute arthritis produced by the deposition of crystals of sodium urate (a product of purine metabolism) in the synovial tissue of joints. An inflammatory response is evoked, involving activation of the kinin, complement and plasmin systems (see Ch. 15 and Fig. 15.1), generation of lipoxygenase products such as leukotriene B_4 (Fig. 15.5) and local accumulation of neutrophil granulocytes. These engulf the crystals by phagocytosis, which causes generation of tissue-damaging toxic oxygen metabolites and subsequently lysis of the cells with release of proteolytic enzymes. Urate crystals also induce the production of IL-1 (p. 218).

Drugs used to treat gout may act in the following ways:

- by inhibiting uric acid synthesis (**allopurinol**)
- by increasing uric acid excretion (uricosuric agents: **probenecid, sulfinpyrazone**)
- by inhibiting leucocyte migration into the joint (**colchicine**)
- by general anti-inflammatory and analgesic effects (**NSAIDs**; see pp. 246–247).

ALLOPURINOL

Allopurinol reduces the synthesis of uric acid by inhibiting xanthine oxidase (Fig. 16.4). It is an analogue of hypoxanthine and inhibits the enzyme mainly by substrate competition. Some degree of inhibition of de novo purine synthesis also occurs. Allopurinol is converted to alloxanthine by xanthine oxidase, and this metabolite, which remains in the tissue for a considerable time, is an effective non-competitive inhibitor of the enzyme. The pharmacological action of allopurinol is largely due to alloxanthine.

Allopurinol reduces the concentration of the relatively insoluble urates and uric acid in tissues, plasma and urine, while increasing the concentration of the more soluble xanthines and hypoxanthines. The deposition of urate crystals in tissues ('tophi') is reversed and the formation of renal stones is inhibited.

Allopurinol is the drug of choice in the long-term treatment of gout, but it is ineffective in the treatment of an acute attack and indeed makes this worse.

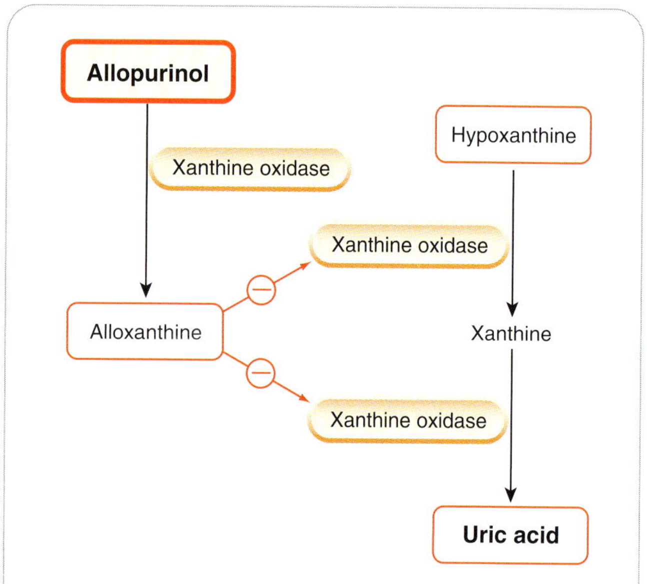

Fig. 16.4 **Inhibition of uric acid synthesis by allopurinol.** (See text for details.)

Pharmacokinetic aspects

Allopurinol is given orally and is well absorbed in the gastrointestinal tract. Its half-life is 2–3 hours; it is converted to alloxanthine (Fig. 16.4), which has a half-life of 18–30 hours. Renal excretion is a balance between glomerular filtration and probenecid-sensitive tubular reabsorption.

Unwanted effects

Unwanted effects are few. Gastrointestinal disturbances and allergic reactions (mainly skin rashes) can occur but disappear if the drug is stopped. Acute attacks of gout sometimes occur during the early stages of therapy.

Drug interactions

Allopurinol increases the effect of **mercaptopurine**, an antimetabolite used in cancer chemotherapy, and also that of **azathioprine** (an immunosuppressant used to prevent transplant rejection; see below), which is metabolised to mercaptopurine. Allopurinol also enhances the effect of another anticancer drug, **cyclophosphamide** (Ch. 50). The effect of oral anticoagulants is increased because of the inhibition of their metabolism.

URICOSURIC AGENTS

Uricosuric agents are drugs that increase uric acid excretion by a direct action on the renal tubule. Examples are **probenecid** and **sulfinpyrazone**.

COLCHICINE

Colchicine has a specific effect in gouty arthritis and can be used both to prevent and to relieve acute attacks. It prevents migration

Drugs used in gout

- Allopurinol inhibits uric acid synthesis.
- Probenecid increases uric acid excretion.
- Colchicine reduces leucocyte migration into joints.
- NSAIDs have anti-inflammatory action and reduce pain.

of neutrophils into the joint by binding to tubulin, resulting in the depolymerisation of the microtubules and interference with cell motility. Colchicine-treated neutrophils develop a 'drunken walk'. Colchicine may also prevent the production of a putative inflammatory glycoprotein by neutrophils that have phagocytosed urate crystals.

Pharmacokinetic aspects

Colchicine is given orally, is well absorbed and reaches peak concentrations in about 1 hour. It is excreted partly in the gastrointestinal tract and partly in the urine.

Unwanted effects

The unwanted effects of colchicine are largely gastrointestinal: nausea, vomiting and abdominal pain. Severe diarrhoea may be a problem and with large doses may be associated with gastrointestinal haemorrhage and kidney damage. Rashes sometimes occur, also peripheral neuropathy. Long courses of treatment have occasionally resulted in blood dyscrasias.

ANTIRHEUMATOID DRUGS

Rheumatoid disease is one of the commonest chronic inflammatory conditions in developed countries and rheumatoid arthritis is a common cause of disability. One in three patients with rheumatoid arthritis is likely eventually to be severely disabled. The joint changes, which probably represent an autoimmune reaction, comprise inflammation, proliferation of the synovium and erosion of cartilage and bone. The primary inflammatory cytokines, IL-1, TNF-α have a major role in pathogenesis (Ch. 15).

The drugs most frequently used in therapy are *the disease-modifying antirheumatoid drugs** (DMARDs) and the **NSAIDs**—the former so-called to point up the comparison with the NSAIDs—which reduce the symptoms of rheumatoid disease but do not retard the progress of the disease. Some *immunosuppressants* (e.g. **azathioprine**, **ciclosporin**; see below and Ch. 50) are also used as are the **glucocorticoids** (covered in Ch. 27). Newer agents, with more specific action against the disease processes of rheumatoid, are the *anticytokine drugs*.

*It is not at all clear that the DMARDs do what their name implies; the name seems to have been thought up by a spin-doctor.

DISEASE-MODIFYING DRUGS (DMARDS)

The term DMARD is a latex concept that can be stretched to cover a variety of agents with different chemical structures and mechanisms of action. Included in this category are **methotrexate**, **sulfasalazine**, **gold compounds**, **penicillamine** and **chloroquine**.

The antirheumatoid action of these agents was discovered by serendipity and clinical intuition. When the drugs were introduced, nothing was known about their mechanism of action in these conditions, and decades of in vitro experiments have resulted in bewilderment rather than understanding.

DMARDs improve symptoms and can reduce disease activity in rheumatoid arthritis, as measured by reduction in number of swollen and tender joints, pain score, disability score, articular index on radiology and the serum concentration of acute-phase proteins and of rheumatoid factor (an IgM antibody against host IgG); however, whether they halt the long-term progress of the disease is controversial, so the term disease-modifying may be overoptimistic.

DMARDs are often referred to as second-line drugs, and some have a place in the treatment of other chronic inflammatory diseases. The effects of this group of drugs on rheumatoid conditions are slow in onset and some (e.g. penicillamine) are not thought to have a general anti-inflammatory action.

Mechanisms of action of DMARDs are reviewed by Bondeson (1997).

SULFASALAZINE

Sulfasalazine, commonly a first choice DMARD in the UK, produces remission in active rheumatoid arthritis. It is also used for chronic inflammatory bowel disease.

It may act by scavenging the toxic oxygen metabolites produced by neutrophils.

It is a combination of sulfonamide (sulfapyridine) with a salicylate. It is split into its component parts by bacteria in the colon, the 5-aminosalicylic acid being the radical scavenger. It is poorly absorbed after oral administration. The common side-effects are gastrointestinal disturbances, malaise and headache. Skin reactions and leucopenia can occur but are reversible on stopping the drug. The absorption of folic acid is sometimes impaired; this can be countered by giving folic acid supplements. A reversible decrease in sperm count has also been reported.

As with other sulfonamides, blood dyscrasias and anaphylactic-type reactions may occur in a few patients.

GOLD COMPOUNDS

The gold compounds used are **sodium aurothiomalate** and **auranofin**.

Actions and mechanism of action

The effect of gold compounds develops slowly, the maximum action occurring after 3–4 months. Pain and joint swelling subside and the progression of bone and joint damage diminishes.

The mechanism of action is not clear. **Auranofin**, but not **aurothiomalate**, inhibits the induction of IL-1 and TNF-α.

Pharmacokinetic aspects

Sodium aurothiomalate is given by deep intramuscular injection; auranofin is given orally. Peak plasma concentrations of aurothiomalate are reached in 2–6 hours. The compounds gradually become concentrated in the tissues, not only in synovial cells in joints (where the concentration is 50% of the plasma concentration) but also in macrophages throughout the body, and in liver cells, kidney tubules and the adrenal cortex. The gold complexes remain in the tissues for some time after treatment is stopped. Excretion is mostly renal, but some is excreted in the gastrointestinal tract. The half-life is 7 days initially but increases with treatment, so the drug is usually given first at weekly then at monthly intervals.

Unwanted effects

Unwanted effects with aurothiomalate are seen in about one third of patients treated, and serious toxic effects in about 1 patient in 10. Unwanted effects with auranofin are less frequent and less severe.

Important unwanted effects are skin rashes (which can be severe), mouth ulcers, proteinuria and blood dyscrasias. Encephalopathy, peripheral neuropathy and hepatitis can occur. If therapy is stopped when the early symptoms appear, the incidence of serious toxic effects is relatively low.

PENICILLAMINE

Penicillamine is dimethylcysteine and is one of the substances produced by hydrolysis of penicillin. The D-isomer is used in the therapy of rheumatoid disease.

Actions and mechanism of action

About 75% of patients with rheumatoid arthritis respond to penicillamine. The effects take weeks to start and the main response is not seen for several months.

Penicillamine is thought to modify rheumatoid disease partly by decreasing IL-1 generation and/or partly by an effect on collagen synthesis, preventing the maturation of newly synthesised collagen. However, the mechanism of action is still a matter of conjecture.

Penicillamine is a highly reactive thiol compound and also has metal-chelating properties.

Pharmacokinetic aspects

Penicillamine is given orally and only half the dose administered is absorbed. It reaches peak plasma concentrations in 1–2 hours and is excreted in the urine. Dosage is started low and increased only gradually to avoid unwanted effects.

Unwanted effects

Unwanted effects occur in about 40% of patients treated and may necessitate cessation of therapy. Anorexia, nausea and vomiting and disturbances of taste (the last related to the chelation of zinc) are seen but often disappear with continued treatment. Proteinuria occurs in 20% of patients. Rashes and stomatitis are the most common unwanted effects and may resolve if the dosage is lowered, as may dose-related thrombocytopenia. Other bone marrow disorders (leucopenia, aplastic anaemia) are absolute indications for stopping therapy, as are the various autoimmune conditions (e.g. thyroiditis, myasthenia gravis) that sometimes supervene.

Since penicillamine is a metal chelator, it should not be given with gold compounds.

CHLOROQUINE

Chloroquine is a 4-aminoquinoline drug used mainly in prevention and treatment of malaria (Ch. 48). It has been shown to cause remission of rheumatoid arthritis but it does not retard the progression of bone damage. It is also used in both systemic and discoid lupus erythematosus. Pharmacological effects do not appear until a month or more after the drug is started, and about half the patients treated respond.

The pharmacokinetic aspects and unwanted effects of chloroquine are dealt with in Chapter 48.

METHOTREXATE

Methotrexate is a folic acid antagonist with cytotoxic and immunosuppressant activity (see below and Chs 44 and 50) and potent antirheumatoid action. It is commonly a first-choice DMARD. It has a more rapid onset of action than other DMARDs and is also said to have fewer adverse effects (Bondeson, 1997), though pulmonary fibrosis may be a problem. More than 50% of patients continue with it for 5 years or more, whereas about half stop other DMARDs within 2 years because of unwanted effects and lack of efficacy.

ANTICYTOKINE THERAPY

With anticytokine agents, treatment can for the first time be aimed at specific aspects of the disease processes in rheumatoid arthritis. The drugs available are **infliximab** (a chimeric (mouse/human) monoclonal antibody against TNF-α) and **etanercept** (a TNF receptor joined to the Fc domain of a human IgG molecule).

Mechanism of action

Both infliximab and etenacept bind TNF and inhibit its effects (Fig. 16.5). Etanercept can also bind to lymphotoxin-α, which may be of relevance for the treatment of juvenile arthritis since this cytokine is found in inflamed tissues in this condition.

Parmacokinetic aspects

Etanercept is given subcutaneously twice a week. Infliximab is used with methotrexate therapy and is given intravenously every 2 months.

Antirheumatoid drugs

- The drugs used in rheumatoid disease are the NSAIDs, the disease-modifying antirheumatoid drugs (DMARDs) and the anticytokine agents.
- DMARDs:
  —include sulfasalazine, methotrexate (a folate antagonist), gold compounds, chloroquine (an antimalarial), penicillamine and azathioprine (an immunosuppressant)
  —are slow-acting drugs and can improve symptoms and reduce the inflammatory process
  —retard progress of the disease but do not halt it entirely.
- *The anticytokine agents* (infliximab, etanercept) are biological preparations that target the action of tumour necrosis factor-α— an important mediator of the rheumatoid inflammation—and inhibit its effects.

Unwanted effects

With etanercept, unwanted effects have in general been minimal and consisted mainly of reactions at the injection site; but there have been reports of blood dyscrasias and demyelinating CNS disorders. Infliximab has been associated with recurrence of tuberculosis and there is evidence that its long-term use can cause the development of anti-infliximab antibodies. TNF has a key role in host defence and it was thought that prolonged inhibition of its action might substantially increase infections or malignancies; but so far there have been few instances of this occurring.

LEFLUNOMIDE

Leflunomide has a relatively specific inhibitory effect on activated T cells. It gives rise to a metabolite that inhibits de novo pyrimidine synthesis by inhibiting dihydroorotate dehydrogenase.

It is orally active and well absorbed from the gastrointestinal tract. It has a long plasma half-life and the active metabolite undergoes enterohepatic circulation. Unwanted effects include diarrhoea, raised liver enzymes and alopecia. The long half-life means that there is a risk of cumulative toxicity.

IMMUNOSUPPRESSANT DRUGS

Most immunosuppressants act in the induction phase of the immunological response (see Fig. 15.3), reducing lymphocyte proliferation; some also inhibit aspects of the effector phase. The drugs used for immunosuppression can be roughly divided into agents that:

- inhibit IL-2 production or action, e.g. **ciclosporin, tacrolimus**
- inhibit cytokine gene expression, e.g. the *corticosteroids*
- inhibit purine or pyrimidine synthesis, e.g. **azathioprine, myclophenolate mofetil**
- block the T cell surface molecules involved in signalling, e.g. *monoclonal antibodies*.

Clinical use of immunosuppressants

- Immunosuppressants are used for three main purposes:
  —to suppress rejection of transplanted organs and tissues (kidneys, bone marrow, heart, liver, etc.)
  —to suppress graft-versus-host disease (i.e. the response of lymphocytes in the graft to host antigens) in bone marrow transplants
  —to treat a variety of conditions that, while not completely understood, are believed to have an important autoimmune component in their pathogenesis: idiopathic thrombocytopenic purpura, some forms of haemolytic anaemia, some forms of of glomerulonephritis, myasthenia gravis, systemic lupus erythematosus, rheumatoid arthritis, psoriasis and ulcerative colitis.
- Therapy for this third category often involves a combination of glucocorticoid and cytotoxic agents.
- For transplantation of organs or bone marrow, ciclosporin is usually combined with a glucocorticoid, a cytotoxic drug or an antilymphocyte immunoglobulin.

Immunosuppressants are used in the therapy of autoimmune disease and to prevent and/or treat transplant rejection. Because they impair immune responses, they carry the hazard of a decreased response to infections and may facilitate the emergence of malignant cells. However, the relationship between these adverse effects and potency in preventing graft rejection varies with different drugs (Morris, 1995).

The clinical use of immunosuppressants is summarised in the clinical box.

CICLOSPORIN

Ciclosporin is a cyclic peptide of 11 amino acid residues with potent immunosuppressive activity but no effect on the acute inflammatory reaction per se. For a detailed review, see Borel et al. (1996).

Mechanism of action

Ciclosporin has numerous actions on various cell types; in general, the actions of relevance for immunosuppression are:

- decreased clonal proliferation of T cells, primarily by inhibiting IL-2 release and possibly also by decreasing expression of IL-2 receptors

- reduced induction of and clonal proliferation of cytotoxic T cells from $CD8^+$ precursor T cells
- reduced function of the effector T cells that mediate cell-mediated responses (e.g. decreased delayed-type hypersensitivity)
- some reduction of T-cell-dependent B cell responses.

The main action is a relatively selective inhibitory effect on IL-2 gene transcription, though an effect on the transcription of the genes for interferon-γ (IFNγ) and IL-3 has also been reported. Normally, interaction of antigen with a Th cell receptor results in increased intracellular Ca^{2+} (Ch. 2). Calcium (complexed with calmodulin) stimulates a phosphatase, calcineurin, that activates various transcription factors;* these, in turn, set in motion the transcription of the gene for IL-2. Ciclosporin binds with a cytosolic protein, termed *cyclophilin* (a member of a group now called immunophilins).** The drug–immunophilin complex binds to and inhibits calcineurin and thus interferes with activation of Th cells and production of IL-2 (Fig. 15.3).

Pharmacokinetic aspects

Ciclosporin can be given orally or by intravenous infusion. After oral administration, peak plasma concentrations are usually attained in about 3–4 hours. The plasma half-life is approximately 24 hours. Metabolism occurs in the liver and most of the metabolites are excreted in the bile. Ciclosporin accumulates in most tissues at concentrations three to four times that seen in the plasma. Some of the drug remains in lymphomyeloid tissue and later in fat depots for some time after administration has stopped.

Unwanted effects

The commonest and most serious unwanted effect of ciclosporin is nephrotoxicity: which is not thought to be associated with calcineurin inhibition. It may be a limiting factor in the use of the drug in some patients (see also Ch. 52). Hepatotoxicity and hypertension can also occur. Less important unwanted effects are anorexia, lethargy, hirsutism, tremor, paraesthesia (tingling sensation), gum hypertrophy and gastrointestinal disturbances. Ciclosporin has no depressant effects on the bone marrow.

TACROLIMUS

Tacrolimus is a macrolide antibiotic with a very similar mechanism of action to ciclosporin, but considerably more potency. The main difference is that the internal receptor for this drug is not cyclophilin but a protein termed FKBP (FK-binding protein, because tacrolimus was initially called FK506). The tacrolimus–FKBP complex inhibits calcineurin with the effects described above.

*For example NF-AT, the 'nuclear factor of activated T cells'.

**The term immunophilin was coined to describe the intracellular proteins that function as receptors for immunosuppressants such as ciclosporin and tacrolimus. It is now known that immunophilin molecules are implicated in several signal transduction mechanisms. Recent work has shown that the human immunodeficiency virus (HIV-1; see Ch. 46) also binds to intracellular cyclophilins.

Pharmacokinetic aspects

Tacrolimus can be given orally or by intravenous injection. It is 99% metabolised by the liver and has a half-life of approximately 7 hours.

Unwanted effects

The unwanted effects of tacrolimus are similar to those of ciclosporin but are more severe. The incidence of nephrotoxicity and neurotoxicity is higher but that of hirsuitism is lower. Gastrointestinal disturbances and metabolic disturbances (hyperglycaemia) can occur. Thrombocytopenia and hyperlipidaemia have been reported but are reversible by reducing the dosage.

GLUCOCORTICOIDS

Immunosuppression by glucocorticoids involves both their effects on the immune response and their anti-inflammatory actions. These are described in Chapter 27, and the sites of action of the agents on cell-mediated immune reactions are indicated in Figure 15.5.

Glucocorticoids are immunosuppressant mainly because, like ciclosporin, they restrain the clonal proliferation of Th cells, through decreasing transcription of the gene for IL-2; however, they also decrease the transcription of many other cytokine genes (including those for TNF-α, IFNγ, IL-1 and many other interleukins) in both the induction and effector phases of the immune response. These effects on transcription are mediated through inhibition of the action of transcription factors, such as AP-1 and NF-κB (p. 413).

AZATHIOPRINE

Azathioprine interferes with purine synthesis and is cytotoxic. It is widely used for immunosuppression particularly for control of tissue rejection in transplant surgery. This drug is metabolised to give mercaptopurine, a purine analogue that inhibits DNA synthesis (see Ch. 50).

Both cell-mediated and antibody-mediated immune reactions are depressed by this drug since it inhibits clonal proliferation in the induction phase of the immune response (see Fig. 15.3) by a cytotoxic action on dividing cells.

As is the case with mercaptopurine itself, the main unwanted effect is depression of the bone marrow. Other toxic effects are nausea and vomiting, skin eruptions and a mild hepatotoxicity.

MYCOPHENOLATE MOFETIL

Mycophenolate mofetil is a semisynthetic derivative of a fungal antibiotic. In the body it is converted to mycophenolic acid, which restrains proliferation of both T and B lymphocytes and reduces the production of cytotoxic T cells by inhibiting inosine monophosphate dehydrogenase, an enzyme crucial for de novo

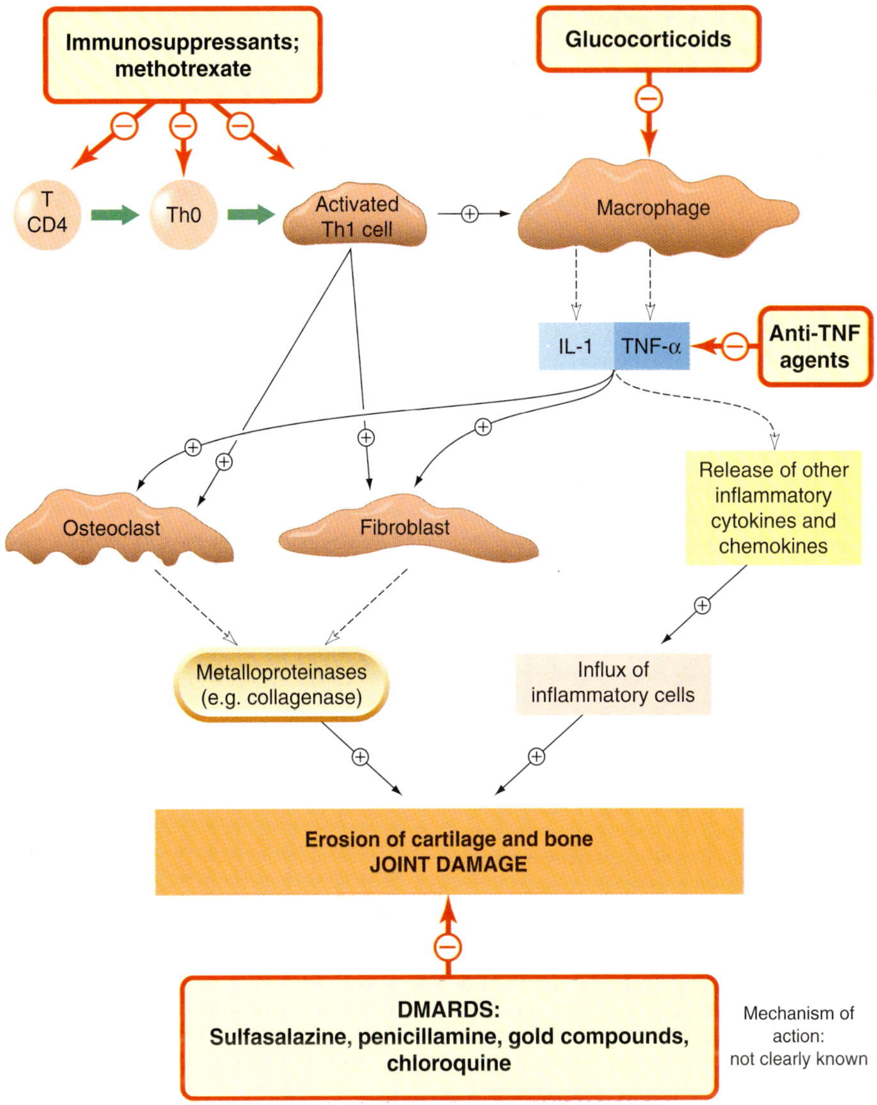

Fig. 16.5 A schematic diagram of the cells and mediators involved in the pathogenesis of rheumatoid joint damage indicating the action of antirheumatoid drugs. The anti-TNF agents are etanercept and infliximab. (IL-1, interleukin-1, TNF-α, tumour necrosis factor-α; DMARDs, disease-modifying antirheumatoid drugs.)

purine biosynthesis. T and B cells are particularly dependent on this pathway* so the drug has a fairly selective action on these cells.

Pharmacokinetic aspects and unwanted effects

Mycophenolate mofetil is given orally and is well absorbed. Magnesium and aluminium hydroxides impair absorption and colestyramine reduces plasma concentrations. The metabolite mycophenolic acid undergoes enterohepatic cycling and is eliminated by the kidney as the inactive glucuronide. Unwanted gastrointestinal effects are common.

MONOCLONAL ANTIBODIES

Basiliximab and **daclizumab** are monoclonal antibodies against the α-chain of the IL-2 receptor. They have immunosuppressant action by blocking this receptor on Th cells (see Fig. 15.3). They

*T and B cells are unique in obtaining the purines needed for DNA synthesis by synthesising them de novo whereas other cells can obtain purines by an alternative pathway.

Immunosuppressants

- Clonal proliferation of Th cells can be decreased through inhibition of transcription of interleukin-2: ciclosporin, tacrolimus and glucocorticoids act in this way
  - —ciclosporin and tacrolimus are given orally or i.v.; common adverse effect is nephrotoxicity
  - —for glucocorticoids see pp. 411–418
- DNA synthesis is inhibited by:
  - —azathioprine through its active metabolite mercaptopurine (Ch. 50)
  - —mycophenolate mofetil through inhibition of de novo purine synthesis.
- T cell signal transduction events are blocked by basiliximab and daclizumab, which are monoclonal antibodies against the α-chain of the interleukin-2 receptor.

are given by intravenous infusion and can cause serious hypersensitivity reactions.

The clinical use of immunosuppressants is summarised on page 257.

POSSIBLE FUTURE DEVELOPMENTS

NO–NSAIDS

As with prostaglandins, NO has a dual role in the body, participating in both tissue homeostasis and inflammation. NO synthase, like COX, is present in both constitutive and inducible isoforms. NO has gastroprotective actions by increasing mucosal blood flow and mucus secretion and inhibiting neutrophil activities. Furthermore, NO inhibits Th1 cytokine generation, possibly by inhibiting the members of the caspase family involved in cytokine release (see Ch. 8).

On the basis of these facts, agents have been produced in which an NO-releasing moiety is coupled to a classical NSAID such as diclofenac, naproxen or flurbiprofen. Several NO–NSAIDs are in phase II trials. They have less gastrointestinal toxicity than the parent compounds. They also have more anti-inflammatory action on the whole, which suggests some COX-independent anti-inflammatory action. (For more information on this topic see Wolfe (1998), Fiorucci (2001) and Sautebin (2000).)

DRUGS BASED ON CYTOKINES OR TRANSCRIPTION FACTORS

IL-1 is a key mediator in chronic inflammatory conditions and is thus clearly an important target for new anti-inflammatory drugs. Preparations of soluble IL-1 receptor (to mop up IL-1), and of recombinant IL-1ra (the endogenous IL-1-receptor antagonist), are in development. The results of clinical trials appear promising (Maini & Taylor, 2000).

The transcription factor NF-κB controls the expression of IL-1 and TNF-α. Administration of selective inhibitors of NF-κB has been shown to abrogate the expression of these cytokines in animal models of chronic inflammation. It is suggested that such inhibitors could eventually be of value in the clinic (Makarov, 2000).

REFERENCES AND FURTHER READING

Basan N G 2001 COX-2 as a multifunctional neuronal modulator. Nat. Med 7: 414–415 (*Succinct treatment of possible role of COX-2 in the CNS. Useful diagrams*)

Basan N G, Flower R J 2002 Lipid signals in pain control. Nature 420: 135–138 (*Succinct article describing the findings of Chandrasekharan et al. (2002) on COX-3*)

Boers M 2001 NSAIDs and selective COX-2 inhibitors: competition between gastroprotection and cardioprotection. Lancet 357: 1222–1223 (*Editorial analysing crisply the results of two major randomised double-blind studies of gastrointestinal toxicity of selective COX-2 inhibitors as compared with non-selective NSAIDs*)

Bondeson J 1997 The mechanisms of action of disease-modifying antirheumatic drugs: a review with emphasis on macrophage signal transduction and the induction of proinflammatory cytokines. Gen Pharmacol 29: 127–150 (*Good detailed review*)

Borel J F, Baumann G et al. 1996 In vivo pharmacological effects of ciclosporin and some analogues. Adv Pharmacol 35: 115–246 (*Borel was instrumental in the development of ciclosporin*)

Breedeveld F C 2000 Therapeutic monoclonal antibodies. Lancet 355: 735–740 (*Good review on the clinical potential of monoclonal antibodies*)

Carterton N L 2000 Cytokines in rheumatoid arthritis: trials and tribulations. Mol Med Today 6: 315–323 (*Good review of agents modulating the action of TNF-α and IL-1. Simple clear diagram of cellular action of these cytokines. Summaries of the clinical trials of the agents in tabular form*)

Catella-Lawson F, Reilly M P et al. 2001 Cyclooxygenase inhibitors and the anti-platelet effects of aspirin. N Engl J Med 345: 1809–1817 (*Points out that ibuprofen, but not rofecoxib, paracetamol or diclfenac, given simultaneously with aspirin reduces the antiplatelet effect of aspirin. Excellent diagram. This problem is discussed by Crofford L J, pp. 1844–1845 in the same issue of the journal*)

Cash J M, Klippel J M 1994 Second-line drug therapy for rheumatoid arthritis. N Engl J Med 330: 1368–1376 (*Good review of DMARDs*)

Chandrasekharan N V et al. 2002 COX-3, a cyclooxygenase-1 variant inhibited by acetaminophen and other analgesic/antipyretic drugs: cloning, structure, and expression. Proc Natl Acad Sci 2002 99: 13926–13931 (*A new COX isozyme is described: COX-3. In humans, the COX-3 mRNA is expressed as most abundantly in cerebral cortex and heart. It is selectively inhibited by analgesic/antipyretic drugs such as paracetamol (acetaminophen) and is inhibited by some other NSAIDs*)

Choy E H S, Panayi G S 2001 Cytokine pathways and joint inflammation in rheumatoid arthritis. N Engl J Med 344: 907–916 (*Clear description of the pathogenesis of rheumatoid arthritis emphasising the cells and mediators involved in joint damage. Excellent diagrams of the interaction of inflammatory cells and of the mechanism of action of anticytokine agents*)

Dale M M, Foreman J C, Fan T-P (eds) 1994 Textbook of

immunopharmacology, 3rd edn. Blackwell Scientific, Oxford (*Simple textbook intended for second and third year medical and science students*)

de Broe M E, Elseviers M M 1998 Current concepts: analgesic nephropathy. N Engl J Med 338: 446–452 (*Useful review*)

Feldman 2002 Development of anti-TFN therapy for rheumatoid arthritis. Nat Rev Immunol 2: 364–371 (*Excellent review covering the role of cytokines in rheumatoid arthritis, the effects of anti-TFN therapy*)

Fiorucci S 2001 NO-releasing NSAIDs re caspase inhibitors. Trends Immunol 22: 232–235 (*Describes modulation of the immune response by NSAIDs and the possible mechanism of their action in downregulating inflammatory cytokines*)

FitzGerald G A, Patrono C 2001 The coxibs, selective inhibitors of cyclooxygenase-2. N Engl J Med 345: 433–442 (*Excellent coverage of the selective COX-2 inhibitors*)

Gummert J F, Ikonen T, Morris R E 1999 Newer immunosuppressive drugs: a review. J Am Soc Nephrol 10: 1366–1380 (*Comprehensive review covering leflunomide, mycophenolate mofetil, sirolinus, tacrolimus and IL-2 receptor antibodies*)

Hawkey C J 1999 COX-2 inhibitors. Lancet 353: 307–314 (*Excellent review. Clear, simple description of the structures of COX-1 and COX-2 and the mechanism of action of selective and non-selective inhibitors. Gives details of results with the COX-2-preferential and COX-2-selective inhibitors. Brief coverage of NO–NSAIDS*)

Hawkey C J 2001 Gastrointestinal toxicity of non-steroid anti-inflammatory drugs. In: Vane J R, Botting R M (eds) Therapeutic roles of selective COX-2 inhibitors. William Harvey Press, London, Ch. 16, pp. 355–394 (*Clear, detailed account of the adverse effects of NSAIDs*)

Henry D, Lim L L-Y et al. 1996 Variability in risk of gastrointestinal complications with individual non-steroidal anti-inflammatory drugs: results of a collaborative meta-analysis. Br Med J 312: 1563–1566 (*Substantial analysis of the gastrointestinal effects of non-selective NSAIDs*)

Jones R 2002 Efficacy and safety of COX-2 inhibitors: new data are encouraging but the risk:benefit ratio remains unclear. Br Med J 325: 607–608 (*Editorial in September 2002*)

Klippel J H K 2000 Biologic therapy for rheumatoid arthritis. N Engl J Med 343: 1640–1641 (*Pithy editorial dealing with the significance of the introduction of the anti-TNF-α agents*)

Leurs R, Blandina P, Tedford C, Timmerm N H 1998 Therapeutic potential of histamine H_3 receptor agonists and antagonists (*Describes the available H_3-receptor agonists and antagonists and their effects in a variety of pharmacological models with discussion of possible therapeutic applications*)

Lipsky J J 1996 Mycophenolate mofetil. Lancet 348: 1357–1359

MacDonald T M, Morant S V et al. 1997 Association of upper gastrointestinal toxicity of non-steroidal anti-inflammatory drugs with continued exposure: cohort study. Br Med J 315: 1333–1338

Mackay I R Rosen F S 2001 Immunomodulation of autoimmune and inflammatory diseases with intravenous globulin. N Engl J Med 345: 747–755 (*Clear review of mechanisms of action and clinical use of immunoglobins: simple, clear diagrams*)

Madhok R, Kerr H, Capell H A 2000 Br Med J 321: 882–885 (*Clinical review of recent advances in the treatment of musculoskeletal diseases*)

Maini R N, Taylor P C 2000 Anti-cytokine therapy for rheumatoid arthritis, Annu Rev Med 51: 207–229 (*Detailed review describing the role of cytokines in the pathogenesis of rheumatoid arthritis and the results of clinical trials with anti-TNF and anti-IL-1 therapy*)

Makarov S S 2000 NF-κB as a therapeutic target in chronic inflammation: recent advances. Mol Med Today 6: 441–448 (*This article gives an overview of the NF-κB signalling pathway and its role in chronic inflammation; and discusses the feasibility of treatment based on selective suppression of this pathway*)

Mitchell J A, Warner T D 1999 Cyclo-oxygenase-2: pharmacology, physiology, biochemistry and relevance to NSAID therapy. Br J Pharmacol 128: 1121–1132 (*Lucid review article. Covers homeostatic roles of COX-2*)

Morris R E 1995 Mechanisms of action of new immunosuppressive drugs. Ther Drug Monit 17: 564–569 (*Succinct, edifying review*)

O'Dell J R 1999 Anticytokine therapy—a new era in the treatment of rheumatoid arthritis. N Engl J Med 340: 310–312 (*Editorial. Excellent coverage of the role of TNF-α in rheumatoid arthritis; Summarises the differences between infliximab and etanercept*)

Rainsford K D, Velo G P (eds) 1992 Side-effects of antiinflammatory/analgesic drugs. Kluwer Academic, Lancaster (*Comprehensive coverage of adverse effects of NSAIDs*)

Rodriguez L A G, Jick H 1994 Risk of gastrointestinal bleeding and perforation associated with non-steroidal anti-inflammatory drugs. Lancet 343: 769–772

Sautebin L 2000 Prostaglandins and nitric oxide as molecular targets for anti-inflammatory therapy. Fitoterapia 71: S48–S57 (*Compares the COX and NO synthase enzymes and their role in physiology and the pathogenesis of disease*)

Simons F E R, Simons K J 1994 Drug therapy: the pharmacology and use of H_1-receptor-antagonist drugs. N Engl J Med 23: 1663–1670 (*Effective coverage*)

Skjelbred et al. 1984 Post-operative administration of acetaminophen to reduce swelling and other inflammatory events. Curr Ther Res 35: 377–385

Smolen J S, Kalden J R et al. 1999 Efficacy and safety of leflunomide compare with placebo and sulphsalazine in active rheumatoid arthritis: a double-blind, randomised, multiventre trial. Lancet 353: 259–260 (*Gives details of the results of a clinical trial showing the efficacy of leflunomide*)

Snyder S H, Sabatini D M 1995 Immunophilins and the nervous system. Nat Med 1: 32–37 (*Good coverage of mechanism of action of ciclosporin and related drugs*)

Suthantharin M, Morris R E, Strom T 1996 Immunosuppressants: cellular and molecular mechanisms of action. Am J Kidney Dis 28: 159–172 (*In-depth review*)

Ulrich H, von Andrian U H, Englehardt B 2003 α4 Integrins as therapeutic targets in autoimmune disease. N Engl J Med 348: 68–70 (*Editorial commenting on two articles in the journal that describe the use of natalizumab, a recombinant monoclonal antibody, for the treatment of the inflammatory/immune diseases: multiple sclerosis and Crohn's disease. Natalizumab binds to α4 integrins on haemopoietic cells and prevents them from binding to their endothelial receptors.*)

Vane J R 1971 Inhibition of prostaglandin synthesis as a mechanism of action for aspirin-like drugs. Nat New Biol 231: 232–239 (*Definitive, seminal article*)

Vane J R, Botting R M (eds) 2001 Therapeutic roles of selective COX-2 inhibitors. William Harvey Press, London, pp. 584 (*Outstanding multiauthor book covering all aspects of the mechanisms of action, actions, adverse effects and clinical role of COX-2 inhibitors in a range of tissues. Excellent up-to-date coverage*)

Vincent F, Kirkman R et al. 1998 Interleukin-2-receptor blockade with daclizaumab to prevent acute rejection in renal transplantation. N Engl J Med 338: 161–165

Whittle B J R 2001 Basis of gastrointestinal toxicity of non-steroid anti-inflammatory drugs. In: Vane J R, Botting R M (eds) Therapeutic roles of selective COX-2 inhibitors. William Harvey Press, London, Ch. 15, pp. 329–354 (*Excellent coverage; very good diagrams*)

Wolfe M M 1998 Future trends in the development of safer nonsteroidal anti-inflammatory drugs. Am J Med 105: 44S–52S (*Discusses various trends emphasising specific COX-2 inhibitors and NO-releasing NSAIDs*)

Wolfe M M, Lichtenstein D R, Singh G 1999 Gastrointestinal toxicity of nonsteroidal antiinflammatory drugs. N Engl J Med 340: 1888–1899 (*Reviews epidemiology of the gastrointestinal complications of NSAIDs, covering the risk factors, the pathogenesis of GIT damage, and treatment. Brief discussion of COX-2 selective drugs and NO–NSAIDs*)

SECTION

3

DRUGS AFFECTING MAJOR ORGAN SYSTEMS

17 The heart

Overview 264

Physiology of cardiac function 264
- Cardiac rate and rhythm 264
- Cardiac contraction 268
- Myocardial oxygen consumption and coronary blood flow 270
- Cardiac natriuretic peptides 272

Drugs that affect cardiac function 272
- Autonomic transmitters and related drugs 272
- Antidysrhythmic drugs 274
- Drugs that increase myocardial contraction 278
- Antianginal drugs 279

OVERVIEW

In this chapter we consider the effects of drugs on the heart under three main headings:

- **rate and rhythm**
- **myocardial contraction**
- **metabolism and blood flow.**

The effects of drugs on these aspects of cardiac function are not, of course, independent of each other. For example, if a drug affects the electrical properties of the myocardial cell membrane, it is likely to influence both cardiac rhythm and myocardial contraction. Similarly, a drug that affects contraction will inevitably alter metabolism and blood flow as well. Nevertheless, from a therapeutic point of view, these three classes of effect represent distinct clinical objectives in relation to the treatment, respectively, of cardiac dysrhythmias, cardiac failure and coronary insufficiency (as occurs during angina pectoris or myocardial infarction). We also give a short account of natriuretic peptides made in the heart and secreted into the blood. We first consider functional aspects to provide a basis for understanding the effects of drugs on the heart and their place in treating cardiac disease. The main drugs considered are:

1. **Antidysrhythmic drugs**
2. **Drugs that increase the force of contraction of the heart (especially digoxin)**
3. **Antianginal drugs.**

PHYSIOLOGY OF CARDIAC FUNCTION

CARDIAC RATE AND RHYTHM

The chambers of the heart normally contract in a coordinated manner, pumping blood efficiently by a route determined by the valves. Coordination of contraction is achieved by a specialised conducting system. Sinus rhythm, which is physiological, is characterised by impulses arising in the sinoatrial (SA) node and conducted in sequence through the atria, the atrioventricular (AV) node, bundle of His, Purkinje fibres and ventricles. Cardiac cells owe their electrical excitability to voltage-sensitive plasma membrane channels selective for various ions including Na^+, K^+ and Ca^{2+}; the structure and function of these channels are described in Chapter 4. Electrophysiological features of cardiac muscle that distinguish it from other excitable tissues include:

- the spontaneous, intrinsic rhythm generated normally by specialised cells in the SA node (i.e. pacemaker activity)
- absence of fast Na^+ current in SA and AV nodes, where slow inward Ca^{2+} current is responsible for initiation and propagation of the action potential
- a long duration of the action potential and long refractory period
- a large influx of Ca^{2+} during the plateau of the action potential.

Thus several of the special features of cardiac rhythm relate to Ca^{2+} currents. There are two distinct kinds of calcium channel in the heart: *intracellular* channels (i.e. the large ryanodine receptors and smaller inositol trisphosphate-activated calcium channels described in Chapter 4 and important in myocardial contraction) and *voltage-dependent plasma membrane calcium channels*, which are important in controlling cardiac rate and rhythm. The main type of voltage-dependent calcium channel in adult working myocardium is the L-type channel, which is also important in vascular smooth muscle; L-type channels are important in specialised conducting regions as well as in working myocardium.

▼ *Voltage-dependent plasma membrane calcium channels* are expressed in many distinct types (including L-, T-, N-, P-, Q- and R-types) in different tissues, classified by their electrophysiological properties and responses to drugs (e.g. dihydropyridines; see below), toxins (e.g. ω-agatoxin, ω-conotoxin) and ions (e.g. Ni^{2+}, Cd^{2+}). T-channels are important in cardiac conduction and are also prominent during fetal development and during cardiac myocyte proliferation, as well as being abundant in the central nervous system.

The action potential of an idealised cardiac muscle cell is shown in Figure 17.1A and is divided into five phases: 0 (fast depolarisation), I (partial repolarisation), II (plateau), III (repolarisation) and IV (pacemaker).

▼ Ionic mechanisms underlying these phases can be summarised as follows.

Phase 0, rapid depolarisation, occurs when the membrane potential reaches a critical firing threshold (about −60 mV) at which the inward current of Na^+ flowing through the voltage-dependent sodium channels becomes large enough to produce a regenerative ('all-or-nothing') depolarisation. This mechanism is the same as that responsible for action potential generation in neurons (see Ch. 4). Activation of sodium channels by membrane depolarisation is transient, and if the membrane remains depolarised for more than a few milliseconds, they close again (inactivation). They are, therefore, closed during the plateau of the action potential and remain unavailable for the initiation of another action potential until the membrane repolarises.

Phase 1, partial repolarisation, occurs as the Na^+ current is inactivated. There may also be a transient voltage-sensitive outward current.

Phase 2, the plateau, results from an inward Ca^{2+} current. Calcium channels show a pattern of voltage-sensitive activation and inactivation qualitatively similar to sodium channels, but with a much slower time course. The plateau is assisted by a special property of the cardiac muscle membrane, known as inward-going rectification, which means that the K^+ conductance falls to a low level when the membrane is depolarised. Because of this, there is little tendency for outward K^+ current to restore the resting membrane potential during the plateau, so a relatively small inward Ca^{2+} current suffices to maintain the plateau.

Phase 3, repolarisation, occurs as the Ca^{2+} current inactivates and a delayed outwardly rectifying K^+ current (analogous to but much slower than the K^+ current that causes repolarisation in nerve fibres; Ch. 4) activates, causing outward K^+ current. This is augmented by another K^+ current, which is activated by high intracellular Ca^{2+} concentrations, $[Ca^{2+}]_i$, during the plateau, and sometimes also by other K^+ currents, including one through channels activated by acetylcholine (see below) and another that is activated by arachidonic acid, which is liberated under pathological conditions such as myocardial infarction.

Phase 4, the pacemaker potential, is a gradual depolarisation during diastole. Pacemaker activity is normally found only in nodal and conducting tissue. The pacemaker potential is caused by a combination of *increasing inward currents* and *reduced outward currents* during diastole. It is usually most rapid in cells of the SA node, which, therefore, acts as pacemaker for the whole heart. Cells in the SA node have a greater background conductance to Na^+ than do atrial or ventricular myocytes, leading to a greater background *inward current.* In addition, inactivation of voltage-dependent calcium channels wears off during diastole resulting in increasing inward Ca^{2+} current during late diastole. Activation of T-type calcium channels during late diastole contributes to pacemaker activity in the SA node. The negative membrane potential early in diastole activates a cation channel that is permeable to Na^+ and K^+, giving rise to another inward current called $I(f)$.*

Several voltage- and time-dependent *outward currents* play a part as well: delayed rectifier K^+ current (I_K), which is activated during the action potential, is turned off by the negative membrane potential early in diastole. Current from the electrogenic Na^+/K^+ pump also contributes to the outward current during the pacemaker potential.

Figure 17.1B shows the action potential configuration in different parts of the heart. Phase 0 is absent in the nodal regions, where the conduction velocity is correspondingly slow (~5 cm/s) compared with other regions such as the Purkinje fibres (conduction velocity ~200 cm/s), which propagate the action potential rapidly to the ventricles. Regions that lack a fast inward current have a much longer refractory period than fast-conducting regions. This is because recovery of the slow inward current following its inactivation during the action potential takes a considerable time (a few hundred milliseconds), and the refractory period outlasts the action potential. With fast-conducting fibres, recovery from inactivation of the Na^+ current is quick, and the cell becomes excitable again as soon as it is repolarised.

The orderly pattern of sinus rhythm can become disrupted either by heart disease or by the action of drugs or circulating hormones, and an important therapeutic use of drugs is to restore a normal cardiac rhythm where it has become disturbed. The commonest cause of cardiac dysrhythmia is ischaemic heart disease, and many deaths following myocardial infarction result from ventricular fibrillation rather than directly from contractile failure.

DISTURBANCES OF CARDIAC RHYTHM

Clinically, dysrhythmias are classified according to:

- the site of origin of the abnormality—atrial, junctional or ventricular
- whether the rate is increased (tachycardia) or decreased (bradycardia).

They may cause palpitations (awareness of the heartbeat) or symptoms from cerebral hypoperfusion (feeling faint or losing consciousness). Their diagnosis depends on the surface electrocardiogram (ECG), and details are beyond the scope of this book. The commonest types of tachyarrhythmia are atrial fibrillation (AF) where the heartbeat is completely irregular, and supraventriacular tachycardia (SVT) where the heart beat is rapid but regular. Occasional ectopic beats (ventricular as well as supraventricular) are common. Sustained ventricular tachyarrhythmias are much less common but much more serious: they include ventricular tachycardia and ventricular fibrillation, where the electrical activity in the ventricles is completely chaotic and cardiac output ceases. Bradyarrhthmias include various kinds of heart block (e.g. at the AV or SA node), and complete cessation of electrical activity ('asystolic arrest'). It is often unclear which of the various mechanisms discussed below are responsible. These mechanisms nevertheless provide a useful starting point for understanding how antidysrhythmic drugs

*'f' for 'funny', because it is unusual for cation channels to be activated by hyperpolarisation; electrophysiologists are renowned for a peculiar sense of humour!

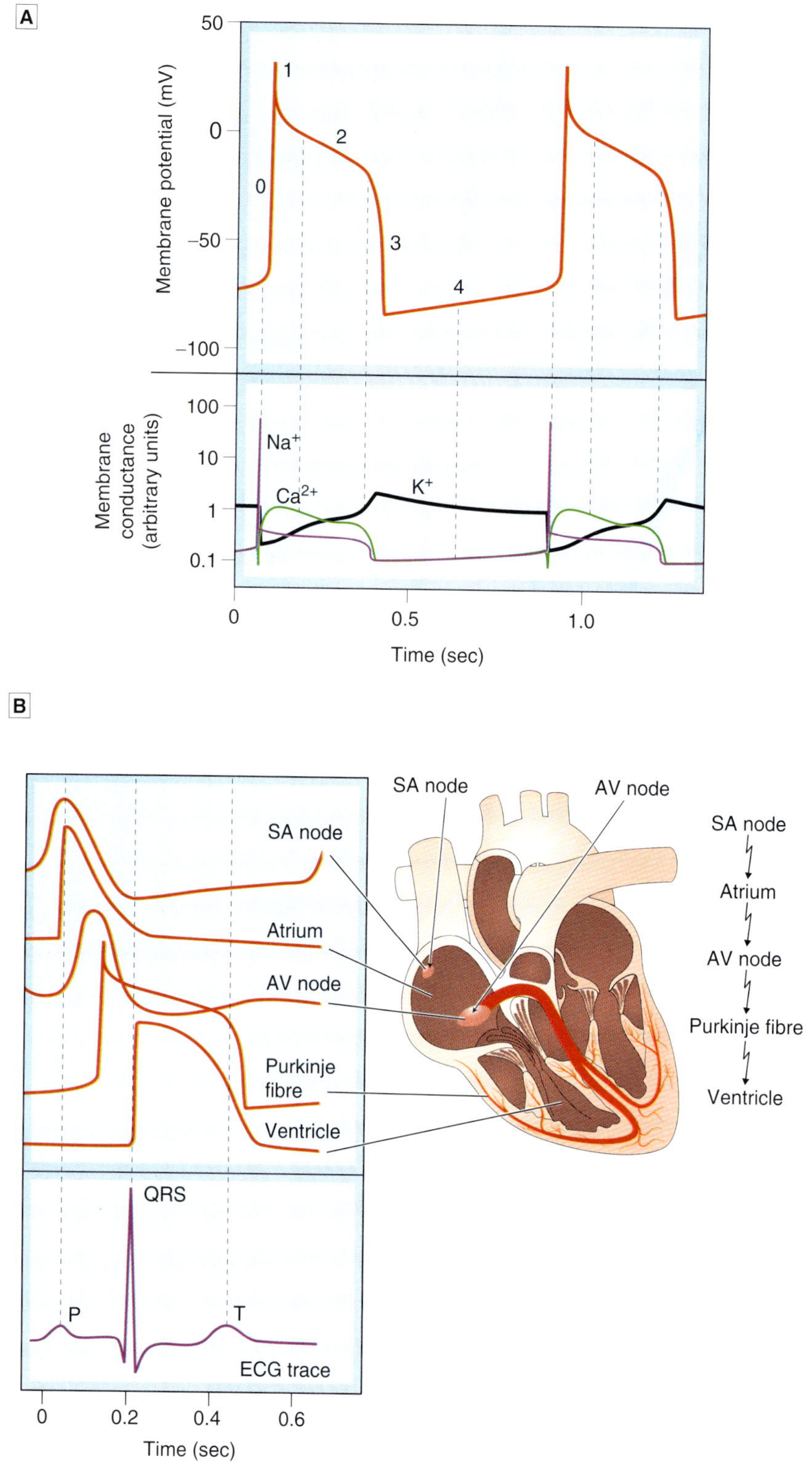

Fig. 17.1 The cardiac action potential. A Phases of the action potential: 0, rapid depolarisation; 1, partial repolarisation; 2, plateau; 3, repolarisation; 4, pacemaker depolarisation. The lower panel shows the accompanying changes in membrane conductance for Na^+, K^+ and Ca^{2+}. B Conduction of the impulse through the heart, with the corresponding electrocardiogram (ECG) trace. Note that the longest delay occurs at the atrioventricular (AV) node, where the action potential has a characteristically slow waveform. (Adapted from: (A) Noble D 1975 The initiation of the heartbeat. Oxford University Press, Oxford.)

work. Four basic phenomena underlie pathological or drug-induced disturbances of cardiac rhythm:

- delayed after-depolarisation
- re-entry
- ectopic pacemaker activity
- heart block.

The main cause of delayed after-depolarisation in ventricular muscle is abnormally raised $[Ca^{2+}]_i$, which triggers inward current and hence a train of abnormal action potentials ('ventricular tachycardia') (Fig. 17.2).

In normal cardiac rhythm, the conducted impulse dies out after it has activated the ventricles because it is surrounded by refractory tissue, which it has just traversed. Re-entry (Fig. 17.3) describes the situation in which the impulse succeeds in re-exciting regions of the myocardium after the refractory period has subsided and can cause the continuous circulation of action potentials. It can result from anatomical anomalies or, more commonly, from myocardial damage, which leads to deplarisation and a disturbed pattern of conductance.

Although the physiological pacemaker resides in the SA node, other cardiac tissues have the ability to take on pacemaker activity. This provides a safety mechanism in the event of failure of the SA node but can also trigger tachyarrhythmias. Such ectopic pacemaker activity is encouraged by sympathetic activity and by partial depolarisation, which may occur during ischaemia. Re-entry underlies many types of dysrhythmia, the pattern depending on the site of the re-entrant circuit, which may be in the atria, ventricles or nodal tissue.

Heart block

Heart block results from fibrosis or ischaemic damage of the conducting system, most commonly the AV node. In complete heart block, the atria and ventricles beat independently of one another, the ventricles beating at a slow rate determined by whatever pacemaker picks up distal to the block. Sporadic complete failure of AV conduction causes sudden periods of unconsciousness (*Stokes–Adams attacks*) and is treated by implanting an artificial pacemaker.

More detailed descriptions of the possible mechanisms underlying some of these basic phenomena are described below.

Delayed after-depolarisation

▼ Normal pacemaker activity, as described above, involves a spontaneous diastolic depolarisation, which initiates an action potential when it reaches threshold. Non-pacemaker cells do not normally undergo this diastolic depolarisation and remain quiescent if not excited by the arrival of an impulse from elsewhere in the heart. Under certain circumstances, however, a phenomenon called delayed after-depolarisation occurs, which can lead to a repetitive discharge that does not depend on the arrival of an impulse from elsewhere (Fig. 17.2). After-depolarisation follows an action potential if $[Ca^{2+}]_i$ increases excessively. It is accentuated if the extracellular Ca^{2+} concentration (and hence the amount of Ca^{2+} entering the cell during the plateau) is increased, and also by agents such as cardiac glycosides, noradrenaline (norepinephrine) or phosphodiesterase inhibitors that increase intracellular Ca^{2+}. After-depolarisation is the result of a net inward current (known as the *transient inward current*). How does a rise in $[Ca^{2+}]_i$ cause an inward current? One possibility is that it activates Na^+–Ca^{2+} exchange (see Fig. 17.4). This transfers one Ca^{2+} out of the cell in exchange for entry of three Na^+, resulting in a net influx of one positive charge and hence membrane depolarisation. Additionally, Ca^{2+} opens non-selective cation channels in the plasma membrane, allowing entry of Na^+ and other ions, analogous to the endplate potential at the neuromuscular junction (Ch. 10).

Re-entry

▼ A simple ring of tissue can give rise to a re-entrant rhythm if a transient or unidirectional conduction block is present (Fig. 17.3). Normally, an impulse originating at any point in the ring will propagate in both directions and die out when the two impulses meet, but if a damaged area

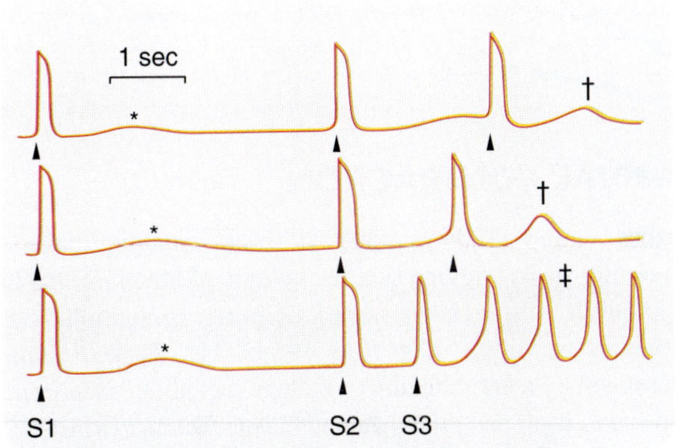

Fig. 17.2 After-depolarisation in cardiac muscle recorded from a dog coronary sinus in the presence of noradrenaline (norepinephrine). The first stimulus (S1) causes an action potential followed by a small after-depolarisation. As the interval S2–S3 is decreased, the after-depolarisation gets larger (†) until it triggers an indefinite train of action potentials (‡). (Adapted from: Wit A L, Cranefield P F 1977 Circ Res 41: 435.)

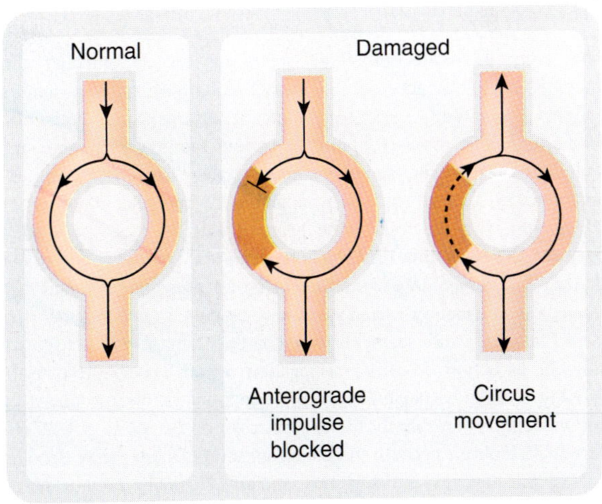

Fig. 17.3 Generation of a re-entrant rhythm by a damaged area of myocardium. The damaged area (brown) conducts in one direction only. This disturbs the normal pattern of conduction and permits continuous circulation of the impulse to occur.

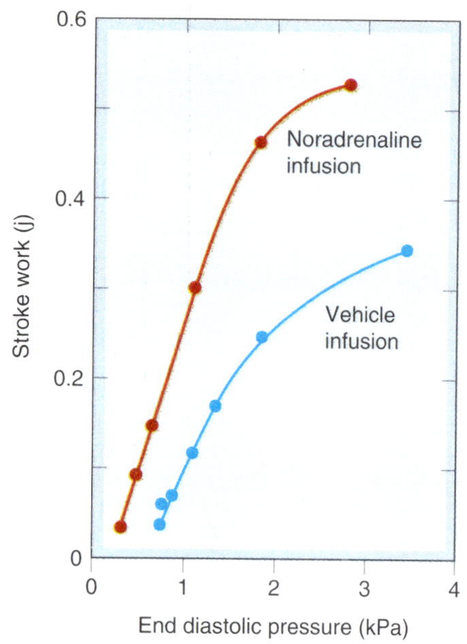

Fig. 17.4 Ventricular function curves in the dog. Infusion of physiological saline increases blood volume and hence end-diastolic pressure. This increases stroke work ('extrinsic' control) by increasing the force of contraction of the heart. This relationship is called the Starling curve. Noradrenaline (norepinephrine) has a direct action on the heart ('intrinsic' control), increasing the slope of the Starling curve. (Redrawn from: Sarnoff S J et al. 1960 Circ Res 8: 1108.)

causes either a transient block (so that one impulse is blocked but the second can get through; Fig. 17.3) or a unidirectional block, continuous circulation of the impulse can occur. This is known as circus movement and was first demonstrated experimentally on rings of jellyfish tissue many years ago.

The 'ring' of tissue sometimes represents an anatomically distinct anomaly such as an accessory pathway linking atria and ventricles, as in patients with Wolff–Parkinson–White syndrome. Such pathways are increasingly accessible to ablation by various minimally invasive surgical techniques. However, more commonly, the 'ring' of tissue is not anatomically distinct but only functionally separate. If it retains a connection with the rest of the heart, it can act as a focus for high frequency re-excitation of the whole atrium or ventricle. The re-entrant rhythm will persist only if the time taken for propagation round the ring exceeds the refractory period, so it may be halted by drugs that prolong the refractory period (see below). Myocardial damage may cause extreme slowing of action potential propagation, which favours re-entry. This slowing is often associated with the attenuation or disappearance of the Na^+ current responsible for the fast upstroke of the action potential. This current is reduced because the compromised cells are partly depolarised during diastole; as a result fast sodium channels remain partly or completely inactivated, leaving only the slow inward current to support propagation of the action potential.

Abnormal pacemaker activity

▼ Under pathological conditions, pacemaker activity can arise in other parts of the heart than the SA node and conducting tissues. The main predisposing factors are: catecholamine action and partial depolarisation, such as may occur in ischaemic damage.

Catecholamines, acting on β_1-adrenoceptors (see below), increase the rate of depolarisation during phase 4 and can cause normally quiescent parts of the heart to take on a spontaneous rhythm. Several tachyarrhythmias (e.g. paroxysmal atrial fibrillation) can be triggered by circumstances associated with increased sympathetic activity. Pain (e.g. during myocardial infarction) increases sympathetic discharge and releases adrenaline from the adrenal gland. Partial depolarisation resulting from ischaemic damage is probably caused by decreased activity of the electrogenic Na^+ pump, and it will also cause abnormal pacemaker activity.

Cardiac dysrhythmias

- Dysrhythmias arise because of:
  —delayed after-depolarisation, which triggers ectopic beats
  —re-entry, resulting from partial conduction block
  —ectopic pacemaker activity
  —heart block.
- Delayed after-depolarisation is caused by an inward current associated with abnormally raised intracellular Ca^{2+}.
- Re-entry is facilitated when parts of the myocardium are depolarised, conduction then depending on slow Ca^{2+} current.
- Ectopic pacemaker activity is encouraged by sympathetic activity.
- Heart block results from damage to the atrioventricular node or ventricular conducting system.
- Clinically, dysrhythmias are divided:
  —according to their site of origin (supraventricular and ventricular)
  —according to whether the heart rate is increased or decreased (tachycardia or bradycardia).

CARDIAC CONTRACTION

Cardiac output is the product of heart rate and mean left ventricular stroke volume (i.e. the volume of blood ejected from the ventricle with each heart beat). Heart rate is controlled by the autonomic nervous system (Chs 10 and 11). Stroke volume is determined by a combination of factors, including some intrinsic to the heart itself and other haemodynamic factors extrinsic to the heart. *Intrinsic factors* regulate *myocardial contractility* via $[Ca^{2+}]_i$ and ATP and are sensitive to various drugs and pathological processes. *Extrinsic circulatory factors* include the contractile state of arteries and veins and the volume and viscosity of the blood, which together determine cardiac load (preload and afterload). Drugs that influence these circulatory factors are of paramount importance in treating patients with heart failure. They are covered in Chapter 18.

MYOCARDIAL CONTRACTILITY AND VIABILITY

The contractile machinery of myocardial cells is basically the same as that of voluntary muscle (Ch. 4). It involves binding of Ca^{2+} to troponin C; this changes the conformation of the troponin complex, permitting cross-bridging of myosin to actin and initiating contraction.

Many effects of drugs on cardiac contractility can be explained in terms of actions on $[Ca^{2+}]_i$, secondary to effects on voltage-sensitive calcium channels in plasma membrane or sarcoplasmic reticulum or on the Na^+/K^+ pump. Other factors that affect the force of contraction are the availability of oxygen and a source of metabolic energy such as free fatty acids. Myocardial 'stunning'—contractile dysfunction that persists after ischaemia and reperfusion despite restoration of blood flow and absence of cardiac necrosis—is incompletely understood but can be clinically important. Its converse is known as 'ischaemic preconditioning': this means an improved ability to withstand ischaemia following previous ischaemic episodes. This potentially beneficial state could also be clinically important. There is some evidence that it is mediated by *adenosine* (see Ch. 12), which accumulates as ATP is depleted. Exogenous adenosine affords protection similar to that caused by ischaemic preconditioning, and blockade of adenosine receptors prevents the protective effect of preconditioning. There is considerable interest in developing strategies to minimise harmful effects of ischaemia while maximising preconditioning.

VENTRICULAR FUNCTION CURVES AND HEART FAILURE

The force of contraction of the heart is determined partly by its intrinsic *contractility* (which, as described above, depends on $[Ca^{2+}]_i$ and availability of ATP) and partly by extrinsic haemodynamic factors that affect *end-diastolic volume* and, hence, the resting length of the muscle fibres. The end-diastolic volume is determined by the end-diastolic pressure, and its effect on stroke work is expressed in the Frank–Starling law of the heart, which reflects an inherent property of the contractile system. The Frank–Starling law can be represented as a *ventricular function curve* (Fig. 17.4). The area enclosed by the pressure–volume curve during the cardiac cycle provides a measure of ventricular *stroke work*. It is approximated by the product of stroke volume and mean arterial pressure. As Starling showed, factors extrinsic to the heart affect its performance in various ways, two patterns of response to increased load being particularly important.

- Increased cardiac filling pressure (*pre-load*), whether caused by increased blood volume or by venoconstriction, increases ventricular end-diastolic volume. This increases stroke volume and hence cardiac output and mean arterial pressure. Cardiac work and cardiac oxygen consumption both increase.
- Arterial and arteriolar vasoconstriction increases *after-load*. End-diastolic volume, and hence stroke work, are initially unchanged but constant stroke work in the face of increased vascular resistance causes reduced stroke volume and hence increased end-diastolic volume. This in turn increases stroke work, until a steady state is re-established with increased end-diastolic volume and the same cardiac output as before. As with increased pre-load, cardiac work and cardiac oxygen consumption both increase.

Normal ventricular filling pressure is only a few centimetres of water, on the steep part of the ventricular function curve, so a large increase in stroke work can be achieved with only a small increase in filling pressure. The Starling mechanism plays little part in controlling cardiac output in healthy subjects (e.g. during exercise), because changes in contractility, mainly as a result of changes in sympathetic activity, achieve the necessary regulation without any increase in ventricular filling pressure (Fig. 17.4). In contrast, the denervated heart in patients who have received a heart transplant relies on the Starling mechanism to increase cardiac output during exercise.

Heart failure is a condition in which the cardiac output is insufficient to meet the circulatory needs of the body (at rest or during exercise). It has many causes, most commonly ischaemic heart disease. In patients with heart failure (see Ch. 18) the heart may be unable to deliver as much blood as the tissues require even when its contractility is increased by sympathetic activity. Under these conditions the basal (i.e. at rest) ventricular function curve is greatly depressed, and there is insufficient reserve, in the sense of extra contractility that can be achieved by sympathetic activity, to enable cardiac output to be maintained during exercise without a large increase in central venous pressure (Fig. 17.4). Oedema of peripheral tissues (causing swelling of the legs) and the lungs (causing breathlessness) is an important consequence of cardiac failure. It is caused by the increased venous pressure, and retention of Na^+ (see Ch. 18).

Myocardial contraction

- Controlling factors are:
  —intrinsic contractility
  —extrinsic circulatory factors.
- Contractility depends critically on control of intracellular Ca^{2+}, and hence on:
  —Ca^{2+} entry across the cell membrane
  —Ca^{2+} storage in the sarcoplasmic reticulum.
- The main factors controlling Ca^{2+} entry are:
  —activity of voltage-gated calcium channels
  —intracellular Na^+, which affects Ca^{2+}–Na^+ exchange.
- Catecholamines, cardiac gycosides and other drugs and mediators influence these factors.
- Extrinsic control of cardiac contraction is through the dependence of stroke work on the end-diastolic volume, expressed in the Frank–Starling law.
- Cardiac work is affected independently by after-load (i.e. peripheral resistance and arterial compliance) and pre-load (i.e. central venous pressure).

pathology is basically the same as that involved in myocardial infarction, namely platelet–fibrin thrombus associated with a ruptured atheromatous plaque, but without complete occlusion of the vessel. The risk of infarction is substantial, and the main aim of therapy is to reduce this. **Aspirin** approximately halves the risk of myocardial infarction in this setting, and **heparin** and **platelet glycoprotein receptor antagonists** add to this benefit (Ch. 20).

Variant angina This is uncommon. It occurs at rest and is caused by coronary artery spasm, again usually in association with atheromatous disease. Therapy is with coronary artery vasodilators (e.g. organic nitrates, calcium antagonists).

Myocardial infarction

Myocardial infarction occurs after a coronary artery has been blocked by thrombus. This may be fatal and is the commonest cause of death in many parts of the world, usually as a result of mechanical failure of the ventricle or from dysrhythmia. Cardiac myocytes rely on aerobic metabolism. If the supply of oxygen remains below a critical value, a sequence of events leading to cell death (by *necrosis* or *apoptosis*) ensues (see Ch. 6 for a fuller account of apoptosis). The sequences leading from vascular occlusion to cell death via the two pathways is illustrated in Figure 17.6. The relative importance of necrosis and apoptosis in myocardial cell death in clinically distinct settings is unknown, but it has been suggested that apoptosis may be an adaptive process in hypoperfused regions, sacrificing some jeopardised myocytes but thereby avoiding the dysrhythmogenic disturbance of membrane function inherent in necrosis. Consequently, it is currently unknown if pharmacological approaches to promote or inhibit this pathway could be clinically beneficial.

Prevention of irreversible ischaemic damage following an episode of coronary thrombosis is nonetheless an important therapeutic aim. The main possibilities among existing therapeutic drugs, shown in Figure 17.6, are:

- thrombolytic and antiplatelet drugs to open the blocked artery (see Ch. 20)
- oxygen
- opioids to prevent pain and reduce excessive sympathetic activity
- β-adrenoceptor antagonists
- angiotensin-converting enzyme inhibitors.

The latter two classes of drug reduce cardiac work and thereby the metabolic needs of the heart. Beta-adrenoceptor antagonists had only a small beneficial effect when given acutely to patients with acute myocardial infarction in the ISIS-1 study (although they have an important longer-term benefit during chronic treatment in reducing dysrhythmic deaths) but are widely used in patients with unstable angina. Several clinical trials have demonstrated that angiotensin-converting enzyme inhibitors improve survival if given to patients shortly after myocardial infarction, especially if there is even a modest degree of

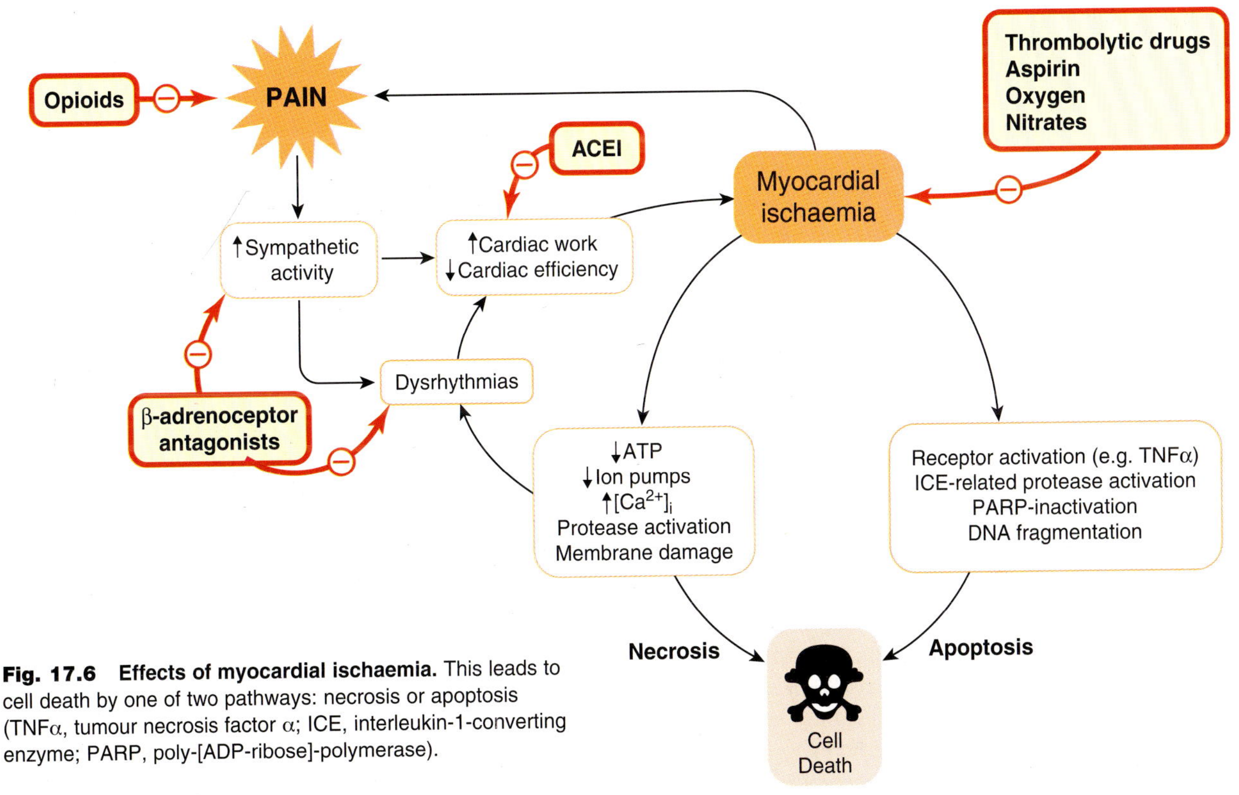

Fig. 17.6 Effects of myocardial ischaemia. This leads to cell death by one of two pathways: necrosis or apoptosis (TNFα, tumour necrosis factor α; ICE, interleukin-1-converting enzyme; PARP, poly-[ADP-ribose]-polymerase).

Coronary flow, ischaemia and infarction

- The heart has a smaller blood supply in relation to its oxygen consumption than most organs.
- Coronary flow is controlled mainly by:
  —physical factors, including transmural pressure during systole
  —vasodilator metabolites.
- Autonomic innervation is less important.
- Coronary ischaemia is usually the result of atherosclerosis, and causes anginal pain. Sudden ischaemia is usually caused by thrombosis and may result in cardiac infarction.
- Coronary spasm sometimes causes angina (variant angina).
- Cellular Ca^{2+} overload results from ischaemia and may be responsible for:
  —cell death
  —initiation of dysrhythmias.

myocardial dysfunction. It is possible (but so far unproven—see Ch. 18 for a discussion of the differences between angiotensin receptor antagonists (*'sartans'*) and angiotensin-converting enzyme inhibitors) that sartans could prove similarly beneficial.

Despite several small trials of *organic nitrates* that appeared encouraging, a large randomised controlled trial (ISIS-4) showed that they do not improve outcome in patients with myocardial infarction, although they are useful in preventing or treating anginal pain (see below). *Calcium antagonists,* which reduce cardiac work (via arteriolar vasodilatation and after-load reduction) and block Ca^{2+} entry into cardiac myocytes, have been disappointing, and several clinical trials of short-acting dihydropyridines (e.g. **nifedipine**) were halted when adverse trends were evident.

CARDIAC NATRIURETIC PEPTIDES

Atrial cells have a specialised endocrine function in relation to the cardiovascular system. They contain secretory granules and store and release atrial natriuretic peptide (ANP). This has powerful effects on the kidney and vascular system. Release of ANP occurs during volume overload in response to stretching of the atria. Saline infusion is sufficient to evoke ANP release. Two related natriuretic peptides (B and C: found, respectively, in ventricular muscle and vascular endothelium) are also known.

The main effects of natriuretic peptides are to increase Na^+ and water excretion by the kidney, relax vascular smooth muscle (except efferent arterioles of renal glomeruli, see below), increase vascular permeability and inhibit the release and/or actions of several hormones and mediators including aldosterone, angiotensin II, endothelin and antidiuretic hormone. They exert their effects by combining with membrane receptors (natriuretic peptide receptors (NPR), which exist in at least two subtypes designated A and B).* NPR-A and NPR-B both incorporate a catalytic guanylate cyclase moiety. Binding of one of the natriuretic peptides to either receptor leads to generation of cGMP. This is the same response as that produced by organic nitrates (see later) and endothelium-derived nitric oxide (NO; Ch. 14), which, however, achieve this by interacting with soluble rather than membrane-bound guanylate cyclase. Renal glomerular afferent arterioles are dilated by ANP but efferent arterioles are constricted, so filtration pressure is increased, leading to increased glomerular filtration and enhanced Na^+ excretion. Elsewhere, natriuretic peptides cause vasorelaxation and reduce blood pressure. Their therapeutic potential is considered in Chapter 18.

DRUGS THAT AFFECT CARDIAC FUNCTION

Drugs that have a major action on the heart can be divided into three groups.

- *Drugs that directly affect myocardial cells.* These include:
  —autonomic neurotransmitters and related drugs
  —antidysrhythmic drugs
  —cardiac glycosides and other inotropic drugs
  —miscellaneous drugs and endogenous substances; those are dealt with elsewhere (e.g. **doxorubicin**, Ch. 50; thyroxine, Ch. 28; glucagon, Ch. 25).
- *Drugs that affect cardiac function indirectly.* These have actions elsewhere in the vascular system. Some antianginal drugs (e.g. nitrates) fall into this category, as do most drugs that are used to treat heart failure (e.g. diuretics and angiotensin-converting enzyme inhibitors).
- *Calcium antagonists.* These affect cardiac function by a direct action on myocardial cells and also indirectly by relaxing arterioles.

AUTONOMIC TRANSMITTERS AND RELATED DRUGS

Many aspects of autonomic pharmacology have been discussed in Chapters 9–11; here we mention only aspects that particularly concern the heart.

AUTONOMIC CONTROL OF THE HEART

The sympathetic and parasympathetic systems each normally exert a tonic effect on the heart at rest.

*The nomenclature of natriuretic peptides and their receptors is peculiarly obtuse. The peptides are named 'A' for atrial, 'B' for brain—despite being present mainly in cardiac ventricle—and 'C' for A,B,C...; NPRs are named NPR-A, which preferentially binds ANP, NPR-B, which binds *C* natriuretic peptide preferentially, and NPR-C for 'clearance' receptor, since until recently clearance via cellular uptake and degradation by lysosomal enzymes was the only definite known function of this binding site.

Sympathetic system

The main effects of sympathetic activity on the heart are:

- increased force of contraction (*positive inotropic effect*; Fig. 17.7)
- increased heart rate (*positive chronotropic effect*; Fig. 17.8)
- increased automaticity
- *repolarisation* and restoration of function following generalised cardiac depolarisation
- *reduced cardiac efficiency* (i.e. oxygen consumption is increased more than cardiac work).

These effects all result from activation of β_1-adrenoceptors. The β_1-effects of catecholamines on the heart, though complex, probably all occur through increased intracellular cAMP (see Ch. 3). cAMP activates protein kinase A, which phosphorylates sites on the α_1-subunits of calcium channels. This increases the probability that the channels will open, increasing inward Ca^{2+} current and hence force of cardiac contraction (Fig. 17.7). Activation of β_1-adrenoceptors activation also increases the Ca^{2+} sensitivity of the contractile machinery, possibly by phosphorylating troponin C; furthermore, it facilitates Ca^{2+} capture by the sarcoplasmic reticulum, thereby increasing the amount of Ca^{2+} available for release by the action potential. The net result of catecholamine action is to elevate and steepen the ventricular function curve (Fig. 17.4). The increase in heart rate results from an increased slope of the pacemaker potential (Figs 17.1 and 17.8) owing to a shift in the voltage dependence of the conductances underlying the pacemaker currents so that they are switched on and reach the firing threshold, earlier. Increased Ca^{2+} entry also causes increased automaticity because of the effect of $[Ca^{2+}]_i$ on the transient inward current, which can result in a train of action potentials following a single stimulus (Fig. 17.2).

Activation of β_1-adrenoceptors repolarises damaged or hypoxic myocardium by stimulating the Na^+/K^+ pump. This can restore function if asystole has occurred following myocardial infarction, and **adrenaline** (**epinephrine**) is one of the most important drugs during cardiac arrest.

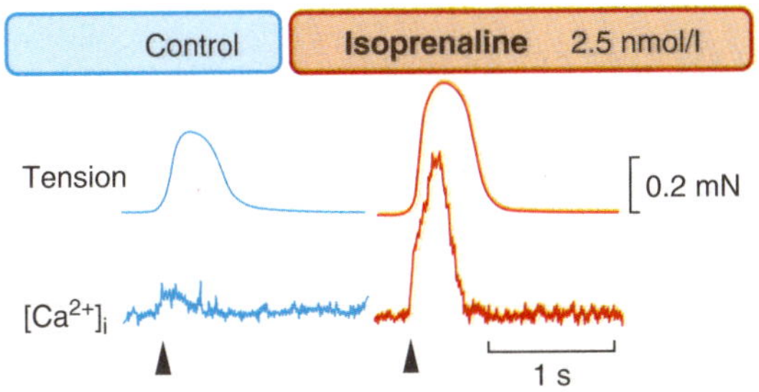

Fig. 17.7 The calcium transient in frog cardiac muscle. A group of cells was injected with the phosphorescent Ca^{2+} indicator aequorin, which allows $[Ca^{2+}]_i$ to be monitored optically. Isoprenaline causes a large increase in the tension and in the $[Ca^{2+}]_i$ transient caused by an electrical stimulus (▲). (From: Allen D G, Blinks J R 1978 Nature 273: 509.)

The reduction of cardiac efficiency by catecholamines is important because it means that the oxygen requirement of the myocardium increases even if the work of the heart is unchanged. This limits the use of β-agonists such as adrenaline (epinephrine) and **dobutamine** for shock (Ch. 18). Myocardial infarction causes sympathetic activation (Fig. 17.6), which has the undesirable effect of increasing the oxygen needs of the damaged myocardium.

Parasympathetic system

Parasympathetic activity produces effects that are, in general, opposite to those of sympathetic activation, namely:

- cardiac slowing and reduced automaticity
- inhibition of AV conduction.

These effects result from occupation of muscarinic (M_2) acetylcholine receptors, which are abundant in nodal and atrial tissue but sparse in the ventricles. These receptors are negatively coupled to adenylate cyclase and thus reduce cAMP formation, acting to inhibit the slow Ca^{2+} current, in opposition to β_1-adrenoceptors. M_2-receptors also open a potassium channel (called K_{ACh}). The resulting increase in K^+ permeability produces a hyperpolarising current that opposes the inward pacemaker current, slowing the heart and reducing automaticity (see Fig.

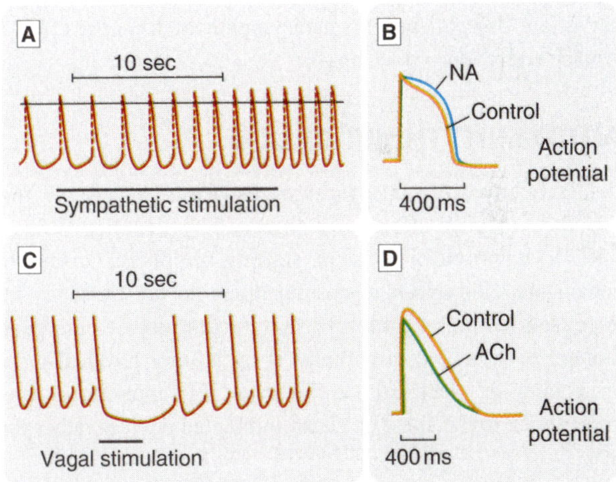

Fig. 17.8 Autonomic regulation of the heartbeat. A and B Effects of sympathetic stimulation and noradrenaline (NA; norepinephrine). C and D Effects of parasympathetic stimulation and acetylcholine (ACh). Sympathetic stimulation (A) increases the slope of the pacemaker potential and increases heart rate, whereas parasympathetic stimulation (C) abolishes the pacemaker potential, hyperpolarises the membrane and temporarily stops the heart (frog sinus venosus). NA (B) prolongs the action potential, while ACh (D) shortens it (frog atrium). (From: (A and C) Hutter O F, Trautwein W 1956 J Gen Physiol 39: 715; (B) Reuter H 1974 J Physiol 242: 429; (D) Giles W R, Noble S J 1976 J Physiol 261: 103.)

Autonomic control of the heart

- Sympathetic activity, acting through β_1-adrenoceptors, increases heart rate, contractility and automaticity, but reduces cardiac efficiency (in relation to oxygen consumption).
- The β_1-adrenoceptors act by increasing cAMP formation, which increases Ca^{2+} currents.
- Parasympathetic activity, acting through muscarinic M_2-receptors, causes cardiac slowing, decreased force of contraction (atria only) and inhibition of atrioventricular conduction.
- M_2-receptors inhibit cAMP formation and also open potassium channels, causing hyperpolarisation.

17.8). Vagal activity is often increased during myocardial infarction, both in association with vagal afferent stimulation and also as a side-effect of opioids used to control the pain, and parasympathetic effects are important in predisposing to acute dysrhythmias.

Vagal stimulation decreases the force of contraction of the atria associated with marked shortening of the action potential (Fig. 17.8). Increased K^+ permeability and reduced Ca^{2+} current both contribute to conduction block at the AV node, where propagation depends on the Ca^{2+} current. Shortening the atrial action potential reduces the refractory period, which can lead to re-entrant arrhythmias. Coronary *vessels* lack cholinergic innervation; consequently the parasympathetic has little effect on coronary artery tone (see Ch. 10).*

ANTIDYSRHYTHMIC DRUGS

A classification of antidysrhythmic drugs based on their electrophysiological effects was proposed by Vaughan Williams in 1970. It provides a good starting point for discussing mechanisms, although many useful drugs do not fit neatly into this classification (Table 17.1). Furthermore, emergency treatment of serious dysrhythmias is usually by physical means (e.g. pacing or electrical cardioversion by applying a direct current shock to the chest or via an implanted device) rather than drugs.

There are four classes (see Table 17.2).

Class I: drugs that block voltage-sensitive sodium channels. They are subdivided: Ia, Ib and Ic (see below).
Class II: β-adrenoceptor antagonists.
Class III: drugs that substantially prolong the cardiac action potential
Class IV: calcium antagonists.

*The creator has, however, thoughtfully provided coronary *endothelium* with muscarinic receptors linked to NO synthesis (see Chs 14 and 18), presumably for the delectation of vascular pharmacologists.

Table 17.1 Antidysrhythmic drugs unclassified in the Vaughan Williams' system

Drug	Use
Atropine	Sinus bradycardia
Adrenaline (epinephrine)	Cardiac arrest
Isoprenaline	Heart block
Digoxin	Rapid atrial fibrillation
Adenosine	Supraventricular tachycardia
Calcium chloride	Ventricular tachycardia due to hyperkalaemia
Magnesium chloride	Ventricular fibrillation, digoxin toxicity

Table 17.2 Summary of antidysrhythmic drugs (Vaughan Williams' classification)

Class	Example(s)	Mechanism
Ia	Disopyramide	Sodium channel block (intermediate dissociation)
Ib	Lidocaine	Sodium channel block (fast dissociation)
Ic	Flecainide	Sodium channel block (slow dissociation)
II	Propranolol	Beta-adrenoceptor antagonism
III	Amiodarone, sotalol	Potassium channel block
IV	Verapamil	Calcium channel block

The phase of the action potential on which each of these classes of drug have their main effect is shown in Figure 17.9.

MECHANISMS OF ACTION

Class I drugs

Class I drugs *block sodium channels*, just as local anaesthetics do, by binding to sites in the α-subunit (see Chs 4 and 43). Because this inhibits action potential propagation in many excitable cells, it has been referred to as 'membrane stabilising' activity, a phrase best avoided now that the ionic mechanism is understood. Their characteristic effect on the action potential is to reduce the maximum rate of depolarisation during phase 0.

The reason for further subdivision of these drugs into classes Ia, Ib and Ic is that the earliest examples, **quinidine** and **procainamide** (class Ia), have different effects from many of the more recently developed drugs, even though all share the same basic mechanism of action. A partial explanation for these

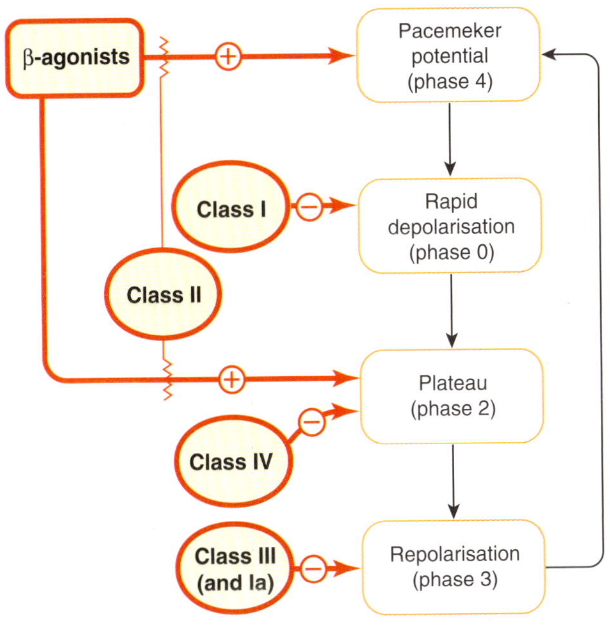

Fig. 17.9 Effects of antidysrhythmic drugs on the different phases (as defined in Fig. 17.1) of the cardiac action potential.

functional differences comes from electrophysiological studies of the characteristics of the sodium channel block produced by different class I drugs.

The central concept is of *use-dependent channel block*. It is this characteristic that enables all class I drugs to block the high-frequency excitation of the myocardium that occurs in tachyarrhythmias, without preventing the heart from beating at normal frequencies. Sodium channels exist in three distinct functional states: *resting*, *open* and *refractory*. Channels switch rapidly from resting to open in response to depolarisation; this is known as activation. Maintained depolarisation, as in ischaemic muscle, causes channels to change more slowly from open to refractory (inactivation) and the membrane must then be repolarised for a time to restore the channel to the resting state before it can be activated again. Class I drugs bind to channels most strongly when they are in either the open or refractory state, less strongly to channels in the resting state. Their action, therefore, shows the property of 'use dependence' (i.e. the more frequently the channels are activated, the greater the degree of block produced).

Class Ib drugs, e.g. **lidocaine**, associate and dissociate rapidly within the time-frame of the normal heartbeat. Drug binds to open channels during phase 0 of the action potential (affecting the rate of rise very little, but leaving many of the channels blocked by the time the action potential reaches its peak). Dissociation occurs in time for the next action potential, provided the cardiac rhythm is normal. A premature beat, however, will be aborted because the channels are still blocked. Furthermore, class Ib drugs bind selectively to refractory channels and thus block preferentially when the cells are depolarised, for example in ischaemia.

Class Ic drugs, such as **flecainide** and **encainide**, associate and dissociate much more slowly, thus reaching a steady-state level of block that does not vary appreciably during the cardiac cycle; they also show only a marginal preference for refractory channels so are not specific for damaged myocardium. Therefore, they cause a rather general reduction in excitability and do not discriminate particularly against occasional premature beats, as class Ib drugs do, but will suppress re-entrant rhythms that depend on unidirectional or intermittent conduction pathways operating at a low margin of safety (e.g. some forms of paroxysmal AF). They markedly inhibit conduction through the His–Purkinje system.

Class Ia, the oldest group (e.g. **quinidine**, **procainamide**, **disopyramide**), lies midway in its properties between Ib and Ic but, in addition, prolongs repolarisation, albeit less markedly than class III drugs (see below).

Class II drugs

Class II drugs comprise the β-adrenoceptor antagonists (e.g. **propranolol**).

Adrenaline (epinephrine) can cause dysrhythmias by its effects on the pacemaker potential and on the slow inward Ca^{2+} current (see above). Ventricular dysrhythmias following myocardial infarction are partly the result of increased sympathetic activity (see Fig. 17.6), providing a rationale for using β-adrenoceptor antagonists in this setting. AV conduction depends critically on sympathetic activity, and β-adrenoceptor antagonists increase the refractory period of the AV node and can, therefore, prevent recurrent attacks of SVT. Beta-adrenoceptor antagonists are also used to prevent paroxysmal attacks of AF when these occur in the setting of sympathetic activation.

Class III drugs

The class III category was originally based on the unusual behaviour of a single drug, **amiodarone** (see below), although others with similar properties (e.g. **sotalol**) have since been described. Both amiodarone and sotalol have more than one class of antidysrhythmic action. The special feature that defines them as class III drugs is that they substantially prolong the cardiac action potential. The mechanism of this effect is not fully understood, but it involves blocking some of the potassium channels involved in cardiac repolarisation, including the outward (delayed) rectifier. Action potential prolongation increases the refractory period, accounting for powerful and varied antidysrhythmic activity, e.g. by interrupting re-entrant tachycardias and suppressing ectopic activity. However, all drugs that prolong the cardiac action potential (detected clinically as prolonged Q–T interval on the electrocardiogram) can paradoxically also have pro-arrhythmic effects, notably a polymorphic form of ventricular tachycardia called (somewhat whimsically) '*torsade de pointes*' (because the appearance of the ECG trace is said to be reminiscent of this ballet sequence). This occurs particularly in patients taking other drugs that can prolong Q–T, including several antipsychotic drugs, those with disturbances of electrolytes involved in repolarisation (e.g. hypokalaemia, hypercalcaemia), or individuals with hereditary prolonged Q–T (Ward–Romano syndrome).* The mechanism of prodysrhythmia is not fully understood; possibilities include increased dispersion of repolarisation and increased Ca^{2+} entry during the prolonged action potential, leading to increased after-depolarisation.

Class IV drugs

Class IV agents act by blocking voltage-sensitive calcium channels. Class IV drugs in therapeutic use as antidysrhythmic drugs (e.g. **verapamil**) act on L-type channels. Class IV drugs slow conduction in the SA and AV nodes where action potential propagation depends on slow inward Ca^{2+} current, slowing the heart and terminating SVT by causing partial AV block. They shorten the plateau of the action potential and reduce the force of contraction. Reduced Ca^{2+} entry reduces after-depolarisation and thus suppresses premature ectopic beats.

DETAILS OF INDIVIDUAL DRUGS

Quinidine, procainamide and disopyramide (class Ia)

Quinidine and **procainamide** are pharmacologically similar. They are now mainly of historical interest. **Disopyramide** resembles quinidine in its antidysrhythmic effects, as well as in its marked atropine-like effects, which result in blurred vision, dry mouth, constipation and urinary retention. It is more negatively inotropic than quinidine but is less likely to cause hypersensitivity reactions.

Lidocaine (class Ib)

Lidocaine is given by intravenous infusion to treat and prevent ventricular dysrhythmias in the immediate aftermath of myocardial infarction. It is almost completely extracted from the portal circulation by hepatic first-pass metabolism (Ch. 8) and so cannot be administered orally. Its plasma half-life is normally about 2 hours, but its elimination is slowed if hepatic blood flow is reduced, for example by reduced cardiac output following myocardial infarction or by negative inotropes (e.g. β-adrenoceptor antagonists). Accumulation and toxicity may result if this is not anticipated and the rate of administration reduced accordingly. Indeed its clearance has been used to estimate hepatic blood flow, analogous to the use of *para*-aminohippurate clearance to measure renal blood flow.

The adverse effects of lidocaine are mainly manifestations of actions on the central nervous system and include drowsiness, disorientation and convulsions. Because of its relatively short half-life, the plasma concentration can be adjusted fairly rapidly by varying the infusion rate.

Phenytoin (class Ib)

Phenytoin is an anticonvulsant (Ch. 39); it has antidysrhythmic actions on the heart, but its clinical use for this indication is obsolete.

Flecainide and encainide (class Ic)

Flecainide and **encainide** suppress ventricular ectopic beats. They are long acting and are effective at reducing the frequency of ventricular ectopic beats when administered orally. However, they were found, in a well-controlled trial, actually to *increase* the incidence of sudden death associated with ventricular fibrillation after myocardial infarction, so they are no longer used in this setting. This study had a profound impact on the way clinicians and drug regulators view the use of seemingly reasonable intermediate end-points (in this case reduction of frequency of ventricular ectopic beats) as evidence of efficacy in clinical trials. Currently, the main use of flecainide is in prophylaxis against paroxysmal atrial fibrillation.

Beta-adrenoceptor antagonists (class II)

The most important β-adrenoceptor antagonists are described in Chapter 11. Their clinical use for rhythm disorders is shown in the clinical box. **Propranolol**, like several other drugs of this type, has some class I action in addition to blocking β-adrenoceptors. This may contribute to its antidysrhythmic effects, though probably not very much since an isomer with little β-antagonist activity has little antidysrhythmic activity, despite similar activity as a class I agent.

Adverse effects are described in Chapter 11, the most important being bronchospasm in patients with asthma or other forms of obstructive airways disease, a negative inotropic effect and increased fatigue. It was hoped that the use of β_1-selective drugs (e.g. **metoprolol**, **atenolol**) would reduce the risk of bronchospasm, but their degree of selectivity is inadequate to

Clinical uses of class I antidysrhythmic drugs

- **Class Ia (e.g. disopyramide)**
  - —ventricular dysrhythmias
  - —prevention of recurrent paroxysmal atrial fibrillation triggered by vagal overactivity.
- **Class Ib (intravenous lidocaine)**
  - —treatment and prevention of ventricular tachycardia and fibrillation during and immediately after myocardial infarction.
- **Class Ic**
  - —to prevent paroxysmal atrial fibrillation (flecainide)
  - —recurrent tachyarrhythmias associated with abnormal conducting pathways (e.g. Wolff–Parkinson–White syndrome).

*'A 3-year-old girl began to have blackouts, which decreased in frequency with age. Her ECG showed a prolonged Q–T interval. When 18 years of age, she lost consciousness running for a bus. When she was 19, she became quite emotional as a participant in a live television audience and died suddenly.' The molecular basis of this rare inherited disorder is now known. It is caused by a mutation in either the gene coding for a particular potassium channel—called *HERG*—or another gene, *SCN5A*, which codes for the sodium channel and disruption of which results in a loss of inactivation of the Na^+ current (see Welsh & Hoshi 1995, for a commentary).

achieve this goal in clinical practice, although their once-a-day convenience has led to their widespread use in patients without lung disease.

Amiodarone and sotalol (class III)

Amiodarone is highly effective at suppressing dysrhythmias (see the clinical box). Unfortunately, it has several peculiarities that complicate its use. It is extensively bound in tissues, has a long elimination half-life (10–100 days) and accumulates in the body during repeated dosing (see p. 97); consequently its action normally takes days or weeks to develop. For this reason, a loading dose is used, and for life-threatening dysrhythmias this is given intravenously via a central vein (it causes phlebitis if given into a peripheral vessel). Adverse effects are numerous and important; they include photosensitive skin rashes and a slate-grey/bluish discoloration of the skin; thyroid abnormalities (hypo- and hyper-, connected with its high iodine content); pulmonary fibrosis, which is slow in onset but may be irreversible; corneal deposits; and neurological and gastrointestinal disturbances.

Sotalol is a non-selective β-adrenoceptor antagonist, this activity residing in the L-isomer. Unlike other β-antagonists, it prolongs the cardiac action potential and the Q–T interval by delaying the slow outward K^+ current. This class III activity is present in both L- and D-isomers. Racemic sotalol (the form prescribed) appears to be somewhat less effective than amiodarone in preventing chronic malignant ventricular tachyarrhythmias. It shares the ability of amiodarone to cause *torsades de pointes* but lacks its other adverse effects; it is valuable in patients in whom β-adrenoceptor antagonists are not contraindicated.

Clinical uses of class II antidysrhythmic drugs (e.g. propranolol, timolol)

- To reduce mortality following myocardial infarction.
- To prevent recurrence of tachyarrhythmias (e.g. paroxysmal atrial fibrillation) provoked by increased sympathetic activity.

Clinical uses of class III antidysrhythmic drugs

- Amiodarone is used to treat tachycardia associated with the Wolff–Parkinson–White syndrome (caused by an anatomically abnormal conducting pathway that can effectively short-circuit the atrioventricular node). It is also effective in a wide range of other supraventricular and ventricular tachyarrhythmias but is reserved for patients in whom other drugs are ineffective or contraindicated, because of its serious adverse effects.
- (Racemic) sotalol (i.e. the form available for prescription) combines class III with class II actions and adverse effects. It is used in paroxysmal supraventricular dysrhythmias and suppresses ventricular ectopic beats and short runs of ventricular tachycardia.

Verapamil and diltiazem (class IV)

Verapamil is given by mouth. (Intravenous preparations are available but are dangerous and almost never needed.) It has a plasma half-life of 6–8 hours and is subject to quite extensive first-pass metabolism, which is more marked for the isomer that is responsible for its cardiac effects. A slow-release preparation is available for once daily use but is less effective when used for prevention of dysrhythmia than the regular preparation because the bioavailability of the cardioactive isomer is reduced through the presention of a steady low concentration to the drug-metabolising enzymes in the liver. If verapamil is added to **digoxin** in patients with poorly controlled AF, the dose of digoxin should be reduced and plasma digoxin concentration checked after a few days because verapamil both displaces digoxin from tissue-binding sites and reduces its renal elimination, hence predisposing to digoxin accumulation and toxicity (see Ch. 51).

Verapamil is contraindicated in patients with Wolff–Parkinson–White syndrome and is ineffective and dangerous in ventricular dysrhythmias. Adverse effects of verapamil and **diltiazem** are described below in the section on calcium channel antagonists.

Diltiazem is similar to verapamil but has relatively more smooth-muscle-relaxing effect and produces less bradycardia.

Adenosine (unclassified in the Vaughan-Williams' classification)

Adenosine is produced endogenously and is an important chemical mediator (Ch. 12), with effects on breathing, cardiac muscle and afferent nerves and on platelets in addition to the effects on cardiac conducting tissue that underlie its therapeutic use. The A_1 receptor is responsible for its effect on the AV node. These receptors are linked to the same cardiac K^+ channel (K_{ACh}) that is activated by acetylcholine, and adenosine hyperpolarises

Clinical uses of class IV antidysrhythmic drugs

- Verapamil is the main drug. It is used:
  - —to prevent recurrence of paroxysmal supraventricular tachycardia (SVT)
  - —to reduce the ventricular rate in patients with atrial fibrillation (especially if inadequately controlled with digoxin), provided they do not have Wolff–Parkinson–White or a related disorder
- Verapamil was previously given intravenously to terminate SVT; it is now seldom used for this because adenosine is safer.

cardiac conducting tissue and slows the rate of rise of the pacemaker potential accordingly. It is used intravenously to terminate SVT if this rhythm persists despite manoeuvres such as carotid artery massage designed to increase vagal tone. It has largely replaced **verapamil** for this purpose because it is safer owing to its effect being short lived. This is a consequence of its pharmacokinetics: it is taken up via a specific nucleoside transporter by red blood cells and is metabolised by enzymes on the lumenal surface of vascular endothelium. Consequently, the effects of a bolus dose of adenosine last only 20–30 seconds. Once SVT has terminated, the patient usually remains in sinus rhythm, even though adenosine is no longer present in plasma, but the unwanted effects resolve very rapidly. These include chest pain, shortness of breath, dizziness and nausea. **Theophylline** and other xanthine alkaloids block adenosine receptors and inhibit the actions of intravenous adenosine, whereas **dipyridamole** (a vasodilator and antiplatelet drug; see below and Ch. 20) blocks the nucleoside uptake mechanism, potentiating adenosine and prolonging its adverse effects. Both of these interactions are clinically important.

DRUGS THAT INCREASE MYOCARDIAL CONTRACTION

CARDIAC GLYCOSIDES

Cardiac glycosides come from foxgloves (*Digitalis* spp.) and related plants. Withering (1775) wrote on the use of the foxglove: 'it has a power over the motion of the heart to a degree yet unobserved in any other medicine...'. There is evidence in mammals of an endogenous digitalis-like factor closely similar to another cardiac glycoside, **ouabain**, although this is of uncertain physiological significance.

Chemistry

▼ Foxgloves contain several cardiac glycosides with similar actions. **Digoxin** is the most important therapeutically. **Ouabain** is similar but shorter acting. The basic chemical structure of glycosides consists of three components, a *sugar moiety*, a *steroid* and a *lactone*. The sugar moiety consists of unusual 1–4 linked monosaccharides. The lactone ring is essential for activity, and substituted lactones can retain biological activity even when the steroid moiety is removed.

Actions and adverse effects

The main actions of glycosides are on the heart, but some of their adverse effects are extracardiac, including nausea, vomiting, diarrhoea and confusion. The cardiac effects are:

- cardiac slowing and reduced rate of conduction through the AV node
- increased force of contraction
- disturbances of rhythm, especially:
  —block of AV conduction
  —increased ectopic pacemaker activity.

Adverse effects are common and can be severe. One of the main drawbacks of glycosides in clinical use is the narrow margin between effectiveness and toxicity.

Mechanism of action

The main mechanisms of action of cardiac glycosides are increased vagal activity and inhibition of the Na^+/K^+ pump. Cardiac glycosides bind to a site on the extracellular aspect of the α subunit of the Na^+/K^+ ATPase (which is an αβ-heterodimer) and are useful experimental tools for studying this important transport system.

Rate and rhythm

Cardiac glycosides *slow AV conduction* by increasing vagal activity via an action on the central nervous system. Their beneficial effect in established rapid atrial fibrillation results partly from this. If ventricular rate is excessively rapid, the time available for diastolic filling is inadequate. Increasing the refractory period of the AV node increases the minimum interval between impulses and reduces ventricular rate. The atrial dysrhythmia is unaffected, but the pumping efficiency of the heart improves owing to improved ventricular filling. SVT can be terminated by cardiac glycosides, which slow AV conduction, although other drugs are usually employed for this indication (see below).

Larger doses of glycosides cause disturbances of rhythm. These may occur at plasma concentrations within, or only slightly above, the therapeutic range. Slowing of AV conduction can progress to AV block. In addition to depressing AV conduction, glycosides cause ectopic beats. Because Na^+–K^+ exchange is electrogenic, inhibition of the pump by glycosides causes depolarisation, predisposing to disturbances of cardiac rhythm. Furthermore, the increased $[Ca^{2+}]_i$ causes increased after-depolarisation, leading first to coupled beats (*bigeminy*), in which a normal ventricular beat is followed by an ectopic beat; this is followed by ventricular tachycardia where there is a continuous succession of such triggered ectopic beats, and eventually by ventricular fibrillation.

Force of contraction

Glycosides cause a large increase in twitch tension in isolated preparations of cardiac muscle. Unlike catecholamines they do not accelerate relaxation (compare Fig. 17.7 with Fig. 17.10). Increased tension is caused by an increased $[Ca^{2+}]_i$ transient (Fig. 17.10). The action potential is only slightly affected and the slow inward current little changed, so the increased $[Ca^{2+}]_i$ transient probably reflects a greater release of Ca^{2+} from intracellular stores. The most likely mechanism is as follows (see also Ch. 4).

1. Glycosides inhibit the Na^+/K^+ pump.
2. Increased $[Na^+]_i$ slows extrusion of Ca^{2+} via the Na^+/Ca^{2+} exchange transporter. Increasing $[Na^+]_i$ reduces the inwardly directed gradient for Na^+; the smaller this gradient the slower is extrusion of Ca^{2+} by Na^+–Ca^{2+} exchange.
3. Increased $[Ca^{2+}]_i$ is stored in the sarcoplasmic reticulum, and thus increases the amount of Ca^{2+} released by each action potential.

The effect of extracellular potassium

Effects of cardiac glycosides are increased if plasma $[K^+]$ decreases, because of reduced competition at the K^+ binding site

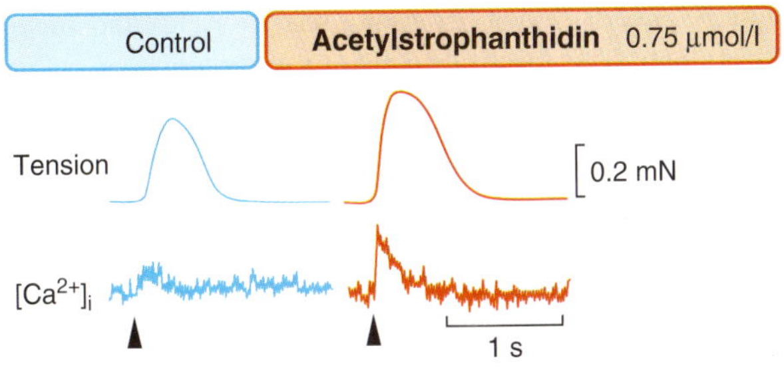

Fig. 17.10 Effect of a cardiac glycoside (acetylstrophanthidin) on the Ca^{2+} transient and tension produced by frog cardiac muscle. The effect was recorded as in Figure. 17.7. (From: Allen D G, Blinks JR 1978 Nature 273: 509.)

on the Na^+/K^+ ATPase. This is clinically important because diuretics (Ch. 23) are often used together with glycosides to treat heart failure, and most of them decrease plasma $[K^+]$ thereby increasing the risk of dysrhythmia.

Pharmacokinetic aspects

Digoxin is administered by mouth or, in urgent situations, intravenously. It is a very polar molecule and elimination is mainly by renal excretion; elimination half-time is approximately 36 hours in patients with normal renal function, considerably longer in elderly patients and those with overt renal failure in whom reduced doses are needed. A loading dose is used in urgent situations. The therapeutic range of plasma concentrations, below which digoxin is unlikely to be effective and above which the risk of toxicity increases substantially, is fairly well defined (1–2.6 nmol/l). Determination of plasma digoxin concentration is useful when lack of efficacy or toxicity is suspected. Clinically important pharmacokinetic interactions occur with drugs that simultaneously reduce digoxin excretion and tissue binding (e.g. **amiodarone**, **verapamil**).

Clinical use

Clinical uses of digoxin are summarised in the box.

Clinical uses of cardiac glycosides (e.g. digoxin)

- To slow ventricular rate in rapid persistent atrial fibrillation
- Treatment of heart failure in patients who remain symptomatic despite optimal use of diuretics and angiotensin-converting enzyme inhibitors.

OTHER DRUGS THAT INCREASE MYOCARDIAL CONTRACTILITY

Certain β_1-adrenoceptor agonists, e.g. **dobutamine**, are used to treat acute but potentially reversible heart failure (e.g. following cardiac surgery or in some cases of cardiogenic or septic shock) on the basis of their positive inotropic action. Dobutamine, for reasons that are not well understood, produces less tachycardia than other β_1-agonists. It is administered intravenously. **Glucagon** also increases myocardial contractility by increasing synthesis of cAMP and has been used in patients with acute cardiac dysfunction owing to overdosage of β-adrenoceptor antagonists (see the glucagon clinical box on p. 385).

Inhibitors of the heart-specific subtype (type III) of phosphodiesterase, the enzyme responsible for the intracellular degradation of cAMP, increase myocardial contractility. Consequently, like β-adrenoceptor agonists they increase intracellular cAMP but are prodysrhythmic for the same reason. Compounds in this group include **amrinone** and **milrinone**, which are chemically and pharmacologically very similar. They improve haemodynamic indices in patients with heart failure but paradoxically worsen survival, presumably because of their prodysrhythmic effect. This dichotomy has had a sobering effect on clinicians and drug regulatory authorities.

ANTIANGINAL DRUGS

The mechanism of anginal pain is discussed above (p. 270). Angina is managed by using drugs that either improve perfusion of the myocardium or reduce its metabolic demand, or both. Two of the main groups of drugs, *organic nitrates* and *calcium antagonists*, are vasodilators and produce both of these effects. The third group, *β-adrenoceptor antagonists*, slow heart rate and hence reduce metabolic demand. Organic nitrates and calcium antagonists are described below. Beta-adrenoceptor antagonists are covered in Chapter 11, except for their antidysrhythmic actions, which are described above.

ORGANIC NITRATES

The ability of organic nitrates (see also Chs 14 and 18) to relieve angina was discovered by Lauder Brunton, a distinguished British physician, in 1867. He had found that angina could be partly relieved by bleeding and also knew that **amyl nitrite**, which had been synthesised 10 years earlier, caused flushing and tachycardia, with a fall in blood pressure, when its vapour was inhaled. He thought that the effect of bleeding resulted from hypotension and found that amyl nitrite inhalation worked much better. Amyl nitrite has now been replaced by **glyceryl trinitrate** (nitroglycerin).* Efforts to increase the duration of action of glyceryl trinitrate have led to the synthesis of several related

*Nobel discovered how to stabilise nitroglycerin with kieselguhr, enabling him to exploit its explosive properties in dynamite, manufacture of which earned him the fortune with which he endowed the eponymous prizes.

organic nitrates, of which the most important is **isosorbide mononitrate**.

Actions

Organic nitrates relax vascular and some other (e.g. oesophageal and biliary) smooth muscles. They cause marked venorelaxation, with a consequent reduction in central venous pressure (reduced pre-load). In healthy subjects, this reduces stroke volume. Venous pooling occurs on standing and can cause postural hypotension and dizziness. Therapeutic doses have less effect on small-resistance arteries than on veins but there is a marked effect on larger muscular arteries. This reduces pulse wave reflection from arterial branches (as appreciated in the 19th century by Murrell but neglected for many years thereafter) and, consequently, reduces central (aortic) pressure and cardiac after-load (see Ch. 18 for more detail on the role of these factors in determining cardiac work). The direct effect on coronary artery tone opposes coronary artery spasm in variant angina. With larger doses, resistance arteries and arterioles dilate, and arterial pressure falls. Nevertheless, coronary flow is *increased* via coronary vasodilatation. Myocardial oxygen consumption is reduced because of the reductions both in cardiac pre-load and after-load. This, together with the increased coronary blood flow, causes a large increase in the oxygen content of coronary sinus blood. Studies in experimental animals have shown that glyceryl trinitrate diverts blood from normal to ischaemic areas of myocardium. The mechanism involves *dilatation of collateral vessels* that bypass narrowed coronary artery segments (Fig. 17.11).

▼ It is interesting to compare this effect with that of other vasodilators (e.g. **dipyridamole**) that dilate arterioles but not collaterals. Dipyridamole is at least as effective as nitrates in increasing coronary flow in normal subjects but actually worsens angina. This is probably because arterioles in an ischaemic region are fully dilated by the ischaemia, and drug-induced dilatation of the arterioles in normal areas has the effect of diverting blood away from the ischaemic areas (Fig. 17.11), producing what is termed a vascular 'steal'. This effect is exploited in a pharmacological 'stress' test for coronary arterial disease in which dipyridamole is administered intravenously to patients in whom this diagnosis is suspected but who cannot exercise.

In summary, the antianginal action of nitrates involves:

- reduction of cardiac oxygen consumption, secondary to reduced cardiac pre-load and after-load
- redistribution of coronary flow towards ischaemic areas via collaterals
- relief of coronary spasm.

In addition to its effects on smooth muscle, NO increases the rate of relaxation of *cardiac* muscle (dubbed a 'lusiotropic' action). It

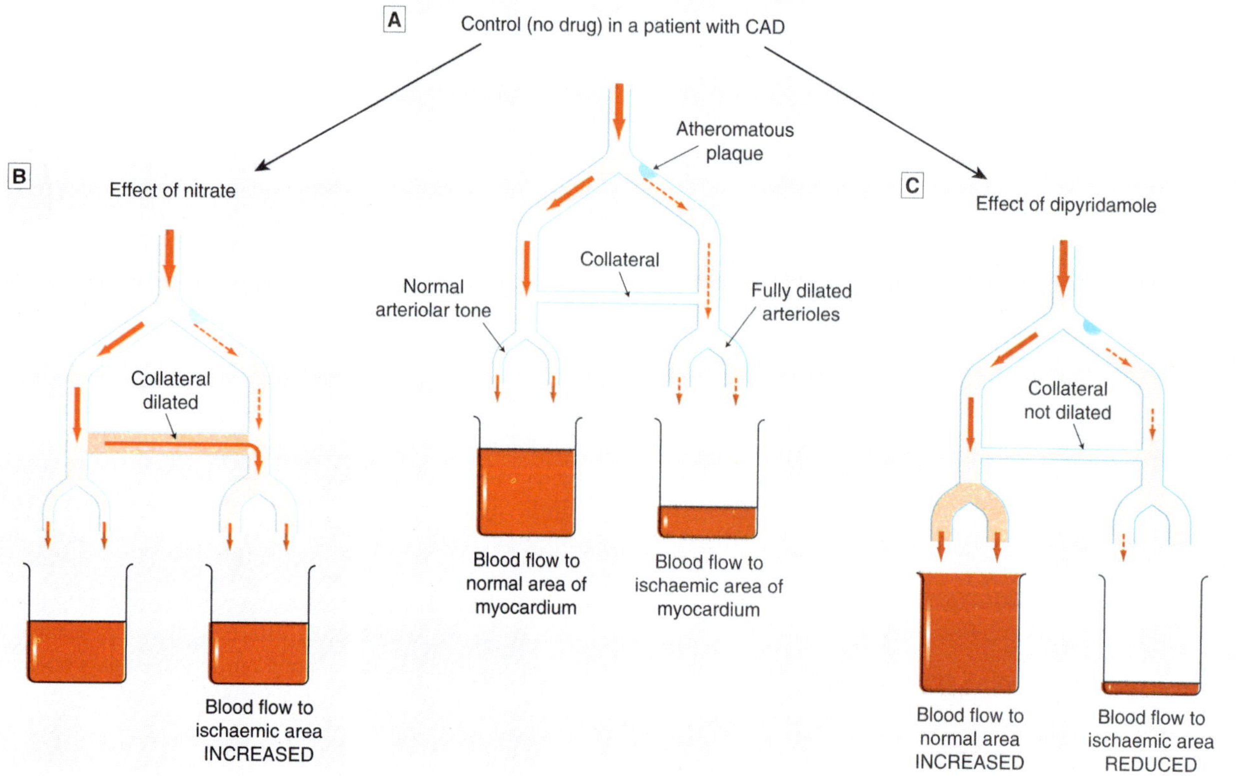

Fig. 17.11 Comparison of the effects of organic nitrates and an arteriolar vasodilator (dipyridamole) on the coronary circulation. [A] Control. [B] Nitrates dilate the collateral vessel, thus allowing more blood through to the underperfused region (mostly by diversion from the adequately perfused area). [C] Dipyridamole dilates arterioles, increasing flow through the normal area at the expense of the ischaemic area (in which the arterioles are anyway fully dilated). (CAD, coronary artery disease.)

is probable that organic nitrates mimic this action, which could be important in patients with impaired diastolic function, a common accompaniment of hypertension and of heart failure.

Mechanism of action

Organic nitrates are metabolised with release of NO. At concentrations achieved during therapeutic use, this involves an enzymic step and possibly a reaction with tissue sulfhydryl (–SH) groups. NO activates soluble guanylate cyclase (see Ch. 14), increasing formation of cGMP, which activates protein kinase G and leads to a cascade of effects in smooth muscle culminating in dephosphorylation of myosin light chains and sequestration of intracellular Ca^{2+}, with consequent relaxation.

Tolerance and unwanted effects

Repeated administration of nitrates to smooth muscle preparations in vitro results in diminished relaxation, possibly partly because of *depletion of free –SH groups*, although attempts to prevent tolerance by agents that restore tissue –SH groups have not been clinically useful. Tolerance to the antianginal effect of nitrates does not occur to a clinically important extent with ordinary formulations of short-acting drugs (e.g. **glyceryl trinitrate**) but does occur with longer-acting drugs (e.g. **isosorbide mononitrate**) or when glyceryl trinitrate is administered by prolonged intravenous infusion or by frequent application of slow-release transdermal patches (see below).

The main *adverse effects* of nitrates are a direct consequence of their main pharmacological actions and include postural hypotension and headache. This was the cause of 'Monday morning sickness' among workers in explosives factories. Tolerance to these effects develops quite quickly but wears off after a brief nitrate-free interval (which is why the symptoms appeared on Mondays and not later in the week). Formation of *methaemoglobin*, an oxidation product of haemoglobin that is ineffective as an oxygen carrier, seldom occurs when nitrates are used clinically but is induced deliberately with **amyl nitrite** in the treatment of cyanide poisoning because methaemoglobin binds cyanide ions.

Pharmacokinetic and pharmaceutic aspects

Glyceryl trinitrate is rapidly inactivated by hepatic metabolism. It is well absorbed from the mouth and is taken as a tablet under the tongue or as a sublingual spray, producing its effects within a few minutes. If swallowed, it is ineffective because of first-pass metabolism. Given sublingually, the trinitrate is converted to di- and mononitrates. Its effective duration of action is approximately 30 minutes. It is quite well absorbed through the skin, and a more sustained effect can be achieved by applying it as a *transdermal patch*. Once a bottle of the tablets has been opened, its shelf life is quite short because the volatile active substance evaporates; spray preparations avoid this problem.

Isosorbide mononitrate is longer acting than glyceryl trinitrate (half-life approximately 4 hours) but has similar pharmacological actions. It is swallowed rather than taken sublingually and is taken twice a day for prophylaxis (usually in the morning and at lunch, to allow a nitrate-free period during the night, when patients are not exerting themselves, to avoid tolerance). It is also available in slow-release form for once daily use in the morning.

Clinical use

The clinical use of organic nitrates is summarised in the box.

Organic nitrates

- Important compounds include glyceryl trinitrate and longer-acting isosorbide mononitrate.
- These drugs are powerful vasodilators, acting on veins to reduce cardiac pre-load and reducing arterial wave reflection to reduce after-load.
- Act via nitric oxide (NO), to which they are metabolised. NO stimulates cGMP formation and hence activates protein kinase G, affecting both contractile proteins (myosin light chains) and Ca^{2+} regulation.
- Tolerance occurs experimentally and is important clinically with frequent use of long-acting drugs or sustained-release preparations.
- Effectiveness in angina results partly from reduced cardiac load and partly from dilatation of collateral coronary vessels, causing more effective distribution of coronary flow. Dilatation of constricted coronary vessels is particularly beneficial in variant angina.
- Serious unwanted effects are uncommon; headache and postural hypotension may occur initially. Overdose can, rarely, cause methaemoglobinaemia.

POTASSIUM CHANNEL ACTIVATORS

Nicorandil combines activation of the potassium K_{ATP} channel (see Chs 4 and 25) with nitrovasodilator (NO donor) actions. It is

Clinical uses of organic nitrates

- Stable angina:
  —prevention (e.g. regular isosorbide mononitrate or glyceryl trinitrate sublingually immediately before exertion)
  —treatment (sublingual glyceryl trinitrate)
- Unstable angina: intravenous glyceryl trinitrate
- Acute heart failure: intravenous glyceryl trinitrate
- Chronic heart failure: isosorbide mononitrate,with hydralazine (Ch. 18) when angiotensin-converting enzyme inhibitors (which are more effective) are contraindicated,
- Uses related to relaxation of other smooth muscles (e.g. uterine, biliary) are being investigated.

both an arterial and a venous dilator and causes the expected unwanted effects of headache, flushing and dizziness. It is used for patients who remain symptomatic despite optimal management with other drugs, often while they await surgery or angioplasty.

BETA-ADRENOCEPTOR ANTAGONISTS

Beta-adrenoceptor antagonists (see Ch. 11) are important in prophylaxis of angina. They work by reducing cardiac oxygen consumption. Their effects on coronary vessels are of minor importance, although these drugs are avoided in variant angina because of the theoretical risk that they will increase coronary spasm. Their very diverse clinical uses are summarised in the box on p. 175.

CALCIUM ANTAGONISTS

The term 'calcium antagonists' is often used for drugs that block cellular entry of Ca^{2+} through calcium channels rather than its intracellular actions (Ch. 4). Some authors use the terms Ca^{2+}-entry blockers or calcium channel blockers to make this distinction clearer. Therapeutically important calcium antagonists act on L-type channels. L-type calcium antagonists comprise three chemically distinct classes: *phenylalkylamines* (e.g. **verapamil**), *dihydropyridines* (e.g. **nifedipine**, **amlodipine**) and *benzothiazepines* (e.g. **diltiazem**).

Mechanism of action: types of calcium channel

The properties of voltage-gated calcium channels have been studied in great detail by voltage-clamp and patch-clamp techniques (see Ch. 2). Drugs of each of the three chemical classes mentioned above all bind the α_1-subunit of the cardiac L-type calcium channel but to distinct sites, each of which interacts allosterically with each other and with the gating machinery of the channel, indirectly preventing diffusion of Ca^{2+} through its pore in the open channel. Many calcium antagonists show properties of use-dependence (i.e. they block more effectively in those cells in which the calcium channels are most active; see the discussion of class I antidysrhythmic drugs above). For the same reason, they also show voltage-dependent blocking actions, blocking more strongly when the membrane is depolarised, causing calcium channel opening and inactivation.

▼ Dihydropyridines affect calcium channel function in a complex way, not simply by physical plugging of the pore. This became clear when some dihydropyridines, exemplified by **Bay K 8644**, were found to bind to the same site but to act in the converse way, that is, to promote the opening of voltage-gated calcium channels. Thus Bay K 8644 produces effects opposite to those of the clinically used dihydropyridines, namely an increase in the force of cardiac contraction, and constriction of blood vessels; it is competitively antagonised by nifedipine. Studies on the response of single calcium channels to a step depolarisation of the membrane suggest that channels can exist in one of three distinct states, termed 'modes' (Fig. 17.12). When a channel is in mode 0 it does not open in response to depolarisation; in mode 1, depolarisation produces a low opening probability, and each opening is brief. In mode 2, depolarisation produces a very high opening probability, and single openings are prolonged. Under normal conditions, about 70% of the channels at any one moment exist in mode 1, with only 1% or less in mode 2; each channel switches randomly and quite slowly between the three modes. Dihydropyridines of the antagonist type bind selectively to channels in mode 0, thus favouring this non-opening state, whereas agonists bind selectively to channels in mode 2 (Fig. 17.12). This type of two-directional modulation resembles the phenomenon seen with the gamma-aminobutyric acid (GABA)/benzodiazepine interaction (Ch. 36) and invites speculation about possible endogenous dihydropyridine-like mediator(s) with a regulatory effect on Ca^{2+} entry.

Mibefradil is distinctive in that it blocks T- as well as L-type channels at therapeutic concentrations, but it was withdrawn from therapeutic use because it caused adverse drug interactions by interfering with drug metabolism.

Pharmacological effects

The main effects of calcium antagonists, as used therapeutically, are on cardiac and smooth muscle. **Verapamil** preferentially affects the heart, whereas most of the dihydropyridines (e.g. **nifedipine**) exert a greater effect on smooth muscle than on the heart. **Diltiazem** is intermediate in its actions.

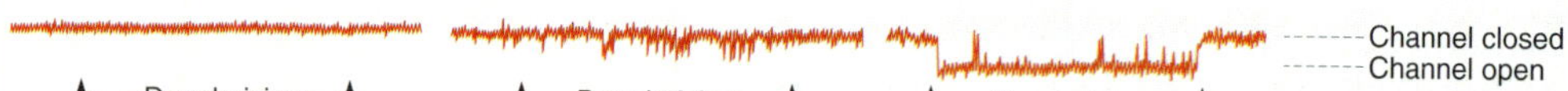

Mode	Mode 0	Mode 1	Mode 2
	▲—Depolarizing—▲ step	▲—Depolarizing—▲ step	▲—Depolarizing—▲ step
Opening probability	Zero	Low	High
Favoured by	DHP antagonists		DHP agonists
% of time normally spent in this mode	<1%	~70%	~30%

Fig. 17.12 Mode of behaviour of calcium channels. The traces are patch-clamp recordings (see Ch. 2) of the opening of single calcium channels (downward deflections) in a patch of membrane from a cardiac muscle cell. A depolarising step is imposed close to the start of each trace, causing an increase in the opening probability of the channel. When the channel is in mode 1 (centre), this causes a few brief openings to occur; in mode 2 (right) the channel stays open for most of the time during the depolarising step; in mode 0 (left), it fails to open at all. Under normal conditions the channel spends most of its time in modes 1 and 2 and only rarely enters mode 0. (Redrawn from Hess et al. 1984 Nature 311: 538–544.)

Cardiac actions

The antidysrhythmic effects of **verapamil** and **diltiazem** have been discussed above. Calcium antagonists can cause AV block and cardiac slowing by their actions on conducting tissues, but this is offset by a reflex increase in sympathetic activity secondary to their vasodilator action. For example, **nifedipine** typically causes reflex tachycardia; **diltiazem** causes little or no change in heart rate and **verapamil** slows the heart rate. Calcium antagonists also have a negative inotropic effect, which results from the inhibition of the slow inward current during the action potential plateau. In spite of this, the cardiac output usually stays constant or increases because of the reduction in peripheral resistance. Again, there are clinically important differences between the different classes of drug, with **verapamil** having the most marked negative inotropic action and, therefore, being contraindicated in heart failure, as are most other calcium antagonists, although **amlodipine** does not worsen cardiovascular mortality in patients with severe chronic heart failure.

Vascular smooth muscle

Calcium antagonists cause generalised arterial/arteriolar dilatation, thereby reducing blood pressure, but do not much affect the veins. They affect all vascular beds, though regional effects vary considerably between different drugs. They cause coronary vasodilatation and are used in patients with coronary artery spasm (variant angina). Other types of smooth muscle (e.g. biliary tract, urinary tract and uterus) are also relaxed by calcium antagonists, but these effects are less important therapeutically than their actions on vascular smooth muscle, although they do cause adverse effects (see below).

Protection of ischaemic tissues

There are theoretical reasons (see Fig. 17.6) why calcium antagonists might exert a cytoprotective effect in ischaemic tissues and thus be of use in treating heart attack and stroke (see Ch. 34), but clinical trials have been disappointing. There is as yet little or no evidence from randomised clinical trials of beneficial (or harmful) effects of calcium antagonists on cardiovascular morbidity or mortality in any patient group. The answers to these questions await the outcome of large ongoing trials. **Nimodipine** has some selectivity for cerebral vasculature and is sometimes used in the hope of reducing cerebral vasospasm following subarachnoid haemorrhage.

Pharmacokinetics

Calcium antagonists in clinical use are all well absorbed from the gastrointestinal tract, and are given by mouth except for some special indications, such as following subarachnoid haemorrhage, for which intravenous preparations are available. They are extensively metabolised. Pharmacokinetic differences between different drugs and different pharmaceutical preparations are clinically important, because they determine the dose interval, and also the intensity of some of the unwanted effects such as headache and flushing (see below). **Amlodipine** has a long elimination half-life and is given once daily, whereas **nifedipine**, **diltiazem** and **verapamil** have shorter elimination half-lives and are either given more frequently or are formulated in various slow-release preparations to permit once daily dosing.

Unwanted effects

Most of the unwanted effects of calcium antagonists are extensions of their main pharmacological actions. Short-acting dihydropyridines cause flushing and headache because of their vasodilator action, and in chronic use dihydropyridines often

Calcium antagonists

- Block Ca^{2+} entry by preventing opening of voltage-gated L-type and T-type calcium channels.
- There are three main L-type antagonists, typified by verapamil, diltiazem and dihydropyridines (e.g. nifedipine).
- Mainly affect heart and smooth muscle, inhibiting the Ca^{2+} entry caused by depolarisation in these tissues.
- Selectivity between heart and smooth muscle varies: verapamil is relatively cardioselective; nifedipine is relatively smooth-muscle selective and diltiazem is intermediate.
- Vasodilator effect (mainly dihydropyridines) is mainly on resistance vessels, causing reduced after-load. Calcium antagonists also dilate coronary vessels, which is important in variant angina.
- Effects on heart (verapamil, diltiazem): antidysrhythmic action (mainly atrial tachycardias), because of impaired atrioventricular conduction, and reduced contractility.
- Clinical uses include antidysrhythmic therapy (mainly verapamil, especially atrial tachycardias), angina (by reducing cardiac work) and hypertension.
- Unwanted effects include headache, constipation (verapamil) and ankle oedema (dihydropyridines). There is a risk of causing cardiac failure or heart block, especially with verapamil.

Clinical uses of calcium antagonists

- Dysrhythmias (verapamil):
  - —to slow ventricular rate in rapid atrial fibrillation
  - —to prevent recurrence of supravenricular tachycardia (SVT) (intravenous administration of verapamil to terminate SVT attacks has been replaced by adenosine)
- Hypertension: usually a dihydropyridine drug, e.g. amlodipine (Ch. 18)
- To prevent angina (usually a dihydropyridine or diltiazem).

cause ankle swelling, related to arteriolar dilatation and increased permeability of postcapillary venules. **Verapamil** can cause constipation, probably because of effects on calcium channels in gastrointestinal nerves or smooth muscle. Effects on cardiac rhythm (e.g. heart block) and force of contraction (e.g. worsening heart failure) are discussed above.

Apart from these predictable effects, which cause tiresome but not usually very severe problems, calcium channel antagonists, as a class, appear rather free from idiosyncratic adverse effects, although long-term safety data are still being collected in ongoing clinical trials.

Clinical uses

The main clinical uses of calcium antagonists are summarised in the clinical box on page 283.

REFERENCES AND FURTHER READING

Camm A J, Garratt C J 1991 Adenosine and supraventricular tachycardia. N Engl J Med 325: 1621–1628 (*Discusses its role as an endogenous mediator and its pharmacology and clinical use*)

Digitalis Investigation Group 1997 The effect of digoxin on mortality and morbidity in patients with heart failure. N Engl J Med 336: 525–533 (*Digoxin did not affect overall mortality, but reduced hospitalisations over an average follow-up of approximately 3 years*)

Falk R H 2001 Atrial fibrillation. N Engl J Med 344:1067–1078 (*Reviews medical progress, including drug therapy*)

ISIS-4 collaborative group 1995 ISIS-4: a randomised factorial trial assessing early oral captopril, oral mononitrate, and intravenous magnesium sulphate in 58 050 patients with suspected acute myocardial infarction. Lancet 345: 669–685 (*Impressive trial: disappointing results! Magnesium was ineffective; oral nitrate did not reduce 1-month mortality*)

Katz A M 1996 Calcium channel diversity in the cardiovascular system. J Am Coll Cardiol 28: 522–528 (*Reviews the diverse calcium channels that participate in signal transduction in the cardiovascular system*)

Linden J 2001 Molecular approach to adenosine receptors: receptor-mediated mechanisms of tissue protection. Annu Rev Pharmacol Toxicol 41: 775–787 (*Adenosine in cardiac ischaemic preconditioning*)

Murad F, Leitman D, Waldman S, Chang C-H, Hirata M, Kohse K 1988 Effects of nitrovasodilators, endothelium-dependent vasodilators and atrial peptides on cGMP. Cold Spring Harb Symp Quant Biol 53: 1005–1009 (*Cellular mechanisms*)

Podrid P J 1999 Redefining the role of antiarrhythmic drugs. N Engl J Med 340: 1910–1911 (*Discusses studies with ibutilide and sotalol, which 'highlight what may become the primary indication for anti-arrhythmic drug therapy; as an adjunct to non-pharmacologic therapy for relief of symptoms and improvement in the quality of life.'*)

Prospective Randomised Amlodipine Survival Evaluation Study Group 1996 Effect of amlodipine on morbidity and mortality in severe chronic heart failure. N Engl J Med 335: 1107–1114 (*No adverse or beneficial effect on survival in the group as a whole*)

Rockman H A, Koch W J, Lefkowitz R J 2002 Seven-transmembrane-spanning receptors and heart function. Nature 415: 206–212 (*Review*)

Roy D, Talajic M, Dorian P et al. 2000 Amiodarone to prevent recurrence of atrial fibrillation. N Engl J Med 342: 913–920 (*Low dose amiodarone was more effective than sotalol or propafenone*)

Ruskin J N 1989 The cardiac arrhythmia suppression trial (CAST). N Engl J Med 321: 386–388 (*Enormously influential trial showing increased mortality with active treatment despite suppression of dysrhythmia*)

Saurin A T, Rakhit R D, Marber M S 2000 Therapeutic potential of ischaemic preconditioning. Br J Clin Pharmac 50: 87–97 (*Adenosine etc.*)

Suzuki T, Yamazaki T, Yazaki Y 2001 The role of the natriuretic peptides in the cardiovascular system. Cardiovasc Res 51: 489–494

Vaughan Williams E M 1989 Classification of antiarrhythmic actions. In: Vaughan Williams E M (ed) Antiarrhythmic drugs. Handbook of experimental pharmacology. Springer-Verlag, Berlin, vol. 89 (*For a different approach see Circulation 1994, 84: 1848*)

Ward D E, Camm A J 1993 Dangerous ventricular arrhythmias—can we predict drug efficacy? N Engl J Med 329: 498–499 (*Commentary on the seemingly logical but problematic strategy of deliberately provoking dysrhythmias in susceptible patients in order to select therapy individualised to their needs*)

Welsh M J, Hoshi T 1995 Molecular cardiology – ion channels lose the rhythm. Nature 376: 640-641 (*Commentary on Ward–Romano syndrome*)

The vascular system

18

Overview 285

Vascular structure and function 285

Control of vascular smooth muscle tone 286
- The vascular endothelium 286
- The renin–angiotensin system 290

Vasoactive drugs 292
- Vasoconstrictor drugs 292
- Vasodilator drugs 293

Clinical uses of vasoactive drugs 298
- Hypertension 298
- Cardiac failure 300
- Shock and hypotensive states 302
- Peripheral vascular disease 303
- Raynaud's disease 304

OVERVIEW

This chapter is concerned with the pharmacology of blood vessels. The walls of arteries, arterioles, venules and veins contain smooth muscle the contractile state of which is controlled by circulating hormones and by mediators released locally from sympathetic nerve terminals and endothelial cells. Regulation of intracellular Ca^{2+} concentrations $[Ca^{2+}]_i$, in vascular smooth muscle is described in Chapter 4. In this chapter, we first consider the control of vascular smooth muscle by the endothelium and by the renin–angiotensin system, followed by the actions of vasoconstrictor and vasodilator drugs. Finally, we briefly consider clinical uses of vasoactive drugs in some important disease states, namely hypertension, heart failure, shock, peripheral vascular disease and Raynaud's disease. The use of vasoactive drugs to treat angina is covered in Chapter 17.

VASCULAR STRUCTURE AND FUNCTION

Blood is ejected with each heartbeat from the left ventricle into the aorta, whence it flows rapidly to the organs via conduit arteries rich in elastin and collagen. Successive branching leads via progressively more muscular arteries to arterioles and capillaries, where gas and nutrient exchange occur. Capillaries coalesce to form postcapillary venules, venules and progressively larger veins leading via the vena cava to the right heart. Deoxygenated blood ejected from the right ventricle travels through the pulmonary artery, pulmonary capillaries and pulmonary veins back to the left atrium.* Arterioles and small muscular arteries are the main resistance vessels in the circulation, while veins are capacity vessels. In terms of cardiac function, therefore, arteries and arterioles regulate the *after-load*, while veins and pulmonary vessels regulate the *pre-load* of the ventricles.

Viscoelastic properties of large conduit arteries determine arterial compliance (i.e. the degree to which the volume of the arterial system increases as the pressure increases). This is an important factor in a circulatory system that is driven by an intermittent, rather than continuous, pump. Blood ejected from the left ventricle is accommodated, in the first instance, by distension of the arterial system, which absorbs the pulsations in cardiac output and delivers a relatively steady flow to the tissues. The greater the compliance of the system, the more effectively are fluctuations damped out,** and the smaller the oscillations of arterial pressure with each heartbeat (i.e. the difference between the systolic and diastolic pressure or 'pulse pressure'). Reflection of the pressure wave from branch points in the vascular tree also sustains arterial pressure during diastole. This helps to preserve a steady perfusion of vital organs, such as the kidney, during diastole. However, excessive reflection can pathologically augment aortic systolic pressure. Excessively rapid reflection results from stiffening of the aorta as a result of loss of elastin during ageing, especially in people with hypertension. Cardiac work (see Ch. 17) can be reduced by introducing additional compliance into the arterial system or by reducing arterial wave

*William Harvey (physician to King Charles I) inferred the circulation of the blood on the basis of superbly elegant quantitative experiments long before the invention of the microscope enabled visual confirmation of the tiny vessels he had predicted. This intellectual triumph did his medical standing no good at all, and Aubrey wrote that 'he fell mightily in his practice, and was regarded by the vulgar as crack-brained'. Plus ça change....

**This cushioning action is called the 'windkessel' effect. The same principle was used to deliver a steady rather than intermittent flow from old-fashioned fire pumps.

reflection, even if the cardiac output and mean arterial pressure are unchanged. In older persons (over around 55 years) pulse pressure and aortic stiffness are important risk factors for cardiac disease.

Actions of drugs on the vascular system can be broken down into effects on:

- total peripheral resistance, which is one of the main determinants of arterial pressure and is relevant to the treatment of hypertension
- the resistance of individual vascular beds, which determines the local distribution of blood flow to and within different organs; such effects are relevant to the drug treatment of angina (Ch. 17), Raynaud's phenomenon and circulatory shock
- aortic compliance and pulse wave reflection, which are relevant to the treatment of cardiac failure and angina
- venous tone and blood volume (the 'fullness' of the circulation), which together determine the central venous pressure and are relevant to the treatment of cardiac failure and angina; diuretics (which reduce blood volume) are discussed in Chapter 23
- atheroma (Ch. 19) and thrombosis (Ch. 20).

Vascular smooth muscle

- Vascular smooth muscle is controlled by mediators secreted by sympathetic nerves and vascular endothelium, and by circulating hormones.
- Smooth muscle cell contraction is initiated by a rise in $[Ca^{2+}]_i$, which activates myosin-light-chain kinase, causing phosphorylation of myosin, or by sensitisation of the myofilaments to Ca^{2+} by inhibition of myosin phosphatase (see Ch. 4).
- Agents causing contraction may:
  - —release intracellular Ca^{2+}, secondary to receptor-mediated inositol trisphosphate formation
  - —depolarise the membrane and thus allow Ca^{2+} entry through voltage-gated calcium channels
  - —allow Ca^{2+} entry through receptor-operated calcium channels.
- Agents causing relaxation may:
  - —inhibit Ca^{2+} entry through voltage-gated calcium channels either directly (e.g. nifedipine) or indirectly by hyperpolarising the membrane (K^+ activators, e.g. cromokalim)
  - —increase intracellular cAMP or cGMP concentration; cAMP causes inactivation of myosin-light-chain kinase and may facilitate Ca^{2+} efflux; cGMP opposes agonist-induced increases in $[Ca^{2+}]_i$

CONTROL OF VASCULAR SMOOTH MUSCLE TONE

Like other muscle cells, vascular smooth muscle contracts when $[Ca^{2+}]_i$ rises, but the coupling between $[Ca^{2+}]_i$ and contraction is less tight than in striated or cardiac muscle (Ch. 4). Vasoconstrictors and vasodilators act by increasing or reducing $[Ca^{2+}]_i$, and/or by altering the sensitivity of the contractile machinery to $[Ca^{2+}]_i$. Figure 4.10 summarises cellular mechanisms that are involved in the control of smooth muscle contraction.

THE VASCULAR ENDOTHELIUM

A new chapter in our understanding of vascular control opened with the discovery that vascular endothelium acts not only as a passive barrier between plasma and extracellular fluid but also as a source of numerous potent chemical mediators. These actively control the contraction of the underlying smooth muscle as well as influencing platelet and mononuclear cell function: the important roles of the endothelium in haemostasis and thrombosis are discussed in Chapter 20. Several distinct classes of mediator are involved (Fig. 18.1).

- *Prostanoids* (see Ch. 15) The discovery by Bunting, Gryglewski, Moncada & Vane in 1976 of *prostaglandin* I_2 (PGI_2, also known as prostacyclin) ushered in this era. This mediator relaxes smooth muscle and inhibits platelet aggregation by activating adenylate cyclase. Endothelial cells from microvessels synthesise PGE_2, which is a direct vasodilator and also inhibits noradrenaline release from sympathetic nerve terminals, while lacking the effect of PGI_2 on platelets. Prostaglandin endoperoxide intermediates (PGG_2, PGH_2) are endothelium-derived contracting factors, acting via thromboxane receptors.
- *Nitric oxide* Endothelium-derived relaxing factor (EDRF) was discovered by Furchgott & Zawadzki in 1980 and was subsequently identified as nitric oxide (NO) by the groups of Moncada and of Ignarro (see Fig. 14.2, p. 209). Awareness of this mediator (see Ch. 14) enormously expanded our understanding of the role of the endothelium. NO activates guanylate cyclase. It is especially important in resistance vessels because it is released continuously, giving rise to vasodilator tone and contributing to the physiological control of blood pressure. As well as causing vascular relaxation, it inhibits vascular smooth muscle cell proliferation, inhibits platelet adhesion and aggregation and inhibits monocyte adhesion and migration; consequently, it may protect blood vessels from developing atheroma and from thrombosis (see Chs 19 and 20).
- *Peptides* The endothelium secretes several vasoactive peptides. *C natriuretic peptide,* which is related to atrial natriuretic peptide (Ch. 17) and *adrenomedulin* (a vasodilator peptide originally discovered in an adrenal tumour—phaeochromocytoma—but expressed in many tissues including vascular endothelium) are vasodilators. *Angiotensin II,* formed by *angiotensin-converting enzyme* (ACE) on the

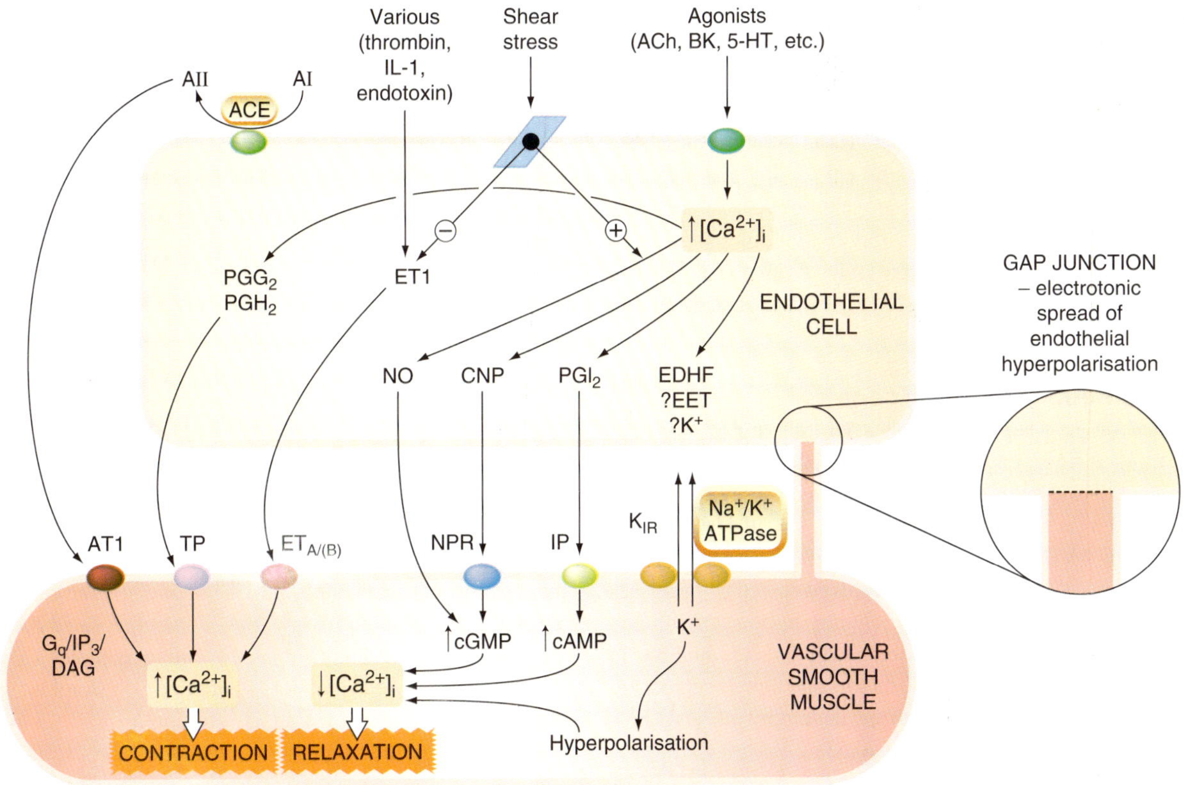

Fig. 18.1 **Endothelium-derived mediators.** The schematic shows some of the more important endothelium-derived contracting and relaxing mediators; many (if not all) of the vasoconstrictors also cause smooth muscle mitogenesis while vasodilators commonly inhibit mitogenesis. (A, angiotensin; ACE, angiotensin-converting enzyme; AT_1, angiotensin AT1-receptor; TP, T prostanoid receptor; $ET_{A/(B)}$, endothelium A (and B) receptors; NPR, natriuretic peptide receptor; IP, I prostanoid receptor; K_{IR}, inward rectifying potassium channel; Na^+/K^+ ATPase, electrogenic pump; G_q, G-protein; IP_3, inosinol 1,4,5-trisphosphate; DAG, diacylglycerol; IL-1, interleukin 1; ACh, acetylcholine; BK, bradykinin; 5-HT, 5-hydroxytryptamine; 'EDHF', endothelium-derived hyperpolarising factor; EET, epoxyeicosatetraenoic acid; PG, prostaglandin; CNP, C-natriuretic peptide; ET-1, endothelin 1.)

surface of endothelial cells (see below), and *endothelin* are potent endothelium-derived vasoconstrictor peptides.

- *Endothelium-derived hyperpolarising factor(s) (EDHF)* Endothelium-dependent dilatation in response to several mediators (including acetylcholine and bradykinin) can persist despite complete inhibition of prostaglandin and NO synthesis. Such relaxation is accompanied by endothelium-dependent hyperpolarisation of vascular smooth muscle and is abolished by an unusual combination of Ca^{2+}-dependent potassium channel blockers (*apamin* plus *charybdotoxin*) but not by these toxins individually or by related inhibitors. These hyperpolarising/relaxant responses are caused by EDHF distinct from prostanoids and NO. EDHF becomes progressively important, compared with NO, in smaller and smaller arteries. Its chemical identity (or identities) remains elusive, but there are currently three main contenders, which are not necessarily mutually exclusive. These are (i) epoxyeicosanoids synthesised from arachidonic acid by an isoform of cytochrome P450; (ii) electrotonic spread of hyperpolarisation from endothelium to vascular smooth muscle by gap junctions; and (iii) K^+ released from endothelium, which paradoxically hyperpolarises vascular smooth muscle by activating inwardly rectifying potassium channels (which can be blocked by barium ions) and the electrogenic Na^+/K^+ pump (which can be blocked by **ouabain**).

In addition to secreting this array of vasoactive mediators, endothelial cells express several enzymes and transport mechanisms on their plasma membranes that act on circulating hormones and are important targets of drug action. ACE is a particularly important example (see below).

Many endothelium-derived mediators are mutually antagonistic, conjuring an image of opposing rugby football players swaying back and forth in a scrum: in moments of exasperation one sometimes wonders whether all this makes sense or whether the designer simply could not make up his mind! An important distinction is made between mechanisms that are tonically active in resistance vessels under basal conditions, as is the case with the *noradrenergic nervous system* (Ch. 11), NO (Ch. 14) and, possibly, *endothelin*, and those that operate

MYOCARDIAL OXYGEN CONSUMPTION AND CORONARY BLOOD FLOW

Relative to its large metabolic needs, the heart is one of the most poorly perfused tissues in the body. Coronary flow is, under normal circumstances, closely related to myocardial oxygen consumption, and both change over a nearly 101-fold range between conditions of rest and maximal exercise.

PHYSIOLOGICAL FACTORS

The main physiological factors that regulate coronary flow are:

- physical factors
- vascular control by metabolites
- neural and humoral control.

Physical factors

During systole, the pressure exerted by the myocardium on vessels that pass through it equals or exceeds the perfusion pressure, so coronary flow occurs only during diastole. Diastole is shortened more than systole during tachycardia, reducing the period available for myocardial perfusion. During diastole, the effective perfusion pressure is equal to the difference between the aortic and ventricular pressures (Fig. 17.5). If diastolic aortic pressure falls or diastolic ventricular pressure increases, perfusion pressure falls and so (unless other control mechanisms can compensate) does coronary blood flow. Stenosis of the aortic valve produces both these effects and often causes ischaemic chest pain ('*angina*') even in the absence of coronary artery disease.

Vascular control by metabolites/mediators

Vascular control by metabolites is the most important mechanism by which coronary flow is regulated. A reduction in arterial partial pressure of oxygen (Po_2) causes marked vasodilatation of coronary vessels in situ but has little effect on isolated strips of coronary artery. This suggests that it is a change in the pattern of metabolites produced by the myocardial cells, rather than the change in Po_2 per se, that controls the state of the coronary vessels, the most popular candidate for the dilator metabolite being *adenosine* (see Ch. 12).

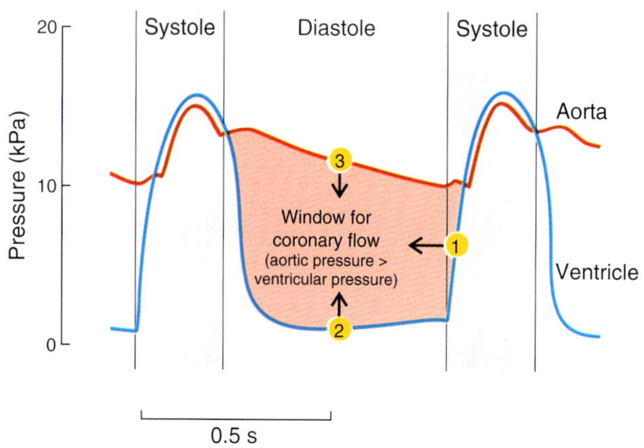

Fig. 17.5 Mechanical factors affecting coronary blood flow. The 'window' for coronary flow may be encroached upon by: (1) shortening diastole, when heart rate increases; (2) increased ventricular end-diastolic pressure; and (3) reduced diastolic arterial pressure.

Neural and humoral control

Coronary vessels have a dense sympathetic innervation, but sympathetic nerves (like circulating catecholamines) exert only a small direct effect on the coronary circulation. Large coronary vessels possess α-adrenoceptors that mediate vasoconstriction, whereas smaller vessels have β_2-adrenoceptors that have a dilator effect. Coronary vessels are also innervated by purinergic, peptidergic and nitrergic nerves. Normally, neural and endocrine effects on coronary vasculature are overshadowed by the vascular response to altered mechanical and metabolic activity.

CORONARY ATHEROSCLEROSIS AND ITS CONSEQUENCES

Atheromatous deposits are ubiquitous in the coronary arteries of adults living in developed countries, but are asymptomatic for most of the natural history of the disease (see Ch. 19). Important consequences of coronary atherosclerosis are:

angina (ischaemic chest pain)
myocardial infarction.

Angina

Angina occurs when the oxygen supply to the myocardium is insufficient for its needs. The pain has a characteristic distribution in the chest, arm and neck and is brought on by exertion or excitement. It is an important target for therapeutic intervention (see below). A similar type of pain occurs in skeletal muscle when it is made to contract while its blood supply is interrupted, and Lewis showed many years ago that chemical factors released by ischaemic muscle are responsible. Possible candidates include K^+, H^+ (Ch. 15) and *adenosine* (Ch. 12), all of which stimulate nociceptors (see Ch. 40). It is possible that the same mediator that causes coronary vasodilatation is responsible, at higher concentration, for initiating pain.

Three kinds of angina are recognised clinically: stable, unstable and variant.

Stable angina This is characterised by predictable pain on exertion. It is produced by an increased demand on the heart and is caused by a fixed narrowing of the coronary vessels, almost always by atheroma. Symptomatic therapy is directed at altering cardiac work with organic nitrates, β-adrenoceptor antagonists and/or calcium antagonists (as described below), together with treatment of the underlying atheromatous disease, usually including a statin (Ch. 19), and prophylaxis against thrombosis with an antiplatelet drug, usually **aspirin** (Ch. 20).

Unstable angina This is characterised by pain that occurs with less and less exertion, culminating in pain at rest. The

only in response to injury, inflammation, etc., as with PGI_2. Some of the latter group may be functionally redundant, perhaps representing vestiges of mechanisms that were important to our evolutionary forebears, or they may simply be taking a breather on the touch-line and are ready to rejoin the fray if called on by the occurrence of some vascular insult. Such redundancy complicates interpretation of experiments using mutant gene 'knockout' animals. For example, acetylcholine relaxes arterioles (from muscle) of wild-type mice mainly by releasing NO; it also relaxes vessels from 'eNOS knockout' mice (which lack the gene for the endothelial NO synthase (NOS)) by releasing EDHF in place of NO.

The endothelium in angiogenesis

As touched on in Chapter 7, the barrier function of vascular endothelium differs markedly in different organs, and its development during angiogenesis is controlled by several growth factors including non-specific ones such as vascular endothelial growth factor (VEGF) and tissue specific factors such as endocrine gland VEGF. These are involved in repair processes but also in pathological situations including tumour growth and neovascularisation in the eye in patients with diabetes mellitus, in whom it can cause blindness. These factors and their receptors are potentially fruitful targets for drug development and new therapies (including gene therapies: Ch. 53).

ENDOTHELIN

Discovery, biosynthesis and secretion

Hickey et al. described a vasoconstrictor factor produced by cultured endothelial cells in 1985. This was identified as endothelin, a 21-residue peptide, by Yanagisawa et al. (1988), who achieved the isolation, analysis and cloning of the gene for this peptide in a very short space of time. Three genes encode different sequences (ET-1, ET-2 and ET-3), each with a distinctive 'shepherd's crook' appearance produced by two internal disulfide bonds. These three isoforms are diversely distributed (Table 18.1) suggesting that endothelin has functions beyond the cardiovascular system, and this is supported by observations of mice in which the gene coding for ET-1 is disrupted (see below). ET-1 is the only endothelin present in endothelial cells and is also expressed in many other tissues. Its synthesis and actions are summarised schematically in Figure 18.2. ET-2 is much less widely distributed but is present in kidney and intestine. ET-3 is present in brain, lung, intestine and adrenal gland. ET-1 is synthesised from a 212-residue precursor molecule (prepro-ET), which is processed to 'big ET-1' and finally cleaved by an endothelin-converting enzyme to ET-1. Cleavage occurs not at the usual Lys–Arg or Arg–Arg position but at a Trp–Val pair, implying a very atypical endopeptidase. The converting enzyme is a metalloprotease and is inhibited by **phosphoramidon**. Big ET-1 is converted to ET-1 intracellularly and also on the surface of endothelial and smooth muscle cells. Stimuli to endothelin synthesis include many noxious, vasoconstrictor mediators released during pathological insults, including activated platelets, endotoxin, thrombin, various cytokines and growth factors, angiotensin II, antidiuretic hormone (arginine-vasopressin), adrenaline, insulin, hypoxia and low shear stress. Inhibitors include NO, natriuretic peptides, PGE_2, PGI_2, heparin and high shear stress. It was originally believed that ET-1 is generated de novo and not stored intracellularly, but secretion of ET-1 can occur more rapidly than would be expected if it were always freshly synthesised (for example, in response to stretch), and there is evidence that preformed ET-1 can be stored in endothelial cells, although probably not in granules. Release mechanisms of such stored

Table 18.1 Distribution of endogenous endothelins and subtypes of endothelin receptors in various tissues

Tissues	Endothelins			Endothelin receptors	
	1	2	3	ET_A	ET_B
Vascular tissue					
Endothelium	++++				+
Smooth muscle	+			++	
Brain	+++		+	+	+++
Kidney	++	++	+	+	++
Intestines	+	+	+++	+	+++
Adrenal gland	+		+++	+	++

Levels of expression of endothelins or the receptor mRNA and/or immunoreactive endothelins: ++++, highest; +++, high; ++, moderate; +, low.
Adapted from: Masaki, 1993.

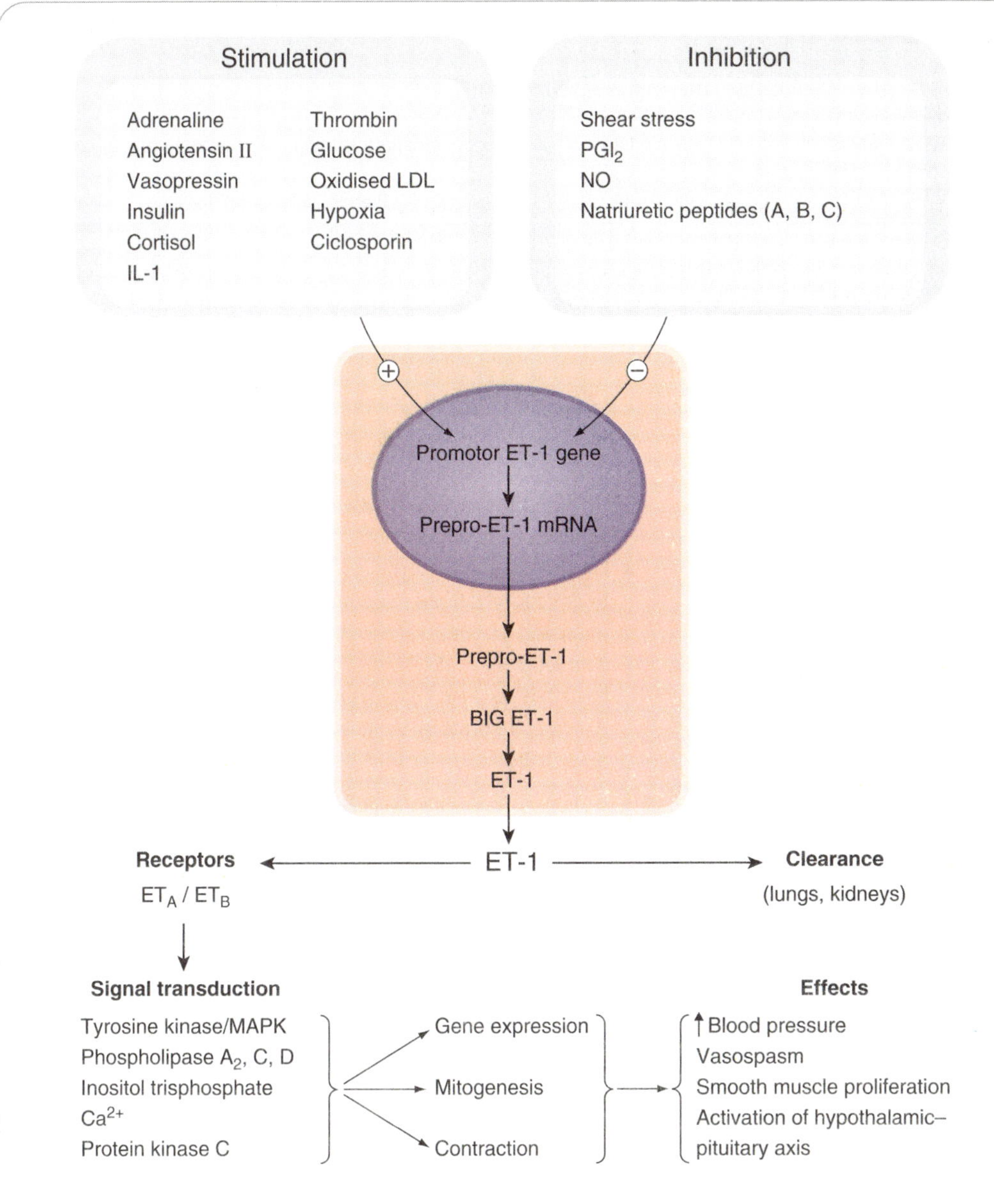

Fig. 18.2 Endothelin-1 (ET-1) synthesis and actions. The schematic shows some of the more important actions only. IL-1, interleukin 1; LDL, low density lipoprotein; PGI_2, prostaglandin I_2; NO, nitric oxide.

ET-1 are poorly understood. ET-1 concentration in plasma is low (<5 pmol/l) compared with concentrations that activate endothelin receptors, but concentrations in the extracellular space between endothelium and vascular smooth muscle are presumably much higher, and endothelin receptor antagonists (see below) cause vasodilatation when infused directly into the brachial artery, consistent with tonic ET-1-mediated vasoconstrictor activity in resistance vasculature. ET-1 has an elimination half life of <5 minutes, despite a much longer duration of action, and clearance occurs mainly in the lung and kidneys. Urinary ET-1 excretion is believed to reflect renal synthesis.

Endothelin receptors and responses

There are at least two types of endothelin receptor, designated ET_A and ET_B (Table 18.2). Both belong to the superfamily of G-protein-coupled receptors (Ch. 3). ET-1 preferentially activates ET_A-receptors. Messenger RNA for the ET_A-receptor is expressed in many human tissues, including vascular smooth muscle, heart, lung and kidney. It is not expressed in endothelium. ET_A-mediated responses include vasoconstriction, bronchoconstriction and aldosterone secretion. ET_A-receptors are coupled to phospholipase C, which stimulates Na^+–H^+ exchange, protein kinase C and mitogenesis as well as causing vasoconstriction through inositol trisphosphate (IP_3) (Ch. 3). There are several selective ET_A-receptor antagonists including **BQ-123** (a cyclic pentapeptide) and several orally active non-peptide drugs (e.g. **BMS 182874**, which is a sulfonamide derivative). ET_B-receptors are activated to a similar extent by each of the three endothelin isoforms but **sarafotoxin S6c** (a 21-residue peptide that shares the shepherd's crook structure of the endothelins and was isolated from the venom of the burrowing

Table 18.2 Subtypes of endothelin receptor

Receptor	Affinity	Pharmacological response
ET_A	ET-1 = ET-2 > ET-3	Vasoconstriction, bronchoconstriction, stimulation of aldosterone secretion
ET_B	ET-1 = ET-2 = ET-3	Vasodilatation, inhibition of ex vivo platelet aggregation

From: Masaki, 1993.

asp) is a selective agonist and has proved useful as a pharmacological tool for studying the ET_B-receptor. Messenger RNA for the ET_B-receptor is mainly expressed in brain (especially cerebral cortex and cerebellum) with moderate expression in aorta, heart, lung, kidney and adrenals. In contrast to the ET_A-receptor, it is highly expressed in endothelium, but it is also present in vascular smooth muscle as is the ET_A-receptor. The receptor on endothelium has been called ET_{B1} while the vascular smooth muscle subtype is termed ET_{B2}, based on subtype-selective antagonists. Agonists acting on ET_{B1}-receptors cause vasodilatation by stimulating NO and PGI_2 production. In contrast, ET_{B2}-mediated responses are vasoconstrictor.

Functions of endothelin

ET-1 is a paracrine mediator rather than a circulating hormone, although it stimulates secretion of several hormones (see below). Administration of ET_A-receptor antagonists into the brachial artery increases forearm blood flow, suggesting that ET-1 may be formed continuously in resistance vessels and contribute to vasoconstrictor tone and the control of peripheral vascular resistance. Endothelins have several other possible functions, including roles in:

- release of various hormones, including atrial natriuretic peptide, aldosterone, adrenaline and hypothalamic and pituitary hormones
- thyroglobulin synthesis (the concentration of ET-1 in thyroid follicles is extremely high)
- control of uteroplacental blood flow (ET-1 is present in very high concentrations in amniotic fluid)
- renal and cerebral vasospasm (Fig. 18.3)
- development of the cardiorespiratory systems (the *ET-1* gene has been disrupted experimentally; pharyngeal arch tissues develop abnormally in such mice and homozygotes die of respiratory failure at birth).

The role of the endothelium in controlling vascular smooth muscle

- Endothelial cells release various vasoactive substances, including prostaglandin I_2 (vasodilator), nitric oxide (NO vasodilator) and endothelin (vasoconstrictor).
- Many vasodilator substances (e.g. acetylcholine and bradykinin) act via endothelial NO production. The NO derives from arginine and is produced when $[Ca^{2+}]_i$ increases in the endothelial cell.
- NO causes smooth muscle relaxation by increasing cGMP formation.
- Endothelin is a potent and long-acting vasoconstrictor peptide, released from endothelial cells by many chemical and physical factors. It is not confined to blood vessels, and its physiological role is not yet clear.

THE RENIN–ANGIOTENSIN SYSTEM

The renin–angiotensin system acts synergistically with the sympathetic nervous system. It also stimulates aldosterone secretion and plays a central role in the control of Na^+ excretion and fluid volume as well as of vascular tone.

Renin is a proteolytic enzyme that is secreted by the *juxtaglomerular apparatus* (see Fig. 23.2). The control of renin secretion (Fig. 18.4) is only partly understood. It is secreted in response to various physiological stimuli, including a fall in Na^+ concentration in the distal tubule, and a fall in renal perfusion pressure. Renal sympathetic nerve activity, β-adrenoceptor agonists and PGI_2 all stimulate renin secretion directly, whereas angiotensin II causes feedback inhibition. Atrial natriuretic peptide also inhibits renin secretion. The macula densa (a specialised part of the distal tubule apposed to the juxtaglomerular apparatus) is rich in NOS, but the effect of NO on renin release is controversial, with conflicting claims that it either inhibits or stimulates this. Renin is cleared rapidly from plasma. It acts on angiotensinogen (a plasma globulin made in the liver) splitting off a decapeptide, *angiotensin I*, from the N-terminal end of the protein.

Angiotensin I has no appreciable activity per se but is converted by ACE to an octapeptide, *angiotensin II*, which is a potent vasoconstrictor. Angiotensin II can be broken down further by enzymes (aminopeptidase A and N) that remove single amino acids residues, giving rise, respectively, to angiotensin III and angiotensin IV (Fig. 18.5). These had been regarded as of little importance, but it is now known that angiotensin III stimulates aldosterone secretion and is involved in thirst.

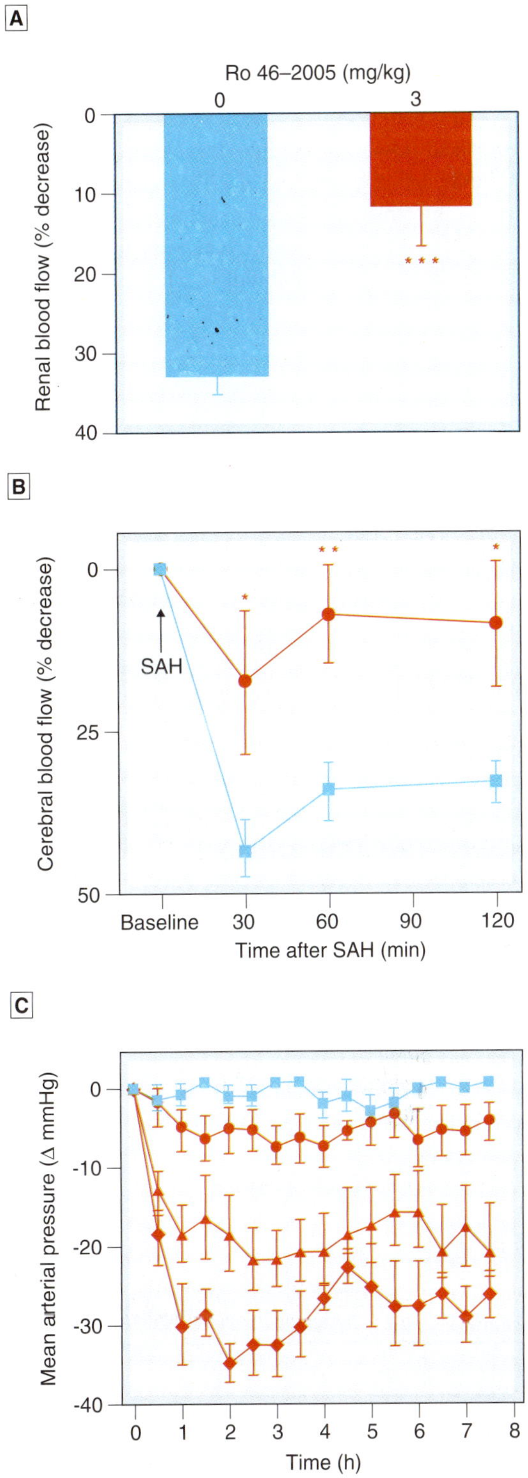

Fig. 18.3 In vivo effects of a potent non-peptide endothelin-1 ET_A- and ET_B-receptor antagonist, Ro 46-2005, in three animal models. A Prevention by Ro 46-2005 of post-ischaemic renal vasoconstriction in rats. B Prevention by Ro 46-2005 of the decrease in cerebral blood flow after subarachnoid haemorrhage (SAH) in rats treated with placebo (blue) or with Ro 46-2005 (red). C Effect of orally administered Ro 46-2005 on mean arterial pressure in sodium-depleted squirrel monkeys treated with placebo (blue) or increasing doses of antagonist (red: ● < ▲ < ◆). (From: Clozel M et al. 1993 Nature 365: 759–761.)

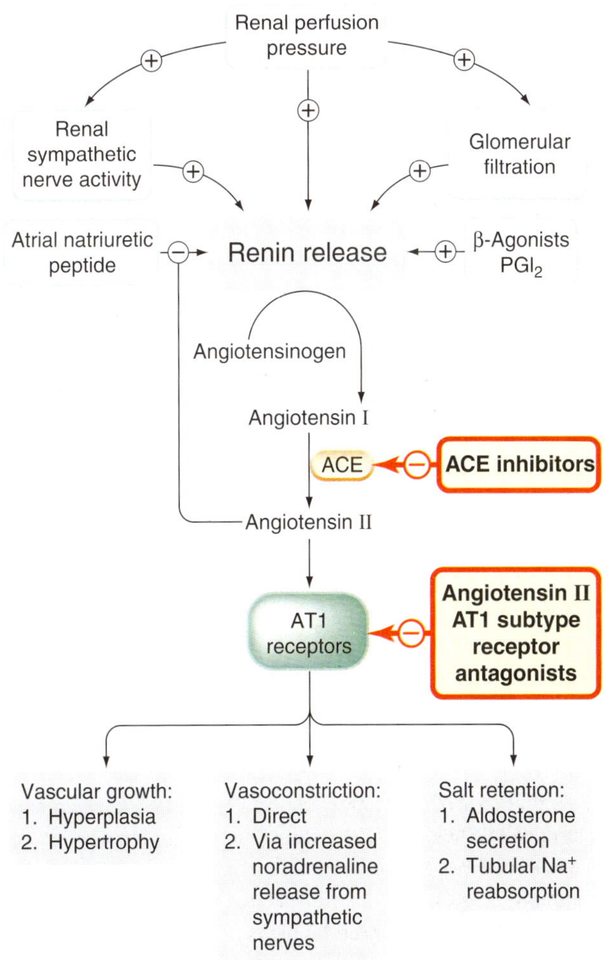

Fig. 18.4 Control of renin release and formation and action of angiotensin II. Sites of action of drugs that inhibit the cascade are shown. (ACE, angiotensin-converting enzyme; AT1, angiotensin II receptor subtype 1.)

Angiotensin IV also has distinct actions, probably via its own receptor, including release of plasminogen activator inhibitor-1 (PAI-1) from the endothelium (Ch. 20). Receptors for angiotensin IV have a distinctive distribution, including the hypothalamus.

ACE is a membrane-bound enzyme on the surface of endothelial cells and is particularly abundant in the lung, which has a vast surface area of vascular endothelium.* The common isoform of ACE is also present in other vascular tissues including heart, brain, striated muscle and kidney and is not restricted to endothelial cells.** Consequently, local formation of angiotensin II can occur in different vascular beds, and it provides local control

*Approximately that of a football field.

**A different isoform of ACE is also present in testis, and male mice lacking ACE have markedly reduced fertility.

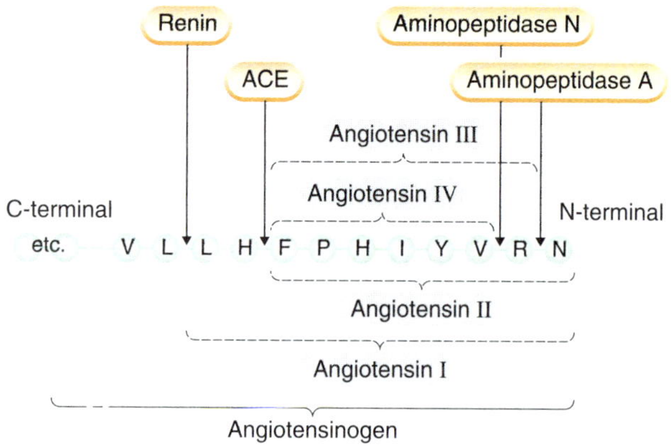

Fig. 18.5 Formation of angiotensins I–IV from the N-terminal of the precursor protein angiotensinogen.

independent of blood-borne angiotensin II. ACE inactivates bradykinin (see Ch. 15) and several other peptides. This may contribute to the pharmacological actions of ACE inhibitors (ACEI), as discussed below. The main actions of angiotensin II are mediated via receptors AT1 and AT2. AT1 is a specific membrane-bound G-protein-coupled receptor; these actions include:

- generalised vasoconstriction, especially marked in efferent arterioles of the kidney
- increased release of noradrenaline from sympathetic nerve terminals, reinforcing vasoconstriction and increasing the rate and force of contraction of the heart
- stimulation of proximal tubular reabsorption of Na^+
- secretion of aldosterone from the adrenal cortex (see Ch. 27)
- cell growth in the heart and in arteries.*

*These effects are initiated by the G-protein-coupled AT1-receptor acting via the same intracellular tyrosine phosphorylation pathways as are used by cytokines, for example the 'Jak/Stat' pathway (Ch. 3; Marrero et al., 1995).

AT2-receptors have also been cloned. They are expressed during fetal life and in distinct brain regions. Studies of mice in which the gene for the AT2-receptor has been disrupted suggest that it may be involved in growth, development and exploratory behaviour. Cardiovascular effects of AT2 receptors (inhibition of cell growth and lowering of blood pressure) appear to be relatively subtle and oppose those of AT1-receptors.

The renin–angiotensin–aldosterone pathway is important in the pathogenesis of heart failure, and several very important classes of therapeutic drug act by inhibiting it at various points (see below).

VASOACTIVE DRUGS

Drugs can affect vascular smooth muscle either directly, by acting on the smooth muscle cells themselves, or indirectly, by acting on endothelial cells or on sympathetic nerve terminals. Another type of indirect action is exemplified by ACEI. Mechanisms of action of directly acting vasoconstrictors and vasodilators are summarised in Figure 4.10 (p. 64). Table 18.3 shows indirectly acting vasoactive drugs, many of which are discussed in other chapters. We concentrate here on agents that are not covered elsewhere.

VASOCONSTRICTOR DRUGS

The α_1-adrenoceptor agonists and drugs that release noradrenaline from sympathetic nerve terminals or inhibit its reuptake (*sympathomimetic amines*) cause vasoconstriction and are discussed in Chapter 11. Some eicosanoids (e.g. *thromboxane* A_2; see Ch. 20) and several peptides, notably *endothelin*, *angiotensin* and *antidiuretic hormone* are also predominantly vasoconstrictor. **Sumatriptan** and ergot alkaloids acting through 5-hydroxytryptamine (5-HT) type 2 and 1D receptors also cause vasoconstriction (Ch. 12).

Table 18.3 Classification of vasoactive drugs that act indirectly

Site	Mechanism	Examples	Further details
Vasoconstrictors			
Sympathetic nerves	NA release	Tyramine	Ch. 11
	Block NA reuptake	Cocaine	Chs 11 and 52
Endothelium	Endothelin release	Thrombin, tumour necrosis factor, angiotensin II	This chapter
Vasodilators			
Sympathetic nerves	Inhibition of NA release	Prostaglandin E_2, α_2-agonists, guanethidine	Chs 9,11 and15
Endothelium	Increase NO release	Acetylcholine, substance P	Ch.14.
CNS	Vasomotor inhibition	Anaesthetics, methyldopa	Chs 11 and 35
Enzymes	ACE inhibition	Captopril	This chapter

NA, noradrenaline; NO, nitric oxide; ACE, angiotensin-converting enzyme.

ANGIOTENSIN

The physiological role of the renin–angiotensin system is described above. Angiotensin II is an extremely powerful vasoconstrictor, being roughly 40 times as potent as noradrenaline in raising blood pressure. Its peripheral effects resemble those of α_1-adrenoceptor agonists, in that it mainly affects cutaneous, splanchnic and renal blood flow, with less effect on blood flow to brain and skeletal muscle. It has no routine clinical uses, its pharmacological importance lying in the fact that other drugs (e.g. **captopril** and **losartan**; see below) affect the cardiovascular system by reducing its production or action.

ANTIDIURETIC HORMONE

Antidiuretic hormone is a posterior pituitary peptide hormone (Ch. 27). It is important for its actions on the kidney (discussed in Ch. 23) but is also a powerful vasoconstrictor in skin and some other vascular beds. Its effects are initiated by two distinct receptors (V_1 and V_2). Water retention is mediated through V_2-receptors, occurs at low plasma concentrations of antidiuretic hormone and involves activation of adenylate cyclase in renal collecting ducts. Vasoconstriction is mediated through V_1-receptors, requires higher concentrations of antidiuretic hormone and involves activation of phospholipase C (see Ch. 3). Antidiuretic hormone causes generalised vasoconstriction, including the coeliac, mesenteric and coronary vessels. It also affects other (e.g. gastrointestinal and uterine) smooth muscle and causes abdominal cramps for this reason. It is sometimes used to treat patients with bleeding oesophageal varices and portal hypertension before more definitive treatment, although many gastroenterologists prefer to use **octreotide** (unlicensed indication; see Ch. 27) for this.

ENDOTHELIN

Endothelins are discussed above; as explained, they have vasodilator and vasoconstrictor actions, but vasoconstriction predominates. Intravenous administration causes transient vasodilatation followed by profound and very long-lived vasoconstriction. The endothelins are even more potent vasoconstrictors than angiotensin II. As yet they have no clinical uses and their pharmacological importance, like that of angiotensin II, will probably lie in drugs that affect the cardiovascular system by reducing their production or actions.

VASODILATOR DRUGS

Many vasodilators are clinically important, being used to treat common conditions including hypertension, cardiac failure and angina pectoris.

DIRECTLY ACTING VASODILATORS

There are several points at which drugs act to relax vascular smooth muscle. These include Ca^{2+} entry, either by blocking directly voltage-dependent calcium channels or by causing hyperpolarisation, Ca^{2+} release from sarcoplasmic reticulum or reuptake into it, and enzymes that determine Ca^{2+} sensitivity. Calcium antagonists, potassium channel activators and drugs that influence cytoplasmic concentrations of cyclic nucleotides exemplify these mechanisms. A pyridine drug, **Y27632**, causes vasorelaxation by inhibiting a Rho-associated protein kinase, thereby selectively inhibiting smooth muscle contraction by inhibiting Ca^{2+} sensitisation, so a whole new group of vasodilators may be on the way!

Calcium antagonists

L-type calcium antagonists are discussed in detail in Chapter 17. They cause generalised arterial vasodilatation, though individual agents exhibit distinct patterns of regional potency. Dihydropyridines (e.g. **nifedipine**) act preferentially on vascular smooth muscle, whereas **verapamil** acts also on the heart; **diltiazem** is intermediate in specificity. Consequently, rapid acting dihydropyridines usually produce reflex tachycardia as a result of lowering the blood pressure, whereas verapamil and

Vasoconstrictor substances

- The main groups are sympathomimetic amines (direct and indirect), certain eicosanoids (thromboxanes), peptides (angiotensin, antidiuretic hormone and endothelin) and a group of miscellaneous other drugs (e.g. ergot alkaloids).
- Clinical uses are limited mainly to local applications (e.g. nasal decongestion, coadministration with local anaesthetics). Usefulness in hypotensive states is not proven, apart from adrenaline (epinephrine) in anaphylactic shock and in cardiac arrest. Antidiuretic hormone may be used to stop bleeding from oesophageal varices in patients with portal hypertension caused by liver disease.

Vasodilator drugs

- Vasodilators act:
  —to increase local tissue blood flow
  —to reduce arterial pressure
  —to reduce central venous pressure.
- Net effect is a reduction of cardiac pre-load (reduced filling pressure) and after-load (reduced vascular resistance), hence reduction of cardiac work.
- Main uses are:
  —antihypertensive therapy (e.g. angiotensin-converting enzyme inhibitors (ACEI), α_1-antagonists)
  —treatment of angina (e.g. calcium antagonists)
  —treatment of cardiac failure (e.g. ACEI).

diltiazem do not, because although they also lower blood pressure they slow the cardiac pacemaker by their direct action on the heart.

Drugs that activate potassium channels

Some drugs (e.g. **cromokalim** and **minoxidil**) relax smooth muscle by selectively increasing the membrane permeability to K^+. This hyperpolarises the cells and switches off voltage-dependent calcium channels. Patch-clamp recording (see Ch. 6) demonstrated that these drugs open a high-conductance potassium channel. This discovery coincided with studies demonstrating the existence of ATP-sensitive potassium channels in various cells. In cardiac muscle and pancreatic islet insulin-secreting B-cells, for example, intracellular ATP closes these potassium channels, thus causing depolarisation.* Potassium channel activators work by antagonising the action of intracellular ATP on these channels (Fig. 18.6), thus opening them and causing hyperpolarisation and relaxation.

Minoxidil is a very potent and long-acting vasodilator, used as a drug of last resort in treating severe hypertension unresponsive to other drugs. It causes hirsutism (its active metabolite is actually used as a rub-on cream to treat baldness). This is unacceptable to most women. It also causes marked salt and water retention and is usually prescribed with a loop diuretic. It causes reflex tachycardia, and a β-adrenoceptor antagonist is used to prevent this. **Cromokalim** and its active isomer **lemakalim** are more recently developed potassium channel activators. Drugs of this type relax most kinds of smooth muscle but have yet to establish a therapeutic niche. **Nicorandil** (Ch. 17) combines potassium channel activation with NO-donor activity and is used in refractory angina.

*This mechanism forms an important link between the metabolic state of the cell and membrane function, and sulfonylurea drugs cause insulin secretion by mimicking the action of ATP on these channels (see Ch. 25). Conversely, some potassium channel activators increase blood glucose by inhibiting insulin secretion from the pancreas.

Drugs that act via cyclic nucleotides

Cyclase activation

Many drugs relax vascular smooth muscle by increasing the cellular concentration of either cGMP or cAMP. For example NO, nitrates and the natriuretic peptides act through cGMP (see Chs 14 and 17); recently, a pyrazolopyridine drug (**BAY41-2272**) has been described that activates soluble guanylate cyclase via an NO-independent site. The β_2-agonists, adenosine and PGI_2 increase cytoplasmic cAMP (see Chs 11, 12 and 15). **Dopamine** has mixed vasodilator and vasoconstrictor actions. It selectively dilates renal vessels where it increases cAMP by activating adenylate cyclase. It is the precursor of noradrenaline (Ch. 11) and is also a transmitter in its own right in the brain (Ch. 31) and probably also in the periphery (Ch. 9). The proposal that dopamine might serve a role as a peripheral transmitter came from observations that stimulation of sympathetic nerves to the kidney causes vasodilatation that is not affected by adrenoceptor antagonists but is blocked by dopamine-receptor antagonists such as **haloperidol** (see Ch. 31). Dopamine produces a mixture of cardiovascular effects resulting from agonist actions on α- and β-adrenoceptors, as well as on dopamine receptors, when administered as an intravenous infusion. Blood pressure increases slightly, but the main effects are vasodilatation in the renal circulation and increased cardiac output. Dopamine was widely used in intensive care units in patients in whom renal failure associated with decreased renal perfusion appeared imminent; despite its beneficial effect on renal haemodynamics, it does not, however, improve survival in these circumstances and this use is obsolete.

Nitroprusside (nitroferricyanide) is a very powerful vasodilator with little effect outside the vascular system. It reacts with tissue sulfhydryl groups under physiological conditions to yield NO. Unlike the organic nitrates, which preferentially dilate capacitance vessels and muscular arteries, it acts equally on arterial and venous smooth muscle. Its clinical usefulness is limited because it must be given intravenously. In solution, particularly when exposed to light, nitroprusside is hydrolysed to cyanide. The intravenous solution must, therefore, be made up freshly from dry

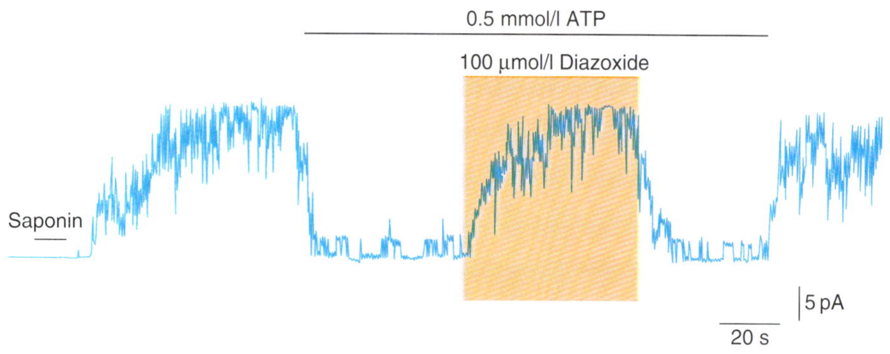

Fig. 18.6 ATP-sensitive potassium channels. Patch-clamp (see Ch. 3) record from insulin-secreting pancreatic B-cell: saponin permeabilised the cell, with loss of intracellular ATP, causing the channels to open (upward deflection) until they were inhibited by ATP. Addition of diazoxide, a vasodilator drug (which also inhibits insulin secretion; see text) reopens the channels. In smooth muscle, this causes hyperpolarisation and relaxation. (Redrawn from: Dunne et al. 1990 Br J Pharmacol 99: 169.)

powder and protected from light (usually by covering the container with foil). Nitroprusside is rapidly converted to thiocyanate, its plasma half-life being only a few minutes, so it must be given as a continuous infusion with careful monitoring to avoid hypotension. Continued use can lead to thiocyanate toxicity (weakness, nausea and inhibition of thyroid function) because thiocyanate is cleared only slowly from the bloodstream; consequently, nitroprusside is only useful for short-term treatment (usually up to 72 hours maximum). It is used in intensive care units for hypertensive crises, to produce controlled hypotension during surgery and to reduce cardiac work during the reversible cardiac dysfunction that occurs after cardiopulmonary bypass surgery.

Natriuretic peptides (atrial, B and C natriuretic peptides; see Ch. 17) also cause vasodilatation by activating guanylate cyclase. They act on the membrane-bound form of this enzyme, which is directly linked with natriuretic peptide receptors. **Anaritide**, a 25-residue synthetic form of atrial natriuretic peptide, increases glomerular filtration rate by dilating afferent arterioles while constricting efferent arterioles. It has been investigated in critically ill patients with acute renal failure: it did not improve the overall rate of dialysis-free survival but appeared to benefit patients who had *oliguria* (reduced urine formation) but be harmful in those who did not, so it is currently undergoing further evaluation. Natriuretic peptides have not found a therapeutic use thus far; the alternative strategy of inhibiting their clearance or metabolism (e.g. with **candoxatril**, a neutral endopeptidase inhibitor) is still being evaluated. **Omapatrilat**, a combined neutral endopeptidase inhibitor and ACEI, has a profound effect on blood pressure and encouraging results have been observed in heart failure, but its development has been slowed by concerns over the occurrence of *angio-oedema*,* especially in Black Afro-Caribean patients.

Phosphodiesterase inhibition

Phosphodiesterases (PDE) include at least 14 distinct isoenzymes. Methylxanthines (e.g. **theophylline**) and **papaverine** are non-selective PDE inhibitors (and have other actions too). Methylxanthines exert their main effects on non-vascular smooth muscle and on the central nervous system (CNS) and are discussed in Chapters 22 and 41. In addition to inhibiting PDE, some methylxanthines are also purine-receptor antagonists, which may partly account for their smooth muscle relaxant effects. They are not used clinically as vasodilators. Papaverine is closely related to **morphine** (see Ch. 40) (and indeed is produced by opium poppies). Pharmacologically, it is quite unlike morphine, however, its main action being to relax smooth muscle in blood vessels and elsewhere. Its mechanism is poorly understood but seems to involve a combination of PDE inhibition (as with methylxanthines) and block of calcium channels. Selective PDE type III inhibitors (e.g. **milrinone, cilostazol**) increase cytoplasmic cAMP by blocking its breakdown. They increase mortality in heart failure (despite short-term haemodynamic improvement), but cilostazol is of symptomatic benefit in patients with peripheral vascular disease (see below). Selective PDE type V inhibitors (e.g. **sildenafil**) inhibit the breakdown of cGMP. Penile erection is caused by increased activity in nitrergic nerves in the pelvis. These release NO, which activates guanylate cyclase in smooth muscle in the corpora cavernosa. Taken by mouth about an hour before sexual stimulation, sildenafil increases penile erection by potentiating this pathway. It has revolutionised treatment of erectile dysfunction (see Ch. 29) and has therapeutic potential via potentiation of other NO-mediated activities (Ch. 14). For example, it abolishes acute effects of hypoxia on pulmonary artery pressure, and trials in treatment of pulmonary hypertension are underway.

*Angio-oedema is localised swelling occurring unpredictably; it can affect the larynx with dire consequences!

VASODILATORS WITH UNKNOWN MECHANISM OF ACTION

Hydralazine

Hydralazine acts mainly on arteries and arterioles, causing a fall in blood pressure accompanied by reflex tachycardia and an increased cardiac output. It interferes with the action of IP_3 on Ca^{2+} release from the sarcoplasmic reticulum. Its main clinical uses were in hypertension and in heart failure (see below). It is still used for short-term treatment of severe hypertension in pregnancy, but it can cause an immune disorder resembling *systemic lupus erythematosus*** so alternative agents are now usually preferred for indications that require prolonged treatment.

Ethanol

Ethanol (see Ch. 52) dilates cutaneous vessels, causing the familiar drunkard's flush. Several general anaesthetics (e.g. propofol) cause vasodilatation as an unwanted effect (Ch. 35).

INDIRECTLY ACTING VASODILATOR DRUGS

The two main groups of indirectly acting vasodilator drugs are inhibitors of:

- sympathetic vasoconstriction
- the renin–angiotensin system.

The central control of sympathetically mediated vasoconstriction is believed to involve not only catecholamine receptors but also another class of receptor, termed the *imidazoline I_1-receptor,* which is present in the brainstem in the rostral ventrolateral medulla. Drugs can inhibit the sympathetic pathway at any point from the CNS to the peripheral sympathetic nerve terminal (see Ch 11). In addition, many vasodilators (e.g. acetylcholine, bradykinin, substance P) exert some or all of their effects by stimulating biosynthesis of vasodilator prostaglandins or of NO (or of both) by vascular endothelium (see above and Ch. 14), thereby causing functional antagonism of the constrictor tone caused by sympathetic nerves and angiotensin II. Recently, endothelin receptor antagonists including **bosentan** have been

**An autoimmune disease affecting one or more tissues, including joints, skin, pleural membranes. It is characterised by antibodies directed against DNA.

shown to lower systemic blood pressure in essential hypertension and pulmonary artery pressure in pulmonary hypertension, where they also improve exercise capacity. These drugs also have promise in heart failure, and other indications for vasodilator drugs, especially when the endothelin system is inappropriately activated. Applications to license them for such uses will doubtless follow.

We concentrate here on the renin–angiotensin–aldosterone system. This can be inhibited at several points:

- renin release: β-adrenoceptor antagonists inhibit renin release (although their other actions can result in a small *increase* in peripheral vascular resistance)
- renin activity: renin inhibitors
- ACE: ACEI
- angiotensin II type 1 (AT1) receptors: AT1-receptor antagonists
- aldosterone receptors: aldosterone receptor antagonists.

All such drugs can increase plasma K^+ concentration by reducing aldosterone secretion or action.

Renin inhibitors

Orally active renin inhibitors (e.g. **enalkiren**) reduce plasma renin activity, but their effects on blood pressure in patients with hypertension have been disappointing.

Angiotensin-converting enzyme inhibitors

Several specific ACEI have been developed, the first of which was **captopril** (Fig. 18.7). ACE cleaves the C-terminal pair of amino acids from peptide substrates. Its active site contains a zinc atom. The development of captopril was one of the first examples of successful drug design based on a chemical knowledge of the target molecule. Various small peptides had been found to be weak inhibitors of the enzyme,* but these were unsuitable as drugs because of their low potency and poor oral absorption. Captopril was designed to combine the steric properties of such peptide antagonists in a non-peptide molecule. It contains a sulfhydryl group appropriately placed to bind the zinc atom, coupled to a proline residue that binds the site on the enzyme which normally accommodates the terminal leucine of angiotensin I (Fig. 18.7). Several ACEI are now used widely, including **enalapril**, **lisinopril**, **ramipril**, **perindopril** and **trandolapril**, each of which differ in their durations of action and tissue distribution.

Pharmacological effects

Captopril is a powerful inhibitor of the effects of angiotensin I in the whole animal. It causes only a small fall in arterial pressure in normal animals or human subjects who are consuming the

*The lead compound was a nonapeptide derived from the venom of *Bothrops jacaraca*—a South American snake.

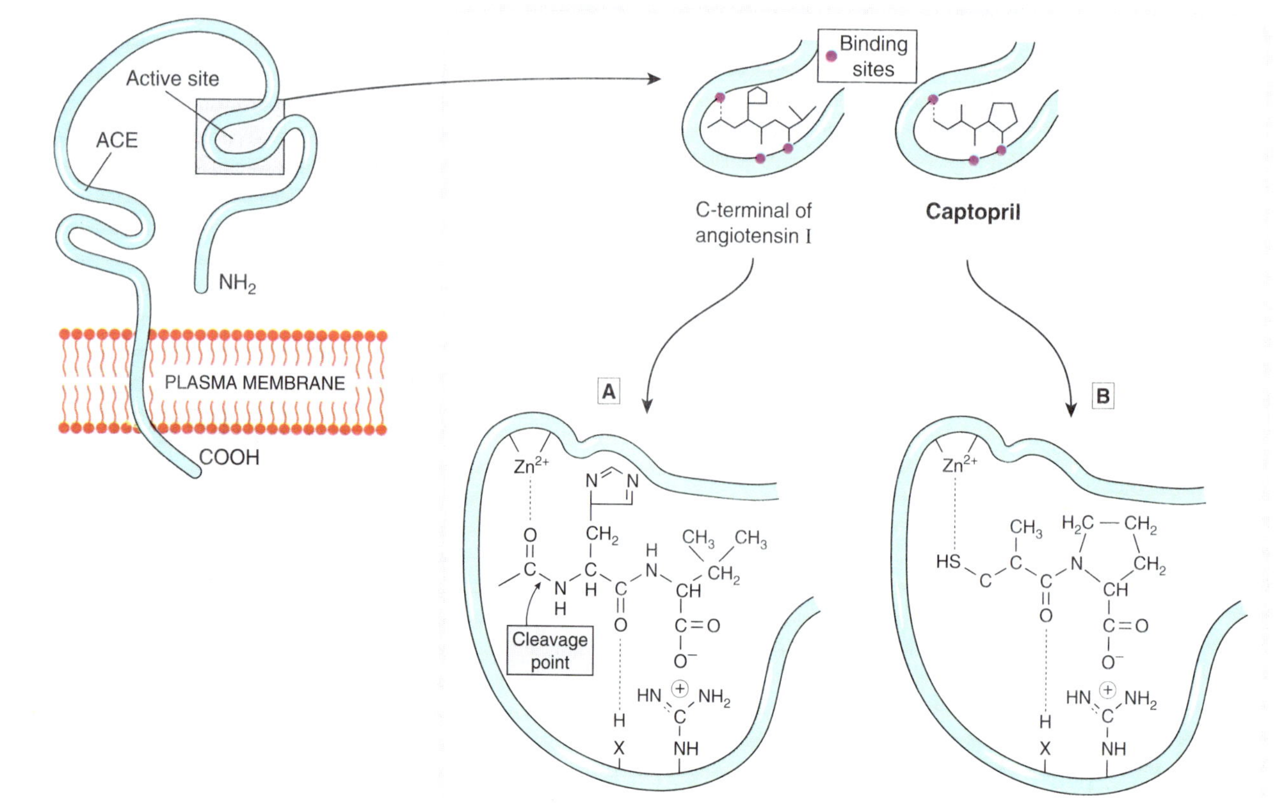

Fig. 18.7 The active site of angiotensin-converting enzyme. A Binding of angiotensin I. B Binding of the inhibitor captopril, which is an analogue of the terminal dipeptide of angiotensin I.

Clinical uses of angiotensin-converting enzyme (ACE) inhibitors

- Hypertension
- Cardiac failure
- Following myocardial infarction (especially when there is ventricular dysfunction, even when this is mild)
- Patients at high risk of ischaemic heart disease
- Diabetic nephropathy
- Progressive renal insufficiency.

amount of salt contained in a usual Western diet, but a much larger fall in hypertensive patients, particularly those in whom renin secretion is enhanced (e.g. in patients receiving diuretics). ACEIs affect capacitance and resistance vessels and reduce cardiac load as well as arterial pressure. They do not affect cardiac contractility, so cardiac output normally increases. They act preferentially on angiotensin-sensitive vascular beds, which include those of the kidney, heart and brain. This selectivity may be important in sustaining adequate perfusion of these vital organs in the face of reduced perfusion pressure. Critical *renal artery stenosis** represents an exception to this, where ACE inhibition results in a fall of glomerular filtration rate (see below).

Clinical uses

Clinical uses of ACEI are summarised in the box.

Unwanted effects

Captopril was initially used in doses that, in retrospect, were excessive. In these large doses, it caused rashes, taste disturbance, neutropenia and heavy proteinuria. This pattern of adverse effects is also seen during treatment with **penicillamine** (Ch. 16) which also contains a sulfhydryl group, and it has been argued that these effects are attributable to this chemical feature of the molecule rather than to ACE inhibition as such. Other ACEI that do not possess a sulfhydryl group do not cause these effects. In contrast, adverse effects that are directly related to ACE inhibition are common to all drugs of this class. These include hypotension, especially after the first dose and especially in patients with heart failure who have been treated with loop diuretics, in whom the renin–angiotensin system is highly activated. A dry cough, possibly the result of accumulation of bradykinin (Ch. 15) in the bronchial mucosa, is the commonest persistent adverse effect. Patients with bilateral renal artery stenosis predictably develop renal failure if treated with ACEI, because glomerular filtration in the face of low afferent arteriolar pressure is maintained by angiotensin II-mediated constriction of the efferent arteriole. Such renal failure is reversible provided it is recognised promptly and the ACEI stopped. If such renal failure occurs, hyperkalaemia may be severe owing to reduced angiotensin-stimulated aldosterone secretion.

*Severe narrowing of the renal artery, usually caused by an atheromatous plaque (Ch. 19) in older patients.

Angiotensin II receptor subtype 1 antagonists

Saralasin, a peptide analogue of angiotensin II, inhibits the vasoconstrictor effect of angiotensin II. It is a partial agonist and must be administered parenterally so it is not used clinically. Attention has again focussed on angiotensin II receptor antagonists with the development of many non-peptide, orally active pure antagonists of the AT1-receptor (e.g. **losartan**; Fig. 18.8). ACE is not the only enzyme capable of forming angiotensin II, *chymase* (which is not inhibited by ACEI) providing one alternative route. It is not known if alternative pathways of angiotensin II formation are important in vivo, but if so, then AT1-receptor antagonists could be more effective than

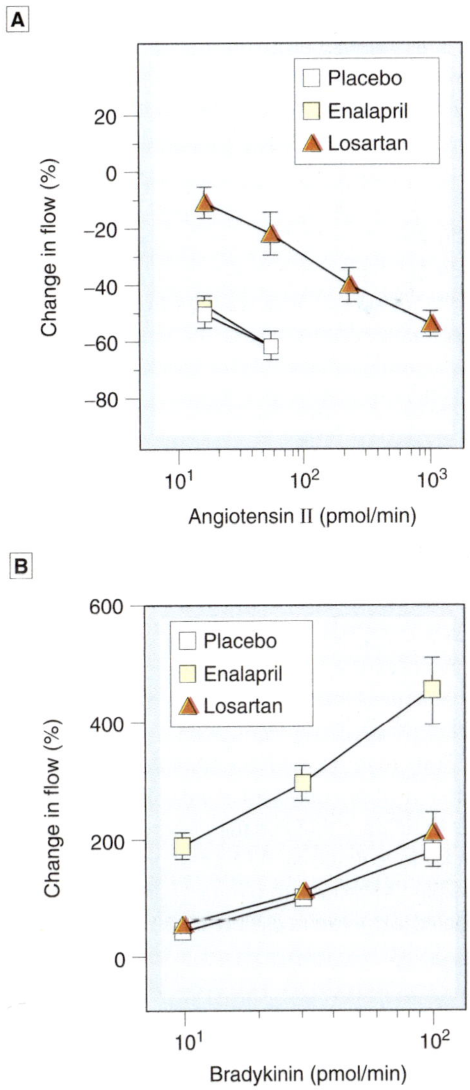

Fig. 18.8 Comparison of effects of angiotensin-converting enzyme inhibition and angiotensin-receptor blockade in the human forearm vasculature. A Effect of brachial artery infusion of angiotensin II on forearm blood flow after oral administration of placebo, enalapril (10 mg) or losartan (100 mg). B Effect of brachial artery infusion of bradykinin as in A. (From: Cockcroft J R et al. 1993 J Cardiovasc Pharmacol 22: 579–584.)

Types of vasodilator drug

- Angiotensin-converting enzyme inhibitors (ACEI, e.g. captopril, enalapril): prevent conversion of angiotensin I to angiotensin II; therefore most effective when renin release is increased.
- Nitrates (e.g. glyceryl trinitrate, nitroprusside): act like endogenous nitric oxide (NO), causing increased cGMP formation.
- Calcium antagonists (diltiazem, nifedipine and many other dihydropyridines): act by blocking Ca^{2+} entry in response to depolarisation; dilate both resistance and capacitance vessels.
- Drugs that interfere with sympathetic transmission (e.g. α_1-adrenoceptor antagonists).
- Potassium channel activators (e.g. diazoxide, cromokalim): open membrane potassium channels, thus causing hyperpolarisation; thought to affect insulin-secreting cells and neurons, as well as smooth muscle, so produce various side-effects.
- Angiotensin II subtype 1 (AT1) receptor antagonists (e.g. losartan).
- Other agents include β_2-adrenoceptor agonists, adenosine, methylxanthines (e.g. theophylline), various diuretics and numerous agents that stimulate endothelial NO production (Ch. 14).

Clinical uses of angiotensin II subtype 1 (AT1) receptor antagonists

- Experience with AT1 antagonists is less than with angiotensin-converting enzyme inhibitors (ACEI), and it cannot be assumed that these classes of drug will prove to be therapeutically equivalent.
- Many clinicians reserve them for patients with hypertension in whom an ACEI is indicated, but who are unable to tolerate this because of dry cough. (This side-effect is not caused by AT1 antagonists.)
- Other possible indications (e.g. heart failure) are currently being explored in clinical trials.

ACEI in such situations. **Losartan** does not cause the dry cough that is sometimes caused by ACEI, consistent with the 'bradykinin accumulation' explanation of this side-effect, mentioned above. It is useful in hypertensive patients who experience this side-effect with ACEI. Conversely, it is not known whether any of the beneficial effects of ACEI (e.g. reversal of left ventricular hypertrophy and improvement of endothelial dysfunction) are bradykinin/NO mediated, so it is unwise to assume that AT1-receptor antagonists will share all of the therapeutic properties of ACEI. Initial experience with losartan and **valsartan** in patients with heart failure has not shown them to be inferior to ACEI, but their efficacy for this indication remains to be fully established.

CLINICAL USES OF VASOACTIVE DRUGS

It is beyond the scope of this book to provide a detailed account of the clinical uses of vasoactive drugs, but it is, nonetheless, useful to consider the various pharmacological approaches that are used to treat certain important clinical states. The conditions that will be briefly discussed are:

- hypertension
- cardiac failure
- shock
- peripheral vascular disease
- Raynaud's disease.

HYPERTENSION

Hypertension is a common disorder that, if not effectively treated, results in a greatly increased probability of coronary thrombosis, strokes and renal failure. Until about 1950, there was no effective treatment, and the development of antihypertensive drugs, which restore healthy life expectancy, has been a major therapeutic success story.

There are a few recognisable and surgically treatable causes of hypertension, such as *phaeochromocytoma*,* steroid-secreting tumours of the adrenal cortex, renal artery stenosis and so on, but most cases involve no obvious cause and are grouped as *essential hypertension* (so-called because it was originally thought that the raised blood pressure was essential to maintain adequate tissue perfusion). Increased cardiac output may be an early feature, followed by increased peripheral resistance and normalisation of cardiac output. Blood pressure control is intimately related to the kidneys, as demonstrated by transplantation experiments in which kidneys are transplanted from or to animals with genetic hypertension, or to humans requiring renal transplantation: hypertension 'goes with' the kidney from a hypertensive donor and vice versa. Persistently raised arterial pressure leads to hypertrophy of the left ventricle and of the media of resistance arteries, with narrowing of the lumen. The raised peripheral vascular resistance calls into play various physiological responses involving the cardiovascular system, nervous system and kidney. Such vicious circles provide targets for pharmacological attack.

Figure 18.9 summarises physiological mechanisms that control arterial blood pressure and shows sites at which antihypertensive drugs act. The main systems include the *sympathetic nervous system*, the *renin–angiotensin–aldosterone* system and *tonically active endothelium-derived autacoids* (NO and probably ET-1; see above). One of the ways in which an unknown primary process leads to progressively worsening hypertension is that remodelling and hypertrophy, associated with proliferation of

*Catecholamine-secreting tumours, usually of the adrenal medulla (Ch. 11).

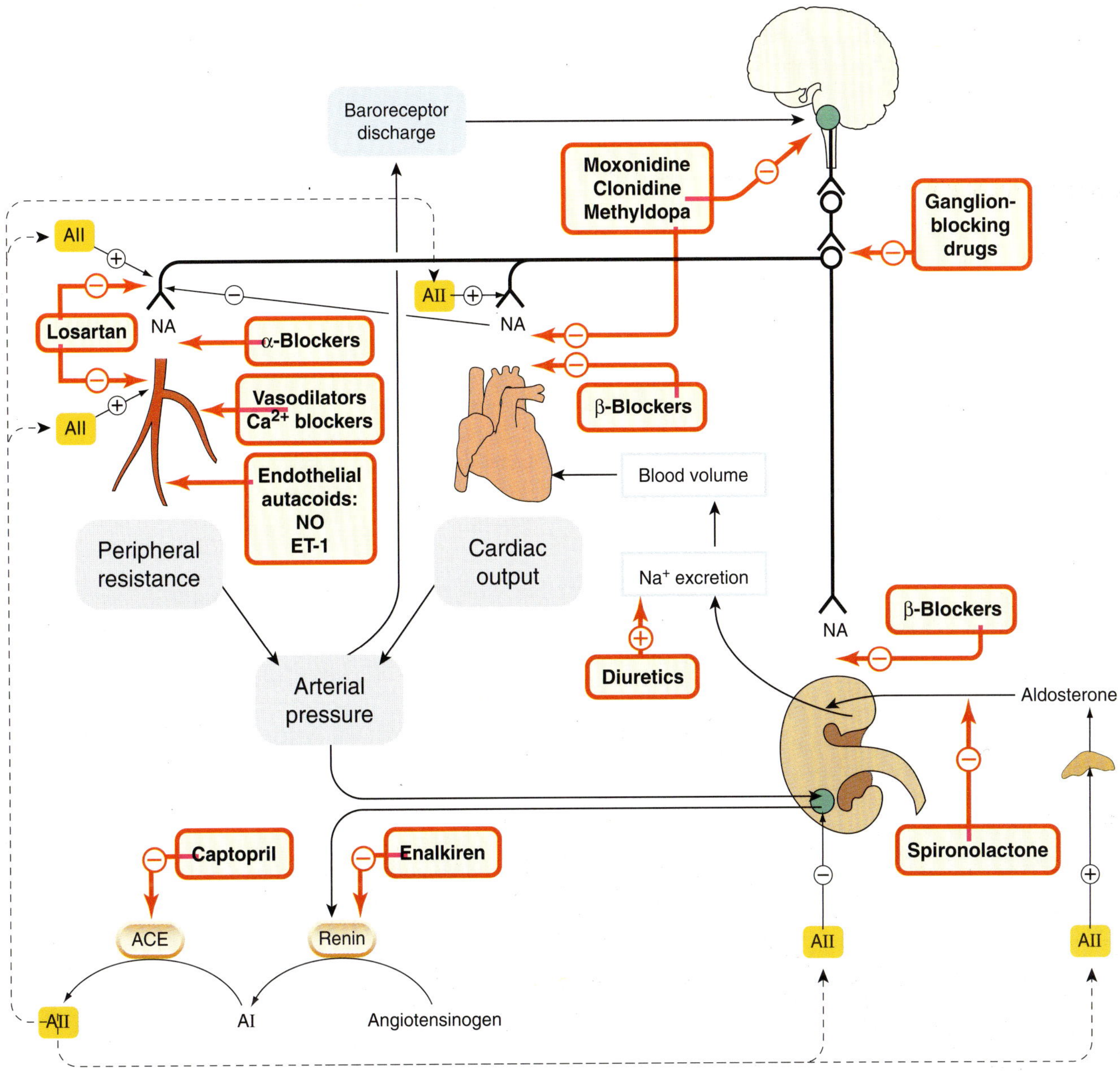

Fig. 18.9 Diagram showing the main mechanisms involved in arterial blood pressure regulation (black lines), and the sites of action of antihypertensive drugs (hatched boxes + orange lines). (NA, noradrenaline; AI, angiotensin I; AII, angiotensin II; ACE, angiotensin-converting enzyme; NO, nitric oxide; ET-1, endothelin-1.)

smooth muscle cells in the media of resistance arteries, occurs in response to the raised pressure, reducing the ratio of lumen diameter to wall thickness and increasing the peripheral vascular resistance. The role of cellular growth factors (including angiotensin II) and inhibitors of growth (e.g. NO) in the evolution of these structural changes is currently of great interest to vascular biologists and is potentially of importance to the therapeutic use of drugs such as ACEI.

Contrary to the earlier view that hypertension was 'essential' to sustain life, reducing arterial blood pressure greatly improves the prognosis of patients with hypertension. The use of drugs to control mild hypertension (which is asymptomatic), without producing unacceptable side-effects, is, therefore, an important clinical need, and much effort has gone into devising satisfactory therapeutic regimens.* Treatment involves non-pharmacological measures (e.g. increased exercise, reduced dietary salt and saturated fat with increased fruit and fibre, weight and alcohol reduction) followed by the staged introduction of drugs, starting

*The harsh realities of life on antihypertensive drugs are graphically described in an article entitled '80,000 pills: a personal history of hypertension' (Mills, 1989).

with those of proven benefit and least likely to produce side-effects. Some of the drugs that were used to lower blood pressure in the early days of antihypertensive therapy, including *ganglion blockers, adrenergic neuron blockers* and **reserpine** (see Ch. 11), produced a fearsome array of adverse effects at the doses used and are now obsolete. The preferred regimens have changed progressively as better-tolerated drugs have become available. *Thiazide diuretics* or *β-adrenoceptor antagonists* remain common starting points for patients who are otherwise healthy. They abolish the excess risk of stroke conferred by hypertension and reduce the risk of myocardial infarction. Their unwanted effects are much less severe than those of drugs such as **methyldopa** or **guanethidine**. In patients with moderate or severe hypertension, it is often possible to control the pressure without causing side-effects by combining low doses of different drugs with complementary mechanisms of action (e.g. a diuretic, with efficacy limited by the increased plasma renin activity that it causes, with an ACEI, which blocks the renin–angiotensin system), rather than increasing the dose of a single agent, the effectiveness of which is often limited by homeostatic mechanisms. High doses of antihypertensive drugs are often not very effective during chronic administration, and they often cause side-effects.

ACEI and calcium channel antagonists (calcium antagonists) are used, alone or in combination, and AT1-receptor antagonists are useful especially in patients who do not tolerate ACEI because of cough; combined ACEI/neutral endopeptidase inhibition with **omapatrilat** (see above) is more effective than ACE inhibition alone. The α_1-adrenoceptor antagonists have also staged something of a comeback with longer-acting drugs such as **doxazosin,** which are well tolerated, used once daily and have theoretically desirable effects on plasma lipids (reducing the ratio of low to high density lipoproteins, see Ch. 19). **Moxonidine** is a centrally acting antihypertensive drug that is an agonist at imidazoline I_1-receptors. It causes less drowsiness than α_2-agonists. **Fenoldopam**, a selective dopamine D_1-receptor agonist, was recently approved by the US Federal Drugs Agency (FDA) for the short-term management in hospital of severe hypertension.

The main categories of antihypertensive drugs are summarised in Table 18.4.

CARDIAC FAILURE

The underlying abnormality in *cardiac failure* (see Ch 17) is a cardiac output that is inadequate to meet the metabolic demands of the body during exercise (and ultimately also at rest). It may be caused by disease of the myocardium itself (most commonly ischaemic heart disease), or by circulatory factors such as volume overload (e.g. leaky valves, or arteriovenous shunts caused by congenital defects)* or pressure overload (e.g. stenosed—narrowed—valves, hypertension). When cardiac output decreases, an increase in fluid volume occurs, partly because increased venous pressure causes increased formation of tissue fluid, and partly because reduced renal blood flow activates the renin–angiotensin–aldosterone system, causing Na^+ and water retention. Irrespective of the cause, the outlook for adults with cardiac failure is grim: 50% of those with the most severe grade are dead in 6 months, and of those with 'mild/moderate' disease 50% are dead in 5 years.

A highly simplified diagram of the sequence of events is shown in Figure 18.10. Non-drug measures, including dietary salt restriction, are important but drugs are needed to improve symptoms of oedema, fatigue and breathlessness and to improve prognosis. ACEI, β-adrenoceptor antagonists and **spironolactone** have each been shown to prolong life in heart failure, although prognosis remains poor despite optimal management. Drugs can act in several ways.

Increase natriuresis Divertics (Ch. 23) are important in increasing salt and water excretion, especially if there is

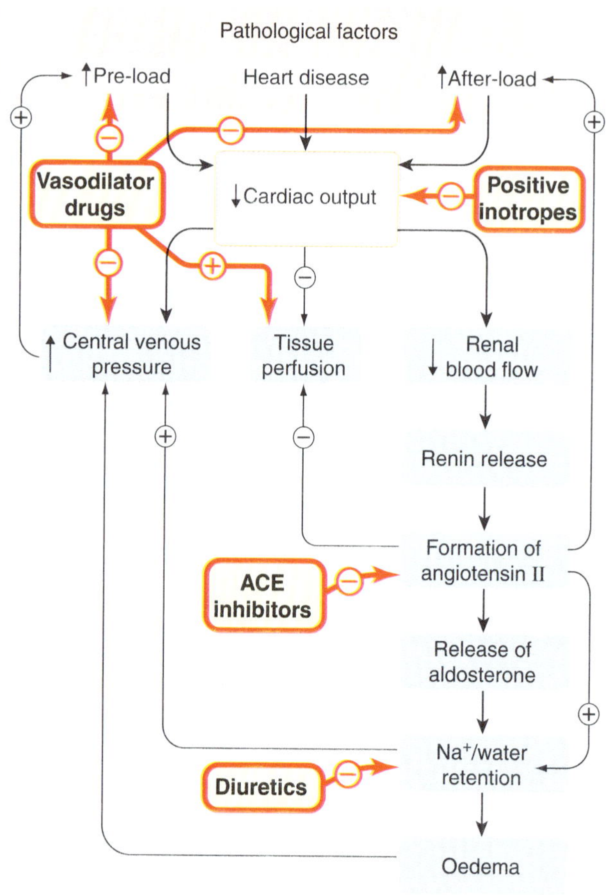

Fig. 18.10 Simplified scheme showing the pathogenesis of heart failure, and the sites of action of some of the drugs used to treat it. The symptoms of heart failure are produced by reduced tissue perfusion, oedema and increased central venous pressure. (ACE, angiotensin-converting enzyme.)

*So-called 'hole-in-the-heart' babies have a defect in the atrial or ventricular septum, leading to shunting of blood from high- to low-pressure parts of the circulation.

Table 15.4 Commonly used antihypertensive drugs

Mode of action	Drugs	Adverse effects			Special features
		Postural hypotension	Impotence	Other	
Reduction of blood volume/indirect vasodilatation	Thiazide diuretics[a]	–	++	Urinary frequency, gout, glucose intolerance, hypokalaemia, hyponatraemia, thrombocytopenia	Reduce stroke in clinical trials, inexpensive
Block of β-adrenoceptors[b]	Atenolol Metoprolol	–	±	Fatigue, cold peripheries	Reduce stroke in clinical trials, inexpensive; additional benefit after MI. Contraindications: asthma, heart block, peripheral vascular disease
ACE inhibition	Captopril Enalapril Lisinopril Trandolapril Ramipril	–	–	First dose hypotension, dry cough, reversible renal failure in patients with bilateral renal artery stenosis Additional benefit in insulin-dependent diabetics with proteinuria, following MI, and in patients with heart failure; cause regression of left ventricular hypertrophy	
Arteriolar vasodilatation	Calcium antagonists, e.g. nifedipine, amlodipine, nicardipine	–	±	Flushing, headache, ankle oedema	–
Block of α_1-adrenoceptors[b]	Prazosin Terazosin Doxazosin	+	–	First dose hypotension Longer-acting drugs (e.g. terazosin, doxazosin) better tolerated than prazosin. Improve plasma lipids. Useful addition to other drugs when two drugs needed	

MI, myocardial infarction.
[a]See Chapter 23.
[b]See Chapter 11.

pulmonary oedema. In chronic heart failure, drugs that have been shown to improve prognosis were all studied in patients treated with diuretics.

Inhibit the renin–angiotensin–aldosterone system The renin–angiotensin–aldosterone system is inappropriately activated in patients with cardiac failure, especially when they are treated with diuretics. ACEI counteract this. By blocking the formation of angiotensin II, they reduce vascular resistance, thus improving tissue perfusion and reducing cardiac after-load. They also cause natriuresis by inhibiting secretion of aldosterone and by reducing the direct stimulatory effect of angiotensin II on reabsorption of Na^+ and HCO_3^- in the early part of the proximal convoluted tubule. Most important of all, they prolong life. Trials to determine whether AT1 antagonists (alone or in combination with ACEI) are as good as (or better than) ACEI alone are in progress. Angiotensin II is not the only stimulus to aldosterone secretion, and during chronic treatment with ACEI, circulating aldosterone concentrations return toward pretreatment values (a process known as 'aldosterone escape'). This provided a rationale for studying the effect of combining **spironolactone** (an aldosterone antagonist, see Ch. 23) with ACEI treatment, and this further reduces mortality.

Beta-adrenoceptor antagonists Heart failure is accompanied by potentially harmful activation of the sympathetic nervous system as well as of the renin–angiotensin system, providing a rationale for using β-adrenoceptor antagonists for this disorder. Most clinicians have been very wary of this approach, because of the negative inotropic action of these drugs, but when started in low doses that are increased slowly, **metoprolol**, **carvedilol** and **bisoprolol** have each been shown convincingly to improve survival when added to other effective drugs in double-blind placebo-controlled trials.

Relax vascular smooth muscle **Glyceryl trinitrate** is used to treat acute cardiac failure, especially if there is associated ischaemic pain. Its venodilator effect reduces venous pressure, and its effects on arterial compliance and wave reflection reduce cardiac work. The combination of **hydralazine** (to reduce after-load) with a long-acting organic nitrate (to reduce pre-load) in patients with chronic heart failure improves survival, albeit less well than treatment with an ACEI. This combination is useful in patients in whom ACEI are contraindicated or are not tolerated.

Increase the force of cardiac contraction Cardiac glycosides (see Ch. 17) are mainly used either in patients who also have chronic rapid atrial fibrillation or in patients who remain symptomatic despite treatment with diuretic and ACEI.

Drugs used in chronic heart failure

- Loop diuretics, e.g. furosemide (frusemide; Ch. 23)
- Angiotensin-converting enzyme inhibitors (ACEI, e.g. captopril, enalapril)
- Beta-adrenoceptor antagonists (e.g. metoprolol), introduced in low dose in stable patients
- Spironolactone (Ch. 23)
- Digoxin (see Ch.17), especially for heart failure associated with established rapid atrial fibrillation. It is also indicated in patients who remain symptomatic despite treatment with loop diuretics and ACEI.
- Organic nitrates (e.g. isosorbide mononitrate) reduce pre-load, and hydralazine reduces after-load. Used in combination, these prolong life, but less effectively than ACEI. They are used when ACEI are contraindicated or not tolerated.

Digoxin does not reduce mortality in this latter group of patients but does improve symptoms and reduces the need for hospital admission. In contrast, PDE inhibitors (e.g. **amrinone**, **milrinone**) increase cardiac output acutely but increase mortality in heart failure probably through cardiac dysrhythmias. **Dobutamine** (a β_1-selective adrenoceptor agonist; see Ch. 17) is used intravenously when a rapid response is needed in the short term, for example following heart surgery.

SHOCK AND HYPOTENSIVE STATES

Shock is a medical emergency characterised by inadequate perfusion of vital organs, usually because of a very low arterial blood pressure. This leads to anaerobic metabolism and hence to increased lactate production. Mortality is extremely high, even with optimal treatment in an intensive care unit. Shock can be caused by various insults, including haemorrhage, burns, bacterial infections, anaphylaxis (Ch. 11) and myocardial infarction (Fig. 18.11). Reduced effective circulating blood volume (hypovolaemia) may be caused either directly by loss of blood or by movement of fluid from the plasma to the tissues. The physiological (homeostatic) response to this is complex: vasodilatation in a vital organ (e.g. brain, heart or kidney) favours perfusion of that organ, but at the expense of a further reduction in blood pressure, which leads to reduced perfusion of other organs. Ideally, there is a balance between vasoconstriction in non-essential vascular beds and vasodilatation in vital ones. The dividing line between the normal physiological response to blood loss and clinical shock is that tissue hypoxia produces secondary effects in the latter which tend to magnify rather than correct the primary disturbance. Therefore, patients with established shock have profound and inappropriate vasodilatation in non-essential organs, and this is difficult to correct with vasoconstrictor drugs. The release of mediators (e.g. histamine, 5-HT, bradykinin, prostaglandins, cytokines including interleukins and tumour necrosis factor (TNF), NO and, undoubtedly, many more as yet unidentified substances) that cause capillary dilatation and leakiness, is the opposite of what is required to improve function in this setting. Mediators promoting vasodilation in vasodilatory shock converge on two main mechanisms:

- activation of ATP-sensitive potassium channels in vascular smooth muscle by reduced cytoplasmic ATP and increased lactate and protons
- increased synthesis of NO, which activates myosin-light-chain phosphatase and activates K_{Ca} channels, thereby hyperpolarising vascular smooth muscle membranes.

A third key mechanism seems to be a relative deficiency of antidiuretic hormone, which is secreted acutely in response to haemorrhage but subsequently declines, probably because of depletion from the neurohypophysis.

Patients with shock are not a homogeneous population, making it hard to perform valid clinical trials, and in contrast to hypertension and heart failure there is very little evidence to support treatment strategies based on hard clinical end-points (such as improved survival). Hypoperfusion leads to multiple

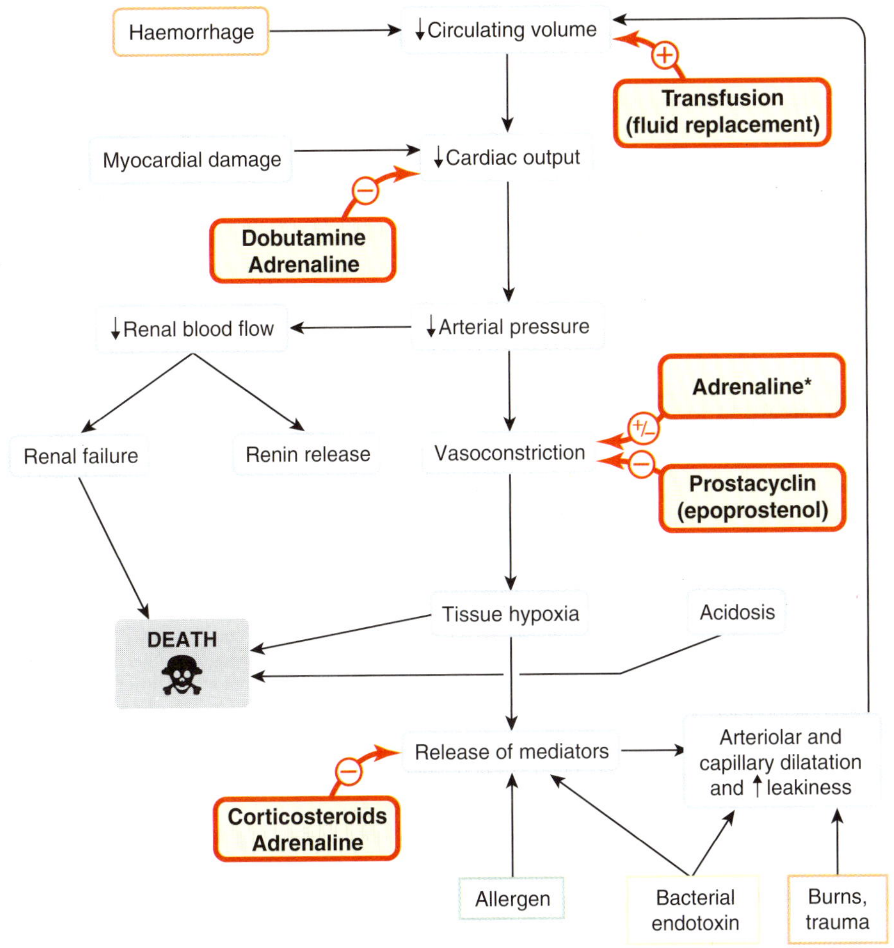

Fig. 18.11 Simplified scheme showing the pathogenesis of hypovolaemic shock. Adrenaline (epinephrine) causes vasodilation in some vascular beds, vasoconstriction in others.

organ failure, and intensive therapy specialists spend much effort supporting the circulations of such patients with cocktails of vasoactive drugs designed to optimise flow to vital organs. There is great interest in antagonists of mediators that may be contributing to the hypotensive state. Clinical trials are in progress with drugs and macromolecules (including monoclonal antibodies and soluble fragments of receptors) designed to block or neutralise endotoxin, interleukins, TNF and the inducible form of NOS among others. So far, these efforts have not yielded fruit. Experimental work strongly suggests that dose will be critical since small amounts of mediators such as NO appear to be beneficial while larger amounts are harmful (Ch. 14). Clinical trials in this setting are extremely difficult because of the unique and distinctive haemodynamic features of each patient. *Volume replacement* is of benefit if there is hypovolaemia; *antibiotics* are essential if there is persistent infection; **adrenaline** (**epinephrine**) can be lifesaving in anaphylaxis; recombinant *activated protein C* improves mortality and was recently licensed for this indication; *antidiuretic hormone* may be effective in increasing blood pressure even when there is resistance to adrenaline; *corticosteroids* suppress the formation of NO and of prostaglandins but are not of proven benefit once shock is established; vasoactive (PGI_2, **epoprostenol**) and positively inotropic (**adrenaline**, (**epinephrine**), **dobutamine**) drugs may help in individual patients but have not been proved to improve the ultimate clinical outcome.

PERIPHERAL VASCULAR DISEASE

When atheroma involves peripheral arteries, the commonest symptom is pain in the legs on walking ('*claudication*'), followed by pain at rest and, in severe cases, gangrene of the feet or legs. Treatment is often surgical (surgical reconstruction or amputation) or by *angioplasty* (disruption of atheroma by inflation of a balloon surrounding the tip of a catheter). Other vascular beds (e.g. coronary, cerebral and renal) are often also affected by atheromatous disease. Drug treatment includes antiplatelet drugs (e.g. **aspirin**, **clopidogrel;** see Ch. 20), a statin (e.g. **simvastatin**; see Ch. 19) and an ACEI (e.g. **ramipril**, see above). These reduce the excess risk of ischaemic coronary events. Additionally, several placebo-controlled studies have demonstrated that **cilostazol**, a type III PDE inhibitor, improves pain-free and maximum walking distance in such patients, but its effect on mortality is unknown.

RAYNAUD'S DISEASE

Inappropriate vasoconstriction of small arteries and arterioles gives rise to Raynaud's phenomenon (blanching of the fingers during vasoconstriction, followed by blueness owing to deoxygenation of the static blood and redness from reactive hyperaemia following return of blood flow). This can be mild but if severe causes ulceration and gangrene of the fingers. It can occur in isolation ('Raynaud's disease') or in association with a number of other diseases including several so-called connective tissue diseases (e.g. systemic sclerosis, systemic lupus erythematosus). Treatment of Raynaud's phenomenon involves stopping smoking and avoiding the cold; β-adrenoceptor antagonists are contraindicated. Vasodilators (e.g. **nifedipine**) are of some benefit in severe cases, but treatment is difficult.

REFERENCES AND FURTHER READING

Control of vascular smooth muscle tone

Chitaley K, Weber D, Webb R C 2001 RhoA/Rho-kinase, vascular changes, and hypertension. Curr Hypertens Rep 3: 139–144

Guimarães S, Moura D 2001 Vascular adrenoceptors: an update. Pharmacol Rev 53: 319–356 (*Functional perspective*)

Quayle J M, Nelson M T, Standen N B 1997 ATP-sensitive and inwardly rectifying potassium channels in smooth muscle. Physiol Rev 77: 1165–1232 (*Reviews these potassium channels, both of which are important in controlling the contractile state of vascular smooth muscle*)

Vascular endothelium (see Ch. 14 for further reading on NO)

Busse R, Edwards G, Feletou M, Fleming I, van Houte P M, Weston A H 2002 EDHF: bringing the concepts together. Trends Pharmacol Sci 23: 374–380 (*Consensus on EDHF? Potassium ions are important*)

Carmeliet P, Jain R K 2000 Angiogenesis in cancer and other diseases. Nature 407: 249–257 (*New approaches to treatment of cancer and other diseases, via a growing number of pro- and anti-angiogenic molecules. See also (in same issue) Yancopoulos GD et al. 2000 Vascular specific growth factors and blood vessel formation. Nature 407: 242–248*)

Hickey K A, Rubanyi G, Paul R J, Highsmith R F 1985 Characterization of a coronary vasoconstrictor produced by cultured endothelial cells. Am J Physiol 248(5 Pt 1): C550–C556

Huang A, Sun D, Smith C J et al. 2000 In eNOS knockout mice skeletal muscle arteriolar dilation to acetylcholine is mediated by EDHF. Am J Physiol 278: H762–H768 (*Where NO is absent, EDHF compensates*)

Kedzierski R M, Yanagisawa M 2001 Endothelin system: the double-edged sword in health and disease. Annu Rev Pharmacol Toxicol 41: 851–876 (*Topical review by one of the discoverers of endothelin*)

Masaki T 1993 Endothelins: homeostatic and compensatory actions in the circulatory and endocrine systems. Endocr Rev 14: 256–268 (*Particularly useful on roles in endocrine—reproductive, neuroendocrine—systems*)

Yanagisawa M, Kurihara H, Kimura S et al. 1988 A novel potent vasoconstrictor peptide produced by vascular endothelial cells. Nature 332: 411–415 (*Tour de force*)

Renin–angiotensin system

Burnier M, Brunner H R 2000 Angiotensin II receptor antagonists. Lancet 355: 637–645 (*Reviews this new class of drugs, which are similar in antihypertensive effect to ACEI; if they also reduce mortality they may one day replace ACEI*)

Hein L, Barsh G S, Pratt R E, Dzau V J, Kobilks B K 1995 Behavioural and cardiovascular effects of disrupting the angiotensin II type-2 receptor gene in mice. Nature 377: 744–747 (*'The AT2 receptor plays a role in the central nervous system and in cardiovascular functions that are mediated by the renin–angiotensin system.' Pause for thought for clinicians inclined to prescribe ACEI and ATI-receptor antagonists interchangeably*)

Ichiki T, Labosky P A, Shiota C et al. 1995 Effects on blood pressure and exploratory behaviour of mice lacking angiotensin II type-2 receptor Nature 377: 748–750 (*Angiotensin II activates AT1 and AT2, which have mutually counteracting haemodynamic effects… AT2 regulates CNS functions, including behaviour*)

Marrero M B et al. 1995 Direct stimulation of Jak/Stat pathway by the angiotensin II AT1 receptor. Nature 375: 247–250.

Drugs (and clinical uses)

Allgren R A for the Auriculin Anaritide Acute Renal Failure Study Group 1997 Anaritide in acute tubular necrosis. N Engl J Med 336: 828–834 (*A synthetic analogue of atrial natriuretic peptide may have improved survival in those patients with oliguria but worsened it in those with non-oliguric renal failure*)

Australian and New Zealand Intensive Care Society (ANZICS) Clinical Trials Group 2000 Low-dose dopamine in patients with early renal dysfunction: a placebo-controlled randomized trial. Lancet 356: 2139–2143 (*No clinically significant protection. See also accompanying editorial: Renal-dose dopamine: will the message now get through?*)

Bagnall A J, Webb D J 2000 The endothelin system: physiology. In: Vallance P J T, Webb D J (eds) Vascular endothelium in human physiology and pathophysiology. Harwood Academic, Singapore, pp. 31–60

Bernard G R et al. 2001 Efficacy and safety of recombinant human activated protein C for severe sepsis. N Engl J Med 344: 699–709 (*Continuous intravenous infusion of activated protein C, a vitamin K-dependent anticoagulant that promotes fibrinolysis, inhibits thrombosis and is anti-inflammatory, significantly reduced risk of death at 28 days, from 30.8 to 24.7%*)

Channick R N et al. 2001 Effects of the dual endothelin-receptor antagonist bosentan in patients with pulmonary hypertension. Lancet 358: 1119–1123 (*Bosentan increased exercise capacity and reduced pulmonary vascular resistance in a 12 week double-blind placebo-controlled study of 32 patients with this serious disorder for which previous therapies have been unsatisfactory*)

Heart Outcomes Prevention Evaluation Study Investigators 2000 Effects of an angiotensin-converting enzyme inhibitor, ramipril, on cardiovascular events in high-risk patients. N Engl J Med 342: 145–153 (*Ramipril significantly lowers rates of death, myocardial infarction and stroke in a wide range of high risk patients. See also accompanying editorial (pp. 201–222) entitled ACE inhibition in cardiovascular disease, by G S Francis: 'the results of the HOPE study make it clear that the benefits of ACE inhibitors…exceed our expectations…they have effects on vasculature, heart, and kidneys that go far beyond their rather small blood pressure lowering effects'*)

Hiatt W R 2001 Medical treatment of peripheral arterial disease and claudication. N Engl J Med 344: 1608–1621 (*Discusses risk factor modification, summarises evidence for efficacy of cilostazol and describes rationale for several investigational drugs, e.g. propionyl levocarnitine*)

Landry D W, Oliver J A 2001 Mechanisms of disease: the pathogenesis of vasodilatory shock. N Engl J Med 345: 588–595 (*Reviews mechanisms promoting inappropriate vasodilation in shock, including activation of ATP-sensitive potassium channels, increased synthesis of NO and depletion of antidiuretic hormone*)

Linz W, Scholkens B A 1992 A specific B_2-bradykinin receptor antagonist HOE140 abolishes the antihypertrophic effect of ramipril. Br J Pharmacol 105: 771–772 (*Some desirable effects of ACEI are mediated by bradykinin*)

Murphy M B, Murray C, Shorten G D 2001 Fenoldopam—a selective peripheral dopamine receptor agonist for treatment of severe hypertension. N Engl J Med 345: 1548–1557 (*Similar effectiveness as nitroprusside, but without thiocyanate toxicity or instability in light; however it is slower in onset and offset than nitroprusside*)

Maschio G for the Angiotensin-converting-enzyme Inhibition in Progressive Renal Failure Study Group 1996 Effect of the angiotensin-converting-enzyme inhibitor benazepril on the progression of chronic renal insufficiency. N Engl J Med 334: 939–945 (*ACE inhibition protected against progression of renal insufficiency in patients with various renal diseases*)

MERIT-HF Study Group 1999 Effect of metoprolol CR/XL in chronic heart failure: metoprolol CR/XL randomized intervention trial in congestive heart failure (MERIT-HF). Lancet 353: 2001–2007 (*Randomised trial in 3991 patients: addition of metoprolol to standard optimum treatment substantially improved survival. See also accompanying editorial entitled 'Benefit of β-blockers for heart failure: proven in 1999' by N Sharpe for references to other β-blocker/heart failure trials*)

Stasch J-P et al. 2001 NO-independent regulatory site on soluble guanylate cyclase. Nature 410: 212–415 (*An activator of this site (BAY41–2242) relaxes vascular smooth muscle, inhibits platelet aggregation and lowers blood pressure in the spontaneously hypertensive rat*)

Uehata M, Ishizaki T, Satoh H et al. 1997 Calcium sensitization of smooth muscle mediated by a Rho-associated protein kinase in hypertension. Nature 389: 990–994 (*A pyridine derivative, Y-27632, selectively inhibits smooth muscle contraction by inhibiting calcium sensitisation via the Rho-associated protein kinase pathway, and lowers blood pressure in several experimental models of hypertension*)

van Zwieten P A, Hamilton C A, Julius S, Prichard B N C (eds) 1996 I_1-imidazoline receptor agonist moxonidine: a new antihypertensive, 2nd edn. Royal Society of Medicine Press, London (*Monograph on this centrally acting antihypertensive drug*)

Weber M A 2001 Vasopeptidase inhibitors Lancet 358: 1525–1532 (*Reviews this new class of drug (e.g. omapatrilat) that inhibits both neutral endopeptidase and ACE; omapatrilat is more effective than other antihypertensive drugs and encouraging in heart failure. The frequency of angiooedema 'remains to be established' as do effects on clinical end-points*)

Zhao L, Mason N A, Morrell N W et al. 2001 Sildenafil inhibits hypoxia-induced pulmonary hypertension. Circulation 104: 424–428

19 Atherosclerosis and lipoprotein metabolism

Overview 306

Atherogenesis 306
Prevention of atheromatous disease 307

Lipoprotein transport in the blood 307
Dyslipidaemia 309

Lipid-lowering drugs 309

OVERVIEW

Atheromatous disease is ubiquitous and underlies the commonest causes of death (e.g. myocardial infarction) and disability (e.g. stroke) in industrial societies. Hypertension is one of the most important risk factors for atheromatous disease, and its treatment with drugs is discussed in Chapter 18. Here we consider other such factors, especially dyslipidaemia,* which, like hypertension, is amenable to drug therapy. We describe briefly the pathogenesis of atheroma and the processes of lipid transport that are the basis for understanding the actions of lipid-lowering drugs. These drugs are described, with emphasis on the statins, which can prevent arterial disease and prolong life.

ATHEROGENESIS

Atheroma is a *focal* disease of the intima of large and medium-sized arteries. Its pathogenesis evolves over many decades during most of which time the lesions are clinically silent, the occurrence of symptoms signalling advanced disease or supervening thrombosis. Until recently, there have been no good subprimate models, but transgenic animals deficient in specific enzymes and receptors that play key roles in lipoprotein metabolism (see Ch. 6) are rapidly transforming this scene. Nevertheless, most of our understanding of atherogenesis comes from human epidemiology and pathology, and from experimental studies in humans and other primates.

Epidemiological studies have identified numerous risk factors for atheromatous disease. Some of these cannot be altered (e.g. a family history of ischaemic heart disease) but others can (see Table 19.1) and are potential targets for therapeutic drugs. It is not known which of these epidemiological associations are causal, but evidence from intervention studies supports this view for some modifiable risk factors. For example, drugs that reduce low density lipoprotein (LDL) cholesterol concentration in clinical trials have reduced myocardial infarction and stroke. Many risk factors cause endothelial dysfunction, evidenced by reduced vasodilator responses to acetylcholine or to increased blood flow (so-called 'flow-mediated dilatation', a response that is inhibited by drugs that block nitric oxide (NO) synthesis; Ch. 14). Healthy endothelium produces NO and other mediators that protect against atheroma, so it is likely that the adverse effects on endothelium of many metabolic risk factors represent a common pathway by which they promote formation of atheromatous lesions. It is believed that atherogenesis involves several stages.

1. Endothelial dysfunction occurs with altered prostaglandin I_2 (PGI_2, prostacyclin; Ch. 15) and NO (Ch. 14) biosynthesis.

Table 19.1 Modifiable risk factors for atheromatous disease

Raised low density lipoprotein
Reduced high density lipoprotein
Hypertension (Ch. 18)
Diabetes mellitus (Ch. 25)
Cigarette smoking (Ch. 52)
Obesity (Ch. 26)
Physical inactivity
Raised C-reactive protein
Raised coagulation factors (e.g. factor VII, fibrinogen)
Raised homocysteine
Raised lipoprotein(a)

*The term dyslipidaemia is preferred to hyperlipoproteinaemia because *low* plasma concentrations of some lipids can be harmful.

2. Injury of dysfunctional endothelium encourages monocyte attachment. Turbulence may be responsible for the striking predilection of lesions for regions of disturbed flow such as the origin of vessels from the aorta. A possible role for chronic infection (e.g. with *Chlamydia*) has been mooted but is controversial.
3. Endothelial cells bind LDL. When activated (e.g. by injury), these cells and attached monocytes/macrophages generate free radicals that oxidise LDL, resulting in lipid peroxidation and destruction of the receptor needed for normal receptor-mediated clearance of LDL.
4. Oxidatively modified LDL is taken up by macrophages via 'scavenger receptors'.
5. Having taken up oxidised LDL, these macrophages (now foam cells) migrate subendothelially. Subendothelial collections of foam cells and T lymphocytes form the fatty streaks that presage atheroma.
6. Platelets, macrophages and endothelial cells release cytokines and growth factors. These cause proliferation of smooth muscle and deposition of connective tissue components. The inflammatory fibroproliferative response leads to a dense fibrous cap of connective tissue overlying a core of lipid and necrotic debris, this whole structure being referred to as an 'atheromatous plaque'.
7. The plaque can rupture, forming the substrate on which thromboses develop (see Ch. 20, Figs 20.1 and 20.10). Features that make a plaque liable to rupture include the presence of large numbers of macrophages, whereas vascular smooth muscle and matrix proteins stabilise it.

PREVENTION OF ATHEROMATOUS DISEASE

Several steps in the atherogenic process are potential targets for pharmacological attack. Angiotensin-converting enzyme inhibitors (Ch. 18) improve endothelial function, as do statins, and both these classes of drug prolong life in patients with atheromatous disease. Regular exercise increases high density lipoprotein (HDL) concentration and probably improves survival. Moderate alcohol consumption also increases HDL and there is epidemiological evidence in favour of such moderate consumption in older people.* Plasma homocysteine can be lowered by supplementing the diet with folic acid and it will be interesting to see whether countries such as the USA, which have introduced such supplements for other reasons (e.g. prevention of neural tube defects), experience a change in pattern of atheromatous disease. Antioxidants (e.g. vitamin C and vitamin E) are of interest, both because of evidence that they improve endothelial function in patients with increased oxidant stress and because of epidemiological evidence that a diet rich in antioxidants is associated with reduced risk of coronary artery disease. Results from clinical trials have been negative, however. Estrogen, used to prevent symptoms of the menopause (Ch. 29) and to prevent postmenopausal osteoporosis, has antioxidant properties and exerts other vascular effects that could be beneficial. Epidemiological evidence suggests that women who use such hormone replacement are at reduced risk of atheromatous disease, but a large controlled trial (called HERS) was negative. In contrast, drugs that lower plasma cholesterol are of proven benefit in preventing coronary artery disease. To understand how such drugs work, it is necessary to know how lipids are handled in the body.

*'Sinful, ginful, rum-soaked men, survive for three score years and ten' — or longer, we rather hope…

LIPOPROTEIN TRANSPORT IN THE BLOOD

Lipids and cholesterol are transported through the bloodstream as macromolecular complexes of lipid and protein known as lipoproteins. These consist of a central core of hydrophobic lipid (triglycerides or cholesteryl esters) encased in a more hydrophilic coat of polar substances—phospholipids, free cholesterol and associated apolipoproteins. There are four main classes of lipoprotein differing in the relative proportion of the core lipids and in the type of apoprotein. They also differ in size and density, and this latter property, as measured by ultracentrifugation, is the basis for their classification into:

- high density lipoproteins (HDL)
- low density lipoproteins (LDL)
- very low density lipoproteins (VLDL)
- chylomicrons.

Each of these lipoprotein classes has a specific role in lipid transport in the circulation, and there are different pathways for exogenous and for endogenous lipids. In the exogenous pathway (see Fig. 19.1), cholesterol and triglycerides absorbed from the gastrointestinal tract are transported in the lymph and then in the plasma as chylomicrons (diameter 100–1000 nm) to capillaries in muscle and adipose tissue. Here the core triglycerides are hydrolysed by lipoprotein lipase, and the tissues take up the resulting free fatty acids. The chylomicron remnants (diameter 30–50 nm), still containing their full complement of cholesteryl esters, pass to the liver, bind to receptors on hepatocytes and undergo endocytosis. Cholesterol is liberated within the liver cell and may be stored, oxidised to bile acids or secreted in the bile unaltered. Alternatively, it may enter the endogenous pathway of lipid transport in VLDL.

In the endogenous pathway, cholesterol and newly synthesised triglycerides are transported from the liver as VLDL (diameter 30–80 nm) to muscle and adipose tissue, where the triglycerides are hydrolysed and the resulting fatty acids enter the tissues as described above. During this process, the lipoprotein particles

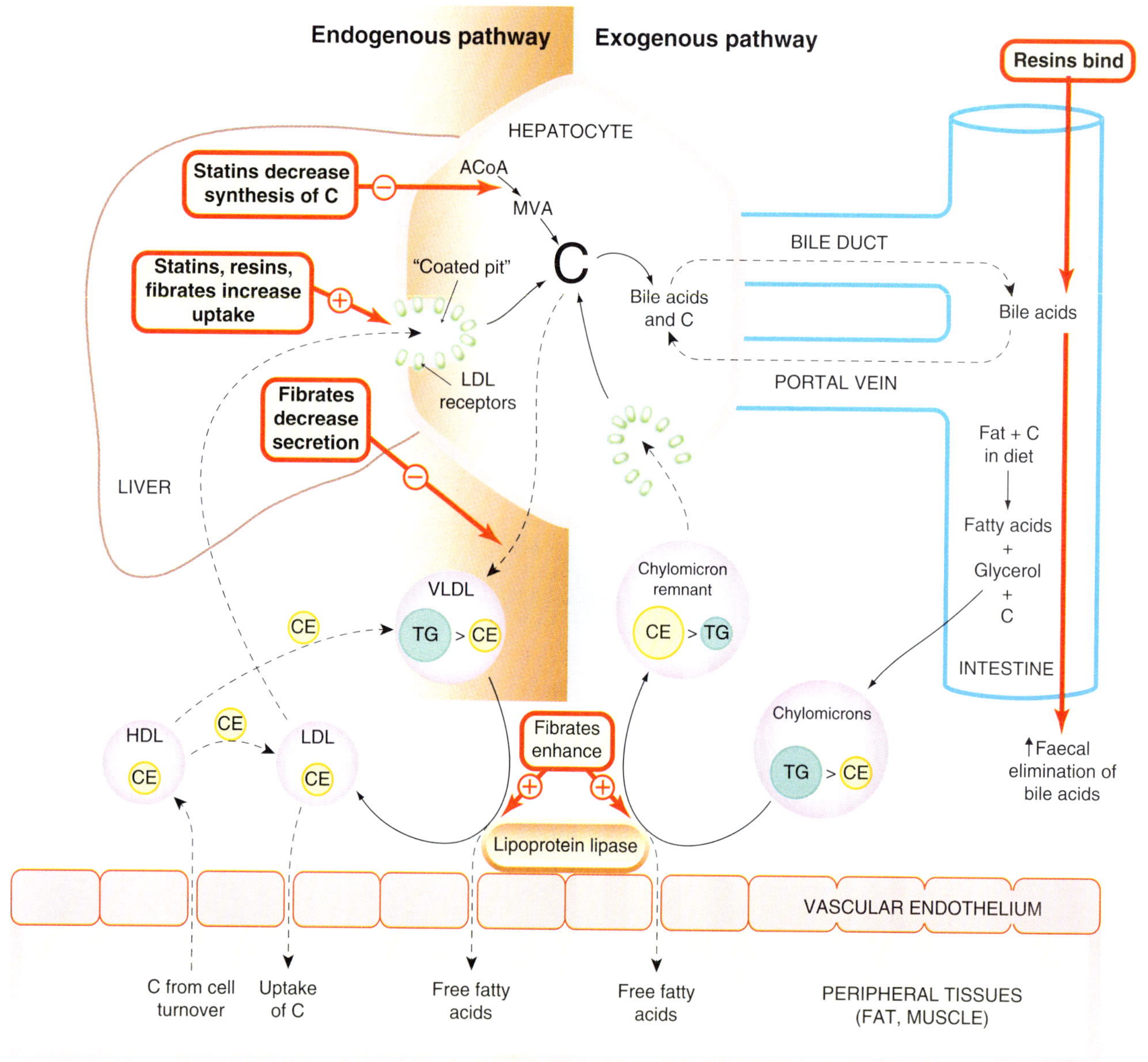

Fig. 19.1 Schematic diagram of cholesterol transport in the tissues, with sites of action of the main drugs affecting lipoprotein metabolism. (ACoA, acetyl-coenzyme A; C, cholesterol; CE, cholesteryl ester; TG, triglyceride; MVA, mevalonate; HMG-CoA reductase, 3-hydroxy-3-methylglutaryl-coenzyme A reductase; VLDL, very low density lipoprotein; LDL, low density lipoprotein; HDL, high density lipoprotein.)

become smaller (diameter 20–30 nm) but still have a full complement of cholesteryl esters and ultimately become LDL, which provides the source of cholesterol for incorporation into cell membranes and for synthesis of steroids (see Chs 27 and 29) and bile acids (Ch. 24). Cells take up LDL by endocytosis via LDL receptors that recognise LDL apolipoproteins. Some drugs (notably statins; see below) reduce the LDL concentration in the blood by stimulating the synthesis of these receptors in hepatocytes. Cholesterol can return to plasma from the tissues in HDL particles (diameter 7–20 nm). Cholesterol is esterified with long-chain fatty acids in HDL particles, and the resulting cholesteryl esters are subsequently transferred to VLDL or LDL particles by a transfer protein present in the plasma. One species of LDL, lipoprotein(a), which is associated with atherosclerosis (and is localised in atherosclerotic lesions), contains a unique apoprotein, apo(a) and is similar in structure to plasminogen. Hence lipoprotein(a) competes with and inhibits the binding of plasminogen to its receptors on the endothelial cell. Plasminogen is normally the substrate for plasminogen activator. Plasminogen activator is secreted by and bound to endothelial cells, generating the fibrinolytic enzyme plasmin (see Fig. 20.10). The effect of the binding of lipoprotein(a) is that less plasmin is generated, fibrinolysis is inhibited and thrombosis promoted. LDL can also activate platelets, constituting a further thrombogenic effect.

DYSLIPIDAEMIA

The normal range of plasma total cholesterol concentration varies in different populations (e.g. in the UK 25–30% of middle-aged people have serum cholesterol concentrations > 6.5 mmol/l in contrast to countries such as China). There are smooth gradations of increased risk with increased LDL cholesterol concentration and with reduced HDL cholesterol concentration. Dyslipidaemia may be primary or secondary. The primary forms are genetically determined. They are classified, according to which lipoprotein particle is raised, into six phenotypes (the Frederickson classification; Table 19.2). This has prognostic and therapeutic implications but is not a diagnostic classification. An especially great risk of ischaemic heart disease occurs in a subset of primary type IIa hyperlipoproteinaemia caused by a monogenic defect of LDL receptors; this is known as familial hypercholesterolaemia and in affected individuals, the serum cholesterol concentration in adults is typically 9–11 mmol/l in heterozygotes. Study of this disorder enabled Brown & Goldstein (1986) to define the LDL-receptor pathway of cholesterol homeostasis.

Secondary forms of dyslipidaemia are a consequence of other conditions such as diabetes mellitus, alcoholism, nephrotic syndrome, chronic renal failure, hypothyroidism, liver disease and administration of drugs, for example **isotretinoin** (an isomer of vitamin A given by mouth as well as topically in the treatment of severe acne) and protease inhibitors used to treat infection with human immunodeficiency virus (Ch. 46).

Lipoprotein metabolism and dyslipidaemia

- Lipids, including cholesterol (C) and triglycerides (TG), are transported in the plasma as lipoproteins, of which there are four classes:
  - —chylomicrons transport TG and C from the gastrointestinal tract to the tissues, where they are split by lipoprotein lipase, releasing free fatty acids (FFA). These are taken up in muscle and adipose tissue. Chylomicron remnants are taken up in the liver, where C is stored, oxidised to bile acids, or released into
  - —very low density lipoproteins (VLDL), which transport C and newly synthesised TG to the tissues, where TGs are removed as before, leaving:
  - —low density lipoproteins (LDL) with a large component of C, some of which is taken up by the tissues and some by the liver, by endocytosis via specific LDL receptors
  - —high density lipoproteins (HDL), which adsorb cholesterol derived from cell breakdown in tissues (including arteries) and transfer it to VLDL and LDL.
- Dyslipidaemias can be primary, or secondary to some generalised disease (e.g. hypothyroidism). They are classified according to which lipoprotein particle is raised, into six phenotypes (the Frederickson classification). The higher the plasma concentration of LDL-cholesterol, and the lower the concentration of HDL-cholesterol, the higher the risk of ischaemic heart disease.

LIPID-LOWERING DRUGS

Several drugs are used to decrease plasma LDL-cholesterol. Drug therapy to lower plasma lipids is only one approach to treatment and is used in addition to dietary management and correction of other modifiable cardiovascular risk factors. The selection of patients to be treated with drugs remains controversial, not least for reasons of cost: the benefit is greatest for those who are at

Table 19.2 Frederickson/WHO classification of hyperlipoproteinaemia

Type	Lipoprotein elevated	Cholesterol	Triglycerides	Atherosclerosis risk	Drug treatment
I	Chylomicrons	+	+++	NE	None
IIa	LDL	++	NE	High	HMG-CoA reductase ± resins
IIb	LDL + VLDL	++	++	High	Fibrates, HMG-CoA reductase inhibitor, nicotinic acid
III	βVLDL	++	++	Moderate	Fibrates
IV	VLDL	+	++	Moderate	Fibrates
V	Chylomicrons + VLDL	+	++	NE	None

HMG-CoA, 3-hydroxy-3-methylglutaryl-coenzyme A; LDL, low density lipoprotein; VLDL, very low density lipoprotein; βVDL, a qualitatively abnormal form of VLDL identified by its pattern on electrophoresis; +, increased concentration; NE, not elevated.

greatest risk, including those with symptomatic atherosclerotic disease and with many cardiovascular risk factors, as well as those with the highest plasma concentrations of cholesterol.

The main classes of drug used clinically are:

- statins: HMG-CoA (3-hydroxy-3-methylglutaryl-coenzyme A) reductase inhibitors
- fibrates
- bile acid-binding resins.

Other drugs include **nicotinic acid** (or one of its derivatives) and **probucol**. Fish oil can lower plasma triglyceride concentration but can increase plasma cholesterol.

STATINS: HMG-CoA REDUCTASE INHIBITORS

The rate-limiting enzyme in cholesterol synthesis is HMG-CoA reductase, which catalyses the conversion of HMG-CoA to mevalonic acid (see Fig. 19.1). **Simvastatin**, **lovostatin** and **pravastatin** are specific, reversible, competitive inhibitors with K_i values of approximately 1 nmol/l. The resulting decrease in hepatic cholesterol synthesis leads to *increased synthesis of LDL receptors* and increased clearance of LDL. The main biochemical effect of statins is, therefore, to reduce plasma LDL-cholesterol concentration. Statins also reduce plasma triglyceride and increase HDL-cholesterol. **Atorvastatin** causes long-lasting inhibition of HMG-CoA reductase. Its effect on coronary events and survival has not been reported. Several large randomised placebo-controlled clinical trials to determine the effects of HMG-CoA reductase inhibitors on morbidity and mortality have been positive.

The Scandinavian Simvastatin Survival Study (4S) This study involved 4444 patients with ischaemic heart disease and whose plasma cholesterol was 5.5–8.0 mmol/l; serum LDL-cholesterol was lowered by simvastatin by 35% (Fig. 19.2). Treatment continued for a median 5.4 years and produced a 30% reduction in risk of death, accounted for by a 42% reduction in death from coronary disease.

The West of Scotland Coronary Prevention Study (WOSCOPS) This study randomised over 6500 45- to 64-year-old healthy men to placebo or pravastatin; the statin reduced LDL-cholesterol by 26%, overall mortality by 22% and the risk of heart attack or death from coronary disease by 31%.

The Cholesterol and Recurrent Events ('CARE') Trial Over 4000 patients who had recovered from myocardial infarction and in whom plasma cholesterol concentration was less than 6.2 mmol/l were allocated to treatment with placebo or pravastatin. Pravastatin lowered LDL-cholesterol by 28%, the risk of either death from coronary disease or recurrent myocardial infarction by 24%, and the risk of stroke by 31%.

The Heart Protection Study This study showed that simvastatin (40 mg daily) improved outcome in a broadly defined high-risk population, including people with normal/low plasma LDL cholesterol, and that simvastatin was extremely safe.

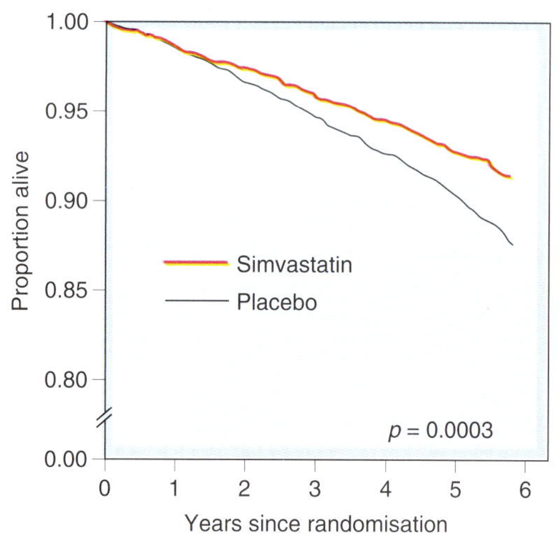

Fig. 19.2 Survival in patients with coronary heart disease and serum cholesterol 5.5–8.0 mmol/l treated either with placebo or with simvastatin. The relative risk of death in the simvastatin group was 0.70 (95% confidence intervals 0.58–0.85). (Based on: 4S study 1994 Lancet 344: 1383–1389.)

Other actions of statins

Products of the mevalonate pathway are involved in prenylation or farnesylation of the amino acid chain of several important membrane-bound enzymes (e.g. endothelial NO synthase; see Ch. 14). These fatty groups then serve as anchors, localising the enzyme in the membrane of intracellular organelles such as caveoli or the Golgi apparatus. Consequently, there is currently great interest in actions of statins that are unrelated, or indirectly related, to their main effect of lowering LDL. Some of these actions are undesirable (for example, HMG-CoA reductase guides migrating primordial germ cells, and statin use is contraindicated during pregnancy), but many offer therapeutic promise. Such actions include:

- improved endothelial function
- reduced vascular inflammation
- reduced platelet aggregability
- increased neovascularisation of ischaemic tissue
- increased circulating endothelial progenitor cells
- stabilisation of atherosclerotic plaque
- antithrombotic actions
- enhanced fibrinolysis
- osteoclast apoptosis and increased synthetic activity in osteoblasts
- inhibition of germ cell migration during development
- immune suppression.

The extent to which these effects contribute to the anti-atheromatous actions of statins, and whether any of them will lead to effective new therapies, are still unknown but it is a promising area.

Clinical uses of HMG-CoA reductase inhibitors ('statins', e.g. simvastatin, pravastatin)

- Secondary prevention of myocardial infarction and stroke in patients who have symptomatic atherosclerotic disease (e.g. angina, transient ischaemic attacks, following acute myocardial infarction or stroke).
- Primary prevention of arterial disease in patients who are at high risk because of elevated serum cholesterol concentration, especially if there are other risk factors for atherosclerosis. Tables (available for example in the British National Formulary) are used to target treatment to those at greatest risk.
- **Atorvastatin** lowers serum cholesterol in patients with homozygous familial hypercholesterolaemia.
- In severe drug-resistant dyslipidaemia (e.g. heterozygous familial hypercholesterolaemia), a bile acid-binding resin is added to treatment with a statin.

Pharmacokinetics

HMG-CoA reductase inhibitors are given by mouth last thing before going to bed at night. They are well absorbed and extracted by the liver, their site of action, and are subject to extensive presystemic metabolism. Simvastatin is an inactive lactone pro-drug; it is metabolised in the liver to its active form, the corresponding β-hydroxy fatty acid.

Adverse effects

HMG-CoA reductase inhibitors are well tolerated: mild unwanted effects include gastrointestinal disturbance, increased plasma concentrations of liver enzymes, insomnia and rash. More serious adverse effects are rare but include severe myositis ('rhabdomyolysis') and angio-oedema.

Clinical uses

See the clinical box on this page.

FIBRATES

Several fibric acid derivatives ('fibrates') are available including **bezafibrate**, **ciprofibrate**, **gemfibrozil**, **fenofibrate** and **clofibrate**. These cause a marked reduction in circulating VLDL, and hence triglyceride, with a modest (approximately 10%) reduction in LDL and an approximately 10% increase in HDL. In one study, gemfibrozil reduced coronary heart disease by approximately one third compared with placebo in middle-aged men with primary hyperlipoproteinaemia. An important recent development has been an HDL intervention trial performed by the US Veterans Affairs Department (VA-HIT) in some 2500 men with coronary heart disease and low HDL together with *low* LDL. This showed that increasing HDL with gemfibrozil reduced subsequent coronary disease and stroke over a median follow-up period of approximately 5 years. Event rates were linked to changes in HDL but not to triglycerides or to LDL, suggesting that increasing HDL with a fibrate reduces vascular risk.

The mechanism of action of fibrates (see Fig. 19.1) is complex. They are agonists at peroxisome proliferator-activated receptor α (PPARα), a receptor that belongs to the superfamily of nuclear receptors (Ch. 3); it stimulates the β-oxidative degradation of fatty acids. Fibrates stimulate lipoprotein lipase, hence increasing hydrolysis of triglyceride in chylomicrons and VLDL particles, and liberate free fatty acid for storage in fat or for metabolism in striated muscle. They also probably reduce hepatic VLDL production and increase hepatic LDL uptake. In addition to these effects on lipoproteins, fibrates reduce plasma fibrinogen, improve glucose tolerance and inhibit vascular smooth muscle inflammation by inhibiting the expression of the transcription factor NF-κB. As with the non-LDL-lowering effects of statins, there is great interest in these actions although it is not yet known if they are clinically important.

Adverse effects

Myositis is unusual but can be severe (rhabdomyolysis), leading to myoglobinuria and acute renal failure. It occurs particularly in patients with renal impairment, because of reduced protein binding and impaired elimination of the drug. Fibrates should be avoided in such patients and also in alcoholics, who are predisposed to hypertriglyceridaemia and are at risk of rhabdomyolysis.* Myositis can also be caused (rarely) by statins (see above) and the combined use of fibrates with this class of drugs is, therefore, generally inadvisable. Fibrates can cause a variety of mild gastrointestinal symptoms. Clofibrate predisposes to gallstones and its use is, therefore, limited to patients who have had a cholecystectomy.

Clinical uses of fibrates (e.g. gemfibrozil, fenofibrate)

- Mixed dyslipidaemia (i.e. raised serum triglyceride as well as cholesterol), provided this is not caused by excessive alcohol consumption. **Fenofibrate** is *uricosuric*, which may be useful where hyperuricaemia coexists with mixed dyslipidaemia.
- Patients with low HDL and high risk of atheromatous disease (often type 2 diabetic patients, see Ch. 25).
- Combined with other lipid-lowering drugs in patients with severe treatment-resistant dyslipidaemia. This may, however, increase the risk of rhabdomyolysis. (**Cerivastatin** was withdrawn because of this adverse event when it was coadminstered with **gemfibrozil**.)

*For several reasons, including a tendency to lie immobile for prolonged periods followed by generalised convulsions—'rum fits'—and *delirium tremens*.

Clinical use

See the clinical box.

BILE ACID BINDING RESINS

Colestyramine and **colestipol** are anion exchange resins. When taken by mouth, they sequester bile acids in the intestine and prevent their reabsorption and enterohepatic recirculation (Fig. 19.1). The result is decreased absorption of exogenous cholesterol and increased metabolism of endogenous cholesterol into bile acids in the liver. This leads to increased expression of LDL receptors on liver cells, and hence to increased removal of LDL from the blood and a reduced concentration of LDL-cholesterol in plasma. The concentration of HDL-cholesterol is unchanged and there may be an unwanted increase in triglycerides. The American Lipid Research Clinics' trial of middle-aged men with primary hypercholesterolaemia showed that addition of a resin to dietary treatment caused a mean 13% fall in plasma cholesterol and a 20–25% fall in coronary heart disease over 7 years.

Unwanted effects

Since resins are not absorbed, systemic toxicity is low, but gastrointestinal symptoms of nausea, abdominal bloating, constipation or diarrhoea are common and dose related. Resins are bulky and unappetising. This can be minimised by suspending them in fruit juice, but even so they remain very inconvenient in comparison to statins or fibrates and their use has declined relative to these agents in consequence. They interfere with the absorption of fat-soluble vitamins, and of drugs such as **chlorothiazide**, **digoxin** and **warfarin**, which should, therefore, be taken at least 1 hour before or 4–6 hours after the resin.

Clinical use

See the clinical box below.

OTHER LIPID-LOWERING DRUGS

Nicotinic acid

Nicotinic acid is a vitamin that has been used in gram quantities as a lipid-lowering agent. **Acipimox** is a derivative of nicotinic acid that is used in lower dose and may have less marked adverse effects, although it is unclear whether the recommended dose is as effective as are standard doses of nicotinic acid. These drugs inhibit hepatic triglyceride production and VLDL secretion (see Fig. 19.1), which leads indirectly to a modest reduction in LDL and increase in HDL. Long-term administration is associated with reduced mortality, but unwanted effects limit their clinical use. Adverse effects include flushing, palpitations and gastrointestinal disturbances. Flushing is associated with production of prostaglandin D_2 (Ch. 15) and is reduced by taking the dose 30 minutes after **aspirin**. High doses can cause disorders of liver function, impair glucose tolerance and precipitate gout.

> **Clinical uses of bile acid-binding resins (e.g. colestyramine)**
>
> - As an addition to a statin when response has been inadequate, e.g. in patients with heterozygous familial hypercholesterolaemia.
> - For hypercholesterolaemia when a statin is contraindicated.
> - Uses unrelated to atherosclerosis, including
>   —pruritus in patients with partial biliary obstruction
>   —bile acid diarrhoea (e.g. caused by diabetic neuropathy).

> **Drugs in dyslipidaemia**
>
> The main drugs used in patients with dsylipidaemias are:
> - HMG-CoA reductase inhibitors (statins, e.g. simvastatin): inhibit de novo synthesis of cholesterol in the liver. This increases expression of LDL receptors on hepatocytes, increasing LDL uptake from plasma and markedly lowering circulating LDL and total cholesterol.
> - Fibrates (e.g. gemfibrozil): activate PPARα receptors, decrease VLDL production, increase activity of lipoprotein lipase, increasing breakdown of chylomicra and VLDL in muscle and adipose tissue, and enhance clearance of LDL by the liver. They markedly lower serum triglycerides, and increase HDL.
> - Bile acid-binding resins (e.g. colestyramine): sequester bile acids in the intestine. This reduces the absorption of exogenous cholesterol and increases the metabolism of endogenous cholesterol into bile acids. Resins modestly lower serum cholesterol but increase triglyceride.

Probucol

Probucol lowers the concentration in the plasma of both LDL and HDL. Its place in therapy has not been defined—it has distinctive properties that could be either desirable (e.g. antioxidant properties) or the reverse (e.g. lowering HDL and prolonging the cardiac action potential). A large clinical trial of its quantitative effects on atheroma in the femoral arteries (trial known as PQRST) did not show any significant improvement in vessel narrowing. Its mechanism of action is not understood. Probucol has unusual pharmacokinetic properties: it is markedly lipophilic, and most of the circulating drug is associated with LDL. It remains in body fat for several months after chronic administration is discontinued. Its peak effect on plasma cholesterol occurs only after 1–3 months of administration. Gastrointestinal disturbances occur in 10% of patients. Probucol should be avoided in patients with a long Q–T interval on the electrocardiogram (see Ch. 17). It is best to avoid drugs that influence cardiac repolarisation, such as **amiodarone**, **sotalol** and **flecainide**, in patients who have received probucol within the past few months to avoid precipitating a form of ventricular tachycardia known as torsades de pointes (p. 275).

Fish oil

The omega-3 marine triglycerides reduce plasma triglyceride concentrations but increase cholesterol. Plasma triglyceride concentrations are less strongly associated with coronary artery disease than is cholesterol, and an effect of fish oil on cardiac morbidity or mortality is unproven, although there is epidemiological evidence that eating fish regularly does reduce ischaemic heart disease. The mechanism of action of fish oil on plasma triglyceride concentrations is unknown. Fish oil is rich in highly unsaturated fatty acids including eicosapentaenoic and docosahexaenoic acids, and it has other potentially important effects including inhibition of platelet function, prolongation of bleeding time, anti-inflammatory effects and reduction of plasma fibrinogen. Eicosapentaenoic acid substitutes for arachidonic acid in cell membranes and gives rise to 3-series prostaglandins and thromboxanes (that is, prostanoids with three double bonds in their side-chains rather than the usual two), and 5-series leukotrienes. This probably accounts for their effects on haemostasis, since thromboxane A_3 is much less active as a platelet-aggregating agent than is thromboxane A_2, whereas prostaglandin I_3 is similar in potency to PGI_2 as an inhibitor of platelet function. The alteration in leukotriene biosynthesis probably underlies the anti-inflammatory effects of fish oil. Fish oil is contraindicated in patients with type IIa hyperlipoproteinaemia because of the increase in LDL-cholesterol that it causes.

REFERENCES AND FURTHER READING

Brown M S, Goldstein J L 1986 A receptor-mediated pathway for cholesterol homeostasis. Science 232: 34–47 (*Classic from these Nobel Prize winners: see also Goldstein J L, Brown M S 1990 Regulation of the mevalonate pathway. Nature 343: 425–430*)

Davies M J, Woolf N 1993 Atherosclerosis: what is it and why does it occur? Br Heart J 69: S3–S11 (*Review of pathology/pathogenesis*)

Durrington P N 1989 Hyperlipidaemia: diagnosis and management. Wright, London (*Extremely readable, authoritative book; for a more recent review of lipid and lipoprotein disorders by the same author see Weatherall D J, Ledingham G G, Warrel D A (eds) 1996 Oxford textbook of medicine, 3rd edn. Oxford University Press, Oxford, vol. 2, pp. 1399–1415*)

Gupta G, Leatham E W, Carrington D, Mendall M A, Kaski J C, Camm A J 1997 Elevated *Chlamydia pneumoniae* antibodies, cardiovascular events, and azithromycin in male survivors of myocardial infarction. Circulation 96: 404–407 (*Controversial study showing that a short course of azithromycin may lower risk of recurrent myocardial infarction*)

McCully K S 1996 Homocysteine and vascular disease. Nat Med 2: 386–389 (*Discusses therapeutic promise of increased dietary folate and vitamin B_6*)

Miles L A, Fless G M, Levin E G, Scann A M, Plow E F 1989 A potential basis for the thrombotic risks associated with lipoprotein(a). Nature 339: 301–303 (*See also comment: Scott J 1989 Thrombogenesis linked to atherogenesis at last? Nature 341: 22–33*)

Nathan L, Chaudhuri G 1997 Estrogens and atherosclerosis. Annu Rev Pharmacol Toxicol 37: 477–515 (*Actions include effects on endothelium and vascular smooth muscle*)

Ramsay L E, Haq I U, Jackson P R, Yeo W W, Pickin D M, Payne J N 1996 Targeting lipid-lowering drug therapy for primary prevention of coronary disease: an updated Sheffield table. Lancet 348: 387–388 (*Tables based on targeting treatment to individuals with a coronary heart disease event rate of 3% per year or greater*)

Reid I R et al. 2001 Effect of pravastatin on the frequency of fracture in the LIPID study. Lancet 357: 509–512 (*No support for the hypothesis that statins reduce fracture risk. Clinical trials aimed primarily at osteoporosis in at-risk subjects and using more sensitive measures of bone density are awaited*)

Ridker P M for the Air Force/Texas Coronary Atherosclerosis Prevention Study Investigators 2001 Measurement of C-reactive protein for the targeting of statin therapy in the primary prevention of acute events. N Engl J Med 344: 1959–1965 (*Statins may be effective in preventing coronary events in people with unremarkable serum lipid concentrations but with elevated C-reactive protein, a marker of inflammation and risk factor for coronary disease. See also accompanying editorial: Munford R S, Statins and the acute phase response, pp. 2016–2018*)

Ross R 1993 The pathogenesis of atherosclerosis: a perspective for the 1990s. Nature 362: 801–809 (*Profoundly influential review*)

Rubins H B et al. 2001 Reduction in stroke with gemfibrozil in men with coronary heart disease and low HDL cholesterol. The Veterans Affairs HDL Intervention Trial (VA-HIT). Circulation 103: 2828–2833 (*Evidence that increasing HDL reduces stroke*)

Staels R et al. 1998 Activation of human aortic smooth-muscle cells is inhibited by PPARα but not by PPARγ activators. Nature 293: 790–793 (*PPARα in the vascular wall is activated by fibrates and may influence atherosclerosis and restenosis*)

Steinberg D, Parthasarathy S, Carew T E, Khoo J C, Witztum J L 1989 Beyond cholesterol: modifications of low-density lipoprotein that increase its atherogenicity. N Engl J Med 320: 915–924 (*The oxidised LDL hypothesis*)

Treasure C B et al. 1995 Beneficial effects of cholesterol-lowering therapy on the coronary endothelium in patients with coronary artery disease N Engl J Med 332: 481–487 (*See also accompanying review discussing studies of plaque rupture and endothelial function: Levine G N, Keaney J F, Vita J A N, pp. 512–519*)

Undas A, Brummel K E, Musial J, Mann K G, Szczeklik A 2001 Simvastatin depresses blood clotting by activation of prothrombin, factor V, and factor XIII and by enhancing factor Va inactivation. Circulation 103: 2248–2253 (*Simvastatin effects on blood clotting independent of cholesterol reduction*)

van Doren M, Broihier H T, Moore L A, Lehman R 1998 HMG-CoA reductase guides migrating primordial germ cells Nature 396: 466–469 (*Regulated expression of HMG-CoA reductase provides spatial guide to migrating primordial germ cells*)

Vasa M et al. 2001 Increase in circulating endothelial progenitor cells by statin therapy in patients with stable coronary artery disease. Circulation 103: 2885–2890 (*May participate in repair after ischaemic injury*)

Walldius G, Erikson U, Olsson A G et al. 1994 The effect of probucol on femoral atherosclerosis: the Probucol Quantitative Regression Swedish Trial. Am J Cardiol 74: 875–883 (*Failed to detect a beneficial effect of this antioxidant lipid-lowering drug. The acronym PQRST brings to mind the electrocardiogram: perhaps a salutary reminder in view of the prodysrhythmic effect of probucol!*)

20 Haemostasis and thrombosis

Overview 314

Introduction 314

Blood coagulation 315
— Coagulation cascade 315
— Vascular endothelium in haemostasis and thrombosis 317

Drugs that act on the coagulation cascade 317
— Coagulation defects 318
— Thrombosis 319

Platelet adhesion and activation 323
— Antiplatelet drugs 323

Fibrinolysis (thrombolysis) 327
— Fibrinolytic drugs 328
— Antifibrinolytic and haemostatic drugs 328

OVERVIEW

This chapter summarises the main features of blood coagulation, platelet function and fibrinolysis. These are the processes that underlie haemostasis and thrombosis and which, when deranged, cause haemorrhagic or thrombotic diseases. This account forms the basis for understanding drugs that act on the coagulation cascade, on platelets and on fibrinolysis. Anticoagulants, antiplatelet drugs and fibrinolytic drugs are especially important clinically because of the prevalence of thrombotic disease and are emphasised for this reason.

INTRODUCTION

Haemostasis is the arrest of blood loss from damaged blood vessels and is essential to life. A wound causes vasoconstriction, accompanied by:

- adhesion and activation of platelets
- fibrin formation.

Platelet activation leads to the formation of a haemostatic plug, which stops the bleeding and is subsequently reinforced by fibrin. The relative importance of each process depends on the type of vessel (arterial, venous or capillary) that has been injured.

Thrombosis is the pathological formation of a 'haemostatic' plug within the vasculature in the absence of bleeding. Over a century ago, Rudolph Virchow defined three predisposing factors still known as Virchow's triad. This comprises: *injury to the vessel wall*—for example when an atheromatous plaque ruptures or becomes eroded; *altered blood flow*—for example in the left atrial appendage of the heart during atrial fibrillation or in the veins of the legs while sitting cramped up on a long journey; and *abnormal coagulability of the blood*—as occurs, for example, in the later stages of pregnancy or during treatment with certain oral contraceptives (see Ch. 29). Increased coagulability of the blood can be inherited and is referred to as thrombophilia. A *thrombus*, which forms in vivo, should be distinguished from a *clot*, which forms in static blood in vitro. Clots are amorphous, consisting of a diffuse fibrin meshwork in which red and white blood cells are trapped indiscriminately. By contrast, arterial and venous thrombi each have a distinct structure.

An *arterial thrombus* (see Fig. 20.1) is composed of so-called 'white thrombus' consisting mainly of platelets and leucocytes in

Haemostasis and thrombosis

- Haemostasis is the arrest of blood loss from damaged vessels and is essential to life. The main phenomena are:
  —platelet adhesion and activation
  —blood coagulation (fibrin formation).
- Thrombosis is a pathological condition resulting from inappropriate activation of haemostatic mechanisms:
  —venous thrombosis is usually associated with stasis of blood; a venous thrombus has a small platelet component and a large component of fibrin
  —arterial thrombosis is usually associated with atherosclerosis, and the thrombus has a large platelet component.
- A portion of a thrombus may break away, travel as an embolus and lodge downstream, causing ischaemia and infarction.

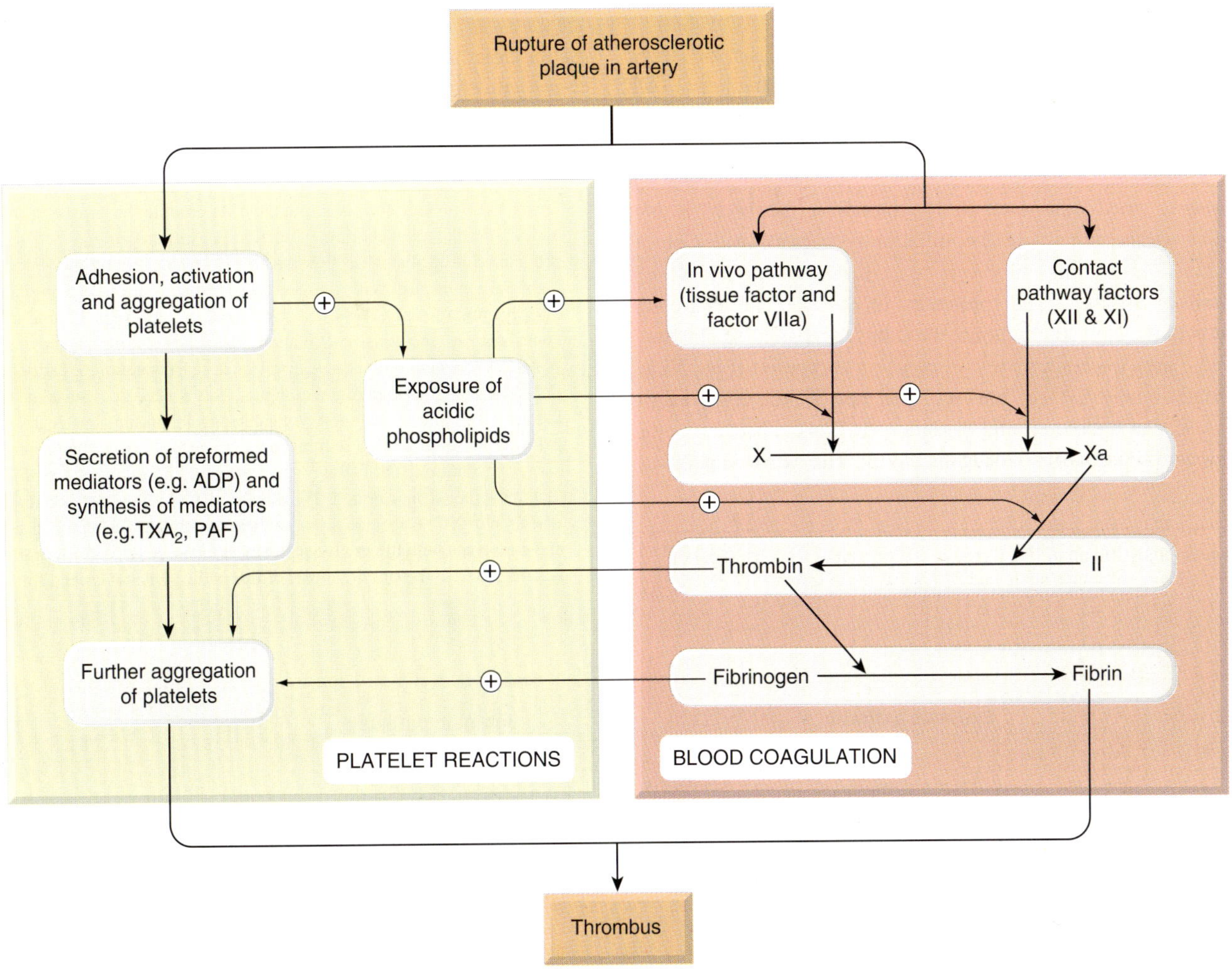

Fig. 20.1 The main events in the formation of an arterial thrombus. Exposure of acidic phospholipids during platelet activation provides a surface on which factors IXa and VIIa interact with factor X; factor Xa then interacts with factor II, as illustrated in more detail in Figure 20.4. Activation of factor XII also initiates the fibrinolytic pathway, which is shown in Figure 20.10. (A similar series of events occurs when there is vascular damage, leading to haemostasis.) (TXA_2, thromboxane A_2; PAF, platelet activating factor.)

a fibrin mesh. It is usually associated with *atherosclerosis*. It interrupts blood flow, causing ischaemia or death (infarction) of the tissue beyond. *Venous thrombus* is composed of 'red thrombus' and consists of a small white head and a large jelly-like red tail, similar in composition to a blood clot, which streams away in the flow. Thrombus can break away, forming an *embolus*; this may lodge in the lungs or, if it comes from the left heart or a carotid artery, in the brain or other organs, causing death or other disaster.

Drug therapy to promote haemostasis is rarely necessary, being required only when this essential process is defective (e.g. coagulation factors in haemophilia or following excessive anticoagulant therapy) or when it proves difficult to staunch haemorrhage following surgery or for menorrhagia (e.g. antifibrinolytic and haemostatic drugs; see below). Drug therapy to treat or prevent thrombosis or thromboembolism, by comparison, is extensively used because such diseases are common as well as serious. Drugs affect haemostasis and thrombosis in three distinct ways, by affecting:

- blood coagulation (fibrin formation)
- platelet function
- fibrin removal (fibrinolysis).

BLOOD COAGULATION

COAGULATION CASCADE

Blood coagulation means the conversion of fluid blood to a solid gel or clot. The main event is the conversion by thrombin of soluble fibrinogen to insoluble strands of fibrin, the last step in a complex enzyme cascade. The components (called factors) are present in blood as inactive precursors (zymogens) of proteolytic enzymes and cofactors. They are activated by proteolysis, the active forms being designated by the suffix 'a'. Factors XIIa, XIa, Xa, IXa and thrombin (IIa) are all serine proteases. Activation of a small amount of one factor catalyses the formation of larger amounts of the next factor, which catalyses the formation of still larger amounts of the next, and so on; consequently, the cascade provides a mechanism of amplification.* As might be expected, this accelerating enzyme cascade has to be controlled by inhibitors, since otherwise all the blood in the body would solidify within minutes of the initiation of haemostasis. One of the most important inhibitors is *antithrombin III*, which neutralises all the serine proteases in the cascade. Vascular endothelium also actively limits thrombus extension (see below).

There are two main pathways of fibrin formation (Fig. 20.2), one traditionally termed 'intrinsic' (because all the components are present in the blood) and the other 'extrinsic' (because some components come from outside the blood). The extrinsic pathway is especially important in controlling blood coagulation and can accurately be called the in vivo pathway. The intrinsic pathway (better called the contact pathway) is activated when shed blood comes into contact with an artificial surface such as glass.

▼ The in vivo (extrinsic) pathway is initiated by 'tissue factor'. This is the cellular receptor for factor VII, which, in the presence of Ca^{2+}, undergoes an active site transition. This results in rapid autocatalytic activation of factor VII to VIIa. The tissue factor–VIIa complex activates factors IX and X. Acidic phospholipids function as *surface catalysts*. They are provided during platelet activation, which exposes acidic phospholipids (especially phosphatidylserine) and these activate various clotting factors, closely juxtaposing them in functional complexes. Platelets also contribute by secreting coagulation factors, including factor Va and fibrinogen. Coagulation is sustained by further generation of factor Xa by IXa–VIIIa–Ca^{2+}–phospholipid complex. This is needed because the tissue factor–VIIa complex is rapidly inactivated in plasma by tissue factor pathway inhibitor and by antithrombin III. Factor Xa, in the presence of Ca^{2+}, phospholipid and factor Va, activates prothrombin to *thrombin*, the main enzyme of the cascade. The *contact* (intrinsic) pathway commences when factor XII (Hageman factor) adheres to a negatively charged surface and converges with the in vivo pathway at the stage of factor X activation (see Fig. 20.2). The proximal part of this pathway is not crucial for blood

*Coagulation of 100 ml of blood requires 0.2 mg of factor VIII, 2 mg of factor X, 15 mg of prothrombin and 250 mg of fibrinogen.

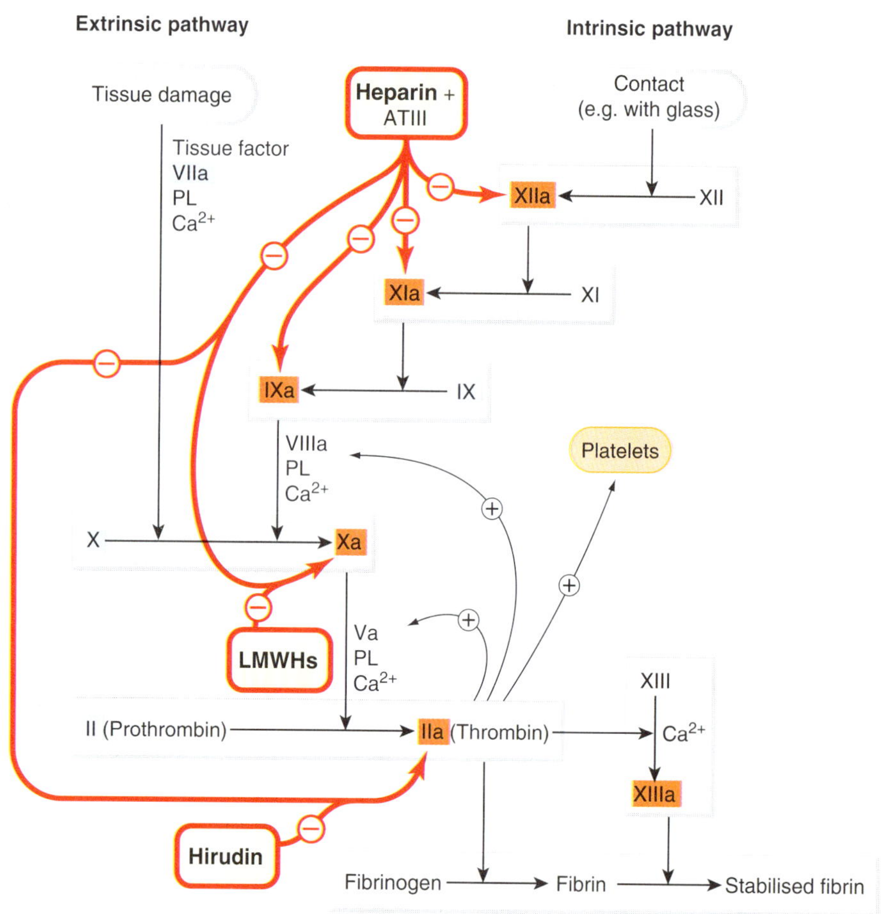

Fig. 20.2 The coagulation cascade: sites of action of anticoagulant drugs. Oral anticoagulants interfere with post-translational γ-carboxylation of factors II, VII, IX and X (shown in blue boxes), see Figure 20.4. Heparins activate antithrombin III. (PL, negatively charged phospholipid supplied by activated platelets; ATIII, antithrombin III; LMWHs, low-molecular-weight heparins.)

coagulation in vivo. The two pathways are not entirely separate even before they converge, and various positive feedbacks promote coagulation.

The role of thrombin

Thrombin (factor IIa) cleaves fibrinogen, producing fragments that polymerise to form fibrin. It also activates factor XIII, a fibrinoligase, which strengthens fibrin-to-fibrin links, thereby stabilising the coagulum. In addition to coagulation, thrombin also causes platelet aggregation, stimulates cell proliferation and modulates smooth muscle contraction. Paradoxically, it can inhibit as well as promote coagulation (see below). Effects of thrombin on platelets and smooth muscle are initiated by interaction with specific protease-activated receptors (PAR), which belong to the superfamily of G-protein-coupled receptors. PAR initiate cellular responses that contribute not only to haemostasis and thrombosis but also to inflammation and perhaps angiogenesis. The signal transduction mechanism is unusual: receptor activation requires proteolysis by thrombin of the extracellular N-terminal domain of the receptor, revealing a new N-terminal sequence that acts as a 'tethered agonist' (see Fig. 3.7, p. 34).

VASCULAR ENDOTHELIUM IN HAEMOSTASIS AND THROMBOSIS

Vascular endothelium, the container of the circulating blood, can change from a non-thrombogenic to a thrombogenic structure in response to different demands. Normally, it provides a non-thrombogenic surface by virtue of surface *heparan sulfate*, a glycosaminoglycan related to **heparin**, which is, like heparin, a cofactor for antithrombin III. Endothelium thus plays an essential role in preventing intravascular platelet activation and coagulation. However, it also plays an active part in haemostasis, synthesising and storing several key haemostatic components: von Willebrand factor,* tissue factor and plasminogen activator inhibitor 1 (PAI-1) are particularly important. PAI-1 is secreted in response to *angiotensin IV*, receptors which are present on endothelial cells, providing a link between the renin–angiotensin system and thrombosis (see Ch. 18). These *prothrombotic factors* are involved, respectively, in platelet adhesion and in coagulation and clot stabilisation. However, the endothelium is also implicated in *thrombus limitation*. Thus it generates *prostaglandin I_2* (PGI_2, *prostacyclin*; Ch. 15) and *nitric oxide* (NO; ch14), converts the platelet agonist ADP to *adenosine*, which inhibits platelet function (Ch. 12), synthesises *tissue plasminogen activator* (tPA; see below) and expresses *thrombomodulin*, a receptor for thrombin. After combination with thrombomodulin, thrombin activates *protein C*, a vitamin K-dependent anticoagulant. Activated protein C helped by its cofactor protein S inactivates factors Va and VIIa. This is known to be physiologically important because a naturally occurring mutation of the gene coding for factor V (factor V Leiden), which confers resistance to activated protein C, results in the commonest recognised form of inherited thrombophilia. A synthetic form of activated protein C was recently licensed for the treament of septic shock (Ch. 18).

Endotoxin and cytokines, including tumour necrosis factor, tilt the balance of prothrombotic and antithrombotic endothelial functions toward thrombosis by causing loss of heparan and expression of tissue factor, and impair endothelial NO function. If other mechanisms limiting coagulation are also faulty or become exhausted, *disseminated intravascular coagulation* can result. This is a serious complication of sepsis and of certain malignancies, and the main treatment is to correct the underlying disease.

Blood coagulation (fibrin formation)

The clotting system consists of a cascade of proteolytic enzymes and cofactors.

- Inactive precursors are activated in series, each giving rise to more of the next.
- The last enzyme, thrombin, derived from prothrombin (II), converts soluble fibrinogen (I) to an insoluble meshwork of fibrin in which blood cells are trapped, forming the clot.
- There are two pathways in the cascade:
  —the extrinsic pathway, which operates in vivo
  —the intrinsic or contact pathway, which operates in vitro.
- Both pathways result in activation of factor X, which then converts prothrombin to thrombin.
- Calcium ions and a negatively charged phospholipid (PL) are essential for three steps, namely the actions of:
  —factor IXa on X
  —factor VIIa on X
  —factor Xa on II.
- PL is provided by activated platelets adhering to the damaged vessel.
- Some factors promote coagulation by binding to PL and a serine protease factor, e.g. factor Va in the activation of II by Xa; VIIIa in the activation of X by IXa.
- Blood coagulation is controlled by:
  —enzyme inhibitors, e.g. antithrombin III
  —fibrinolysis.

DRUGS THAT ACT ON THE COAGULATION CASCADE

Drugs are used to modify the cascade either when there is a *defect in coagulation* or when there is *unwanted coagulation*.

*Von Willebrand factor is a glycoprotein that is missing in a hereditary haemorrhagic disorder called von Willebrand's disease. It is synthesised by vascular endothelial cells (the presence of immunoreactive von Willebrand factor is an identifying feature of these cells in culture) and is also present in platelets.

COAGULATION DEFECTS

Genetically determined deficiencies of clotting factors are rare. Examples are *classical haemophilia*, caused by lack of factor VIII, and an even rarer form of haemophilia (haemophilia B or Christmas disease) caused by lack of factor IX (also called Christmas factor). Missing factors can be supplied by giving fresh plasma or concentrated preparations of factor VIII or factor IX. In the past, these have transmitted viral infections including human immonodeficiency virus and hepatitis B and C (Ch. 45). Pure forms of several human factors are now available, synthesised by recombinant technology, but are difficult to manufacture because of the need for post-translational modification in mammalian cells and are expensive.*

Acquired clotting defects are more common than hereditary ones. These include liver disease, vitamin K deficiency (universal in neonates) and excessive oral anticoagulant therapy, each of which may require treatment with vitamin K.

VITAMIN K

Vitamin K (for 'Koagulation' in German) is a fat-soluble vitamin occurring naturally in plants (Fig. 20.3). It is essential for the formation of clotting factors II, VII, IX and X. These are all glycoproteins with several *γ-carboxyglutamic acid* (Gla) residues. Gamma-carboxylation occurs *after* the synthesis of the chain and the carboxylase enzyme requires vitamin K as a cofactor. The role of the vitamin is clarified by considering the interaction of factors Xa and prothrombin (factor II) with Ca^{2+} and phospholipid as shown in Figure 20.4. Binding does not occur in the absence of γ-carboxylation. Reduced vitamin K is an essential cofactor in the carboxylation of glutamate residues (Fig. 20.5). Similar considerations apply to the proteolytic activation of factor X by IXa and by VIIa (see Fig. 20.2).

There are several other vitamin K-dependent Gla-proteins, including proteins C and S (see above) and osteocalcin in bone. The effect of the vitamin on osteoporosis is under investigation.

Administration and pharmacokinetic aspects

Natural vitamin K (*phytomenadione*) may be given orally or by intravenous injection. If given by mouth, it requires bile salts for

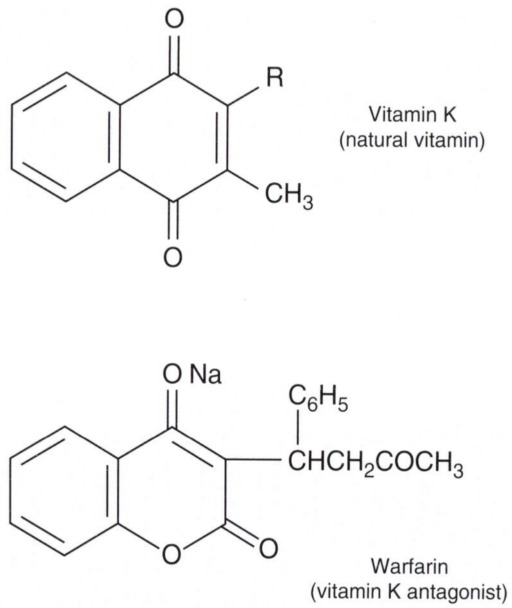

Fig. 20.3 Vitamin K and warfarin. Warfarin, a vitamin K antagonist, is an oral anticoagulant . It competes with vitamin K (note the similarity in their structures) for the reductase enzyme that activates vitamin K (see Fig. 20.5).

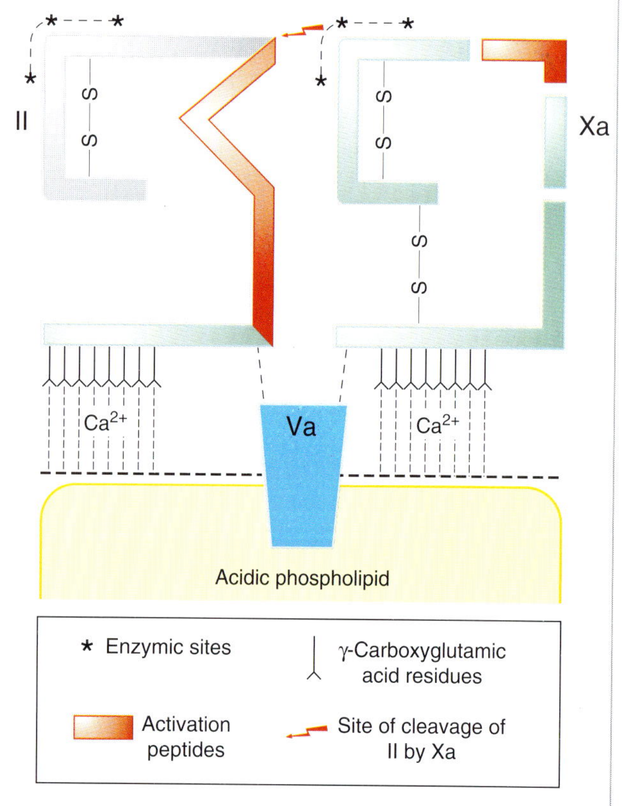

Fig. 20.4 Activation of prothrombin (factor II) by factor Xa. The complex of factor Va with a negatively charged phospholipid surface (supplied by aggregating platelets) forms a binding site for factor Xa and prothrombin (II), which have peptide chains (shown schematically) that are similar to one another. Platelets thus serve as a localising focus. Calcium ions are essential for binding. Xa activates prothrombin, liberating thrombin (shown in grey). (Modified from: Jackson C M 1978 Br J Haematol 39: 1.)

*The first publicly announced cloned sheep with a human transgene—Polly—contains the gene for human factor IX; if she and her clones secrete this in their milk, production costs will be dramatically reduced!

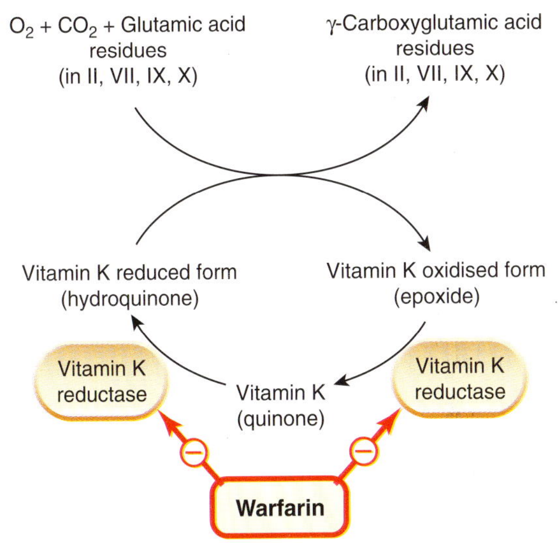

Fig. 20.5 Mechanism of vitamin K and of warfarin. After the peptide chains in clotting factors II, VII, IX and X have been synthesised, reduced vitamin K (the hydroquinone) acts as a cofactor in the conversion of glutamic acid (Glu) to γ-carboxyglutamic acid (Gla). During this reaction, the reduced form of vitamin K is converted to the epoxide, which in turn is reduced to the quinone and then the hydroquinone.

absorption and this occurs by a saturable energy-requiring process in the top part of the small intestine. A synthetic preparation, menadiol sodium phosphate, is also available. It is water soluble and does not require bile salts for its absorption. This synthetic compound takes longer to act than phytomenadione. There is very little storage of vitamin K in the body. It is metabolised to more polar substances that are excreted in the urine and the bile.

Clinical uses

Clinical uses of vitamin K are summarised in the clinical box.

THROMBOSIS

Thrombotic and thromboembolic disease is common and has severe consequences including myocardial infarction, stroke,

Clinical use of vitamin K

- Treatment and/or prevention of bleeding:
  - —resulting from use of oral anticoagulant drugs (e.g. warfarin)
  - —babies: to prevent haemorrhagic disease of the newborn.
- For vitamin K deficiencies in adults:
  - —sprue, coeliac disease, steatorrhoea
  - —lack of bile (e.g. with obstructive jaundice).

Clinical use of anticoagulants

- Heparin (often as low-molecular-weight heparin) is used acutely for short-term action.
- Warfarin is used for prolonged therapy.
- Anticoagulants are used for the prevention of:
  - —deep vein thrombosis (e.g. perioperatively)
  - —extension of established deep vein thrombosis or recurrence of pulmonary embolus
  - —thrombosis and embolisation in patients with atrial fibrillation (Ch. 17)
  - —thrombosis on prosthetic heart valves
  - —clotting in extracorporeal circulations (e.g. during haemodialysis or bypass surgery)
  - —cardiac events in patients with unstable coronary syndromes (e.g. unstable angina).

deep vein thrombosis and pulmonary embolus. The main drugs used for platelet-rich 'white' thrombi are the antiplatelet drugs (notably **aspirin**) and fibrinolytic drugs, which are considered below. The main drugs used to prevent or treat red thrombus are:

- injectable anticoagulants (**heparin** and newer thrombin inhibitors)
- oral anticoagulants (**warfarin** and related compounds).

Heparins act immediately whereas oral anticoagulants take several days to exert their effect. Consequently patients with venous thrombosis are treated immediately with an injectable anticoagulant, which is continued until the effect of warfarin has become established.

INJECTABLE ANTICOAGULANTS

Heparin and low-molecular-weight heparins

Heparin was discovered in 1916 by a second-year medical student at Johns Hopkins Hospital. He was attempting to extract thromboplastic (i.e. coagulant) substances from various tissues during a vacation project but found instead a powerful anticoagulant activity.* This was named 'heparin' because it was first extracted from liver.

Heparin is not a single substance but a family of sulfated glycosaminoglycans (mucopolysaccharides). It is present together with histamine in the granules of mast cells. Commercial preparations are extracted from beef lung or hog intestine and, since preparations differ in potency, assayed biologically against an agreed international standard: doses are specified in units of activity rather than of mass.

*This kind of good fortune also favoured Vane and his colleagues in their discovery of PGI_2 (Ch. 15 and 18), where they were looking for one kind of biological activity and found another. More specific chemical assays (Ch. 6), for all their strengths, cannot throw up this kind of unexpected discovery.

Heparin fragments, referred to as low-molecular-weight heparins (LMWHs), are used increasingly in place of unfractionated heparin.

Mechanism

Heparin inhibits coagulation both in vivo and in vitro, by activating antithrombin III (see above). Antithrombin III inhibits thrombin and other serine proteases by binding to the active serine site. Heparin modifies this interaction by binding, via a unique pentasaccharide sequence, to antithrombin III, changing its conformation and accelerating its rate of action.

Thrombin is considerably more sensitive to the inhibitory effect of the heparin–antithrombin III complex than is factor X. To inhibit thrombin, it is necessary for heparin to bind to the enzyme as well as to antithrombin III; to inhibit factor X it is only necessary for heparin to bind to antithrombin III (Fig. 20.6). Antithrombin III deficiency is very rare but can cause thrombophilia and resistance to heparin therapy.

LMWHs increase the action of antithrombin III on factor Xa but not its action on thrombin, since the molecules are too small to bind to both enzyme and inhibitor, essential for inhibition of thrombin but not for that of factor Xa (Fig. 20.6).

Administration and pharmacokinetic aspects

Heparin is not absorbed from the gut because of its charge and large size and is, therefore, given intravenously or subcutaneously (intramuscular injections would cause haematomas).

▼ After intravenous injection of a bolus dose, there is a phase of rapid elimination followed by a more gradual disappearance owing both to saturable processes (involving binding to sites on endothelial cells and macrophages) and slower first-order processes including renal excretion. As a result, once the dose exceeds the saturating concentration, a greater proportion is dealt with by these slower processes and the apparent half-life increases with increasing dose (saturation kinetics; see Ch. 8).

Heparin acts immediately following intravenous administration, but the onset is delayed by up to 60 minutes when it is given subcutaneously. The elimination half-life is approximately 40–90 minutes. In urgent situations, it is, therefore, usual to start treatment with a bolus intravenous dose, followed by a constant-rate infusion. The activated partial thromboplastin time (APTT), or some other in vitro clotting test, is measured and the dose of unfractionated heparin adjusted to achieve a value within a target range (e.g. 1.5–2.5 times control).

LMWHs are given subcutaneously. They have a longer elimination half-life than unfractionated heparin and this is independent of dose (first-order kinetics), so the effects are more predictable and dosing less frequent (once or twice a day). LMWHs do not prolong the APTT; unlike unfractionated heparin, the effect of a standard dose is sufficiently predictable that monitoring is not required routinely. They are eliminated mainly by renal excretion. They are at least as safe and effective as unfractionated heparin and are more convenient to use, since patients can be taught to inject themselves at home and there is generally no need for blood tests and dose adjustment.

Unwanted effects

Haemorrhage The main hazard is haemorrhage, which is treated by stopping therapy and, if necessary, giving **protamine** sulfate. This heparin antagonist is a strongly basic protein that forms an inactive complex with heparin; it is given intravenously. The dose is estimated from the dose of heparin that has been administered recently, and it is important not to give too much as this can itself cause bleeding. If necessary, an in vitro neutralisation test is performed on a sample of blood from the patient to provide a more precise indication of the required dose.

Thrombosis This is an uncommon but serious adverse effect of heparin and, as with warfarin necrosis (see below), may be misattributed to the natural history of the disease for which heparin is being administered. Paradoxically, it is associated with thrombocytopenia. A transitory early decrease in platelet numbers is not uncommon and is not clinically important. More serious thrombocytopenia occurring 2–14 days after the start of therapy is uncommon and is caused by IgM or IgG antibodies against complexes of heparin and platelet factor 4. Circulating immune complexes bind to Fc receptors (see Ch. 15) on circulating platelets, thereby activating them and releasing more platelet factor 4 and causing thrombocytopenia. Antibody also binds to platelet factor 4 complexed with glycosaminoglycans on the surface of endothelial cells, leading to immune injury of the vessel wall, thrombosis and disseminated intravascular coagulation. LMWHs are less liable than standard heparin to activate platelets to release platelet factor 4, and they bind less

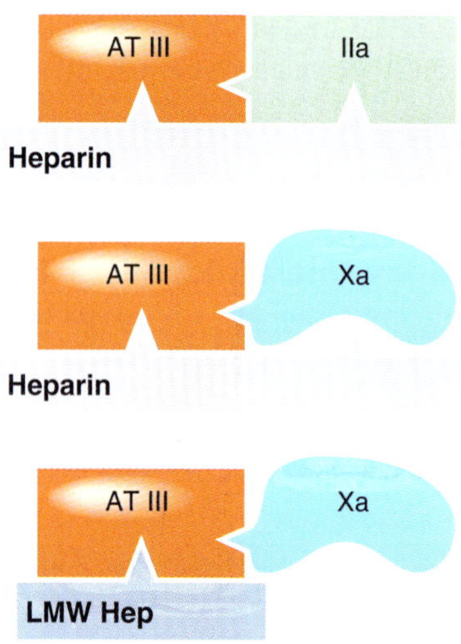

Fig. 20.6 Action of heparins. The schematic shows interactions of heparins, antithrombin III (AT III) and clotting factors. To increase the inactivation of thrombin (IIa) by AT III, heparin needs to interact with both substances (top), but to speed up its effect on factor Xa it need only interact with AT III (middle). Low-molecular-weight heparins (LMW Hep) increase the action of AT III on factor Xa (bottom) but cannot increase the action of AT III on thrombin because they cannot bind both simultaneously. (Modified from: Hirsh J & Levine M 1992 Blood 79: 1–17.)

avidly to platelet factor 4. Consequently, LMWHs are less likely than unfractionated heparin to cause thrombocytopenia and thrombosis. If antibodies to heparin–platelet factor 4 complexes have formed, however, it is to be expected that LMWHs could trigger these immunologically mediated adverse effects.

Osteoporosis Osteoporosis with spontaneous fractures has been reported with long-term (6 months or more) treatment with heparin (usually during pregnancy). Its explanation is unknown.

Hypoaldosteronism This (with consequent hyperkalaemia) has been described.

Hypersensitivity reactions These are rare with heparin but are more common with protamine. (Protamine sensitivity also occurs in patients treated with protamine zinc insulin. It is extracted from fish roe, and sensitivity to protamine occurs in some people with fish allergy.)

ANTITHROMBIN-III-INDEPENDENT ANTICOAGULANTS

▼ Several direct inhibitors of thrombin are under investigation, including **hirudin**, **hirugen**, **argatroban** and a tripeptide chloromethyl ketone, PPACK.

Hirudin, the anticoagulant from the medicinal leech, has been synthesised by recombinant DNA techniques. Clinical trials, including GUSTO-2 and TIMI-9, have been somewhat disappointing. Hirugen is a synthetic dodecapeptide derived from hirudin. Argatroban, an arginine-based compound, is a weak competitive inhibitor of thrombin. PPACK alkylates the active site in thrombin, inhibiting it irreversibly. The latter three compounds can reach and inactivate thrombin that is bound to fibrin, but it is unknown whether this will prove clinically advantageous. These drugs have a niche in the treatment of patients who have developed immune thrombocytopenia/thrombosis during treatment with heparin, from which they are immunologically quite distinct.

Various other approaches are being explored. These include several naturally occurring anticoagulants (tissue factor pathway inhibitor, thrombomodulin and protein C) synthesised by recombinant technology. A particularly ingenious approach is the development of thrombin agonists that are selective for the anticoagulant properties of thrombin. One such modified thrombin, differing by a single amino acid substitution, has substrate specificity for protein C. It produces anticoagulation in monkeys without prolonging bleeding times, suggesting that it may be less likely than standard anticoagulants to cause complications owing to bleeding.

ORAL ANTICOAGULANTS: WARFARIN

▼ Oral anticoagulants became available as an indirect result of a change in agricultural policy in North America in the 1920s. Sweet clover was substituted for corn in cattle-feed, and an epidemic of deaths of cattle from haemorrhage ensued. This turned out to be caused by *bishydroxycoumarin* in spoiled sweet clover, and it led to the discovery of **warfarin** (named for the Wisconsin Alumni Research Foundation). One of the first uses to which this was put was as a rat poison.

Warfarin (Fig. 20.3) is the most important oral anticoagulant; alternatives, e.g. **phenindione**, are now used only in rare patients who experience idiosyncratic adverse reactions to warfarin.

Mechanism of action

Oral anticoagulants act only in vivo and have no effect on clotting if added to blood in vitro. They interfere with the post-translational γ-carboxylation of glutamic acid residues in clotting factors II, VII, IX and X. They do this by inhibiting enzymic reduction of vitamin K to its active hydroquinone form (Fig. 20.5). Inhibition is competitive (reflecting the structural similarity between warfarin and vitamin K; Fig. 20.3). Their effect takes several days to develop because of the time taken for degradation of carboxylated factors. Their onset of action thus depends on the elimination half-lives of the relevant factors. Factor VII, with a half-life of 6 hours, is affected first, then IX, X and II with half-lives of 24, 40 and 60 hours, respectively.

Administration and pharmacokinetic aspects

Warfarin is given orally and is absorbed quickly and totally from the gastrointestinal tract. It has a small distribution volume, being strongly bound to plasma albumin (see Ch. 7). The peak concentration in the blood occurs within an hour of ingestion, but because of the mechanism of action this does not coincide with the peak pharmacological effect, which occurs about 48 hours later. The effect on *prothrombin time* (PT, see below) of a single dose does not start for 12–16 hours, and it lasts 4–5 days. Warfarin is metabolised by hepatic mixed function oxidase P450 system and its half-life is very variable, being of the order of 40 hours in many individuals.

Warfarin crosses the placenta and is not given in the first months of pregnancy because it is teratogenic, nor in the later stages because it can cause intracranial haemorrhage in the baby during delivery. It appears in milk during lactation. This could theoretically be important because newborn infants are naturally deficient in vitamin K. However, infants are routinely prescribed vitamin K to prevent haemorrhagic disease (see above), so warfarin treatment of the mother does not generally pose a risk to the breast-fed infant.

The therapeutic use of warfarin requires a careful balance between giving too little, leaving unwanted coagulation unchecked, and giving too much thereby causing haemorrhage. Therapy is complicated not only because the effect of a particular dose is only seen 2 days after giving it but also because of numerous conditions that modify sensitivity to warfarin, including interactions with other drugs. The effect of warfarin is monitored by measuring PT, which is expressed as an *International Normalised Ratio* (INR).

▼ The PT is the time taken for clotting of citrated plasma after the addition of Ca^{2+} and standardised reference thromboplastin; it is expressed as the ratio (PT ratio) of the PT of the patient to the PT of a pool of plasma from healthy subjects on no medication. Because of the variability of thromboplastins, different results can be obtained in different laboratories. To standardise PT measurements internationally, each thromboplastin is assigned an International Sensitivity Index (ISI) and the patient's PT is expressed as an INR, where INR = $(\text{PT ratio})^{\text{ISI}}$. This kind of normalisation procedure shocks purists but provides similar results when a patient moves from, say, Birmingham to Baltimore, permitting warfarin dose adjustment independent of laboratory. Pragmatic haematologists argue that the proof of the pudding is in the eating!

The dose of warfarin is usually adjusted to give an INR of 2–4, the precise target depending on the clinical situation. The duration of treatment also varies, but for several indications (e.g.

to prevent thromboembolism in chronic atrial fibrillation) treatment is long term.

Factors that potentiate oral anticoagulants

Various diseases and drugs potentiate warfarin, increasing the risk of haemorrhage.

Disease

Liver disease interferes with the synthesis of clotting factors; conditions in which there is a high metabolic rate, such as fever and thyrotoxicosis, increase the effect of anticoagulants by increasing degradation of clotting factors.

Drugs (see also Chs 8 and 51)

Many drugs potentiate warfarin.

Agents that inhibit hepatic drug metabolism Examples include **cimetidine, imipramine, co-trimoxazole, chloramphenicol, ciprofloxacin, metronidazole, amiodarone** and many antifungal azoles. Stereoselective effects (warfarin is a racemate, and its isomers are metabolised differently from one another) are described in Chapter 51.

Drugs that inhibit platelet function Non-steroidal anti-inflammatory drugs (NSAIDs) are particularly evident but some antibiotics incuding **moxalactam** and **carbenicillin** also alter platelet function. **Aspirin** increases the risk of bleeding if given during warfarin therapy, although this combination can be used safely with careful monitoring.

Drugs that displace warfarin from binding sites on plasma albumin Some of the NSAIDs and **chloral hydrate**, for example, result in a transient increase in the concentration of free warfarin in plasma. This mechanism seldom causes clinically important effects, unless accompanied by an additional effect on warfarin metabolism (Ch. 51).

Drugs that inhibit reduction of vitamin K Such drugs include the cephalosporins.

Drugs that decrease the availability of vitamin K Broad-spectrum antibiotics and some sulfonamides (see Ch. 45) depress the intestinal flora, which normally synthesise vitamin K_2 (a form of vitamin K made by gut bacteria), but this has little effect unless there is a concurrent dietary deficiency.

Factors that lessen the effect of oral anticoagulants

Physiological state/disease

There is a decreased response to warfarin in conditions (e.g. *pregnancy*) where there is increased coagulation factor synthesis. Similarly, the effect of oral anticoagulants is lessened in *hypothyroidism*, which is associated with reduced degradation of coagulation factors.

Drugs (see also Chs 8 and 51)

Several drugs reduce the effectiveness of warfarin; this leads to increased doses being used to achieve the target INR. If the dose of warfarin is not reduced when the interacting drug is discontinued, this can result in over-anticoagulation and haemorrhage.

Vitamin K This vitamin is present in some parenteral feeds and vitamin preparations.

Drugs that induce hepatic P450 enzymes Such induction will increase the degradation of warfarin (e.g. **rifampicin, carbamazepine, barbiturates, griseofulvin**). Induction may wane only slowly after the inducing drug is discontinued, making it difficult to adjust the dose appropriately.

Drugs that reduce absorption Drugs that alter passage through the gastrointestinal tract, for example **colestyramine**, will affect absorption of warfarin.

Drugs affecting blood coagulation

Procoagulant drugs: vitamin K

- The reduced form of vitamin K is a cofactor in the post-translational γ-carboxylation of a cluster of glutamic acid (glu) residues in each of factors II, VII, IX and X; vitamin K is oxidised during the reaction. The γ-carboxylated glutamic acid (gla) residues are essential for the interaction of these factors with Ca^{2+} and negatively charged phospholipid.

Injectable anticoagulants, e.g. heparin, low-molecular-weight heparins (LMWHs)

- These increase the rate of action of antithrombin III (AT III), a natural inhibitor that inactivates Xa and thrombin.
- They act both in vivo and in vitro.
- Anticoagulant activity results from a unique pentasaccharide sequence with high affinity for AT III.
- The effect of heparin is monitored by the APTT (activated partial thromboplastin time) and the dose is individualised.
- LMWHs have the same effect on factor X as heparin but less effect on thrombin; however, their anticoagulant effects are similar to heparin.
- LMWHs are given subcutaneously or intravenously and the onset of action is rapid. A standard dose (on a body weight basis) is given without the need for monitoring or individual dose adjustment. Patients can administer them at home.

Oral anticoagulants, e.g. warfarin

- These inhibit the reduction of vitamin K, thus inhibiting the γ-carboxylation of glu in II, VII, IX and X.
- They act only in vivo and the effect is delayed.
- Many factors modify their action; drug interactions are especially important.
- There is wide variation in response; their effect is monitored by measuring the INR (international normalised ratio) and the dose individualised accordingly.

Unwanted effects

Haemorrhage (especially into the bowel or the brain) is the main hazard. Depending on the urgency of the situation, treatment may consist of withholding warfarin (for minor problems), administration of vitamin K, fresh plasma or coagulation factor concentrates (for life-threatening bleeding). Oral anticoagulants are teratogenic. Hepatotoxicity occurs but is uncommon. Necrosis of soft tissues (for example breast or buttock) owing to thrombosis in venules occurs rarely shortly after starting treatment and is attributed to inhibition of biosynthesis of protein C, which has a shorter elimination half-life than do the vitamin K-dependent coagulation factors; this results in a procoagulant state soon after starting treatment. Treatment with heparin is usually started before warfarin, avoiding this problem.

Clinical use

The clinical use of anticoagulants is summarised in the box on page 319.

Platelet function

- Healthy vascular endothelium prevents platelet adhesion.
- Platelets adhere to diseased or damaged areas and become activated, i.e. they change shape, exposing negatively charged phospholipids and glycoprotein (GP) IIb/IIIa receptors, and synthesise and release various mediators, e.g. thromboxane, ADP, which stimulate other platelets to aggregate.
- Aggregation entails fibrinogen binding to GPIIb/IIIa receptors on adjacent platelets.
- Activated platelets constitute the focus for fibrin formation.
- Chemotactic factors and growth factors necessary for repair, but also implicated in atherogenesis, are released during platelet activation.

PLATELET ADHESION AND ACTIVATION

Platelets maintain the integrity of the circulation: a low platelet count results in *thrombocytopenic purpura*.*

When platelets are activated, they undergo a sequence of reactions that is essential for haemostasis, important for the healing of damaged blood vessels and plays a part in inflammation (see Ch. 15). These reactions, of which several are redundant (in the sense that if one pathway of activation is blocked another is available) and several are autocatalytic, include:

- *adhesion* following vascular damage (via von Willebrand factor bridging between subendothelial macromolecules and glycoprotein (GP) Ib receptors on the platelet surface)**
- *shape change* (from smooth discs to spiny spheres with protruding pseudopodia)
- *secretion* of the granule contents (including platelet agonists, such as ADP and 5-hydroxytryptamine (5-HT), and coagulation factors and growth factors such as platelet-derived growth factor)
- *biosynthesis of labile mediators* such as platelet-activating factor and thromboxane (TX) A_2 (see Fig. 20.7)
- *aggregation*, which is promoted by various agonists, including collagen, thrombin, ADP and TXA_2, acting on specific receptors on the platelet surface: activation by agonists leads to expression of GPIIb/IIIa receptors which bind fibrinogen and this links adjacent platelets sticking them together (aggregation).
- *exposure of acidic phospholipid* on the platelet outer surface, promoting thrombin formation (and hence further platelet activation via thrombin receptors and fibrin formation via cleavage of fibrinogen; see above).

These processes are essential for haemostasis but may be inappropriately triggered if the vessel wall is diseased, most commonly with atherosclerosis, resulting in thrombosis (Fig. 20.7).

ANTIPLATELET DRUGS

Platelets play such a critical role in thromboembolic disease that it is no surprise that antiplatelet drugs are of immense therapeutic value. Advances in this area, particularly clinical trials of **aspirin**, have radically altered clinical practice. Sites of action of antiplatelet drugs are shown in Figure 20.7.

ASPIRIN

Aspirin (see Ch. 16) alters the balance between TXA_2, which promotes aggregation, and PGI_2 which inhibits it. Aspirin inactivates cyclooxygenase—acting mainly on the constitutive form COX-1—by irreversibly acetylating a serine residue in its active site. This reduces both TXA_2 synthesis in platelets and PGI_2 synthesis in endothelium. Vascular endothelial cells, however, can synthesise new enzyme whereas platelets cannot. After administration of aspirin, TXA_2 synthesis does not recover until the affected cohort of platelets is replaced in 7–10 days. Furthermore, higher doses of aspirin are needed to inhibit cyclooxygenase in vascular endothelium than in platelets, especially when administered by mouth. This is because platelets are exposed to aspirin in the portal blood, whereas systemic vasculature is partly protected by presystemic metabolism of aspirin to salicylate by esterases in the liver. Consequently, low doses of aspirin given intermittently decrease the synthesis of

*'Purpura' means a purple rash caused by spontaneous bleeding in the skin. Bleeding can occur into other organs including the gut and brain.

**Various platelet membrane glycoproteins are receptors or binding sites for adhesive proteins such as von Willebrand factor or fibrinogen.

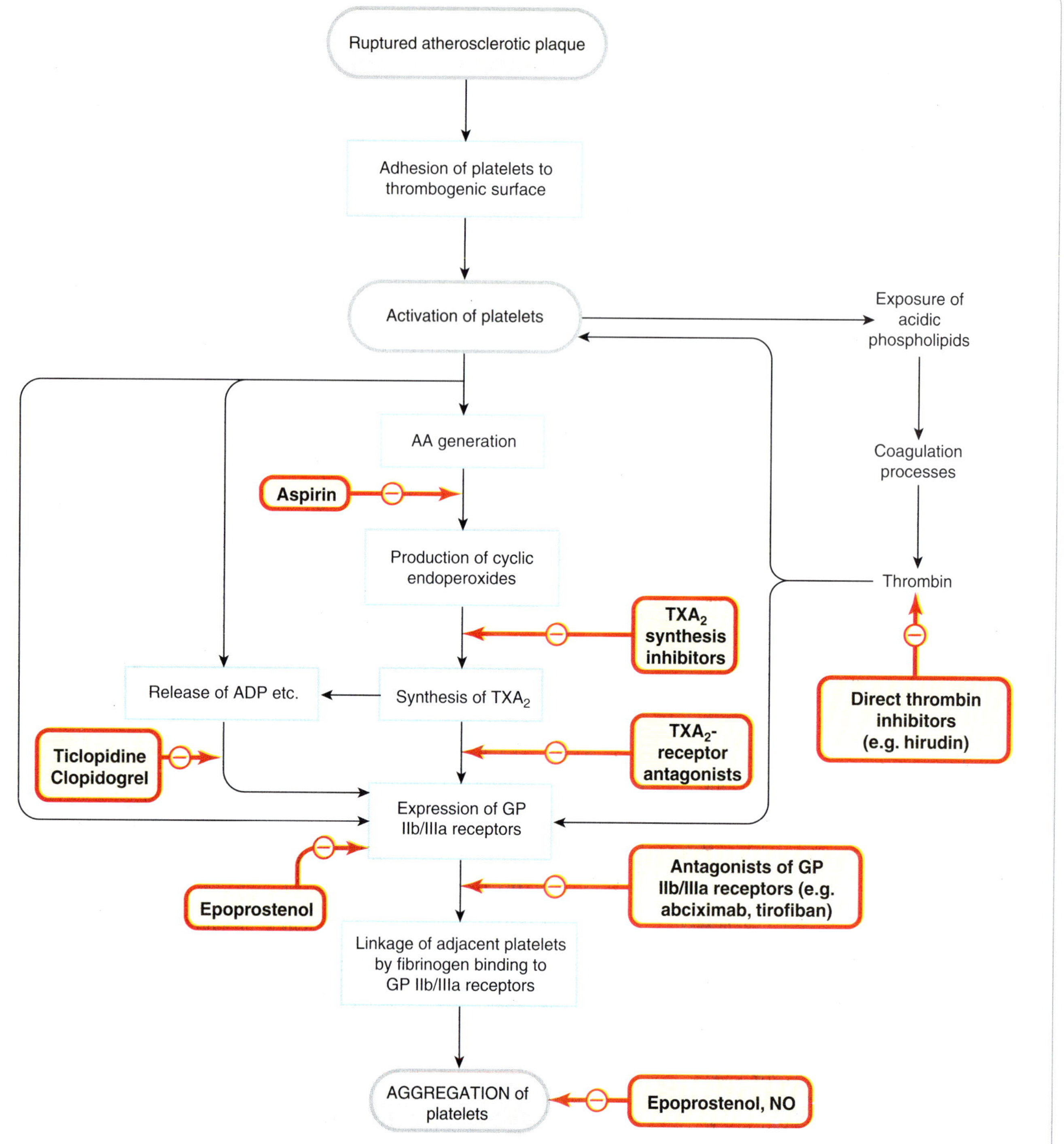

Fig. 20.7 Platelet activation. Events involved in platelet adhesion and aggregation are shown, with the sites of action of drugs and endogenous mediators. (AA, arachidonic acid; ADP, adenosine bisphosphate; GP, glycoprotein; NO, nitric oxide; TXA_2, thromboxane A_2.)

TXA_2 without drastically reducing PGI_2 synthesis. Clinical trials have demonstrated the efficacy of aspirin in several clinical settings (see the clinical box on p. 326). Treatment of acute myocardial infarction involves fibrinolytic drugs as well as aspirin (see Fig. 20.8 and below). Other non-steroidal drugs (e.g. **sulfinpyrazone**, for which there is supportive trial evidence) could have similar effects to aspirin but they differ from aspirin in several potentially important ways (notably in being reversible rather than irreversible inhibitors of cyclooxygenase), so it is unwise to assume this in the absence of clinical trials.

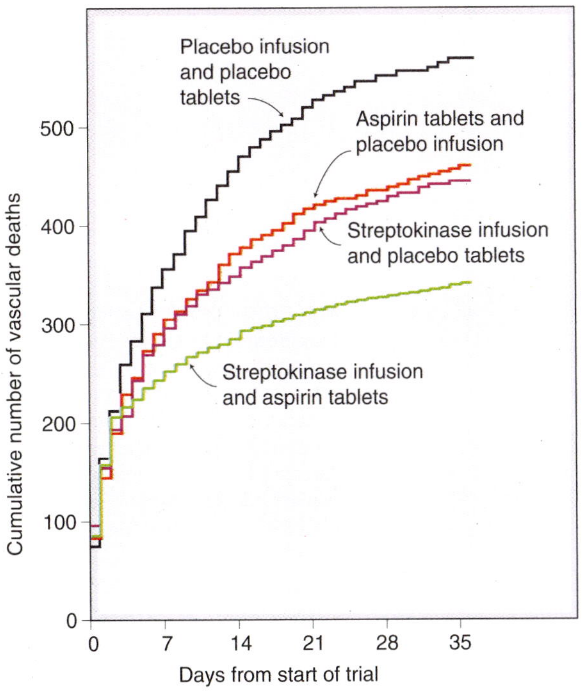

Fig. 20.8 Efficacy of aspirin and streptokinase for myocardial infarction. The curves show cumulative vascular mortality in patients treated with placebo, aspirin alone, streptokinase alone or a combined aspirin–streptokinase regimen. (ISIS-2 trial 1988 Lancet ii: 350–360.)

DIPYRIDAMOLE

The value of **dipyridamole**—a phosphodiesterase inhibitor, see Chapter 18—has been clarified by a European stroke prevention trial (ESPS-2) in patients with a history of ischaemic stroke or transient cerebral ischaemic attack. This showed that a modified release form of dipyridamole reduced the risk of stroke and death in such patients by around 15%—a similar effect to that of aspirin (25 mg twice daily).* The beneficial effects of aspirin and dipyridamole were additive. Headache was the commonest adverse effect of dipyridamole; unlike aspirin it caused no excess risk of bleeding.

THIENOPYRIDINE DERIVATIVES

Ticlopidine inhibits ADP-dependent aggregation. Its action is slow in onset, taking 3–7 days to reach maximal effect, and it works through an active metabolite. Its efficacy in reducing stroke is similar to that of aspirin but idiosyncratic unwanted effects, including severe blood dyscrasias (especially neutropenia), have limited its long-term use.

Clopidogrel is structurally related to ticlopidine and also inhibits ADP-induced aggregation through an active metabolite. Like ticlopidine, it can cause rash or diarrhoea, but neutropenia is no more common than with aspirin. Clopidogrel was slightly more effective than aspirin (in the unconventionally large dose of 325 mg/day) in reducing a composite outcome of ischaemic stroke, myocardial infarction or vascular death in one large trial. Since ADP antagonists inhibit a separate pathway of platelet activation than that which is inhibited by aspirin, it is possible that their effects may be additive with those of aspirin. This has been tested in a recent large (approximately 12 500 patients) trial in patients with acute coronary syndromes without the electrocardiographic changes that accompany acute transmural myocardial infarction (and which indicate a need for immediate treatment to reopen the blocked artery—see below), such as those with unstable angina or infarction that has not extended through the wall of the heart (Ch. 17). Patients randomly allocated to treatment (for 6–9 months) with clopidogrel (plus aspirin) had fewer vascular events than did those allocated to placebo (plus aspirin)—see Figure 20.9. More patients treated with clopidogrel had serious bleeds, but life-threatening bleeds and haemorrhagic strokes were similar in the two groups. Pretreatment with clopidorel and aspirin followed by long-term therapy is also effective in patients with ischaemic heart disease undergoing percutaneous coronary interventions. These findings are likely to change usual clinical practice radically in the next few years.

GLYCOPROTEIN IIB/IIIA RECEPTOR ANTAGONISTS

Antagonists of the GPIIb/IIIa receptor have the theoretical attraction that they inhibit all pathways of platelet activation (since these all converge on activation of GP IIb/IIIa receptors). A hybrid murine/human monoclonal antibody Fab fragment directed against the GPIIb/IIIa receptor, which rejoices in the catchy little name of **abciximab**, is licensed for use in high-risk patients undergoing coronary angioplasty, as an adjunct to heparin and aspirin. It reduces the risk of restenosis at the expense of an increased risk of bleeding. Immunogenicity limits its use to a single administration.

Tirofiban and **eptifibatide** are cyclic peptides based on the Arg–Gly–Asp ('RGD') sequence that is common to ligands for GP IIb/IIIa receptors. Given intravenously, these agents reduce early events in unstable coronary syndrome patients treated invasively,** but long-term oral therapy is not effective and may be harmful.

OTHER ANTIPLATELET DRUGS

Epoprostenol (PGI_2) is sometimes administered parenterally (into blood entering the dialysis circuit) to prevent thrombosis

*This dose of aspirin is unconventional, being somewhat lower than the 75 mg per day that is the lowest dose commonly used in thromboprophylaxis.

**The UK National Institute for Clinical Excellence (NICE) has belied suspicions that it was actually an institute for rationing by endorsing use of these drugs.

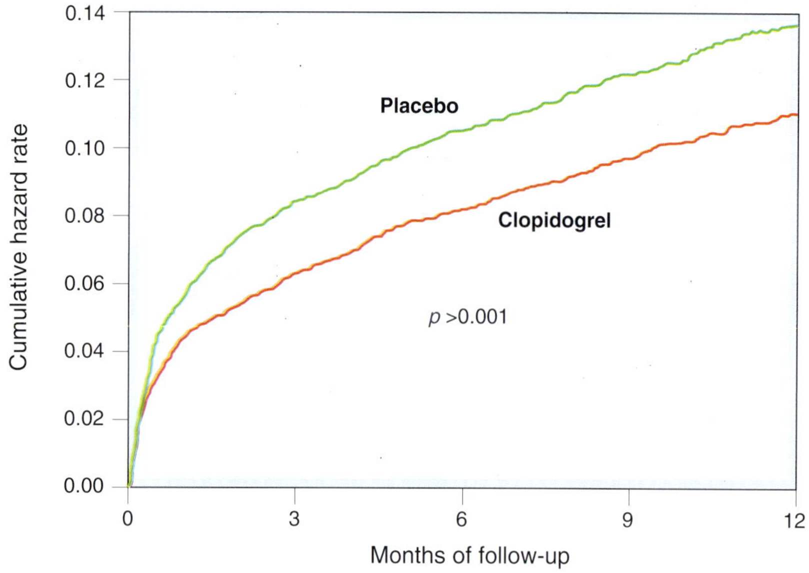

Fig. 20.9 Effect of adding clopidogrel to aspirin. The curves show cumulative hazard rates for major vascular events in patients with acute coronary syndromes treated either with placebo + aspirin or clopidogrel + aspirin. (Modified from N Engl J Med 2001 345: 494–502.)

Clinical uses of antiplatelet drugs

- The main drug is aspirin. Other drugs with different actions (e.g. dipyridamole, clopidogrel) can be additive in their effects. Uses of antiplatelet drugs mainly relate to arterial thrombosis and include:
  - —acute myocardial infarction
  - —high risk of myocardial infarction, including: patients who have recovered from myocardial infarction and patients with symptoms from atherosclerosis, including angina, transient cerebral ischaemic attacks, intermittent claudication
  - —following coronary artery bypass grafting
  - —unstable coronary syndromes (clopidogrel can be added to aspirin)
  - —following coronary artery angioplasty ± stenting (intravenous glycoprotein IIb/IIIa antagonists, e.g. abciximab, are used in some patients in addition to aspirin; long-term therapy with clopidogrel in addition to aspirin reduces major cardiovascular events)
  - —transient cerebral ischaemic attack (TIA) or thrombotic stroke, to prevent recurrence (dipyridamole can be added to aspirin)
  - —atrial fibrillation, if oral anticoagulation is contraindicated.
- Other antiplatelet drugs (e.g. epoprostenol (PGI_2), see Ch 15) have limited specialised clinical applications.

Antiplatelet drugs

- Aspirin inhibits cyclooxygenase irreversibly. The balance between prostaglandin I_2 (an inhibitor of aggregation generated by vascular endothelium) and thromboxane (TX) (a stimulant of aggregation generated by platelets) is thus altered, since the endothelium can synthesise more enzyme but platelets cannot. Synthesis of the latter only recovers when new platelets are formed. It is very important clinically.
- Clopidogrel is a pro-drug. Given by mouth, it inhibits platelet responses to ADP. Its actions are additive with aspirin.
- Antagonists of glycoprotein (GP) IIb/IIIa receptors include a monoclonal antibody (abciximab) and several oligopeptides (e.g. tirofiban). They inhibit diverse agonists (e.g. ADP, TXA_2, etc.), since different pathways of activation converge on GPIIb/IIIa receptors. They are used intravenously for short-term treatment.
- Dipyridamole is a phosphodiesterase inhibitor. It is used in addition to aspirin.
- Epoprostenol (synthetic prostaglandin I_2) is chemically unstable. Given as an intravenous infusion it acts on inositol phosphate receptors on vascular smooth muscle and platelets (Ch. 15), stimulating adenylate cyclase thereby causing vasodilatation and inhibiting aggregation caused by any pathway (eg ADP, TXA_2, etc.).
- Agents that either inhibit TXA_2 synthesis or block TXA_2 receptors, or have both actions, are available but are not used clinically.

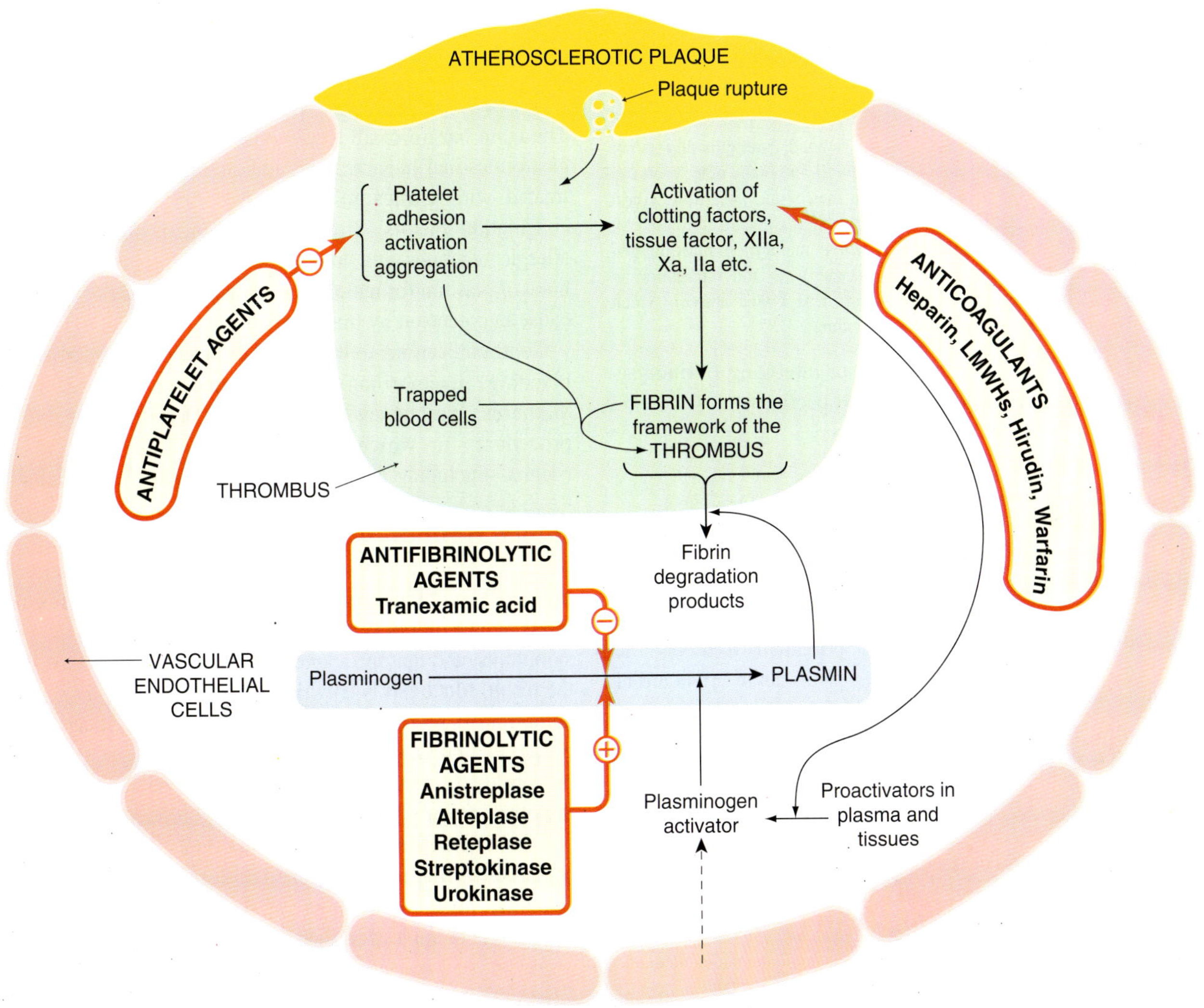

Fig. 20.10 Fibrinolytic system. The schematic shows interactions with coagulation and platelet pathways and sites of action of drugs that modify these systems. (LMHs, low-molecular-weight heparins.) For more details of platelet activation and the coagulation cascade refer to Figures 20.1, 20.2 and 20.7.

during haemodialysis in patients in whom heparin is contraindicated.

▼ *TXA_2-receptor ('TP') antagonists* (e.g. GR32191) are unlikely to be more effective than low-dose aspirin but could have less adverse effects. *TXA_2-synthesis inhibitors* ('TXSI' e.g. dazoxiben, an analogue of imidazole) increase PGI_2 synthesis, as a consequence of diversion of endoperoxide intermediates from TXA_2 synthesis to PGI_2 synthesis, as well as reducing TXA_2 production. However, they only weakly inhibit platelet function in vitro, probably because prostaglandin endoperoxides (e.g. PGH_2) are agonists at thromboxane receptors. Compounds that have both TXA_2 synthetase inhibition as well as TXA_2-receptor blocking activity offer a better possibility of selectively inhibiting thromboxane synthesis while increasing PGI_2 synthesis, and drugs with this combination of activities (e.g. **ridogrel**) are in development.

Clinical use of antiplatelet drugs

The clinical use of antiplatelet drugs is summarised in the box on p. 326.

FIBRINOLYSIS (THROMBOLYSIS)

When the coagulation system is activated, the fibrinolytic system is also set in motion via several endogenous *plasminogen activators*, including tPA, urokinase-type plasminogen activator (uPA), kallikrein and neutrophil elastase. tPA is inhibited by a structurally related lipoprotein, lipoprotein(a), increased concentrations of which constitute an independent risk factor for myocardial infarction (Ch. 19). Plasminogen is deposited on the fibrin strands within a thrombus. Plasminogen activators are serine proteases and are unstable in circulating blood. They diffuse into thrombus and cleave plasminogen to release plasmin (see Fig. 20.10).

▼ Plasmin is trypsin-like, acting on Arg–Lys bonds, and thus digests not only fibrin but fibrinogen, factors II, V and VIII and many other proteins. It is formed locally and acts on the fibrin meshwork, generating fibrin degradation products and lysing the clot. Its action is localised to the clot because plasminogen activators are effective mainly on plasminogen adsorbed to fibrin; any plasmin that escapes into the circulation is inactivated by plasmin inhibitors, including PAI-1 (see above), which protect us from digesting ourselves from within.

Drugs affect this system by increasing or inhibiting fibrinolysis (*fibrinolytic* and *antifibrinolytic* drugs, respectively).

FIBRINOLYTIC DRUGS

Figure 20.10 summarises the interaction of the fibrinolytic system with the coagulation cascade and platelet activation, and the action of drugs that modify this. Several fibrinolytic (thrombolytic) drugs are used clinically, principally to reopen the occluded coronary artery in patients with acute myocardial infarction.

Streptokinase is a protein extracted from cultures of streptococci. It activates plasminogen. Infused intravenously, it reduces mortality in acute myocardial infarction and this beneficial effect is additive with aspirin (Fig. 20.8). Its action is blocked by antistreptococcal antibodies, which appear about 4 days or more after the initial dose. At least 1 year must elapse before it is used again.

Alteplase and **duteplase** are, respectively, single- and double-chain recombinant tPA. They are more active on fibrin-bound plasminogen than on plasma plasminogen and are, therefore, said to be 'clot selective'. Recombinant tPA is not antigenic and can be used in patients likely to have antibodies to streptokinase. Because of their short half-lives, they must be given as intravenous infusions. **Reteplase** is similar but has a longer elimination half-life, allowing for bolus administration and making for simplicity of administration. It is available for clinical use in myocardial infarction.

Unwanted effects and contraindications

The main hazard of all fibrinolytic agents is bleeding, including gastrointestinal haemorrhage and stroke. If serious, this can be treated with **tranexamic acid** (see below), fresh plasma or coagulation factors. Streptokinase and anistreplase can cause allergic reactions and low-grade fever. Streptokinase causes a burst of plasmin formation, generating kinins (see Ch. 15) and can cause hypotension by this mechanism.

Contraindications to the use of these agents are active internal bleeding, haemorrhagic cerebrovascular disease, bleeding diatheses, pregnancy, uncontrolled hypertension, invasive procedures in which haemostasis is important and recent trauma—including vigorous cardiopulmonary resuscitation.

Which fibrinolytic agent is best?

Several large placebo-controlled studies in patients with myocardial infarction have shown convincingly that fibrinolytic drugs reduce mortality if given within 12 hours from the onset of symptoms, and that the sooner they are administered the better is the result. Much has been written as to which drug is best, but an authoritative review (Collins et al., 1997) concluded that: 'the choice of fibrinolytic drug makes little difference to the overall probability of stroke-free survival, because the regimens that dissolve coronary thrombi more rapidly produce greater risks of cerebral haemorrhage … It is … important that any uncertainties about which fibrinolytic regimen or dose of aspirin to use do not engender uncertainty about whether to use fibrinolytic and antiplatelet therapies routinely.'

Clinical use

The clinical use of fibrinolytic agents is summarised in the box.

ANTIFIBRINOLYTIC AND HAEMOSTATIC DRUGS

Tranexamic acid inhibits plasminogen activation and thus prevents fibrinolysis. It can be given orally or by intravenous

Fibrinolysis and drugs modifying fibrinolysis

- A fibrinolytic cascade is initiated concomitantly with the coagulation cascade, resulting in the formation within the coagulum of plasmin, which digests fibrin.
- Various agents promote the formation of plasmin from its precursor plasminogen, e.g. streptokinase, and tissue plasminogen activators such as alteplase, duteplase and reteplase. Most are infused; reteplase can be given as a bolus injection.
- Some drugs (e.g. tranexamic acid, aprotinin) inhibit fibrinolysis.

Clinical uses of fibrinolytic drugs

- The main drugs are streptokinase and tissue plasminogen activators (tPA), e.g. tenecteplase.
- The main use is in acute myocardial infarction, within 12 hours of onset (the earlier the better!)
- Other uses include:
  —acute thrombotic stroke within 3 hours of onset (tPA), in selected patients
  —clearing thrombosed shunts and cannulae
  —acute arterial thromboembolism.

injection. It is used to treat various conditions in which there is bleeding or risk of bleeding, such as haemorrhage following prostatectomy or dental extraction, in menorrhagia (excessive menstrual blood loss) and for life-threatening bleeding following thrombolytic drug administration. It is also used in patients with the rare disorder of hereditary angioedema.

Aprotinin inhibits proteolytic enzymes and is used for hyperplasminaemia caused by fibrinolytic drug overdose and in patients at risk of major blood loss during cardiac surgery.

REFERENCES AND FURTHER READING

Antiplatelet Trialists' Collaboration 1994 Collaborative overview of randomised trials of antiplatelet therapy I, II, III. Br Med J 308: 81–105, 159–168, 235–246 (*Overview of large number of randomised trials, leaves no room for doubt regarding the efficacy of aspirin—well hardly any: 2p < 0.00001 in many comparisons!*)

Aster R H 1995 Heparin-induced thrombocytopenia and thrombosis. N Engl J Med 332: 1374–1376 (*Succinct and lucid editorial; see also accompanying paper, pp. 1330–1335*)

CAPRIE Steering Committee 1996 A randomised, blinded trial of clopidogrel versus aspirin in patients at risk of ischaemic events (CAPRIE). Lancet 348: 1329–1339 (*19 185 patients randomised. Clopidogrel was marginally more effective than aspirin, with an overall safety profile at least as good as that of aspirin*)

Chew D P, Bhatt D, Sapp S, Topol EJ 2001 Increased mortality with oral platelet glycoprotein IIb/IIIa antagonists: a meta-analysis of phase III multicenter trials. Circulation 103: 201–206

Clouse LH, Comp P C 1987 The regulation of hemostasis: the protein C system. N Engl J Med 314: 1298–1304

Collins R, Peto R, Baigent C, Sleight P 1997 Aspirin, heparin and thrombolytic therapy in suspected acute myocardial infarction. N Engl J Med 336: 847–860 (*Unbiased and authoritative overview. Includes a section on 'general problems of unduly selective emphasis'—fighting stuff!*)

Coughlin S R 2000 Thrombin signalling and protease-activated receptors. Nature 407: 258–264 (*Reviews cellular actions of thrombin via protease-activated receptors. See also Brass S 2001 Platelets and proteases Nature 413: 26–27*)

CURE Investigators 2001 Effects of clopidogrel in addition to aspirin in patients with acute coronary syndromes without ST-segment elevation. N Engl J Med 345: 494–502 (*12 562 patients randomised; primary outcome occurred in 9.4% of patients in the clopidogrel + aspirin group and in 11.3% of those in the placebo + aspirin group, a relative risk of 0.72–0.90, p < 0.001*)

Diener H, Cunha L, Forbes C, Sivenius J, Smets P, Lowenthal A 1996 European stroke prevention study 2. Dipyridamole and acetylsalicylic acid in the secondary prevention of stroke. J Neurol Sci 143: 1–14 (*Slow-release dipyridamole 200 mg twice daily was as effective as aspirin 25 mg twice daily, and the effects of aspirin and dipyridamole were additive*)

EPIC Investigators 1994 Use of a monoclonal antibody directed against the platelet glycoprotein IIb/IIIa receptor in high-risk coronary angioplasty. N Engl J Med 330: 956–961 (*Ischaemic complications were reduced by 35% at the cost of increased bleeding*)

Fears R 1990 Biochemical pharmacology and therapeutic aspects of thrombolytic agents. Pharmacol Rev 42: 201–224

Fiorucci S et al. 2001 Proteinase-activated receptor 2 is an anti-inflammatory signal for colonic lamina propria lymphocytes in a mouse model of colitis. Proc Natl Acad Sci USA 98: 13936–13941 (*Elegant demonstration of the diversity of cellular responses initiated by PAR*)

Furie B, Furie B C 1992 Molecular and cellular biology of blood coagulation. N Engl J Med 326: 800–806

Gibbs C S 1995 Conversion of thrombin into an anticoagulant by protein engineering. Nature 387: 413–416 (*A single amino acid substitution shifts thrombin's specificity in favour of the anticoagulant protein C. See also accompanying editorial: Griffin JH 1992 The thrombin paradox. Nature 387: 337–338*)

Hirsh J 1991 Heparin. N Engl J Med 324: 1565–1574

Hirsh J 1991 Oral anticoagulant drugs. N Engl J Med 324: 1865–1873 (*See also subsequent editorial by the same author on the optimal duration of anticoagulant therapy for venous thrombosis: Hirsh J 1995 N Engl J Med 332: 1710–1711*)

Levine M 1995 A comparison of low-molecular-weight heparin administered primarily at home with unfractionated heparin administered in the hospital for proximal deep vein thrombosis. N Engl J Med 334: 677–681 (*Concludes that LMWH can be used safely and effectively at home. This has potentially very important implications for patient care*)

Mannuccio M 1998 Hemostatic drugs. N Engl J Med 333: 245–253

Mehta S R for the CURE Investigators 2001 Effects of pretreatment with clopidogrel and aspirin followed by long-term therapy in patients undergoing percutaneous coronary intervention: the PCI–CURE study. N Engl J Med 345: 494–502 (*Positive study showing additive effect of clopidogrel + aspirin*)

Patrono C 1994 Aspirin as an antiplatelet drug. N Engl J Med 330: 1287–1294

Salzman E W 1992 Low-molecular-weight heparin and other new antithrombotic drugs. N Engl J Med 326: 1017–1019 (*Review*)

Schömig A 1996 A randomized comparison of antiplatelet and anticoagulant therapy after the placement of coronary-artery stents. N Engl J Med 334: 1084–1089 (*Combined therapy with aspirin and ticlopidine was safer and more effective than conventional treatment with aspirin plus anticoagulant*)

Suttie J W 1980 Vitamin K-dependent carboxylation. Trends Biochem Sci 5: 302–304

Special Writing Group of the Stroke Council of the American Health Association 1996 Guidelines for thrombolytic therapy for acute stroke: a supplement to the guidelines for the management of patients with acute ischemic stroke. Stroke 27: 1711–1718 (*Recommends using tPA in selected patients within the first 3 hours of ischaemic stroke. Remains contentious—see for example editorial comment by Dorman & Sandercock in Lancet 1996; 348: 1600–1601*)

Turpie A G G 1993 A comparison of aspirin with placebo in patients treated with warfarin after heart-valve replacement. N Engl J Med 329: 524–529 (*Considerable benefit of combined treatment with aspirin and warfarin. Meticulous monitoring mandatory!*)

Vane J 1994 Towards a better aspirin. Nature 367: 215–216

Vermeer C, Hamulyak K 1991 Pathophysiology of vitamin K deficiency and oral anticoagulants. Thromb Haemost 66: 153–159

Ware J A, Heisted D D 1993 Platelet–endothelium interactions. N Engl J Med 328: 628–635

Weitz J I, Hirsh J 1992 Antithrombins: their potential as antithrombotic agents. Annu Rev Med 43: 9–16

21 The haemopoietic system

Overview 330

The haemopoietic system 330
— Types of anaemia 330

Haematinic agents 331
— Iron 331
— Folic acid and vitamin B_{12} 333

Haemopoietic growth factors 336
— Erythropoietin 336
— Colony-stimulating factors 337

OVERVIEW

In this chapter we summarise the different kinds of anaemia and cover the main haematinic agents used to treat them, namely iron, folic acid and vitamin B_{12}. We also cover erythropoietin, a growth factor specific for red blood cells used to treat anaemia of chronic disease, and several other haemopoietic factors, known as colony-stimulating factors, which are used to increase numbers of circulating white blood cells.

THE HAEMOPOIETIC SYSTEM

The main components of the haemopoietic system are the blood, bone marrow, lymph nodes and thymus, with the spleen, liver and kidneys as important accessory organs. Blood consists of formed elements (red and white blood cells and platelets) and plasma. It has diverse functions, including key roles in host defence (Ch. 15) and haemostasis (Ch. 20). This present chapter deals mainly with red cells, which have the principal function of carrying oxygen. Their oxygen-carrying power depends on their haemoglobin content. The most important site of formation of red blood cells in adults is the bone marrow, whereas the spleen acts as their graveyard. Red cell loss in healthy adults is precisely balanced by production of new cells. The liver stores vitamin B_{12} and is involved in the process of breakdown of the haemoglobin liberated when red blood cells are destroyed. The kidney manufactures erythropoietin. Cells from various other organs synthesise and release colony-stimulating factors (CSFs), which regulate the production of leucocytes and platelets. The function of platelets is discussed in Chapter 20 and that of leucocytes in Chapter 15.

TYPES OF ANAEMIA

Anaemia is defined as a reduced concentration of haemoglobin in the blood. It may give rise to fatigue but, especially if it is chronic, is often surprisingly asymptomatic. The commonest cause is blood loss related to menstruation and child bearing, but there are several different types of anaemia, and several different diagnostic levels. Determining indices of red cell size and haemoglobin content and microscopical examination of a stained blood smear of blood allows characterisation into:

- hypochromic, microcytic anaemia (small red cells with low haemoglobin; caused by iron deficiency)
- macrocytic anaemia (large red cells, few in number)
- normochromic normocytic anaemia (fewer normal-sized red cells, each with a normal haemoglobin content)
- mixed pictures.

Further evaluation may include determination of concentrations of ferritin, iron, vitamin B_{12} and folic acid in serum, and microscopic examination of smears of bone marrow. This leads to more precise diagnostic groupings of anaemias into:

- deficiency of nutrients necessary for haemopoiesis, most importantly:
  —iron
  —folic acid and vitamin B_{12}
  —pyridoxine, vitamin C
- depression of the bone marrow, caused by:
  —toxins (e.g. drugs used in chemotherapy)
  —radiation therapy
  —diseases of the bone marrow of unknown origin (e.g. idiopathic aplastic anaemia, leukaemias)
  —reduced production of, or responsiveness to, erythropoietin (e.g. chronic renal failure, rheumatoid arthritis, acquired immunodeficiency disease (AIDS))
- excessive destruction of red blood cells (i.e. haemolytic anaemia); this has many causes including haemoglobinopathies (such as sickle cell anaemia), adverse reactions to drugs and inappropriate immune reactions.

It is important to note that the use of haematinic agents is often only an adjunct to treatment of the underlying cause of the anaemia—for example surgery for colon cancer (a common cause of iron deficiency) or anthelminthic drugs for patients with hookworm (a frequent cause of anaemia in parts of Africa and Asia; Ch. 49). Sometimes treatment consists of stopping an offending drug, e.g. a non-steroidal anti-inflammatory drug that causes blood loss from the stomach (Ch. 16).

HAEMATINIC AGENTS

IRON

Iron is a transition metal with two important properties relevant to its biological role:

- ability to exist in several oxidation states
- ability to form stable coordination complexes.

The body of a 70 kg man contains about 4 g of iron, 65% of which circulates in the blood as haemoglobin. About one half of the remainder is stored in the liver, spleen and bone marrow, chiefly as *ferritin* and *haemosiderin*. The iron in these molecules is available for fresh haemoglobin synthesis. The rest, which is not available for haemoglobin synthesis, is present in myoglobin, cytochromes and various enzymes.

The distribution of iron in an average adult male is shown in Table 21.1. The corresponding values for a woman would be about 55% of these. Since most of the iron in the body is either part of—or destined to be part of—haemoglobin, the most obvious clinical result of iron deficiency is anaemia, and the only indication for therapy with iron is to provide material for haemoglobin synthesis.

Haemoglobin is made up of four protein chain subunits (globins), each of which contains one haem moiety. Haem consists of a tetrapyrrole porphyrin ring containing ferrous (Fe^{2+}) iron. Each haem group can carry one oxygen molecule, which is bound reversibly to Fe^{2+} and to a histidine residue in the globin chain. This reversible binding is the basis of oxygen transport.

Iron turnover and balance

Both the normal physiological turnover of iron and *pharmacokinetic factors* affecting iron when it is given therapeutically will be dealt with here. The normal daily requirement for iron is approximately 5 mg for men, and 15 mg for growing children and for menstruating women. A pregnant woman needs between two and ten times this amount because of the demands of the fetus and increased requirements of the mother.* The average diet in Western Europe provides 15–20 mg of iron daily, mostly in meat. Iron in meat is generally present as haem and about 20–40% of haem iron is available for absorption.

▼ Humans are adapted to absorb iron in the form of haem. It is thought that one reason why modern humans have problems in maintaining iron balance (there are an estimated 500 million people with iron deficiency in the world) is that the change from hunting to grain cultivation 10 000 years ago led to cereals, which have a relatively small amount of utilisable iron, constituting a significant proportion of the diet.

Non-haem iron in food is mainly in the ferric state and this needs to be converted to ferrous iron for absorption. Ferric iron, and to a lesser extent ferrous iron, has low solubility at the neutral pH of the intestine; however, in the stomach, iron dissolves and binds to mucoprotein. In the presence of ascorbic acid, fructose and various amino acids, iron is detached from the carrier, forming soluble low-molecular-weight complexes that enable it to remain in soluble form in the intestine. Ascorbic acid stimulates iron absorption partly by forming soluble iron–ascorbate chelates and partly by reducing ferric iron to the more soluble ferrous form.

*Each pregnancy 'costs' the mother 680 mg iron, equivalent to 1300 ml of blood, owing to the demands of the fetus, plus requirements of the expanded blood volume and blood loss at delivery.

Table 21.1 The distribution of iron in the body of a healthy 70 kg male

Protein	Tissue	Iron content (mg)
Haemoglobin	Erythrocytes	2600
Myoglobin	Muscle	400
Enzymes (cytochromes, catalase, guanylate cyclase etc.)	Liver and other tissues	25
Transferrin	Plasma and extracellular fluid	8
Ferritin and haemosiderin	Liver	410
	Spleen	48
	Bone marrow	300

Data from: Jacobs A, Worwood M 1982 In: Hardisty R M, Weatherall D J (eds) Blood and its disorders. Blackwell Scientific, Oxford, ch. 5.

Tetracycline forms an insoluble iron chelate, resulting in impaired uptake of both substances.

The amount of iron in the diet and the various factors affecting its availability are thus important determinants in absorption, but the regulation of iron absorption is a function of the intestinal mucosa, influenced by the body's iron stores. Because there is no mechanism whereby iron excretion is regulated, the absorptive mechanism has a central role in iron balance since it is the sole mechanism by which body iron is controlled.

The site of iron absorption is the duodenum and upper jejunum, and absorption is a two-stage process involving first a rapid uptake across the brush border and then transfer into the plasma from the interior of the epithelial cells. The second stage, which is rate limiting, is energy dependent. Haem iron in the diet is absorbed as intact haem and the iron is released in the mucosal cell by the action of haem oxidase. Non-haem iron is absorbed in the ferrous state. Within the cell, ferrous iron is oxidised to ferric iron, which is bound to an intracellular carrier, a transferrin-like protein; the iron is then either held in storage in the mucosal cell as ferritin (if body stores of iron are high) or passed on to the plasma (if iron stores are low).

Iron is carried in the plasma bound to *transferrin*, a β-globulin with two binding sites for ferric iron, which is normally only 30% saturated. Plasma contains 4 mg iron at any one time, but the daily turnover is about 30 mg (Fig. 21.1). Most of the iron that enters the plasma is derived from mononuclear phagocytes, following the degradation of time-expired erythrocytes. Intestinal absorption and mobilisation of iron from storage depots contribute only small amounts. Most of the iron that leaves the plasma each day is used for haemoglobin synthesis by red cell precursors. These cells have receptors that bind transferrin molecules, releasing them after the iron has been taken up.

Iron is stored in two forms—soluble *ferritin* and insoluble *haemosiderin*. Ferritin is found in all cells, the mononuclear phagocytes of liver, spleen and bone marrow containing especially high concentrations. It is also present in plasma. The precursor of ferritin, *apoferritin*, is a large protein of molecular weight 450 000, composed of 24 identical polypeptide subunits that enclose a cavity in which up to 4500 iron molecules can be stored. Apoferritin takes up ferrous iron, oxidises it and deposits the ferric iron in its core. In this form, it constitutes ferritin, the primary storage form of iron, from which the iron is most readily available. The lifespan of this iron-laden protein is only a few days. Haemosiderin is a degraded form of ferritin in which the iron cores of several ferritin molecules have aggregated, following partial disintegration of the outer protein shells.

The ferritin in plasma has virtually no iron associated with it. It is in equilibrium with the storage ferritin in cells and its concentration in plasma provides an estimate of total body iron stores.

The body has no means of actively excreting iron. Small amounts leave the body through *desquamation* (peeling off) of mucosal cells containing ferritin, and even smaller amounts leave in the bile, sweat and urine. A total of about 1 mg is lost daily. Iron balance is, therefore, critically dependent on the active absorption mechanism in the intestinal mucosa. This absorption is influenced by the iron stores in the body, but the precise mechanism of this control is still a matter of debate: the amount of ferritin in the intestinal mucosa may be important, as may the balance between ferritin and the transferrin-like carrier molecule in these cells. The daily movement of iron in the body is illustrated in Figure 21.1.

The clinical use of iron is given in the box below.

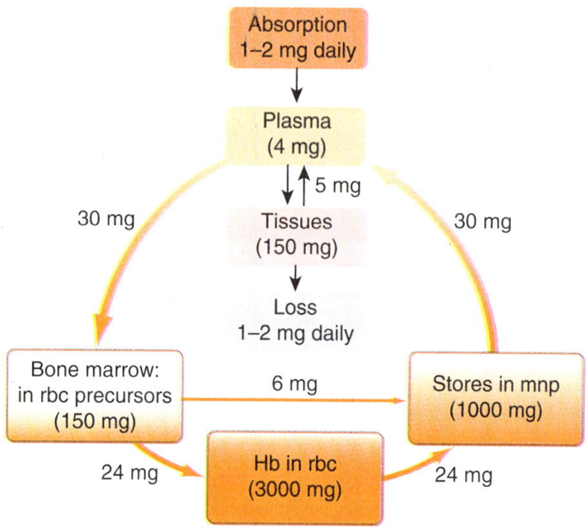

Fig. 21.1 Schematic illustration of the distribution of iron in the body. The quantities by the arrows indicate the usual amounts transferred each day. (Hb, haemoglobin; rbc, red blood cells; mnp, mononuclear phagocytes.)

Administration

Iron is usually given orally but may be given parenterally in special circumstances.

Several different preparations of ferrous iron salts are available for oral administration. The main one is **ferrous sulfate**, which has an elemental iron content of 200 μg/mg. Others are ferrous

Clinical uses of iron

- To treat iron deficiency anaemia, which can be caused by:
  - —chronic blood loss (e.g. with menorrhagia, hook worm, colon cancer)
  - —increased demand (e.g. in pregnancy and early infancy)
  - —inadequate dietary intake (uncommon in developed countries)
  - —inadequate absorption (e.g. following gastrectomy).

succinate, ferrous gluconate and ferrous fumarate. These are all absorbed to a comparable extent.

Parenteral iron is rarely given but may be necessary in individuals who are not able to absorb oral iron because of malabsorption syndromes or as a result of surgical procedures or inflammatory conditions involving the gastrointestinal tract. The preparations used are iron-dextran or iron-sorbitol, both given by deep intramuscular injection. **Iron-dextran** (but not **iron-sorbitol**) can be given by slow intravenous infusion, but this method of administration should only be used if absolutely necessary because of the risk of anaphylactoid reactions.

Unwanted effects

The unwanted effects of oral iron administration are dose related and include nausea, abdominal cramps and diarrhoea.

Acute iron toxicity, usually seen in young children who have swallowed attractively coloured iron tablets in mistake for sweets, occurs after ingestion of large quantities of iron salts. This can result in severe necrotising gastritis with vomiting, haemorrhage and diarrhoea, followed by circulatory collapse.

Chronic iron toxicity or iron overload is virtually always caused by conditions other than ingestion of iron salts, for example chronic haemolytic anaemias such as the thalassaemias (a large group of genetic disorders of globin chain synthesis) or repeated blood transfusions.

The treatment of acute and chronic iron toxicity involves the use of iron chelators, such as **desferrioxamine**. This is not absorbed from the gut but is nonetheless given intragastrically following acute overdose (to bind iron in the bowel lumen and prevent its absorption) as well as intramuscularly and, if necessary, intravenously. In severe poisoning, it is given by slow intravenous infusion. Desferrioxamine forms a complex with ferric iron, and, unlike unbound iron, this is excreted in the urine. A new, orally absorbed iron chelator, **deferiprone** (L1), was recently licensed in the UK to treat iron overload in patients with thalassaemia major, in whom desferrioxamine is contraindicated or not tolerated. Agranulocytosis and other blood dyscrasias have been described, so its use requires careful monitoring.

> **Iron**
>
> - Iron is important for the synthesis of haemoglobin; it is also present in myoglobin, and in the cytochromes and other enzymes.
> - Ferric iron (Fe^{3+}) must be converted to ferrous iron (Fe^{2+}) for absorption in the gastrointestinal tract.
> - Absorption involves active transport into mucosal cells in jejunum and upper ileum, from where it can be transported into the plasma and/or stored intracellularly as ferritin.
> - Total body iron is controlled exclusively by absorption; in iron deficiency, more is transported into plasma than is stored as ferritin in jejunal mucosa.
> - Iron loss occurs mainly by sloughing of ferritin-containing mucosal cells; iron is not excreted in the urine.
> - Iron in plasma is bound to transferrin, and most is used for erythropoiesis. Some is stored as ferritin in other tissues. Iron from time-expired erythrocytes enters the plasma for re-use.
> - The main therapeutic preparation is ferrous sulfate.
> - Unwanted effects include gastrointestinal disturbances. Severe toxic effects occur if large doses are ingested; these can be countered by desferrioxamine, an iron chelator.

FOLIC ACID AND VITAMIN B_{12}

Vitamin B_{12} and **folic acid** are necessary constituents of the human diet, being essential for DNA synthesis and, consequently, for cell proliferation. Their biochemical actions are interdependent (see below), and treatment of vitamin B_{12} deficiency with folic acid corrects some, but not all, of the features of vitamin B_{12} deficiency. Deficiency of either vitamin B_{12} or folic acid affects tissues with a rapid cell turnover, particularly bone marrow, but vitamin B_{12} deficiency also causes important disorders of nerves, which are not corrected (or may even be made worse) by treatment with folic acid. Deficiency of either vitamin causes *megaloblastic haemopoiesis* in which there is disordered erythroblast differentiation and defective erythropoiesis in the bone marrow. Large abnormal erythrocyte precursors appear in the marrow, each with a high RNA:DNA ratio as a result of decreased DNA synthesis. The circulating erythrocytes ('macrocytes') are large fragile cells, often distorted in shape. Mild leucopenia and thrombocytopenia usually accompany the anaemia, and the nuclei of polymorphonuclear leucocytes are abnormal (hypersegmented). Neurological disorders caused by deficiency of B_{12} include *peripheral neuropathy* and *dementia*, as well as *subacute combined** *degeneration* of the spinal cord.

Folic acid deficiency is caused by dietary insufficiency, especially in settings of increased demand (e.g. during pregnancy, or because of chronic haemolysis in patients with haemoglobinopathies). Vitamin B_{12} deficiency, however, is usually caused by decreased absorption, caused either by a lack of intrinsic factor (see below) or conditions that interfere with its absorption in the terminal ileum, for example resection of diseased ileum in patients with Crohn's disease (a chronic inflammatory bowel disease that can affect this part of the gut). Intrinsic factor is a glycoprotein secreted by the stomach and is essential for vitamin B_{12} absorption. It is lacking in patients with *pernicious anaemia* and in individuals who have had total gastrectomies. In pernicious anaemia there is atrophic gastritis caused by autoimmune injury of the stomach, and antibodies to gastric parietal cells are often present in the plasma of such patients.

*'Combined' because the lateral columns as well as the dorsal columns are involved, giving rise to motor as well as sensory symptoms.

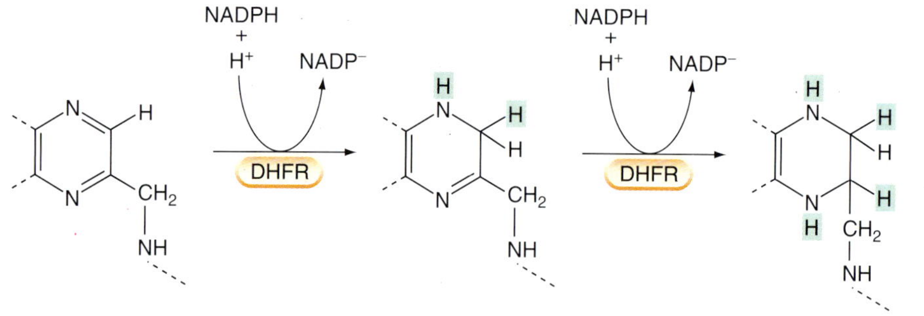

Fig. 21.2 Reduction of folate (F) to dihydrofolate (FH_2) then to tetrahydrofolate (FH_4) by the enzyme dihydrofolate reductase (DHFR).

FOLIC ACID

Folic acid (pteroylglutamic acid) consists of a pteridine ring, *para*-aminobenzoic acid and glutamic acid. Some aspects of folate structure and metabolism are dealt with in Chapters 45 and 50, because several important antibacterial and anticancer drugs are antimetabolites that interfere with folate synthesis in microorganisms. Liver and green vegetables are rich sources of folate. In healthy non-pregnant adults the daily requirement is about 200 μg daily, but this is increased during pregnancy.

Actions

Dihydrofolate (FH_2) and tetrahydrofolate (FH_4) act as carriers and donors of methyl groups (1-carbon transfers) in a number of important metabolic pathways. The latter is essential for DNA synthesis as cofactor in the synthesis of purines and pyrimidines. It is also necessary for reactions involved in amino acid metabolism. For activity, folate must be in the FH_4 form, in which it is maintained by *dihydrofolate reductase*. This enzyme reduces dietary folic acid to FH_4 and also regenerates FH_4 from FH_2 produced from FH_4 during thymidylate synthesis (see Figs 21.2 and 21.3). Folate antagonists act by inhibiting dihydrofolate reductase (see also Chs 45 and 50).

Folates are especially important for the conversion of deoxyuridylate monophosphate to deoxythymidylate monophosphate. This is rate limiting in mammalian DNA synthesis and is catalysed by thymidylate synthetase, with folate acting as methyl donor (Fig. 21.3).

The clinical use of folic acid is given in the box.

Pharmacokinetic aspects

Folates in food are in the form of polyglutamates. These are converted to monoglutamates before absorption and are transported in blood as such. They are converted back into polyglutamates, which are considerably more active than monoglutamates, in the tissues. Therapeutically, folic acid is given orally (or, in exceptional circumstances, parenterally) and is absorbed in the ileum. Methyl-FH_4 is the form in which folate is usually carried in blood and which enters cells. It is functionally inactive until it is demethylated in a vitamin B_{12}-dependent reaction (see below). This is because unlike FH_2, FH_4 and formyl-FH_4, methyl-FH_4 is a poor substrate for polyglutamate formation. This has relevance for the effect of vitamin B_{12} deficiency on folate metabolism, as is explained below. Folate is taken up into hepatocytes and bone marrow cells by active transport. Within the cells, folic acid is reduced and formylated before being converted to the active polyglutamate form. **Folinic acid**, a synthetic FH_4, is converted much more rapidly to the polyglutamate form.

The clinical use of folic acid is given in the box on p. 335.

Unwanted effects

Unwanted effects do not occur even with large doses of folic acid—except possibly in the presence of vitamin B_{12} deficiency, because if the vitamin deficiency is treated with folic acid, the

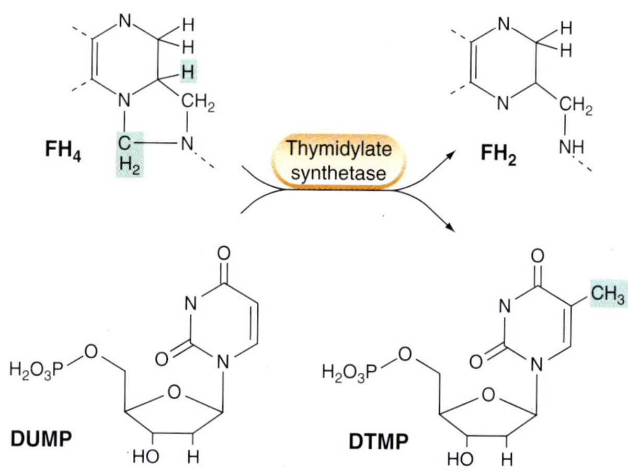

Fig. 21.3 The synthesis of 2-deoxythymidylate (DTMP). DTMP is synthesised by the transfer of a methyl group from tetrahydrofolate (FH_4) to 2-deoxyuridylate (DUMP), the FH_4 being oxidised to dihydrofolate (FH_2) in the process.

Clinical uses of folic acid and hydroxocobalamin

Folic acid

- Treatment of megaloblastic anaemia resulting from folate deficiency, which can be caused by:
  - —poor diet (common in alcoholics)
  - —malabsorption syndromes
  - —drugs, e.g. phenytoin.
- Treatment or prevention of toxicity from methotrexate, a folate antagonist, see Ch. 50
- prophylactically in individuals at hazard from developing folate deficiency, for example:
  - —pregnant women and before conception (especially if there is a risk of birth defects)
  - —premature infants
  - —patients with severe chronic haemolytic anaemias, including haemoglobinopathies (e.g. sickle cell anaemia).

Hydroxocobalamin (vitamin B_{12}) is used:

- Treatment of pernicious anaemia and other causes of vitamin B_{12} deficiency.
- Prophylactically after surgical operations that remove the site of production of intrinsic factor (the stomach) or of vitamin B_{12} absorption (the terminal ileum).

blood picture may improve and give the appearance of cure while the neurological lesions get worse. It is, therefore, important to determine whether a megaloblastic anaemia is caused by a folate or a vitamin B_{12} deficiency. This could be important in the setting of supplementation of bread with folate, which is used in the USA as a public health measure to reduce the number of neural tube defects. There is a theoretical risk of precipitating neuropathy in the small group of people with undiagnosed pernicious anaemia, by such measures.

VITAMIN B_{12}

Vitamin B_{12} is a complex cobalamin compound. The vitamin B_{12} used medically is **hydroxocobalamin**. The principal dietary sources of vitamin B_{12} are meat (particularly liver), eggs and dairy products. All cobalamins, dietary and therapeutic, must be converted to *methylcobalamin* (methyl-B_{12}) or *5′-deoxyadenosylcobalamin* (ado-B_{12}) for activity in the body. The average daily diet in Western Europe contains 5–25 µg of vitamin B_{12} and the daily requirement is 2–3 µg. Absorption requires intrinsic factor (p. 333), which forms a one-to-one complex with vitamin B_{12}. The stomach secretes a huge excess of intrinsic factor—what normally limits absorption is the amount the ileum is capable of absorbing. Vitamin B_{12} is taken up by active transport, intrinsic factor being removed on the way.

Vitamin B_{12} is carried in the plasma by binding proteins called *transcobalamins* (TCs). The vitamin is stored mainly in the liver, the total amount in the body being about 4 mg. This store is so large compared with the daily requirement that if vitamin B_{12} absorption is stopped suddenly—as after a total gastrectomy—it takes 2–4 years for evidence of deficiency to become manifest.

Actions

Vitamin B_{12} is required for two main biochemical reactions in humans:

- the conversion of methyl-FH_4 to FH_4
- isomerisation of methylmalonyl-CoA to succinyl-CoA.

The conversion of methyl-FH_4 to FH_4

The role of vitamin B_{12} in folate coenzyme synthesis is illustrated in Figure 21.4. It is through these mechanisms that the metabolic activities of vitamin B_{12} and folic acid are linked and implicated in the synthesis of DNA. It is also through this pathway that folate/vitamin B_{12} treatment can lower plasma homocysteine concentration. Since increased homocysteine concentrations may have undesirable vascular effects (Ch. 18), this has potential therapeutic implications.

▼ The reaction involves conversion of both methyl-FH_4 to FH_4 and homocysteine to methionine. The enzyme that accomplishes this is homocysteine–methionine methyltransferase; the reaction requires

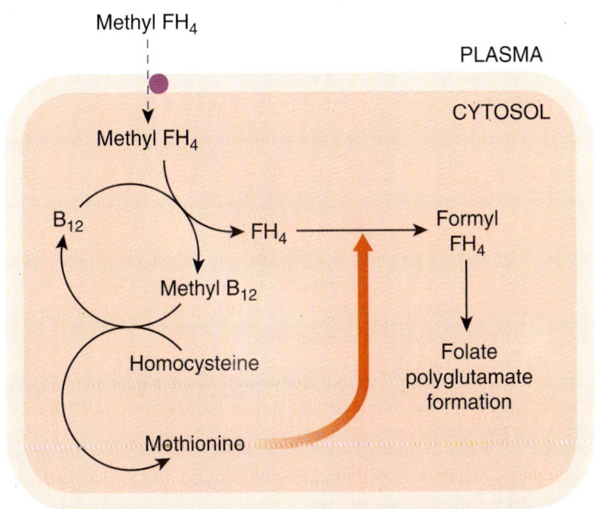

Fig. 21.4 The role of vitamin B_{12} in the synthesis of folate polyglutamate. Methyltetrahydrofolate (Methyl FH_4) enters cells by active transport. The methyl group is transferred to homocysteine to form methionine via vitamin B_{12}, which is bound to the apoenzyme homocysteine–methionine methyltransferase. (Vitamin B_{12} is shown as 'B_{12}' and as 'methyl B_{12}', but the enzyme is not shown.) Methionine is important in the donation of formate (shown by the curved red arrow) for the conversion of tetrahydrofolate (FH_4) to formyl tetrahydrofolate (formyl FH_4), which is the preferred substrate for the formation of folate polyglutamates.

Vitamin B_{12} and folic acid

Both vitamin B_{12} and folic acid are needed for DNA synthesis. Deficiencies particularly affect erythropoiesis, causing macrocytic megaloblastic anaemia.

Folic acid

- Folic acid consists of a pteridine ring, *p*-aminobenzoic acid and a glutamate residue.
- There is active uptake into cells and reduction to tetrahydrofolate (FH_4) by dihydrofolate reductase; extra glutamates are then added.
- Folate polyglutamate is a cofactor (a carrier of one-carbon units) in the synthesis of purines and pyrimidines (especially thymidylate).

Vitamin B_{12} (hydroxocobalamin)

- Vitamin B_{12} needs an 'intrinsic factor' (a glycoprotein) secreted by gastric parietal cells for absorption in terminal ileum. It is stored in the liver.
- It is required for:
  —conversion of methyl-FH_4 (inactive form of FH_4) to active formyl-FH_4 which, after polyglutamation, is a cofactor in the synthesis of purines and pyrimidines (see above)
  —isomerisation of methylmalonyl-CoA to succinyl-CoA.
- Deficiency occurs most often in pernicious anaemia, which results from malabsorption caused by lack of intrinsic factor from the stomach. It causes neurological disease as well as anaemia.
- Vitamin B_{12} is given by injection to treat pernicious anaemia.

vitamin B_{12} as cofactor and methyl-FH_4 as methyl donor. Methyl-FH_4 donates the methyl group to B_{12}, the cofactor. The methyl group is then transferred to homocysteine to form methionine (Fig. 21.4). This vitamin-B_{12}-dependent reaction generates active FH_4 from inactive methyl-FH_4 and converts homocysteine to methionine.

Vitamin B_{12} deficiency thus traps folate in the inactive methyl-FH_4 form, thereby depleting the folate polyglutamate coenzymes needed for DNA synthesis (see above).

Vitamin B_{12}-dependent methionine synthesis also affects the synthesis of folate polyglutamate coenzymes by an additional mechanism. The preferred substrate for polyglutamate synthesis is formyl-FH_4, and the conversion of FH_4 to formyl-FH_4 requires a formate donor such as methionine.

Isomerisation of methylmalonyl-CoA to succinyl-CoA

This isomerisation reaction is part of a route by which propionate is converted to succinate. Through this pathway, cholesterol, odd-chain fatty acids, some amino acids and thymine can be used for gluconeogenesis or for energy production via the tricarboxylic acid cycle. Ado-B_{12} is an essential cofactor, so methylmalonyl-CoA accumulates in vitamin B_{12} deficiency. This distorts fatty acid synthesis in neural tissue and may be the basis of neuropathy in vitamin B_{12} deficiency.

Administration and pharmacokinetic aspects

When vitamin B_{12} is used therapeutically (as hydroxocobalamin), it is almost always given by intramuscular injection, since, as explained above, vitamin B_{12} deficiency is a result of malabsorption. Plasma transport and distribution of therapeutically administered vitamin B_{12} are described above (p. 335).

Patients with pernicious anaemia require lifelong therapy. Unwanted effects do not occur. Clinical use of vitamin B_{12} is summarised in the box.

HAEMOPOIETIC GROWTH FACTORS

Every 60 seconds, a human being must generate about 120 million granulocytes and 150 million erythrocytes, as well as numerous mononuclear cells and platelets. The cells responsible for this remarkable productivity are derived from a relatively small number of self-renewing, pluripotent stem cells laid down during embryogenesis. Maintenance of haemopoiesis necessitates a balance between self-renewal on the one hand, and differentiation into the various types of blood cell on the other. The factors involved in controlling this balance are the *haemopoietic growth factors*, which direct the division and maturation of the progeny of these cells down eight possible lines of development (Fig 21.5). These cytokine growth factors are glycoproteins with high potency, acting at concentrations of 10^{-12}–10^{-10} mol/l. They are present at very low concentrations in plasma, under basal conditions, but their concentrations can increase by 1000-fold or more within hours in response to stimulation. *Erythropoietin* regulates the red cell line and the signal for its production is blood loss and/or low tissue oxygen tension. The CSFs regulate the myeloid divisions of the white cell line, and the main stimulus for their production is infection (see also Ch. 15).

The genes for several haemopoietic factors have been cloned, and recombinant erythropoietin (**epoetin**), recombinant granulocyte colony-stimulating factor (G-CSF: **filgrastim,** lenograstim) and granulocyte–macrophage colony-stimulating factor (GM-CSF: **molgrasmostim**) are being used clinically; **thrombopoietin** is in development. Some of the other haemopoietic growth factors (e.g. interleukin-1, interleukin-2 and various other cytokines) are covered in Chapter 15.

ERYTHROPOIETIN

Erythropoietin is produced in juxtatubular cells in the kidney and also in macrophages; its action is to stimulate committed erythroid progenitor cells to proliferate and generate erythrocytes (Fig. 21.5). Two forms of recombinant human erythropoietin, **epoetin alfa** and **epoetin beta** are available. These are clinically indistinguishable and are referred to here as simply as epoetin.

The clinical use of epoietin is given in the box (p. 337).

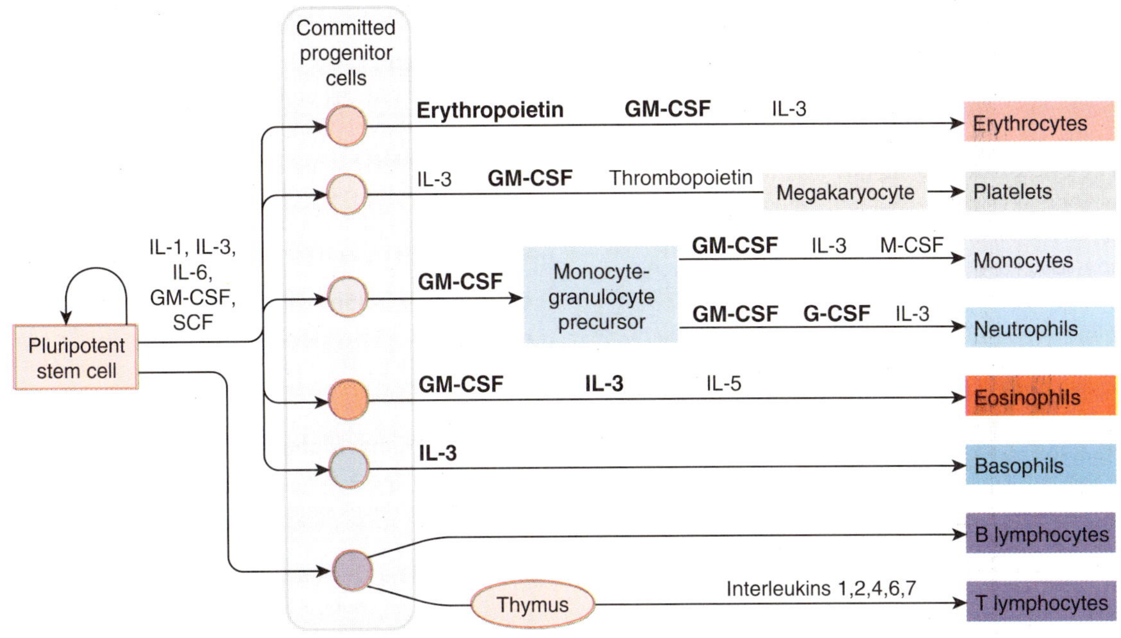

Fig. 21.5 Simplified diagram of the role of endogenous haemopoietic growth factors in blood cell differentiation. The factors shown in **bold** are in clinical use under different names (see text). Most T cells generated in the thymus die by apoptosis; those that emerge are either CD4 or CD8 T cells. The colours used for the mature blood cells reflect how they appear in common staining preparations (and after which some are named). (CSF, colony-stimulating factor; GM-CSF, granulocyte–macrophage CSF; G-CSF, granulocyte CSF; M-CSF, macrophage CSF; IL-3, interleukin-3, or multi-CSF; IL-1, interleukin-1; SCF, stem cell factor.) (See also Ch. 15.)

Pharmacokinetic aspects

Epoetin can be given intravenously, subcutaneously or intraperitoneally, the response being greatest after subcutaneous injection and fastest after intravenous injection.

Unwanted effects

Transient influenza-like symptoms are common. Hypertension is also common and can cause encephalopathy with headache, disorientation and sometimes convulsions. Iron deficiency can be induced because more iron is required for the enhanced erythropoiesis. Blood viscosity increases as the haematocrit (i.e. the fraction of the blood that is occupied by red blood cells) rises, increasing the risk of thrombosis, especially during dialysis.

Clinical uses of epoietin

- Anaemia of chronic renal failure
- Anaemia during chemotherapy for cancer
- Prevention of the anaemia that occurs in premature infants
- To increase the yield of autologous blood before donation
- Anaemia of AIDS (which is exacerbated by zidovudine treatment)
- Anaemia of chronic inflammatory conditions such as rheumatoid arthritis (investigational).

COLONY-STIMULATING FACTORS

The CSFs are so called because they were found to stimulate the formation of maturing colonies of leucocytes in semi-solid medium in vitro. CSFs are classified as cytokines (see Ch. 15). They not only stimulate particular committed progenitor cells to proliferate (Fig. 21.5) but also cause irreversible differentiation. The responding precursor cells have membrane receptors to CSFs and may express receptors for more than one factor, thus permitting collaborative interactions between factors.

GM-CSF is produced by many cell types and influences at least five of the eight lines of blood cell development. G-CSF is produced mainly by monocytes, fibroblasts and endothelial cells, and it controls primarily the development of neutrophils.

Actions

GM-CSF stimulates the development of the progenitors of neutrophils, monocytes, eosinophils, and (under some circumstances) megakaryocytes and erythrocytes (Fig. 21.5). It also enhances the functional activity and survival of the mature cells. GM-CSF may increase the production of other cytokines.

Clinical uses of the colony-stimulating factors (CSFs)

CSFs are used in specialist centres:

- to reduce the severity and duration of the neutropenia induced by cytotoxic drugs during:
  - —conventional anticancer chemotherapy
  - —intensive courses of chemotherapy that damage the haemopoietic tissue, necessitating autologous bone marrow rescue
  - —following bone marrow transplant
- to stimulate release into the circulation of progenitor cells, which can then be harvested and infused with, or instead of, bone marrow cells after high-dose, intensive chemotherapy
- to expand the number of harvested progenitor cells ex vivo before re-infusing them
- for persistent neutropenia in advanced HIV infection
- they may have a role in treatment of aplastic anaemia.

Haemopoietic growth factors

Erythropoietin
- Regulates red cell production.
- Is given intravenously, subcutaneously, intraperitoneally.
- Can cause transient 'flu-like symptoms, hypertension, iron deficiency and increased blood viscosity.
- Is available as epoietin.

Granulocyte colony-stimulating factor (G-CSF)
- Stimulates neutrophil progenitors.
- Is available as filgrastim; it is given intravenously or subcutaneously.

Granulocyte-macrophage colony-stimulating factor (GM-CSF)
- Stimulates development of many types of progenitor cell.
- Is available as molgramostim and is given intravenously, subcutaneously.
- Can cause fever, rashes, bone pain, hypotension, gastrointestinal symptoms and arterial oxygen desaturation.

G-CSF acts only on the neutrophil line (Fig. 21.5)—increasing the proliferation and maturation of neutrophils, stimulating their release from bone marrow storage pools and enhancing their function.

The clinical use of CSFs is given in the box.

Pharmacokinetic aspects and unwanted effects

Both GM-CSF and G-CSF can be given either subcutaneously or by intravenous infusion.

Both CSFs are well tolerated. Bone pain occurs in 10–20% of patients.

GM-CSF frequently produces fever and can cause skin rashes, muscle pain and lethargy. There may be pain and reddening at the site of the injection. With intravenous infusion, a syndrome of flushing, hypotension, tachycardia, breathlessness, nausea and vomiting and arterial oxygen desaturation has occurred; this is reversed by giving oxygen and intravenous fluids. At high doses (> 20 mg/kg per day) pleural and pericardial effusions, venous thrombosis and pulmonary embolism have been reported.

G-CSF has produced mild dysuria (rare) and reversible abnormalities in liver function tests. Vasculitis has been reported with long-term use.

THROMBOPOIETIN

Thrombopoietin stimulates proliferation of the progenitor cells of the platelet lineage and strikingly increases platelet production. Recombinant thrombopoietin is being tested clinically.

REFERENCES AND FURTHER READING

Andrews N C 1999 Disorders of iron metabolism N Engl J Med 341: 1986–1995

Clarke R, Armitage J 2000 Vitamin supplements and cardiovascular risk: review of the randomized trials of homocysteine-lowering vitamin supplements. Sem Thromb Hemostas 26: 341–348

Dale D C 1995 Where now for colony-stimulating factors? Lancet 346: 135–136

Finch C A, Hueber S H 1982 Perspectives in iron metabolism. N Engl J Med 306: 1520–1528 (*Good background article on iron*)

Fishman S M, Christian P, West K P 2000 The role of vitamins in the prevention and control of anaemia. Public Health Nutrit 3: 125–150

Frewin R, Henson A, Provan D 1997 ABC of clinical haematology: iron deficiency anaemia. Br Med J 314: 360–363

Goodenough L T, Monk T G, Andriole G L 1997 Erythropoietin therapy. N Engl J Med 336: 933–938 (*A useful 'Current Concepts' article*)

Hoelzer D 1997 Haemopoietic growth factors—not whether, but when and where. N Engl J Med 336: 1822–1824 (*An edifying editorial comment*)

Hoffbrand A V, Herbert V 1999 Nutritional anemias. Semin Hematol 36(suppl 7): 13–23

Levin J 1997 Thrombopoietin—clinically realised? N Engl J Med 336: 434–436 (*A useful editorial*)

Lieschke G J, Burges A W 1992 Granulocyte colony-stimulating factor and granulocyte-macrophage colony-stimulating factor. N Engl J Med 327: 1–35, 99–106 (*Worthwhile, comprehensive reviews*)

Lieu P T, Heiskala M, Peterson P A, Yang Y 2001 The roles of iron in health and disease. Mol Aspects Med 22: 1–87

Nimer S D 1997 Platelet stimulating agents—off the launch pad. Nature Med 3: 154–155 (*Thrombopoietic growth factors prove useful in clinical trials*)

Petros W P 1996 Colony-stimulating factors. In: Chabner B A, Longo D L

(eds) Cancer chemotherapy and biotherapy, 2nd edn. Lippincott-Raven, Philadelphia, pp. 639–654 (*Covers mechanism of action, biological effects and clinical pharmacology*)
Provan D, Weatherall D 2000 Red cells II: acquired anaemias and polycythaemia. Lancet 355: 1260–1268
Refsum H 2001 Folate, vitamin B_{12} and homocysteine in relation to birth defects and pregnancy outcome. Br J Nutr 85 (Suppl 2): S109–S113
Spivak J L 1993 Recombinant erythropoietin. Annu Rev Med 44: 243–253
Steinberg S E 1984 Mechanisms of folate homeostasis. Am J Physiol 246: G319–G324 (*Good background article on folate*)
Toh B-H, van Driel I R, Gleeson P A 1997 Pernicious anaemia. N Engl J Med 337: 1441–1448 (*Immunopathogenesis of pernicious anaemia; excellent figures*)
Wald N J, Bower C 1994 Folic acid. pernicious anaemia, and prevention of neural tube defects. Lancet 343: 307

22 The respiratory system

Overview 340

The regulation of respiration 340
- The regulation of the musculature, blood vessels and glands of the airways 340

Disorders of respiration 341
- Bronchial asthma 341
- Drugs used to treat asthma 345
- Severe acute asthma (status asthmaticus) 349
- Chronic obstructive pulmonary disease 349
- Cough 350
- Drugs used for cough 350

OVERVIEW

In this chapter we cover some basic aspects of the physiology of the respiratory system before going on to the main disorders of respiratory function—asthma, chronic obstructive pulmonary disease and cough—and the drugs used in their treatment. We devote most of the chapter to asthma, dealing first with the factors involved in its pathogenesis and then the main drugs used in treatment—the bronchdilators and anti-inflammatory agents.

THE REGULATION OF RESPIRATION

Respiration is controlled by spontaneous rhythmic discharges from the respiratory centre in the medulla, modulated by input from pontine and higher central nervous system (CNS) centres and vagal afferents from the lungs. Various chemical factors affect the respiratory centre including the blood partial pressure of carbon dioxide ($P\text{CO}_2$), by an action on medullary chemoreceptors, and the blood partial pressure of oxygen ($P\text{O}_2$), by an action on the chemoreceptors in the aortic and carotid bodies.

A moderate degree of voluntary control can be superimposed on the automatic regulation of breathing, and this implies connections between the cortex and the motor neurons innervating the muscles of respiration. Bulbar poliomyelitis and certain lesions in the brainstem result in loss of the automatic regulation of respiration without loss of voluntary regulation. (This has been referred to as 'Ondine's curse'. Ondine was a water nymph who fell in love with a mortal. When he was unfaithful to her, the king of the water nymphs put a curse on him—that he must stay awake in order to breathe. When exhaustion finally supervened and he fell asleep, he died.)

THE REGULATION OF THE MUSCULATURE, BLOOD VESSELS AND GLANDS OF THE AIRWAYS

In the normal neurohumoral control of the airways, the efferent pathways are the acetylcholine-releasing parasympathetic nerves, the noradrenaline-releasing sympathetic nerves, circulating adrenaline and the non-noradrenergic, non-cholinergic (NANC) inhibitory neurons. The afferent pathways include three different types of sensory receptor, described below.

In pathological conditions such as asthma and bronchitis, other mediators—the inflammatory mediators (see Ch. 15) and, possibly, the NANC contractile mediators—have a significant role.

The signal transduction mechanisms for the various receptors mediating contraction and relaxation of bronchiolar muscle are discussed by Dale & Hirst (1993).

The tone of the bronchial muscle affects the airways resistance, and in asthma and bronchitis the state of the mucosa and the activity of the glands also contribute. The airways resistance can be measured indirectly by instruments which record the volume or flow of forced expiration. FEV_1 is the forced expiratory volume in 1 second. The peak expiratory flow rate (PEFR) is the maximal flow (expressed as litres per minute) after a full inhalation.

EFFERENT PATHWAYS

Parasympathetic innervation

Parasympathetic ganglia are embedded in the walls of the bronchi and bronchioles, and the postganglionic fibres innervate airway smooth muscle, vascular smooth muscle and glands. There are three types of muscarinic (M) receptors present (see Ch. 10, Table 10.1). M_1-receptors are localised in ganglia, on the postsynaptic cells, and their stimulation facilitates neurotransmission mediated by acetylcholine acting on nicotinic receptors. M_2-receptors are inhibitory 'autoreceptors' mediating negative feedback effects on acetylcholine release by postganglionic cholinergic nerves. M_3-receptors are found on bronchial smooth muscle and glands and mediate contraction of the former and secretion from the latter. Stimulation of the vagus causes bronchoconstriction—mainly in the larger airways. The possible clinical relevance of the heterogeneity of muscarinic receptors in the airways is discussed below on page 347.

Sympathetic innervation and catecholamines

Sympathetic nerves innervate blood vessels and glands, the released noradrenaline causing constriction of the former and inhibiting secretion by the latter (Ch. 11). There is no sympathetic innervation of the bronchial smooth muscle; all 'sympathetic' *effects caused by circulating catecholamines.*

Autoradiography shows that β-adrenoceptors occur in the smooth muscle, the epithelium and glands, and also, in very large numbers, in the alveoli (though what they are doing in this last site is anybody's guess). They are also found on mast cells. In humans, virtually all the β-adrenoceptors in the airways are β_2; those in the alveoli are both β_1 and β_2.

Stimulation of the airway β-adrenoceptors with drugs results in relaxation of smooth muscle, inhibition of mediator release from mast cells and increased mucociliary clearance.

Agonists at α-adrenoceptors have no effect on normal airways but cause contraction if the airways are diseased.

Non-noradrenergic, non-cholinergic mediators

There is evidence that airway function is influenced by neuronal mediators other than acetylcholine and noradrenaline; these are referred to as NANC mediators (p. 130).

The inhibitory NANC mediator—the main neurotransmitter relaxant in the airways—is now believed to be nitric oxide (NO; see Ch. 14). Inducible nitric oxide synthase (NOS) and both forms of constitutive NOS are present in human airways; the inducible form is implicated in asthma and other types of airway inflammation.

The stimulant NANC mediators are thought to be excitatory neuropeptides* (see Chs 13 and 15) that are released from sensory C fibres when stimulated by inflammatory mediators and irritant chemicals. The main neuropeptides in the lung are substance P (which increases vascular permeability and induces mucus secretion), and neurokinin A (a potent spasmogen).

The inflammatory mediators are dealt with below.

SENSORY RECEPTORS AND AFFERENT PATHWAYS

The receptors involved in the central regulation of respiration by the respiratory centre are the slowly adapting stretch receptors. In addition, there are unmyelinated sensory C fibres and rapidly adapting irritant receptors associated with myelinated vagal fibres.

*These peptides are considered to be the mediators of neurogenic inflammation, which may also be a contributing factor in various inflammatory conditions

Regulation of airway muscle, blood vessels and glands

Afferent pathways

- Irritant receptors and C-fibres respond to exogenous chemicals, inflammatory mediators and physical stimuli (e.g. cold air) by causing bronchoconstriction and mucus secretion through acetylcholine release in the upper airway and release of excitatory neuropeptides in the lower.

Efferent pathways

- The parasympathetic nerves mediate bronchial constriction and mucus secretion through an action on muscarinic M_3-receptors.
- Sympathetic nerves innervate blood vessels (causing constriction) and glands (inhibiting secretion), but not airway smooth muscle.
- Circulating adrenaline acts on β_2-adrenoceptors to relax airway smooth muscle.
- The main neurotransmitter causing relaxation of airway smooth muscle is the NANC (non-adrenergic, non-cholinergic) inhibitory transmitter, thought to be nitric oxide.
- NANC excitatory transmitters are peptides released from sensory neurons.

Chemical stimuli, acting on irritant receptors on myelinated fibres in the upper airways and/or C-fibre receptors in the lower airways, cause coughing, bronchoconstriction and an increase in mucus secretion. The stimuli that produce these effects include both exogenous agents, such as ammonia, sulfur dioxide, cigarette smoke and the experimental tool capsaicin (Ch. 40), and endogenous stimuli such as the inflammatory mediators.

DISORDERS OF RESPIRATION

Two of the main disorders of the respiratory system are bronchial asthma and cough. Others, less susceptible to treatment, are chronic bronchitis, with resultant chronic obstructive airway disease, and the adult respiratory distress syndrome

BRONCHIAL ASTHMA

Asthma may be loosely defined as a condition in which there is recurrent 'reversible' obstruction of the airflow in the airways in response to stimuli which are not in themselves noxious and which do not affect non-asthmatic subjects. Reversal of the obstruction generally requires drug treatment. This contrasts with the obstructive airway disease mentioned above, which is not reversible. The condition affects over 5–10% of the population in industrialised countries. Most authorities agree that it is increasing in prevalence and severity.

THE CHARACTERISTICS OF ASTHMA

Asthma may be chronic or acute.

In chronic* asthma, the individual has intermittent attacks of dyspnoea (disorder of breathing), wheezing, and cough, the dyspnoea consisting of difficulty in breathing *out*. Note that the term reversible as applied to chronic asthma needs to be qualified since it is only the acute attack of dyspnoea that is reversible—the underlying pathological change may not be reversible and indeed can progress.

Acute severe asthma (also known as *status asthmaticus*) is not easily reversed. It can be fatal and requires prompt and energetic treatment. Hospitalisation may be necessary.

It is currently recognised that the characteristic features of most cases of asthma are:

- inflammatory changes in the airways associated with
- bronchial hyper-reactivity.

In allergic asthma, these are related to, and follow from, prior sensitisation.

The term bronchial hyper-reactivity (or hyper-responsiveness) refers to abnormal sensitivity to a wide range of stimuli such as irritant chemicals, cold air, stimulant drugs, etc., all of which can result in bronchoconstriction. Stimuli that cause the actual asthma attacks are many and varied and include allergens (in sensitised individuals), exercise (in which the stimulus may be cold air), respiratory infections and atmospheric pollutants such as sulfur dioxide. The non-steroidal anti-inflammatory drugs (NSAIDs), especially aspirin, can precipitate asthma in sensitive individuals.

The development of allergic asthma probably involves both genetic and environmental factors, and the asthmatic attack itself consists, in many subjects, of two main phases—the immediate phase and the late (or delayed) phase. These phases can be demonstrated by tests of FEV_1 after allergen challenge (Fig. 22.1). This division into two phases is fairly arbitrary—indeed, in some subjects, only one of the phases may be obvious—but it provides a useful basis for discussing the physiopathological changes in the bronchi as well as the locus of action and the effects of drugs used in treatment.

Numerous cells and mediators play a part in the pathogenesis of asthma and the full details of the complex events involved are still a matter of debate. The following account is, therefore, necessarily simplified. Nevertheless, it should provide a useful basis for understanding the rational use of current (and future) drugs in the treatment of asthma.

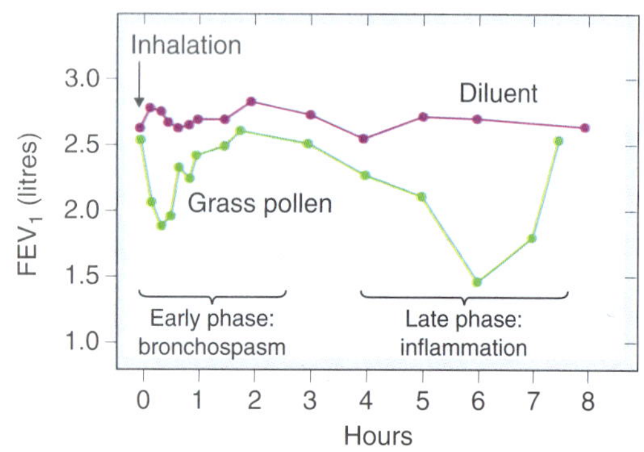

Fig. 22.1 The two phases of asthma as demonstrated by the changes in the forced expiratory volume in 1 second (FEV_1) after inhalation of grass pollen in an allergic subject. (From: Cockcroft D W 1983 Lancet ii: 253.)

THE DEVELOPMENT OF ALLERGIC ASTHMA

In allergic asthma, there is predominant activation of the T helper (Th) type 2 cell wing of the immune response (see Ch. 15 and Fig. 15.3). Sensitisation involves exposure of genetically predisposed individuals to allergens such as pollen or proteins of the house dust mite; environmental factors (e.g. atmospheric pollutants) may contribute. The allergens interact with dendritic cells and Th0 helper lymphocytes giving rise to a clone of Th2** lymphocytes, which then:

- generate a cytokine environment that switches B cells/plasma cells to the production and release of IgE***
- generate cytokines such as interleukin-5 (IL-5), which promote differentiation and activation of eosinophils
- generate various cytokines (e.g. IL-4**** and IL-13) that induce expression of IgE receptors, mainly on mast cells but also on eosinophils; IL-4 also induces endothelium to express receptors that specifically attract eosinophils.

The system thus becomes primed so that subsequent re-exposure to the relevant allergen will cause an asthmatic attack (Fig. 22.2).

The immediate phase of the asthmatic attack

In allergic asthma, the immediate phase (i.e. the initial response to allergen provocation) occurs abruptly and is mainly caused by spasm of the bronchial smooth muscle. Allergen interaction with mast cell-fixed IgE causes release of several spasmogens: histamine, the cysteinyl-leukotrienes (LTC_4 and LTD_4; Ch. 15) and prostaglandin D_2 (PGD_2).

*The term 'chronic asthma' is sometimes used rather indiscriminately to mean the propensity for repeated attacks and/or a state of semicontinuous low-grade asthma.

**A current hypothesis for this dominance of the Th2 wing is based partly on the high asthma incidence in the developed world compared with the Third World. It is known that infectious diseases such as measles, whooping cough, etc. induce potent Th1 responses and it is suggested that, in the presence of the Th1 cytokine environment that supervenes, the development of allergen-specific Th2 cells is hampered. The decrease of these childhood diseases in the developed world has allowed the development of atopy-orientated Th2 cell dominance in genetically susceptible individuals.

***Some types of asthma are not associated with the development of IgE antibodies; these are referred to as non-atopic asthma.

****The genes for both IL-4 and IL-4 receptors have been shown to be linked to asthma.

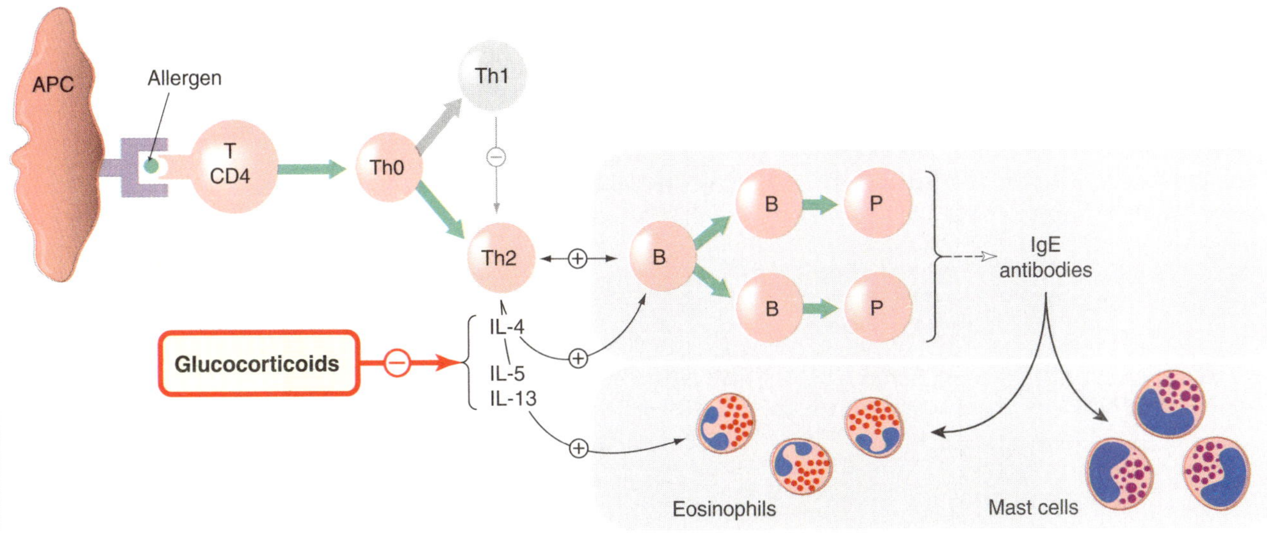

Fig. 22.2 The part played by T lymphocytes in asthma. In genetically susceptible individuals, allergen (green circle) interacts with dendritic cells and CD4+ T cells, leading to the development of Th0 helper lymphocytes, which give rise to a clone of helper Th2 lymphocytes. These then (i) generate a cytokine environment that switches B cells/plasma cells to the production and release of IgE; (ii) generate cytokines such as interleukin (IL)-5, which promote differentiation and activation of eosinophils; and (iii) generate various cytokines (e.g. IL-4 and IL-13) that induce expression of IgE receptors, mainly on mast cells but also on eosinophils. The role of these cells and cytokines in asthma is depicted in Figure 22.3. It is believed that a decrease in activation of the Th1 wing of the response (shown greyed) allows for the allergen-induced priming of the immune response for asthma. Glucocorticoids inhibit the action of the cytokines specified. (APC, antigen-presenting dendritic cell; B, B cell; Th, T helper cell; P, plasma cell.)

Bronchial asthma

- Asthma is defined as recurrent reversible airway obstruction of airflow through the airway. The asthmatic attack comprises wheezing, cough and difficulty in breathing out; the airways resistance is increased—manifest as a decrease in the 'forced expiratory volume in 1 second' (FEV_1). Severe attacks are life threatening.
- Two characteristic features are:
  - —underlying inflammatory changes in the airways
  - —underlying bronchial hyper-responsiveness, i.e. abnormal sensitivity to stimuli.
- The development of allergic asthma involves exposure of genetically sensitive individuals to allergens; these cause activation of Th2 lymphocytes, which in turn generate cytokines that promote:
  - —differentiation and activation of eosinophils
  - —IgE production and release
  - —expression of IgE receptors on mast cells and eosinophils.
- In many subjects, the asthmatic attack consists of two phases:
  - —an immediate phase on exposure to eliciting agent, consisting mainly of bronchospasm
  - —a later phase consisting of a special type of inflammation in the brochioles comprising: vasodilatation, oedema, mucus secretion and bronchospasm caused by inflammatory mediators released from eosinophils and other cells. Activated, cytokine-releasing Th2 cells have an important role.
- Important mediators include leukotrienes C_4 and D_4, various chemotaxins and chemokines (in both phases) and tissue-damaging eosinophil proteins (delayed phase).
- In acute severe asthma (status asthmaticus), the airway obstruction can be fatal.
- Anti-asthmatic drugs include:
  - —bronchodilators
  - —anti-inflammatory agents.

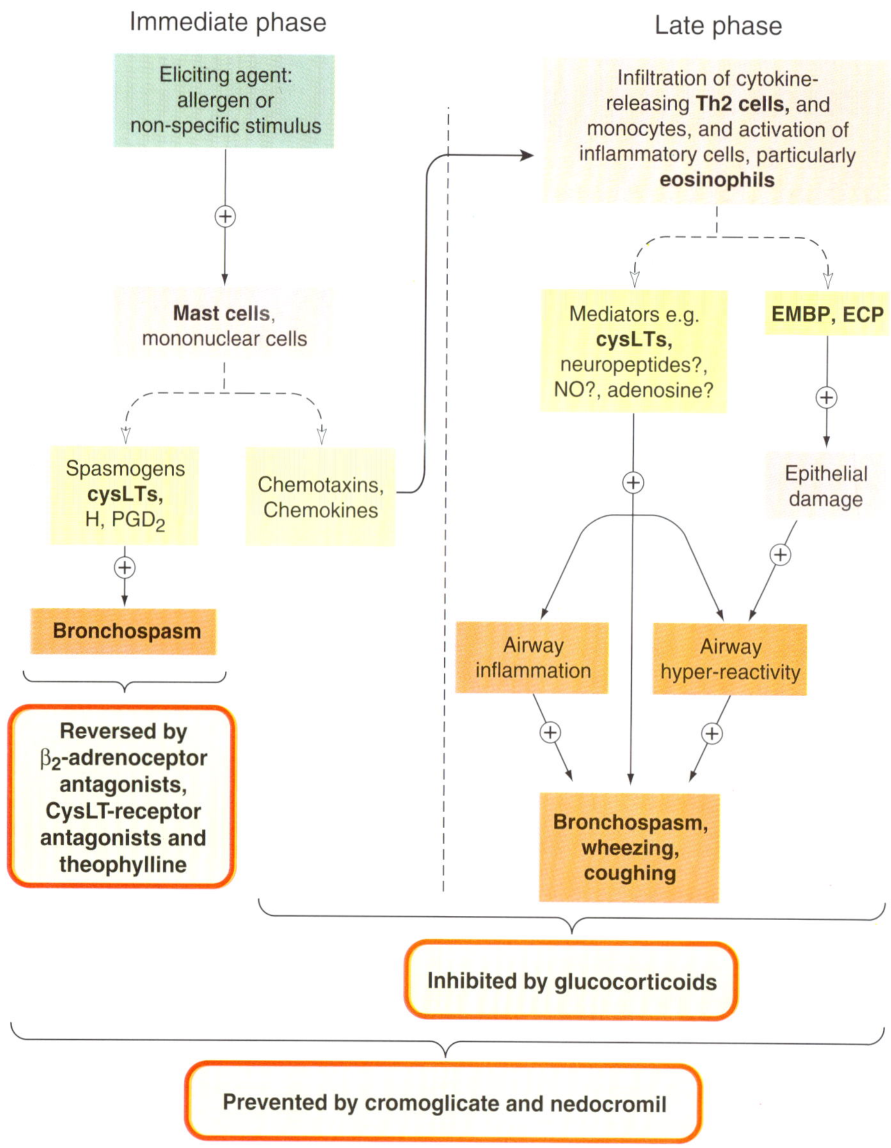

Fig. 22.3 Outline of the reactions thought to occur in asthma, with the actions of the main drugs. Important mediators and cells are emphasised. (CysLTs, cysteinyl-leukotrienes (leukotrienes C_4 and D_4); H, histamine; EMBP, eosinophil major basic protein; ECP, eosinophil cationic protein; iNO, induced nitric oxide.) For more detail of the Th2-derived cytokines and chemokines, see Chapter 15, page 225 and Figure 15.4. Note that not all asthmatic subjects respond to cromoglicate or nedocromil, and that theophylline and the cysteinyl-leukotriene receptor antagonists are only second-line drugs.

Other mediators released include IL-4, IL-5, IL-13, macrophage inflammatory protein-1α and tumour necrosis factor-α (TNF-α).

Various chemotaxins and chemokines (see Ch. 15) attract leucocytes—particularly eosinophils and mononuclear cells—into the area, setting the stage for the delayed phase (Fig. 22.3).

Once IgE binds to mast cells (or activated eosinophils), an amplification system operates since the cells not only release the spasmogens and other mediators specified but also can stimulate B cells to produce more IgE. Furthermore, the production of IL-4, IL-5 and IL-13 amplifies the Th2-mediated events described above.

Most exercise-induced asthma appears to involve mainly the phenomena of this first phase.

The late phase

The second, late phase or delayed response (see Figs 22.1 and 22.3) occurs at a variable time after exposure to the eliciting stimulus and may be nocturnal. This phase is in essence a progressing inflammatory reaction, initiation of which occurred

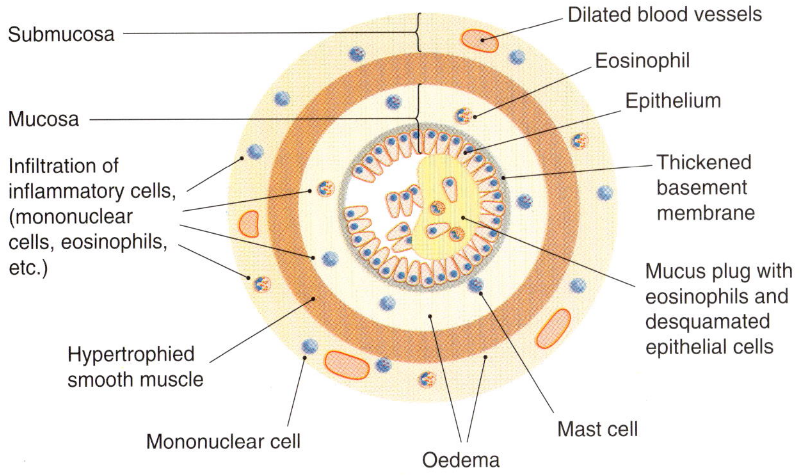

Fig 22.4 Schematic diagram of a cross-section of a bronchiole showing the changes that can occur with severe chronic asthma. The individual elements depicted are not of course drawn to scale.

during the first phase, the influx of Th2 lymphocytes being of particular importance. The inflammation is different from that seen, for example, in bronchitis. It has special characteristics in that there is infiltration not only by the usual inflammatory cells (Ch. 15) but also, and more specifically, by activated cytokine-releasing Th2 cells and by activated eosinophils. The physiological importance of these latter cells is in the defence against invading organisms, particularly helminths. But in the context of asthma they are inappropriately activated and release cysteinyl-leukotrienes, cytokines IL-3 and IL-5, chemokine IL-8 and the toxic proteins, eosinophil cationic protein, major basic protein and eosinophil-derived neurotoxin. These substances play an important part in the events of the late phase, the toxic proteins causing damage and loss of epithelium (reviewed by Corrigan & Kay, 1992).

Growth factors released from inflammatory cells act on smooth muscle cells, causing hypertrophy and hyperplasia, and the smooth muscle can itself release pro-inflammatory mediators and autocrine growth factors (Chs. 5 and 15). Figure 22.4 shows schematically the changes that take place in the bronchioles.

The epithelial loss means that irritant receptors and C fibres are more accessible to irritant stimuli; this is thought to be the main basis of the hyper-reactivity.

Other factors that have been put forward as putative mediators of the inflammatory process in the delayed phase are adenosine (acting on the A_1-receptor, see Ch. 12), induced NO (see Ch. 14) and the neuropeptides (see Chs 13 and 15).

DRUGS USED TO TREAT ASTHMA

There are two categories of anti-asthma drugs: *bronchodilators* and *anti-inflammatory agents*. Bronchodilators are effective in reversing the bronchospasm of the immediate phase; anti-inflammatory agents are effective in inhibiting or preventing the inflammatory components of both phases (Fig. 22.3). But note that these two categories are not mutually exclusive: some drugs classified as bronchodilators may also have some effect on inflammatory cells.

The problem of how to use the above two categories of drug in the clinical treatment of asthma is complex. A recent set of guidelines (see British Thoracic Society, 1997) specifies five therapeutic steps. The first involves only a short-acting β-agonist; progressing, if this type of agent is needed more than once daily, to subsequent steps involving both bronchodilators and anti-inflammatory drugs. There is now general agreement on the need to implement early anti-inflammatory treatment in many cases, rather than relying on symptomatic treatment with bronchodilators alone, since it is now recognised that progression of the condition, with increase in the severity of the asthmatic attacks, is caused by a gradual increase in the allergic inflammatory reaction in the bronchi and bronchioles.

BRONCHODILATORS

Drugs used as bronchodilators include β_2-adrenoceptor agonists, xanthines, cysteinyl-leukotriene receptor antagonists and muscarinic receptor antagonists.

The β_2-adrenoceptor agonists

The β_2-adrenoceptor agonists are dealt with in detail in Chapter 11. Their primary effect in asthma is to dilate the bronchi by a direct action on the β_2-adrenoceptors on the smooth muscle. Being physiological antagonists (see Ch. 2, pp. 14–15), they relax the bronchial muscle whatever the spasmogens involved. They also inhibit mediator release from mast cells and the release from monocytes of one of the primary mediators of inflammation (see Ch. 15)—TNF-α. In addition, they may increase mucus clearance by an action on cilia.

These drugs are usually given by inhalation of aerosol, powder or nebulised solution, but some may be given orally or by injection. A metered-dose inhaler is used for aerosol preparations. If patients (e.g. children, the elderly) have problems using these, a 'spacer' device* can be used instead.

Two categories of β_2-adrenoceptor agonists are used in asthma.

- Short-acting agents: **salbutamol** and **terbutaline**. These are given by inhalation, the maximum effect occurs within 30 minutes and the duration of action is 4–6 hours; they are usually used on an 'as needed' basis to control symptoms. **Bambuterol**, a pro-drug of terbutaline, is also now available.
- Longer-acting agents: e.g. **salmeterol**. These are given by inhalation and the duration of action is 12 hours. They are not used 'as needed' but are given regularly, twice daily, as adjunctive therapy in patients whose asthma is inadequately controlled by glucocorticoids. Other long-acting agents are **formoterol**, **fenoterol**, **pirbuterol** and **reprotelol**.

Unwanted affects

The unwanted effects of β_2-adrenoceptor agonists result from systemic absorption and are given in Chapter 11. In the context of their use in asthma, the commonest adverse effect is tremor. There is some evidence that β_2-agonist tolerance can occur in asthmatic airways (see Cockroft et al., 1993) and that steroids can reduce the development of tolerance because they inhibit β_2-adrenoceptor downregulation.

The β_2-adrenoceptor agonists are also used to improve respiratory function in chronic obstructive lung disease.

The β_2-adrenoceptor *antagonists*, such as propranolol, though having no effect on airway function in normal individuals, cause wheezing in asthmatics and can precipitate a potentially serious acute asthmatic attack by abrogating the compensatory effect of endogenous adrenaline.

Xanthine drugs

There are three pharmacologically active, naturally occurring methylxanthines: theophylline, theobromine and caffeine (see also Chs 17 and 41). The xanthine usually employed in clinical medicine is **theophylline** (1,3-dimethylxanthine), which can also be used as theophylline ethylenediamine, known as **aminophylline**. Caffeine and theophylline are constituents of coffee and tea, and theobromine is a constituent of cocoa. Theophylline has bronchodilator action, though it is rather less effective than the β_2-adrenoceptor agonists.

Actions

Anti-asthmatic actions Xanthines have long been used as bronchodilators.** Actions in addition to bronchodilatation seem to be involved since there is some evidence that theophylline can inhibit some aspects of the late phase, as shown by measurement of FEV_1 after bronchial allergen challenge (Pauwels, 1989); however, it does not appear to prevent bronchial hyper-responsiveness.

Actions on the central nervous system The methylxanthines have a stimulant effect on the CNS, causing increased alertness (see Ch. 41). They can cause tremor and nervousness and can interfere with sleep and have a stimulant action on respiration.

Actions on the cardiovascular system All the xanthines stimulate the heart (see Ch. 17), having positive chronotropic and inotropic actions. They cause vasodilatation in most blood vessels, though some can cause constriction in some vascular beds, more particularly cerebral blood vessels.

Actions on the renal system Methylxanthines have a weak diuretic effect, involving both increased glomerular filtration rate and reduced reabsorption in the tubules.

Mechanisms of action

The way in which the xanthine drugs produce effects in asthma is still unclear.

The relaxant effect on smooth muscle has been attributed to inhibition of the phosphodiesterase (PDE) isoenzymes, with resultant increase in cAMP (see Fig. 18.1). However, the concentrations necessary to inhibit the isolated enzyme greatly exceed the therapeutic range.

There is some evidence that the smooth muscle relaxation could be related to an effect on a cGMP PDE.

Another proposed mode of action is competitive antagonism of adenosine at adenosine receptors (Ch. 12), but the PDE inhibitor **enprofylline**, which is a more potent bronchodilator, is not an adenosine antagonist.

Unwanted effects

When theophylline is used in asthma, most of its other effects, such as those on the CNS, cardiovascular system and gastrointestinal tract, are unwanted side-effects. Furthermore, the plasma concentration range for an optimum therapeutic effect is 30–100 μmol/l, and adverse effects are likely to occur with concentrations greater than 110 μmol/l; thus, there is a relatively small therapeutic window. Measurements of the plasma concentration are necessary when the drug is given intravenously for treatment of status asthmaticus and are advisable to optimise therapy at high oral doses.

Gastrointestinal symptoms (anorexia, nausea and vomiting) and nervousness and tremor are sometimes seen with

Clinical use of β_2-adrenoceptor agonists as bronchodilators

- Short-acting drugs (salbutamol or terbutaline, usually by inhalation) to prevent or treat wheeze in patients with reversible obstructive airways disease.
- Salmeterol (long-acting bronchodilator) to prevent bronchospasm (e.g. at night or with exercise) in patients requiring long-term bronchodilator therapy.

*An extension tube between the aerosol source and the patient's mouth that prevents dispersion of the aerosol before the patient inhales.

**Over 200 years ago, William Withering recommended 'coffee made very strong' as a remedy for asthma; belief in its efficacy was reinforced by Salter in 1859.

Clinical use of theophylline

- As a second-line drug, in additon to steroids, in patients whose asthma does not respond adequately to β_2-adrenoceptor agonists.
- Intravenously in acute severe asthma.
- To reduce symptoms of chronic obstructive pulmonary disease.

Clinical use of ipratropium bromide

- As an adjunct to β_2-adrenoceptor antagonists and steroids when these on their own do not control asthma.
- As a bronchodilator in some patients with chronic bronchitis, and in bronchospasm precipitated by β_2-adrenoceptor antagonists.

concentrations only slightly higher than the clinically effective levels. Serious cardiovascular and CNS effects can occur when the plasma concentration exceeds 200 μmol/l. The most serious cardiovascular effect is dysrhythmia, which can be fatal. In children, seizures can occur with theophylline concentrations at or slightly above the upper limit of the therapeutic range. Seizures can be fatal in patients with respiratory compromise due to severe asthma.

Pharmacokinetic aspects

Xanthine drugs are given orally in sustained-release preparations; it is not feasible to give them by inhalation. Aminophylline can also be given by slow intravenous injection of a loading dose followed by intravenous infusion.

Theophylline is well absorbed from the gastrointestinal tract. It is metabolised in the liver and the plasma half-life is about 8 hours in adults but varies widely in different subjects.

The half-life of theophylline is increased in liver disease, cardiac failure and viral infections and is decreased in heavy cigarette smokers and drinkers. Theophylline is implicated as a culprit in many unwanted drug interactions. Its plasma concentration is decreased by drugs that increase P450 enzymes, such as rifampicin, phenobarbital, phenytoin and carbamazepine. The concentration is increased by drugs that inhibit P450 enzymes such as oral contraceptives, erythromycin, ciprofloxacin, calcium-channel blockers, fluconazole and cimetidine (but not ranitidine). These factors should be borne in mind in view of the narrowness of the range of safe and effective therapeutic concentrations.

The clinical use of theophylline is summarised in the box.

Muscarinic receptor antagonists

Muscarinic receptor antagonists are dealt with in detail in Chapter 10. The main compound used specifically as an anti-asthmatic is **ipratropium**. Oxitropium is also available. Ipratropium relaxes bronchial constriction caused by parasympathetic stimulation, which occurs particularly in asthma produced by irritant stimuli (see p. 342) and can occur in allergic asthma.

Ipratropium is a quaternary derivative of *N*-isopropylatropine. It does not discriminate between muscarinic receptor subtypes (see Ch. 10), and it is possible that its blockade of M_2-autoreceptors on the cholinergic nerves increases acetylcholine release and reduces the effectiveness of its antagonism at the M_3-receptors on the smooth muscle. It is not particularly effective against allergen challenge but it inhibits the augmentation of mucus secretion that occurs in asthma and may increase the mucociliary clearance of bronchial secretions. It has no effect on the late inflammatory phase of asthma.

It is given by aerosol inhalation. It is not well absorbed into the circulation and thus does not have much action at muscarinic receptors other than those in the bronchi. The maximum effect occurs after 30 minutes or so but then lasts for 3–5 hours. It has few unwanted effects and is, in general, safe and well tolerated. It can be used with β_2-adrenoceptor agonists.

The cysteinyl-leukotriene receptor antagonists

Cysteinyl-leukotriene receptor antagonists include **montelucast** and **zafirlukast** (who thinks up these names?). Note that all the leukotrienes (LTC_4, LTD_4 and LTE_4) act on the same high-affinity cysteinyl-leukotriene receptor (see Chs 15 and 16), which has been cloned.

Pharmacological actions

The cysteinyl-leukotriene receptor antagonists prevent aspirin-sensitive asthma, inhibit exercise-induced asthma and decrease both early and late responses to inhaled allergen. They relax the airways in mild asthma, the bronchodilator activity being one third that of salbutamol. Their action is additive with β_2-adrenoceptor agonists. They also reduce sputum eosinophilia, but so far there is no clear evidence that they modify the underlying inflammatory process in chronic asthma.

Unwanted effects

These are in general few, consisting mainly of headache and gastrointestinal disturbances. A few subjects have developed Churg–Strauss syndrome* possibly precipitated by withdrawal of the concomitant corticosteroid.

Pharmacokinetic aspects

Both drugs are given orally, montelukast once daily, zafirlukast twice.

Clinical use

Early reports of the actions of these agents led to some perhaps unrealistic expectations. The drugs are not a cure-all for asthma;

*This syndrome is characterised by systemic vasculitis, eosinophilia and a history of asthma, sinusitis and rhinitis.

their main use is as add-on therapy for mild-to-moderate asthma that is not controlled by an 'as required' short-acting β_2-agonist taken together with an inhaled glucocorticoid. It was expected that they would also be important as add-on therapy in the difficult situation of asthma not controlled by long-acting β_2-agonists, theophylline and glucocorticoids (inhaled or oral). However, a recent well-controlled trial has shown that they do not add any benefit.

Anti-asthma drugs: bronchodilators

- The β_2-adrenoceptor agonists (e.g. salbutamol) are first-line drugs (for details see Ch. 11).
  - —they act as physiological antagonists of the spasmogenic mediators but have little or no effect on the bronchial hyper-reactivity.
  - —salbutamol is given by inhalation; its effects start immediately and last 3–5 hours; it can also be given by intravenous infusion in status asthmaticus
  - —salmeterol is given by inhalation; its duration of action is 12 hours.
- Theophylline is a second-line drug; theophylline:
  - —is a xanthine compound; the mechanism of action is uncertain but may be by inhibition of GMP or cAMP phosphodiesterase
  - —has a narrow therapeutic window; unwanted effects include chronotropic and inotropic effects on the heart, CNS stimulation and gastrointestinal disturbances
  - —is given intravenously (by slow infusion) for status asthmaticus, or orally (as a sustained-release preparation) as a second-line treatment
  - —is metabolised in the liver, and liver dysfunction and viral infections increase its plasma concentration and half-life (normally 12 hours with sustained-release preparation)
  - —has interactions with other drugs that are important; some (e.g. some antibiotics) increase the half-life of theophylline, others (e.g. antiepileptic drugs) decrease it.
- Muscarinic receptor antagonists (e.g. ipratropium bromide) are second-line drugs (see Ch. 10 for details). Ipratropium bromide:
  - —inhibits acetylcholine-mediated bronchospasm
  - —binds to all muscarinic receptor subtypes (M_1, M_2 and M_3)
  - —is given by aerosol inhalation.
- Cysteinyl-leukotriene receptor antagonists (e.g. montelukast):
  - —competitively inhibit cysteinyl leukotriene receptors
  - —inhibit exercise-induced bronchospasm and aspirin-induced asthma
  - —have a bronchodilator action that is additive with β_2-adrenoceptor agonists
  - —are of use mainly as add-on therapy for mild-to-moderate asthma

Histamine H_1-receptor antagonists

Although mast cell mediators are thought to play a part in the immediate phase of allergic asthma (Fig. 22.3) and in some types of exercise-induced asthma, histamine H_1-receptor antagonists have had no place in therapy. Recently, clinical trials have shown that some newer, non-sedating antihistamines, such as **loratidine**, may be moderately effective in mild atopic asthma.

ANTI-INFLAMMATORY AGENTS

The main drugs used for their anti-inflammatory action in asthma are the **glucocorticoids**. **Cromoglicate** and nedocromil also have some anti-inflammatory action.

Glucocorticoids

Glucocorticoids are dealt with in detail in Chapter 27. They are not bronchodilators and are not effective in the treatment of the immediate response to the eliciting agent. In the management of chronic asthma, in which there is a predominant inflammatory component, their efficacy is unequivocal.*

Actions and mechanism of action

The basis of the anti-inflammatory action of glucocorticoids is discussed on page 416. An important action, of relevance for asthma, is that they decrease formation of cytokines (Fig. 15.3), in particular the Th2 cytokines that recruit and activate eosinophils and are responsible for promoting the production of IgE and the expression of IgE receptors (p. 342 above and Ch. 15). Glucocorticoids also inhibit the generation of the vasodilators PGE_2 and PGI_2, by inhibiting induction of cyclooxygenase-2 (Fig. 15.5). In addition, by virtue of inducing lipocortin, they may inhibit production of the spasmogens LTC_4 and LTD_4 and decrease synthesis of the leucocyte chemotaxins LTB_4 and platelet-activating factor, thus reducing recruitment and activation of inflammatory cells (Fig. 15.5). Bronchoalveolar lavage studies have shown that they inhibit the allergen-induced influx of eosinophils into the lung. Glucocorticoids can upregulate β_2-adrenoceptors, decrease microvascular permeability and reduce mediator release from eosinophils. The reduction in the synthesis of IL-3 (the cytokine that regulates mast cell production) may explain why long-term steroid treatment eventually reduces the early-phase response to allergens and prevents exercise-induced asthma.

The main compounds used are **beclometasone dipropionate**, **budesonide** and **fluticasone propionate**, which are given by inhalation with a metered-dose inhaler, the full effect being attained only after several days of therapy.

*In 1900, Solis-Cohen reported that dried bovine adrenals had anti-asthma action. He noted that the extract did not serve acutely 'to cut short the paroxysm' but was 'useful in averting recurrence of paroxysms'. Mistaken for the first report on the effect of adrenaline, his astute observation was probably the first on the efficacy of steroids in asthma (see Persson, 1997).

> **Clinical use of glucocorticoids in asthma**
>
> - Patients who require regular bronchodilators should be considered for glucocorticoid treatment (e.g. with inhaled beclometasone).
> - More severely affected patients are treated with high-potency inhaled drugs (e.g. budesonide) and additional agents (e.g. slow release theophylline).
> - Patients with acute exacerbations of asthma may require intravenous hydocortisone and oral prednisolone.
> - A 'rescue course' of oral prednisolone may be needed at any stage of severity if the clinical condition is deteriorating.
> - Prolonged treatment with oral prednisolone, in addition to inhaled bronchodilators and steroids, is needed by a few severe asthmatics.

For chronic asthma and severe or rapidly deteriorating asthma, a short course of an oral glucocorticoid (e.g. prednisolone) is indicated, combined with an inhaled steroid to reduce the oral dose required. In status asthmaticus, hydrocortisone is given intravenously followed by oral prednisolone.

Unwanted effects

Unwanted effects are uncommon with inhaled steroids. Oropharyngeal candidiasis (thrush; Ch. 47), can occur, as can dysphonia (voice problems), but these are less likely to occur if 'spacing' devices are used, which decrease oropharyngeal deposition of the drug and increase airway deposition. Regular large doses can produce adrenal suppression, particularly in children, and necessitate the carrying of a 'steroid card' (Ch. 27). The unwanted effects of oral glucocorticoids are given in Chapter 27, page 417; these can sometimes occur with inhaled steroids if part of an inhaled dose is ingested. This is less likely with fluticasone propionate as it has limited absorption from the gastrointestinal tract and undergoes almost complete first-pass metabolism.

Cromoglicate

Cromoglicate is unique in that it was first tested—and its efficacy demonstrated—in allergic asthma in humans, without prior testing in animals.

Actions and mechanisms of action

Cromoglicate and the related drug **nedocromil sodium** are not bronchodilators; they do not have any direct effects on smooth muscle, nor do they inhibit the actions of any of the known smooth muscle stimulants. If given prophylactically, they can reduce both the immediate and the late-phase asthmatic responses and reduce bronchial hyper-reactivity. They are effective in antigen-induced, exercise-induced and irritant-induced asthma, though not all asthmatic subjects respond, and it is not possible to predict which patients will benefit. Children are more likely to respond than adults.

The mechanism of action is not fully understood. Cromoglicate was originally thought to act as a 'mast cell stabiliser', preventing histamine release from mast cells. However, although it has this effect it is clearly not the basis of its action in asthma because many other compounds have been produced which are equally or more potent than cromoglicate at inhibiting mast cell histamine release but none has proved to have any anti-asthmatic effect at all in humans.

There is evidence that cromoglicate depresses the exaggerated neuronal reflexes that are triggered by stimulation of the 'irritant receptors'; it suppresses the response of sensory C fibres to the irritant capsaicin and may inhibit the release of preformed T cell cytokines. Various other effects on the inflammatory cells and mediators involved in asthma have been described. (See review by Garland, 1991.)

Pharmacokinetic aspects

Cromoglicate is extremely poorly absorbed from the gastrointestinal tract. It is given by inhalation as an aerosol, as a nebulised solution or in powder form; about 10% is absorbed into the circulation when it is given in this way. It is excreted unchanged: 50% in the bile and 50% in the urine. Its half-life in the plasma is 90 minutes.

Nedocromil is also given by inhalation and is rather better absorbed.

Unwanted effects

Unwanted effects are few and consist mostly of the effects of irritation in the upper respiratory tract. Hypersensitivity reactions have been reported (urticaria, anaphylaxis), but are rare.

SEVERE ACUTE ASTHMA (STATUS ASTHMATICUS)

Severe acute asthma is a medical emergency requiring hospitalisation. Treatment includes oxygen, inhalation of salbutamol in oxygen given by nebuliser, and intravenous hydrocortisone followed by a course of oral prednisolone. Additional measures include nebulised ipratropium, intravenous salbutamol or aminophylline and antibiotics (if bacterial infection is present).

CHRONIC OBSTRUCTIVE PULMONARY DISEASE

Chronic obstructive pulmonary disease (COPD) is the name given to a syndrome consisting of chronic bronchitis and emphysema.

Chronic bronchitis is inflammation of the bronchi and bronchioles, the inflammatory process being similar to inflammation in other tissues and unlike that seen in the bronchioles in asthma (p. 342). It can be caused by air pollution but is more usually associated with cigarette smoking. The symptoms are cough in the early stages and in the later stages productive cough, wheezing and breathlessness owing to airflow limitation. *Emphysema* is distension and damage of lung tissue

Anti-asthma drugs: anti-inflammatory agents

Glucocorticoids (for details see Ch. 27)

- These reduce the inflammatory component in chronic asthma and are life saving in status asthmaticus (acute severe asthma).
- They are not effective in the treatment of the immediate response to the eliciting agent.
- The mechanism of action involves decreased formation of cytokines, particularly those generated by Th2 lymphocytes (see Key Points Box on p. 413), decreased activation of eosinophils and other inflammatory cells, and decreased formation of prostaglandins and possibly of platelet-activating factor and leukotrienes C_4 and D_4.
- They are given by inhalation (e.g. beclometasone); systemic unwanted effects are rare, but oral thrush and voice problems can occur. In deteriorating asthma, an oral glucocorticoid (e.g. prednisolone) or intravenous hydrocortisone is also given.

Cromoglicate

- Given prophylactically this can prevent both phases of asthma and reduce bronchial hyper-responsiveness in many but not all patients. Children are more likely to respond than adults.
- The mechanism of action is uncertain. Depression of release of neuropeptides, antagonism of tachykinin receptors, inhibition of cytokine release and inhibition of platelet-activating factor interaction with platelets and eosinophils may be important; mast cell stabilisation is not.
- It is given by inhalation and acts locally; 10% is absorbed and is excreted unchanged.
- Unwanted effects are minor respiratory tract irritation and (rarely) hypersensitivity.

beyond the respiratory bronchioles; it supervenes after years of coughing. The airflow limitation is partially reversible in the early stages.

Drug treatment is palliative, the main drug being **ipratropium bromide** (see p. 347). **Salbutamol** is also used and **corticosteroids** (inhaled or oral) can be of value in some cases.

COUGH

Cough is a protective reflex mechanism that removes foreign material and secretions from the bronchi and bronchioles. It can be inappropriately stimulated by inflammation in the respiratory tract or by neoplasia. In these cases, antitussive (or cough suppressant) drugs are sometimes used, for example for the dry painful cough associated with bronchial carcinoma or with inflammation of the pleura. It should be understood that these drugs merely suppress the symptom without influencing the underlying condition. In cough associated with bronchiectasis (suppurating bronchial inflammation) or chronic bronchitis, antitussive drugs can cause harmful sputum thickening and retention. They should not be used for the cough associated with asthma.

DRUGS USED FOR COUGH

Antitussive drugs act by an ill-defined effect in the brainstem, depressing an even more poorly defined 'cough centre'. The narcotic analgesics (see Ch. 40) have effective antitussive action in doses below those required for pain relief, and various isomers of these agents, which are neither analgesic nor addictive, are also effective against cough. New opioid analogues that suppress cough by inhibiting release of excitatory neuropeptides through an action on μ-receptors (see Table 40.1) on sensory nerves in the bronchi are being assessed.

CODEINE

Codeine, or methylmorphine, is an opiate (see Ch. 40) that has considerably less addiction liability than the main opioid analgesics and is an effective cough suppressant. However, it also decreases secretions in the bronchioles, which thickens sputum and inhibits ciliary activity; this reduces clearance of the thickened sputum. Constipation also occurs because of the well-known action of opiates on the gastrointestinal tract (see Chs 24 and 40).

DEXTROMETHORPHAN

Dextromethorphan is related to levorphanol, a synthetic narcotic analgesic. Its antitussive potency is equivalent to that of codeine and it produces only marginally less constipation and inhibition of mucociliary clearance.

PHOLCODINE

Pholcodine is a non-analgesic opiate of the same chemical class as papaverine; it is also used as a cough suppressant.

REFERENCES AND FURTHER READING

Anderson G P, Coyle A J 1994 Th2 and 'Th2-like' cells in asthma: pharmacological perspectives. Trends Pharmacol Sci 15: 324–331 (*Perceptive article on the contribution of Th2 cells and the Th2 profile of cytokines to allergic disease. Excellent diagrams*)

Barnes P J, Chung K F, Page C P 1998 Inflammatory mediators of asthma: an update. Pharmacol Rev 50: 515–596 (*Clearly written review giving exhaustive coverage of all possible inflammatory mediators that could have a role in asthma, giving for each mediator: synthesis and metabolism, receptors, effect on airways and role in asthma*)

British Thoracic Society 1997 The British guidelines on asthma management. Thorax 52(suppl): S1–S21 (*Important precepts for asthma treatment*)

Chauhan A J, Krishna M T, Holgate S 1996 Aetiology of asthma. Mol Med Today (May): 192–197 (*Valuable analysis of asthma aetiology*)

Cockcroft D W, McParland C P et al. 1993 Regular inhaled salbutamol and airway responsiveness to allergen. Lancet 342: 833–837

Corrigan C J, Kay A B 1992 T cells and eosinophils in the pathogenesis of asthma. Immunol Today 13: 501–507 (*Discusses the initiation of inflammation by activated T cells; and the role of eosinophils*)

Corry D B 2002 Emerging immune targets for the therapy of asthma. Nat Rev: Drug Disc 1: 55–64 (*Outstanding review. Considers the pathophysiology of asthma and discuss potential immune targets. Excellent diagrams. Annotated references.*)

Dale M M, Hirst S J 1993 Advances in receptor biochemistry. In: Weiss E B, Stein M S 1993 (eds) Bronchial asthma: mechanisms and therapeutics, 3rd edn. Little Brown, Boston, ch. 16, pp. 203–216 (*Covers signal transduction mechanisms in smooth muscle*)

Erb K J 1999 Atopic disorders: a default pathway in the absence of infection. Immunol Today 20: 317–322 (*Discusses the hypothesis that the decline of infectious diseases in the developed world could account for an increase in atopic disorders, stressing the role of the Th1-type immune response to infection in inhibiting the development of atopy. Useful diagrams*)

Gale E A M 2002 The role of mast cells in the pathophysiology of asthma. N Engl J Med 346: 1742–1743 (*Stresses the role of smooth muscle in the pathophysiology of asthma and discusses the inter-relationship of mast cells and smooth muscle*)

Garland L G 1991 Pharmacology of prophylactic anti-asthma drugs. In: Page C P, Barnes P J (eds) Handbook of experimental pharmacology. Springer-Verlag, Berlin, vol. 98, ch. 9, pp. 261–290 (*Excellent review*)

Green R H, Pavord I D 2001 Leukotriene antagonists and symptom control in chronic persistent asthma. Lancet 357: 1991–1992 (*Editorial discussing briefly the significance of studies of leukotriene receptor antagonists for drug treatment of asthma*)

Hall I P 1997 The future of asthma. Br Med J 314: 45–49 (*Thought-provoking article on future developments in therapy*)

Hay D P, Torphy T J, Undem B J 1995 Cysteinyl leukotrienes in asthma: old mediators up to new tricks. Trends Pharmacol Sci 16: 304–309 (*Discusses role in asthma and lists potential new compounds*)

Holgate S 1993 Mediator and cytokine mechanisms in asthma. Thorax 48: 103–109

Johnson D C 2001 A role for phosphodiesterase type-4 inhibitors in COPD? Lancet 358: 256–257 (*Editorial assessing possible role of these drugs in chronic obstructive pulmonary disease*)

Kollef M H, Schuster D P 1995 The acute respiratory distress syndrome. N Engl J Med 332: 27–37

Leff A R 2001 Regulation of leukotrienes in the management of asthma: biology and clinical therapy. Annu Rev Med 52: 1–14 (*Discusses the role of leukotrienes in the pathogenesis of bronchoconstriction and the pharmacology of antagonists at the cysteinyl-leukotriene receptor*)

Lucaks N W 2001 Role of chemokines in the pathogenesis of asthma. Nat Immunol 1: 108–116 (*Excellent coverage of the chemokines involved in asthma, with detailed table of chemokines and good diagrams*)

McFadden E R, Gilbert I A 1994 Exercise-induced asthma. N Engl J Med 330: 1362–1366 (*Effective coverage*)

Misson J, Clark W, Kendall M J 1999 Therapeutic advances: leukotriene antagonists for the treatment of asthma. J Clin Pharm Ther 24: 17–22 (*Neat summary of the characteristics of asthma and current asthma therapy. Clear outline of clinical efficacy of and adverse events with montelukast and zafirlukast*)

Nelson H S 1995 β-Adrenergic bronchodilators. N Engl J Med 333: 499–506 (*Worthwhile coverage*)

Pauwels R A 1989 New aspects of the therapeutic potential of theophylline in asthma. J Allergy Clin Immunol 83: 548–553

Persson C G A 1997 Centennial notions of asthma as an eosinophilic, desquamative, exudative, and steroid-sensitive disease. Lancet 349: 1021–1024 (*A review of astute early observations of the pathogenesis of asthma that foreshadowed modern understanding of the disease*)

Puchelle E, Vargaftig B B 2001 Chronic obstructive pulmonary disease: an old disease with novel concepts and drug strategies. Trends Pharmacol Sci 22: 495–498 (*Report of meeting on chronic lung disease*)

Spina D, Page C P 2002 Asthma—time for a rethink. Trends Pharmacol Sci 23: 311–315 (*Discusses the role of alterations in the function of the afferent nerves to the airways in bronchial hyper-responsiveness*)

Spina D, Landells L J, Page C P 1998 The role of phosphodiesterase enzymes in allergy and asthma. Adv Pharmacol 44: 33–89 (*Good review*)

Tattersfield A E, Harrison T W 2001 Exacerbations of asthma—still room for improvement. Lancet 358: 599–601 (*Editorial discussing optimal treatment of acute asthma*)

Texeira M M, Gristwood R W et al. 1997 Phosphodiesterase (PDE) 4 inhibitors: anti-inflammatory drugs of the future. Trends Pharmacol Sci 18: 164–170 (*Thought provoking review*)

Torphy T J 1998 Phosphodiesterase isozymes. Am J Respir Crit Care Med 157: 351–370 (*Considers phosphodiesterase isozymes as potential targets for new anti-asthma drugs*)

Walker C, Zuany-Amorim C 2001 New trends in immunotherapy to prevent atopic diseases. Trends in Pharmacol Sci 22: 84–90 (*Discerning article on the possible development of new treatments for atopic diseases based on recent understanding of the role of Th2 cells and Th2 cytokines in allergy. Very clear diagram*)

Weinberger M E, Hendeles L 1996 Theophylline in asthma. N Engl J Med 334: 1380–1388 (*Addresses the possible role of theophylline in asthma therapy*)

Wills-Karp M 1999 Immunologic basis of antigen-induced airway hyperresponsiveness. Annu Rev Immunol 17: 255–281 (*Detailed review discussing current understanding of the mechanisms whereby Th2 cytokines induce airway disease*)

23 The kidney

Overview 352

Outline of renal function 352

The structure and function of the nephron 352
- Tubular function 354
- Acid–base balance 360
- Potassium balance 360
- Excretion of organic molecules 361
- Arachidonic acid metabolites and renal function 361

Drugs acting on the kidney 362
- Diuretics 362

Drugs which alter the pH of the urine 365

Drugs which alter the excretion of organic molecules 365

OVERVIEW

In this chapter we deal with drugs that affect kidney function, the most important of these being the diuretics—agents that increase the excretion of NaCl and water. These are important in the therapy of cardiovascular diseases, disorders of fluid and electrolyte balance and pathological conditions of the kidney itself. We set the scene for describing these drugs with a brief outline of the overall functions of the kidney and then go on to a more detailed consideration of the functional unit of the kidney—the nephron.

OUTLINE OF RENAL FUNCTION

The main function of the kidney is the excretion of waste products such as urea, uric acid and creatinine. In the course of this activity, it fulfils another function crucially important in homeostasis—the regulation of the NaCl and electrolyte content and the volume of the extracellular fluid. It also plays a part in acid–base balance.

The kidneys receive about a quarter of the cardiac output. From the several hundred litres of plasma which flow through them each day, they filter an amount equivalent to about 11 times the extracellular fluid volume. This filtrate is similar in composition to plasma, the main difference being that it has very little protein or protein-bound substances. As it passes through the renal tubule, about 99% of it is reabsorbed while some substances are secreted, and eventually about 1.5 litres of the filtered fluid are voided as urine (Table 23.1).

In structure, each kidney consists of an outer cortex, an inner medulla and a hollow pelvis, which empties into the ureter. The functional unit is the nephron, of which there are about 1.3×10^6 in each kidney.

THE STRUCTURE AND FUNCTION OF THE NEPHRON

The nephron consists of a glomerulus, proximal convoluted tubule, loop of Henle, distal tubule and collecting duct (Fig. 23.1). The glomerulus comprises a tuft of capillaries projecting into a dilated end of the renal tubule. Most nephrons lie largely or entirely in the cortex. The remaining 12%, called the juxtamedullary nephrons, have their glomeruli and convoluted tubules next to the junction of the medulla and cortex, and their loops of Henle pass deep into the medulla.

THE BLOOD SUPPLY TO THE NEPHRON

The nephron possesses the special characteristic of having two capillary beds in series with each other (see Fig. 23.1). For those nephrons that lie entirely in the cortex, the afferent arterioles branch to form the capillaries of the glomerulus; these empty into the efferent arterioles, which, in turn, branch to form a second capillary network in the cortex, around the convoluted tubules and loops of Henle, before emptying into the veins. In the case of the juxtamedullary nephrons, some of the branches of the afferent arterioles bypass the convoluted tubules and instead form bundles of vessels that pass deep into the medulla with the thin loops of Henle. These loops of vessels are called *vasa recta* and they have a role in counter-current exchange (see pp. 359–360).

THE JUXTAGLOMERULAR APPARATUS

A conjunction of afferent arteriole, efferent arteriole and distal convoluted tubule near the glomerulus forms the juxtaglomerular

Table 23.1 Reabsorption of fluid and solute in the kidney

	Filtered/day	Excreted/day[a]	Percentage reabsorbed
Na^+ (mEq)	25 000	150	99+
K^+ (mEq)	600	90	93+
Cl^- (mEq)	18 000	150	99+
HCO_3^- (mEq)	4900	0	100
Total solute (mosmol)	54 000	700	87
H_2O (litres)	180	~1.5	99+

1 mEq = 1 mmol for univalent ions.
Typical values for a healthy young adult: renal blood flow, 1200 ml/min (20–25% of cardiac output); renal plasma flow, 660 ml/min; glomerular filtration rate, 125 ml/min.
[a]These are typical figures for an individual eating a Western diet. The kidney excretes more or less of each of these substances to maintain the constancy of the internal milieu, so on a low-sodium diet (for instance), NaCl excretion may be reduced to as low as 20 mmol/day.

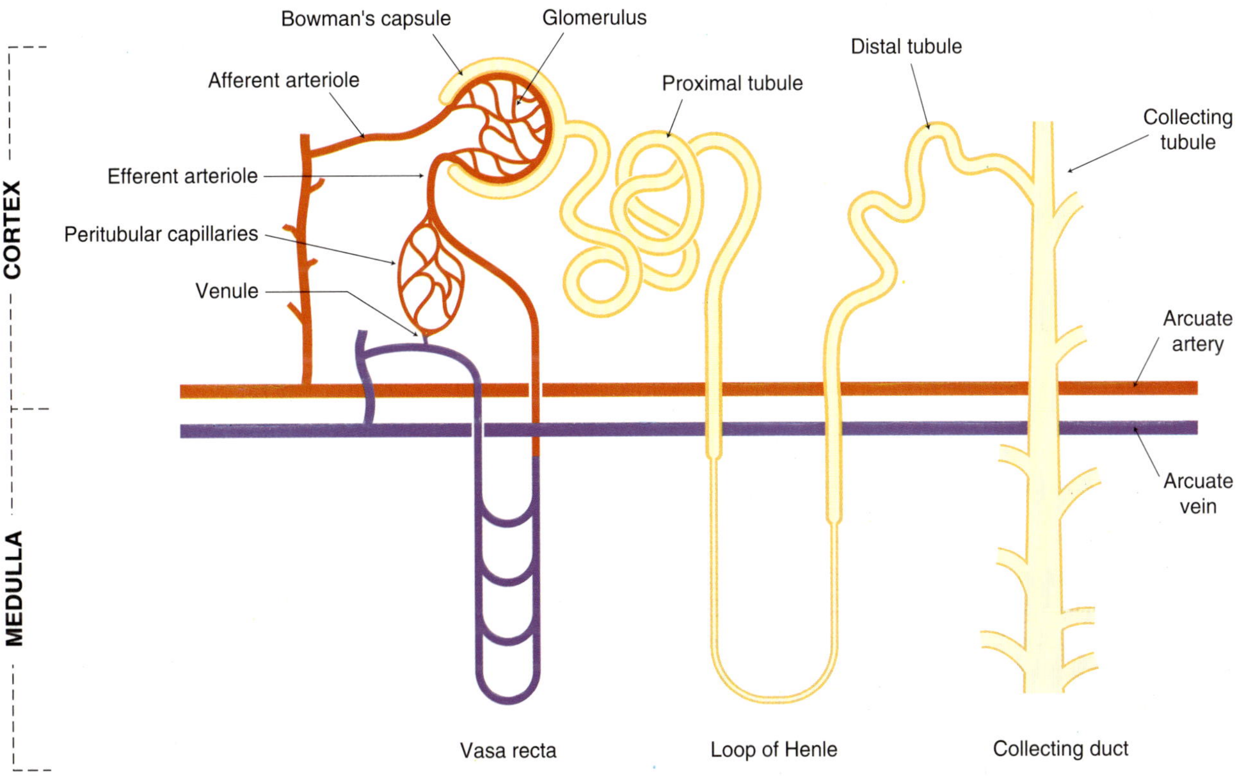

Fig. 23.1 Simplified diagram of a juxtamedullary nephron and its blood supply. The tubules and the blood vessels are shown separately for clarity. In the kidney, the peritubular capillary network surrounds the convoluted tubules, and the distal convoluted tubule passes close to the glomerulus, between the afferent and efferent arterioles. (This last is shown in more detail in Fig. 23.2.)

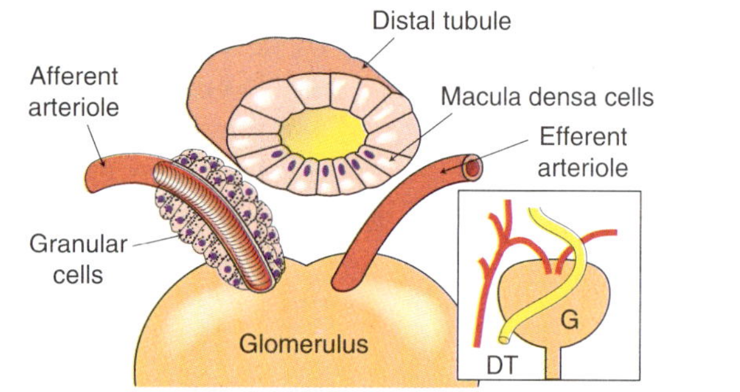

Fig. 23.2 The juxtaglomerular apparatus. The cutaway sections show the granular renin-containing cells round the afferent arteriole, and the *macula densa* cells in the distal convoluted tubule. The inset shows the general relationships between the structures. (G, glomerulus; DT, distal tubule.) (Modified from: Sullivan & Grantham 1982.)

apparatus (Fig. 23.2). At this site, there are specialised cells in both the afferent arteriole and in the tubule. The latter, termed *macula densa* cells, respond to changes in the rate of flow and the composition of tubule fluid, and they control renin release from the specialised granular renin-containing cells in the afferent arteriole (Ch. 18). The juxtaglomerular apparatus is important in controlling the blood flow to the nephron and the glomerular filtration rate. Factors extrinsic to the kidney can influence these processes through circulating hormones and through noradrenergic sympathetic fibres, which supply the afferent and efferent arterioles and the specialised cells. They will thus influence the generation of angiotensin I and II. The role of the juxtaglomerular apparatus in the control of Na^+ balance is dealt with below, and its role in cardiovascular dynamics is considered in Chapter 18.

GLOMERULAR FILTRATION

Fluid is driven from the capillaries into the tubular capsule (Bowman's capsule) by hydrodynamic force. It crosses three layers: the capillary endothelium, the basement membrane and the epithelial cell layer of the capsule. These form a complex filter that excludes large molecules. Normally, all constituents in the plasma, except the plasma proteins, appear in the filtrate, and the blood which passes on through the efferent arteriole to the peritubular capillaries has a higher concentration of plasma proteins and thus a higher oncotic pressure than normal. (The term 'oncotic pressure' refers to osmotic pressure contributed by large molecules such as the plasma proteins.)

TUBULAR FUNCTION

In the epithelium of the tubules, as in all epithelia, the apex or luminal surface of each cell is surrounded by a *zonula occludens*, a specialised region of membrane that forms a tight junction between it and neighbouring cells, and which separates the intercellular space from the lumen (see Fig. 23.7, below). The movement of ions and water across the epithelium can occur both through the cells (the transcellular pathway) and between the cells through the *zonulae occludentes* (the paracellular pathway). The zonulae in different parts of the nephron vary in their degree of functional tightness, i.e. their relative permeability to ions. The tightness or leakiness of the epithelium of various portions of the nephron is an important factor in their function (see Taylor & Palmer, 1982). Tight epithelium is found in the distal portion of the nephron, which is the site of action of the major hormones involved in the control of NaCl and water excretion.

THE PROXIMAL CONVOLUTED TUBULE

The epithelium of the proximal convoluted tubule is 'leaky', i.e. the *zonula occludens* is permeable to ions and water and permits passive flows in either direction. This prevents the build-up of significant ionic or osmotic gradients; separate regulation of the movements of ions and water occurs mainly in the distal part of the tubule.

About 60–70% of the filtered load of Na^+ and water is reabsorbed in the proximal tubule. Some of the transport processes in the proximal tubule are shown in Figure 23.3 and below in Figure 23.10. In quantitative terms, the most important mechanism for Na^+ entry into the cell from the filtrate is the Na^+/H^+ exchanger (see below; also shown in Fig. 23.10). Some

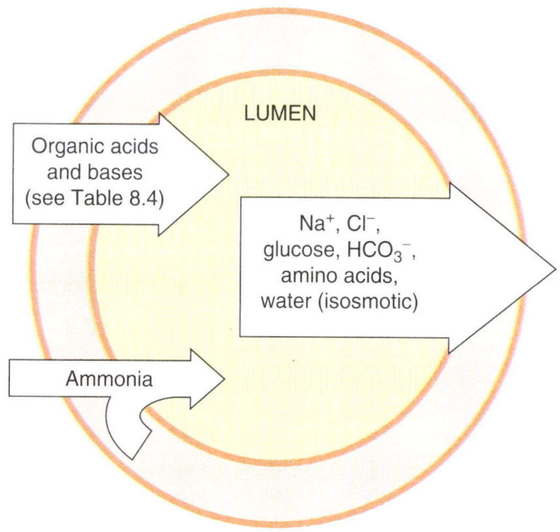

Fig. 23.3 The main transport processes in the proximal convoluted tubule. The main driving force for the absorption of solutes and water from the lumen is the Na^+/K^+-ATPase in the basolateral membrane of the tubule cells. Many drugs are secreted into the proximal tubule (see Ch. 8). (Redrawn from: Burg 1985.)

Na^+ entry is coupled to that of other solutes (glucose, amino acids) by symport mechanisms.* Sodium is transported out of the cells into the interstitia and thence into the blood by *the primary active transport mechanism of the nephron,* the Na^+/K^+ ATPase (the sodium pump) in the basolateral membrane.

Water is reabsorbed as a result of the osmotic pressure gradient generated by this solute reabsorption, the increased oncotic pressure in the peritubular capillaries contributing to this effect.

Chloride absorption is largely passive. Some diffuses through the *zonula occludens.*

Many organic acids and bases are actively secreted by specific transporters into the tubule from the blood (see below, Fig. 23.3 and Ch. 7).

Bicarbonate is returned to the plasma—mainly in the proximal tubule—by an indirect method involving the action of carbonic anhydrase (for detail see Fig. 23.10. below). Drugs, such as acetazolamide, which inhibit carbonic anhydrase, increase the volume of urine flow (i.e. are diuretic) by preventing bicarbonate reabsorption (Fig. 23.10). They also result in a depletion of extracellular bicarbonate.

After passage through the proximal tubule, the remaining 30–40% of the filtrate, which is still isosmotic with plasma, passes on to the loop of Henle.

*In a symport or co-transport system, the transport of one substance is coupled to that of another, both being transported across a membrane in the same direction (see the Na^+/Cl^+ symport in Fig. 23. 8, below), as opposed to an antiport system in which two substances are exchanged with each other across a membrane (see the Na^+/H^+ exchanger in Fig. 23.10, below).

THE LOOP OF HENLE

The loop consists of a descending and an ascending portion (Figs 23.1 and 23.4), the ascending portion having both thick and thin segments. During passage through the loop of Henle, up to 20–30% of the Na^+ in the tubule is reabsorbed. This part of the nephron plays an important part in regulating the osmolarity of the urine, and hence in regulating the osmotic balance of the body as a whole. Its function is summarised in Figure 23.5.

The *descending* limb is highly permeable to water, which moves out passively. This happens because the interstitial fluid of the medulla is kept hypertonic by the countercurrent concentrating system (see below and p. 359). In juxtamedullary nephrons with long loops, there is extensive movement of water out of the tubule (and also movement of urea in) so that the fluid eventually reaching the tip of the loop has a high osmolarity—normally approximately 1200 mosmol/l, but up to 1500 mosmol/l under conditions of dehydration—compared with plasma and extracellular fluid, which is approximately 300 mosmol/l.

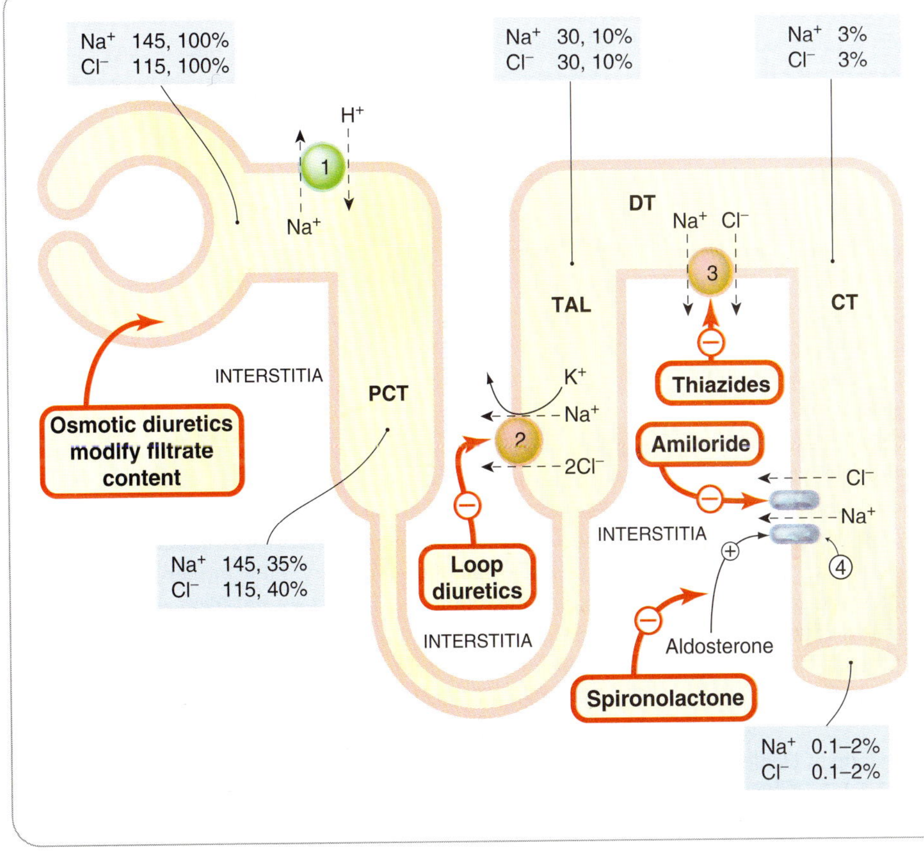

Fig. 23.4 Schematic summary diagram showing the absorption of sodium and chloride in the nephron and the main sites of action of drugs. The tubule cells are depicted as an orange border round the yellow tubular lumen. Mechanisms of ion absorption at the apical margin of the tubule cell (not of course shown to scale): (1) Na^+/H^+ exchange; (2) $Na^+/K^+/2Cl^-$ co-transport; (3) Na^+/Cl^- co-transport, (4) Na^+ entry through sodium channels (see Fig. 23.5 for detail). Sodium is pumped out of the cells into the interstitia by the Na^+/K^+ ATPase in the basolateral margin of the tubular cells (not shown). Chloride ions may pass out of the tubule through the paracellular pathway. The numbers in the boxes give the concentration of ions as millimoles per litre of filtrate and the percentage of filtered ions at the sites specified. No absolute concentrations are given for the DT and CT because they can vary considerably. (PCT, proximal convoluted tubule; TAL, thick ascending loop; DT, distal tubule; CT, collecting tubule.) (Data from Greger 2000.)

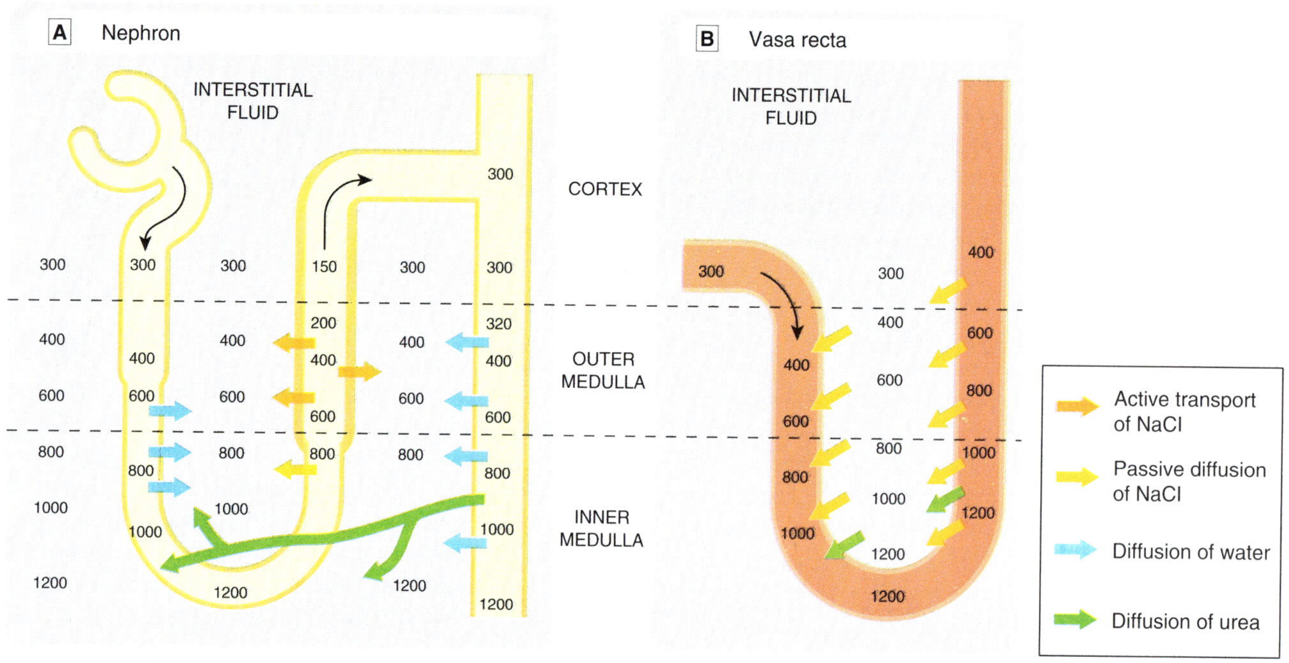

Fig. 23.5 Schematic diagram of the counter-current mechanisms for concentrating the urine. (The figures are in milliosmoles per litre.) A Renal tubules. B Vasa recta. The main factors are:

- a counter-current multiplier mechanism involving the tubules and a counter-current exchange mechanism involving the vasa recta
- a source of energy, which is supplied by the Na^+ pump and the active transport of NaCl in the ascending loop of Henle. (Loop diuretics act by inhibiting this active transport, thus interfering with the counter-current concentrating mechanism.)
- differences in permeability between tubules carrying fluid in opposite directions; the thickened outline of the ascending limb of Henle's loop indicates decreased permeability to water in contrast to the water-permeable descending loop
- diffusion of NaCl into the vessels taking blood down into the medulla and out of vessels passing back up to the cortex, maintaining hypertonicity in the medulla.

The absorption of water in the collecting ducts is controlled by antidiuretic hormone. Additional active reabsorption of NaCl occurs in the distal tubule and is controlled by aldosterone.

The *ascending* limb has very low permeability to water. It is here, in the thick segment of this limb, that the 20–30% of filtered Na^+ is reabsorbed. There is active reabsorption of NaCl, not accompanied by water, which reduces the osmolarity of the tubular fluid and makes the interstitial fluid of the medulla hypertonic (Figs 23.4 and 23.5). Both Na^+ and Cl^- move into the cell by a co-transport system involving $Na^+/K^+/2Cl^-$, this process being driven by the electrochemical gradient for Na^+ produced by the Na^+/K^+-ATPase in the basolateral membrane (Fig. 23.6). **Loop diuretics** inhibit this process, as shown in Figures 23.4 and 23.7. Chloride then passes out of the cell into the circulation, partly by diffusion through chloride channels and partly by a symport mechanism with K^+ (see Fig. 23.6). Most of the K^+ taken into the cell by the co-transport system cycles back to the lumen through potassium channels but some K^+ is reabsorbed along with Mg^{2+} and Ca^{2+}.

The tubular fluid, after passage through the loop of Henle, will have been reduced in volume by a further 5% and, because of the absorption of NaCl, it is hypotonic with respect to plasma as it enters the distal convoluted tubule (Fig. 23.4). The thick ascending limb of the loop of Henle is sometimes referred to as the 'diluting segment' because the absorption of NaCl with very little water results in this marked dilution of the filtrate.

THE DISTAL TUBULE

In the early distal tubule, active NaCl transport, coupled with impermeability of the *zonula occludens*, continues to dilute the tubular fluid—and the osmolarity falls further below that of plasma. At this point, K^+ and H^+ are added to the filtrate. The transport is driven by the Na^+/ K^+ pump in the basolateral membrane, Na^+ entering the cell from the lumen, accompanied by Cl^- by means of an electroneutral Na^+/Cl^- carrier (Fig. 23.8). **Thiazide diuretics** act by inhibiting this carrier.

This part of the nephron is where Ca^{2+} excretion is regulated. Parathormone and calcitriol both increase Ca^{2+} reabsorption (see Ch. 30).

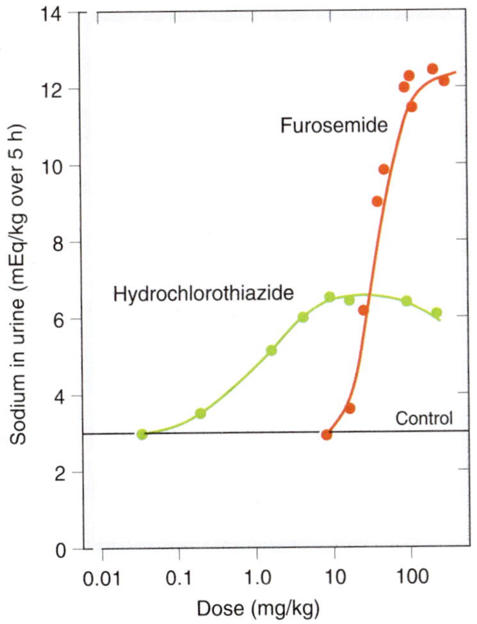

Fig. 23.6 The dose–response curves for furosemide (frusemide) and hydrochlorothiazide, showing differences in potency and 'ceiling'. Note that these doses are not used clinically. (Adapted from: Timmerman R J et al. 1964 Curr Ther Res 6: 88.)

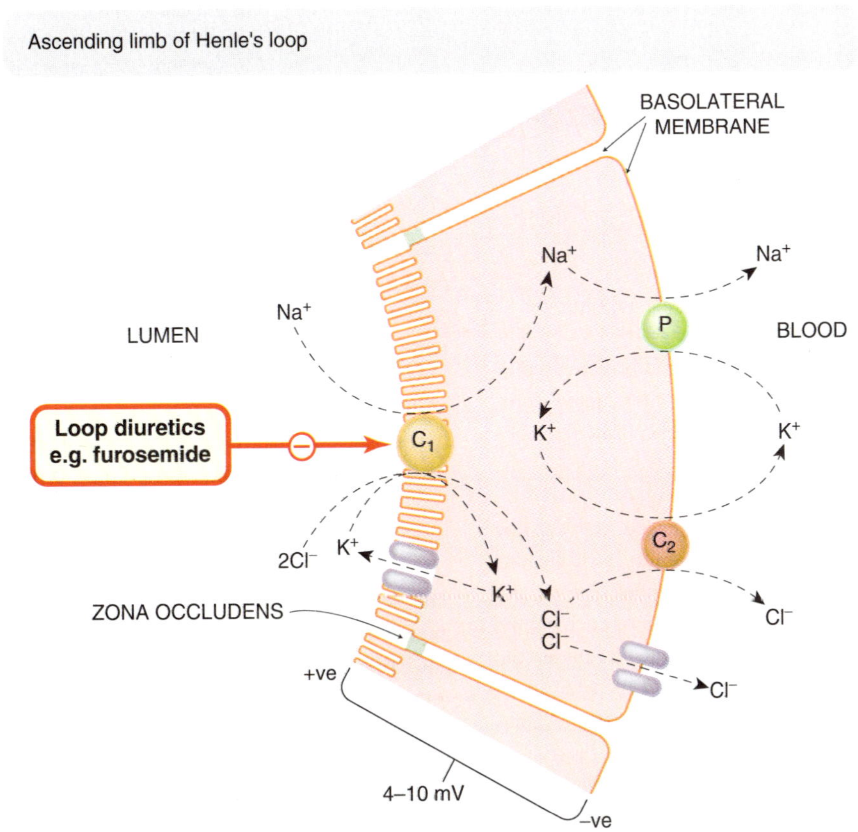

Fig. 23.7 Ion transport in the cells of the thick ascending limb of Henle's loop, showing the site of action of loop diuretics. The sodium pump (P) is the main primary active transport mechanism and Na^+, K^+ and Cl^- enter by a co-transport system (C_1). Chloride leaves the cell both through basolateral chloride channels and by an electroneutral K^+/Cl^- co-transport system (C_2). Some K^+ returns to the lumen via potassium channels in the apical membrane and some Na^+ is absorbed paracellularly, through the *zonula occludens*. Note that the diagram is simplified; consequently, the stoichiometry is not accurate; e.g. each time the sodium pump works, it exchanges $3Na^+$ for $2K^+$. (Based on Greger 2000.)

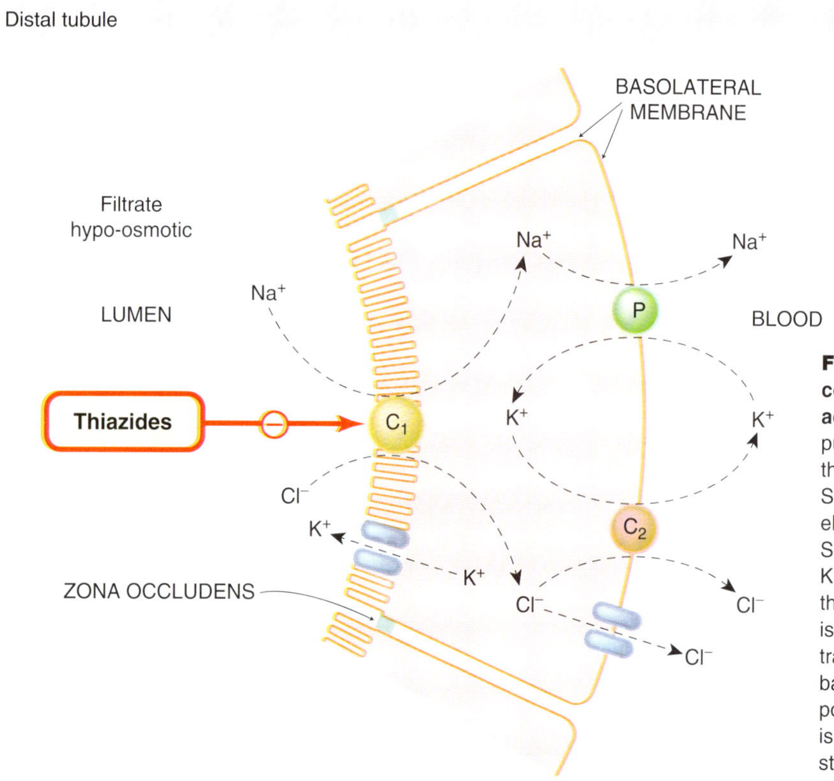

Fig. 23.8 Salt transport in the distal convoluted tubule showing the site of action of thiazide diuretics. The sodium pump (P) in the basolateral membrane is the primary active transport mechanism. Sodium and chloride ions enter by an electroneutral co-transport carrier (C_1). Some Cl^- is transported out of the cell by a K^+/Cl^- co-transport carrier (C_2); some leaves the cell through chloride channels. Some K^+ is transported out of the cell by the co-transport carrier (C_2), and some passes back into the tubule lumen through potassium channels. Note that the diagram is simplified; consequently, the stoichiometry is not accurate; e.g. each time the sodium pump works, it exchanges $3Na^+$ for $2K^+$. (Based on Greger 2000.)

THE COLLECTING TUBULE AND THE COLLECTING DUCT

Several distal tubules empty into each collecting tubule and the collecting tubules join to form collecting ducts (Fig. 23.1). The collecting tubule has two different cell types: the principal cells, which reabsorb Na^+ and secrete K^+ and the intercalated cells, which are involved mainly in H^+ secretion. The principal cells have sodium and potassium channels, not co-transporters, in the luminal membrane.

This portion of the nephron has 'tight' junctions between the cells, i.e. the *zona occludens* has low permeability to both ions and water. Because of this property, the movement of ions and water can be dissociated and individual regulation of each can be influenced by hormones. The absorption of NaCl is under the control of the mineralocorticoid **aldosterone**, and the absorption of water is under the control of **antidiuretic hormone** (ADH), also termed **vasopressin** (see Chs 18 and 27).

Aldosterone enhances Na^+ reabsorption and promotes K^+ excretion. It has a threefold action on Na^+ reabsorption. First, it has a rapid effect through stimulation of the Na^+/H^+ exchanger by an action on membrane aldosterone receptors.* Second, it has a delayed effect by binding to receptors within the cell (see Chs 3 and 27) and directing the synthesis of a specific mediator protein that activates sodium channels in the apical membrane, which allow transcellular passage of Na^+. **Amiloride** and **triamterene** inhibit these channels, as shown in Figures 23.4 and 23.9. Third, it exerts long-term effects by increasing the number of basolateral Na^+ pumps.

Aldosterone secretion is controlled indirectly by the juxtaglomerular apparatus (Fig. 23.2), which is sensitive to the composition of the fluid in the distal tubule. A decrease in the NaCl concentration of the filtrate is sensed by the *macula densa* cells of the distal tubule, which stimulate renin release (p. 354). This leads to the formation of angiotensin I and, subsequently, angiotensin II (see Ch. 18), which in turn stimulates the synthesis and release of aldosterone by the adrenal cortex. The renin–angiotensin system and the mechanism of action of aldosterone are considered in more detail in Chapters 18 and 27. **Spironolactone** exerts a diuretic effect by antagonising the action of aldosterone in this part of the nephron; shown in Figure 23.9.

ADH produces a sustained increase in the permeability to water in this part of the nephron, allowing its passive reabsorption. This hormone is secreted by the posterior pituitary gland (Ch. 27) and binds to receptors in the basolateral membrane. These receptors, which are different from those involved in vascular responses (p. 293), are termed V_2-receptors.

*A mechanism distinct from regulation of gene transcription, which is the normal transduction mechanism for steroid hormones (Chs 3 and 27).

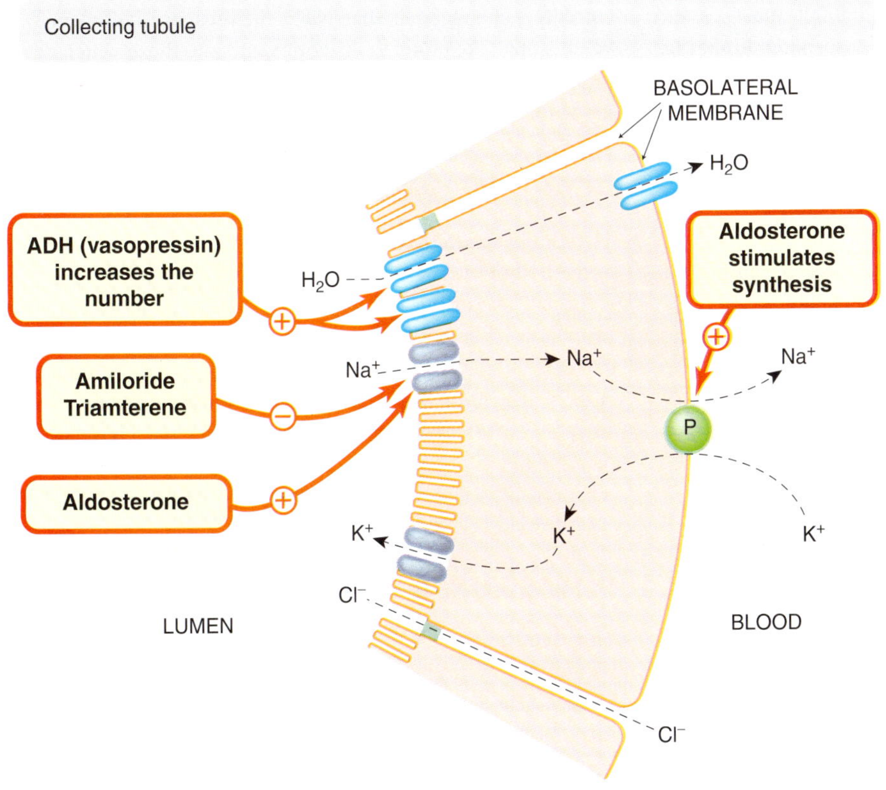

Fig. 23.9 Simplified diagram of the action of hormones and drugs on the principal cells of the collecting tubule. The cells are normally impermeable to water in the absence of antidiuretic hormone (ADH), and to Na^+ in the absence of aldosterone. Sodium chloride and water reabsorption in this part of the tubule are controlled physiologically by these two hormones, through their respective effects on the water channels and sodium channels. Aldosterone acts within the tubule (see p. 358). Spironolactone antagonises aldosterone action. Chloride ions may pass out of the tubule through the paracellular pathway. Potassium ions are added to the filtrate, as is H^+ (not shown). The Na^+ pump (P) in the basolateral membrane is the main source of energy for ion movement. Note that the diagram is simplified; consequently, the stoichiometry is not accurate; e.g. each time the sodium pump works, it exchanges $3Na^+$ for $2K^+$. (Adapted from: Greger 2000.)

The eventual result of stimulation of the V_2-receptors is an increase in the number of *aquaporins* (water channels) in the apical membrane.

Inhibition of the action of ADH occurs as a side-effect of some drugs—lithium carbonate (used in psychiatric disorders; see Ch. 38), demeclocycline (an antibiotic; see Ch. 45) and agents that affect the microtubules, such as colchicine (Ch. 16) and the vinca alkaloids (see Ch. 50).

Urea is reabsorbed from the medullary section of the collecting tubule and passes into the interstitial tissue, where it plays a part in increasing the osmolarity of this area (see Fig. 23.5).

The main site at which the urine is concentrated is in the collecting tubule as it passes into the medulla, where there is passive reabsorption of water owing to the increasing osmolarity of the interstitial fluid. This absorption depends on ADH and, in its absence, the low water permeability of the collecting ducts means that the hypo-osmolarity of the distal tubular fluid is maintained as the fluid traverses the collecting ducts, and a large volume of hypotonic urine is excreted.

NATRIURETIC PEPTIDES

Endogenous natriuretic peptides are involved in the regulation of Na^+ excretion in the distal nephron. The *atrial natriuretic peptide* (aka atriopeptin) (see Ch. 17) is released when the atrial pressure is high. It causes solute and water diuresis by both renal haemodynamic effects (increasing glomerular capillary pressure by dilating afferent and constricting efferent arterioles) and direct tubular actions. The tubular actions include the inhibition of angiotensin II-stimulated Na^+ and water reabsorption in the proximal convoluted tubule and antidiuretic-mediated water reabsorption in the collecting tubule (Levin et al., 1998). The effect is to decrease blood volume and, therefore, to reduce atrial pressure.

Another peptide, similar to atriopeptin and termed urodilatin, is now thought to be produced in the distal tubule and is believed to promote Na^+ excretion and produce diuresis by action on receptors on the luminal side of the collecting duct cells.

THE COUNTER-CURRENT MULTIPLIER AND EXCHANGE SYSTEM IN THE MEDULLA

The loops of Henle function as counter-current multipliers and the vasa recta as counter-current exchangers. In the ascending limb, NaCl is actively absorbed in the thick part and passively absorbed in the thin part. This results in hypertonicity of the interstitial tissue. In the descending limb, water moves out of the tubule and the fluid becomes more concentrated as it reaches the bend. There is, consequently, an osmotic gradient in the medulla, which ranges from isotonicity (300 mosmol/l) at the cortical boundary to 1200–1500 mosmol/l or more in the innermost area (see Fig. 23.5). Urea contributes to this gradient because it is more slowly reabsorbed than water throughout most of the nephron (it may be added to the fluid in the descending limb; Fig. 23.5) and so its concentration rises until it reaches the collecting tubules in the medulla, where it diffuses out into the interstitia. It is thus 'trapped' in the inner medulla.

These differences in NaCl concentration are the basis of the counter-current multiplier system, the main principle being that a small horizontal osmotic gradient is multiplied vertically (see Fig. 23.5). The primary generating force is the active reabsorption of NaCl in the ascending limb of the loop of Henle.

The osmotic gradient would be dissipated if all the excess NaCl in the medulla were carried away by the blood vessels. This does not happen because the vasa recta function as counter-current exchangers in that NaCl diffuses passively out of the vessels that take blood to the cortex and into those which descend into the medulla (Fig. 23.5), while water diffuses out of the descending and into the ascending vessels.

Renal tubular function

- All the constituents of the plasma, other than proteins, are filtered into the tubules.
- Transport of Na^+ out of the tubules by the Na^+/K^+-ATPase in the basolateral membrane is the main primary active transport process throughout the tubules.
- In the proximal tubules, 60–70% of the filtered NaCl and water is reabsorbed isosmotically and organic acids and bases are secreted into the tubular lumen, as is 90% of bicarbonate.
- In the descending limb of Henle's loop, water is reabsorbed owing to hypertonicity in the medulla; fluid of high osmolarity, therefore, reaches the thick ascending limb.
- The thick ascending limb is impermeable to water, and within it 20–30% of the filtered NaCl is reabsorbed (the major factor in producing hypertonicity in the medulla). The ions are transported by a $Na^+/2Cl^-/K^+$ carrier (inhibited by loop diuretics), the co-transport being driven by the Na^+ pump in the basolateral membrane. The filtrate is diluted.
- Counter-current mechanisms maintain hypertonicity in the medulla.
- In the distal convoluted tubule, an electroneutral co-transport carrier (inhibited by thiazides) is responsible for the reabsorption of 5–10% of the filtered load of NaCl, the reabsorption being driven by the Na^+ pump in the basolateral membrane. Potassium ions are secreted into the tubule.
- The collecting tubules and ducts have low permeability to salts and water. Sodium ions are absorbed through sodium channels, which are stimulated by the aldosterone mediator (and inhibited by amiloride). Aldosterone also increases the number of basolateral Na^+ pumps. Water absorption through water channels is stimulated by antidiuretic hormone. Both K^+ and H^+ are secreted into the tubule.

ACID–BASE BALANCE

The kidneys participate in the regulation of the H^+ concentration of the body fluids. Though either an acid or alkaline urine can be excreted according to need, the usual requirement is the formation of an acid urine to compensate for the tendency to a decrease in body pH consequent on the metabolic production of carbon dioxide. The compensating renal mechanism is the secretion of H^+ into the tubular fluid and the conservation of bicarbonate. This depends on the carbonic anhydrase-catalysed reactions illustrated in Figure 23.10.

POTASSIUM BALANCE

The extracellular K^+ concentration is controlled rapidly and within narrow limits through regulation of K^+ excretion by the kidney. This regulation is very important because small changes in extracellular $[K^+]$ affect the function of many excitable tissues, particularly the heart, brain and skeletal muscle. Urinary K^+ excretion is normally about 50–100 mEq (50–100 mmol) in 24 hours, but can be as low as 5 mEq or as high as 1000 mEq. The amount that normally appears in the urine represents mainly K^+ secreted into the filtrate in the collecting tubule, as much of the filtered K^+ is reabsorbed in the proximal tubule and loop of Henle. Some diuretics cause significant K^+ loss (see below). This may be particularly important if such K^+-losing agents are administered at the same time as cardiac glycosides or class II antidysrhythmic drugs (for which toxicity is increased by low plasma K^+; see Ch. 17).

In the collecting duct, K^+ is transported into the cell from the blood and the interstitial fluid by the Na^+/K^+-ATPase in the basolateral membrane; it then leaks into the tubule through a K^+-selective ion channel. Sodium passes through sodium channels in the apical membrane down the electrochemical gradient for Na^+ created by the Na^+/K^+-ATPase; this influx results in depolarisation of the luminal, but not the basolateral membrane, and generates a lumen-negative potential difference across the cell, which increases the driving force for K^+ secretion. Thus the K^+ secretory flux is regulated by the extent to which Na^+ is reabsorbed.

It follows that K^+ loss will be *increased* in the following circumstances:

- when more Na^+ reaches the collecting duct: as occurs with the **thiazide** (p. 363) and *loop diuretics* (p. 362), which decrease Na^+ absorption in earlier parts of the nephron and, therefore, increase its delivery to the collecting ducts (the high flow rate of filtrate produced by these diuretics will also favour K^+ excretion by continually flushing it away, increasing the gradient from cell to lumen)

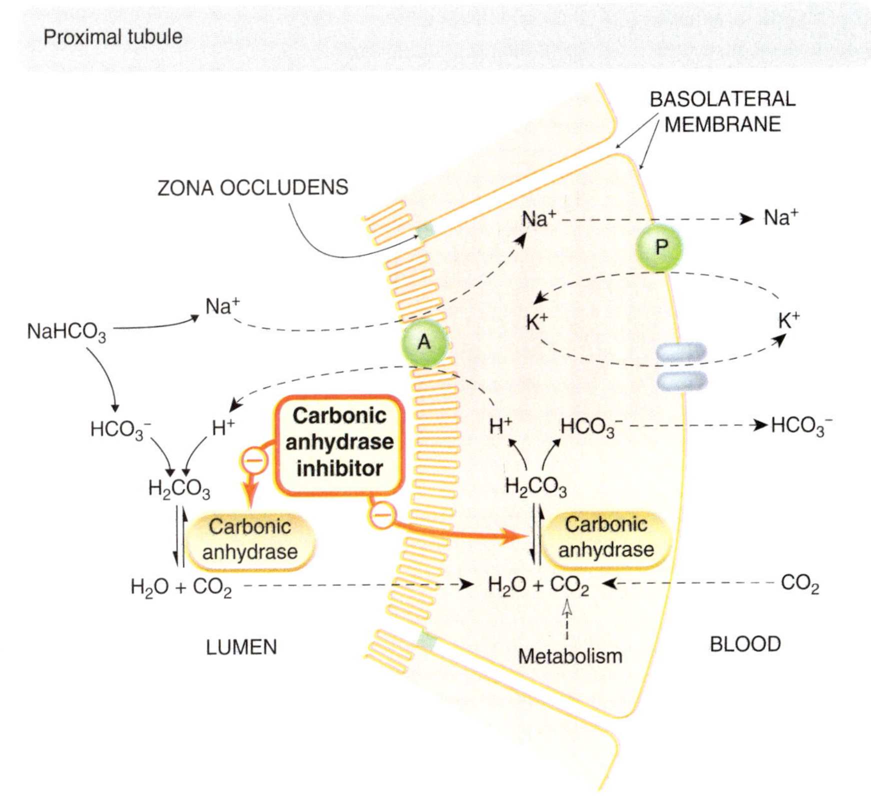

Fig. 23.10 Renal mechanisms for conserving base showing the action of carbonic anhydrase inhibitors. Sodium ions are absorbed and H^+ secreted at the luminal surface by an antiport mechanism (A). Most bicarbonate in the filtrate is 'reabsorbed' in this way in the proximal tubule. In the distal tubule, bicarbonate is added to the plasma, and monobasic phosphate or ammonium chloride is added to the urine (not shown). The primary active transport mechanism is the Na^+ pump (P). Potassium ions pass out of the cell through potassium channels. (Amiloride inhibits the Na^+/H^+ exchange or antiport, but this is not a major factor in its diuretic action.) Note that the diagram is simplified; consequently, the stoichiometry is not accurate; e.g. each time the sodium pump works, it exchanges $3Na^+$ for $2K^+$. (Adapted from Hendry & Ellory, 1988.)

- when Na^+ reabsorption in the collecting ducts is markedly increased—as occurs in hyperaldosteronism: this indirectly increases K^+ excretion but aldosterone may also directly increase luminal membrane K^+ permeability.

Potassium loss will be *reduced* in the following circumstances:

- when Na^+ reabsorption in the collecting ducts is decreased—as occurs with **amiloride** and **triamterene**, which block the sodium channel in this part of the nephron (see p. 364) and with spironolactone, which blocks the action of aldosterone (see p. 364).

Recent work suggests that the kidney has a previously unsuspected mechanism for primary, active K^+ absorption in the collecting duct, possibly by a luminal membrane H^+/K^+-ATPase similar to that on gastric parietal cells.

EXCRETION OF ORGANIC MOLECULES

There are different mechanisms for the excretion of organic anions and organic cations (see Ch. 8) but both involve active transport, the energy being derived from the action of the basolateral Na^+/K^+-ATPase in the basolateral membrane.

Organic anions bound to plasma albumin do not pass into the glomerular filtrate, but when the blood from the glomerulus passes into the peritubular capillary plexus they may be secreted into the proximal convoluted tubule. They are exchanged with α-ketoglutarate by an antiport in the basolateral membrane and diffuse passively into the tubular lumen (Fig. 23.3). Among the drugs excreted in this way are the thiazides, furosemide (frusemide), salicylates and most penicillins and cephalosporins.

Organic cations are thought to diffuse into the cell from the interstitia and are then actively transported into the tubular lumen in exchange for H^+. Some diuretics (triamterene, amiloride) are added to the tubular fluid in this way and many drugs are eliminated by this route, including atropine, morphine and quinine.

This topic is dealt with in more detail in Chapter 8 (Table 8.4).

ARACHIDONIC ACID METABOLITES AND RENAL FUNCTION

The metabolites of arachidonic acid, the *eicosanoids*, which are generated in the kidney, modulate its haemodynamics and excretory functions. Details of the eicosanoids are given in Chapter 15.

Prostanoids, the products of the cylcooxygenase pathway, are synthesised in all parts of the kidney, the predominant products being prostaglandin (PG) E_2 in the medulla and PGI_2 (prostacyclin) in the glomeruli. Factors that stimulate their synthesis include ischaemia, mechanical trauma, circulating angiotensin II, catecholamines, ADH and bradykinin.

Influence on haemodynamics

Under basal conditions, prostaglandins probably do not have much effect. However, in circumstances in which vasoconstrictor agents (angiotensin II, noradrenaline) are generated and released, the vasodilator prostaglandins PGE_2 and PGI_2 modulate the effects of these agents in the kidney by causing compensatory vasodilatation. Prostaglandins play a part in the control of renin release under basal conditions, and also in conditions of intravascular volume depletion.

Influence on the renal control of NaCl and water

The overall effect of the renal prostaglandins is to increase renal blood flow and cause natriuresis. This can, in some circumstances, be an important consideration, for example, when non-steroidal anti-inflammatory agents (NSAIDs, which inhibit prostaglandin production; see Ch. 16) are used in therapy. These agents (both traditional NSAIDs and cyclooxygenase-2 inhibitors) can cause a decline in renal perfusion and decreased excretion of both Na^+ and K^+ (Brater, 1999). NSAIDs can cause renal failure in several clinical conditions in which renal blood flow depends on vasodilator prostaglandins, for example cirrhosis of the liver, heart failure, nephrotic syndrome and glomerulonephritis. They can also exacerbate NaCl and water retention in patients with heart failure.

DRUGS ACTING ON THE KIDNEY

DIURETICS

Diuretics are drugs that increase the excretion of Na^+ and water from the body by an action on the kidney. Their primary effect is to decrease the reabsorption of Na^+ and Cl^- from the filtrate, increased water loss being secondary to the increased excretion of NaCl. This can be achieved by:

- a direct action on the cells of the nephron
- indirectly modifying the content of the filtrate.

Since a very large proportion of the NaCl and water that passes into the tubule in the glomerulus is reabsorbed (Table 23.1), a small decrease in reabsorption can result in a marked increase in excretion. A summary diagram of the mechanisms and sites of action of various diuretics is given in Figure 23.4.

Note that the diuretics which have a direct action on the cells of the nephron (with the exception of spironolactone) act from within the tubular lumen and reach their sites of action by being secreted into the proximal tubule.

DIURETICS ACTING DIRECTLY ON THE CELLS OF THE NEPHRON

Drugs that cause NaCl loss by an action on cells must obviously affect those parts of the nephron where most of the active and selective solute reabsorption occurs:

- the ascending loop of Henle
- the early distal tubule
- the collecting tubules and ducts.

Loop diuretics

Loop diuretics are the most powerful of all diuretics, capable of causing 15–25% of the Na^+ in the filtrate to be excreted (see Fig. 23.6 for comparison with a thiazide). They are termed 'high ceiling' diuretics and their action is often described—in a phrase that conjures up a rather uncomfortable picture—as causing 'torrential urine flow'. The main example is **furosemide**; others are **bumetanide**, **piretanide**, **torasemide** and **etacrynic acid**. These drugs act primarily on the thick segment of the ascending loop of Henle, inhibiting the transport of NaCl out of the tubule into the interstitial tissue by inhibiting the $Na^+/K^+/2Cl^-$ carrier in the luminal membrane (see Figs 23.4 and 23.7). Furosemide, bumetanide and torasemide have a direct inhibiting effect on the carrier, acting on the Cl^--binding site.

As has been explained above, the reabsorption of solute at this site is the basis for the ability of the kidney to concentrate the urine by creating a hypertonic interstitial area in the medulla, which provides the osmotic pressure gradient by which water is reabsorbed from the collecting tubules under the influence of the ADH. The action of the loop diuretics has the additional effect that more solute is delivered to the distal portions of the nephron, where its osmotic pressure further reduces water reabsorption. Essentially, some of the solute which normally passes into the medullary interstitium and draws water out of the collecting ducts now remains in the tubular fluid and holds water with it. As much as 25% of the glomerular filtrate may pass out of the nephron (compared with the normal loss of about 1%), resulting in a profuse diuresis.

Loop diuretics appear to have a venodilator action, directly and/or indirectly through the release of a renal factor. After intravenous administration to patients with acute heart failure (see Ch. 17), a therapeutically useful vascular effect is seen before the onset of the diuretic effect.

The increased Na^+ concentration that reaches the distal tubule results in increased loss of H^+ and K^+ (see p. 356). Loop diuretics may thus produce a metabolic alkalosis.

There is an increase in the excretion of Ca^{2+} and Mg^{2+} and a decreased excretion of uric acid. The effect on Na^+ is beneficial in the treatment of hypercalcaemia. Torasemide causes less loss of K^+ and Na^+.

Pharmacokinetic aspects

The loop diuretics are readily absorbed from the gastrointestinal tract and may also be given by injection. They are strongly bound to plasma protein and so do not pass into the glomerular filtrate to any marked degree. They reach their site of action—the luminal membrane of the cells of the thick ascending loop—by being secreted in the proximal convoluted tubule by the organic acid transport mechanism; the fraction thus secreted will pass out in the urine. The fraction not secreted is metabolised in the liver—bumetanide and torasemide being metabolised by cytochrome P450 pathways and furosemide being glucuronidated. Given orally, they act within 1 hour; given intravenously, they produce a peak effect within 30 minutes. The plasma half-lives are about 90 minutes (longer in renal failure) and the duration of action 3–6 hours, except in the case of torasemide, which has a longer half-life and longer duration of action and can, therefore, be given once a day. The clinical use of loop diuretics is given in the box.

Unwanted effects

Some unwanted effects are common with loop diuretics and are directly related to their renal actions. Potassium loss (see p. 360), resulting in low plasma K^+ (hypokalaemia), and metabolic alkalosis owing to H^+ excretion are both very likely to occur. Hypokalaemia can be averted or treated by concomitant use of K^+-sparing diuretics (see below) or by potassium supplements. Depletion of Mg^{2+} and Na^+ is common, and in elderly patients, hypovolaemia and hypotension, with collapse as a result of the sudden loss of extracellular fluid volume, can follow the profuse diuresis produced by these agents.

Unwanted effects that are not related to the renal actions of the drugs are rare. They include nausea, allergic reactions (more common in those agents related to sulfonamides) and, infrequently, deafness (compounded by concomitant use of an aminoglycoside antibiotic).

Diuretics acting on the distal tubule

The diuretics acting at on the distal tubule include the thiazides and related drugs.

The main thiazide is **bendroflumethiazide** (bendrofluazide). Others are **hydrochlorothiazide** and **cyclopenthiazide**, but many similar drugs are available. Drugs with similar actions include **chlortalidone**, and newer ones such as **indapamide**, **xipamide** and **metolazone**.

This group of drugs has a moderately powerful diuretic action (see comparison with loop diuretics in Fig. 23.6). They decrease active reabsorption of Na^+ and accompanying Cl^- by binding to the Cl^- site of the electroneutral Na^+/Cl^- co-transport system and inhibiting its action (Figs 23.4 and 23.8). They do not have any action on the thick ascending loop of Henle. Potassium loss with these drugs is significant (by mechanisms explained on p. 360) and can be serious. Excretion of uric acid and Na^+ is decreased; that of Mg^{2+} is increased.

Hypochloraemic alkalosis can occur.

Thiazide diuretics have a paradoxical effect in diabetes insipidus, where they reduce the volume of urine.

They have some extrarenal actions—they produce vasodilatation and can cause hyperglycaemia. When used in the treatment of hypertension (Ch. 18), the initial fall in blood pressure results from the decreased blood volume caused by diuresis, but the later phase seems to be caused by a direct action on the blood vessels. Note that diazoxide, a non-diuretic thiazide, (now seldom used) has powerful vasodilator effects and also increases the blood sugar. It also inhibits insulin secretion from the pancreatic islet cells, both effects being mediated by the same mechanism, namely the opening of ATP-sensitive potassium channels. **Indapamide** is said to lower blood pressure at subdiuretic doses with less metabolic disturbance.

There is evidence that thiazides may reduce bone loss in postmenopausal women (Reid et al., 2000)

Pharmacokinetic aspects

The thiazides and related drugs are all effective orally, being well absorbed from the gastrointestinal tract. All are excreted in the urine, mainly by tubular secretion (see p. 361). Their tendency to increase plasma uric acid results from competition with uric acid for tubular secretion mechanisms. With the shorter-acting drugs such as bendroflumethiazide, hydrochlorothiazide, chlorothiazide and cyclopenthiazide, the maximum effect is at about 4–6 hours and duration between 8 and 12 hours. Chlortalidone has a longer duration of action (up to 48 hours) and can be given on alternate days. The clinical use of thiazide diuretics is given in the clinical box.

Unwanted effects

Serious unwanted effects are relatively rare. The main adverse effects of thiazides are the result of some of the renal actions, K^+ depletion being the most important. Others are metabolic alkalosis and increased plasma uric acid (with the possibility of gout). Indapamide has little obvious effect on K^+, uric acid and glucose excretion.

Clinical uses of loop diuretics

- Loop diuretics are used (cautiously!) usually in conjunction with dietary salt restriction and often with other classes of diuretic drug in the treatment of salt and water overload associated with:
  - —acute pulmonary oedema
  - —chronic heart failure
  - —cirrhosis of the liver complicated by ascites
  - —nephrotic syndrome
  - —renal failure.
- The treatment of hypertension (thiazides are usually preferred), especially if this is complicated by renal impairment.
- An additional distinct use is in acute treatment of hypercalcaemia after replacement of plasma volume with intravenous isotonic NaCl solution.

Clinical uses of thiazide diuretics

- Hypertension.
- Mild heart failure (loop diuretics are usually needed).
- Severe resistant oedema (metolazone, especially, is used, together with loop diuretics).
- To prevent recurrent stone formation in idiopathic hypercalciuria.
- Nephrogenic diabetes insipidus.

- the motility of the bowel and the expulsion of the faeces
- the formation and excretion of bile.

GASTRIC SECRETION

The stomach secretes about 2.5 litres of gastric juice daily. The principal exocrine secretions are pepsinogens, from the *chief* or *peptic cells*, and hydrochloric acid (HCl) and intrinsic factor (see Ch. 21) from the *parietal* or *oxyntic cells*. Mucus is secreted by mucus-secreting cells found amongst the surface cells throughout the gastric mucosa. Bicarbonate ions are also secreted and are trapped in the mucus, creating a gradient of pH from 1–2 in the lumen to 6–7 at the mucosal surface. The mucus and bicarbonate form an unstirred gel-like layer protecting the mucosa from the gastric juice. Alcohol and bile can disrupt this layer. Locally produced prostaglandins stimulate the secretion of both mucus and bicarbonate.

Disturbances in the above secretory functions are thought to be involved in the pathogenesis of peptic ulcer, and the therapy of this condition involves drugs that modify each of these factors.

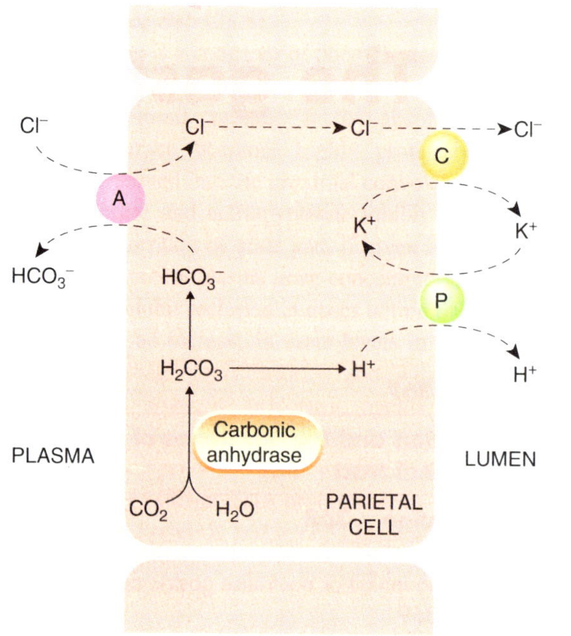

Fig. 24.1 A schematic illustration of the secretion of hydrochloric acid by the gastric parietal cell. Secretion involves a proton pump (P) which is a H^+/K^+-ATPase, a symport carrier (C) for K^+ and Cl^-, and an antiport (A), which exchanges Cl^- and HCO_3^-. A Na^+/H^+ antiport at the interface with the plasma may also have a role (not shown).

THE REGULATION OF ACID SECRETION BY PARIETAL CELLS

The regulation of acid secretion by parietal cells is especially important in peptic ulcer and constitutes a particular target for drug action. The secretion of the parietal cells is an isotonic solution of HCl (150 mmol/l) with a pH less than 1, the concentration of H^+ being more than a million times higher than that of the plasma.

The Cl^- is actively transported into canaliculi in the cells which communicate with the lumen of the gastric glands and thus with the lumen of the stomach. This Cl^- secretion is accompanied by K^+, which is then exchanged for H^+ from within the cell by a K^+/H^+-ATPase (Fig. 24.1). Carbonic anhydrase catalyses the combination of carbon dioxide and water to give carbonic acid, which dissociates into H^+ and bicarbonate ions. The latter exchanges across the basal membrane for Cl^-. Three main stimuli act on the parietal cells:

- gastrin (a hormone)
- acetylcholine (a neurotransmitter)
- histamine (a local hormone).

Prostaglandins E_2 and I_2 inhibit acid secretion. Figure 24.2 summarises the actions of these chemical mediators.

Gastrin

Gastrin is a peptide hormone synthesised in endocrine cells of the mucosa of the gastric antrum and duodenum; it is secreted into the portal blood. Its main action is stimulation of the secretion of acid by the parietal cells, but there is controversy as to the mechanism of action (discussed below). Gastrin receptors on the parietal cells have been demonstrated with radioactively labelled gastrin. The receptors are blocked by **proglumide** (Fig. 24.2)—a drug used only as an experimental tool.

Gastrin also indirectly increases pepsinogen secretion and stimulates blood flow and gastric motility. Control of gastrin release involves both neuronal transmitters and blood-borne mediators, and the direct effects of the stomach contents. Within

Secretion of gastric acid, mucus and bicarbonate

- Acid is secreted from gastric parietal cells by a proton pump (K^+/H^+-ATPase).
- The three endogenous secretagogues for acid are histamine, acetylcholine and gastrin.
- Prostaglandins E_2 and I_2 inhibit acid, stimulate mucus and bicarbonate secretion and dilate mucosal blood vessels.
- The genesis of peptic ulcers involves:
  —infection of the gastric mucosa with *Helicobacter pylori* plus
  —other factors such as an imbalance between the mucosal-damaging mechanisms (acid, pepsin), and the mucosal-protecting mechanisms (mucus, bicarbonate, local synthesis of prostaglandins E_2 and I_2 and nitric oxide).

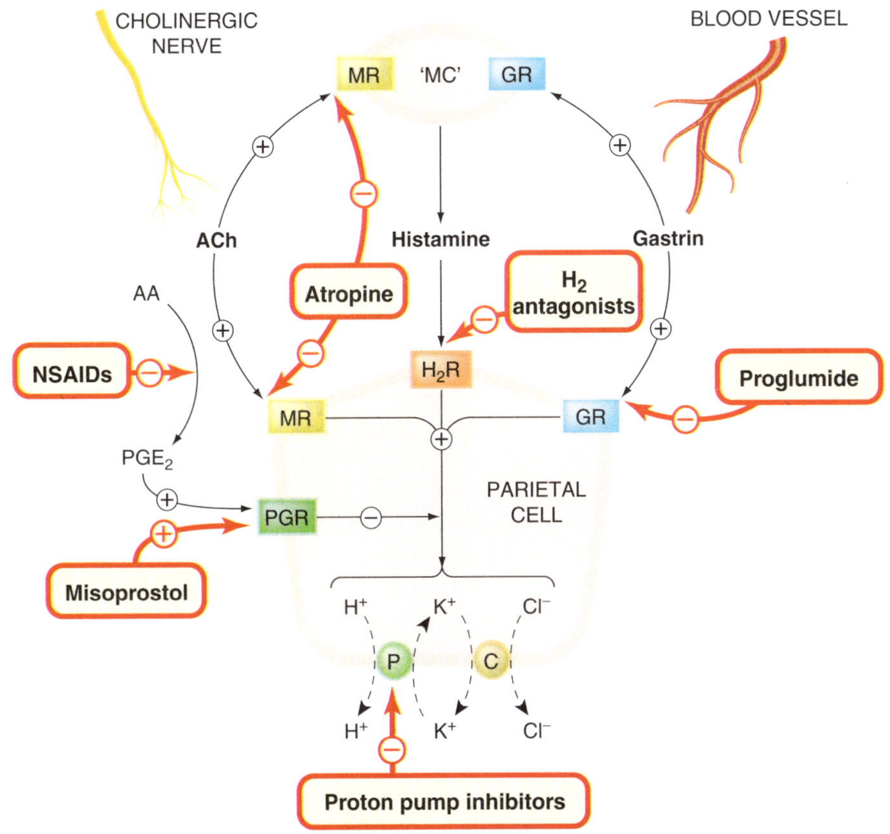

Fig. 24.2 Schematic diagram showing the one-cell and two-cell hypotheses of the action of secretagogues on the acid-secreting gastric parietal cell, giving the site of action of drugs influencing acid secretion. Acetylcholine and gastrin may act mainly directly on their receptors (the one-cell hypothesis) or partly directly and partly by releasing histamine (the two-cell hypothesis). ('MC', mast-cell-like, histamine-secreting cell; Hist, histamine; ACh, acetylcholine; MR, muscarinic receptor; H_2R, histamine H_2-receptor; GR, gastrin receptor; PGR, prostaglandin E_2 (PGE_2) receptor; AA, arachidonic acid; NSAIDs, non-steroidal anti-inflammatory drugs; P, proton pump (H^+/K^+-ATPase); C, symport carrier for K^+ and Cl^-.)

the stomach, the important stimuli are amino acids and small peptides, which act directly on the gastrin-secreting cells. Milk and solutions of calcium salts are also effective stimulants, so it is inappropriate to use calcium-containing salts as antacids.

Acetylcholine

Acetylcholine is released from neurons and stimulates specific muscarinic receptors on the surface of the parietal cells and on the surface of histamine-containing cells, as determined by studies with competitive antagonists (see Ch. 10).

Histamine

Histamine is discussed in Chapter 15. Only those aspects of its pharmacology relevant to gastric secretion will be dealt with here. The parietal cells are stimulated by histamine acting on H_2-receptors. They respond to amounts that are below the threshold concentration that acts on H_2-receptors in blood vessels. The histamine is derived from mast cells (or histamine-containing cells similar to mast cells) that lie close to the parietal cell. There is a steady basal release of histamine, which is increased by gastrin and acetylcholine.

The role of acetylcholine, histamine and gastrin in acid secretion

The exact mechanism of action of the three secretagogues on the parietal cell is not entirely clear. A general scheme is given in Figure 24.2, which summarises the two main theories: the *single-cell* hypothesis and the *two-cell* hypothesis.

According to the *single-cell hypothesis*, the parietal cell has H_2-receptors for histamine, muscarinic M_2-receptors for acetylcholine, and also gastrin receptors. Stimulation of the H_2-receptors increases cAMP, and stimulation of the M_2- and gastrin receptors increases cytosolic Ca^{2+}; these intracellular messengers synergise to produce acid secretion. In this scheme, all three secretagogues act directly on the parietal cell. Evidence for independent action of all three secretagogues comes from experiments with isolated canine parietal cells. However, the situation in vivo is more complicated, in that **cimetidine**, (an H_2-receptor antagonist) and atropine (a muscarinic receptor antagonist) can block gastrin action.

According to the *two-cell hypothesis*, gastrin and acetylcholine act either only by releasing histamine, or partly by releasing histamine and partly by direct action on their respective receptors on the parietal cell. This is discussed by Black & Shankley (1987), Soll & Berglindh (1987) and Sandvik & Waldrum (1991).

DRUGS USED TO INHIBIT OR NEUTRALISE GASTRIC ACID SECRETION

The principal pathological conditions in which it is useful to reduce acid secretion are peptic ulceration (both duodenal and gastric), reflux oesophagitis (in which gastric juice causes damage to the oesophagus) and the Zollinger–Ellison syndrome (a rare condition which is caused by a gastrin-producing tumour).

The reason why peptic ulcers develop is not fully understood. Infection of the stomach mucosa with *Helicobacter pylori**—a Gram-negative bacillus that causes chronic gastritis—is now generally considered to be a major cause, especially of duodenal ulcer. Treatment of *H. pylori* infection is discussed below.

Prostaglandins, synthesised in the mucosa, stimulate mucus and bicarbonate secretion, decrease acid secretion and cause vasodilatation, all of which serves to protect the stomach against damage. This explains the ability of non-steroidal anti-inflammatory drugs (NSAIDs: inhibitors of prostaglandin formation, Ch. 16) to cause gastric bleeding and erosions. More selective cyclooxygenase-2 inhibitors such as **celecoxib** and **rofecoxib** appear to cause less stomach damage.

Therapy of peptic ulcer and reflux oesophagitis involves decreasing the secretion of acid with H_2-receptor antagonists or proton-pump inhibitors, and/or neutralising secreted acid with antacids (see Colin-Jones, 1990; Huang & Hunt, 2001). These treatments are often coupled to eradication of *H. pylori* (see Horn, 2000).

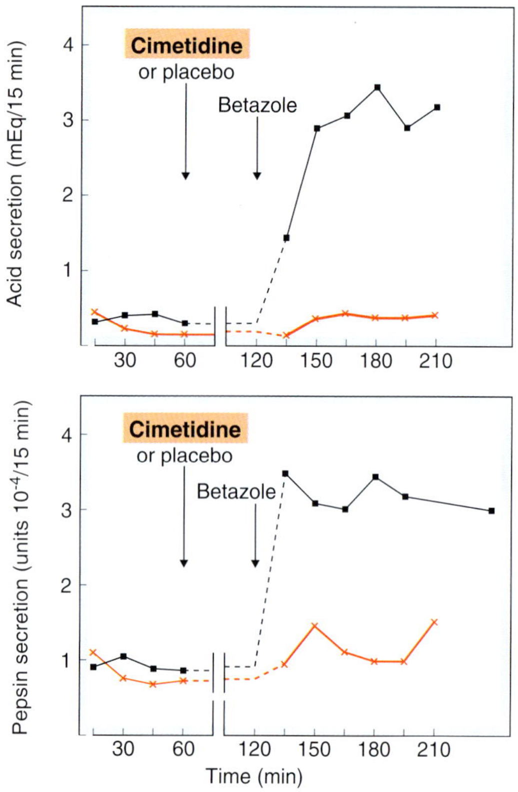

Fig. 24.3 The effect of cimetidine on betazole-stimulated gastric acid and pepsin secretion in humans. Either cimetidine or a placebo was given orally 60 minutes prior to injecting betazole (1.5 mg/kg) subcutaneously. (Betazole, an isomer of histamine that is a relatively specific histamine H_2-receptor agonist; it stimulates gastric acid secretion.) (Modified from: Binder H J, Donaldson R M 1978 Gastroenterology 74: 371–375.)

HISTAMINE H_2-RECEPTOR ANTAGONISTS

The histamine H_2-receptor antagonists competitively inhibit histamine actions at all H_2-receptors, but their main clinical use is as inhibitors of gastric acid secretion. They inhibit histamine-, gastrin- and acetylcholine-stimulated acid secretion; pepsin secretion also falls with the reduction in volume of gastric juice. These agents not only decrease both basal and food-stimulated acid secretion by 90% or more but also promote healing of duodenal ulcers, as shown by numerous clinical trials. Relapses are likely to follow when treatment with H_2-receptor antagonists is stopped.

The drugs used are **cimetidine** (Table 15.2) and **ranitidine**. Newer H_2-receptor antagonists, such as **nizatidine** and **famotidine**, are also available. The results of experiments with cimetidine on gastric secretion in humans are given in Figure 24.3. The clinical use of H_2-receptor antagonists is given in the clinical box on page 372.

Pharmacokinetic aspects and unwanted effects

The drugs are given orally and are well absorbed. Preparations of cimetidine and ranitidine for intramuscular and intravenous use are also available. With these two preparations, oral doses twice daily, even single doses nocturnally, are effective. Famotidine and nizatidine need only be given once a day.

Unwanted effects are rare. Diarrhoea, dizziness, muscle pains, transient rashes and hypergastrinaemia have been reported. Cimetidine sometimes causes gynaecomastia in men and, rarely, decrease in sexual function. This is probably caused by a modest affinity for androgen receptors. Cimetidine also inhibits cytochrome P450 and can retard the metabolism (and thus potentiate the action) of a range of drugs including oral anticoagulants and tricyclic antidepressants. It can also cause confusion in the elderly.

PROTON-PUMP INHIBITORS

The first proton-pump inhibitor was the substituted benzimidazole **omeprazole**. It acts by irreversible inhibition of the H^+/K^+-ATPase (the proton pump), the terminal step in the acid secretory pathway (see Figs 24.1 and 24.2). It markedly inhibits both basal and stimulated gastric acid secretion (Fig. 24.4). It is inactive at neutral pH, but, being a weak base, accumulates in the acid environment of the canaliculi of the stimulated parietal cell where it is activated. This preferential accumulation in areas of very low pH, such as occur uniquely in the secretory canaliculi of gastric parietal cells, means that it has a specific effect on these cells. Other proton-pump inhibitors include **lansoprazole, pantoprazole** and **rabeprazole.**

**H. pylori* infection in the stomach is an important risk factor for gastric cancer. *H. pylori* has been classified as a class 1 (definite) carcinogen for this type of malignancy.

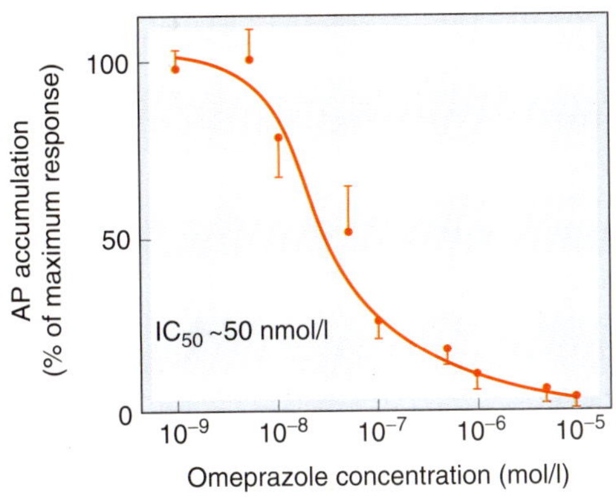

Fig. 24.4 The inhibitory action of omeprazole on acid secretion from isolated human gastric glands stimulated by 50 μmol/l histamine. Mean and standard error for tissue from eight patients. Acid secretion was measured by the accumulation of a radiolabelled weak base, aminopyrine (AP), in the secretory channels. (Adapted from: Lindberg P et al. 1987 Trends Pharmacol Sci 8: 399–402.)

The clinical use of proton-pump inhibitors is given in the clinical box on p. 372.

Pharmacokinetic aspects and unwanted effects

Omeprazole is given orally but as it degrades rapidly at low pH, it is administered as capsules containing enteric-coated granules. It is absorbed and from the blood passes into the parietal cells and then into the canaliculi. Increased doses give disproportionately higher increases in plasma concentration (possibly because its inhibitory effect on acid secretion improves its own relative bioavailability). Although its half-life is about 1 hour, a single daily dose affects acid secretion for 2–3 days because it accumulates in the canaliculi. With daily dosage, there is an increasing antisecretory effect for up to 5 days, after which a plateau is reached.

Unwanted effects are not common. They include headache, diarrhoea (both sometimes severe) and rashes. Dizziness, somnolence, mental confusion, impotence, gynaecomastia, and pain in muscles and joints have been reported.

ANTACIDS

Antacids act by neutralising gastric acid and thus raising the gastric pH. This has the effect of inhibiting peptic activity, which practically ceases at pH 5. Given in sufficient quantity for long enough they can produce healing of duodenal ulcers but are less effective for gastric ulcers.

The antacids in common use are salts of magnesium and aluminium. Magnesium salts cause diarrhoea and aluminium salts constipation, so mixtures of these two can, happily, be used to preserve normal bowel function. Some preparations of these substances (e.g. magnesium trisilicate mixture and some proprietary aluminium preparations) contain high concentrations of sodium and should not be given to patients on a sodium-restricted diet.

Numerous antacid preparations are available; a few of the main ones are given below.

Magnesium hydroxide is an insoluble powder that forms magnesium chloride in the stomach. It does not produce systemic alkalosis since Mg^{2+} is poorly absorbed from the gut.

Magnesium trisilicate is an insoluble powder that reacts slowly with the gastric juice forming magnesium chloride and colloidal silica. This agent has a prolonged antacid effect, and it also adsorbs pepsin.

Aluminium hydroxide gel forms aluminium chloride in the stomach; when this reaches the intestine, the chloride is released and is reabsorbed. Aluminium hydroxide raises the pH of the gastric juice to about 4; it also adsorbs pepsin. It acts gradually and its effect continues for several hours.* Colloidal aluminium hydroxide combines with phosphates in the gastrointestinal tract and the increased excretion of phosphate in the faeces that occurs results in decreased excretion of phosphate via the kidney. This is important in the management of patients with chronic renal failure.

Sodium bicarbonate acts rapidly and is said to raise the pH of gastric juice to about 7.4. Carbon dioxide is liberated and this causes belching. The carbon dioxide stimulates gastrin secretion and can result in a secondary rise in acid secretion. Since some sodium bicarbonate is absorbed in the intestine, large doses or frequent administration of this antacid can cause alkalosis, the onset of which can be insidious. This agent should, therefore, not be prescribed for long-term treatment; nor should it be given to patients who are on a sodium-restricted diet.

Alginates are sometimes combined with antacids for use in reflux oesophagitis, because they are believed to increase adherence of mucus to the oesophageal mucosa.

The clinical use of antacids is given in the box on page 372.

TREATMENT OF *HELICOBACTER PYLORI* INFECTION

As specified above, *H. pylori* is implicated in the production of gastric and, more particularly, duodenal ulcers and is a risk factor for gastric cancer.**

Combination therapy with three drugs is employed to eradicate *H. pylori*, usually **omeprazole, amoxicillin** and **metronidazole**. Other combinations used are **omeprazole**, **clarythromycin**, and amoxicillin or **tetracycline**, **metronidazole** and **bismuth chelates**. The antibiotics are covered in Chapter 45 and bismuth chelates are considered below.

*There was a suggestion—no longer widely believed—that aluminium, if absorbed, could be involved in the pathogenesis of Alzheimer's disease. In fact, aluminium is said not to be absorbed to any significant extent during administration of aluminium hydroxide, but some perhaps overly cautious practitioners may prefer to use other antacids.

**Some authorities have proposed that *H. pylori*-induced gastroduodenitis should be considered as a disease in its own right, with peptic ulcer and gastric cancer as its important complications.

Elimination of the bacillus can produce long-term remission of ulcers but reinfection with the organism can occur.

DRUGS THAT PROTECT THE MUCOSA

Some agents, termed 'cytoprotective', are said to enhance the mucosal protection mechanisms (see above) and/or provide a physical barrier over the surface of the ulcer.

Bismuth chelate

Bismuth chelate (**colloidal bismuth subcitrate, tripotassium dicitratobismuthate**) is used in combination regimens to treat *H. pylori* involvement in peptic ulcer. It has toxic effects on the bacillus and may also prevent its adherence to the mucosa or inhibit its proteolytic enzymes. It is also believed to have other mucosal-protecting actions: coating the ulcer base, adsorbing pepsin, enhancing local prostaglandin synthesis and stimulating bicarbonate secretion.

The small amount of bismuth that is absorbed is excreted in the urine. If renal excretion is impaired, the raised plasma concentrations of bismuth can result in encephalopathy.

Unwanted effects include nausea and vomiting, and blackening of the tongue and faeces.

Sucralfate

Sucralfate is a complex of aluminium hydroxide and sulfated sucrose, which, in the presence of acid, releases aluminium, acquires a strong negative charge and binds to positively charged groups in proteins, glycoproteins, etc. It can form complex gels with mucus, an action that is thought to decrease the degradation of mucus by pepsin and to limit the diffusion of H^+. In vitro studies indicate that it can inhibit the action of pepsin. It also stimulates the mucosal-protecting mechanisms—mucus and bicarbonate secretion and prostaglandin production.

Sucralfate is given orally and in the acid environment of the stomach the polymerised product forms a viscous paste; about 30% is still present in the stomach 3 hours after administration. It reduces the absorption of a number of other drugs, including **fluoroquinolone** antibiotics, **theophylline**, **tetracycline**, **digoxin** and **amitriptyline.** Since it requires an acid environment for activation, antacids given concurrently or prior to its administration will reduce its efficacy.

Unwanted effects are few, the most common being constipation, which occurs in up to 15% of patients treated. Less common are dry mouth, nausea, vomiting, headache and rashes.

Carbenoxolone

Carbenoxolone is derived from a natural product found in liquorice root. It promotes the production of mucus, which lines and protects the stomach.

Misoprostol

A deficiency in prostaglandin production (after ingestion of a NSAID, for example) may contribute to ulcer formation. **Misoprostol** is a stable analogue of PGE_1. It inhibits gastric acid secretion, both basal and in response to food, histamine, pentagastrin and caffeine, by a direct action on the parietal cell (Fig. 24.2). It increases mucosal blood flow and augments the secretion of mucus and bicarbonate.

It is given orally and is used to prevent the gastric damage that can occur with chronic use of NSAIDs.

Unwanted effects are diarrhoea and abdominal cramps; uterine contractions can also occur (see Ch. 29). Prostaglandins and NSAIDs are discussed in Chapters 15 and 16.

Clinical use of agents affecting gastric acidity

- Histamine H_2-receptor antagonists, e.g. ranitidine:
  —peptic ulcer
  —reflux oesophagitis.
- Proton-pump inhibitors, e.g. omeprazole, lansoprazole:
  —peptic ulcer
  —reflux oesophagitis
  —as one component of therapy for *Helicobacter pylori* infection
  —Zollinger–Ellison syndrome (a rare condition caused by gastrin-secreting tumours).
- Antacids, e.g. magnesium trisilicate, aluminium hydroxide, alginates:
  —dyspepsia
  —symptomatic relief in peptic ulcer or (alginates) oesophageal reflux.
- Bismuth chelate:
  —as one component of therapy for *H. pylori* infection.

VOMITING

The act of vomiting is a physical event that results in the forceful evacuation of gastric contents through the mouth. It is often preceded by *nausea* (a feeling of 'queaziness' or of impending vomiting) and can be accompanied by *retching* (repetitive contraction of the abdominal muscles with or without actual discharge of vomit). Vomiting can be a valuable (indeed life-saving) physiological response to the ingestion of a toxic substance (e.g. alcohol), but it is also an unwanted side-effect of many clinically used drugs, notably in patients receiving cancer chemotherapy. Vomiting also occurs in early pregnancy, in the form of motion sickness and accompanies numerous disease states (e.g. migraine) and also bacterial and viral infections.

THE REFLEX MECHANISM OF VOMITING

The central neural regulation of vomiting is vested in two separate units in the medulla. These are the *vomiting centre* and the *chemoreceptor trigger zone* (CTZ).

The CTZ is sensitive to chemical stimuli and is the main site of action of many emetic and antiemetic drugs. The blood–brain

The reflex mechanism of vomiting

- Emetic stimuli include
  —chemicals in blood
  —neuronal input from gastrointestinal tract, labyrinth and CNS.
- Impulses from chemoreceptor trigger zone, and various CNS centres relay to the vomiting centre.
- Chemical transmitters include: histamine, acetylcholine, dopamine and 5-hydroxytryptamine, acting on H_1-, muscarinic, D_2- and 5-HT_3-receptors, respectively.
- Antiemetic drugs:
  —H_1-receptor antagonists (e.g. cyclizine)
  —muscarinic antagonists (e.g. hyoscine)
  —5-HT_3-receptor antagonists (e.g. ondansetron)
  —D_2-receptor antagonists (e.g. thiethylperazine, metoclopramide)
  —cannabinoids (e.g. nabilone).
  —neurokinin-1 antagonists.
- Main side-effects of principal antiemetics include:
  —drowsiness and antiparasympathetic effects (hyoscine, nabilone > cinnarizine)
  —dystonic reactions (thiethylperazine > metoclopramide)
  —general CNS disturbances (nabilone)
  —headache, gastrointestinal tract upsets (ondansetron).

barrier is relatively permeable in the neighbourhood of the CTZ, allowing circulating mediators to act on it directly. The CTZ is also concerned in the mediation of motion sickness, a condition caused by stimulation of the vestibular apparatus triggered by certain types of movement. Impulses from the CTZ pass to those areas of the brainstem—known collectively as the vomiting centre—that control and integrate the visceral and somatic functions involved in vomiting. An outline of the suggested inter-relationships is given in Figure 24.5 and reviewed in detail by Hornby (2001).

The main neurotransmitters considered to be involved in the control of vomiting are acetylcholine, histamine, 5-HT and dopamine. Receptors for these transmitters have been demonstrated in the relevant areas and are illustrated in Figure 24.5. It has been hypothesised that enkephalins (see Ch. 13) are also implicated in the mediation of vomiting, acting possibly at δ- (CTZ) or μ- (vomiting centre) opioid receptors. Substance P (see Ch. 40) acting at neurokinin-1 receptors in the CTZ may also play a role in vomiting.

EMETIC DRUGS

In some circumstances, such as when a toxic substance has been swallowed, it may be necessary to stimulate vomiting. This should never be attempted if the patient is not fully conscious or if the substance is corrosive. The drug usually used to produce vomiting is **ipecacuanha**, which acts locally in the stomach. Its irritant action results from the presence of two alkaloids *emetine* and *cephaeline*. In cases of poisoning, activated charcoal can also be given to sequester the toxic drug.

ANTIEMETIC DRUGS

Different antiemetic agents are used for different conditions, though there may be some overlap. Antiemetic drugs are of particular importance as an adjunct to cancer chemotherapy to combat the nausea and vomiting produced by many cytotoxic drugs (see Ch. 50). These agents can cause almost unendurable nausea and vomiting.*

In using drugs to treat the morning sickness of pregnancy, the problem of potential damage to the fetus has to be borne in mind. In general, all drugs should be avoided, if possible, during the first 3 months of pregnancy.

Details of the main categories of agents are given below and a summary of the main clinical uses of antiemetic drugs is given in the box.

Receptor antagonists

Antagonists at H_1 (see Ch. 16), muscarinic (see Ch. 10) and 5-HT_3 (see Ch. 12) receptors all exhibit clinically useful antiemetic activity. H_1 antagonists such as **meclizine, cinnarizine, cyclizine, dimenhydrinate, promethazine** and **diphenydramine** and muscarinic antagonists such as **hyoscine** (**scopolamine**) are effective treatments for motion sickness and vomiting caused by the presence of irritants in the stomach but have little effect against substances that act directly on the CTZ.

Hyoscine is the most widely used antimuscarinic agent. It is employed principally for prophylaxis and treatment of motion sickness and is often administered as a transdermal patch. Promethazine has proven of particular benefit for morning sickness of pregnancy and has been used by NASA to treat space motion sickness. Selective 5-HT_3-receptor antagonists, including **ondansetron, granisetron, tropisetron** and **dolasetron**, are of particular value in preventing and treating vomiting caused either by radiation therapy in cancer patients or by administration of cytotoxic drugs such as cisplatin. The primary site of action of these drugs is the CTZ. They are given orally, and unwanted effects such as headache and gastrointestinal upsets are relatively uncommon.

Phenothiazines and butyrophenones

Phenothiazines are dealt with in Chapter 37; only those aspects relevant to the control of vomiting will be considered here.

*It was reported that a young medically qualified patient being treated by combination chemotherapy for sarcoma stated that 'the severity of vomiting at times made the thought of death seem like a welcome relief'.

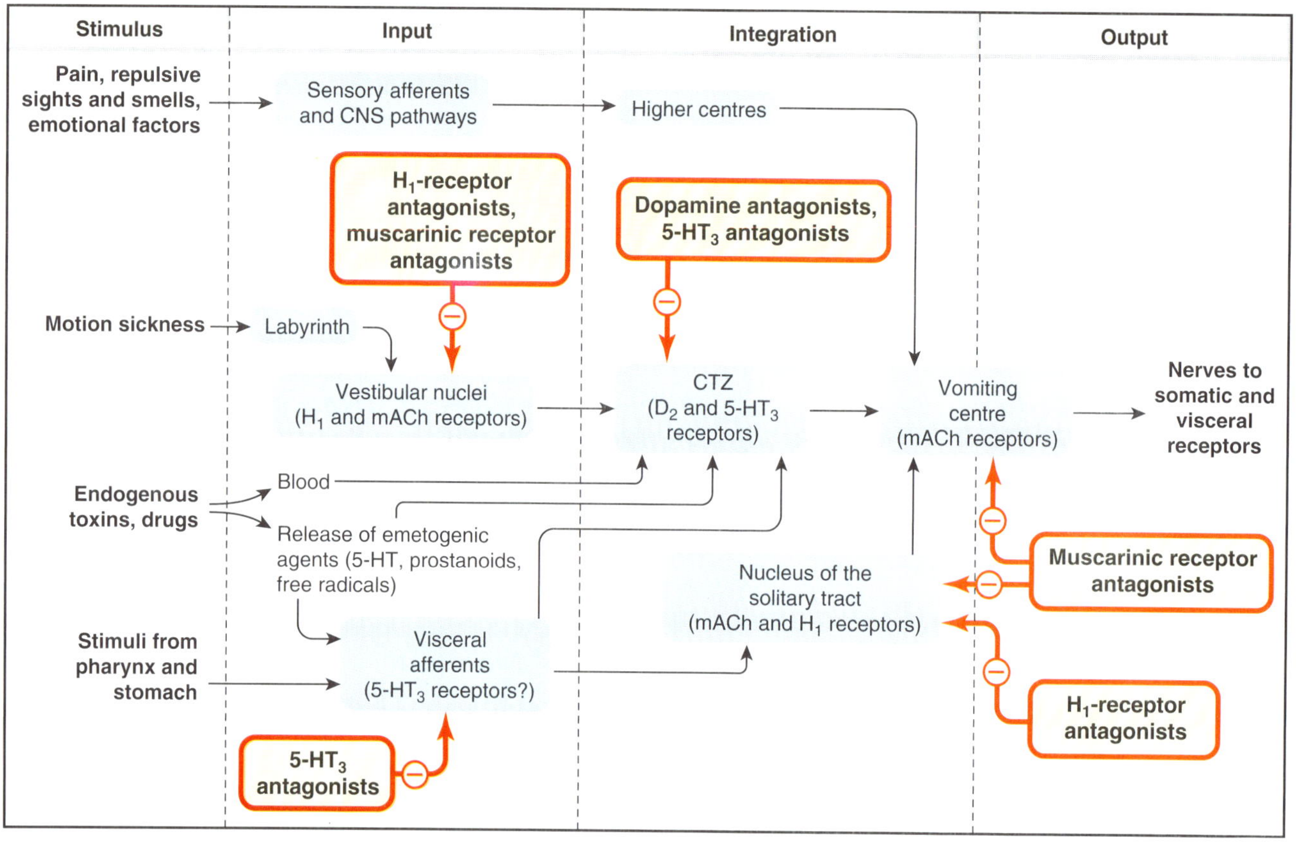

Fig. 24.5 Schematic diagram of the factors involved in the control of vomiting, with the probable sites of action of antiemetic drugs. The cerebellum may function as a second relay or gating mechanism in the link between labyrinth and CTZ (not shown). (ACh, acetylcholine; CTZ, chemoreceptor trigger zone; H_1, histamine H_1; M, muscarinic; D_2, dopamine D_2; 5-HT_3, 5-hydroxytryptamine type 3.) (Based partly on a diagram from Borison H L et al. 1981 J Clin Pharmacol 21: 235–295.)

Antipsychotic phenothiazines, such as **chlorpromazine, prochlorperazine** and **trifluoperazine**, are effective antiemetics, while some phenothiazines, such as **thiethylperazine**, are employed only as antiemetic drugs. They can be administered orally, intravenously or by suppository and are commonly used for severe episodes of nausea and vomiting associated with vertigo, motion sickness and migraine. They act mainly as antagonists of the dopamine D_2-receptors in the CTZ (see Fig. 24.5). However, they also have some degree of blocking action at histamine and muscarinic receptors and may have other sites of action.

Unwanted effects are relatively frequent and include sedation, hypotension and extrapyramidal symptoms including dystonias and tardive dyskinesia (Ch. 37).

Antipsychotic butyrophenones such as **haloperidol** and **droperidol** (Ch. 37) can be used for acute chemotherapy-induced emesis and also act as D_2-antagonists in the CTZ.

Metoclopramide and domperidone

Metoclopramide and domperidone are D_2-receptor antagonists (Fig. 24.5) that act in the CTZ. Both drugs also have a peripheral *prokinetic* action to increase the motility of the oesophagus, stomach and intestine. This not only adds to their antiemetic effect but explains their use to treat conditions such as gastro-oesophageal reflux (see below). The two drugs differ in that domperidone does not penetrate the blood–brain barrier to any extent and, although an effective antiemetic (the CTZ is on the blood side of the barrier), it is free from central side-effects. In contrast, metoclopramide blocks dopamine receptors (see Ch. 37) elsewhere in the central nervous system (CNS), resulting in a number of unwanted effects including disorders of movement, (more common in children and young adults), fatigue, motor restlessness, spasmodic torticollis (involuntary twisting of the neck) and occulogyric crises (rapid involuntary eye movements). Metoclopramide also stimulates prolactin release (see Ch. 27) and can cause galactorrhoea and disorders of menstruation. Both drugs are given orally, have plasma half lives of 4–5 hours and are excreted in the urine.

Benzoquimanide, trimethobenzamide and **alizapride** are similar in structure to metoclopramide and domperidone and have been used in the treatment of moderate to severe nausea and vomiting.

Cannabinoids

Anecdotal evidence originally suggested the possibility of using cannabinoids as antiemetics. Since that time, synthetic cannabinol derivatives such as **nabilone** and **dronabinol** have been found to decrease vomiting caused by agents which stimulate the CTZ. The antiemetic effect of these agents are antagonised by **naloxone**, which implies that opioid receptors may be important in the action of these drugs.

Nabilone is given orally, is well absorbed from the gastrointestinal tract and is metabolised in many tissues. Its plasma half-life is approximately 120 minutes, and its metabolites are excreted in the urine and faeces.

Unwanted effects are common, especially drowsiness, dizziness and dry mouth. Mood changes and postural hypotension are also fairly frequent. Some patients experience hallucinations and psychotic reactions, resembling the effect of other cannabinoids (see Ch. 42).

Steroids

High-dose glucocorticoids (particularly **dexamethasone** and **methylprednisolone**; see Ch. 27) can have antiemetic action. The mechanism of action is not clear but may involve inhibition of prostaglandin synthesis. They can be used alone or in combination with a phenothiazine or ondansetron.

Neurokinin-1 antagonists

The finding that substance P causes vomiting when injected intravenously and is found both in gastrointestinal vagal afferent nerves and in the vomiting centre suggested that neurokinin-1 antagonists may be effective antiemetics. Early clinical trials with agents such as vofopitant (GR-205171) suggest that this approach may be effective in the control of both chemotherapy-induced and postoperative nausea and vomiting. To date, no major unwanted effects have been reported.

Clinical use of anti-emetic drugs

- Histamine H_1-receptor antagonists:
  - —cyclizine: motion sickness
  - —cinnarizine: motion sickness, vestibular disorders (e.g. Ménière's disease)
  - —promethazine: severe morning sickness of pregnancy (but only if absolutely essential).
- Muscarinic receptor antagonists:
  - —hyoscine: motion sickness
- Dopamine D_2-receptor antagonists:
  - —phenothiazines (e.g. prochlorperazine): vomiting caused by uraemia, radiation, viral gastroenteritis; severe morning sickness of pregnancy (but only if absolutely essential)
  - —metoclopramide: vomiting caused by uraemia, radiation, gastrointestinal disorders, cytotoxic drugs.
- 5-Hydroxytryptamine 5-HT_3-receptor antagonists (e.g. ondansetron): vomiting caused by cytotoxic anticancer drugs; postoperative vomiting; radiation-induced vomiting.
- Cannabinoids (e.g. nabilone) for vomiting caused by cytotoxic anticancer drugs.

THE MOTILITY OF THE GASTROINTESTINAL TRACT

Drugs that alter movement through the gastrointestinal tract include:

- purgatives, which accelerate the passage of food through the intestine
- agents that increase the motility of the gastrointestinal smooth muscle without causing purgation
- antidiarrhoeal drugs, which decrease movement
- antispasmodic drugs, which decrease movement.

PURGATIVES

The transit of food through the intestine may be hastened by several different methods. These include *laxatives, faecal softeners* and *stimulant purgatives.*

Bulk and osmotic laxatives

The bulk laxatives include **methylcellulose** and certain plant gums, for example **sterculia, agar, bran** and **ispaghula husk**. These agents are polysaccharide polymers that are not broken down by the normal processes of digestion in the upper part of the gastrointestinal tract. They act by virtue of their capacity to retain water in the gut lumen and so promote peristalsis. They take several days to work but have no serious unwanted effects.

The osmotic laxatives consist of poorly absorbed solutes—the **saline purgatives** and **lactulose**. These maintain an increased volume of fluid in the lumen of the bowel by osmosis, which accelerates the transfer of the gut contents through the small intestine and results in an abnormally large volume entering the colon. This leads to distension and purgation about an hour later. Abdominal cramps can occur. Isotonic or hypotonic solutions of saline purgatives cause purgation; hypertonic solutions can cause vomiting.

The main salts in use are **magnesium sulfate** and **magnesium hydroxide**. These are virtually insoluble; they remain in the lumen and retain water, increasing the volume of the faeces. The amount of magnesium absorbed after an oral dose is usually too small to have adverse systemic effects but these salts should be avoided in small children and in patients with poor renal function, in whom they can cause heart block, neuromuscular block or CNS depression.

Lactulose is a semisynthetic disaccharide of fructose and galactose. In the colon, bacteria convert it to its two component sugars, which are poorly absorbed; when these are fermented, the lactic and acetic acids formed function as osmotic laxatives. It takes 2–3 days to act. *Unwanted effects*, with high doses, are flatulence, cramps, diarrhoea and electrolyte disturbance. Tolerance can develop.

Faecal softeners

Docusate sodium is a surface-active compound that acts in the gastrointestinal tract in a manner similar to a detergent and produces softer faeces. It is also a weak stimulant laxative.

Stimulant purgatives

The stimulant purgative drugs act mainly by increasing water and electrolyte secretion by the mucosa and also by increasing peristalsis—possibly by stimulating enteric nerves.

Bisacodyl is usually given by suppository, causing stimulation of the rectal mucosa, which results in peristaltic action and defaecation in 15–30 minutes. **Sodium picosulfate** has a similar action; it is given orally and is often used in preparation for intestinal surgery.

Senna has laxative activity because it contains derivatives of anthracene (e.g. **emodin**) combined with sugars to form glycosides. The drug passes unchanged into the colon, where bacteria hydrolyse the glycoside bond, releasing the free anthracene derivatives. These are absorbed and have a direct stimulant effect on the myenteric plexus, resulting in smooth muscle activity and thus defaecation. Some emodin is excreted in the urine and some may appear in the milk of women who are breast-feeding.

DRUGS THAT INCREASE GASTROINTESTINAL MOTILITY

Domperidone is primarily a dopamine receptor antagonist acting at D_2-receptors and is used as an antiemetic as described above. It increases gastrointestinal motility by an unknown mechanism. Clinically, it increases lower oesophageal sphincter pressure (thus inhibiting gastro-oesophageal reflux), increases gastric emptying and enhances duodenal peristalsis.

It is useful in disorders of gastric emptying and in chronic gastric reflux. Its main unwanted effect is hyperprolactinaemia, consistent with its action on dopamine receptors.

Metoclopramide (also an antiemetic, see above) stimulates gastric motility, causing a marked acceleration of gastric emptying. It is useful in gastro-oesophageal reflux and in disorders of gastric emptying but is ineffective in paralytic ileus.

Cisapride stimulates acetylcholine release in the myenteric plexus in the upper gastrointestinal tract through a 5-HT_4-receptor-mediated effect. This raises oesophageal sphincter pressure and increases gut motility. It is used in reflux oesophagitis and in disorders of gastric emptying. Unwanted effects such as diarrhoea and abdominal cramps are generally rare but it may also have a prodysrhythmic effect in some individuals.

ANTIDIARRHOEAL AGENTS

Diarrhoea is the frequent passage of liquid faeces. There are numerous causes including infectious agents, toxins, anxiety, drugs, etc. Repercussions range from discomfort and inconvenience in a healthy well-nourished adult, to a medical emergency requiring hospitalisation and parenteral fluid and electrolyte therapy. On a worldwide basis, acute diarrhoeal disease is one of the principal causes of death in malnourished infants; this is particularly important in developing countries.

Diarrhoea involves both an increase in the motility of the gastrointestinal tract, along with increased secretion, and a decrease in the absorption of fluid, and thus a loss of electrolytes (particularly Na^+) and water. Cholera toxins and some other bacterial toxins produce not only loss of gut contents but also a profound increase in secretion through their effect on the guanine nucleotide regulatory proteins that couple the surface receptors of the mucosal cells to adenylate cyclase (see Ch. 3).

There are three approaches to the treatment of severe acute diarrhoea:

- maintenance of fluid and electrolyte balance
- use of anti-infective agents
- use of non-antimicrobial antidiarrhoeal agents.

The maintenance of fluid and electrolyte balance by means of oral rehydration is the first priority, and wider appreciation of this could save the lives of many infants in the developing world. Many patients require no other treatment. In the ileum, as in parts of the nephron, there is co-transport of Na^+ and glucose across the epithelial cell and, therefore, glucose enhances Na^+ absorption and thus water uptake; amino acids have a similar effect. Preparations of sodium chloride and glucose for oral use are available in powder form, ready to be dissolved in water before use.

The use of anti-infective agents is usually not necessary in simple gastroenteritis since most infections are usually viral in origin, and those that are bacterial generally resolve without antibacterial drug therapy. *Campylobacter* sp. is the commonest bacterial organism causing gastroenteritis in the UK, and severe infections may require **erythromycin** or **ciprofloxacin** (Ch. 45). Chemotherapy may be necessary in some types of enteritis (e.g. typhoid, amoebic dysentery and cholera).

The *use of non-antimicrobial antidiarrhoeal agents* is dealt with below; these include antimotility agents, adsorbents and agents that modify fluid and electrolyte transport.

Traveller's diarrhoea

More than 3 million people cross international borders each year. Many travel hopefully but come back ill, having encountered enterotoxin-producing *Escherichia coli*, *Cyclospora cayetanensis* or other organisms. Most infections are self-limiting and require only oral replacement of fluid and salt as detailed above. General principles for the treatment of traveller's diarrhoea are detailed by Gorbach (1987), who makes the pertinent remark 'travel broadens the mind and loosens the bowels'.

Antimotility agents

The main pharmacological agents that decrease motility are **opiates** (details in Ch. 40) and **muscarinic receptor antagonists** (details in Ch. 10). Agents in this latter group are seldom employed as primary therapy for diarrhoea because of their actions on other systems; but small doses of atropine are used combined with diphenoxylate (see below).

The action of **morphine**, the archetypal opiate, on the alimentary tract is complex; it increases the tone and rhythmic contractions of the intestine but diminishes propulsive activity. Its overall effect is constipating. The pyloric, ileocolic and anal sphincters are contracted and the tone of the large intestine is markedly increased.

The main opiates used in diarrhoea are **codeine** (a morphine congener), **diphenoxylate** and **loperamide** (both pethidine congeners that do not readily penetrate the blood–brain barrier and are used only for their actions in the gut). All may have unwanted effects including constipation, abdominal cramps, drowsiness and dizziness. Paralytic ileus can also occur. They should not be used in young children.

Loperamide has a relatively selective action on the gastrointestinal tract and undergoes significant enterohepatic cycling. In traveller's diarrhoea, loperamide reduces the frequency of passage of faeces and the duration of the illness.

Diphenoxylate, given once in the therapeutic dose suitable for diarrhoea, does not have morphine-like activity in the CNS, though large doses (25-fold higher) produce typical opioid effects. Preparations of diphenoxylate usually contain atropine as well.

Codeine and **loperamide** have antisecretory actions in addition to their effects on intestinal motility.

Bismuth subsalicylate, which is used for traveller's diarrhoea, is said to be safe in healthy young adults and is reported to prevent up to 65% of cases of diarrhoea in areas of high risk. It decreases fluid secretion in the bowel and may work largely by virtue of its salicylate component. Bismuth subsalicylate can cause tinnitus and blackening of the faeces.

Cannabinoid receptor agonists also reduce gut motility in animals most probably by decreasing acetylcholine release from enteric nerves. There have been anecdotal reports of a beneficial effect of cannabis against dysentery and cholera.

Adsorbents

Adsorbent agents are used extensively in the treatment of diarrhoea, although properly controlled trials proving adequacy have not been carried out.

The main preparations used are kaolin, pectin, chalk, charcoal, methyl cellulose and activated attapulgite (magnesium aluminium silicate).

It has been suggested that these agents may act by adsorbing microorganisms or toxins, by altering the intestinal flora or by coating and protecting the intestinal mucosa, but there is no hard evidence for this.

ANTISPASMODIC AGENTS

Drugs that reduce spasm in the gut are of value in irritable bowel syndrome and diverticular disease.

Muscarinic receptor antagonists are dealt with in Chapter 10. They decrease spasm by inhibiting parasympathetic activity.

Drugs and gastrointestinal tract motility

- Purgatives are:
  - —bulk laxatives, e.g. ispaghula husk (first choice for slow action)
  - —osmotic laxatives, e.g. lactulose
  - —faecal softeners, e.g. docusate sodium
  - —stimulant purgatives, e.g. senna.
- Drugs which increase motility without purgation:
  - —domperidone, used in disorders of gastric emptying.
- Drugs used to treat diarrhoea:
  - —oral rehydration with isotonic solutions of NaCl plus glucose or starch-based cereal (important in infants)
  - —antimotility agents, e.g. loperamide (unwanted effects: drowsiness and nausea)
  - —absorbents, e.g. magnesium aluminium silicate.

Agents available include **propantheline** and **dicycloxerine** (**dicyclomine**). The last named is thought to have some additional direct relaxant action on smooth muscle.

Mebeverine, a derivative of reserpine, has a direct relaxant action on gastrointestinal smooth muscle. *Unwanted effects* are few.

DRUGS FOR CHRONIC INFLAMMATORY BOWEL DISEASE

Chronic inflammatory bowel disease comprises ulcerative colitis and Crohn's disease (a granulomatous condition affecting especially the terminal ileum and the colon), both of uncertain aetiology. The following agents are used.

Glucocorticoids

Glucocorticoids are anti-inflammatory agents and are dealt with in Chapter 27. Prednisolone is given locally in the bowel by suppository or enema.

Sulfasalazine

Sulfasalazine is a combination of the sulfonamide sulfapyridine with 5-aminosalicylic acid. The latter is the active moiety; it is released in the colon and is not absorbed. Its mechanism of action is not known. It may act by scavenging free radicals, inhibiting prostaglandin and leukotriene production and/or by decreasing neutrophil chemotaxis and superoxide generation. Its unwanted effects are diarrhoea, salicylate sensitivity and interstitial nephritis.

The sulfapyridine moiety is absorbed and its unwanted effects are those associated with the sulfonamides (see Ch. 45).

Sulfasalazine is not useful for the actual attack of inflammatory bowel disease but is valuable in preventing recurrence in patients who are in remission. Sulfasalazine has also been used to treat arthritis.

Newer compounds are **mesalazine** (5-aminosalicylic acid itself), **olsalazine** (two molecules of 5-aminosalicylic acid linked by a diazo bond, which is broken by colonic bacteria) and **balsalazide** (4-aminosalicylic acid).

The immunosuppressants **azathioprine** and **6-mercaptopurine** (see Ch. 16) are used in patients with severe disease.

DRUGS AFFECTING THE BILIARY SYSTEM

Drugs used to treat cholesterol cholelithiasis

The commonest pathological condition of the biliary tract is cholesterol cholelithiasis, i.e. the formation of cholesterol gallstones. Drugs that dissolve non-calcified cholesterol gallstones are **chenodeoxycholic acid** (CDCA) and **ursodeoxycholic acid** (UDCA). CDCA is one of the two primary bile acids. UDCA, the 7β-hydroxy epimer of CDCA, occurs in small amounts in human bile and is the main bile acid in the bear (hence 'urso'). Diarrhoea is the main unwanted effect.

The clinical use of these agents is appropriate only in selected patients with gallstones, as surgery is the preferred treatment in most cases when active intervention is indicated.

Drugs affecting biliary spasm

The pain produced by the passage of gallstones down the bile duct (biliary colic) can be very intense, and immediate relief may be required. **Morphine** relieves the pain effectively but it may have an undesirable local effect since it constricts the sphincter of Oddi and raises the pressure in the bile duct. **Buprenorphine** may be preferable. **Pethidine** has similar actions, although it relaxes other smooth muscle, for example that of the ureter. **Atropine** is commonly employed to relieve biliary spasm since it has antispasmodic action. It may be used in conjunction with morphine. The **nitrates** (see Ch. 17) can produce a marked fall of intrabiliary pressure and may relieve biliary spasm.

REFERENCES AND FURTHER READING

Innervation and hormones of the gastrointestinal tract

Del Valle J, Yamada T 1990 The gut as an endocrine organ. Annu Rev Med 41: 447–455

Goyal R K, Hirano I 1996 The enteric nervous system. N Engl J Med 334: 1106–1115

Walsh J H 1988 Peptides as regulators of gastric acid secretion. Annu Rev Physiol 50: 41–63

Gastric secretion

Angus J A, Black J W 1982 The interaction of choline esters, vagal stimulation and H_2-receptor blockade on acid secretion in vitro. Eur J Pharmacol 80: 217–224

Black J W, Shankley N P 1987 How does gastrin act to stimulate oxyntic cell secretion? Trends Pharmacol Sci 8: 486–490

Black J W, Duncan W A M, Durant C J, Ganellin C R, Parsons E M 1972 Definition and antagonism of histamine H_2-receptors. Nature 236: 385–390 (*Seminal paper*)

Blaser M J 1998 *Helicobacter pylori* and gastric disease. Br Med J 316: 1507–1510 (*Succinct review, emphasis on future developments*)

Sachs G, Shin J M et al. 1995 The pharmacology of the gastric acid pump: the H^+,K^+ATPase. Annu Rev Pharmacol Toxicol 35: 277–305 (*Comprehensive review*)

Sandvik A K, Waldrum H L 1991 Gastrin is a potent stimulant of the parietal cell—maybe. Am J Physiol 260: G925–G928

Soll A H, Berglindh T 1987 Physiology of isolated gastric glands and parietal cells: receptors and effectors regulating function. In: Johnson L R (ed) Physiology of the gastrointestinal tract, 2nd edn. Raven Press, New York

Drugs in gastric disorders

Alper J 1993 Ulcers as an infectious disease. Science 260: 159–160

Axon A, Forman D 1997 Helicobacter gastroduodenitis: a serious infectious disease. Br Med J 314: 1430–1431 (*Editorial comment*)

Bateman D N 1997 Proton-pump inhibitors: three of a kind? Lancet 349: 1637–1638 (*Editorial commentary*)

Blaser M J 1996 The bacteria behind ulcers. Sci Am Feb: 92–97 (*Simple coverage, very good diagrams*)

Colin-Jones D G 1990 Acid suppression: how much is needed. Br Med J 301: 564–565

Feldman M, Burton M E 1990 Histamine H_2-receptor antagonists: standard therapy for acid-peptic disease. N Engl J Med 323: 1672–1680, 1749–1755

Horn J H 2000 The proton-pump inhibitors: similarities and differences. Clin Ther 22: 266-280 (*Excellent overview*)

Huang J Q, Hunt R H 2001 Pharmacological and pharmacodynamic essentials of H(2)-receptor antagonists and proton pump inhibitors for the practising physician. Baillières Best Pract Res Clin Gastroenterol 15: 355–370

McCarthy D M 1991 Sucralfate. N Engl J Med 325: 1017–1025

Marks I N, Schmassmann A et al. 1992 Antacid therapy today. Eur J Gastroenterol Hepatol 4: 977–983

Rauws E A J, van der Hulst R W M 1998 The management of *H. pylori* infection. Br Med J 316: 162–163 (*Editorial commentary*)

Walsh J H, Peterson W L 1995 The treatment of *Helicobacter pylori* infection in the management of peptic ulcer disease. N Engl J Med 333: 984–991 (*Useful coverage*)

Walt R P 1992 Misoprostol for the treatment of peptic ulcer and anti-inflammatory-drug-induced gastroduodenal ulceration. N Engl J Med 327: 1575–1580

Yeomans N D, Tulassy Z et al. 1998 A comparison of omeprazole with ranitidine for ulcers associated with nonsteroidal antiinflammatory drugs. N Engl J Med 338: 719–726

Vomiting

American Gastroenterological Association 2001 Technical Review on Nausea and Vomiting. Gastroenterology 120: 263–286

Bunce K, Tyers M, Beranek P 1991 Clinical evaluation of 5-HT_3 receptor antagonists as anti-emetics. Trends Pharmacol Sci 12: 46–48

Hesketh P J 2001 Potential role of the NK1 receptor antagonists in chemotherapy-induced nausea and vomiting. Support Care Cancer 9: 350–354

Hornby P J 2001 Central neurocircuitry associated with emesis. Am J Med 111: 106S–112S (*Comprehensive review of central control of vomiting*)

Tramèr M R, Moore R et al. 1997 A quantitative systematic review of ondansetron in treatment of established postoperative nausea and vomiting. Br Med J 314: 1088–1092

Yates B J, Miller A D, Lucot J B 1998 Physiological basis and pharmacology of motion sickness: an update. Brain Res Bull 5: 395–406 (*Good account of the mechanisms underlying motion sickness and its treatment*)

Motility of the gastrointestinal tract

Avery M E, Snyder J D 1990 Oral therapy for acute diarrhoea. N Engl J Med 323: 891–894

Bateman D N, Smith J M 1989 A policy for laxatives. Br Med J 298: 1420–1421

Costello A M de L, Bhutta T I 1992 Antidiarrhoeal drugs for acute diarrhoea in children: none work, and many may be dangerous. Br Med J 304: 1–2
De Las Casas C, Adachi J, Dupont H, 1999 Travellers' diarrhoea. Aliment Pharmacol Ther 13: 1373–1378 (*Review article*)
Farthing M J G 1993 Travellers diarrhoea: mostly due to bacteria and difficult to prevent. Br Med J 306: 1425–1426
Field M, Rao M C, Chang E B 1989 Intestinal electrolyte transport and diarrhoeal disease. N Engl J Med 321: 800–806, 879–883
Gorbach S L 1987 Bacterial diarrhoea and its treatment. Lancet ii: 1378–1382
Huizinga J D, Thuneberg L et al. 1997 Interstitial cells of Cajal as targets for pharmacological intervention in gastrointestinal motor disorders. Trends Pharmacol Sci 18: 393–403
Pertwee R G 2001 Cannabinoids and the gastrointestinal tract. Gut 48: 859–867

The biliary system

Bateson M C 1997 Bile acid research and applications. Lancet 349: 5–6
Editorial 1992 Bile acid therapy in the 1990s. Lancet 340: 1260–1261
Kumar D, Tandon R K 2001 Use of ursodeoxycholic acid in liver diseases J Gastroenterol Hepatol 16: 3–14

Inflammatory disease

Klotz U 2000 The role of aminosalicylates at the beginning of the new millennium in the treatment of chronic inflammatory bowel disease. Eur J Clin Pharmacol 56: 353–362

25 The endocrine pancreas and the control of blood glucose

Overview 380

Pancreatic islet hormones 380
- Insulin 380
- Glucagon 384
- Somatostatin 385
- Amylin (islet amyloid polypeptide) 385

Control of blood glucose 385

Diabetes mellitus 385
- Treatment of diabetes mellitus 387

OVERVIEW

Insulin is the main hormone controlling intermediary metabolism. Its most obvious acute effect is to lower blood glucose. Reduced (or absent) secretion of insulin, often coupled with reduced sensitivity to its action ('insulin resistance'), causes diabetes mellitus, the prevalence of which is rapidly increasing to epidemic proportions. The consequences of diabetes are dire—especially vascular complications such as myocardial infarction (see Ch. 17), kidney failure and blindness.

In this chapter, we describe pancreatic hormones, emphasising insulin and the control of blood glucose. The second part of the chapter is devoted to diabetes mellitus and its treatment with drugs. This comprises the insulins and the orally active hypoglycaemic agents: biguanides, α-glucosidase inhibitors, sulfonylureas and other drugs that stimulate insulin secretion, and the thiazolidinediones.

PANCREATIC ISLET HORMONES

The islets of Langerhans contain four main cell types: B- (or β-) cells secrete *insulin*, A-cells secrete *glucagon*, D-cells secrete *somatostatin* and PP cells secrete *pancreatic polypeptide* (the function of which is unknown). The core of each islet contains mainly the predominant B-cells surrounded by a mantle of A-cells interspersed with D-cells or PP cells (see Fig. 25.1). B-cells secrete, as well as insulin, a peptide known as *islet amyloid polypeptide* or *amylin*, which delays gastric emptying and opposes insulin by stimulating glycogen breakdown in striated muscle. Glucagon also opposes insulin, increasing blood glucose and stimulating protein breakdown in muscle. Somatostatin inhibits secretion of insulin and of glucagon. It is widely distributed outside the pancreas and is also released from the hypothalamus, inhibiting the release of growth hormone from the pituitary (p. 406).

INSULIN

Insulin was the first protein for which an amino acid sequence was determined (by Sanger's group in Cambridge in 1955). It consists of two peptide chains (A and B, of 21 and 30 amino acid residues, respectively).

SYNTHESIS AND SECRETION

Like other islet hormones, insulin is synthesised as a precursor (preproinsulin) in the rough endoplasmic reticulum. Preproinsulin is transported to the Golgi apparatus where it undergoes proteolytic cleavage first to proinsulin and then to insulin plus a fragment of uncertain function called C-peptide. Insulin and C-peptide are stored in granules in B-cells and are normally cosecreted by exocytosis in equimolar amounts together with smaller and variable amounts of proinsulin. The main factor controlling the synthesis and secretion of insulin is the blood glucose concentration (Fig. 25.1). B-cells respond both to the absolute glucose concentration and also to the rate of change of blood glucose. There is a steady basal release of insulin and also a response to a change in blood glucose. The response to an increase in blood glucose has two phases—an initial rapid phase reflecting release of stored hormone and a slower, delayed phase reflecting both continued release of stored hormone and new synthesis (Fig. 25.2). The response is abnormal in diabetes mellitus, as discussed later.

ATP-sensitive potassium channels ('K_{ATP}') determine the resting membrane potential in B-cells. Glucose enters B-cells via a membrane transporter called Glut-2, and its subsequent metabolism via glucokinase (the rate-limiting enzyme that acts as the 'glucose sensor' linking insulin secretion to extracellular glucose) and glycolysis increases intracellular ATP. This blocks

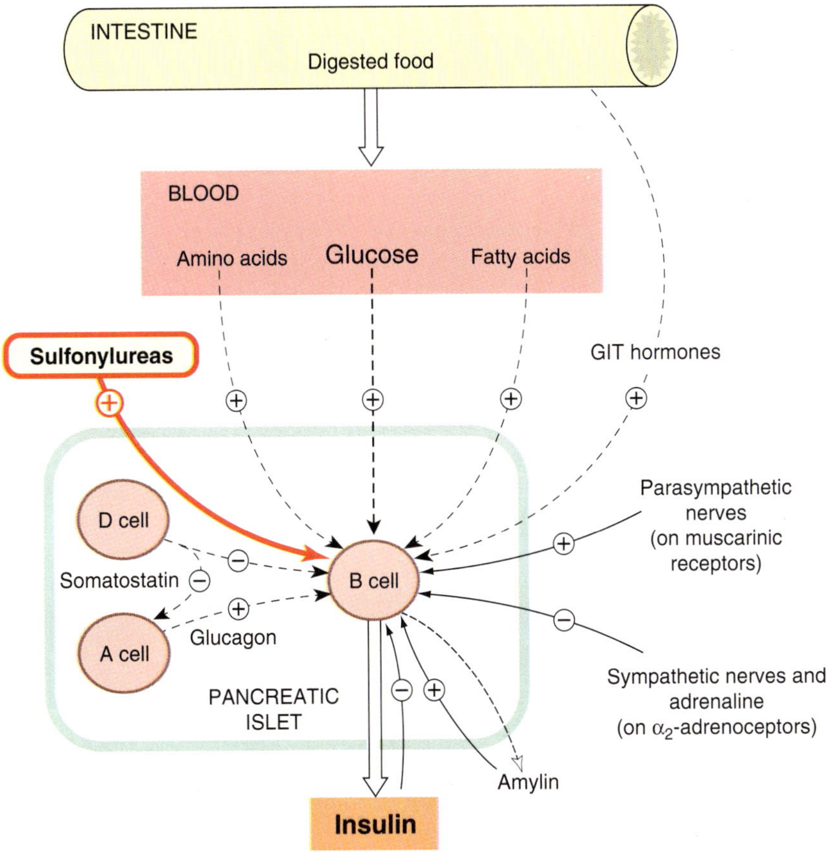

Fig. 25.1 Factors regulating insulin secretion. Blood glucose is the most important factor. Drugs used to stimulate insulin secretion are shown in yellow boxes. Glucagon potentiates insulin release but opposes some of its peripheral actions and increases blood glucose; see Table 22.2. (GIT, gastrointestinal tract.)

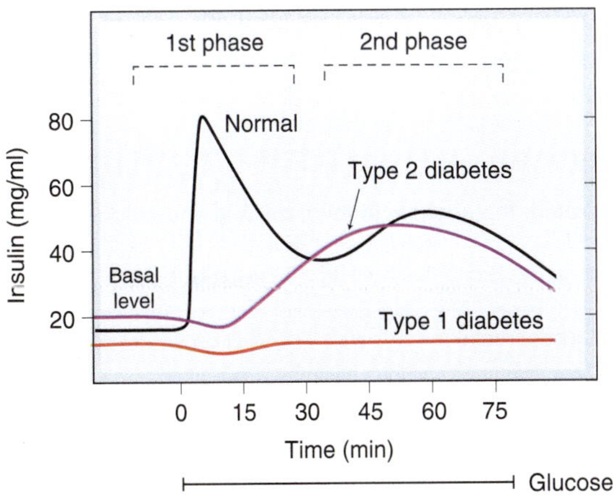

Fig. 25.2 Schematic diagram of the two-phase release of insulin in response to a constant glucose infusion. The first phase is missing in type 2 (non-insulin-dependent) diabetes mellitus and both are missing in type 1 (insulin-dependent) diabetes mellitus. The first phase is also produced by amino acids, sulfonylureas, glucagon and gastrointestinal tract hormones. (Data from: Pfeifer et al. 1981 Am J Med 70: 579–588.)

K_{ATP}, causing membrane depolarisation and opening of voltage-dependent calcium channels, leading to Ca^{2+} influx. This Ca^{2+} signal induces insulin secretion, but only in the presence of amplifying messengers including diacylglycerol (DAG), non-esterified arachidonic acid (which facilitates further Ca^{2+} entry) and 12-lipoxygenase products of arachidonic acid (mainly 12*S*-hydroxyeicosatetraenoic acid (12-*S*-HETE); see Ch. 15). Phospholipases are commonly activated by Ca^{2+}, but free arachidonic acid is liberated in B-cells by an ATP-sensitive Ca^{2+}-insensitive ('ASCI') phospholipase A_2. Consequently, in B-cells, Ca^{2+} entry and arachidonic acid production are both driven by ATP, linking cellular energy status to insulin secretion.

Many gastrointestinal hormones stimulate insulin secretion, including gastrin, secretin, cholecystokinin, gastric inhibitory polypeptide (GIP), glucagon-like peptide (GLP) and GLP_1 (the amide of a fragment of GLP). They are released by eating. This explains why oral glucose causes greater insulin release than does the same amount of glucose administered intravenously. These hormones (in particular GIP and GLP_1) provide an anticipatory signal from the gastrointestinal tract to the islets. Other stimuli to insulin release include amino acids (particularly arginine and leucine), fatty acids, the parasympathetic nervous system and drugs that act on sulfonylurea receptors (see below).

Insulin release is inhibited by the sympathetic nervous system (Fig. 25.1). Adrenaline increases blood glucose by inhibiting insulin release (via α_2-adrenoceptors) and by promoting glycogenolysis via β_2-adrenoceptors in striated muscle and liver. Several peptides, including somatostatin, galanin (an endogenous ATP-sensitive potassium channel activator) and amylin, also inhibit insulin release.

About one fifth of the insulin stored in the pancreas of the human adult is secreted daily. Circulating insulin is measured by immunoassay, but this may give an overestimate because many insulin antibodies cross-react with proinsulin and its less-active degradation products. The plasma insulin concentration after an overnight fast is 20–50 pmol/l. Plasma insulin concentration is reduced in patients with type 1 ('insulin-dependent') diabetes mellitus (see below) and markedly increased in patients with insulinomas (uncommon functioning tumours of B-cells), as is C-peptide, with which it is co-released.* It is also raised in obesity and other normoglycaemic insulin-resistant states.

ACTIONS

Insulin is the main hormone controlling intermediary metabolism, having actions on liver, muscle and fat (Table 25.1). Its overall effect is to conserve fuel by facilitating the uptake and storage of glucose, amino acids and fats after a meal. Acutely, it reduces blood sugar. Consequently, a *fall* in plasma insulin increases blood sugar. The biochemical pathways through which insulin exerts its effects are summarised in Figure 25.3 and molecular aspects of its mechanism are discussed below.

*Insulin for injection does not contain C-peptide, which, therefore, provides a means of distinguishing endogenous from exogenous insulin. This is used to differentiate insulinoma (an insulin-secreting tumour causing high circulating insulin with high C-peptide) from surreptitious injection of insulin (high insulin, normal or low C-peptide). Deliberate induction of hypoglycaemia by self-injection with insulin is a well-recognised, if unusual, manifestation of psychiatric disorder, especially in health professionals—it has also been used in murder.

Effect of insulin on carbohydrate metabolism

Insulin influences glucose metabolism in most tissues, especially the liver where it inhibits glycogenolysis (glycogen breakdown) and gluconeogenesis (synthesis of glucose from non-carbohydrate sources) while stimulating glycogen synthesis. It also increases glucose utilisation (glycolysis), but the overall effect is to increase hepatic glycogen stores.

In muscle, unlike liver, uptake of glucose is slow and is the rate-limiting step in carbohydrate metabolism. The main effect of insulin is to increase facilitated transport of glucose via a transporter called Glut-4, and to stimulate glycogen synthesis and glycolysis.

Insulin increases glucose uptake by Glut-4 in adipose tissue as well as in muscle, enhancing glucose metabolism. One of the main end-products of glucose metabolism in adipose tissue is glycerol, which is esterified with fatty acids to form triglycerides, thereby affecting fat metabolism (see below and Table 25.1).

Effect of insulin on fat metabolism

Insulin increases fatty acid as well as triglyceride synthesis in adipose tissue and liver. It inhibits lipolysis, partly via dephosphorylation (and hence inactivation) of lipases (Table 25.1). It also inhibits the lipolytic actions of adrenaline, growth hormone and glucagon by opposing their actions on adenylate cyclase.

Effect of insulin on protein metabolism

Insulin stimulates uptake of amino acids into muscle and increases protein synthesis. It also decreases protein catabolism and inhibits oxidation of amino acids in the liver.

Table 25.1 **Summary of the effects of insulin on carbohydrate, fat and protein metabolism in liver, muscle and adipose tissue**

Type of metabolism	Liver cells	Fat cell	Muscle
Carbohydrate metabolism	↓↑ Gluconeogenesis ↓ Glycogenolysis ↑ Glycolysis ↑ Glycogenesis	↑ Glucose uptake ↑ Glycerol synthesis	↑ Glucose uptake ↑ Glycolysis ↑ Glycogenesis
Fat metabolism	↑ Lipogenesis ↓ Lipolysis	↑ Synthesis of triglycerides ↑ Fatty acid synthesis ↓ Lipolysis	–
Protein metabolism	↓ Protein breakdown	–	↑ Amino acid uptake ↑ Protein synthesis

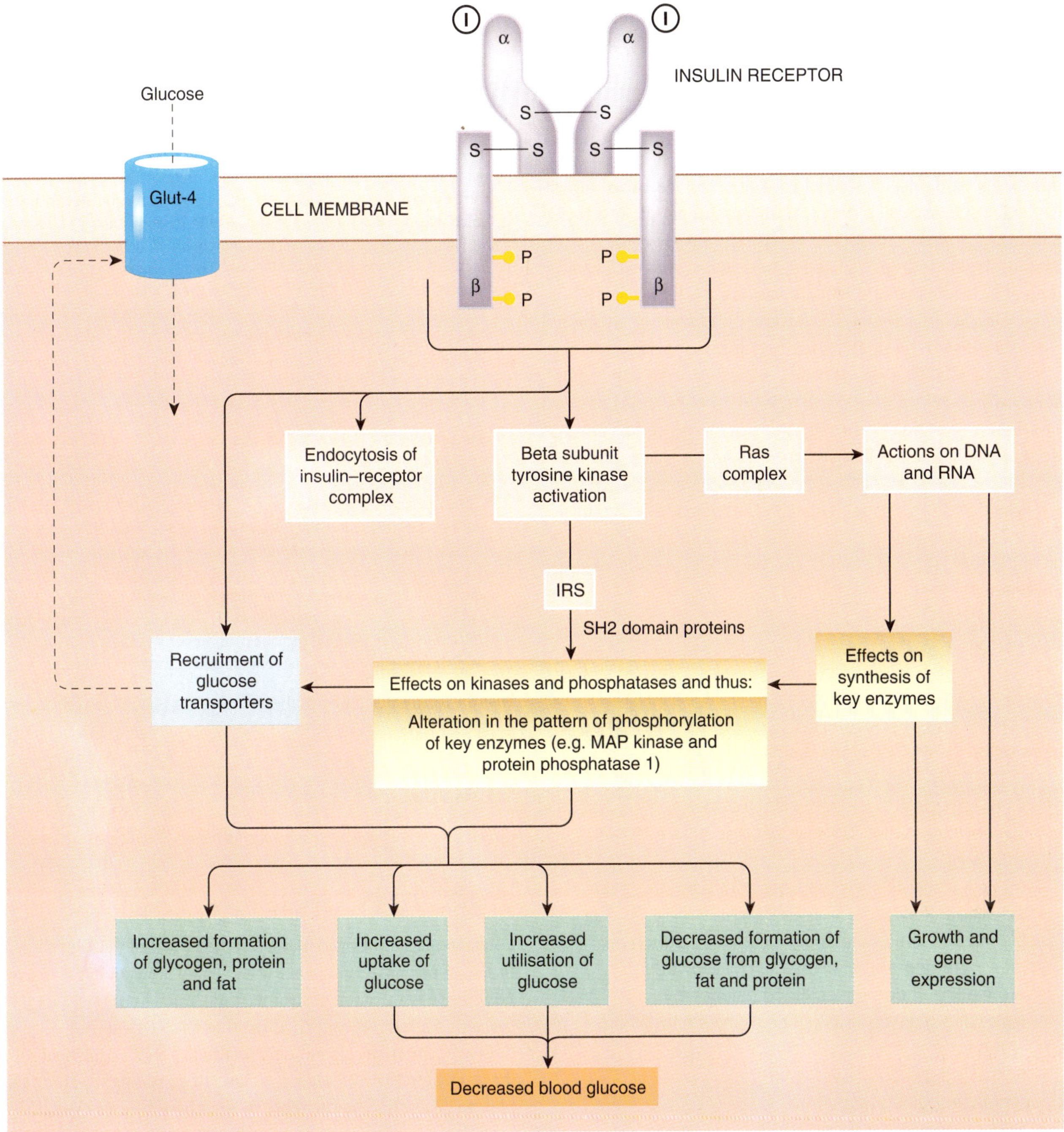

Fig. 25.3 Insulin signalling pathways. (I, insulin; IRS, insulin receptor substrate (several forms: 1–4); Glut-4, an insulin-sensitive glucose transporter present in muscle and fat cells.)

Other metabolic effects of insulin

Other metabolic effects of insulin include transport into cells of K^+,* Ca^{2+}, nucleosides and inorganic phosphate.

*This action is exploited in the emergency treatment of hyperkalaemia by intravenous glucose with insulin.

Long-term effects of insulin

In addition to its rapid effects on metabolism, exerted via altered activity of enzymes and transport proteins, insulin has longer-term actions via altered enzyme synthesis. It is an important anabolic hormone, especially during fetal development. It stimulates cell proliferation and is implicated in somatic and visceral growth and development.

▼ Mitogenic actions of insulin are of great concern in the development of insulin analogues, because these are intended for long-term use and because mammary tumours develop in rats given B10-asp insulin.

MECHANISM OF ACTION

Insulin binds to a specific receptor on the surface of its target cells. The receptor is a large transmembrane glycoprotein complex consisting of two α- and two β-subunits (Fig. 25.3). The α-subunits are entirely extracellular and each carries an insulin-binding site, whereas the β-subunits are transmembrane proteins with tyrosine kinase activity. This activity is suppressed by the α-subunits, but insulin binding causes a conformational change that derepresses (activates) the tyrosine kinase activity of the β-subunits, which act on each other (autophosphorylation) and on other target proteins (see Figure 25.3 and Ch. 2). At concentrations of insulin that produce maximum effects, less than 10% of the receptors are occupied. Occupied receptors aggregate into clusters, which are subsequently internalised in vesicles, resulting in downregulation. Internalised insulin is degraded in lysosomes, but the receptors are recycled to the plasma membrane.

▼ Binding data for insulin and its receptors are not linear when displayed on a Scatchard plot (cf. Fig. 2.2), probably because of 'negative cooperativity' (i.e. binding of insulin to the binding site on one α-subunit reduces the affinity for insulin of the site on the neighbouring α-subunit). The signal transduction mechanisms that link receptor binding to the biological effects of insulin are complex. Insulin receptor substrate (IRS) proteins undergo rapid tyrosine phosphorylation in response to insulin and insulin-like growth factor-1 (IGF-1) but not to other growth factors that act through receptor tyrosine kinases. The best characterised of these is IRS-I, which contains 22 tyrosine residues; these are potential phosphorylation sites and interact with proteins that contain a so-called SH2 domain (see Ch. 3), thereby passing on the insulin signal. Knockout mice lacking IRS-1 are hyporesponsive to insulin ('insulin resistant') but do not become diabetic because of robust B-cell compensation with increased insulin secretion. By contrast, mice lacking IRS-2 fail to compensate and develop overt diabetes, implicating the gene for IRS-2 as a candidate gene for human type 2 diabetes. Activation of phosphatidylinositol 3-kinase by interaction of its SH2 domain with phosphorylated IRS has several important effects, including recruitment of insulin-sensitive glucose transporters (Glut-4) from the Golgi apparatus to the plasma membrane in muscle and fat cells.

The longer-term actions of insulin entail effects on DNA and RNA, mediated partly at least by the Ras signalling complex. Ras is a protein that regulates cell growth and cycles between an active GTP-bound form and an inactive GDP-bound form (see Chs 3 and 50). Insulin shifts the equilibrium in favour of the active form and initiates a phosphorylation cascade that results in activation of mitogen-activated protein kinase (MAP kinase), which in turn activates several nuclear transcription factors leading to the expression of genes that are involved both with cell growth and with intermediary metabolism. Regulation of the rate of mRNA transcription by insulin provides an important means of modulating enzyme activity. IGF can also bind to and activate insulin receptors.

Insulin for treatment of diabetes mellitus is considered below.

Endocrine pancreas and blood glucose

- Islets of Langerhans secrete insulin from B- (or β-) cells, glucagon from A-cells and somatostatin from D-cells.
- Many factors stimulate insulin secretion, but the main one is blood glucose.
- Insulin has essential metabolic actions as a fuel-storage hormone and also affects cell growth and differentiation. It decreases blood glucose by:
  - —increasing glucose uptake into muscle and fat via Glut-4
  - —increasing glycogen synthesis
  - —decreasing gluconeogenesis
  - —decreasing glycogen breakdown.
- Glucagon is a fuel-mobilising hormone, stimulating gluconeogenesis and glycogenolysis, also lipolysis and proteolysis. It increases blood sugar and also increases the force of contraction of the heart.
- Diabetes mellitus is a chronic metabolic disorder in which there is hyperglycaemia. There are two main types:
  - —type 1 (insulin-dependent) diabetes, with an absolute deficiency of insulin
  - —type 2 (non-insulin-dependent) diabetes, with a relative deficiency of insulin associated with reduced sensitivity to its action ('insulin resistance').

GLUCAGON

Glucagon is a single chain polypeptide of 21 amino acid residues.

SYNTHESIS AND SECRETION

Glucagon is synthesised mainly in the A-cell of the islets, but also in the upper gastrointestinal tract. It has considerable structural homology with other gastrointestinal tract hormones, including secretin, vasoactive intestinal peptide and GIP (see Ch. 24).

One of the main physiological stimuli to glucagon secretion is the concentration of amino acids, in particular L-arginine, in plasma. Therefore, an increase in secretion follows ingestion of a high-protein meal, but compared with insulin there is relatively little change in plasma glucagon concentrations throughout the day. Glucagon secretion is stimulated by low and inhibited by high concentrations of glucose and fatty acids in the plasma. Sympathetic nerve activity and circulating adrenaline stimulate glucagon release via β-adrenoceptors. Parasympathetic nerve activity also increases secretion, whereas somatostatin, released from D-cells adjacent to the glucagon-secreting A-cells in the periphery of the islets, inhibits glucagon release.*

*__Octreotide__, a somatostatin analogue (see p. 385), is used to treat the syndrome (which includes relatively mild hyperglycaemia but profound muscle catabolism) caused by rare glucagon-secreting tumours.

ACTIONS

Glucagon increases blood glucose and causes breakdown of fat and protein. It acts on specific receptors to stimulate adenylate cyclase, and consequently its actions are somewhat similar to β-adrenoceptor-mediated actions of adrenaline. Unlike adrenaline, however, its metabolic effects are more pronounced than its cardiovascular actions. Glucagon is proportionately more active on liver, while adrenaline is more active on muscle and fat. Glucagon stimulates glycogen breakdown and gluconeogenesis and inhibits glycogen synthesis and glucose oxidation. Its metabolic actions on target tissues are thus the opposite of those of insulin. Glucagon increases the rate and force of contraction of the heart, though less markedly than adrenaline.

Clinical uses of glucagon are summarised in the box.

SOMATOSTATIN

Somatostatin is secreted by the D-cells of the islets. It is also the growth hormone release-inhibiting factor generated in the hypothalamus (see Ch. 27). It provides local inhibitory regulation of insulin and glucagon release within the islet. **Octreotide** is a long-acting octapeptide analogue of somatostatin. It inhibits release of a number of hormones and is used clinically to relieve symptoms from several uncommon gastroentero-pancreatic endocrine tumours, and for treatment of acromegaly* (the endocrine disorder caused by a functioning tumour of cells that secrete growth hormone from the anterior pituitary—see Ch. 27).

AMYLIN (ISLET AMYLOID POLYPEPTIDE)

▼ Amyloid is an amorphous protein that is deposited in different tissues in a variety of diseases. Amyloid deposits occur in the pancreas of patients with diabetes mellitus, although it is not known if this is functionally important. The major component of pancreatic amyloid is a peptide of 37 amino acid residues, which is known as islet amyloid polypeptide or amylin. This is stored with insulin in secretory granules in B-cells and is cosecreted with insulin. Amylin delays gastric emptying. Supraphysiological concentrations stimulate the breakdown of glycogen to lactate in striated muscle. Amylin also inhibits insulin secretion (Fig. 25.1). It is structurally related to calcitonin and has weak calcitonin-like actions on calcium metabolism and osteoclast activity. It is also about 50% identical with calcitonin gene-related peptide (CGRP; see Ch. 3) and large intravenous doses cause vasodilatation, presumably by an action on CGRP receptors. Whether amylin has a role in the physiological control of glucose metabolism is controversial, but there is interest in the therapeutic potential of amylin agonists (such as **pramlintide**, an analogue with three proline substitutions that reduce its tendency to aggregate into insoluble fibrils). These have been given to supplement insulin in type 1 diabetes mellitus, and to lower postprandial glucose concentrations in such patients. Their role in therapy is not yet established.

Clinical uses of glucagon

- Glucagon can be administered intramuscularly or subcutaneously as well as intravenously.
- Treatment of hypoglycaemia in unconscious patients (who cannot drink); unlike intravenous glucose it can be administered by non-medical personnel (e.g. spouses or ambulance crew). It is also useful if there is difficulty in obtaining intravenous access.
- Treatment of acute cardiac failure precipitated by injudicious use of β-adrenoceptor antagonists where it will increase the force of contraction of the heart (positive inotropic action).

CONTROL OF BLOOD GLUCOSE

Glucose is the obligatory source of energy for the brain, and physiological control of blood glucose reflects the need to maintain adequate fuel supplies in the face of intermittent food intake and variable metabolic demands. More fuel is made available by feeding than is immediately required, and excess calories are stored as glycogen or fat. During fasting, these energy stores need to be mobilised in a regulated manner. The most important regulatory hormone is insulin, the actions of which are described above. Increased blood sugar causes increased insulin secretion, whereas reduced blood sugar reduces insulin secretion. Hypoglycaemia, caused by excessive insulin, not only reduces insulin secretion but also elicits secretion of an array of 'counter-regulatory' hormones, including glucagon, adrenaline, glucocorticoids and growth hormone. These increase blood glucose. Their main effects on glucose uptake and carbohydrate metabolism are summarised and contrasted with those of insulin in Table 25.2.

DIABETES MELLITUS

Diabetes mellitus is a chronic metabolic disorder characterised by a high blood glucose concentration—hyperglycaemia (fasting plasma glucose >7.0 mmol/l, or plasma glucose >11.1 mmol/l 2 hours after a meal)—caused by insulin deficiency, often combined with insulin resistance. Hyperglycaemia occurs because of uncontrolled hepatic glucose output and reduced uptake of glucose by skeletal muscle with reduced glycogen synthesis. When the renal threshold for glucose reabsorption is exceeded, glucose spills over into the urine (glycosuria) and causes an osmotic diuresis (polyuria), which, in turn, results in dehydration, thirst and increased drinking (polydipsia). Insulin deficiency causes wasting through increased breakdown and reduced synthesis of proteins. *Diabetic ketoacidosis* is an acute emergency. It develops in the absence of insulin because of accelerated fat breakdown to acetyl-CoA, which, in the absence of aerobic carbohydrate metabolism, is converted to acetoacetate

*Octreotide is used either short term before surgery on the pituitary tumour while waiting for radiotherapy of the tumour to take effect or if other treatments have been ineffective.

Table 25.2 The effect of hormones on blood glucose

Hormone	Main actions	Main stimulus for secretion	Main effect
Main regulatory hormone			
Insulin	↑ Glucose uptake ↑ Glycogen synthesis ↓ Glycogenolysis ↓ Gluconeogenesis	Acute rise in blood glucose	↓ Blood glucose
Main counter-regulatory hormones			
Glucagon	↑ Glycogenolysis ↑ Gluconeogenesis	Hypoglycaemia, (i.e. blood glucose < 3 mmol/l), e.g. with exercise, stress, high protein meals, etc.	↑ Blood glucose
Adrenaline	↑ Glycogenolysis ↓ Glucose uptake		
Glucocorticoids	↑ Gluconeogenesis ↓ Glucose uptake and utilisation		
Growth hormone	↓ Glucose uptake		

and β-hydroxybutyrate (which cause acidosis) and acetone (a ketone).

Various complications develop as a consequence of the metabolic derangements in diabetes, often over many years. Many of these are the result of disease of blood vessels, either large (macrovascular disease) or small (microangiopathy). Dysfunction of vascular endothelium (see Ch. 18) is an early and critical event in the development of vascular complications. Oxygen-derived free radicals, protein kinase C and non-enzymic products of glucose and albumin (called advanced glycation end-products, or AGE) have been implicated. *Macrovascular disease* consists of accelerated atheroma, which is much more common and severe in diabetic patients. *Microangiopathy* is a distinctive feature of diabetes mellitus and particularly affects the retina, kidney and peripheral nerves. Diabetes mellitus is the commonest cause of chronic renal failure, which itself represents a huge and rapidly increasing problem, the costs of which to society as well as to individual patients are staggering. Coexistent hypertension promotes progressive renal damage, and treatment of hypertension slows the progression of diabetic nephropathy and reduces myocardial infarction. Angiotensin-converting enzyme inhibitors or antagonists of angiotensin AT1 receptors are more effective in preventing diabetic nephropathy than other antihypertensive drugs, perhaps because they prevent fibroproliferative actions of angiotensin II and aldosterone.

Diabetic neuropathy is associated with accumulation of osmotically active metabolites of glucose, produced by the action of aldose reductase, but aldose reductase inhibitors have been disappointing as therapies.

There are two main types of diabetes mellitus:

- type 1 diabetes (previously known as insulin-dependent diabetes mellitus (IDDM) or juvenile-onset diabetes)
- type 2 diabetes (previously known as non-insulin-dependent diabetes mellitus (NIDDM) or maturity-onset diabetes).

In type 1 diabetes, there is an absolute deficiency of insulin resulting from autoimmune destruction of B-cells. Without insulin treatment such patients will ultimately die with diabetic ketoacidosis.

▼ Type 1 diabetic patients are usually young (children or adolescents) and not obese when they first develop symptoms. There is an inherited predisposition, with a 10-fold increased incidence in first-degree relatives of an index case, and strong associations with particular histocompatibility antigens (HLA types). Studies of identical twins have shown that genetically predisposed individuals must additionally be exposed to an environmental factor such as viral infection (e.g. with coxsackie virus or echovirus). Viral infection may damage pancreatic B-cells and expose antigens that initiate a self-perpetuating autoallergic process. The patient becomes overtly diabetic only when more than 90% of the B-cells have been destroyed. This natural history provides a tantalising prospect of intervening in the prediabetic stage, and a variety of strategies have been mooted including immunosuppression, early insulin therapy, antioxidants, nicotinamide and many others, but so far these have been disappointing.

Type 2 diabetes is accompanied both by insulin resistance (which precedes overt disease) and by impaired insulin secretion, each of which are important in its pathogenesis. Such patients are often obese and usually present in adult life, the incidence rising progressively with age as B-cell function declines. Treatment is initially dietary although oral hypoglycaemic drugs usually become necessary, and about one third of patients ultimately require insulin. Prospective studies have demonstrated a relentless deterioration in diabetic control* over the years. This is delayed but not prevented by treatment.

Insulin secretion in the two main forms of diabetes is shown schematically in Figure 25.2, contrasted with the normal response.

There are many other less common forms of diabetes mellitus in addition to the two main ones described above, and hyperglycaemia can also be a clinically important adverse effect of several drugs, including glucocorticoids (Ch. 27), high doses of thiazide diuretics (Ch. 23) and several of the protease inhibitors used to treat human immunodeficiency virus infection (Ch. 46).

TREATMENT OF DIABETES MELLITUS

Insulin is essential for the treatment of type 1 diabetes. For many years it was assumed, as an act of faith, that normalising plasma glucose would prevent diabetic complications. The Diabetes Control and Complications Trial (American Diabetes Association, 1993) showed that this faith was well placed: type 1 diabetic patients were randomly allocated to intensive or conventional management. Mean fasting blood glucose concentration was 2.8 mmol/l lower in the intensively managed group, who had a substantial reduction in the occurrence and progression of retinopathy, nephropathy and neuropathy over a period of 4–9 years. These benefits outweighed a threefold increase in severe hypoglycaemic attacks and modest excess weight gain.

The UK Prospective Diabetes Study (UKPDS) showed that lowering blood pressure markedly improves outcome in type 2 diabetes (see above). Optimal control was not achieved even in intensively treated patients. Better metabolic control did improve outcome, but the magnitude of the benefit was disappointing and only statistically significant for microvascular complications. Consequently, realistic goals in type 2 diabetic patients are usually less ambitious than in younger type 1 patients. Diet is the cornerstone (albeit one with a tendency to crumble), combined with increased exercise. Oral agents are used to control symptoms from hyperglycaemia, as well as to limit microvascular complications. Insulin is often needed as endogenous insulin secretion becomes further impaired with increasing age. Dietary measures to prevent atheromatous disease (specially limitation of saturated fat consumption Ch. 19) are crucial. Details of dietary management are beyond the scope of this book, as is treatment for specific diabetic complications such as laser treatment of the retina, which prevents blindness in some cases.

*Diabetic control is not easily estimated by determination of blood glucose, because this is so variable. Instead, glycated haemoglobin (haemoglobin A_{1C}), is measured. This provides an integrated measure of control over the lifespan of the red cell: approximately 120 days.

INSULIN TREATMENT

Effects of insulin and its mechanism of action have been described above. Here we describe pharmacokinetic aspects and adverse effects, both of which are central to its therapeutic use. Insulin for clinical use was once either porcine or bovine but is now almost entirely human (made by recombinant DNA technology). Few advantages of human insulin emerged during clinical trials, but manufacturing advantages over animal insulins are substantial and the quality of the products much more consistent than when insulins were extracted from pancreases of freshly slaughtered animals. Nevertheless, doses are still quantified in terms of units of activity, with which doctors and patients are familiar, rather than of mass.

Pharmacokinetic aspects and insulin preparations

Insulin is destroyed in the gastrointestinal tract, and must be given parenterally—usually subcutaneously, but intravenously or occasionally intramuscularly in emergencies. Intraperitoneal insulin is used in diabetic patients with end-stage renal failure treated by ambulatory peritoneal dialysis. Pulmonary absorption of insulin occurs and inhalation of an aerosol is a promising route of administration. Other new approaches include incorporation of insulin into biodegradable polymer microspheres, and its encapsulation with a lectin in a glucose-permeable membrane.** Once absorbed, insulin has an elimination half-life of approximately 10 minutes. It is inactivated enzymically in the liver and kidney, and 10% is excreted in the urine. Renal impairment reduces insulin requirement.

One of the main problems in using insulin is to avoid wide fluctuations in plasma concentration and thus in blood glucose. To address this, various formulations are available, varying in the timing of their peak effect and duration of action. Soluble insulin produces a rapid and short-lived effect. Longer-acting preparations are made by precipitating insulin with protamine or zinc, thus forming finely divided amorphous solid or relatively insoluble crystals, which are injected as a suspension from which insulin is slowly absorbed. These preparations include isophane insulin and amorphous or crystalline insulin zinc suspensions. Mixtures of different forms in fixed proportions are available. **Insulin lispro** is an insulin analogue in which a lysine and a proline residue are 'switched'. It acts more rapidly but for a shorter time than natural insulin, enabling patients to inject themselves immediately before the start of a meal. **Insulin glargine** is another modified insulin analogue, designed with the opposite intention, namely to provide a constant basal insulin supply and mimic physiological postabsorptive basal insulin secretion. Insulin glargine, which is a clear solution, forms a microprecipitate at the physiological pH of subcutaneous tissue,

**This could, in theory, provide variable release of insulin controlled by the prevailing glucose concentration, because glucose and glycosylated insulin compete for binding sites on the lectin.

and absorption from the subcutaneous site of injection is prolonged. It is hoped that, used in conjunction with short-acting insulin, it will lower postabsorptive plasma glucose but reduce the risk of night time hypoglycaemia, so it could prove to be a major advance.

Various dosage regimens are used. A common one for type 1 patients involves injecting a combination of short- and intermediate-acting insulins twice daily, before breakfast and before the evening meal. Intensified regimens can improve control of blood glucose; these involve multiple daily injections of short-acting insulins with meals and a longer-acting insulin at night or continuous subcutaneous infusion of a short-acting insulin through a pump. The most sophisticated forms of pump regulate the dose by means of a sensor that continuously measures blood glucose, but these are not routinely available.

Unwanted effects

The main undesirable effect of insulin is hypoglycaemia. This is common and, if very severe, can cause brain damage. Intensive insulin therapy results in a threefold increase in severe hypoglycaemia. The treatment of hypoglycaemia is to take a sweet drink or snack, or, if the patient is unconscious, to give intravenous glucose or intramuscular glucagon (see above). Rebound hyperglycaemia ('Somogyi effect') can follow insulin-induced hypoglycaemia, because of the release of counter-regulatory hormones (see above). This can cause hyperglycaemia before breakfast following an unrecognised hypoglycaemic attack during sleep in the early hours of the morning. It is essential to appreciate this possibility to avoid the mistake of increasing (rather than reducing) the evening dose of insulin in this situation.

Allergy to human insulin is unusual but can occur. It may take the form of local or systemic reactions. Insulin resistance as a consequence of antibody formation is rare.

Clinical uses of insulin are summarised in the box.

Clinical uses of insulin

- Patients with type 1 diabetes require long-term maintenance treatment with insulin. An intermediate-acting preparation (e.g. isophane insulin, to provide a low background level) is often combined with a short-acting preparation (e.g. soluble insulin) taken before meals.
- Soluble insulin is used (intravenously) in emergency treatment of hyperglycaemic diabetic emergencies (e.g. diabetic ketoacidosis).
- Many patients with type 2 diabetes ultimately require insulin treatment.
- Short-term treatment of patients with type 2 diabetes or impaired glucose tolerance during intercurrent events (e.g. operations, infections, myocardial infarction).
- During pregnancy, for gestational diabetes not controlled by diet alone.
- Emergency treatment of hyperkalaemia: insulin is given with glucose to lower extracellular K^+ via redistribution into cells.

ORAL HYPOGLYCAEMIC AGENTS

The main oral hypoglycaemic agents (see the box on p. 391) are **metformin** (a biguanide), sulfonylureas and other drugs that act on the sulfonylurea receptor, and the recently introduced *glitazones*. **Acarbose** is an α-glucosidase inhibitor.

Biguanides

Metformin is the only drug of this class presently available in the UK.

Actions and mechanism

Biguanides lower blood glucose. Their mechanisms are complex and incompletely understood. They increase glucose uptake and utilisation in skeletal muscle (thereby reducing insulin resistance) and reduce hepatic glucose production (gluconeogenesis). Metformin, as well as lowering blood glucose, additionally reduces low density and very low density lipoproteins (LDL and VLDL, respectively).

Pharmacokinetic aspects

Metformin has a half-life of about 3 hours and is excreted unchanged in the urine.

Unwanted effects

The commonest unwanted effects of metformin are dose-related gastrointestinal disturbances (e.g. anorexia, diarrhoea, nausea), which are usually but not always transient. Lactic acidosis is a rare but potentially fatal toxic effect, and metformin should not be given to patients with renal or hepatic disease, hypoxic pulmonary disease, heart failure or shock. Such patients are predisposed to lactic acidosis because of reduced drug elimination or reduced tissue oxygenation. It should also be avoided in other situations that predispose to lactic acidosis and is contraindicated in pregnancy. Long-term use may interfere with absorption of vitamin B_{12}.

Clinical use

Clinical use of metformin is in patients with type 2 diabetes. It does not stimulate appetite (rather the reverse, see above!) and is consequently useful in the majority of type 2 patients who are obese and who fail treatment with diet alone. It does not cause hypoglycaemia and can be combined with sulfonylureas, glitazones or insulin.

Sulfonylureas

The sulfonylureas were developed following the chance observation that a sulfonamide derivative (used to treat typhoid) caused hypoglycaemia. Numerous sulfonylureas are available. The first used therapeutically were **tolbutamide** and **chlorpropamide**. Chlorpropamide has a long duration of action and a substantial fraction is excreted in the urine. Consequently it can cause severe hypoglycaemia, especially in elderly patients in whom renal function declines inevitably but insidiously (Ch. 23). It causes flushing after alcohol because of a disulfiram-like effect (Ch. 42) and has an action like that of antidiuretic hormone on the distal nephron, giving rise to hyponatraemia and water intoxication. Williams (1994) comments that 'time honoured but idiosyncratic chlorpropamide should now be laid to rest'—a sentiment with which we concur. Tolbutamide, however, remains useful. So-called second-generation sulfonylureas (e.g. **glibenclamide**, **glipizide**; see Table 25.3) are more potent (on a milligram basis), but their maximum hypoglycaemic effect is no greater and failure of treatment to control blood sugar is just as common as with tolbutamide. They all contain the sulfonylurea moiety, but different substitutions result in differences in pharmacokinetics and hence in duration of action (see Table 25.3).

Mechanism of action

The principal action of sulfonylureas is on B-cells (Fig. 25.1), stimulating insulin secretion (the equivalent of phase I in Fig. 25.2) and thus reducing plasma glucose. High-affinity receptors for sulfonylureas are present on the K_{ATP} channels in B-cell plasma membranes, and the binding of various sulfonylureas parallels their potency in stimulating insulin release. The drugs reduce the K^+ permeability of B-cells by blocking K_{ATP} channels (pp. 380–381), causing depolarisation, Ca^{2+} entry and insulin secretion.

Pharmacokinetic aspects

Sulfonylureas are well absorbed after oral administration and most reach peak plasma concentrations within 2–4 hours. The duration of action varies (Table 25.3). All bind strongly to plasma albumin and are implicated in interactions with other drugs (e.g. salicylates and sulfonamides) that compete for these binding sites (see below and Ch. 51). Most sulfonylureas (or their active metabolites) are excreted in the urine, so their action is increased in the elderly and in patients with renal disease.

Most sulfonylureas cross the placenta and stimulate fetal B-cells to release insulin, causing severe hypoglycaemia at birth (glibenclamide is an exception in this regard); as a result, use of sulfonylureas is generally contraindicated in pregnancy.

Unwanted effects

The sulfonylureas are usually well tolerated. Unwanted effects are specified in Table 25.3. The commonest adverse effect is hypoglycaemia, which can be severe and prolonged. Its incidence is related to the potency and duration of action of the agent, the highest incidence occurring with chlorpropamide and glibenclamide and the lowest with tolbutamide. Glibenclamide is best avoided in the elderly and in patients with even mild renal impairment because of the risk of hypoglycaemia, since several of its metabolites are excreted in urine and are moderately active. Sulfonylureas stimulate appetite (probably via their effects on

Table 25.3 Oral hypoglycaemic sulfonylurea drugs

Drug	Relative potency[a]	Duration of action and (half-life) in hours	Pharmacokinetic aspects[b]	General comments
Tolbutamide	1	6–12 (4)	Some converted in liver to weakly active hydroxytolbutamide; some carboxylated to inactive compound Renal excretion	A safe drug; least likely to cause hypoglycaemia May decrease iodide uptake by thyroid Contraindicated in liver failure
Glibenclamide[c]	150	18–24 (10)	Some is oxidised in the liver to moderately active products and is excreted in urine; 50% is excreted unchanged in the faeces	May cause hypoglycaemia. The active metabolite accumulates in renal failure
Glipizide	100	16–24 (7)	Peak plasma levels in 1 hour. Most is metabolised in the liver to inactive products, which are excreted in urine; 12% is excreted in faeces.	May cause hypoglycaemia Has diuretic action Only inactive products accumulate in renal failure

[a]Relative to tolbutamide.
[b]All are largely protein bound (90–95%).
[c]Termed gliburide in USA.

insulin secretion and blood glucose) and often cause weight gain. This is a major concern in obese diabetic patients. About 3% of patients experience gastrointestinal upsets. Allergic skin rashes can occur, and bone marrow damage (Ch. 52), though very rare, can be severe.

During acute myocardial infarction sulfonylureas are discontinued and type 2 diabetic patients are treated with insulin. This is associated with a substantial reduction in short-term mortality. A vexing question is whether prolonged therapy with oral hypoglycaemic drugs has adverse effects on the cardiovascular system. A study in the USA in the 1970s found that after 4–5 years of treatment there was an increase in cardiovascular deaths in the group treated with oral drugs compared with the groups treated with insulin or placebo. Blockade of K_{ATP} in heart and vascular tissue could have adverse effects. However, in the US study there was no statistically significant increase in total mortality in the sulfonylurea group and the UKPDS, which included a group randomised to sulfonylureas, did not incriminate these drugs.

Drug interactions

Several drugs augment the hypoglycaemic effect of the sulfonylureas. Non-steroidal anti-inflammatory drugs, coumarins, some uricosuric drugs (e.g. **sulfinpyrazone**), alcohol, monoamine oxidase inhibitors, some antibacterials (including **sulfonamides**, **trimethoprim** and **chloramphenicol**) and some imidazole antifungal drugs have all been reported to produce severe hypoglycaemia when given with the sulfonylureas. The probable basis of most of these interactions is competition for metabolising enzymes, but interference with plasma protein binding or with excretion may also play a part.

Agents that decrease the action of the sulfonylureas include high doses of thiazide diuretics and corticosteroids.

Clinical use

Sulfonylureas require functional B-cells, so they are useful in the early stages of type 2 diabetes. They can be combined with metformin or with thiazolidinediones.

Other drugs that stimulate insulin secretion

Several drugs that lack the sulfonylurea moiety but stimulate insulin secretion have recently been developed. These include **repaglinide** and **nateglinide**. These act, like the sulfonylureas, by blocking the sulfonylurea receptor on K_{ATP} channels in pancreatic B-cell membranes. Thus nateglinide, which is structurally derived from D-phenylalanine ('the first of a new class of insulin secretion enhancers' according to one piece of promotional literature), displaces tritiated glibenclamide from specific binding sites on B-cells. Like sulfonylureas, it inhibits flux of radioactive rubidium ions (which traverse K_{ATP} channels) from B-cells loaded with this isotope and blocks these channels in patch clamp experiments. It is much less potent than most sulfonylureas (with the exception of tolbutamide) and has rapid onset and offset kinetics. These features, coupled with rapid absorption (time to maximal plasma concentration approximately 55 minutes after an oral dose) and elimination (half-life approximately 3 hours), leads to short duration of action and a low risk of hypoglycaemia.* These drugs are administered shortly before a meal to reduce the postprandial glucose rise in type 2 diabetic patients inadequately controlled with diet and exercise. A potential advantage is that they may cause less weight gain than conventional sulfonylureas. Later in the course of the disease they can be combined with other oral agents such as metformin or thiazolidinediones. Unlike glibenclamide, these drugs are relatively selective for K_{ATP} channels on B-cells versus K_{ATP} channels in vascular smooth muscle.

Thiazolidinediones (glitazones)

The thiazolidinediones (or glitazones) were developed following the chance observation that a clofibrate analogue, **ciglitazone**, which was being screened for effects on lipids, unexpectedly lowered blood glucose. Ciglitazone caused liver toxicity, as did **troglitazone**, but currently marketed thiazolidinediones (**rosiglitazone** and **pioglitazone**) lower blood glucose, apparently without causing serious hepatotoxicity.

Effects

The effect of thiazolidinediones on blood glucose is slow in onset, the maximum effect being achieved only after 1–2 months of treatment. Thiazolidinediones reduce hepatic glucose output and increase glucose uptake into muscle, enhancing the effectiveness of endogenous insulin and reducing the amount of exogenous insulin needed to maintain a given level of blood glucose by approximately 30%. The reduction in blood glucose is often accompanied by reductions in circulating insulin and free fatty acids. Triglycerides may decline, while LDL and high density lipoproteins (HDL) are either unchanged or slightly increased, with little alteration in LDL/HDL ratio. The proportion of small dense LDL particles (believed to be the most atherogenic, Ch. 19) is reduced. Weight gain of 1–4 kg is common, usually stabilising in 6–12 months. Some of this is attributable to fluid retention: there is an increase in plasma volume of up to 500 ml with a concomitant reduction in haemoglobin concentration caused by haemodilution; there is also an increase in extravascular fluid, and increased deposition of subcutaneous (as opposed to visceral) fat.

Mechanism of action

Thiazolidinediones bind to a nuclear receptor called the peroxisome proliferator-activated receptor-gamma (PPARγ), which is complexed with retinoid X receptor (RXR; see Ch. 3).** PPARγ occurs mainly in adipose tissue, but also in muscle and liver. It mediates differentiation of adipocytes, increases

*It is ironic that these recently introduced and aggressively marketed drugs share many of the properties of tolbutamide, the oldest, least expensive and least fashionable of the sulfonylureas. Perhaps diabetologists should turn some of their investigative effort to studying how best to use this Cinderella drug!

**Compare with fibrates (to which thiazolidinediones are structurally related) which bind to PPARα (see Ch. 19).

lipogenesis and enhances uptake of fatty acids and glucose. Endogenous agonists include unsaturated fatty acids and various derivatives of these, including prostaglandin J_2. Thiazolidinediones are exogenous agonists. They change the PPARγ–RXR complex so that it binds DNA and promotes transcription of several genes with products that are important in insulin signalling, including lipoprotein lipase, fatty acid transporter protein, adipocyte fatty acid-binding protein, Glut-4, phosphoenolpyruvate carboxykinase, malic enzyme and others. It remains something of a mystery that glucose homeostasis should be so responsive to drugs that bind to receptors found mainly in fat cells; it has been suggested that the explanation may lie in resetting of the glucose–fatty acid (Randle) cycle by the reduction in circulating free fatty acids.

Pharmacokinetic aspects

Both rosiglitazone and pioglitazone are rapidly and nearly completely absorbed, with time to peak plasma concentration of less than 2 hours. Both are highly (>99%) bound to plasma proteins, both are subject to hepatic metabolism and both have a short (<7 hours) elimination half-life for the parent drug, but substantially longer (up to 150 hours for rosiglitazone, up to 24 hours for pioglitazone) for the metabolites. Rosiglitazone is metabolised by CYP2C8 to weakly active metabolites, pioglitazone mainly by a CYP2C isozyme (known as CYP2C*) and CYP3A4 to active metabolites. The metabolites of rosiglitazone are eliminated mainly in urine, and those of pioglitazone mainly in bile.

Unwanted effects

The serious hepatotoxicity of ciglitazone and troglitazone was not encountered during clinical trials of rosiglitazone or pioglitazone, although cases of liver dysfunction of uncertain causality* have been reported since their general release. Regular blood tests of liver function are currently recommended. One (unproven) hypothesis is that the hepatotoxicity of troglitazone is caused by quinone metabolites of its α-tocopherol side-chain, which are not formed from the newer thiazolidinediones. The commonest unwanted effects of rosiglitazone and pioglitazone are weight gain and fluid retention (see above). Fluid retention is a substantial concern since it can precipitate or worsen heart failure, which contraindicates their use. Symptoms of uncertain cause including headache, fatigue and gastrointestinal disturbances have also been reported. Thiazolidinediones are contraindicated in pregnant or breast-feeding women and in

Clinical uses of oral hypoglycaemic drugs

- Type 2 diabetes mellitus, as a supplement to diet and exercise to reduce symptoms from hyperglycaemia (e.g. thirst, excessive urination). Tight control of blood glucose has only a small effect on vascular complications.
- Metformin is preferred for obese patients unless contraindicated by factor(s) that predispose to lactic acidosis (renal or liver failure, heart failure, hypoxaemia).
- Acarbose (α-glucosidase inhibitor) reduces carbohydrate absorption; it causes flatulence and diarrhoea.
- Drugs that act on the sulfonylurea receptor (e.g. tolbutamide, glibenclamide) are well tolerated but often promote weight gain.

Drugs in diabetes

Insulin

- Human insulin is made by recombinant DNA technology. For routine use it is given subcutaneously (by intravenous infusion in emergencies).
- Different formulations of insulin differ in their duration of action:
  - —fast- and short-acting soluble insulin: peak action after subcutaneous dose 2–4 hours and duration 6–8 hours; it can be given intravenously
  - —intermediate-acting insulin (e.g. isophane insulin can be mixed with soluble insulin)
  - —long-acting forms, e.g. insulin zinc suspension.
- The main unwanted effect is hypoglycaemia.
- Altering the amino acid sequence ('designer' insulins, e.g. lispro and glargine) can usefully alter insulin kinetics.

Oral hypoglycaemic drugs

- These are used in type 2 diabetes.
- Biguanides (e.g. metformin):
  - —have complex peripheral actions in the presence of residual insulin, increasing glucose uptake in striated muscle and inhibiting hepatic glucose output and intestinal glucose absorption
  - —cause anorexia and assist in weight loss
  - —are used with sulfonylureas when these have ceased to work adequately.
- Sulfonylureas and other drugs that stimulate insulin secretion (e.g. tolbutamide, glibenclamide, nateglinide):
  - —can cause hypoglycaemia (which stimulates appetite and leads to weight gain)
  - —are only effective if B-cells are functional
  - —block ATP-sensitive potassium channels in B-cells.
- Thiazolidinediones (e.g. rosiglitazone, pioglitazone)
  - —increase insulin sensitivity and lower blood glucose in type 2 diabetes
  - —can cause weight gain and oedema
  - —are PPARγ (a nuclear receptor) agonists.

*A confounding issue is that fatty liver is quite common in patients with type 2 diabetes.

children. It is theoretically possible that these drugs could cause ovulation to resume in women who are anovulatory because of insulin resistance (e.g. with polycystic ovary syndrome).

Interactions

Thiazolidinediones are additive with other oral hypoglycaemic drugs. In Europe, both rosiglitazone and pioglitazone are contraindicated for use with insulin because of concern that these combinations increase the risk of heart failure, although in the USA thiazolidinediones are widely used in combination with insulin.

Clinical use

Since insulin resistance is one important component of the pathogenesis of type 2 diabetes and has been implicated in the excess cardiovascular mortality that accompanies the common 'metabolic syndrome' (visceral obesity, hypertension, dyslipidaemia, insulin resistance, etc.), there is a good rationale for glitazones in type 2 diabetes. This probably explains their widespread adoption into clinical practice, especially in the USA. There is, however, as yet no evidence that this optimism is justified in terms of improved clinical outcomes. Clinical trial evidence to-date is from short-term studies and supports their use in combination with metformin or with a sulfonylurea in patients who are inadequately controlled on one of these drugs and are unsuited to addition of the other. Hopefully evidence to support wider and more useful applications (e.g. as monotherapy or as triple therapy with both metformin and a sulfonylurea) will soon be forthcoming.

Alpha-glucosidase inhibitors

Acarbose, an inhibitor of intestinal α-glucosidase, is used in type 2 patients inadequately controlled by diet with or without other agents. It delays carbohydrate absorption, reducing the postprandial increase in blood glucose. The commonest adverse effects are related to its main action and consist of flatulence, loose stools or diarrhoea and abdominal pain and bloating. Like metformin it may be particularly helpful in obese type 2 patients.

Potential new antidiabetic drugs

Several agents are currently being studied including α_2-antagonists and inhibitors of fatty acid oxidation. Lipolysis in fat cells is controlled by adrenoceptors of the β_3-subtype (see Ch. 11). The possibility of using selective β_3-agonists, currently in development, in the treatment of obese patients with type 2 diabetes is being investigated (see Ch. 26). There is great interest in inhibitors of protein kinase C (e.g. **LY333531**, a specific inhibitor specific for the β isoform), because of evidence implicating activation of this pathway in the development of vascular diabetic complications.

REFERENCES AND FURTHER READING

Several of the references below are to specific chapters of particular relevance in Pickup J C, Williams J (eds) 2002 Textbook of diabetes, 3rd edn. Blackwell Science, Oxford. This extremely readable textbook offers an excellent 'way in' to the original literature.

ACE Inhibitors in Diabetic Nephropathy Trialist Group 2001 Should all patients with type 1 diabetes mellitus and microalbuminuria receive angiotensin converting enzyme inhibitors? A meta-analysis of individual patient data. Ann Intern Med 134: 370–379 (*Probably*)

American Diabetes Association 1993 Implications of the diabetes control and complications trial. Diabetes 42: 1555–1558 (*Landmark clinical trial*)

Anonymous 2001 Pioglitazone and rosiglitazone for diabetes. Drug and Therapeutics Bulletin 39: 65–68 (*Succinct review concluding that the optimal place of the glitazones in the management of patients with type 2 diabetes, and their long-term risks and effects on the complications of diabetes is not yet known*)

Bolli G B, Owens D R 2000 Insulin glargine. Lancet 356: 443–445 (*Balanced, succinct commentary. 'In the 50 years since NPH insulin was devised by Hagedorn and Lente insulin by Hallas-Møller, no improved formulations of intermediate acting or long-acting insulin preparations have been introduced until now.' Insulin glargine could represent a milestone*)

Brenner B M et al. 2001 Effects of losartan on renal and cardiovascular outcomes in patients with type 2 diabetes and nephropathy. N Engl J Med 345: 861–869 (*Significant renal benefits from the AT1 antagonist; see also two adjacent articles Lewis E J et al. pp. 851–860 and Parving H-H et al. pp. 870–878 and an editorial on prevention of renal disease caused by type 2 diabetes by Hostetter T H pp. 910–911*)

de Fronzo R A, Goodman A M 1995 Efficacy of metformin in patients with non-insulin-dependent diabetes mellitus. N Engl J Med 333: 541–549 (*See also accompanying editorial on metformin by Crofford, OB pp. 588–589*)

Dornhorst A 2001 Insulinotropic meglitinide analogues. Lancet 358: 1709–1716 (*Reviews rationale for this class, which includes repaglinide and nateglinide*)

Dunn M J 1997 Familial persistent hyperinsulinemic hypoglycemia of infancy and mutations in the sulfonylurea receptor. N Engl J Med 336: 703–706 (*A rare disease resulting from disorder of potassium channels as a result of mutation in the sulphonylurea receptor*)

Gale E A M 2001 Lessons from the glitazones: a story of drug development. Lancet 357: 1870–1875 (*Fighting stuff: 'Troglitazone was voluntarily withdrawn in Europe, but went on to generate sales of over $2 billion in the USA and caused 90 cases of liver failure before being withdrawn. Rosiglitazone and pioglitazone reached the USA for use alone or in combination with other drugs whereas in Europe the same dossiers were used to apply for a limited licence as second-line agents. How should we use them? How did they achieve blockbuster status without any clear evidence of advantage over existing therapy?'*)

Hu S et al. 2000 Pancreatic β-cell K_{ATP} channel activity and membrane—binding studies with nateglinide: a comparison with sulphonylureas and repaglinide. J Pharmacol Exp Ther 293: 444–452 (*In competition binding studies nateglinide displaced ^{3}H-glibenclamide with lower affinity than all sulphonylureas studied except tolbutamide*)

Maratos-Flier E, Goldstein B J, Kahn C R 2002 The insulin receptor and postreceptor mechanisms. In: Pickup J C, Williams J (eds) Textbook of diabetes, 3rd edn. Blackwell Science, Oxford

Owens D R, Zinman B, Bolli G B 2001 Insulins today and beyond. Lancet 358: 739–746 (*Reviews the physiology of glucose homeostasis, genetically engineered 'designer' insulins and developments in insulin delivery and glucose sensing*)

Saltiel A R, Kahn C R 2001 Insulin signaling and the regulation of glucose and lipid metabolism. Nature 414: 799–806 (*Discusses insulin resistance and related hormonal and signalling events*)

Saltiel A R, Pessin J E 2002 Insulin signaling pathways in space and time. Trends Cell Biol 12: 65–70 (*Up to date review*)

Skyler J S, Cefalu W T, Kourides I A et al. 2001 Efficacy of inhaled human insulin in type 1 diabetes mellitus: a randomized proof-of-concept study. Lancet 357: 324–325 (*Preprandial inhaled insulin is a less invasive alternative to injection. See also a paper on type 2 patients from the same group, showing that 3 months of treatment with inhaled insulin was effective and well tolerated without adverse pulmonary effects Ann Intern Med 2001; 134: 203–207*)

Thompson R G, Peterson J, Gottlieb A, Mullane J 1997 Effects of pramlintide, an analog of human amylin, on plasma glucose profiles in patients with IDDM: results of a multicenter trial. Diabetes 46: 632–636 (*This amylin analogue lowered blood glucose when added to patients' usual insulin*)

Turk J, Gross R W, Ramanadham S 1993 Perspectives in diabetes. Amplification of insulin secretion by lipid messengers. Diabetes 42: 367–374 (*Amplifying intracellular messengers include diacylglycerol, non-esterified arachidonic acid, 12-S-HETE*)

Way K J, Katai N, King G L 2001 Protein kinase C and the development of diabetic vascular complications. Diabet Med 18: 945–959 (*Reviews the considerable evidence implicating protein kinise C activation in the aetiology of diabetic vascular complications*)

Williams G 1994 Management of non-insulin-dependent diabetes mellitus. Lancet 343: 95–100

Withers D J, Gutierrez J S, Towery H et al. 1998 Disruption of IRS-2 causes type 2 diabetes in mice. Nature 391: 900–904 (*Dysfunction of IRS-2 may 'contribute to the pathophysiology of human type 2 diabetes'; see also accompanying commentary by Avruch J, A signal for β-cell failure, pp. 846–847*)

Zimmet P, Alberti K G M M, Shaw J 2001 Global and societal implications of the diabetes epidemic. Nature 414: 782–787 (*Changes in human behaviour have resulted in a dramatic increase in type 2 diabetes worldwide*)

26 Obesity

Overview 394

Background 394
— Definition of obesity 394

The homeostatic mechanisms controlling energy balance 394
— Linking energy stores in body fat with the hypothalamus 395
— Integration of information and effect on energy balance 395
— Regulation of energy expenditure and food intake 396

Obesity as a health problem 397
— The pathophysiology of obesity 399
— Pharmacological approaches to the problem of obesity 401

OVERVIEW

Obesity is a growing health problem in many of the richest nations of the world and should now be considered as a chronic disease that is reaching epidemic proportions. Body fat represents stored energy and obesity occurs when the homeostatic mechanisms controlling energy balance are distorted. In this chapter, we cover first the current understanding of the homeostatic mechanisms that control energy balance. We go on to consider the main health aspects of obesity, then its pathophysiology and then the possible pharmacological agents that might be used in therapy.

BACKGROUND

The survival of an animal species requires a continuous supply of energy for physiological functioning even though the supply of food is intermittent. This requirement has been met by the evolution of a mechanism for storing energy in fuels, mainly the triglycerides of fat, from which it can be quickly mobilised. The mechanism, controlled by the so-called thrifty genes, was an obvious asset to our hunter–gatherer ancestors. However, in affluent societies that combine sedentary lifestyles with an ample supply of calorie-rich foods, it is the cause of an increasing medical problem—obesity.

It had long been thought that the body had a homeostatic system for controlling body fat and that the central nervous system (CNS) was involved. At the beginning of the 20th century it was observed that patients with damage to the hypothalamus tended to get fat. In the 1940s, it was shown that discrete lesions in the hypothalamus of rodents caused them to become obese. In 1953, Kennedy proposed, on the basis of experiments on rats, that the suggested homeostatic mechanism did in fact exist and that it involved a hormone from the adipose tissue acting on the hypothalamus. The details of this homeostatic system are now becoming clear and are leading to an understanding of the problem of obesity.

DEFINITION OF OBESITY

Obesity has been variously defined as 'an excess of body fat' or 'body weight that is 20% over the ideal'. These phrases leave us with the problem of defining what is meant by 'excess' or 'ideal'. The nutritionists achieved more precision, if not more understanding, by defining a new unit: the *body mass index* (BMI). The BMI is body mass (kg) divided by the square of the height (metres); it is highly correlated with body fat. 'Healthy' people have a BMI of 20–25, those with a BMI of 25–30 are deemed to be 'overweight', those with a BMI of >30 are said to be obese and those with a BMI >40 to be morbidly obese.

The level of BMI obviously depends on the energy balance. An operational definition of obesity would be that it is a multifactorial disorder of energy balance in which calorie intake over the long term has been greater than energy output, resulting in an excessively large BMI.

THE HOMEOSTATIC MECHANISMS CONTROLLING ENERGY BALANCE

Energy balance depends on food intake, energy storage in fat and energy expenditure. The regulation of energy balance requires:

- a mechanism for sensing the level of energy stores in body fat and relaying the information to controlling sites in the hypothalamus
- integration of information in the hypothalamus and, in turn, determination of energy balance through control of food intake and energy expenditure.

Many reviews of energy balance control contain spaghetti diagrams of interacting factors—endocrines, autonomic mediators, gastrointestinal peptides, CNS transmitters, etc.—all impinging on the hypothalamus, which, in turn, releases mediators that act on CNS, autonomic and endocrine systems; this then affects food intake and energy balance. In this chapter, we will have to confine ourselves to the main strips of pasta (images of food keep intruding).

LINKING ENERGY STORES IN BODY FAT WITH THE HYPOTHALAMUS

A mechanism for sensing the level of energy stores in fat would involve the generation of a factor (or factors) by the adipose tissue, as proposed by Kennedy in 1953. Does such a factor exist?

There has been phenomenal progress in understanding in this area in recent years. The unravelling of the story started with a study of fat rodents. For many years, it had been known that mice can become obese through mutations of certain genes, at least five of which have been identified—including the *ob* (obesity) gene and the *db* (diabetes) gene.* Mice that are homozygous for mutant forms of these genes—*ob/ob* mice and *db/db* mice—eat excessively and have low energy expenditure; they become grossly fat and have numerous metabolic and other abnormalities. Weight gain in an *ob/ob* mouse is suppressed if its circulation is linked to that of a normal mouse, implying that the obesity is caused by lack of a blood-borne factor.

In 1994, Friedman and his colleagues (see Zhang et al., 1994) cloned the *ob* gene and identified its protein product—*leptin*. (The word leptin is derived from the Greek *leptos* meaning thin.)

LEPTIN AS THE SENSOR OF ENERGY STORES IN FAT

When recombinant leptin is given intravenously or intraperitoneally to *ob/ob* mice, it strikingly reduces food intake and body weight (Fig. 26.1). It has a similar effect if directly injected into the lateral or the third ventricle, implying that it acts on the regions of the brain that control food intake and energy balance.

Leptin mRNA is expressed in fat cells; its synthesis is increased by glucocorticoids, insulin and the oestrogens; and it is reduced by β-adrenoceptor agonists. In humans, the concentration of leptin in the circulation varies according to the fat stores and BMI in normal subjects (Fig. 26.2); the leptin concentration in the plasma is pulsatile and inversely related to hydrocortisone levels.

On reaching the brain, leptin enters by saturable transport, its entry into the CNS being proportional to the plasma level. It acts on hypothalamic nuclei that express specific leptin receptors.

Thus leptin fulfils many criteria for a sensor of body fat.

INSULIN AS THE SENSOR OF ENERGY STORES IN FAT

Insulin also fulfils most of the criteria listed above (see Schwartz et al., 2000) and insulin strongly stimulates leptin expression in fat cells. But insulin's role as a fat sensor is more complex (see below, p. 397) and it is accepted that leptin has the more critical role.

It has become evident that the fat cell is not only a storage depot for fat but an important staging post on the energy information highway. But note that fat cell-derived factors other than leptin (e.g. tumour necrosis factor-α) (TNF-α)) may be part of the traffic on the highway.

Recent work has shown that fat cells secrete a host of other autocrine, paracrine and endocrine mediators, leading some authorities to consider that adipose tissue is a dispersed endocrine organ (Ahima and Flier, 2000a; Früebeck et al 2001).

INTEGRATION OF INFORMATION AND THE EFFECT ON ENERGY BALANCE

Leptin's main targets in the hypothalamus are two groups of neurons in the arcuate nucleus of the hypothalamus. These have opposing actions and energy homeostasis depends, in the first instance, on the balance between these actions. In one group, the peptides neuropeptide (NPY) and agouti-related peptide (AGRP) are colocalised. The other group contains the protein pro-opiomelanocortin (POMC) and releases α-melanocyte-stimulating hormone (α-MSH). Both groups express specific leptin receptors. Activation of the first group—by reduced leptin levels—results in increased food intake* and decreased energy expenditure; activation of the second—by increased leptin levels—has the opposite effect. Insulin receptors also occur in both groups. Leptin and insulin act in concert on the hypothalamic neurons, but leptin is the main regulating factor.

The signal transduction mechanisms following leptin receptor activation are thought to involve the Jak/Stat pathway (Ch. 3).

The integration of the information on fat stores with other information is very complex; leptin, though apparently an important coordinator, is only one part of the process.

Some of the existing information on energy balance and the control of body weight and fat depots has been put together in Figure 26.3 (see also Friedman, 1997). Numerous factors other

*The other genes are termed *agouti yellow*, and (named with geneticist tongue in cheek as usual) *tubby* and *fat*. Versions of all five genes occur in humans.

*NPY also promotes the synthesis and storage of fat by an action on the lipoprotein lipase in adipose tissue.

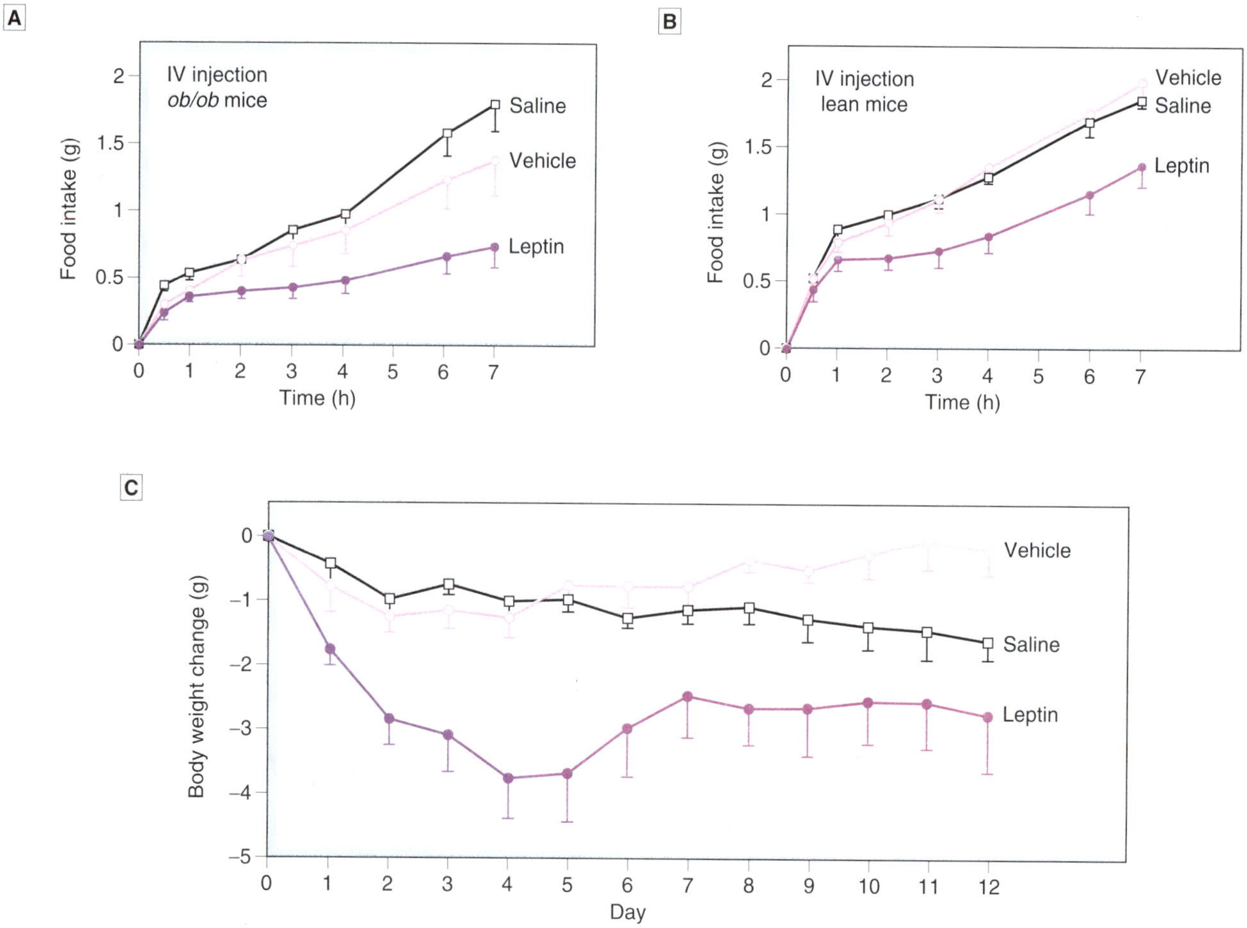

Fig. 26.1 The effect of recombinant leptin on food intake and body weight in mice. *ob/ob* mice are genetically obese mice with a mutation in the gene coding for leptin. A and B The effect of a single intravenous (IV) injection on food intake in *ob/ob* and lean mice, respectively. C The effect on body weight in *ob/ob* mice, of two daily intraperitoneal injections for 5 days. (Data from Campfield et al. 1995 Science 269: 546–549.)

than those included in the figure are involved in regulating food intake and energy expenditure.* Many are being targeted as potential anti-obesity drugs (see below).

REGULATION OF ENERGY EXPENDITURE AND FOOD INTAKE

ENERGY EXPENDITURE

Energy is expended in metabolism, physical activity and thermogenesis (heat production). The metabolic aspects of energy expenditure include, amongst other things, cardiorespiratory work and the actions of a multitude of enzymes. Physical activity increases all these as well as increasing energy expenditure by the skeletal muscles. The sympathetic nervous system plays a significant part in the regulation of energy expenditure not only as regards effects on cardiovascular and skeletal muscle function during physical activity but also in thermogenesis (see below).

Fat cells, both white and brown, but particularly brown, have a major role in thermogenesis. Brown fat cells contain abundant mitochondria and are remarkable heat generators, producing

*Other factors involved include (a) the stimulators of feeding behaviour (orexigenic factors) such as melanin-concentrating hormone (MCH), orexins A and B, galanin, gamma-aminobutyric acid (GABA), growth hormone-releasing hormone (GHRH), ghrelin; and (b) inhibitors of feeding behaviour (anorexigenic factors) such as corticotrophin-releasing hormone (CRH), the 'cocaine and amphetamine-regulated transcript' (CART), neurotensin, TNF-α, interleukin-β (IL-1β), 5-hydroxytryptamine, glucagon-like peptides, bombesin, ciliary neurotrophic factor (CNTF) and the satiety factor cholecystokinin. For more detail see Ahima and Osei (2001.)

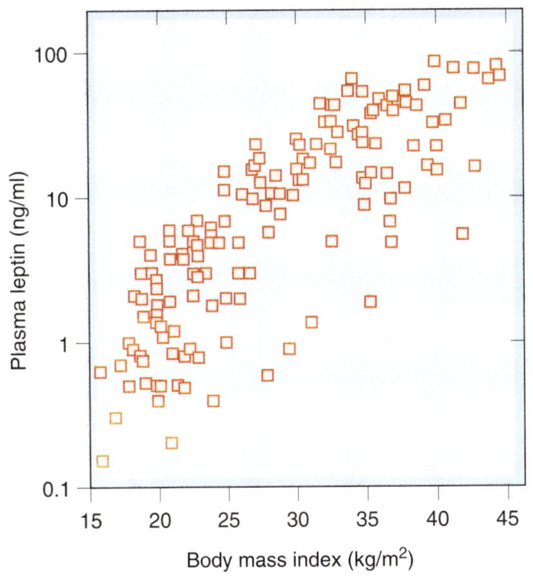

Fig. 26.2 Relation between body mass index and plasma leptin concentration measured by specific radioimmunoassay in 149 lean and obese subjects. (Adapted from Hamann & Matthaei 1996 Exp Clin Endocrinol Diabetes 104: 293-300.)

> **Energy balance**
>
> Energy balance depends on food intake, energy storage in fat, and energy expenditure. The homeostatic control of energy balance involves:
>
> - Mechanisms that signal the level of fat stores, e.g. leptin. Plasma leptin concentrations are proportional to fat stores. Variations in leptin concentration occur when there is increased food intake and/or reduced energy expenditure; fat cells then increase in size and number and their *ob* genes code for an increase in the basal levels of leptin synthesis and release.
> - The relay of the information on fat stores to centres in the hypothalamus (e.g. neurons with leptin receptors).
> - The integration of the signal with other systems. Increased leptin causes release of α-melanocyte-stimulating hormone, which activates systems that result in decreased food intake and increased energy expenditure. Decreased leptin causes release of neuropeptide Y and agouti-related protein, which have the opposite effect.
> - Along with leptin, insulin has a critical role in energy homeostasis but many other factors also play a part: other endocrines, autonomic transmitters, other CNS neuropeptide transmitters and a variety of mediators released from adipose tissue (which is now regarded as an endocrine organ).

more heat and less ATP than white fat cells. The basis for this, as determined in mice, is the presence of a special mitochondrial uncoupling protein, UCP-1, that uncouples oxidative phosphorylation. Another uncoupling protein, UCP-2, occurs in both white and brown fat and is upregulated if mice are fed a high-fat diet. The genes that code for these proteins are known and human fat cells have a gene similar to the mouse gene for UCP-2.

Brown fat cells, more abundant in infants and children than in adults, have an extensive sympathetic innervation. Noradrenaline, acting on β-adrenoceptors (mainly β_3) in brown fat, increases lipolysis and fatty acid oxidation, increasing heat production. It increases the activity of the PPAR-γ (peroxisome proliferator-activated receptor-γ) transcription factor, which, with its co-activator PGC-1, activates the gene for UCP-1 (see below).

The expression of β_3-adrenoceptors is decreased in genetically obese mice.

FOOD INTAKE

Food intake is modified by a multitude of factors—physiological, psychological, social, etc. Meal size seems to be controlled by a feedback loop in which signals from the gastrointestinal tract are transmitted to the hypothalamus after relay in the brainstem. An important afferent signal is *cholecystokinin*—a peptide secreted by the duodenum in response to mechanical and chemical stimuli. Cholecysokinin acts locally on cholecystokinin A receptors in the gastrointestinal tract, the signal being transmitted to the brainstem by the vagus. The effect is to decrease food intake. Circulating cholecystokinin does not cross the blood–brain barrier but the peptide is also a neurotransmitter and acts on cholecystokinin B receptors in the brain to function as a satiety factor.

Insulin, as mentioned above, has a significant role in the control of energy metabolism. It stimulates leptin release from fat cells and it enters the CNS where it can decrease food intake by affecting the actions of NPY (see Fig. 26.3). However, insulin may also, in some circumstances, increase food intake, presumably indirectly, by an effect on blood glucose. Thus patients with type 2 diabetes mellitus usually gain weight when treated with insulin or sulfonylureas—an effect that is clinically important (see Ch. 25).

OBESITY AS A HEALTH PROBLEM

Obesity is a growing and costly health problem in many of the richest nations of the world and it is now considered as a chronic disease that is reaching epidemic proportions in the developed world. Approximately 33% of adults in the USA are said to be

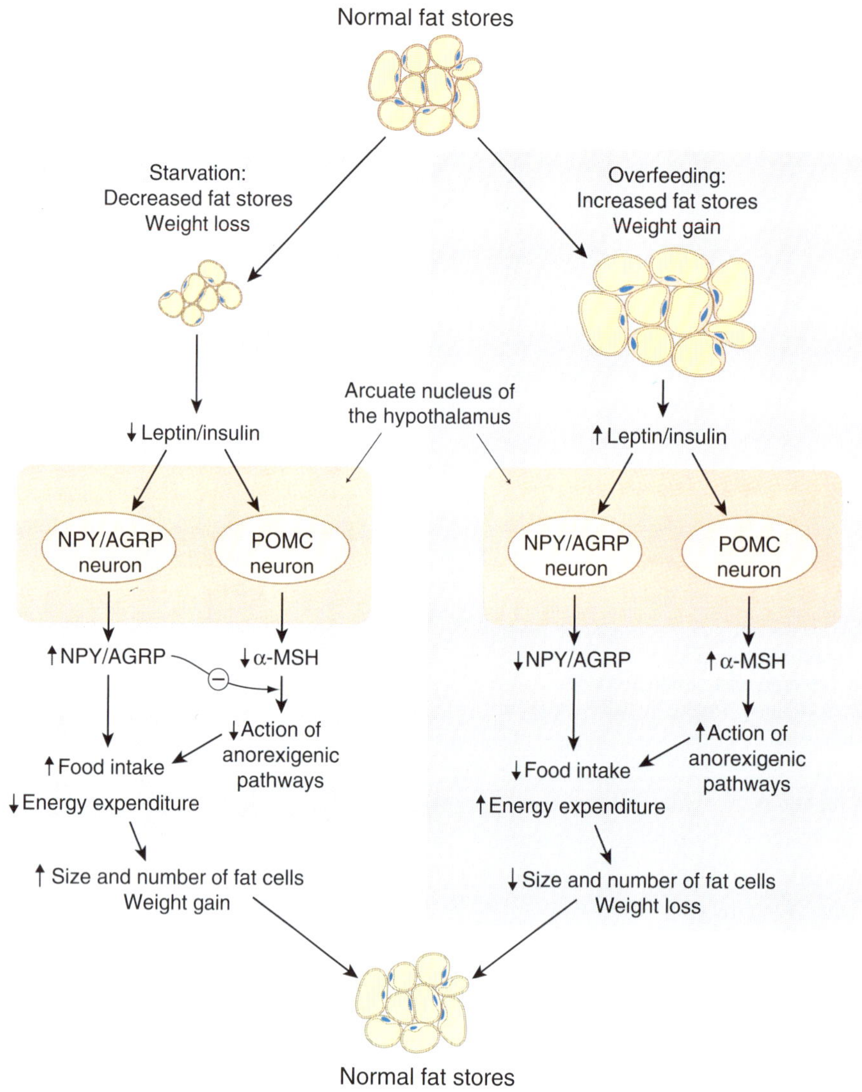

Fig. 26.3 The role of leptin, insulin and hypothalamic peptides in the regulation of energy balance and fat stores. The primary level of hypothalamic control is vested in two groups of neurons, with opposing actions, in the arcuate nucleus. Both groups express leptin receptors. In one group, the peptides neuropeptide Y (NPY) and agouti-related protein (AGRP) are colocalised, the other contains the protein prepro-opiomelanocortin (POMC), which releases α-melanocyte-stimulating hormone (α-MSH). Activation of the first group by fall in leptin levels results in increased food intake and decreased energy expenditure. Increased leptin levels following overfeeding activates the second group and has the opposite effect. Alpha-MSH acts on melanocortin-4 receptors, an action that is inhibited by AGRP. Insulin receptors also occur in both groups. Leptin and insulin act in concert on the hypothalamic neurons, but leptin is the main regulating factor. Many other factors are involved in regulating food intake and energy expenditure; see text and footnote on p. 396.

obese and the incidence in other developed nations is increasing. In Europe, 15–20% of the middle-aged population is obese (Björntorp, 1997).

With a BMI above 30 there is a significant increase in the risk of non-insulin-dependent (type 2) diabetes mellitus. The risk of hypertension, hypertriglyceridaemia, gallstones and ischaemic heart disease is also substantially increased (Fig. 26.4). The relationship between type 2 diabetes, increased BMI and insulin resistance is discussed in Chapter 25; (see also O'Rahilly, 1997). Obese subjects have an increased risk of colon, breast, prostate, gall bladder, ovarian and uterine cancer. Numerous other disorders are associated with excess body weight, including osteoarthritis, hyperuricaemia and male hypogonadism. Gross obesity (BMI over 40) is associated with a 12-fold increase in mortality in the group aged 25–35 years compared with those in this age group with a BMI of 20–25.

The distribution of adipose tissue is also important: a central distribution of fat (visceral fat) is associated with a higher

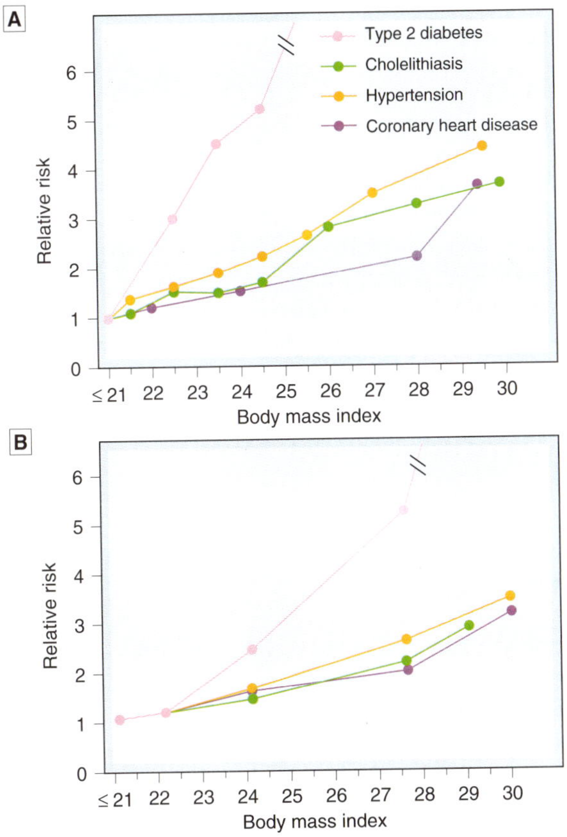

Fig. 26.4 The relation between body mass index (BMI) and the relative risk of the diseases specified. A The figures for females, initially 30–55 years of age, who were followed for 18 years. B The figures for males, initially 40–65 years of age, who were followed up for 10 years. (Adapted from Kopelman P G 2000 Nature 404: 635–643; data from Willet W C, Dietz W H, Colditz G A 1999 N Engl J Med 341: 427–433.)

morbidity and mortality than a peripheral distribution. The waist circumference is a simple clinical measure of visceral fat. The risk of developing cardiovascular disease or type 2 diabetes is high if this is above 88 cm (35 in) in females or 102 cm (40 in) in males.

THE PATHOPHYSIOLOGY OF OBESITY

In most adult subjects, body fat and body weight remain more or less constant over many years, even decades, in the face of very large variations in food intake and energy expenditure—amounting to about a million calories per year. The steady-state body weight and BMI of an individual is, as has been stressed above, the result of the integration of multiple interacting factors; and perturbations—either in the direction of increase or decrease—are resisted by homeostatic mechanisms. How, then, does obesity occur? Why is it so difficult for the obese to lose weight and maintain the lower weight?

The main determinant is manifestly *a disturbance of the homeostatic mechanisms that control energy balance*, but *genetic endowment* underlies this disturbance. Other factors such as *food intake* and *lack of physical activity* contribute and there are, of course, social, cultural and psychological aspects. We will deal below with the imbalance of homeostatic mechanisms and genetic endowment and then briefly mention the role of food intake and physical activity. The role of social, cultural and psychological aspects we will leave, with relief, to the psychosociologists.

OBESITY AS A DISORDER OF THE HOMEOSTATIC CONTROL OF ENERGY BALANCE

Since the homeostatic control of energy balance is extremely complex, it is not easy to determine what goes wrong in obesity.

When the leptin story unfolded, it was thought that alterations in leptin kinetics might provide a simple explanation. But plasma leptin is higher in obese individuals, compared with non-obese subjects, not lower as might be expected (Fig. 26.2); in fact leptin concentrations correlate with body fat mass in both lean and obese subjects.

Resistance to leptin seems to be a characteristic of obesity. Such resistance could be caused by defects in leptin synthesis, in its carriage in the circulation, in its transport into the CNS, in leptin receptors in the hypothalamus (as occurs in *db/db* mice) or in postreceptor signaling. There is some evidence that the action of a member of the family of suppressors of cytokine signalling, SOCS-3, may underlie or contribute to leptin resistance.

Dysfunction of mediators other than leptin could be implicated in obesity. Only a few important ones can be considered here.

TNF-α, another cytokine that relays information from fat to brain, is increased in the adipose tissue of insulin-resistant obese individuals. Another pathophysiological alteration in obesity is a reduced insulin sensitivity of muscle and fat.

Reduced function of β_3-adrenoceptors in brown adipose tissue (see above) could also be implicated (p. 397); alternatively, one of the proteins that uncouple oxidative phosphorylation in fat cells, UCP-2, could be dysfunctional in obese individuals.

A further suggestion is that alteration of function of specific transcription factors, such as the PPAR transcription factors α, β and γ, may have a role in obesity. These transcription factors regulate gene expression of enzymes associated with lipid and glucose homeostasis, and they also promote the genesis of adipose tissue. PPARγ is expressed preferentially in fat cells and synergises with another transcription factor, C/EBPα, to convert precursor cells to fat cells (see Spiegelman & Flier, 1996). The gene for UCP (see above) in white fat cells has regulatory sites that respond to PPARα and C/EBPα. A new class of agents, the thiazoladinediones, bind to and activate PPARγ (see Ch. 25). One of these, **troglitazone**, is licensed in the UK for treatment of type 2 diabetes.

In fact, the pathophysiology of obesity could involve disturbance(s) in any of the multitude of other factors involved in energy balance.

GENETIC FACTORS AND OBESITY

Studies in twins and in adoptees and their families indicate that from 40% to as much as 80% of the variance of BMI can be attributed to genetic factors. It is estimated that heritability is as high as 30–40% for factors relevant to energy balance such as body fat distribution, resting metabolic rate, energy expenditure after overeating, lipoprotein lipase activity and basal rates of lipolysis. It appears that modern populations have a genetic propensity, more manifest in some individuals than others, to increase their fat depots—as a result of the 'thrifty genes' developed during evolution by our forebears to code for proteins that promote fat storage at feasts to sustain them during famine.

There are some rare cases in which obesity is the consequence of a single gene disorder, but, in general, it probably involves the interaction of many genes. So far, 200 genes, gene markers and chromosomal regions have been shown to be associated with human obesity (see Chagnon et al., 2000).

Most obese subjects so far studied have not had any abnormalities in the genes for either leptin or the leptin receptor.

Linkage of human obesity to genes for other factors relevant to energy balance have been reported: β_3-adrenoceptor and the glucocorticoid receptor.

The β_3-adrenoceptor Decreased function of this gene could be associated with impairment of lipolysis in white fat or with thermogenesis in brown fat. A mutation of the gene has been found to be associated with abdominal obesity, insulin resistance and early-onset type 2 diabetes in some subjects and a markedly increased propensity to gain weight in a separate group of morbidly obese subjects.

The glucocorticoid receptor This could be associated with obesity through the permissive effect of glucocorticoids on several aspects of fat metabolism and energy balance.

FOOD INTAKE AND OBESITY

As Spiegelman & Flier (1996) point out 'one need not be a rocket scientist to notice that increased food intake tends to be associated with obesity'. A typical obese subject will usually have put on 20 kg over 10 years. This means that there has been a daily excess of energy input over output of 30–40 kcal initially, increasing gradually to maintain the increased body weight.

The type of food eaten can play a part in upsetting the energy balance. Fat has more calories per gram and it may be that the mechanisms regulating appetite react rapidly to carbohydrate and protein but slowly to fat—too slowly to stop an individual consuming too much high-fat food before the satiety systems come into play.

Obese individuals diet to lose weight. However, when a subject reduces calorie intake, shifts into negative energy balance and loses weight, the resting metabolic rate decreases, and there is a concomitant reduction in energy expenditure. Thus, an individual who was previously obese and is now of normal weight generally needs fewer calories to maintain that weight than an individual who has never been obese. The decrease in energy expenditure appears to be largely caused by an alteration in the conversion efficiency of chemical energy to mechanical work in the skeletal muscles. This adaptation to the caloric reduction contributes to the difficulty of maintaining weight loss by diet.

PHYSICAL EXERCISE AND OBESITY

It used to be said that the only exercise effective in combating obesity was pushing one's chair back from the table. It is now recognised that physical activity—i.e. increased energy expenditure—has a much more positive role in reducing fat storage and adjusting energy balance in the obese, particularly if associated with modification of the diet. An inadvertent, natural population study provides an example. Many years ago, a tribe of Pima Indians split into two groups. One group settled in Mexico and continued to live simply at subsistence level, eating frugally

Obesity

- Obesity is a multifactorial disorder of energy balance in which chronic calorie intake is greater than energy output.
- It is characterised by an excessive body mass index (BMI), which is weight (kg) divided by the square of height (m^2).
- A subject with a BMI of 20–25 is considered as having a healthy body weight, one with a BMI of 25–30 as overweight, and one with a BMI >30 as obese.
- Obesity is a growing problem in most rich nations; the incidence—at present 30% in the USA and 15–20% in Europe—is increasing.
- A BMI >30 significantly increases the risk of type 2 diabetes; the risk of hypercholesterolaemia, hypertension, ischaemic heart disease, gallstones and various cancers is also increased.
- Obesity is primarily an energy balance disorder, the details of which are not clear but may include the following:
  —deficiencies in the genesis of, and/or the response to leptin or other fat depot sensors
  —defects in the hypothalamic neuronal systems responding to leptin or other fat depot sensors
  —defects in the systems controlling energy expenditure (e.g. reduced sympathetic activity), decreased metabolic expenditure of energy, decreased thermogenesis in adipocytes owing to reduction of β_3-adrenoceptor-mediated action on lipid metabolism and/or dysfunction of the proteins that uncouple oxidative phosphorylation
  —a contribution by genetic factors.
- The tendency to develop obesity could be a genetic propensity, developed during evolution, to store fat at feasts for sustenance during famine.

and spending most of the week in hard physical labour. They are generally lean and have a low incidence of type 2 diabetes. The other group moved to the USA—an environment with easy access to calorie-rich food and less need for hard physical work. They are on average, 57 lbs (26 kg) heavier than the Mexican group and have a high incidence of early-onset type 2 diabetes.

PHARMACOLOGICAL APPROACHES TO THE PROBLEM OF OBESITY

Carefully controlled diet and physical exercise are the main therapeutic approaches to obesity, but increasing numbers of patients may also need anti-obesity drugs. Such drugs could aim to suppress food intake, increase energy expenditure or increase lipolysis. A prodigious effort is underway by numerous pharmaceutical companies to provide effective anti-obesity agents.

At present, only two drugs have been shown to reduce the body weight of obese individuals: **orlistat** (which decreases fat absorption by preventing the breakdown of dietary fat in the gastrointestinal tract) and **sibutramine** (which is mainly an inhibitor at the CNS sites that stimulate food intake). Neither is ideal. Many others are in various stages of development, see below.

ORLISTAT

Orlistat is a pancreatic lipase inhibitor, preventing the breakdown of dietary fat to fatty acids and glycerols. It causes a dose-related increase in faecal fat that plateaus at 32% of dietary fat. Given with a low-calorie diet in obese individuals, it produces a modest loss of weight compared with diet plus placebo. In two placebo-controlled trials lasting 2 years and involving over 1500 obese patients, a dose of 120 mg three times a day given with a diet designed to produce a mild hypocaloric deficit of 600 kcal per day caused weight loss of 8.7% and 10.2% as compared with 5.8% and 6.1% with placebo plus diet.

Pharmacokinetic aspects

Most ortistat is excreted in the faeces, only minute amounts being absorbed.

Unwanted effects

Abdominal cramps, flatus with discharge and faecal incontinence can occur, as can intestinal borborygmi (rumbling) and oily spotting. Surprisingly, in view of the possibility of these antisocial effects occurring, the drug is well tolerated. Supplementary therapy with fat-soluble vitamins may be needed and there has been a report of decreased absorption of contraceptive pills.

SIBUTRAMINE

Sibutramine, originally intended to be used as an antidepressant, has recently been shown to have anti-obesity action.

Pharmacological actions

Its main actions are to reduce food intake and cause dose-dependent weight loss (see Fig. 26.5), the weight loss being associated with a decrease in obesity-related risk factors. It enhances satiety and is reported to produce a reduction in waist circumference (i.e. a reduction in visceral fat), a decrease in plasma triglycerides and very low density, lipoproteins but an increase in high density lipoproteins. In addition, beneficial effects on hyperinsulinaemia and the rate of glucose metabolism are said to occur.

There is preliminary evidence that the weight loss is associated with a higher energy expenditure, possibly through an increase in thermogenesis mediated by the sympathetic nervous system.

The weight reduction obtained with sibutramine alone is not easily maintained. To be effective in anti-obesity therapy it may need to be combined with other anti-obesity measures. A recent multicentre trial involving 499 obese patients was designed to assess the efficacy of sibutramine in maintaining weight loss over a period of 2 years (James et al., 2000). With oral sibutramine and an individualised management programme of diet, activity and behavioural advice, 77% of obese patients achieved weight loss and most maintained this with continuing treatment over the following 2 years (Fig. 26.5).

Mechanism of action

Sibutramine is an inhibitor of neuronal 5-hydroxytryptamine (5-HT)/noradrenaline reuptake at the hypothalamic sites that regulate food intake.

Pharmacokinetic aspects

Sibutramine is given orally, is well absorbed and undergoes extensive first-pass metabolism. The metabolites are responsible

Clinical uses of anti-obesity drugs

- The main treatment of obesity is a suitable diet and increased exercise.
- Drugs acting on the gastrointestinal tract (e.g. orlistat, which causes malabsorption of fat) are considered for severely obese individuals who have lost at least 2.5 kg in the previous month by dieting, especially if they have additional cardiovascular risk factors such as diabetes mellitus or hypertension. Treatment with orlistat is short term (never longer than 2 years) and combined with non-drug treatment.
- Many centrally acting appetite suppressants have been withdrawn because of addiction, pulmonary hypertension or other serious adverse effects. Sibutramine is considered for adjunctive treatment of severely obese individuals. An increase in heart rate and blood pressure is reported and the drug is contraindicated if cardiovascular disease is present. Interactions with drugs that are metabolised by one of the P450 isoenzymes can occur.

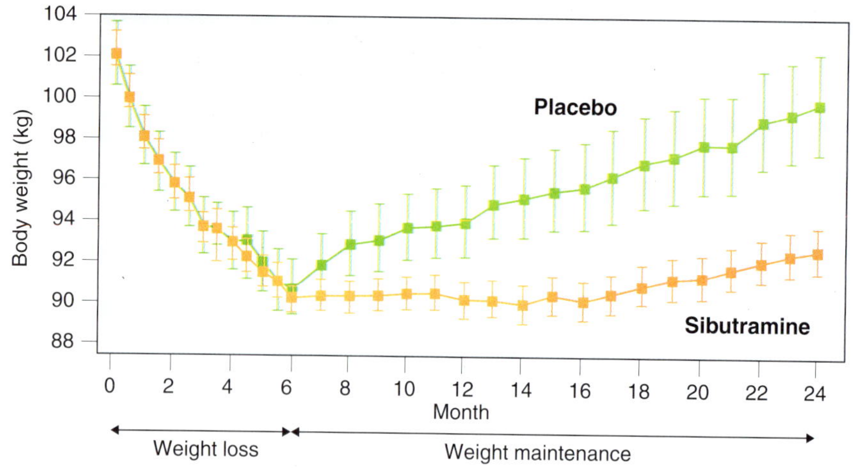

Fig. 26.5 The results of a clinical trial of the efficacy of sibutramine in maintaining weight loss. Patients selected for the trial had a body mass index of 30–45 and were put onto an initial 6 month management programme including oral sibutramine, an individualised 600 kcal/day dietary deficit programme along with activity and behavioural advice. The results are shown in the 'weight loss' section of the graph. (Only patients who had lost 5% of their body weight are represented; 467 of the 499 who completed the 6 month programme). These responders were then entered into a randomised, placebo-controlled, double-blind parallel group trial to evaluate the effect of sibutramine on weight maintenance. Figure adapted from James et al., 2000 The Lancet v. 356 pp. 2119–2125.)

for the pharmacological actions. Steady-state blood levels of the metabolites occur within 4 days. The active metabolites are inactivated in the liver and 85% of the inactive residues are excreted in the urine and faeces.

Unwanted effects

These can include dry mouth, constipation and insomnia. An increase in heart rate and blood pressure is reported and the drug is contraindicated if cardiovascular disease is present. Interactions with drugs that are metabolised by one of the P450 isoenzymes can occur.

POTENTIAL NEW ANTI-OBESITY DRUGS

Some in phase III clinical trial are mazindol (adrenergic agonist), posatirelin (a thyrotrophin-releasing hormone analogue) and sertraline (a selective serotonin uptake inhibitor, Ch. 38). Some in phase II trial are buproprion (a dopamine re-uptake inhibitor, Ch. 38), enterostatin, linitript (cholecystokinin A antagonist), pegylated leptin and AD 9677 (a β_3-adrenoceptor agonist) (see Clapham et al., 2001).

Potential targets for new drugs

Agents that reduce food intake

- reuptake inhibitors of 5-HT and noradrenaline at hypothalamic sites
- antagonists at receptors for melanin-concentrating hormone (MCH),* NPY (Y5), corticotrophin-releasing hormone (CRH), galanin, orexins A and B
- binding proteins for CRH
- agonists at receptors for leptin, AGRP, cholecystokinin A, glucagon-like peptide 1 (GLP-1), bombesin.

Agents that increase energy expenditure or enhance lipolysis

- stimulators of the action or expression of the transcription factors UCP-2 and UCP-3
- agonists at the β_3-adrenoceptor.

For more detail on potential new drugs see Clapham et al. (2001), Ahima and Osei (2001) Chiesi et al. (2001).

CURRENT DRUG AVAILABILITY

There are, at present only two drugs licensed for the treatment of obesity, sibutramine and orlistat. Both are only really effective if given with a controlled diet, the tolerability of neither is ideal and sibutramine can cause an increase in heart rate and blood pressure. However, the understanding of the basis of obesity is progressing rapidly and the pharmaceutical industry is in full cry after effective anti-obesity drugs. When these become available, they will probably be recommended mainly for obese patients who are at risk for obesity-related diseases. To the moderately overweight and those individuals whose problem is dissatisfaction with their chubby body image, the recommendation will be, as at present, 'stick to the diet and keep jogging'.

*MCH is an orexigenic neuropeptide that binds with high affinity to the orphan G-protein-coupled receptor SLC-1, activating it.

REFERENCES AND FURTHER READING

Ahima R S, Flier J S 2000a Adipose tissue as an endocrine organ. Trends Endocrinol Metab 11: 327–332 (*Succinct article on the new view of adipose tissue*)

Ahima R S, Flier J S 2000b Leptin. Annu Rev Physiol 62: 413–437 (*Comprehensive review of leptin, its expression, actions in hypothalamus, role in energy homeostasis and its other actions*)

Ahima R S, Osei S 2001 Molecular regulation of eating behaviour: new insights and prospects for future strategies. Trends Mol Med 7: 205–213 (*Praisworthy short review. Excellent figures and useful tables of the mediators involved in stimulation and inhibition of feeding behaviour*)

Björntorp P 1997 Obesity. Lancet 350: 423–426 (*Clear concise article emphasising the epidemiology of obesity*)

Bray G A, Greenway F L 1999 Current and potential drugs for treatment of obesity. Endocrine Rev 20: 905–875 (*Comprehensive review of agents that affect or could affect food intake, metabolism, energy expenditure with details of drugs in development*)

Collins P, Williams G 2001 Drug treatment of obesity: from past failures to future successes? Br J Clin Pharamcol 51: 13–25 (*Overview—from a clinical perspective—of currently available anti-obesity drugs and potential future drugs. Well written*)

Chagnon Y C, Pérusse C et al. 2000 The human obesity gene map: the 1999 update. Obesity Res 8: 89–117 (*Detailed review of the genes, markers, and chromosomal regions that have been shown to be associated with human obesity*)

Chiesi M, Huppertz C, Hofbauer K G 2001 Pharmacotherapy of obesity: targets and perspectives. Trends Pharmacol Sci 22: 247–254 (*Commendable, succinct review. Table of the potential targets. Useful, simple figures of the central and peripheral pathways of energy regulation and of the regulation of thermogenesis*)

Clapham J C, Arch J R S, Tadayyon M 2001 Anti-obesity drugs: a critical review of current therapies and future opportunities. Pharmacol Ther 89: 81–121 (*Comprehensive review covering, under energy intake: biogenic amines, cannabinoids, neuropeptides, leptin, gastrointestinal tract peptides and inhibitors of fat absorption; and under energy expenditure:* β_3*-adrenoceptor agonists and uncoupling proteins*)

Crowley V E F, Yeo G S H, O'Rahilly S 2002 Obesity therapy: altering the energy intake-and-expenditure balance sheet. Nat Rev Drug Discovery (*Review stressing that pharmacological approaches to obesity therapy necessitate altering the balance between energy intake and expenditure and/or altering the partitioning of nutrients between lean tissue and fat*)

Deprés J-P, Lemieux I, Prud'homme D 2001 Treatment of obesity: need to focus on high risk abdominally obese patients. Br Med J 322: 716–722 (*Succinct review giving simple clear coverage of the clinical approach to obesity therapy with simple clear diagrams*)

Friedman J M 1997 The alphabet of weight control. Nature 385: 119–120 (*Concise article delineating the roles of the main factors involved in energy balance*)

Frühbeck G, Gómez-Ambrosi et al. 2001 The adipocyte: a model for integration of endocrine and metabolic signalling in energy metabolism regulation. Am J Physiol Endocrinol Metab 280: E827–E847 (*Detailed review covering receptors on and the factors secreted by the fat cell and the role of these factors in energy homeostasis*)

Gibbs W W 1996 Gaining on fat. Sci Am Aug: 70–76 (*Simple, well written analysis; very readable*)

James W P T, Finer N, Kopelman P et al. 2000 Effect of sibutramine on weight maintenance after weight loss: a randomised trial. Lancet 256: 2119–2125 (*Report of the results of a multicentre randomised double-blind clinical trial*)

Kennedy G C 1953 The role of depot fat in the hypothalamic control of food intake in the rat. Proc R Soc 140: 578–592 (*The paper that put forward the proposal, based on experiments on rats, that there was a hypothalamus-based homeostatic mechanism for controlling body fat*)

Lowell B B, Spiegelman B M 2000 Towards a molecular understanding of adaptive thermogenesis. Nature 404: 652–660 (*Detailed coverage of the role of the mitochondria, UCP-1 and PPAR in adaptive thermogenesis, emphasising the control of mitochondrial genes*)

Luque C A, Rey J A 1999 Sibutramine: a serotonin–norepinephrine re-uptake inhibitor for the treatment of obesity. Ann Pharmacother 33: 968–978 (*Covers the pharmacology, pharmacokinetic aspects, clinical trials and adverse effects of sibutramine*)

O'Rahilly S 1997 Non-insulin dependent diabetes mellitus: the gathering storm. Br Med J 314: 955–960 (*Clinical review*)

Schwartz M W, Morton G J 2002 Keeping hunger at bay. Nature 418: 595–597 (*Succinct article on factors controlling appetite and weight; good diagram on hormones that control eating*)

Schwartz M W, Woods S C et al. 2000 Central nervous control of food intake. Nature 404: 661–671 (*Outlines a model that delineates the roles of hormones and neuropeptides in the control of food intake. Outstanding diagrams. Note that there are several other excellent articles in this Nature Insight supplement on Obesity*)

Spiegelman B M, Flier J S 1996 Adipogenesis and obesity: rounding out the big picture. Cell 87: 377–389 (*Excellent review, elegantly written, detailing the requirements for a homeostatic system for energy balance. Good coverage of the role of the PPAR transcription factors*)

Spiegelman B M, Flier J S 2001 Obesity regulation and energy balance. Cell 104: 531–543 (*Excellent review with up-to-date coverage of the CNS control of energy intake/body weight, monogenic obesities, leptin physiology, central neural circuits, the melanocortin pathway, the role of insulin, and adaptive thermogenesis*)

Yanovski S Z, Yanovski J A 2002 Obesity. N Engl J Med 346: 591–602 (*Outlines non-pharmacological approaches to promoting weight loss and then discusses in more detail the use of anti-obesity drugs*)

Zhang Y, Proenca R et al. 1994 Positional cloning of the mouse obese gene and its human homologue. Nature 372: 425–432 (*Seminal article describing the cloning of the* ob *gene and the identification of its product—leptin*)

27 The pituitary and adrenal cortex

Overview 404

The pituitary 404
- Anterior pituitary (adenohypophysis) 404
- Hypothalamic hormones 406
- Anterior pituitary hormones 407
- Posterior pituitary (neurohypophysis) 410

The adrenal cortex 411
- Adrenal steroids 411

OVERVIEW

The pituitary and adrenal glands are major sites for the synthesis and release of a number of hormones that exert widespread metabolic effects in the body. The function of the pituitary is controlled by hormones released from the hypothalamus. In turn, the *hypothalamic–pituitary axis* orchestrates the activity of the adrenal (and other endocrine) glands. In the first part of this chapter, we examine the control of pituitary function by hypothalamic hormones and review the physiological roles and clinical uses of both anterior and posterior pituitary hormones. The second part of the chapter concentrates on the actions of adrenal hormones and, in particular, the anti-inflammatory effect of glucocorticoids.

THE PITUITARY

The pituitary gland is composed of three sections arising from two different embryological sites. The *anterior pituitary* is derived from the endoderm of the buccal cavity, as is the *intermediate lobe* (which can thus be considered for practical purposes as part of the anterior pituitary), while the *posterior pituitary* is derived from neural ectoderm. Both main parts of the gland have an intimate functional relationship with the *hypothalamus*, the neurons of which control the anterior and posterior pituitary independently.

ANTERIOR PITUITARY (ADENOHYPOPHYSIS)

The anterior pituitary secretes a number of different hormones vital for normal physiological function, some of which are involved in the regulation of other endocrine glands (Table 27.1). The cells of the anterior pituitary can be classified into corticotrophs, lactotrophs (mammotrophs), somatotrophs, thyrotrophs and gonadotrophs, according to the substances they secrete.

Secretion from the anterior pituitary is largely regulated by factors* (hormones) derived from the hypothalamus, which reach the pituitary through the bloodstream. Blood vessels to the hypothalamus divide in its tissue to form a meshwork of capillaries—the primary plexus (Fig. 27.1), which drains into the

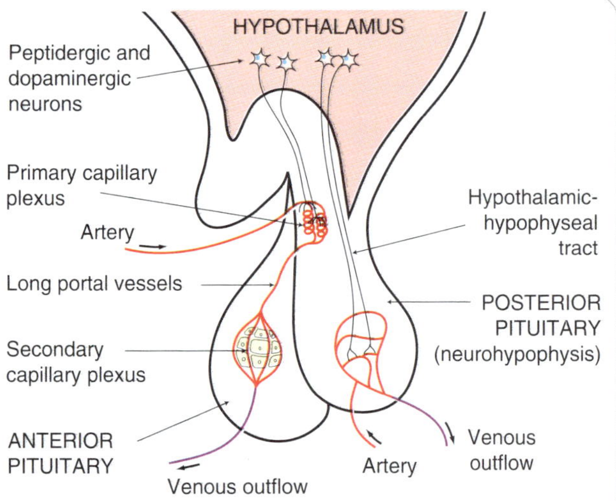

Fig. 27.1 Schematic diagram of vascular and neuronal relationships between the hypothalamus, the posterior pituitary and the anterior pituitary. The main portal vessels to the anterior pituitary lie in the pituitary stalk and arise from the primary plexus in the hypothalamus, but some (the short portal vessels) arise from the vascular bed in the posterior pituitary (not shown).

*The word 'factor' was originally coined at a time when their structure and function were not known. These are blood-borne messengers and as such are clearly hormones. Nevertheless, the term 'factor', however irrational, lingers on.

hypophyseal portal vessels. These pass through the pituitary stalk to feed a secondary plexus of capillaries in the anterior pituitary. Peptidergic neurons in the hypothalamus secrete a variety of releasing or release-inhibiting hormones directly into the capillaries of the primary plexus (Table 27.1 and Fig. 27.1). Most of these regulate the secretion of hormones from the anterior lobe. The melanocyte-stimulating hormones (MSHs) are secreted mainly from the intermediate lobe.

There is a balance—involving various negative feedback pathways—between the hypothalamic hormones, the anterior pituitary hormones whose release they regulate and the secretions of the peripheral endocrine glands. In general, the long negative feedback pathways, in which the mediators are the hormones that are secreted from the peripheral glands, affect both the hypothalamus and the anterior pituitary. The mediators of the short negative feedback pathways are anterior pituitary hormones that act on the hypothalamus.

The peptidergic neurons in the hypothalamus are themselves influenced by other parts of the central nervous system (CNS). This action is mediated through pathways that release dopamine, noradrenaline (norepinephrine), 5-hydroxytryptamine (5-HT) and the opioid peptides, the last being found in very high concentration in the hypothalamus (see Ch. 13). Hypothalamic control of the anterior pituitary is also exerted through the

Table 27.1 Hormones secreted by the hypothalamus and the anterior pituitary

Hypothalamic factor/ hormone (and related drugs)	Hormone affected in anterior pituitary (and related drugs)	Main effects of anterior pituitary hormone
Corticotrophin-releasing factor (CRF)	Adrenocorticotrophic hormone (ACTH; corticotrophin; tetracosactide)	Stimulates secretion of adrenal cortical hormones (mainly glucocorticoids); maintains integrity of adrenal cortex
Thyrotrophin-releasing hormone (TRH; protirelin)	Thyroid-stimulating hormone (TSH; thyrotrophin)	Stimulates synthesis and secretion of thyroid hormones, thyroxine and triiodothyronine; maintains integrity of thyroid gland
Growth hormone-releasing factor (GHRF)	Growth hormone (GH; somatotrophin)	Regulates growth, partly directly, partly through evoking the release of somatomedins from the liver and elsewhere. Increases protein synthesis, increases blood glucose, stimulates lipolysis
Growth hormone-release inhibiting factor (GHRIF; somatostatin, octreotide)	Growth hormone	As above
Gonadotrophin-releasing hormone (GnRH; somatorelin, sermorelin)	Follicle-stimulating hormone (FSH; see Ch. 29)	Stimulates the growth of the ovum and the Graafian follicle in the female and gametogenesis in the male; with LH, stimulates the secretion of oestrogen throughout the menstrual cycle and progesterone in the second half
	Luteinising hormone (LH) or interstitial-cell-stimulating hormone (ICSH) (see Ch. 29)	Stimulates ovulation and the development of the corpus luteum; with FSH, stimulates secretion of oestrogen and progesterone in menstrual cycle. In male, regulates testosterone secretion
Prolactin release-inhibiting factor (PRIF, probably dopamine)	Prolactin	Together with other hormones, prolactin, promotes development of mammary tissue during pregnancy; stimulates milk production in the postpartum period
Prolactin-releasing factor (PRF)	Prolactin	As above
Melanocyte-stimulating hormone (MSH) releasing factor (MSH-RF)	α-, β- and γ-MSH	Promotes formation of melanin, which causes darkening of skin; MSH is anti-inflammatory and helps to regulate feeding
MSH release-inhibiting factor (MSH-RIF)	α-, β- and γ-MSH	As above

tuberohypophyseal dopaminergic pathway, the neurons of which lie in close apposition to the primary capillary plexus (see Ch. 31). Dopamine can be secreted directly into the hypophyseal portal circulation and thus reach the anterior pituitary.

HYPOTHALAMIC HORMONES

There are at least six sets of hormones (also referred to as 'factors') that originate in the hypothalamus and which regulate the secretion of anterior pituitary hormones. These are listed in Table 27.1 and are described in more detail below. Some are used clinically for diagnosis or treatment; some are used as research tools. Many of these hormones also function as neurotransmitters or neuromodulators elsewhere in the CNS (Ch. 31).

GROWTH HORMONE-RELEASING FACTOR (SOMATORELIN)

Growth hormone-releasing factor (GHRF) is a peptide with 40–44 amino acid residues. An analogue, **sermorelin**, has been introduced as a diagnostic test for growth hormone secretion.

The main action of GHRF is summarised in Figure 27.2. Given intravenously, subcutaneously or intranasally, it causes secretion of growth hormone within minutes and peak concentrations in 60 minutes. The action is selective for the somatotrophs in the anterior pituitary, no other pituitary hormones being released.

Unwanted effects are rare.

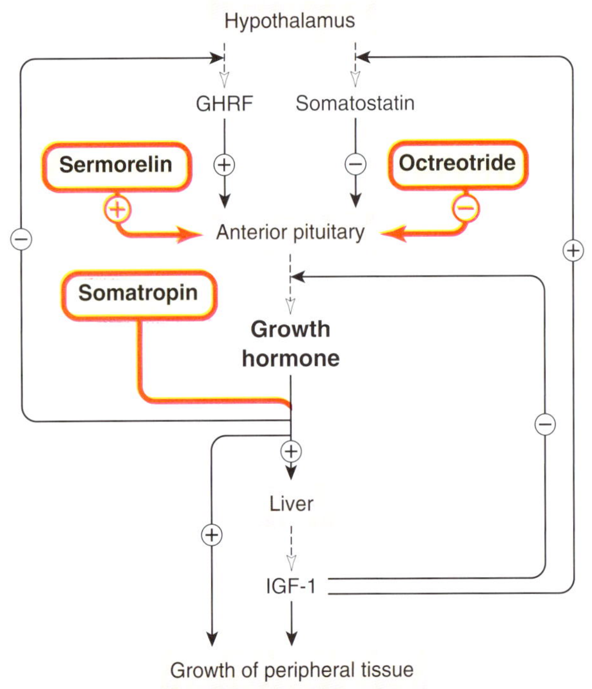

Fig. 27.2 Control of growth hormone secretion and its actions. Drugs are shown in yellow boxes. (GHRF, growth hormone-releasing factor; IGF-1, insulin-like growth factor-1.)

SOMATOSTATIN

Somatostatin is a peptide of 14 amino acid residues. Somatostatin inhibits the release of growth hormone and thyroid-stimulating hormone (TSH, thyrotrophin) from the anterior pituitary (Figs 27.2 and 28.4), and insulin and glucagon from the pancreas; it also decreases the release of most gastrointestinal hormones and reduces gastric acid and pancreatic secretion.

Octreotide is a long-acting analogue of somatostatin. It is used for the treatment of tumours secreting vasoactive intestinal peptide (Ch. 13), carcinoid tumours (Ch. 12), glucagonomas and various pituitary adenomas. It has a place in the therapy of acromegaly (a condition in which there is oversecretion of growth hormone in an adult) and of bleeding oesophageal varices.

It is given subcutaneously, the peak action is at 2 hours and the suppressant effect lasts for up to 8 hours.

Unwanted effects include pain at the injection site and gastrointestinal disturbances. Gallstones and postprandial hyperglycaemia have also been reported and acute hepatitis has occurred in a few cases.

THYROTROPHIN-RELEASING HORMONE (PROTIRELIN)

Thyrotrophin-releasing hormone (TRH) from the hypothalamus releases TSH from the anterior pituitary. **Protirelin** is a synthetic TSH; it is used for the diagnosis of thyroid disorders (see Fig. 28.4). Given intravenously in normal subjects, it causes an increase in plasma TSH concentration, whereas in patients with hyperthyroidism, there is a blunted response to protirelin because the raised blood thyroxine concentration has a negative feedback effect on the anterior pituitary. The opposite occurs with hypothyroidism, in which the defect is in the thyroid itself.

CORTICOTROPHIN-RELEASING FACTOR

Corticotrophin-releasing factor (CRF) is a peptide that releases adrenocorticotrophic hormone (ACTH; corticotrophin) and β-endorphin from the anterior pituitary. Synthetic preparations are available. CRF acts synergistically with antidiuretic hormone (ADH; arginine-vasopressin), and both its action and its release are inhibited by **glucocorticoids** (see Fig. 27.4, below).

Its main use is in diagnostic tests: to assess the ability of the pituitary to secrete ACTH, to assess whether a deficiency of ACTH is caused by a pituitary or a hypothalamic defect, and to evaluate hypothalamic pituitary function after therapy for Cushing's syndrome (see Fig. 27.7, below).

GONADOTROPHIN-RELEASING HORMONE

Gonadotrophin-releasing hormone (GnRH) is a decapeptide that releases both follicle-stimulating hormone and luteinising hormone. It is also available as a preparation called **gonadorelin**. Its actions and uses are described in Chapter 29.

ANTERIOR PITUITARY HORMONES

The main hormones of the anterior pituitary are listed in Table 27.1. The gonadotrophins are dealt with in Chapter 29 and TSH in Chapter 28. The others are dealt with below.

GROWTH HORMONE (SOMATOTROPHIN)

Growth hormone is derived from the somatotroph cells and is found in the anterior pituitary in larger quantities than any other pituitary hormone. Secretion of growth hormone is high in the newborn, decreasing at 4 years to an intermediate level, which is then maintained until after puberty, when there is a further decline.

A preparation of growth hormone, **somatropin**, produced by recombinant DNA technology and identical to growth hormone, is available for clinical use.

Regulation of secretion

Secretion of growth hormone is regulated by the action of hypothalamic GHRF modulated by somatostatin as described above and outlined in Figure 27.2.

One of the mediators of growth hormone action, *insulin-like growth factor1* (IGF-1), which is released from the liver (see below), has an inhibitory effect on growth hormone secretion by stimulating somatostatin release from the hypothalamus (Fig. 27.2).

Growth hormone release, like that of other anterior pituitary secretions, is pulsatile, and its plasma concentration fluctuates 10- to 100-fold. These surges occur repeatedly during the day and night and reflect changes in hypothalamic control. Deep sleep is a potent stimulus to growth hormone secretion, particularly in children.

Actions

The main effect of growth hormone (and its analogues) is to stimulate normal growth and, in doing this, it affects many tissues, acting in conjunction with other hormones secreted from the thyroid, the gonads and the adrenal cortex. It stimulates the production, mainly from the liver, of several polypeptide mediators, the IGFs—also termed somatomedins—which are responsible for most of its anabolic actions (see Fig. 27.2). IGF-1 is the main mediator of growth hormone action. Receptors for IGF-1 exist on many cell types, including liver cells and fat cells.

Protein synthesis is stimulated by growth hormone, and the uptake of amino acids into cells is increased, especially in skeletal muscle. IGF-1 mediates many of these anabolic effects, acting on skeletal muscle and also on the cartilage at the epiphyses of long bones, thus influencing bone growth.

Disorders of production and clinical use

Deficiency of growth hormone results in pituitary dwarfism. In this condition, which can be produced by lack of GHRF or a failure of IGF generation or action, the normal proportions of the body are maintained. The only established clinical use is in patients with growth hormone deficiency and in short stature associated with Turner's syndrome. Satisfactory linear growth can be achieved by giving synthetic growth hormone. *Somatropin* is given subcutaneously, six to seven times per week, and therapy is most successful when started early. Humans are insensitive to growth hormone of other species, so human growth hormone has to be used clinically. This used to be obtained from human cadavers, but this led to the spread of Creutzfeld–Jackob disease, a prion-mediated neurodegenerative disorder (Ch. 34). Human growth hormone is now prepared by recombinant DNA technology, which avoids the risk of prion contamination.

An excessive production of growth hormone in children results in gigantism. An excessive production in adults, which is usually the result of a benign pituitary tumour, results in acromegaly—a condition in which there is enlargement mainly of facial structures and of the hands and feet. The dopamine agonist **bromocriptine** and **octreotide** may ameliorate the condition, but effective treatment consists of removal or irradiation of the tumour.

PROLACTIN

Prolactin is secreted by lactotroph (mammotroph) cells, which are abundant in the anterior pituitary and which increase in number during pregnancy, probably under the influence of oestrogen.

Regulation of secretion

Prolactin secretion is under tonic *inhibitory* control by the hypothalamus (Fig. 27.3 and Table 27.1), the inhibitory mediator being dopamine (acting on D_2 receptors on the lactotrophs).

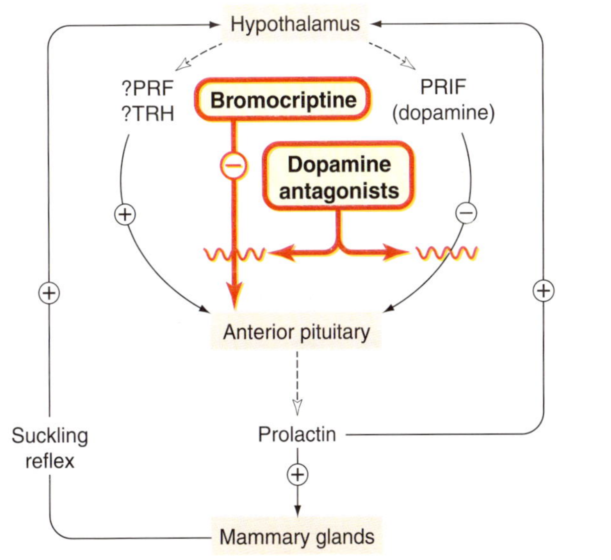

Fig. 27.3 Control of prolactin secretion and the drugs that modify it. (TRH, thyrotrophin-releasing hormone; PRF, prolactin-releasing factor; PRIF, prolactin release-inhibiting factor)

The main stimulus for prolactin release is suckling; in rats, both the smell and the sounds of hungry pups are also effective triggers. Neural reflexes from the breast may stimulate the secretion from the hypothalamus of a *prolactin-releasing factor* (PRF). Possible candidates for PRF include TRH and oxytocin. Oestrogens increase both prolactin secretion and the proliferation of lactotrophs through release, from a subset of lactotrophs, of the neuropeptide, galanin.

Dopamine antagonists (used mainly as antipsychotic drugs; see Ch. 37) are potent stimulants of prolactin release.

Dopamine agonists such as bromocriptine (see below) suppress prolactin release. Bromocriptine is also used in parkinsonism (Ch. 34).

Actions

Prolactin acts via specific receptors. At least three variants of these receptors occur; they are distributed widely in the body, not only in the mammary gland but also throughout the brain and in ovary, heart and lungs.

The main function of prolactin in females is the control of milk production. At parturition, when the blood level of oestrogen falls, the prolactin concentration rises and lactation is initiated. Maintenance of lactation depends on suckling, which stimulates a reflex secretion of prolactin by neural pathways, causing a 10- to 100-fold increase within 30 minutes.

Prolactin, along with other hormones, is responsible for the proliferation and differentiation of mammary tissue during pregnancy. It inhibits gonadotrophin release and/or the response of the ovaries to these trophic hormones. This is one of the reasons why ovulation does not usually occur during breast-feeding, and it is believed to constitute a natural contraceptive mechanism.

According to one rather appealing hypothesis, the high postdelivery concentration of prolactin reflects its biological function of 'parental' hormone. Certainly broodiness and nest-building activity can be induced in birds by prolactin injections, and equivalent 'parental' behaviour can be induced in mice and rabbits. It is rather attractive to think that it might have a similar action in humans, but this is conjectural.

Prolactin is best known for its effects on the mammary gland but it also exerts other unrelated actions including stimulating mitogenesis in lymphocytes. There is some evidence that prolactin may also play a part in regulating immune responses.

Modification of prolactin secretion

Prolactin itself is not used clinically. **Bromocriptine** is used to decrease prolactin secretion. It is well absorbed orally, and peak concentrations occur after 2 hours. Unwanted reactions include nausea and vomiting. Dizziness, constipation and postural hypotension may also occur.

ADRENOCORTICOTROPHIC HORMONE

ACTH (corticotrophin) is the anterior pituitary secretion that controls the synthesis and release of the glucocorticoids of the adrenal cortex (see Table 27.1 and p. 411). It is a polypeptide hormone with 39 amino acid residues. It is rarely used in therapy because its action is less predictable than that of the corticosteroids and it provokes antibody formation. **Tetracosactide,** a synthetic polypeptide that consists of the first 24 N-terminal residues of human ACTH, is now widely used.

Detail of the regulation of ACTH secretion is given on page 412 and shown in Figure 27.4.

The concentration of ACTH in the blood is reduced by glucocorticoids, forming the basis of the dexamethasone suppression test (see p. 418).

Actions

ACTH and tetracosactide have two actions on the adrenal cortex.

- stimulation of the synthesis and release of glucocorticoids. The action is very rapid—a release of glucocorticoids occurs within minutes of injection and the main biological actions are those of the steroids released.
- a trophic action on adrenal cortical cells, and regulation of the levels of key mitochondrial steroidogenic enzymes. The loss of this effect accounts for the adrenal atrophy that results from chronic glucocorticoid administration (see p. 417), which suppresses ACTH secretion.

The main use of tetracosactide is in the diagnosis of adrenal cortical insufficiency. The drug is given intramuscularly, and

Clinical use of bromocriptine

- To prevent lactation
- To treat galactorrhoea (i.e. non-puerperal lactation in either sex) owing to excessive prolactin secretion.
- To treat prolactin-secreting pituitary tumours (prolactinomas).
- In the treatment of parkinsonism (Ch. 34) and of acromegaly.

Adrenocorticotrophic hormone (ACTH; corticotrophin) and the adrenal steroids

- ACTH stimulates synthesis and release of glucocorticoids (e.g. hydrocortisone) from the adrenal cortex (also some androgens).
- Corticotrophin-releasing factor (CRF) from the hypothalamus regulates ACTH release and is, in turn, regulated by neural factors and negative feedback effects of plasma glucocorticoids.
- Mineralocorticoid (e.g. aldosterone) release from the adrenal cortex is controlled by the renin–angiotensin system.

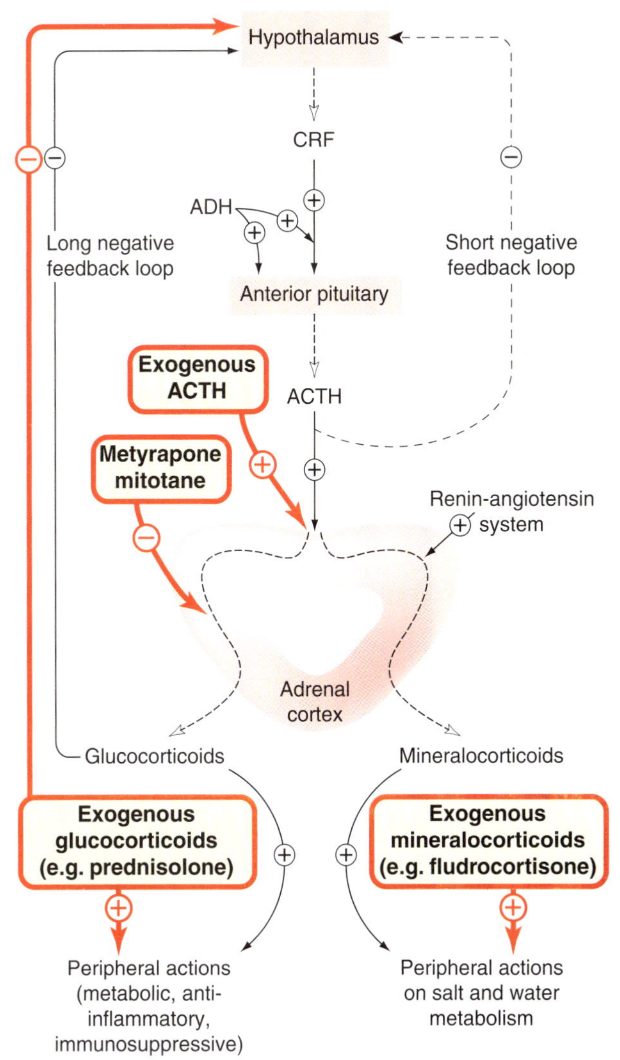

Fig. 27.4 Regulation of synthesis and secretion of adrenal corticosteroids. The long negative feedback loop is more important than the short one (dashed line). ACTH has only a minimal effect on mineralocorticoid production (indicated by dotted line). (ACTH, adrenocorticotrophic hormone (corticotrophin); ADH, antidiuretic hormone (vasopressin); CRF, corticotrophin-releasing factor.)

then the concentration of hydrocortisone in the plasma is measured by radioimmunoassay.

MELANOCYTE-STIMULATING HORMONE

The MSH peptides, α-, β- and γ-MSH are peptide hormones with structural similarity to ACTH. Together these peptides are referred to as *melanocortins* since their first recognised action was to stimulate the production of melanin by specialised skin cells called *melanocytes*. As such, they play an important part in determining skin and hair coloration and tanning ability following exposure to ultraviolet light.

MSH acts on melanocortin receptors of which five (MC_{1-5}) have been cloned. These are G-protein-coupled receptors that activate cAMP synthesis. Melanin formation is under the control of the MC_1-receptor. Excessive α-MSH production can provoke abnormal proliferation of melanocytes and may predispose to melanoma.

Besides their action on melanocytes, melanocortins exhibit numerous other biological effects. For example, α-MSH inhibits cytokine (interleukin (IL)-1β and tumour necrosis factor (TNF)-α) release, reduces neutrophil infiltration and exhibits anti-inflammatory and antipyretic activity. Alpha-MSH levels are increased in synovial fluid of patients with rheumatoid arthritis. MC_1- and MC_3-receptors mediate the immunomodulatory effect of MSH. Antagonists at these receptors with potential anti-inflammatory activity are being sought.

Gamma-MSH increases blood pressure, heart rate and cerebral blood flow following intracerebroventricular or intravenous injection. These effects are likely mediated by the MC_4-receptor. Central injection of α-MSH also causes changes in animal behaviour such as increased grooming and sexual activity and reduced feeding.

Two naturally occurring ligands for MC receptors (*agouti-signalling protein* and *agouti-related peptide,* together called the *agouti*) have been discovered in human tissues. These are proteins that competitively antagonise the effect of MSH at MC receptors. Their precise role in the body is not known.

Anterior pituitary and hypothalamus

- The anterior pituitary secretes hormones which regulate:
  —the release of glucocorticoids from adrenal cortex
  —the release of thyroid hormones
  —ovulation in the female and spermatogenesis in the male, and the release of sex hormones (Ch. 29)
  —growth
  —mammary gland structure and function.
- Each anterior pituitary hormone is regulated by a specific hypothalamic releasing factor. Feedback mechanisms influence the release of these factors. Substances available for clinical use are:
  —growth hormone-releasing factor (sermorelin) and analogues of growth hormone (GH, somatrem, somatropin)
  —thyrotrophin-releasing factor (protirelin) and thyroid-stimulating hormone (thyrotrophin; used to test thyroid function)
  —octreotide, an analogue of somatostatin, which inhibits GH release
  —corticotrophin-releasing factor, used in diagnosis
  —gonadotrophin-releasing factor (see Ch. 29).

POSTERIOR PITUITARY (NEUROHYPOPHYSIS)

The posterior pituitary gland consists largely of the terminals of nerve cells that lie in the supraoptic and paraventricular nuclei of the hypothalamus. Their axons form the hypothalamic–hypophyseal tract, and the fibres terminate in dilated nerve endings in close association with capillaries in the posterior pituitary gland (Fig. 27.1). Peptides, synthesised in the hypothalamic nuclei, pass down the axons into the posterior pituitary, where they are stored and eventually secreted into the bloodstream. See also Chapter 13.

The two main hormones of the posterior pituitary are *oxytocin* (which contracts the smooth muscle of the uterus; see Ch. 29) and *ADH* (also called *vasopressin*; see Chs 18 and 23).

Several similar peptides have been synthesised that vary in their antidiuretic, vasopressor and oxytocic (uterine stimulant) properties.

ANTIDIURETIC HORMONE

Regulation of secretion and physiological role

ADH released from the posterior pituitary has a crucial role in the control of the water content of the body through its action on the cells of the distal part of the nephron and the collecting tubules in the kidney (see Ch. 23). Specific nuclei in the hypothalamus that control water metabolism lie close to the nuclei which synthesise and secrete ADH.

One of the main stimuli to ADH release is an *increase in plasma osmolality* (which produces a sensation of thirst). A decrease in circulating blood volume (hypovolaemia) is another major factor causing secretion of ADH, the stimuli arising from baroreceptors in the cardiovascular system. Angiotensin also releases ADH.

Diabetes insipidus is a condition in which large volumes of dilute urine are produced, resulting from failure of ADH secretion or reduced sensitivity of the kidney to ADH.

The receptors for ADH

There are three classes of receptor for ADH—V_1, V_2 and V_3. V_2-receptors mediate its main physiological actions in the kidney and are coupled to adenylate cyclase; the V_1- and V_3-receptors are coupled to the phospholipase C/inositol trisphosphate system.

Actions

Renal actions

ADH binds to V_2-receptors in the basolateral membrane of the cells of the distal tubule and collecting ducts of the nephron. Its main effect in the collecting duct is to increase the rate of insertion of water channels into the luminal membrane, thus increasing the permeability of the membrane to water. (Details of this action are given in Ch. 23.) It also activates urea transporters and transiently increases Na^+ absorption, particularly in the distal tubule.

Several drugs affect the action of ADH. *Non-steroidal anti-inflammatory drugs* (NSAIDs) and **carbamazepine** increase ADH effects; **lithium, colchicine** and **vinca alkaloids** decrease it, the latter two agents by virtue of their action on microtubules—organelles required for the movement of the water channels. **Demeclocycline** counteracts the action of ADH and can be used to treat patients with hyponatraemia (and thus water retention) caused by excessive secretion of ADH.

Non-renal actions

ADH causes contraction of smooth muscle, particularly in the cardiovascular system, by acting on V_1-receptors (see Ch. 18). The affinity of these receptors for ADH is lower than that of the V_2-receptors, and smooth muscle effects are only seen with doses larger than those affecting the kidney. ADH also stimulates blood platelet aggregation and coagulation factor release.

In the CNS, ADH acts as a neuromodulator and neurotransmitter; released into the pituitary 'portal circulation' it promotes the release of ACTH from the anterior pituitary by an action on V_3-receptors (Fig. 27.4).

Pharmacokinetic aspects

Various analogues of ADH have been developed for clinical use, the aims being (a) to increase the duration of action and (b) to shift the potency between V_1- and V_2-receptors.

The main analogues are **vasopressin** (ADH itself: short duration of action, weak selectivity for V_2-receptors, given by subcutaneous or intramuscular injection, or by intravenous infusion), **desmopressin** (increased duration of action, V_2 selective and usually given as a nasal spray), **terlipressin** (increased duration of action, low but protracted vasopressor action and minimal antidiuretic properties) and **felypressin** (short duration of action, vasoconstrictor effect is used with local anaesthetics such as prilocaine to prolong its action).

Vasopressin is rapidly eliminated with a plasma half-life of 10 minutes and a short duration of action. Metabolism is by tissue peptidases, and 33% is removed by the kidney. Desmopressin is

Clinical use of antidiuretic hormone (vasopressin) and analogues

- Treatment of diabetes insipidus: lypressin, desmopressin.
- The initial treatment of bleeding oesophageal varices: vasopressin, terlipressin, lypressin. (Octreotide is also used but sclerotherapy by direct injection of sclerosant via an endoscope is the main treatment.)
- As prophylactic against bleeding in haemophilia (e.g. before tooth extraction): vasopressin, desmopressin (by increasing the concentration of factor VIII); somatostatin is also effective.
- Felypressin is used as a vasoconstrictor with local anaesthetics (see Ch. 43).
- Desmopressin is used for persistent nocturnal enuresis in older children and adults.

Posterior pituitary

- The posterior pituitary secretes:
  —oxytocin (see Ch. 29)
  —antidiuretic hormone (vasopressin), which acts on V_2-receptors in the distal kidney tubule to increase water reabsorption, and, in higher concentrations, on V_1-receptors to cause vasoconstriction. It also participates in the control of adrenocorticotrophic hormone (ACTH) secretion.
- Substances available for clinical use are vasopressin, and the analogues, desmopressin, terlipressin.

less subject to degradation by peptidases, and its plasma half-life is 75 minutes.

Various synthetic non-peptide agonists and antagonists of ADH have been synthesised and are used as experimental tools. Several orally active V_1-receptor antagonists are under study for the treatment of dysmenorrhoea (for a review of ADH receptor antagonists and their possible clinical uses, see Thibonnier et al., 2001).

Unwanted effects

There are few unwanted effects if the antidiuretic peptides are used intranasally in therapeutic doses, although intravenous vasopressin may cause spasm of the coronary arteries, with resultant angina.

OXYTOCIN

Oxytocin is discussed in Chapter 29.

THE ADRENAL CORTEX

ADRENAL STEROIDS

The steroids secreted by the adrenal cortex have two main actions:

- those seen primarily in the resting state and which are 'permissive' in nature, i.e. they permit or facilitate the actions of other hormones
- those which occur in response to a threatening environment.

These latter actions are crucial for survival, an animal deprived of its adrenal cortex being able to survive only in rigorously controlled conditions.

The principal adrenal steroids are those with *mineralocorticoid* and *glucocorticoid* activity, but some sex steroids—mainly *androgens*—are also secreted. The mineralocorticoids affect water and electrolyte balance and the main endogenous hormone is *aldosterone*. The glucocorticoids affect carbohydrate and protein metabolism and the main endogenous hormones are *hydrocortisone* and *corticosterone*. The two actions are not completely separated in naturally occurring steroids, some glucocorticoids having quite substantial effects on water and electrolyte balance.* In addition to their metabolic effects, glucocorticoids also have anti-inflammatory and immunosuppressive activity, and it is for these actions that they are most commonly used therapeutically. When they are used as anti-inflammatory and immunosuppressive agents, all of their other actions are unwanted side-effects.

Synthetic steroids have been developed in which it has been possible to separate the glucocorticoid from the mineralocorticoid actions (see Table 27.2), but it has not been possible to separate the anti-inflammatory actions from the other actions of the glucocorticoids.

A deficiency in corticosteroid production, *Addison's disease*, is characterised by muscular weakness, low blood pressure, depression, anorexia, loss of weight and hypoglycaemia. Addison's disease may have an autoimmune aetiology, or it may result from destruction of the gland by chronic inflammatory conditions such as tuberculosis. A decreased production of endogenous corticoids also occurs when glucocorticoids are given therapeutically for prolonged periods; this can result in deficiency eventually, when treatment is discontinued.

When corticosteroids are produced in excess, the clinical picture depends on which of the steroids predominate. Excessive glucocorticoid activity results in *Cushing's syndrome*, the manifestations of which are outlined in Figure 27.7, below. This can be caused by hypersecretion from the adrenal glands or by prolonged administration of glucocorticoids. An excessive production of mineralocorticoids results in disturbances of Na^+ and K^+ balance. This may occur with hyperactivity of the adrenals or tumours of the glands (*primary hyperaldosteronism*, or *Conn's syndrome*, an uncommon but important cause of hypertension; see Ch. 18), or with excessive renin–angiotensin action such as occurs in kidney disease, cirrhosis of the liver or congestive cardiac failure (*secondary hyperaldosteronism*).

GLUCOCORTICOIDS

Synthesis and release

Adrenal steroids are synthesised and released as needed under the influence of ACTH, which is secreted from the anterior pituitary gland (see p. 408 and Fig. 27.4). ACTH secretion is regulated partly by CRF derived from the hypothalamus (see Table 27.1 and Fig. 27.4) and partly by the level of glucocorticoids in the blood. (ADH, which may reach the pituitary through short portal vessels from the posterior pituitary, also stimulates ACTH release and may have a physiological role.) The release of CRF, in turn, is inhibited by the level of glucocorticoids in the blood and is influenced by input from the CNS. There is a basal release of

*In fact hydrocortisone and aldosterone are equiactive on mineralocorticoid receptors; but, in mineralocorticoid-sensitive tissues such as the kidney, the action of 11β-hydroxysteroid dehydrogenase converts hydrocortisone to receptor-inactive cortisone.

Table 27.2 Comparison of the main corticosteroid agents (using hydrocortisone as a standard)

Compound	Relative affinity for glucocorticoid receptors[a]	Approximate relative potency in clinical use:		Duration of action after oral dose[b]	Comments
		Anti-inflammatory	Sodium-retaining		
Hydrocortisone (cortisol)	1	1	1	S	Drug of choice for replacement therapy
Cortisone	0.01	0.8	0.8	S	Cheap; inactive until converted to hydrocortisone; not used as anti-inflammatory because of mineralocorticoid effects
Corticosterone	0.85	0.3	15	S	–
Prednisolone	2.2	4	0.8	I	Drug of choice for systemic anti-inflammatory and immunosuppressive effects
Prednisone	0.05	4	0.8	I	Inactive until converted to prednisolone
Methylprednisolone	11.9	5	Minimal	I	Anti-inflammatory and immunosuppressive
Triamcinolone	1.9	5	None	I	Relatively more toxic than others
Dexamethasone	7.1	30	Minimal	L	Anti-inflammatory and immunosuppressive, used especially where water retention is undesirable, e.g. cerebral oedema; drug of choice for suppression of ACTH production
Betamethasone	5.4	30	Negligible	L	Anti-inflammatory and immunosuppressive, used especially where water retention is undesirable
Beclometasone dipropionate		+	–	–	Anti-inflammatory and immunosuppressive; effective topically and as an aerosol
Budesonide		+	–	–	Anti-inflammatory and immunosuppressive; effective topically and as an aerosol
Deoxycortone	0.19	Negligible	50	–	
Fludrocortisone	3.5	15	150	S	Drug of choice for mineralocorticoid effects
Aldosterone	0.38	none	500	–	Endogenous mineralocorticoid

[a]Human fetal lung cells.
Duration of action (half-lives in hours): S, 8–12; I, 12–36; L, 36–72. Data for relative affinity obtained from Baxter & Rousseau (1979).

glucocorticoids. The concentration of endogenous corticosteroids in the blood is high in the morning, at 8 a.m. and low at midnight. Opioid peptides exercise a tonic inhibitory control on the secretion of CRF. Psychological factors can affect the release of CRF, as can stimuli such as excessive heat or cold, injury or infections; this is the mechanism, in fact, by which the pituitary adrenal system is activated in response to a threatening environment.

The inter-relationship of these factors is outlined in Figure 27.4.*

*When released, the corticosteroids pass first through the adrenal medulla because both the medulla and cortex of the adrenal gland have a common blood supply. Glucocorticoids play a part in controlling the conversion of noradrenaline to adrenaline by stimulating expression of the relevant methyltransferase (see Ch. 11).

The starting substance for synthesis of glucocorticoids is *cholesterol* (Fig. 27.5). The first step, the conversion of cholesterol to *pregnenolone* is the rate-limiting step and is regulated by ACTH. Some of the reactions in the synthesis can be inhibited by drugs.

Metyrapone prevents the β-hydroxylation at C11 and thus the formation of hydrocortisone and corticosterone (Fig. 27.5). Synthesis is stopped at the 11-deoxycorticosteroid stage and, as these substances have no negative feedback effects on the hypothalamus and pituitary, there is a marked increase in ACTH in the blood. Metyrapone can, therefore, be used to test ACTH production and may also be used in some patients with Cushing's syndrome. **Trilostane** (of use in Cushing's syndrome and primary hyperaldosteronism) blocks an earlier step in the pathway—the 3β-dehydrogenase.

Aminoglutethimide inhibits an earlier stage in the synthetic pathway and has the same effect as metyrapone (Fig. 27.5). **Ketoconazole**, an antifungal agent (Ch. 47) used in higher doses, inhibits steroidogenesis and can be of value in Cushing's syndrome.

Glucocorticoids

- Drugs used: hydrocortisone, prednisolone and dexamethasone.

Metabolic actions

- On carbohydrates: decreased uptake and utilisation of glucose and increased gluconeogenesis; this causes a tendency to hyperglycaemia.
- On proteins: increased catabolism, reduced anabolism.
- On fat: a permissive effect on lipolytic hormones, and a redistribution of fat, as in Cushing's syndrome.

Regulatory actions

- On hypothalamus and anterior pituitary: a negative feedback action resulting in reduced release of endogenous glucocorticoids.
- On vascular events: reduced vasodilatation, decreased fluid exudation.
- On cellular events:
  - —in areas of acute inflammation: decreased influx and activity of leucocytes
  - —in areas of chronic inflammation: decreased activity of mononuclear cells, decreased proliferation of blood vessels, less fibrosis
  - —in lymphoid areas: decreased clonal expansion of T and B cells and decreased action of cytokine-secreting T cells.
- On inflammatory and immune mediators:
  - —decreased production and action of cytokines including many interleukins, tumour necrosis factor-γ, granulocyte–macrophage colony-stimulating factor
  - —reduced generation of eicosanoids
  - —decreased generation of IgG
  - —decrease in complement components in the blood.
- Overall effects: reduction in chronic inflammation and autoimmune reactions but also decreased healing and diminution in the protective aspects of the inflammatory response.

Mechanism of action

For the most part, glucocorticoid effects involve interactions between the steroids and intracellular receptors that belong to the superfamily of receptors that control gene transcription (see Ch. 3). This superfamily also includes the receptors for mineralocorticoids, the sex steroids, thyroid hormones, vitamin D_3 and retinoic acid. There are believed to be 10–100 steroid-responsive genes in each cell.

The glucocorticoids, after entering cells, bind to specific receptors (GRα and GRβ) in the cytoplasm. These receptors, which have a high affinity for glucocorticoids, are found in virtually all tissues—about 3000 to 10 000 per cell, the number varying in different tissues (Fig. 27.6). GRα has been cloned and contains 777 amino acid residues. After interaction with the steroid, the receptor becomes 'activated', i.e. it undergoes a conformational change that exposes a DNA-binding domain (see Figs 27.6B, 3.2 and 3.3). The steroid–receptor complexes form dimers (pairs), then move to the nucleus and bind to steroid-response elements in the DNA. The effect is either to repress (prevent transcription of) or induce (initiate transcription of) particular genes.

Repression is brought about by inhibition of the action of various transcription factors* such as AP-1** and NF-κB*** (see Tak & Firestein, 2001). These transcription factors normally switch on the genes for cyclooxygenase-2, various cytokines and adhesion factors, as well as the inducible isoform of nitric oxide synthase (see above and Ch. 14). Basal and induced transcription of the genes for collagenase are modified and vitamin D_3 induction of the ostecalcin gene in osteoblasts is inhibited (see Landers & Spelsberg, 1992; Funder, 1997).

Induction involves the formation of specific mRNAs, which direct the synthesis of specific proteins. In addition to the enzymes involved in their metabolic actions (e.g. the cAMP-dependent kinase), glucocorticoids induce the formation of *annexin-1* (previously called *lipocortin-1*). Annexin-1 is important in the negative feedback action of glucocorticoids on the hypothalamus and anterior pituitary and has anti-inflammatory actions (possibly by inhibiting phospholipase A_2). As might be predicted, the anti-inflammatory effect of glucocorticoids take several hours to become evident since formation of annexin-1 (and other active proteins) is relatively slow.

---

*These factors bind to the DNA upstream from the start site of transcription and act as enhancers of transcription.

**AP-1 is a heterodimer of Fos and Jun proteins, which are the products of c-*fos* and c-*jun* proto-oncogenes (Fig. 50.1).

***Glucocorticoids induce the transcription of the gene for the inhibitory factor IF-κBα; this binds NF-κB transcription factor in the cytosol, preventing its translocation to the nucleus.

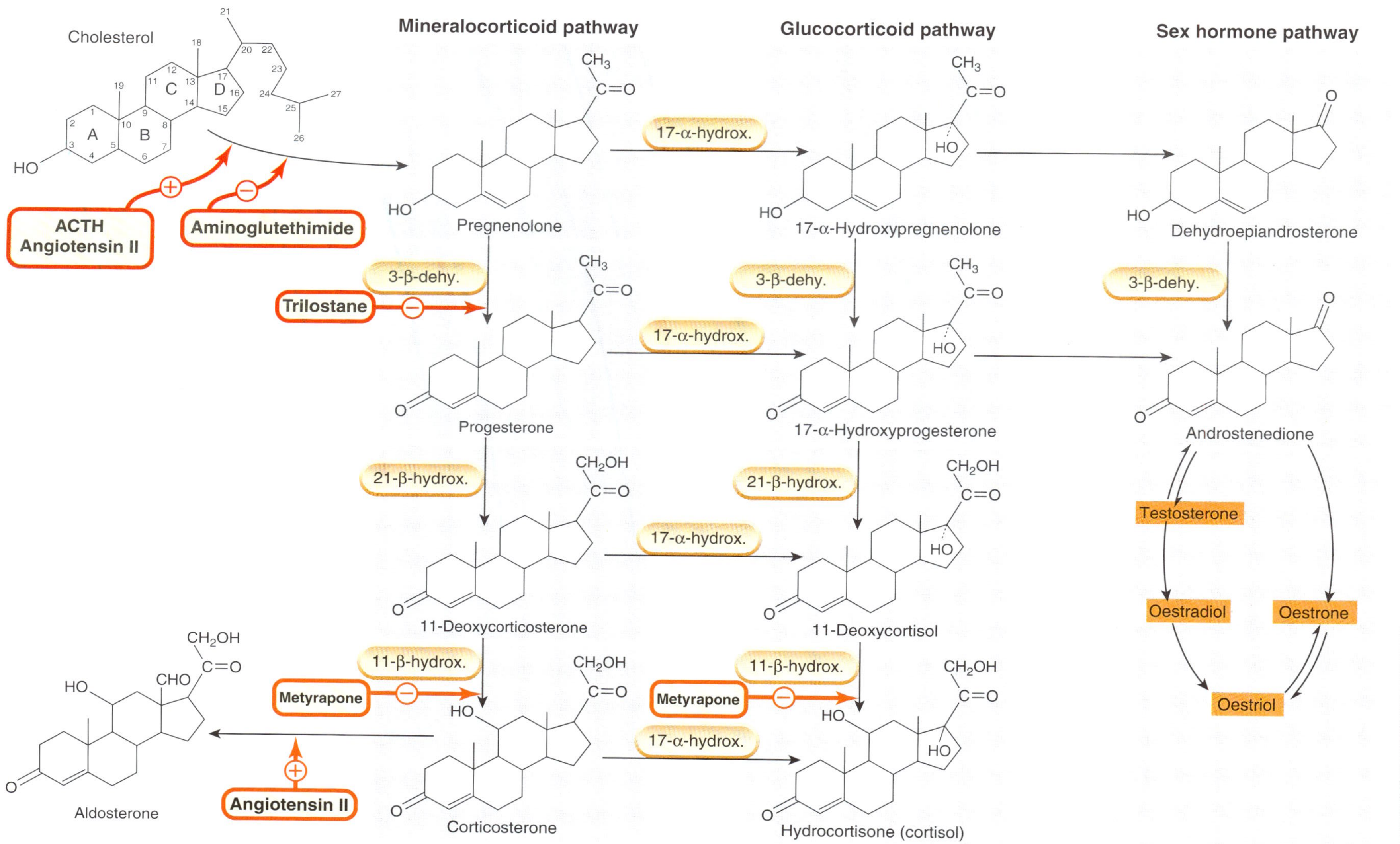

Fig. 27.5 Main pathways in the biosynthesis of corticosteroids and adrenal androgens with sites of action of drugs indicated. Note that the drugs have selective actions on different cortical cell types. Glucocorticoids are produced by cells of the zona fasciculata and their synthesis is stimulated by ACTH; aldosterone is produced by cells of the zona glomerulosa and its synthesis is stimulated by angiotensin II. Metyrapone inhibits glucocorticoid synthesis; aminoglutethimide inhibits both glucocorticoid and sex hormone synthesis, and trilostane blocks synthesis of all three types of adrenal steroid. (Further details of sex steroid biosynthesis are given in Fig. 29.3. (ACTH, adrenocorticotrophic hormone; 3-β-dhy., 3-β-dehydrogenase; 17-β-hydrox., 17-β-hydroxylase; 21-β-hydrox., 21-β-hydroxylase; 11-β-hydrox., 11-β-hydroxylase.)

A

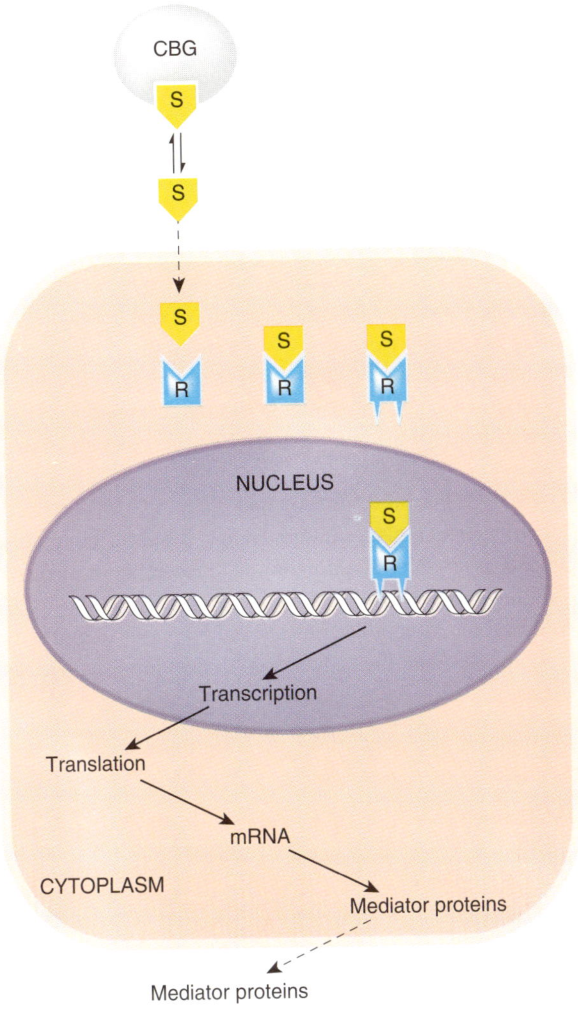

B

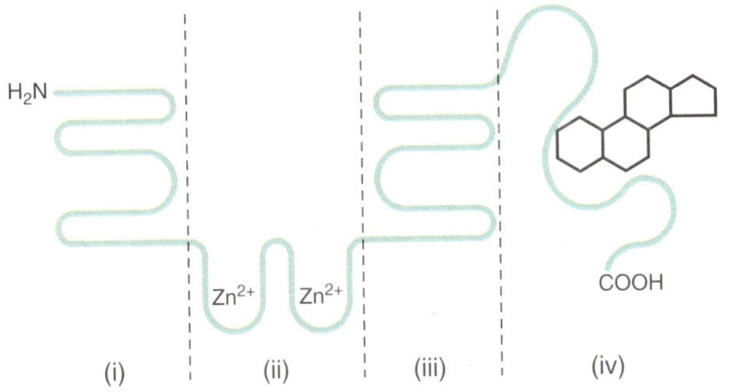

Fig. 27.6 Mechanism of action of glucocorticoids at the cellular level and the functional domains of the glucocorticoid receptor. A Diagram showing glucocorticoid-mediated induction (initiation of transcription). Note that the glucocorticoids can also repress induction by inhibiting transcription factors such as AP-1 and NF-κB. (S, steroid; R, receptor; CBG, corticosteroid-binding globulin.) After the binding of steroid to receptor and before interaction with DNA, there is dimer formation, i.e. the linking of two steroid–receptor complexes (not shown). B Diagram of the glucocorticoid receptor domains with the main functions associated with each domain. Note that three domains are involved in transcription and three in dimer formation. (i) Regulatory domain: activates gene-specific transcription and can bind other protein factors. (ii) The DNA-binding domain: determines which genes will be influenced by the receptor (it contains two 'zinc fingers', which wrap around the DNA helix), controls transcriptional activation (i.e. positive as opposed to negative genomic events) and is involved in dimer formation. (iii) Hinge domain: involved in nuclear localisation, transcription and dimer formation. (iv) Steroid-binding domain: binds steroid and is involved in nuclear localisation and dimer formation. (Modified from: Landers & Spelsberg, 1992.)

Glucocorticoids can, however, produce effects over a very much shorter time frame, For example, corticosterone inhibits Ca^{2+} fluxes in hippocampal neurons more or less instantaneously. These rapid effects of glucocorticoids do not involve interaction with genes (i.e. they are non-genomic) but are mediated instead by interacting with specific membrane receptors to cause changes within the cell (e.g on intracellular Ca^{2+}) that are similar to those triggered by neurotransmitters. The biological significance of most rapid glucocorticoid effects discovered so far are not yet known but they might be important for some of their metabolic effects (see below).

Actions

General metabolic and systemic effects

The main metabolic effects are on carbohydrate and protein metabolism. The hormones cause both a decrease in the uptake and utilisation of glucose and an increase in gluconeogenesis, resulting in a tendency to hyperglycaemia (see Ch. 25). There is a concomitant increase in glycogen storage, which may be a result of insulin secretion in response to the increase in blood sugar. There is decreased protein synthesis and increased protein breakdown, particularly in muscle. Glucocorticoids have a 'permissive' effect on the lipolytic response to catecholamines and other hormones, which act by increasing intracellular cAMP concentration (see Ch. 3). Such hormones cause lipase activation through a cAMP-dependent kinase, the synthesis of which requires the presence of glucocorticoids (see below). Large doses of glucocorticoids given over a long period result in the redistribution of fat characteristic of Cushing's syndrome (Fig. 27.7).

The glucocorticoids, in non-physiological concentrations, have some mineralocorticoid actions (see below), causing Na^+

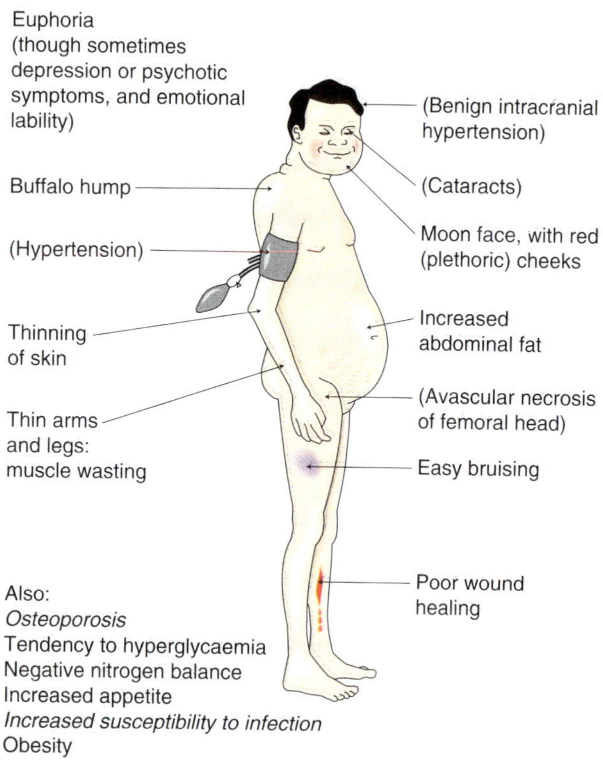

Fig. 27.7 Effects of prolonged glucocorticoid excess: iatrogenic Cushing's syndrome. Italicised effects are particularly common. Less-frequent effects, related to dose and duration of therapy, are shown in parentheses. (Adapted from: Baxter & Rousseau, 1979.)

retention and K^+ loss—possibly by occupying mineralocorticoid receptors.

Glucocorticoids tend to produce a negative calcium balance by decreasing Ca^{2+} absorption in the gastrointestinal tract and increasing its excretion by the kidney. This can result in osteoporosis (see below).

Negative feedback effects on the anterior pituitary and hypothalamus

Both endogenous and exogenous glucocorticoids have a negative feedback effect on the secretion of CRF and ACTH (see Fig. 27.4). Administration of exogenous glucocorticoids depresses the secretion of CRF and ACTH, thus inhibiting the secretion of endogenous glucocorticoids and causing atrophy of the adrenal cortex. If therapy is prolonged, it may take many months to return to normal function when the drugs are stopped.

Anti-inflammatory and immunosuppressive effects

When given therapeutically, glucocorticoids have powerful anti-inflammatory and immunosuppressive effects. They inhibit both the early and the late manifestations of inflammation, i.e. not only the initial redness, heat, pain and swelling, but also the later stages of wound healing and repair and the proliferative reactions seen in chronic inflammation (Ch. 15). They affect all types of inflammatory reaction whether caused by invading pathogens, by chemical or physical stimuli or by inappropriately deployed immune responses such as are seen in hypersensitivity or autoimmune disease. When used clinically to suppress graft rejection, glucocorticoids suppress the initiation and generation of a 'new' immune response more efficiently than a response that is already established and in which clonal proliferation has already occurred.

Actions on inflammatory cells These include:

- decreased egress of neutrophils from blood vessels and reduced activity of neutrophils and macrophages owing to decreased transcription of the genes for cell adhesion factors and the relevant cytokines (see below)
- decreased action of T helper cells and reduced clonal proliferation of T cells, mainly through decreased transcription of the genes for IL-2 and its receptor (see below)
- decreased fibroblast function and, therefore, less production of collagen and glycosaminoglycans; the contribution of these events to chronic inflammation is reduced but so also is healing and repair
- reduced function of osteoblasts and increased activity of osteoclasts—and thus a tendency to develop osteoporosis (see below).

Action on the mediators of inflammatory and immune responses These in include:

- decreased production of prostanoids owing to decreased expression of cyclooxygenase-2 (Fig. 15.5)
- decreased generation of cytokines—IL-1, IL-2, IL-3, IL-4, IL-5, IL-6, IL-8, TNF-γ and cell adhesion factors (see Ch. 15), granulocyte–macrophage colony-stimulating factor (see Ch. 21)—through inhibition of transcription of the relevant genes (see below)
- reduction in the concentration of complement components in the plasma (Ch. 15)
- decreased generation of induced nitric oxide (see below)
- decreased histamine release from basophils
- decreased IgG production.

Significance of the anti-inflammatory and immunosuppressive actions of the glucocorticoids These have generally been considered to be 'pharmacological' actions only, i.e. to be qualitatively different from the physiological effects (namely the metabolic and regulatory actions) of endogenously produced glucocorticoids. However, the anti-inflammatory and immunosuppressive actions may also have a physiological role in that they prevent 'overshoot' of the body's powerful defence reactions, which might otherwise themselves threaten homeostasis (see Munck et al., 1984).

The consequence of these powerful actions of the glucocorticoids is that they can be of great value when used to treat certain conditions in which there is hypersensitivity and unwanted inflammation, but they carry the hazard that they are

Mechanism of action of the glucocorticoids

- Glucocorticoids interact with intracellular receptors; the resulting steroid–receptor complexes dimerise (form pairs) then interact with DNA to modify gene transcription: inducing synthesis of some proteins and inhibiting synthesis of others.
- For metabolic actions, most mediator proteins are enzymes, e.g. cAMP-dependent kinase, but not all actions on genes are known.
- For anti-inflammatory and immunosuppressive actions, some actions at the level of the genes are known:
  - —inhibition of transcription of the genes for cyclooxygenase-2, cytokines (e.g. the interleukins), cell adhesion molecules and the inducible form of nitric oxide synthase
  - —block of vitamin D_3-mediated induction of the osteocalcin gene in osteoblasts and modification of transcription of the collagenase genes
  - —increased synthesis of annexin-1, which is important in negative feedback on the hypothalamus and anterior pituitary and may have anti-inflammatory actions.
- Some non-genomic (rapid) effects of glucocorticoids have also been observed.

able to suppress the necessary protective responses to infection and can decrease essential healing processes.

Unwanted effects

Unwanted effects are likely to occur with large doses or prolonged administration but should not occur with replacement therapy. Possible unwanted effects include *suppression of the response to infection or injury*; an intercurrent infection can be potentially very serious unless quickly treated with antimicrobial agents along with an increase in the dose of steroid. Wound healing may be impaired and peptic ulceration may also occur.

Sudden withdrawal of the drugs after prolonged therapy may result in acute adrenal insufficiency through *suppression of the patient's capacity to synthesise corticosteroids.** Careful procedures for phased withdrawal should be followed. Recovery of full adrenal function usually takes about 2 months, though it can take 18 months or more.

When the drugs are used in anti-inflammatory and immunosuppressive therapy, the metabolic actions and the effects on water and electrolyte balance and organ systems are unwanted side-effects, and Cushing's syndrome may occur (see Fig. 27.7).

Osteoporosis, with the attendant hazard of fractures, is probably one of the main limitations to long-term glucocorticoid therapy. Glucocorticoids influence bone by regulation of calcium and phosphate metabolism and through effects on collagen synthesis by osteoblasts and collagen degradation by collagenase. Glucocorticoids modify transcription of the collagenase genes and inhibit vitamin D_3-mediated induction of genes in osteoblasts (see above). Given long term, glucocorticoids reduce the function of osteoblasts (which lay down bone matrix) and increase the activity of osteoclasts (which digest bone matrix).

The tendency to hyperglycaemia which occurs with exogenous glucocorticoids may develop into actual diabetes. Another limitation is the development of muscle wasting and weakness.

In children, the metabolic effects (particularly those on protein metabolism) may result in inhibition of growth, even with fairly low doses, though this is not likely to occur unless treatment is continued for more than 6 months. An effect on the blood supply to bone can result in avascular necrosis of the head of the femur.

There is often euphoria, but some patients may become depressed or develop psychotic symptoms.

Other toxic effects that have been reported are glaucoma, raised intracranial pressure, hypercoagulability of the blood, fever and disorders of menstruation and an increased incidence of cataracts. Oral thrush (candidiasis, a fungal infection; see Ch. 47) frequently occurs when glucocorticoids are taken by inhalation.

Pharmacokinetic aspects

Glucocorticoids may be given by a variety of routes. Most are active when given orally. All can be given systemically, either intramuscularly or intravenously. They may also be given topically—injected intra-articularly, given by aerosol into the respiratory tract, administered as drops into the eye or the nose, or applied in creams or ointments to the skin. There is much less likelihood of systemic toxic effects after topical administration unless large quantities are used. When prolonged use of systemic glucocorticoids is necessary, therapy on alternate days may decrease the unwanted effects.

The endogenous glucocorticoids are carried in the plasma, bound to corticosteroid-binding globulin (CBG) and to albumin. CBG accounts for about 77% of hydrocortisone bound but it does not bind synthetic steroids. Albumin has a lower affinity for hydrocortisone; it binds both natural and synthetic steroids. Both CBG-bound and albumin-bound steroids are biologically inactive.

Steroids, being small lipophilic molecules, enter their target cells by simple diffusion.

Hydrocortisone has a plasma half-life of 90 minutes, though its main biological effects occur only after 2–8 hours. The main step in inactivation is the reduction of the double bond between C4 and C5. This occurs in liver cells and elsewhere. Cortisone and prednisone are inactive until converted in vivo to hydrocortisone and prednisolone, respectively.

The clinical use of the glucocorticoids is given in the box (p. 418).

*Patients on long-continued glucocorticoid therapy are advised to carry a card stating: 'I am a patient on STEROID TREATMENT which must not be stopped abruptly'. This is because the exogenous glucocorticoids will have suppressed the necessary general hypothalamic–pituitary–adrenal response to the stress of illness or trauma.

Pharmacokinetics and unwanted actions of the glucocorticoids

- Administration can be oral, topical and parenteral. The drugs are bound to corticosteroid-binding globulin in the blood and enter cells by diffusion. They are metabolised in the liver.
- Unwanted effects are seen mainly with prolonged systemic use as anti-inflammatory or immunosuppressive agents (in which case all the metabolic actions are unwanted), but not usually with replacement therapy. The most important are:
  —suppression of response to infection
  —suppression of endogenous glucocorticoid synthesis
  —metabolic actions (see above)
  —osteoporosis
  —iatrogenic Cushing's syndrome (see Fig. 27.7).

Clinical use of glucocorticoids

- Replacement therapy for patients with adrenal failure (Addison's disease).
- Anti-inflammatory/immunosuppressive therapy (see also Ch. 16):
  —in asthma (Ch. 22)
  —topically in various inflammatory conditions of skin, eye, ear or nose (e.g. eczema, allergic conjunctivitis or rhinitis)
  —in hypersensitivity states (e.g. severe allergic reactions)
  —in miscellaneous diseases with autoimmune and inflammatory components (e.g. rheumatoid arthritis and other 'connective tissue' diseases, inflammatory bowel diseases, some forms of haemolytic anaemia, idiopathic thrombocytopenic purpura)
  —to prevent graft-versus-host disease following organ or bone marrow transplantation.
- In neoplastic disease (see also Ch. 50):
  —in combination with cytotoxic drugs in treatment of specific malignancies (e.g. Hodgkin's disease, acute lymphocytic leukaemia)
  —to reduce cerebral oedema in patients with metastatic or primary brain tumours (dexamethasone is the drug used)
  —as a component of antiemetic treatment in conjunction with chemotherapy.

Dexamethasone can be used to test hypothalamic–pituitary–adrenocortical function in the 'dexamethasone suppression test'. A low dose, usually given at night, should suppress the hypothalamus and pituitary, and result in reduced ACTH secretion and hydrocortisone output, the hydrocortisone being measured in the plasma about 9 hours later. Failure of suppression implies hypersecretion of ACTH or of glucocorticoids (Cushing's syndrome).

MINERALOCORTICOIDS

The main endogenous mineralocorticoid is *aldosterone*, which is produced in the outermost of the three zones of the adrenal medulla, the *zona glomerulosa*. Its main action is to increase Na^+ reabsorption by an action on the distal tubules in the kidney, with concomitant increased excretion of K^+ and H^+ (see Ch. 23). An excessive secretion of mineralocorticoids, as in Conn's syndrome, causes marked Na^+ and water retention with resultant increase in the volume of extracellular fluid, hypokalaemia, alkalosis and hypertension. A decreased secretion, as in Addison's disease, causes increased Na^+ loss, which is relatively more pronounced than water loss. The osmotic pressure of the extracellular fluid is thus reduced, resulting in a shift of fluid into the intracellular compartment and a marked decrease in extracellular fluid volume. There is a concomitant decrease in the excretion of K^+, resulting in hyperkalaemia.

Regulation of aldosterone synthesis and release

The control of the synthesis and release of aldosterone is complex. Control depends mainly on the electrolyte composition of the plasma and on the angiotensin II system (Fig. 27.4 and Chs 18 and 23). Low plasma Na^+ or high plasma K^+ concentrations affect the zona glomerulosa cells of the adrenal directly, stimulating aldosterone release. Depletion of body Na^+ also activates the renin–angiotensin system (see Fig. 18.4). One of the effects of angiotensin II is to increase the synthesis and release of aldosterone.

Mechanism of action

Aldosterone, like other steroids, binds to specific intracellular receptors. Unlike the glucocorticoid-binding receptors, which occur in most tissues, aldosterone receptors occur in fewer target tissues, such as the kidney and in the transporting epithelia of the colon and bladder. Cells containing mineralocorticoid receptors also contain 11β–hydroxysteroid dehydrogenase.* This enzyme converts glucocorticoids, but not mineralocorticoids, to metabolites that have only low affinity for the mineralocorticoid receptors, thus ensuring that the cells are affected only by *bona fide* mineralocorticoids.

*This enzyme is inhibited by carbenoxolone (used to treat ulcers; see Ch. 24) and liquorice; marked inhibition allows corticosterone to act on the mineralocorticoid receptor producing a syndrome similar to Conn's syndrome (primary hyperaldosteronism).

Mineralocorticoids

Fludrocortisone is given orally to produce a mineralocorticoid effect. This agent:

- —increases Na^+ reabsorption in distal tubules and increases K^+ and H^+ efflux into the tubules
- —acts, like most steroids, on intracellular receptors that modulate DNA transcription causing synthesis of protein mediators
- —is used with a glucocorticoid in replacement therapy.

As with the glucocorticoids, the interaction of ligand with receptor initiates DNA transcription of specific proteins, resulting in an early increase in the number of sodium channels in the apical membrane of the cell and later on an increase in the number of Na^+/K^+-ATPase molecules in the basolateral membrane (see Fig. 23.9).

The increased K^+ excretion into the tubule produced by aldosterone results from influx of K^+ into the cell by the action of the basal Na^+/K^+-ATPase, coupled with an increased efflux of K^+ through apical potassium channels.

In addition to the effects mediated through DNA, there is evidence for a rapid non-genomic effect of aldosterone on Na^+ influx, by an action on the Na^+–H^+ exchanger in the apical membrane.

Spironolactone is a competitive antagonist of aldosterone, and it also prevents the mineralocorticoid effects of other adrenal steroids on the renal tubule (Ch. 23). Side-effects include gynaecomastia and impotence, since spironolactone also has some blocking effect on androgen and progesterone receptors. **Eplerenone** is currently undergoing clinical trials; it has a similar mechanism of action but lesser side-effects.

Clinical use of mineralocorticoids

The main clinical use of mineralocorticoids is in replacement therapy (Table 27.2). The most commonly used drug is **fludrocortisone** (Table 27.2 and Fig. 27.4), which can be taken orally.

REFERENCES AND FURTHER READING

The hypothalamus and pituitary

Birnbaumer M 2000 Vasopressin receptors. Trends Endocrinol Metab 11: 406–410

Clark R G, Robinson C A F 1996 Up and down the growth hormone cascade. Cytokine Growth Factor Rev 1: 65–80 (*A review covering the cascade that controls the primary regulators of growth and metabolism, namely growth hormone and the insulin-like growth factors*)

Drolet G, Rivest S 2001Corticotropin-releasing hormone and its receptors; an evaluation at the transcription level in vivo. Peptides 22: 761–767

Freeman M E, Kanyicska B, Lerant A, Nagy G 2000 Prolactin: structure, function and regulation of secretion. Physiol Res 80: 1524–1585 (*Comprehensive review of prolactin and its receptors*)

Jørgensen J O L, Christiansen J S 1993 Growth hormone therapy. Lancet 341: 1247–1248

Lamberts S W J, van der Lely A-J et al. 1996 Octreotide. N Engl J Med 334: 246–254 (*A review covering somatostatin receptors, somatostatin analogues, treatment of tumours expressing somatostatin receptors with octreotide*)

Lamberts, S W J, Bruining H A, de Jong F S 1997 Corticosteroid therapy in severe illness. N Engl J Med 337: 1285–1292 (*Review with succinct coverage of normal response of adrenal to illness, followed by more detail on clinical therapy*)

Okada S, Kopchick J J 2001 Biological effects of growth hormone and its antagonist. Trends Mol Med 7: 126–132

Page R B 1982 Pituitary blood flow. Am J Physiol 243: E427–E442

Thibonnier M, Coles P, Thibonnier A et al. 2001 The basic and clinical pharmacology of nonpeptide vasopressin receptor antagonists. Annu Rev Pharmacol 41: 175–202 (*Authoritive account of ADH receptors and the search for new antagonists*)

Vance M L 1994 Hypopituitarism. N Engl J Med 330: 1651–1662 (*Review of causes, clinical features and hormone-replacement therapy of hypopituitarism*)

Wikberg J E S, Muceniece R, Mandrika I et al. 2000 New aspects on the melanocortins and their receptors. Pharmacol Res 42: 393–420 (*Detailed review of the varied biological roles of melanocortins and their receptors*)

ACTH and the adrenal corticosteroids

Barnes P J, Adcock I 1993 Anti-inflammatory actions of steroids: molecular mechanisms. Trends Pharmacol Sci 14: 436–441 (*Clear review covering the binding of glucocorticoid receptor to heat shock protein 90, and AP-1-mediated transcription of genes for inflammatory mediators; useful diagrams*)

Bastl C, Hayslett J P 1992 The cellular action of aldosterone in target epithelia. Kidney Int 42: 250–264 (*A detailed review covering the aldosterone receptor and regulation of gene expression, aldosterone action on electrogenic and electroneutral Na^+ transport, and on K^+ and H^+ secretion*)

Baxter J D, Rousseau G G (eds) 1979 Glucocorticoid hormone action. Monographs on endocrinology. Springer-Verlag, Berlin, vol. 12 (*Early review of glucocorticoid action with memorable diagram of Cushing's syndrome*)

Borski R J (2000) Nongenomic membrane actions of glucocorticoids in vertebrates. Trends Endocrinol Metab 11: 427–436 (*A thought provoking account of the non-genomic effects of glucocorticoids*)

Buckingham J C 1998 Stress and the hypothalamo–pituitary–immune axis. Int J Tissue React 20: 23–34 (*Clear review of the complexities of the effect of stress on HPA function*)

Buckingham J C, Flower R J 1997 Lipocortin 1: a second messenger of glucocorticoid action in the hypothalamic–pituitary–adrenocortical axis. Mol Med Today 3: 296–302 (*Outline of HPA axis function, glucocorticoid action and the possible role of lipocortin-1 in both*)

de Kloet E R 2000 Stress in the brain. Eur J Pharmacol 405: 187–198

Falkenstein E, Tillmann H C, Christ M et al. 2000 Multiple actions of steroid hormones—a focus on rapid, nongenomic effects. Pharmacol Rev 52: 513–556

Funder J W 1997 Glucocorticoid and mineralocorticoid receptors: biology and clinical relevance. Annu Rev Med 48: 231–240 (*Succinct review of glucocorticoid (GR) and mineralocorticoid (MR) receptors, differences in GR- and MR-mediated transcription and responses, and steroid resistance*)

Landers J P, Spelsberg T C 1992 New concepts in steroid hormone action: transcription factors, proto-oncogenes, and the cascade model of gene expression. Crit Rev Eukaryotic Gene Express 2: 19–63 (*Excellent, detailed review on topics in the title, with useful diagrams*)

Munck A, Guyre P M, Holbrook N J 1984 Physiological functions of glucocorticoids in stress and their relation to pharmacological actions. Endocr Rev 5: 25–44 (*Review suggesting that the anti-inflammatory/immunosuppressive actions of the glucocorticoids have a physiological function*)

Ramirerz V D 1996 How do steroids act? Lancet 347: 630–631 (*Short discussion of the non-genomic actions of steroids, with particular reference to aldosterone*)

Rhodes D, Klug A 1993 Zinc fingers. Sci Am Feb: 32–39 (*Clear discussion of the role of zinc fingers in regulating gene transcription; excellent diagrams, of course*)

Smith S F 1996 Lipocortin 1: glucocorticoids caught in the act? Thorax 51: 1057–1059

Tak P P, Firestein G S 2001 NF-kappaB: a key role in inflammatory diseases. J Clin Invest: 107: 7–11 (*Succinct and very readable account of the role of NF-κB in inflammation*)

Tsai M-J, O'Malley B W 1994 Molecular mechanisms of action of steroid/thyroid receptor superfamily members. Annu Rev Biochem 63: 451–486 (*Detailed review of molecular biology of these receptors, including gene activation and gene silencing*)

Wilckens T 1995 Glucocorticoids and immune dysfunction: physiological relevance and pathogenic potential of hormonal dysfunction. Trends Pharmacol Sci 16: 193–197 (*Covers glucocorticoid interaction with Gc receptors, heat shock protein 90, and AP-1 and NF-κB transcription factors; clear diagram*)

The thyroid 28

Overview 421

Synthesis, storage and secretion of thyroid hormones 421

Regulation of thyroid function 422

Actions of the thyroid hormones 423

Transport and metabolism 424

Abnormalities of thyroid function 424

Drugs used in diseases of the thyroid 425
- Hyperthyroidism 425
- Hypothyroidism 427

OVERVIEW

In this chapter we deal with drugs acting on the thyroid. We set the scene by briefly outlining the structure, regulation and physiology of the thyroid and the main abnormalities of thyroid function. We then go on to consider the drugs that replace the thyroid hormones when these cease to function adequately and the drugs that decrease thyroid function when this is excessive.

SYNTHESIS, STORAGE AND SECRETION OF THYROID HORMONES

The thyroid secretes three main hormones: thyroxine (T_4), triiodothyronine (T_3) and calcitonin. T_4 and T_3 are critically important for normal growth and development and for energy metabolism. Calcitonin is involved in the control of plasma Ca^{2+} and is dealt with in Chapter 30. The term 'thyroid hormone' will be used here to refer to T_4 and T_3.

The functional unit of the thyroid is the follicle or acinus. Each follicle consists of a single layer of epithelial cells around a cavity, the follicle lumen, which is filled with a thick colloid containing *thyroglobulin*. Thyroglobulin is a large glycoprotein, each molecule of which contains about 115 tyrosine residues. It is synthesised, glycosylated and then secreted into the lumen of the follicle where iodination of the tyrosine residues occurs. Surrounding the follicles is a rich capillary network, and the rate of blood flow through the gland is very high in comparison with other tissues. The main steps in the synthesis, storage and secretion of thyroid hormone (Fig. 28.1), are as follows:

- uptake of plasma iodide by the follicle cells
- oxidation of iodide and iodination of tyrosine residues in the thyroglobulin of the colloid
- secretion of thyroid hormone.

Uptake of plasma iodide by the follicle cells

Iodide uptake is an energy-dependent process occurring against a gradient, which is normally about 25:1. Iodide is taken up by a Na^+/I^- symporter, which has now been cloned, the energy being provided by the Na^+/K^+-ATPase.

Oxidation of iodide and iodination of tyrosine residues

The oxidation of iodide is brought about by an enzyme, thyroperoxidase, at the inner, apical surface of the cell at the interface with the colloid. It is very rapid—labelled iodide (^{125}I) can be found in the lumen within 40 seconds of intravenous injection—and requires hydrogen peroxide (H_2O_2) as an oxidising agent. Iodination (referred to as 'organification' of iodine) occurs after the tyrosine has been incorporated into thyroglobulin. The process believed to occur is shown in Figure 28.2.

Tyrosine is iodinated first at position 3 on the ring, forming *monoiodotyrosine* (MIT) and then, in some molecules, on position 5 as well, forming *diiodotyrosine* (DIT). Two of these molecules are then coupled—either MIT with DIT to form T_3 or two DIT molecules to form T_4 (Fig. 28.3). The mechanism for coupling is believed to involve a peroxidase system similar to that involved in iodination. About one fifth of the tyrosine residues in thyroglobulin are iodinated.

The iodinated thyroglobulin of the thyroid forms a large store of thyroid hormone and, as is explained below, there is a relatively slow turnover of hormone in the tissues. This is in contrast to other endocrine secretions, such as growth hormone secreted by the anterior pituitary or the hormones of the adrenal cortex, which are synthesised on demand.

Secretion of thyroid hormone

The thyroglobulin molecule is taken up into the follicle cell by endocytosis of some of the colloid in the lumen (Fig. 28.1). The

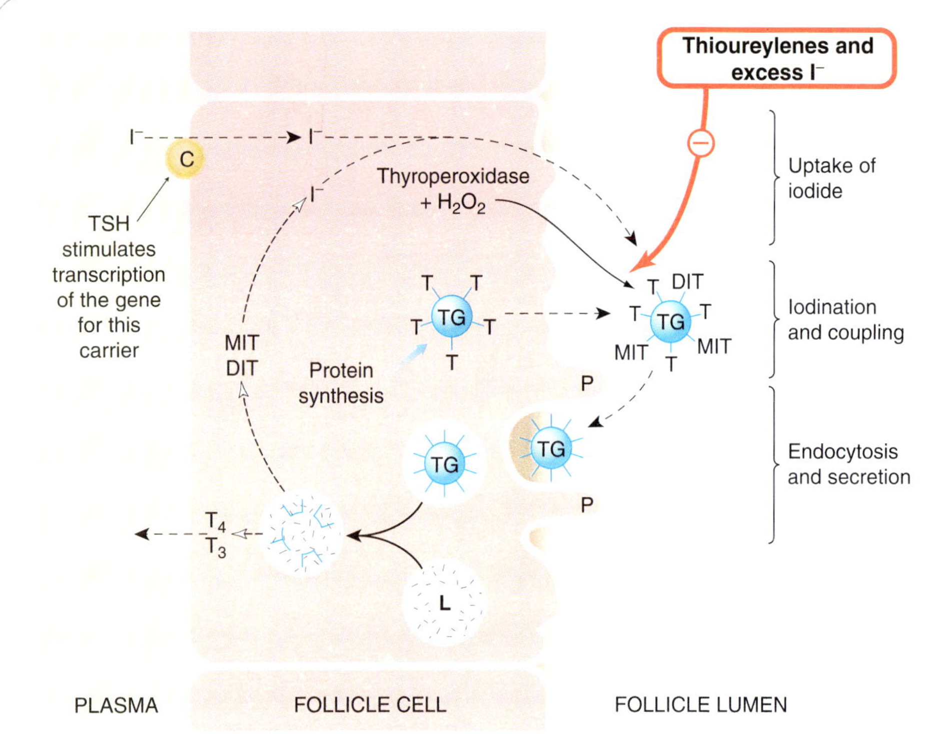

Fig. 28.1 Diagram of thyroid hormone synthesis and secretion with the sites of action of drugs which modify it. The carrier (C) is a symport that transports Na^+ and I^- into the cell. See text for details. (TSH, thyroid-stimulating hormone (thyrotrophin); TG, thyroglobulin; T, tyrosine; MIT, monoiodotyrosine; DIT, diiodotyrosine; T_4, thyroxine; T_3, triiodothyronine; L, lysosome; P, pseudopod.)

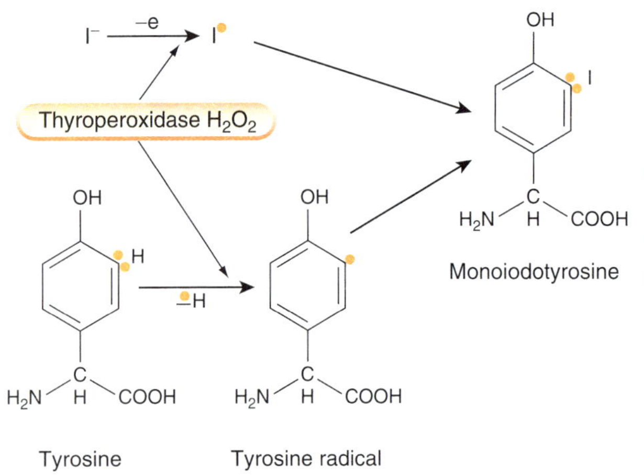

Fig. 28.2 Iodination of tyrosyl by the thyroperoxidase–H_2O_2 complex. This probably involves two sites on the enzyme, one of which removes an electron from iodide to give the free radical, I•; another removes a monohydrogen (monoelectron) from tyrosine to give the tyrosine radical (radical shown by the orange dot). Formation of monoiodotyrosine (MIT) results from addition of the two radicals.

endocytotic vesicles then fuse with lysosomes, proteolytic enzymes act on thyroglobulin, and T_4 and T_3 are released and secreted into the plasma. The MIT and DIT, which are released at the same time, are recaptured and metabolised within the cell, the iodide being removed enzymically and re-used.

REGULATION OF THYROID FUNCTION

Thyrotrophin-releasing hormone (TRH) from the hypothalamus releases thyroid-stimulating hormone (TSH; thyrotrophin) from the anterior pituitary (Fig. 28.4), as does **protirelin**, a synthetic tripeptide (pyroglutamyl-histidyl-proline amide). The actions and uses of protirelin are considered on page 406. Somatostatin (see p. 406) reduces basal TSH release.

The production of TSH is also influenced by a negative feedback effect of thyroid hormones, T_3 being more active than T_4.

The control of the secretion of TSH thus depends on a balance between the actions of T_4 and TRH, and probably also somatostatin, on the pituitary, but even high concentrations of thyroid hormone do not completely inhibit TSH secretion.

TSH acts on receptors on the membrane of thyroid follicle cells and its main second messenger is cAMP. It controls all aspects of thyroid hormone synthesis:

- the uptake of iodide by follicle cells, by stimulating transcription of the Na^+/I^- transporter gene; this is the main mechanism by which it regulates thyroid function
- the synthesis and secretion of thyroglobulin
- the generation of H_2O_2 and the iodination of tyrosine
- endocytosis and proteolysis of thyroglobulin
- secretion of T_3 and T_4
- the blood flow through the gland.

TSH also has a trophic action on the thyroid cells; it stimulates the action of the genes for thyroglobulin, thyroperoxidase (see below) and the Na^+/I^- transporter.

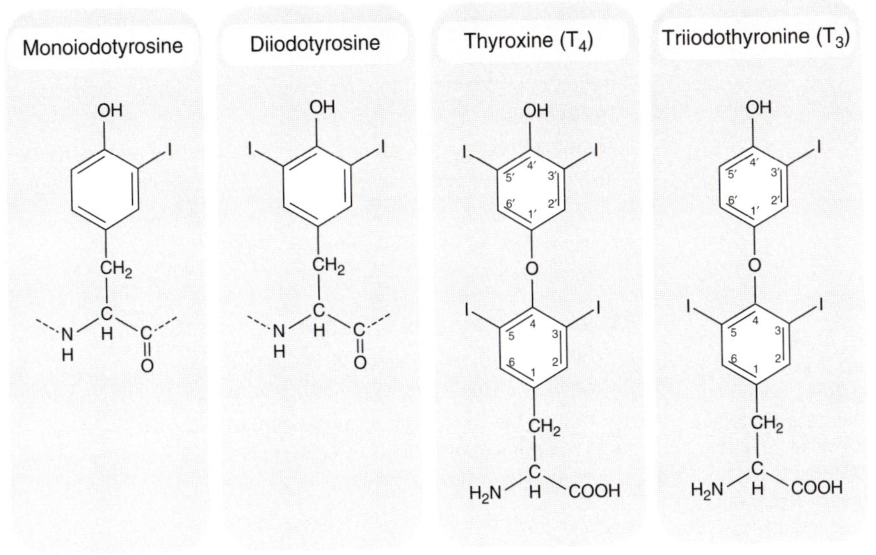

Fig. 28.3 Iodinated tyrosine residues. Monoiodotyrosine and diiodotyrosine are shown in peptide linkage, as in thyroglobulin. When T_4 is used as a drug it is given as the salt of the amino acid.

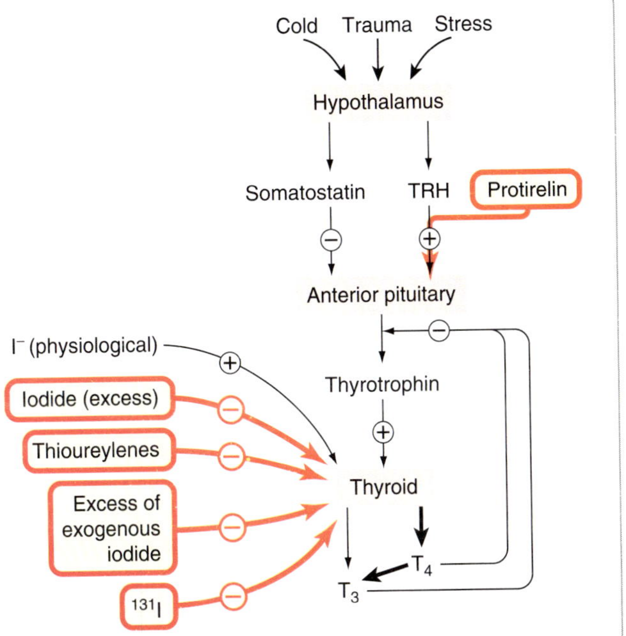

Fig. 28.4 Regulation of thyroid hormone secretion. Agents used clinically are shown in the red-bordered boxes. For the endogenous substances (shown in black) the thickness of the lines indicates the relative importance of each factor. Iodide (I^-) is essential for thyroid hormone synthesis, but excess of exogenous iodide (30× the daily requirement of iodine) inhibits the increased thyroid hormone production, which occurs in thyrotoxicosis. (TRH, thyrotrophin-releasing hormone; T_3, triiodothyronine; T_4, thyroxine.)

The other main factor influencing thyroid function is the plasma iodide concentration. About 100 nmol of T_4 is synthesised daily, necessitating the gland taking up approximately 500 nmol iodide each day (equivalent to about 70 mg iodine). A *reduced* iodine intake, with *reduced* plasma iodide concentration, will result in a decrease of hormone production and an increase in TSH secretion. An *increased* plasma iodide has the opposite effect, though this may be modified by other factors (see below). The overall feedback mechanism responds to changes of iodide only slowly—over fairly long periods, days or weeks, since there is a large reserve capacity for the binding and uptake of iodide in the thyroid. The size and vascularity of the thyroid are reduced by an increase in plasma iodide. A prolonged decrease of iodine in the diet results in a continuous excessive secretion of TSH and eventually in an increase in vascularity, and hypertrophy of the gland.

ACTIONS OF THE THYROID HORMONES

The physiological actions of the thyroid hormones fall into two categories:

- those affecting metabolism
- those affecting growth and development.

EFFECTS ON METABOLISM

The hormones are regulators of metabolism in most tissues, T_3 being three to five times more active than T_4 (Fig. 28.5). They produce a general increase in the metabolism of carbohydrates, fats and proteins. Most of these effects involve modulation of the actions of other hormones such as insulin, glucagon, the glucocorticoids and the catecholamines, although the thyroid hormones also control, directly, the activity of some of the enzymes of carbohydrate metabolism. There is an increase in oxygen consumption and heat production, which is manifested as an increase in the measured basal metabolic rate. This reflects action on some tissues, such as heart, kidney, liver and muscle, but not others, such as the gonads, brain and spleen. The

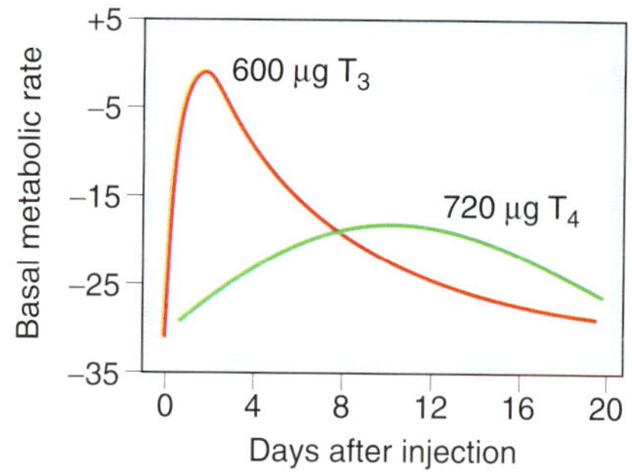

Fig. 28.5 Schematic diagram of the effect of single equimolar doses of triiodothyronine (T_3) and thyroxine (T_4) on basal metabolic rate in a hypothyroid subject. Note that this figure is meant only to illustrate overall differences in effect; thyroxine is not given clinically in a single bolus dose as here but in regular daily doses so that the effect builds up to a plateau. The apparent differences in potency really represent differences in kinetics, reflecting the prehormone role of T_4. (From: Blackburn C M et al. 1954 J Clin Invest 33: 819.)

calorigenic action is important as part of the response to a cold environment. Administration of thyroid hormone results in augmented cardiac rate and output and increased tendency to dysrhythmias such as atrial fibrillation.

EFFECTS ON GROWTH AND DEVELOPMENT

The thyroid hormones have a critical effect on growth, partly by a direct action on cells and partly indirectly by influencing growth hormone production and potentiating its effects. The hormones are important for a normal response to parathormone and calcitonin, and for skeletal development; they are particularly necessary for normal growth and maturation of the central nervous system (CNS).

MECHANISM OF ACTION

The hormones act by a mechanism rather similar to that of the steroids (Ch. 27 p. 413 and Fig. 27.6). After they enter the cell, T_4 is converted to T_3, which binds with high affinity to specific receptors associated with DNA in the nucleus. Consequently, T_4 can be regarded as a prohormone. There are several receptor isoforms, coded for by two distinct genes. Without bound ligand, the receptors repress basal transcription ('gene silencing'); a soluble corepressor complex is involved. When T_3 is bound, the receptors change conformation, the corepressor complex is released, a co-activator complex is recruited, which then activates transcription—resulting in generation of mRNA and protein synthesis.

TRANSPORT AND METABOLISM

The normal plasma concentrations of the hormones, which can be measured by radioimmunoassay, are 1×10^7 mol/l for T_4 and 2×10^9 mol/l for T_3. Both hormones are bound mainly to thyroxine-binding globulin (TBG).

The thyroid hormones are eventually degraded by deiodination, deamination and conjugation with glucuronic and sulfuric acids. This occurs mainly in the liver, and the free and conjugated forms are excreted partly in the bile and partly in the urine. The metabolic clearance of T_3 is 20 times faster than that of T_4 (which is about 6 days). The long half-life of T_4 is a consequence of its strong binding to TBG.

In summary:

- there is a large pool of T_4 in the body; it has a low turnover rate and is found mainly in the circulation
- there is a small pool of T_3 in the body; it has a fast turnover rate and is found mainly intracellularly
- T_3 is the active form at the cellular level, being formed from T_4 in target tissues.

ABNORMALITIES OF THYROID FUNCTION

HYPERTHYROIDISM (THYROTOXICOSIS)

In thyrotoxicosis, there is excessive activity of the thyroid hormones, resulting in a high metabolic rate, an increase in skin temperature and sweating and a marked sensitivity to heat. Nervousness, tremor, tachycardia, fatiguability and increased appetite associated with loss of weight occur. There are several types of hyperthyroidism but only two are common:

- diffuse toxic goitre (also called Graves' disease or exophthalmic goitre)
- toxic nodular goitre.

Diffuse toxic goitre is an organ-specific autoimmune disease caused by thyroid-stimulating immunoglobulins directed at the TSH receptor. Constitutively active mutations of the TRH receptor may be involved. As is indicated by the name, patients with exophthalmic goitre have protrusion of the eyeballs. The pathogenesis of this condition is not fully understood but it is thought to be caused by the presence of TSH receptor-like proteins in the tissues of the orbit. There is also increased sensitivity to catecholamines.

Toxic nodular goitre is caused by a benign neoplasm or adenoma and may develop in patients with long-standing simple goitre (see below). This condition does not usually have concomitant exophthalmos.

The antidysrhythmic drug **amiodarone** (Ch. 17) is rich in iodine and can cause either hyperthyroidism or hypothyroidism.

HYPOTHYROIDISM

A decreased activity of the thyroid results in hypothyroidism, and in severe cases myxoedema. It is immunological in origin and the manifestations are low metabolic rate, slow speech, deep hoarse voice, lethargy, bradycardia, sensitivity to cold and mental

The thyroid

- Thyroid hormones are synthesised by iodination of tyrosine residues on thyroglobulin within the lumen of the thyroid follicle.
- The thyroglobulin is endocytosed and thyroxine (T_4) and triiodothyronine (T_3) are secreted.
- Synthesis and secretion of T_3 and T_4 are regulated by thyroid-stimulating hormone (TSH; thyrotrophin) and influenced by plasma iodide.
- T_3 and T_4 actions are:
  - —o stimulate metabolism generally, causing increased oxygen consumption and increased metabolic rate
  - —to influence growth and development.
- Within cells, the T_4 is converted to T_3, which interacts with a nuclear receptor; the receptor represses basal transcription when not bound to T_3, and activates transcription when bound.
- There is a large pool of T_4 in the body; it has a low turnover rate and is found mainly in the circulation.
- There is a small pool of T_3 in the body; it has a fast turnover rate and is found mainly intracellularly.
- Abnormalities of thyroid function include:
  - —hyperthyroidism (thyrotoxicosis), either diffuse toxic goitre or toxic nodular goitre
  - —hypothyroidism; in adults this causes myxoedema, in infants, cretinism
  - —simple non-toxic goitre, caused by dietary iodine deficiency, usually with normal thyroid function.

impairment. Patients also develop a characteristic thickening of the skin, which gives myxoedema its name. *Hashimoto's thyroiditis*, a chronic autoimmune disease in which there is an immune reaction against thyroglobulin or some other component of thyroid tissue, can lead to hypothyroidism and myxoedema. Therapy of thyroid tumours with **radioiodine** (see below) is another cause of hypothyroidism.

Thyroid deficiency during development, caused by congenital absence or incomplete development of the thyroid, causes *cretinism*, which is characterised by gross retardation of growth and mental deficiency.

SIMPLE, NON-TOXIC GOITRE

A dietary deficiency of iodine, if prolonged, causes a rise in plasma TRH and eventually an increase in the size of the gland. This condition is known as simple or non-toxic goitre. Another cause is ingestion of goitrogens (e.g. from cassava root). The enlarged thyroid usually manages to produce normal amounts of thyroid hormone, though if the iodine deficiency is very severe, hypothyroidism may supervene.

DRUGS USED IN DISEASES OF THE THYROID

Drugs are used to treat both hyperthyroidism and hypothyroidism.

HYPERTHYROIDISM

Hyperthyroidism may be treated pharmacologically or surgically. In general, surgery is only used when there are mechanical problems resulting from compression of the trachea.

Although the condition of hyperthyroidism can be controlled with antithyroid drugs, the disease is not 'cured' since the drugs do not alter the underlying autoimmune mechanisms. Furthermore, there is little evidence that these drugs affect the course of the exophthalmos associated with Graves' disease.

RADIOIODINE

Radioiodine is a first-line treatment for hyperthyroidism (particularly in the USA). The isotope used is ^{131}I. Given orally, it is taken up and processed by the thyroid in the same way as the stable form of iodide, eventually becoming incorporated into thyroglobulin. It emits both β-particles and γ-rays. The γ-rays pass through the tissue, but the β-radiation has a very short range and exerts a cytotoxic action virtually restricted to the cells of the thyroid follicles—resulting in significant destruction. Iodine-131 has a half-life of 8 days; by 2 months its radioactivity has effectively disappeared. It is used in one single dose, but its cytotoxic effect on the gland is delayed for 1–2 months and does not reach its maximum for a further 2 months.

Hypothyroidism will eventually occur after treatment with radioiodine, particularly in patients with Graves' disease, but is easily managed by replacement therapy with thyroxine. Radioiodine is best avoided in children and also in pregnant patients because of potential damage to the fetus.

The uptake of ^{131}I and other isotopes of iodine may be used as a test of thyroid function. A tracer dose of the isotope is given orally or intravenously and the amount accumulated by the thyroid is measured by a gamma scintillation counter placed over the gland.

THIOUREYLENES

The thioureylenes used are **carbimazole**, **methimazole** and **propylthiouracil**. They are related to thiourea, the thiocarbamide group (S–C–N) being essential for antithyroid activity.

Action

Thioureylenes decrease the output of thyroid hormones from the gland and cause a gradual reduction in the signs and symptoms of thyrotoxicosis, the basal metabolic rate and pulse rate returning to normal over a period of 3–4 weeks. Their mode of action is not completely understood, but there is evidence that they inhibit the iodination of tyrosyl residues in thyroglobulin (see Figs 28.1,

28.2 and 28.6). It is thought that they inhibit the thyroperoxidase-catalysed oxidation reactions by acting as substrates for the postulated peroxidase–iodinium complex, thus competitively inhibiting the interaction with tyrosine. Propylthiouracil has the additional effect of reducing the de-iodination of T_4 to T_3 in peripheral tissues.

Pharmacokinetic aspects

Thioureylenes are given orally. **Carbimazole** is rapidly converted to methimazole. **Methimazole** is distributed throughout the body water and has a plasma half-life of 6–15 hours. An average dose of carbimazole produces more than 90% inhibition of thyroid organification of iodine within 12 hours. The clinical response to this and other antithyroid drugs, however, may take several weeks (Fig. 28.7). This is not only because T_4 has a long half-life but also because the thyroid may have large stores of hormone, which need to be depleted before the drug's action can be manifest. Propylthiouracil is thought to act somewhat more rapidly because of its effect in inhibiting peripheral conversion of T_4 to T_3.

Both methimazole and propylthiouracil cross the placenta and also appear in the milk, but this effect is less pronounced with propylthiouracil because it is more strongly bound to plasma protein. After degradation, the metabolites are excreted in the urine, propylthiouracil being excreted more rapidly than methimazole. The thioureylenes are not concentrated in the thyroid.

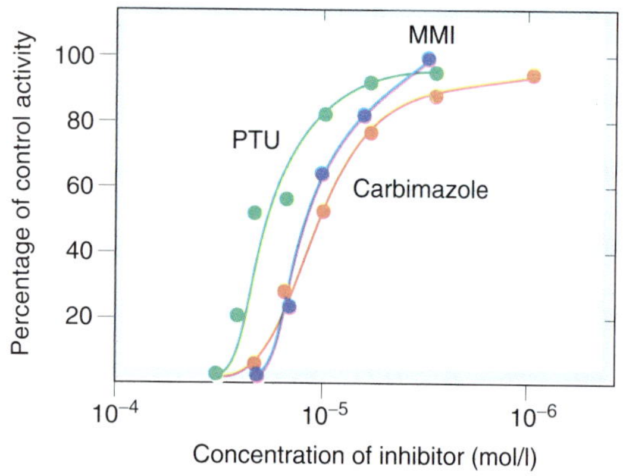

Fig. 28.6 Dose–response curves for inhibition of thyroperoxidase-catalysed iodination of thyroglobulin. The IC_{50} (dose giving 50% inhibition) for carbimazole is 10.5 μmol/l, for methimazole (MMI) is 11.5 μmol/l, and for propylthiouracil (PTU) is 18.5 μmol/l. (Modified from: Taurog A 1976 Endocrinology 98: 1031.)

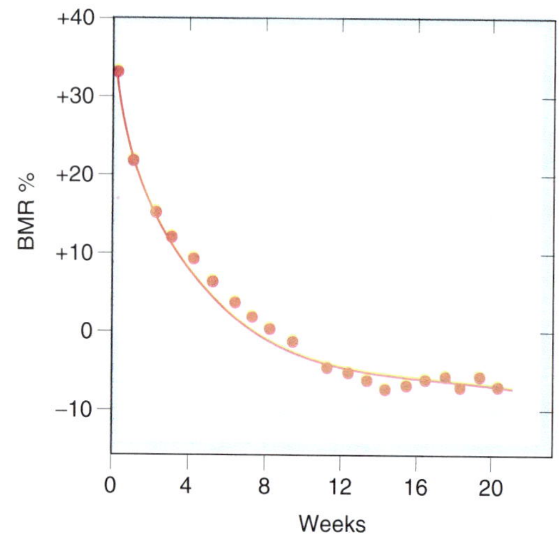

Fig. 28.7 Average time course of fall of basal metabolic rate (BMR) during treatment with an antithyroid drug, carbimazole. The curve is exponential, corresponding to a daily decrease in BMR of 3.4%. (From: Furth E O et al. 1963 J Clin Endocrinol Metab 23: 1130.)

Unwanted effects

The most important unwanted effect is granulocytopenia (see Ch. 52), which, fortunately, is relatively rare, having an incidence of 0.1–1.2% and being reversible if the drug is stopped. Rashes are more common (2–25%), and other symptoms such as headaches, nausea, jaundice and pain in the joints can occur.

IODINE/IODIDE

Iodine is converted in vivo to iodide (I^-), which temporarily inhibits the release of thyroid hormones. When high doses of iodine are given to thyrotoxic patients, the symptoms subside within 1–2 days. There is inhibition of the secretion of thyroid

Drugs in thyroid disease

Drugs for hyperthyroidism

- Radioiodine, given orally, is selectively taken up by thyroid and damages cells; it emits short-range β-radiation, which affects only thyroid follicle cells. Hypothyroidism will eventually occur.
- Thioureylenes (e.g. propylthiouracil) decrease the synthesis of thyroid hormones; the mechanism is through inhibition of thyroperoxidase, thus reducing iodination of thyroglobulin. They are given orally.
- Iodine, given orally in high doses, transiently reduces thyroid hormone secretion and decreases vascularity of the gland.

Drugs for hypothyroidism

- Thyroxine has all the actions of endogenous thyroxine, (see box on p. 425); it is given orally.
- Liothyronine has all the actions of endogenous triiodothyronine (see box on p. 425); it is given intravenously.

hormones and, over a period of 10–14 days, a marked reduction in vascularity of the gland, which becomes smaller and firmer. Iodine solution in potassium iodide ('Lugol's iodine') is given orally. With continuous administration its effect reaches maximum within 10–15 days and then decreases.

The mechanism of action is not entirely clear; it may inhibit iodination of thyroglobulin, possibly by inhibiting the H_2O_2 generation that is necessary for this process.

The main uses are for the preparation of hyperthyroid subjects for surgery and as part of the treatment of severe thyrotoxic crisis (thyroid storm).

Allergic reactions can occur: these include angio-oedema, rashes, drug fever, lacrimation, conjunctivitis, pain in the salivary glands and a cold-like syndrome.

OTHER DRUGS USED

The *β-adrenoceptor antagonists*, for example propranolol (Ch. 11), are not antithyroid agents, but they are useful for decreasing many of the signs and symptoms of hyperthyroidism—the tachycardia, dysrhythmias, tremor and agitation. They are used in preparation for surgery, for the initial treatment of most hyperthyroid patients while the thioureylenes or radioiodine are taking effect, and as part of the treatment of thyroid storm (acute hyperthyroid crisis).

Guanethidine, a noradrenergic-blocking agent (Ch. 10), is used in eye drops to ameliorate the exophthalmos of hyperthyroidism (which is not relieved by antithyroid drugs); it acts by relaxing the sympathetically innervated smooth muscle that causes eyelid retraction.

Glucocorticoids (e.g. prednisolone) or surgical decompression may be needed for the exophthalmia of Graves' disease.

Clinical use of drugs acting on the thyroid

Radioiodine

- As first-line treatment for hyperthyroidism; recurrence is rare provided the dose is adequate.
- For treatment of relapse of hyperthyroidism after carbimazole therapy or surgery.

Carbimazole (or propylthiouracil)

- Hyperthyroidism (diffuse toxic goitre), at least 1 year of treatment being necessary; recurrence occurs eventually in over half the patients but can be managed by a repeat course of treatment. Propylthiouracil can be used in patients who suffer sensitivity reactions to carbimazole.
- Preliminary to surgery for toxic goitre.
- Part of the treatment of thyroid storm (very severe hyperthyroidism); propylthiouracil is preferred because of its action in decreasing the conversion of T_4 to T_3 in the tissues. The β-adrenoceptor antagonists (e.g. propranolol) are also used to treat symptoms.

Thyroid hormones and iodine

- Thyroxine is the standard replacement therapy for hypothyroidism.
- Liothyronine (T_3) is the treatment of choice for myxoedema coma.
- Iodine dissolved in aqueous potassium iodide ('Lugol's iodine') is used short-term to control thyrotoxicosis preoperatively. It reduces the vascularity of the gland.

HYPOTHYROIDISM

There are no drugs that specifically augment the synthesis or release of thyroid hormones. The only effective treatment for hypothyroidism, unless it is caused by iodine deficiency (which is treated with iodide; see above), is to administer the thyroid hormones themselves—used as replacement therapy. **Thyroxine** and **triiodothyronine** (**liothyronine**) are available and are given orally. Thyroxine is the drug of choice, liothyronine being reserved for the rare condition of myxoedema coma, when its more rapid action is required for emergency treatment.

The actions and mechanisms of action of T_4 and T_3 are detailed in the box.

Unwanted effects may occur with overdose, and in addition to the signs and symptoms of hyperthyroidism there is a risk of precipitating angina pectoris, cardiac dysrhythmias or cardiac failure. The effects of less severe overdose are more insidious; the patient feels well but bone resorption is increased leading to osteoporosis.

The use of drugs acting on the thyroid is given in the clinical box.

REFERENCES AND FURTHER READING

Brent G A 1994 The molecular basis of thyroid hormone action. N Engl J Med 331: 847–854 (*A review covering receptor subtypes; T_3 regulation of genes in liver, adipocytes, cardiac and skeletal muscle; resistance to thyroid hormone*)

Franklin J A 1995 The management of hyperthyroidism. N Engl J Med 330: 1731–1738 (*An excellent review of the drug treatment of hyperthyroidism*)

Franklin J F, Sheppard M 1992 Radioiodine for hyperthyroidism: perhaps the best option. Br Med J 305: 728–729 (*An editorial commenting on the role of radioiodine in the treatment of thyrotoxicosis*)

Gittoes N J L, Franklyn J A 1998 Hyperthyroidism: Current treatment guidelines. Drugs 55: 543–553 (*Clinical approach to the therapy of hyperthyroidism*)

Hermus A R, Huysmans D A 1998 Treatment of benign nodular thyroid disease. N Engl J Med 338: 1438–1447

Lazarus J H 1997 Hyperthyroidism. Lancet 349: 339–343 (*A 'seminar' covering aetiology, clinical features, pathophysiology, diagnosis and treatment*)

Lindsay R S 1997 Hypothyroidism. Lancet 349: 413–417 (*A 'seminar' emphasising the management of hypothyroidism*)

Oppenheimer J H Schwartz H L et al. 1987 Advances in our understanding of thyroid action at the cellular level. Endocr Rev 8: 288–308 (*Early, general review of the molecular basis of thyroid hormone action at the nuclear level*)

Paschke R, Ludgate M 1997 The thyrotropin receptor and its diseases. N Engl J Med 337: 1675–1679 (*Up-to-date review on aspects of molecular biology*)

Perlmann T, Vennstrom B 1995 Nuclear receptors: the sound of silence. Nature 377: 387–388 (*A simple commentary on two articles that provide evidence that thyroid hormone silences basal transcription*)

Schmutzler C, Kohrle J 1998 Implications of the molecular characterization of the sodium–iodide symporter (NIS). Exp Clin Endocrinol Diabetes 106(CCV): S1–S10 (*Discusses the diagnostic and therapeutic implications of the information now available as a result of the cloning of NIS*)

Surks M I, Sievert R 1995 Drugs and thyroid function. N Engl J Med 333: 1688–1694 (*Review covering drugs affecting secretion of TSH, secretion of thyroid hormone, T_4 absorption, the transport of T_4 and T_3 in blood, and the metabolism of T_3 and T_4*)

Yen P M 2001 Physiological and molecular basis of thyroid hormone action Physiol Rev 81: 1097–1142 (*Comprehensive review of thyroid hormone–receptor interaction and the effects of thyroid hormone on target tissues*)

Zhang J, Lazar M 2000 The mechanism of action of thyroid hormones. Annu Rev Physiol 62: 439–466 (*Detailed review of the molecular aspects of thyroid hormone/receptor interaction*)

The reproductive system

29

Overview 429

Endocrine control of reproduction and modulating drugs 429
- Neurohormonal control of the female reproductive system 429
- Behavioural effects of sex hormones 431
- Oestrogens 431
- Anti-oestrogens 433
- Progestogens 434
- Antiprogestogens 434
- Postmenopausal hormone replacement therapy 434
- Neurohormonal control of the male reproductive system 435
- Androgens 436
- Anabolic steroids 437
- Anti-androgens 437
- Gonadotrophin-releasing hormone: agonists and antagonists 437
- Gonadotrophins and analogues 438

Drugs used for contraception 439
- Oral contraceptives 439
- Other drug regimens used for contraception 441

The uterus 441
- Drugs that stimulate uterine contraction 441
- Drugs that inhibit uterine contraction 443

Erectile dysfunction 443

OVERVIEW

Drugs that affect reproduction (both by preventing conception and more recently for treating infertility) have had profound consequences for individuals and for society. In this chapter, we describe the endocrine control of the female and male reproductive systems, since this forms the basis for understanding many important drugs. The principle of negative feedback, which is stressed, is central to understanding how hormones interact to control reproduction,* and many drugs, including agents used to prevent or assist conception, work by influencing negative feedback mechanisms. Oestrogen replacement therapy prevents postmenopausal bone loss as well as treating symptoms of oestrogen deficiency, benefits that are somewhat offset by effects on the endometrium and by an increase in thromboembolism. Oestrogen replacement is taken by large numbers of postmenopausal women and is considered in some detail. There is a separate section on drugs that alter the contractile state of the uterus, which are important in obstetrics: drugs that stimulate uterine contraction—'oxytocic' drugs—are used to induce labour or abortion and to prevent postpartum haemorrhage, whereas uterine relaxants are used, much less satisfactorily, to delay labour. There is a short final section on erectile dysfunction, since drugs used to treat this have recently made a remarkable transition from below-the-counter charlatanry to medical orthodoxy.

ENDOCRINE CONTROL OF REPRODUCTION AND MODULATING DRUGS

Hormonal control of the reproductive systems in men and women involves sex steroids from the gonads, hypothalamic peptides and glycoprotein gonadotrophins from the anterior pituitary.

NEUROHORMONAL CONTROL OF THE FEMALE REPRODUCTIVE SYSTEM

At puberty, an increased output of the hormones of the hypothalamus and anterior pituitary stimulates secretion of

*Recognition that negative feedback is central to endocrine control was a profound insight, made in 1930 by Dorothy Price, a laboratory assistant in the University of Chicago experimenting on effects of testosterone in rats. She referred to it as 'reciprocal influence'.

oestrogenic sex steroids. These are responsible for the maturation of the reproductive organs and the development of the secondary sexual characteristics, and also for a phase of accelerated growth followed by closure of the epiphyses of the long bones. Sex steroids are thereafter involved in the regulation of the cyclic changes expressed in the menstrual cycle and are important in pregnancy. A simplified outline of the inter-relationship of these substances in the physiological control of the menstrual cycle is given in Figures 29.1 and 29.2.

The menstrual cycle begins with *menstruation*, which lasts for 3–6 days during which the superficial layer of uterine endometrium is shed. The endometrium regenerates during the *follicular phase* of the cycle after menstrual flow has stopped. A releasing factor, the *gonadotrophin-releasing hormone* (GnRH), is secreted from peptidergic neurons in the hypothalamus in a pulsatile fashion, the frequency being about 1 burst of discharges per hour, and stimulates the anterior pituitary to release gonadotrophic hormones (Fig. 29.1)—*follicle-stimulating hormone* (FSH) and *luteinising hormone* (LH). These act on the ovaries (Fig. 29.2A) to promote development of small groups of follicles, each of which contains an ovum. One follicle develops faster than the others and forms the Graafian follicle (Figs 29.1 and 29.2E), and the rest degenerate. The ripening Graafian follicle consists of thecal and granulosa cells surrounding a fluid-filled centre within which lies an ovum. Oestrogens are produced by the granulosa cells stimulated by FSH, from androgen

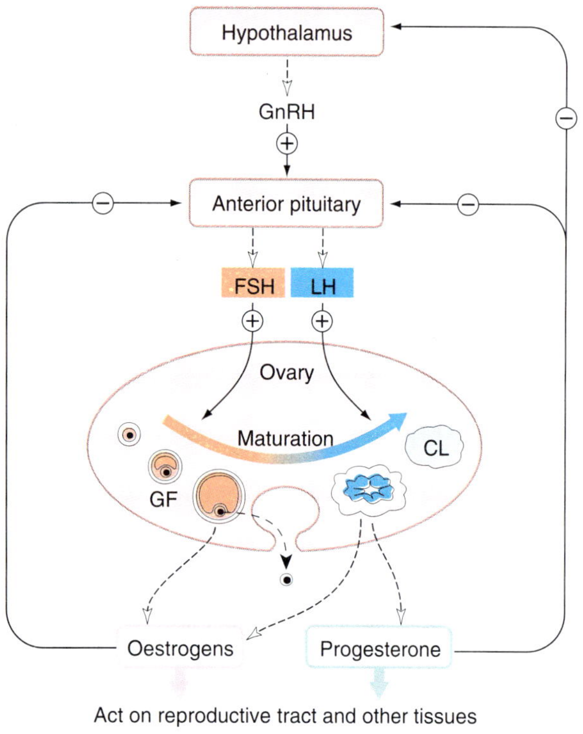

Fig. 29.1 Hormonal inter-relationship in the control of the female reproductive system. The Graafian follicle (GF) is shown developing on the left, then involuting to form the corpus luteum (CL) on the right, after the ovum (•) has been released. (LH, luteinising hormone; FSH, follicle-stimulating hormone; GnRH, gonadotrophin-releasing hormone)

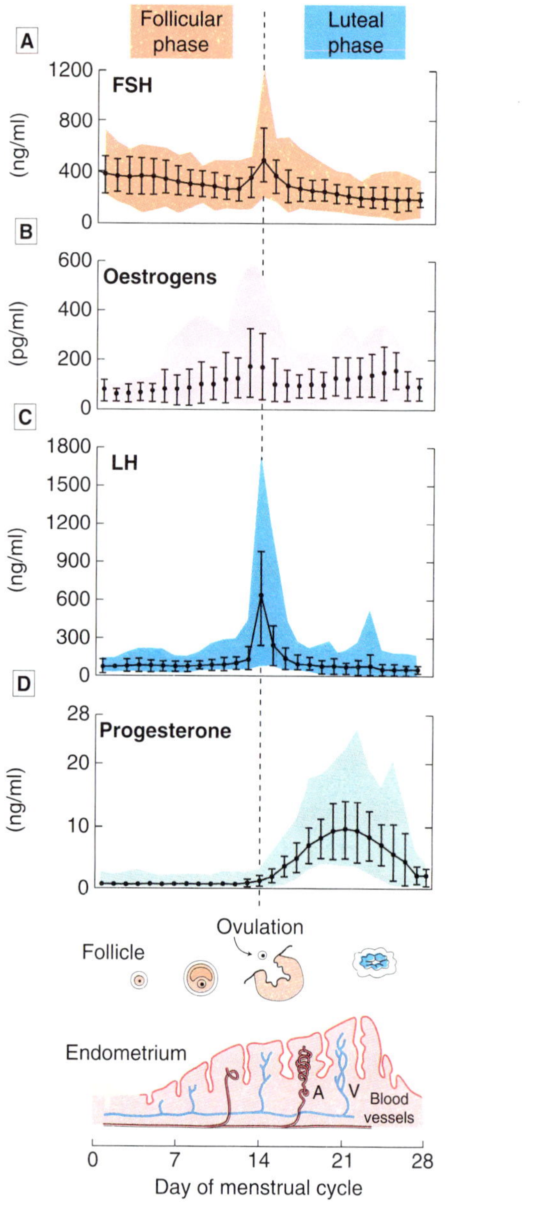

Fig. 29.2 Plasma concentrations of ovarian hormones and gonadotrophins in women during normal menstrual cycles. Values are the mean ± standard deviation of 40 women. The shaded areas indicate the entire range of observations. Day 1 is the onset of menstruation. E and F show diagrammatically the changes in the ovarian follicle and the endometrium during the cycle. Ovulation on day 14 of the menstrual cycle occurs with the midcycle peak of LH, represented by the vertical dashed line. (LH, luteinising hormone; FSH, follicle-stimulating hormone; A, arterioles; V, venules.) (After: van de Wiele R L, Dyrenfurth I 1974 Pharmacol Rev 25: 189–217.)

precursor molecules derived from thecal cells stimulated by LH. Oestrogens are responsible for the proliferative phase of endometrial regeneration, which occurs from day 5 or 6 until midcycle (Fig. 29.2B,F). During this phase, the endometrium increases in thickness and vascularity, and at the peak of oestrogen secretion there is a prolific cervical secretion of mucus of pH 8–9, rich in protein and carbohydrate, which facilitates entry of spermatozoa. Oestrogen has a negative feedback effect on the anterior pituitary, decreasing gonadotrophin release during chronic administration of oestrogen as oral contraception (see below). In contrast, the high endogenous oestrogen secretion just before midcycle sensitises LH-releasing cells of the pituitary to the action of the GnRH and causes the midcycle surge of LH secretion (Fig. 29.2C). This, in turn, causes rapid swelling and rupture of the Graafian follicle, resulting in ovulation. If fertilisation occurs, the fertilised ovum passes down the fallopian tubes to the uterus, starting to divide as it goes.

Stimulated by LH, cells of the ruptured follicle proliferate and develop into the corpus luteum, which secretes progesterone. Progesterone acts, in turn, on oestrogen-primed endometrium, stimulating the *secretory phase* of the cycle, which renders the endometrium suitable for the implantation of a fertilised ovum. During this phase, cervical mucus becomes more viscous, less alkaline, less copious and in general less welcoming for sperm. Progesterone exerts negative feedback on hypothalamus and pituitary, decreasing the release of LH. It also has a thermogenic effect, causing a rise in body temperature of about 0.5°C at ovulation, which is maintained until the end of the cycle.

Hormonal control of the female reproductive system

- The menstrual cycle starts with menstruation.
- Hypothalamic gonadatrophin-releasing hormone (GnRH) acts on the anterior pituitary to release the gonadotrophins follicle-stimulating hormone (FSH) and luteinising hormone (LH), which act on the ovary.
- The gonadotrophins stimulate follicle development. FSH is the main hormone stimulating oestrogen release. LH stimulates ovulation at midcycle and is the main hormone controlling subsequent progesterone secretion from the corpus luteum.
- Oestrogen controls the proliferative phase of the endometrium and has negative feedback effects on the anterior pituitary. Progesterone controls the later secretory phase and has negative feedback effects on both hypothalamus and anterior pituitary.
- If a fertilised ovum is implanted, the corpus luteum continues to secrete progesterone.
- After implantation, human chorionic gonadotrophin (HCG) from the chorion becomes important, and later in pregnancy progesterone and other hormones are secreted by the placenta.

If implantation of the ovum does not occur, progesterone secretion stops, triggering menstruation. If implantation does occur, the corpus luteum continues to secrete progesterone, which, by its effect on the hypothalamus and anterior pituitary, prevents further ovulation. The chorion (an antecedent of the placenta) secretes *human chorionic gonadotrophin* (HCG), which maintains the lining of the womb during pregnancy. For reasons that are not physiologically obvious, HCG has an additional pharmacological action in stimulating ovulation. As pregnancy proceeds, the placenta develops further hormonal functions and secretes a gamut of hormone variants (often with post-translational modifications), including *gonadotrophins* as well as *progesterone* and *oestrogens*. Progesterone secreted during pregnancy controls the development of the secretory alveoli in the mammary gland, while oestrogen stimulates the lactiferous ducts. After parturition, oestrogens, along with *prolactin* (see Ch. 27, pp. 407–408), are responsible for stimulating and maintaining lactation, whereas high doses of exogenous oestrogen suppress this.

Oestrogens are dealt with below, progestogens (progesterone-like drugs) on page 434, androgens on page 436, and the gonadotrophins on page 438.

BEHAVIOURAL EFFECTS OF SEX HORMONES

As well as controlling the menstrual cycle, sex steroids affect sexual behaviour. Two types of control are recognised, namely organisational and activational. The former refers to the fact that sexual differentiation of the brain can be permanently altered by the presence or absence of sex steroids at a key stage in development.

In rats, administration of androgens to females within a few days of birth results in long-term virilisation of behaviour. Conversely, neonatal castration of male rats causes them to develop behaviourally as females. Brain development in the absence of sex steroids follows female lines, but it is switched to the male pattern by exposure of the hypothalamus to androgen at a key stage of development. Similar but less-complete behavioural virilisation of female offspring has been demonstrated following androgen administration in non-human primates and probably also occurs in humans if pregnant women secrete, or are treated with, androgens.

The activational effect of sex steroids refers to their ability to modify sexual behaviour after brain development is complete. In general, oestrogens and androgens increase sexual activity in the appropriate sex. *Oxytocin*, which is important during parturition (see below), also has roles in mating and parenting behaviours, its action in the central nervous system being regulated by oestrogen.

OESTROGENS

Oestrogens are synthesised by the ovary and placenta, and, in small amounts, by the testis and adrenal cortex. As for other steroids the starting substance for oestrogen synthesis is cholesterol. The immediate precursors to the oestrogens are androgenic substances—androstenedione or testosterone (Fig. 29.3). There are three main endogenous oestrogens in humans—*oestradiol*, *oestrone* and *oestriol* (Fig. 29.3). Oestradiol is the most potent and is the principal oestrogen secreted by the ovary. At the beginning of the menstrual cycle, the plasma concentration is 0.2 nmol/l rising to ~2.2 nmol/l in midcycle.

Actions

Oestrogen acts in concert with progesterone and induces synthesis of progesterone receptors in uterus, vagina, anterior pituitary and hypothalamus. Conversely, progesterone *decreases* oestrogen receptor expression in the reproductive tract, by reducing their synthesis. Prolactin (see Ch. 27) also influences oestrogen action by increasing the numbers of oestrogen receptors in the mammary gland but has no effect on oestrogen receptor expression in the uterus.

Effects of exogenous oestrogen depend on the state of sexual maturity when the oestrogen is administered:

- in primary hypogonadism: oestrogen stimulates development of secondary sexual characteristics and accelerates growth
- in adults with primary amenorrhoea: oestrogen, given cyclically with a progestogen, induces an artificial cycle
- in sexually mature women: oestrogen (with a progestagen) is contraceptive
- at or after the menopause: oestrogen replacement prevents menopausal symptoms and bone loss.

Oestrogens have several metabolic actions, including mineralocorticoid (retention of salt and water) and mild anabolic actions. They increase plasma concentrations of high density lipoproteins, a potentially beneficial effect (Ch. 19) that may contribute to the relatively low risk of atheromatous disease in premenopausal women compared with men of the same age. Oestrogens increase the coagulability of blood, and contraceptive pills containing a high oestrogen content increase the risk of thromboembolism. This effect is dose related.

Mechanism of action

As with other steroids, oestrogen binds to intracellular receptors. There are at least two types of oestrogen receptor, termed ER_α and ER_β, the roles of which are currently being investigated using mice in which the gene coding one or other of these has been 'knocked out' (Ch. 53). Binding is followed by interaction of the resultant complexes with nuclear sites and subsequent genomic effects—either gene transcription (i.e. DNA-directed RNA and protein synthesis) or gene repression (inhibition of transcription). More details are given in Chapters 3 and 27; see especially Figure 27.6. In addition to these 'classical' intracellular receptors, evidence is emerging that some oestrogen effects, in particular its rapid vascular actions, may be mediated via membrane receptors. Acute vasodilatation caused by 17-β-oestradiol is mediated by nitric oxide, and a plant-derived ('phyto-') oestrogen called **genistein** (which is selective for ER_β, as well as having quite distinct effects from inhibition of protein kinase C) is as potent as 17-β-oestradiol in this regard. There is considerable therapeutic interest in receptor-selective oestrogen agonists or antagonists for different indications. One drug, **raloxifene**, has been dubbed a 'selective oestrogen receptor modulator' (SERM). It has antioestrogenic effects on breast and endometrial tissue but oestrogenic effects on bone, lipid metabolism and blood coagulation. It is licensed in the UK for treatment and prevention of postmenopausal osteoporosis. Unlike hormone replacement treatment (HRT, see below), raloxifene does not improve menopausal flushing; however, among postmenopausal women with osteoporosis, its use decreased the risk of breast cancer by nearly 80% during a 3 year randomised controlled trial. A related drug, **teripatide,** is being developed for osteoporosis in men as well as women. Other agents with different specificities are in development, and oestrogen receptor pharmacology is a space worth watching!

Preparations

Many preparations (oral, transdermal, intramuscular, implantable and topical) of oestrogens are available for a wide range of

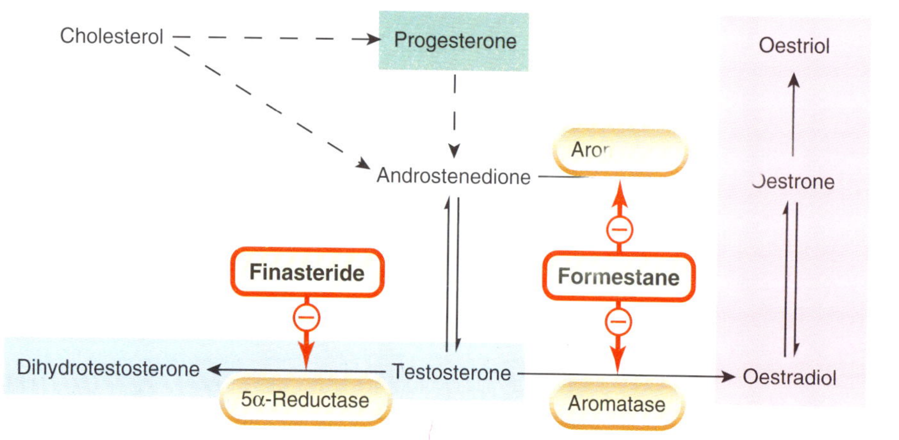

Fig. 29.3 The biosynthetic pathway for the androgens and oestrogens with sites of drug action. (See also Fig. 27.5.) Finasteride is used in benign prostatic hyperplasia and formestane to treat breast cancer in postmenopausal women.

Clinical use of oestrogens and anti-oestrogens

Oestrogens

- Replacement therapy:
  —primary ovarian failure (e.g. Turner's syndrome)
  —secondary ovarian failure (menopause) for flushing, vaginal dryness and to preserve bone mass.
- Contraception
- Prostate and breast cancer (these uses have largely been superseded by other hormonal manipulations; see Ch. 50).

Anti-oestrogens

- To treat oestrogen-sensitive breast cancer (tamoxifen).
- To induce ovulation (clomiphene) in treating infertility.

indications. These preparations include natural (e.g. **estradiol**, **estriol**) and synthetic (e.g. **mestranol**, **ethinylestradiol**, **stilbestrol**) oestrogens. Oestrogens are presented either as single agents or combined with progestagen. Very different doses of oestrogen are used for different conditions, for example ethinylestradiol is used in a dose of 10–20 μg/day for postmenopausal hormone replacement therapy, 20–50 μg/day in the combined contraceptive pill, 1–3 mg/day for breast cancer.

The clinical use of oestrogens and anti-oestrogens is given in the box.

Pharmacokinetic aspects

Natural as well as synthetic oestrogens are well absorbed in the gastrointestinal tract, but after absorption, the natural oestrogens are rapidly metabolised in the liver, whereas synthetic oestrogens are degraded less rapidly. There is a variable amount of enterohepatic cycling, which forms the basis for drug interaction since broad-spectrum antibiotic use alters bowel flora and can thereby render oral contraception ineffective. Most oestrogens are readily absorbed from skin and mucous membranes. They may be given topically in the vagina as creams or pessaries for local effect. In the plasma, natural oestrogens are bound to albumin and to a sex-steroid-binding globulin. Natural oestrogens are excreted in the urine as glucuronides and sulfates.

Unwanted effects

Unwanted effects of oestrogens include tenderness in the breasts, nausea, vomiting, anorexia, retention of salt and water with resultant oedema, and increased risk of thromboembolism. More details of the unwanted effects of oral contraceptives are given on pages 439–440.

Used intermittently for postmenopausal replacement therapy, oestrogens cause menstruation-like bleeding. Oestrogen causes endometrial hyperplasia unless given cyclically with a progestogen. When administered to males, oestrogens result in feminisation.

Oestrogen administration to pregnant women can cause genital abnormalities in their offspring. Carcinoma of the vagina was more common in young women whose mothers were given stilbestrol in early pregnancy in a misguided attempt to prevent miscarriage (see Ch. 52).

ANTI-OESTROGENS

Anti-oestrogens compete with natural oestrogens for receptors in target organs. **Tamoxifen** has anti-oestrogenic action on mammary tissue but oestrogenic actions on plasma lipids, endometrium and bone. It produces mild oestrogen-like adverse effects consistent with partial agonist activity. The tamoxifen–oestrogen receptor complex does not readily dissociate, so there is interference with the recycling of receptors.

Tamoxifen upregulates transforming growth factor-β (TGF-β), decreased function of which is associated with the progression of malignancy; this may play a part in its anticancer action. The anti-osteoporotic action of tamoxifen may also be related to upregulation of TGF-β since this cytokine has a role in controlling the balance between bone-producing osteoblasts and bone-resorbing osteoclasts (Ch. 30).

Tamoxifen is discussed further in Chapter 50.

Clomiphene inhibits oestrogen binding in the anterior pituitary, so preventing the normal modulation by negative feedback and causing increased secretion of GnRH and

Oestrogens and anti-oestrogens

- The endogenous oestrogens are oestradiol (the most potent), oestrone and oestriol; there are numerous exogenous synthetic forms, e.g. ethinylestradiol.
- Mechanism of action involves interaction with intracellular receptors (termed ERα or ERβ) in target tissues, resulting in modification of gene transcription.
- The pharmacological effects depend on the sexual maturity of the recipient:
  —before puberty they stimulate development of the secondary sexual characteristics
  —given cyclically in the adult female they induce an artificial menstrual cycle and are used for contraception
  —given at or after the menopause they prevent menopausal symptoms and protect against osteoporosis.
- Anti-oestrogens are competitive antagonists or partial agonists. Tamoxifen is used in oestrogen-dependent breast cancer. Clomiphene induces ovulation by inhibiting the negative feedback effects on the hypothalamus and anterior pituitary.
- Selective drugs that are oestrogen agonists in some tissues but antagonists in others are being developed. Raloxifene (one such drug) is used to treat and prevent osteoporosis; it also protects against breast cancer.

gonadotrophins. This results in a marked stimulation and enlargement of the ovaries and increased oestrogen secretion. The main effect of their anti-oestrogen action in the pituitary is that they induce ovulation. These compounds are used in treating infertility caused by lack of ovulation. Twins are common, but multiple pregnancy is unusual.

PROGESTOGENS

The natural progestational hormone ('progestogen') is progesterone (see Figs 29.2 and 29.3). This is secreted by the corpus luteum in the second part of the menstrual cycle, and by the placenta during pregnancy. Small amounts are also secreted by testis and adrenal cortex.

Mechanism of action

Progestogens act, as do other steroid hormones, on intracellular receptors. The density of progesterone receptors is controlled by oestrogens (see above).

Preparations

There are two main groups of progestogens.

- The naturally occurring hormone and its derivatives (e.g. **hydroxyprogesterone, medroxyprogesterone, dyhydrogesterone**). Progesterone itself is virtually inactive orally because after absorption it is metabolised in the liver and hepatic extraction is nearly complete. Other preparations are available for oral administration, intramuscular injection or via the vagina or rectum.
- Testosterone derivatives (e.g. **norethisterone**, **norgestrel**, and **ethynodiol**) can be given orally. The first two have some androgenic activity and are metabolised to give oestrogenic products. Newer progestogens used in contraception include **desogestrel** and **gestodene**; they may have less adverse effects on lipids than ethynodiol and may be considered for women who experience side-effects such as acne, depression or breakthrough bleeding with the older drugs. However, these newer drugs have been associated with higher risks of venous thromboembolic disease (see below).

Actions

The pharmacological actions of the progestogens are in essence the same as the physiological actions of progesterone described above. Specific effects relevant to contraception are detailed on pages 439–440.

Pharmacokinetic aspects

Injected progesterone is bound to albumin, not to the sex-steroid-binding globulin. Some is stored in adipose tissue. It is metabolised in the liver, and the products, pregnanolone and pregnanediol, are conjugated with glucuronic acid and excreted in the urine.

Unwanted effects

Unwanted effects of progestagens include weak androgenic actions of some of the progestogens derived from testosterone.

Progestogens and antiprogestogens

- The endogenous hormone is progesterone. Examples of synthetic drugs are the progesterone derivative medroxyprogesterone, and the testosterone derivative norethisterone.
- Mechanism of action involves intracellular receptor/altered gene expression as for other steroid hormones. Oestrogen stimulates synthesis of progesterone receptors, whereas progesterone inhibits synthesis of oestrogen receptors.
- Main therapeutic uses are in oral contraception and oestrogen replacement regimens, and to treat endometriosis.
- The antiprogestogen mifepristone, in combination with prostaglandin analogues, is an effective medical alternative to surgical termination of early pregnancy.

Other unwanted effects include acne, fluid retention, weight change, depression, change in libido, breast discomfort, premenstrual symptoms, irregular menstrual cycles and breakthrough bleeding. There is an increased incidence of thromboembolism.

Clinical use

Clinical uses are summarised in the box on page 435.

ANTIPROGESTOGENS

Mifepristone is a partial agonist at progesterone receptors. It sensitises the uterus to the action of prostaglandins. It is given orally and has a plasma half-life of 21 hours. Mifepristone is used as a medical alternative to surgical termination of pregnancy (see box). If given in the late follicular phase of the menstrual cycle, mifepristone inhibits ovulation and hence has potential as a postcoital contraceptive agent.

POSTMENOPAUSAL HORMONE REPLACEMENT THERAPY

At the menopause, either natural or surgically induced, ovarian function decreases and oestrogen levels fall. Gonadotrophin secretion increases because of loss of negative feedback. Oestrogen replacement (HRT) has some clear-cut benefits:

- improvement of symptoms caused by reduced oestrogen, for example vasomotor symptoms (hot flushes) and vaginitis
- prevention and treatment of osteoporosis.

Additional *possible* benefits of oestrogen replacement have been suggested.

- A possible reduction in the risk of coronary heart disease (the commonest cause of death in postmenopausal women);

Clinical use of progestogens and anti-progestogens

Progestogens
- Contraception:
  - —with oestrogen in combined oral contraceptive pill
  - —as progesterone-only contraceptive pill
  - —as injectable or implantable progesterone-only contraception
  - —as part of an intrauterine contraceptive system.
- Combined with oestrogen for long-term oestrogen replacement therapy in women with an intact uterus, to prevent endometrial hyperplasia and carcinoma.
- For endometriosis.
- As second- or third-line in breast cancer; also in endometrial and renal carcinoma.
- Poorly validated uses have included various menstrual disorders.

Anti-progestogens
- Medical termination of pregnancy: mifepristone (partial agonist) combined with a prostaglandin (e.g. gemeprost).

epidemiological studies suggest that there is a 50% reduction, but a large randomised controlled trial of secondary prevention was negative. Further randomised trials of primary prevention in somewhat younger postmenopausal women are under way.
- Some observational studies have raised the possibility that women on HRT have a reduced incidence and/or a delayed onset of Alzheimer's disease, but other studies have not. There are no data so far from randomised trials.

The use of HRT has some definite drawbacks.

- Uterine bleeding; this occurs if withdrawal of oestrogen and cyclical progestogens are included in the HRT regimen as is needed unless the woman has had a hysterectomy.
- Mood changes and other, usually mild, adverse effects related to progestogen (see above).
- An increased risk of endometrial cancer if oestrogen is given unopposed by progestogen. Progestogens are, therefore, given, usually for 10 days each month, to women with an intact uterus.
- An increase in the risk of breast cancer, related to the duration of HRT use and disappearing within 5 years of stopping. The epidemiological evidence suggests that about 45 women in 1000 aged 50 and not using HRT will have breast cancer diagnosed during the next 20 years; this is increased by 2 cases (in 1000) among those using HRT for 5 years, by 6 for those using it for 10 years and by 12 for those using it for 15 years (BNF, 2001). This contrasts dramatically with **raloxifene**, which prevents postmenopausal osteoporosis without improving vasomotor symptoms of oestrogen deficiency but *reduces* the risk of breast cancer (see above).
- An increased risk of venous thromboembolism. This is not so great as to affect the overall positive balance of benefit to risk of HRT for most women, but shifts this unfavourably in women who have other risk factors for venous thrombosis.

Oestrogens used in HRT can be given orally (conjugated estrogens, estradiol, estriol), vaginally (estriol), by transdermal patch (estradiol) or by subcutaneous implant (estradiol). **Tibolone** is marketed for the treatment of postmenopausal symptoms and prevention of osteoporosis. It has oestrogenic, progestogenic and weak androgenic activity and can be used continuously without cyclical progesterone (avoiding the inconvenience of withdrawal bleeding).

There is still some controversy about the use of HRT—see Toozs-Hobson & Cardozo (1996) versus Jacobs (1996) and Khaw (1998)—but many authorities consider that the benefits outweigh the risks for most women. One 20-year retrospective study using data from 34 000 women showed a 20% reduction in overall mortality for HRT users, the reduction being greater for women with a higher risk of coronary disease. Survival benefit decreases with longer duration of use (see Brinton & Schairer, 1997).

NEUROHORMONAL CONTROL OF THE MALE REPRODUCTIVE SYSTEM

As in the female, endocrine secretions from the hypothalamus, anterior pituitary and gonads control the male reproductive system. A simplified outline of the inter-relationship of these factors is given in Figure 29.4. GnRH controls the secretion of gonadotrophins by the anterior pituitary. This secretion is not cyclical as in menstruating women; in both sexes it is pulsatile (see below). FSH is responsible for the integrity of the seminiferous tubules and, after puberty, is important in gametogenesis through an action on *Sertoli cells,* which nourish and support developing spermatozoa. LH, which in the male is also called interstitial cell stimulating hormone (ICSH), stimulates the interstitial cells (*Leydig cells*) to secrete androgens—in particular *testosterone*. LH/ICSH secretion begins at puberty, and the consequent secretion of testosterone causes maturation of the reproductive organs and development of secondary sexual characteristics. Thereafter, the primary function of testosterone is the maintenance of spermatogenesis and hence fertility—an action mediated by Sertoli cells. Testosterone is also important in the maturation of spermatozoa as they pass through the epididymis and vas deferens. A further action is a feedback effect on the anterior pituitary, modulating its sensitivity to GnRH and thus influencing secretion of LH/ICSH. Testosterone has marked anabolic effects, causing development of the musculature and increased bone growth, resulting in a rapid increase in height (the pubertal growth spurt) at puberty, followed by closure of the epiphyses of the long bones.

Secretion of testosterone is mainly controlled by LH/ICSH, but FSH also plays a part, possibly by releasing a factor similar to

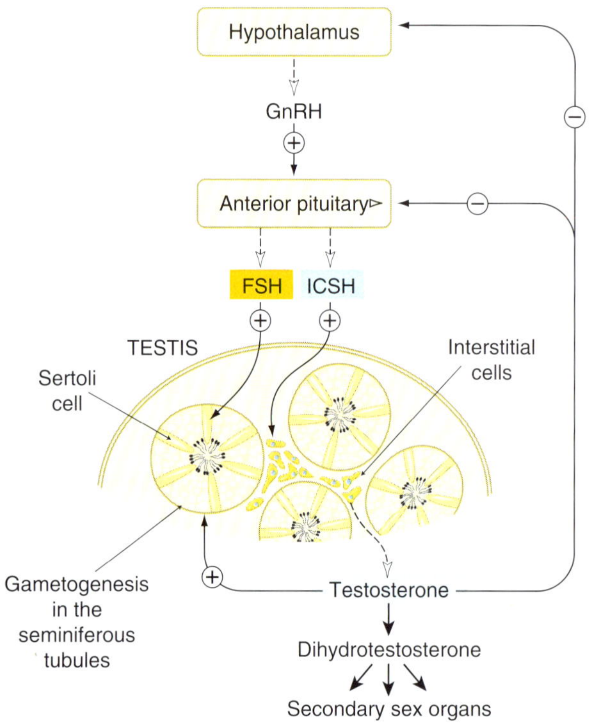

Fig. 29.4 Hormonal inter-relationships in the control of the male reproductive system. (GnRH, gonadotrophin-releasing hormone; FSH, follicle-stimulating hormone; ICSH, interstitial-cell-stimulating hormone (equivalent to luteinising hormone in the female).)

GnRH from the Sertoli cells (which are its primary target). The interstitial cells that synthesise testosterone also have receptors for prolactin, which may influence testosterone production by increasing the number of receptors for LH/ICSH.

ANDROGENS

Testosterone is the main natural androgen. It is synthesised mainly by the interstitial cells of the testis, and in smaller amounts by the ovaries and adrenal cortex. Adrenal production of androgens is under the control of adrenocorticotrophic hormone (ACTH, corticotrophin). As for other steroid hormones, cholesterol is the starting substance. Dehydroepiandrosterone and androstenedione are important intermediates. They are released from the gonads and the adrenal cortex and converted to testosterone in the liver (see Fig. 29.3).

Actions

In general, the effects of exogenous androgens are the same as those of testosterone and depend on the age and sex of the recipient. If administered to boys at the age of puberty, there is rapid development of the secondary sexual characteristics, maturation of the reproductive organs and a marked increase in muscular strength. Height increases more gradually. The anabolic effects can be accompanied by retention of salt and water. The skin thickens and may darken, and sebaceous glands become more active (which can result in acne). There is growth of hair on the face and on pubic and axillary regions. The vocal cords hypertrophy, resulting in a lower pitch to the voice. Androgens cause a feeling of well-being and an increase in physical vigour and may increase libido. Whether they are responsible for sexual behaviour as such is controversial, as is their contribution to aggressive behaviour.

If given to prepubertal males, the individuals concerned do not reach their full predicted height because of premature closure of the epiphyses of the long bones.

Administration to women results in masculinisation.

Androgens and the hormonal control of the male reproductive system

- Gonadatrophin-releasing hormone (GnRH) from the hypothalamus acts on the anterior pituitary to release both follicle-stimulating hormone (FSH), which stimulates gametogenesis, and luteinising hormone (LH; also called interstitial-cell-stimulating hormone), which stimulates androgen secretion.
- The endogenous hormone is testosterone; an exogenous preparation is mesterolone.
- Mechanism of action is via intracellular receptors.
- Effects depend on age/sex and include development of male secondary sexual characteristics in prepubertal boys and masculination in women.

Mechanism of action

In most target cells, testosterone works through an active metabolite, *dihydrotestosterone,* to which it is converted locally by a 5α-reductase enzyme. In contrast, testosterone itself causes virilisation of the genital tract in the male embryo and regulates LH/ICSH production in anterior pituitary cells. Both testosterone and dihydrotestosterone modify gene transcription by interacting with intracellular receptors, in common with other steroids.

Preparations

Testosterone itself can be given by subcutaneous implantation. Various esters (e.g. enanthate and proprionate) are given by intramuscular depot injection. Testosterone undecanoate and mesterolone can be given orally.

Pharmacokinetic aspects

If given orally, testosterone is rapidly metabolised in the liver. It is, therefore, usually injected. Virtually all testosterone in the circulation is bound to plasma protein—mainly to the sex-steroid-binding globulin. The elimination half-life of free testosterone is short (10–20 minutes). It is inactivated in the liver by conversion to androstenedione (see Fig. 29.3). This has weak androgenic activity in its own right and can be reconverted to testosterone, although approximately 90% of testosterone is eliminated as metabolites rather than the parent compound. Synthetic

Clinical use of androgens and anti-androgens

- Androgens (testosterone preparations) are used for replacement therapy in testicular failure and as anabolic agents.
- Anti-androgens (e.g. flutamide, cyproterone) are used as part of the treatment of prostatic cancer.
- 5α-Reductase inhibitors (e.g. finasteride) are used in benign prostatic hypertrophy.

androgens are less rapidly metabolised and some are excreted in the urine unchanged.

Unwanted effects

Unwanted effects of androgens include eventual decrease of gonadotrophin release, with resultant infertility, and salt and water retention leading to oedema. Adenocarcinoma of the liver has been reported. Androgens impair growth in children (via premature fusion of epiphyses) and cause acne and masculinisation in girls.

Clinical use

The clinical use of androgens is given in the box.

ANABOLIC STEROIDS

Androgens can be modified to enhance the anabolic effects and decrease other effects. These anabolic steroids (e.g. **nandrolone**, **stanozolol**) increase protein synthesis and enhance muscle development, resulting in weight gain. They are used to decrease the itching of chronic biliary obstruction and in the therapy of some aplastic anaemias. They may have a place in treating debilitating and wasting conditions and in terminal disease, in which they can improve appetite and promote well-being. They are used in some cases of hormone-dependent metastatic mammary cancer. Unwanted effects can occur, in particular cholestatic jaundice.

Anabolic steroids are used by some athletes to increase strength and athletic performance. When combined with strength training, a short course of weekly 600 mg doses of testosterone (a dose six times higher than that used for replacement therapy) increased fat-free mass and muscle size. As anabolic steroid abusers may take up to 26 times the therapeutic dose, serious unwanted effects can occur—as specified above under Androgens—including testicular atrophy, sterility and gynaecomastia in men, and inhibition of ovulation, hirsutism, deepening of the voice, alopecia and acne in women. Increased aggressiveness and psychotic symptoms have been described. In both sexes, there is increased risk of coronary heart disease, and there have been instances of sudden death in young athletes in which there was a strong suspicion that anabolic steroid use had been contributory.

ANTI-ANDROGENS

Both *oestrogens* and *progestogens* have anti-androgen activity, oestrogens mainly by inhibiting gonadotrophin secretion and progestogens by competing with androgens in target organs. **Cyproterone** is a derivative of progesterone and has weak progestational activity. It is a partial agonist at androgen receptors, competing with dihydrotestosterone for receptors in androgen-sensitive target tissues. Through its effect in the hypothalamus it depresses the synthesis of gonadotrophins. It is used as an adjunct in the treatment of prostatic cancer during initiation of GnRH treatment (see below). It is also used in the therapy of precocious puberty in males, and of masculinisation and acne in women. It also has a CNS effect, decreasing libido, and has been used to treat hypersexuality in male sexual offenders.*

Flutamide is a non-steroidal anti-androgen used with GnRH in the treatment of prostate cancer.

Drugs can have anti-androgen action by inhibiting synthetic enzymes. Finasteride inhibits the enzyme (5α-reductase) that converts testosterone to dihydrotestosterone (Fig. 29.3). Dihydrotestosterone has greater affinity than testoserone for androgen receptors in the prostate gland. It is well absorbed after oral administration, has a half-life of about 7 hours and is excreted in the urine and faeces. It is used to treat benign prostatic hyperplasia, though α_1-adrenoceptor antagonists, **terazosin** or **tamsolusin**, are more effective (working by the entirely different mechanism of relaxing smooth muscle in the capsule of the prostate gland). Surgery is the preferred option (especially by surgeons).

GONADOTROPHIN-RELEASING HORMONE: AGONISTS AND ANTAGONISTS

GnRH is a decapeptide that controls the secretion of FSH and LH by the anterior pituitary. Secretion of GnRH is controlled by neural input from other parts of the brain and through negative feedback by the sex steroids (Figs 29.1 and 29.5). Exogenous androgens, oestrogens and progestogens all inhibit GnRH secretion, but only progestogens exert this effect at doses that do not have marked hormonal actions on peripheral tissues, presumably because progesterone receptors in the reproductive tract are sparse unless they have been induced by previous exposure to oestrogen. **Danazol** (see below) is a synthetic steroid that inhibits release of GnRH and, consequently, of gonadotrophins (FSH and LH). **Clomiphene** is an oestrogen antagonist that stimulates gonadotrophin release by inhibiting the negative feedback effects of endogenous oestrogen; it is used to treat infertility (see above and Fig. 29.5).

Synthetic GnRH is termed **gonadorelin**. Numerous analogues of GnRH, both agonists and antagonists, have been synthesised. **Buserelin**, **leuprorelin**, **goserelin** and **nafarelin** are agonists, the last being 200 times more potent than endogenous GnRH.

*As with the oestrogens, very different doses are used for these different conditions, for example 2 mg/day for acne, 100 mg/day for hypersexuality, 300 mg/day for prostatic cancer.

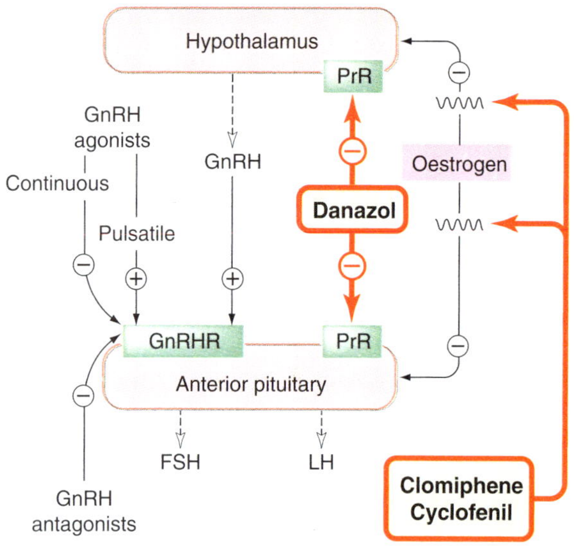

Fig. 29.5 The regulation of gonadotrophin release from the anterior pituitary by endogenous gonadotrophin-releasing hormone (GnRH) and drugs. (GnRHR, GnRH receptor; PrR, progestogen receptor; FSH, follicle-stimulating hormone; LH, luteinising hormone.)

Pharmacokinetics and clinical use

GnRH agonists, given by subcutaneous infusion in pulses to mimic physiological secretion of GnRH, stimulate gonadotrophin release (Fig. 29.5) and induce ovulation. As with some other peptides, they are absorbed intact following nasal administration (Ch. 7). Continuous use, by nasal spray or as depot preparations, stimulates gonadotrophin release transiently but then paradoxically *inhibits* gonadotrophin release (Fig. 29.5), because of downregulation (desensitisation) of GnRH receptors in the pituitary. GnRH analogues are given in this fashion to cause gonadal suppression in various sex hormone-dependent conditions including prostate and breast cancers, endometriosis (endometrial tissue outside the uterine cavity) and uterine fibroids when these have been causing anaemia from menorrhagia (heavy periods). Continuous, non-pulsatile administration inhibits spermatogenesis and ovulation, raising the possibility (which is under investigation) that GnRH analogues could be useful as contraceptives. GnRH agonists are used by specialists in infertility treatment, not to stimulate ovulation (which is achieved using gonadotrophin preparations) but to suppress the pituitary before administration of FSH or HCG (see below). It was originally hoped that GnRH *antagonists* would be useful for contraception, but this has not been realised.

Unwanted effects of GnRH analogues

Unwanted effects of the GnRH agonists in women result from hypo-oestrogenism, which causes menopausal symptoms (e.g. flushing, vaginal dryness) and bone loss. The initial stimulation of gonadotrophin secretion on starting treatment can cause transient worsening of symptoms (e.g. worsening of pain from bone metastases in men with prostate cancer), so treatment of prostate cancer with these agents is only started after the patient has received an androgen receptor antagonist such as **flutamide** (see above and Ch. 50).

DANAZOL

Actions and pharmacokinetics

Danazol inhibits gonadotrophin secretion (especially the midcycle surge) and consequently reduces oestrogen synthesis in the ovary (Fig. 29.5). It is also active in men, reducing androgen synthesis and spermatogenesis. It has androgenic activity. It is orally active and metabolized in the liver.

Clinical uses

Danazol is used in sex-hormone-dependent conditions including endometriosis, breast dysplasia, gynaecomastia. An additional specialist use is to reduce attacks of swelling in an uncommon and miserable disease called hereditary angioedema.*

Unwanted effects

Unwanted effects are common and include gastrointestinal disturbances, weight gain, fluid retention, dizziness, menopausal symptoms, muscle cramps and headache. Danazol has a virilising action in females.

GONADOTROPHINS AND ANALOGUES

Gonadotrophins (FSH, LH and HCG) are glycoproteins produced and secreted by the anterior pituitary (see Ch. 27) or chorion and placenta. Large amounts of gonadotrophins are present in the urine of women following the menopause, in whom oestrogen no longer exerts feedback inhibition on the pituitary, which consequently secretes large amounts of FSH and LH.** The chorion and placenta secretes HCG.

Preparations

Gonadotrophins are extracted from urine of pregnant (HCG) or postmenopausal women (human menopausal gonadotrophin, HMG, which contains a mixture of FSH and LH). Recombinant FSH (**follitrophin**) is also available.

Pharmacokinetics and clinical use

Gonadotrophin preparations are given by injection. They are used to treat infertility caused by lack of ovulation as a result of hypopituitarism, or following failure of treatment with clomiphene; they are also used by specialists to induce ovulation

*Hereditary angioedema is caused by lack of an endogenous inhibitor of the complement pathway and is characterised by recurrent attacks of pain and swelling in soft tissues, including (most dangerously) the larynx.

**This forms the basis for the standard blood test, estimation of plasma LH/FSH concentrations, to confirm whether a woman is postmenopausal.

Gonadotrophin-releasing hormone (GnRH) and gonadotrophins

- GnRH is a decapeptide; gonadorelin is the synthetic form. Nafarelin is a potent analogue.
- Given in pulsatile fashion they stimulate gonadotrophin release; given continuously they inhibit it.
- The gonadotrophins, follicle-stimulating hormone (FSH) and luteinising hormone (LH), are glycoproteins.
- Preparations of gonadotrophins (e.g. chorionic gonadotrophin, extracted from the urine of pregnant women) are used to treat infertility caused by lack of ovulation.
- Danazol is a modified progestogen that inhibits gonadotrophin production by an action on the hypothalamus and anterior pituitary.

to enable eggs to be collected* for in vitro fertilisation and re-implantation into the uterine cavity in women whose infertility is caused by mechanical obstruction of their fallopian tubes. For this use, gonadotrophin is usually administered after endogenous secretion of FSH and LH has been suppressed using a continuously administered GnRH agonist (see above). Gonadotrophins are also sometimes used in men with infertility caused by a low sperm count as a result of hypogonadotrophic hypogonadism (a disorder that is sometimes accompanied by lifelong anosmia, i.e. lack of sense of smell). (Gonadotrophins do not, of course, work for patients whose low sperm count is the result of primary testicular failure.) HCG has been used to stimulate testosterone synthesis in boys with delayed puberty, but testosterone is usually preferred.

DRUGS USED FOR CONTRACEPTION

ORAL CONTRACEPTIVES

There are two main types of oral** contraceptives:

- combinations of an oestrogen with a progestogen (the combined pill)
- progestogen alone (the progestogen-only pill).

The combined pill

The combined oral contraceptive pill is extremely effective, at least in the absence of intercurrent illness and of treatment with potentially interacting drugs (see below). The oestrogen in most combined preparations (second-generation pills)** is ethinylestradiol, though a few preparations contain mestranol instead. The progestogen may be norethisterone, levonorgestrel, ethynodiol, or—in 'third-generation' pills—desogestrel or gestodene, which are more potent, have less androgenic action and cause less change in lipoprotein metabolism but which probably cause a greater risk of thromboembolism than do second-generation preparations. The oestrogen content is generally 20–50 μg ethinylestradiol or its equivalent, and a preparation is chosen with the lowest oestrogen and progestogen content that is well tolerated and gives good cycle control in the individual woman. This combined pill is taken for 21 consecutive days followed by 7 pill-free days, which causes a withdrawal bleed. Normal cycles of menstruation usually commence fairly soon after discontinuing treatment, and permanent loss of fertility (which may be a result of early menopause rather than a long-term consequence of the contraceptive pill) is rare.

The mode of action is as follows:

- oestrogen inhibits secretion of FSH via negative feedback on the anterior pituitary and thus suppresses development of the ovarian follicle
- progestogen inhibits secretion of LH and thus prevents ovulation; it also makes the cervical mucus less suitable for the passage of sperm
- oestrogen and progestogen act in concert to alter the endometrium in such a way as to discourage implantation.

They may also interfere with the coordinated contractions of cervix, uterus and fallopian tubes, which facilitate fertilisation and implantation.

Potential unwanted and beneficial effects of the combined pill

More than 200 million women worldwide have used this method since the 1960s, and, in general, the combined pill constitutes a safe and effective method of contraception. There are distinct health benefits from taking the pill (see below) and serious adverse effects are rare. However, minor unwanted effects constitute drawbacks to its use and several important questions need to be considered.

Common adverse effects

The common effects are:

- weight gain, owing to fluid retention or an anabolic effect or both
- mild nausea, flushing, dizziness, depression or irritability
- skin changes, (e.g. acne and/or an increase in pigmentation)
- amenorrhoea of variable duration on cessation of taking the pill.

* The eggs are harvested using laparoscopy, a technique whereby a flexible fibre optic instrument is inserted under anaesthesia just below the umbilicus, the ovaries inspected at the predicted time of ovulation and eggs retrieved.

**For oral contraceptives to be effective, they must of course be absorbed. Gastrointestinal disturbances may impair absorption. A bout of gastroenteritis, for example, could have unexpected consequences.

**The first-generation pills, containing more than 50 μg oestrogen, were shown, in the 1970s, to be associated with an increased risk of deep vein thrombosis and pulmonary embolism.

Questions that need to be considered

Is there an increased risk of cardiovascular disease (venous thromboembolism, myocardial infarction, stroke)? With second-generation pills (oestrogen content less than 50 μg), the risk of thromboembolism is small (incidence approximately 15 per 100 000 users per year, compared with 5 per 100 000 non-pregnant non-users per year or 60 per 100 000 pregnancies). The risk is greatest in specific subgroups in whom other factors contribute, such as smoking (which increases risk substantially) and long-continued use of the pill, especially in women over 35 years of age. For preparations containing the third-generation progestogens **desogestrel** or **gestodene**, the incidence of thromboembolic disease is approximately 25 per 100 000 users per year, which is still a small absolute risk that is substantially less than that caused by a pregnancy. In general, as stated by Baird & Glasier (1993), 'the evidence suggests…that after risk factors (e.g. smoking, hypertension, and obesity) have been identified, combined oral contraceptives are safe for most women for most of their reproductive lives'.

Is there an increase in the risk of cancer? One large epidemiological study suggests that there may be a duration-related increase in the risk of breast cancer, the risk being 0.5 excess cancers per 10 000 women aged 16–19, and 4.7 excess cancers per 10 000 women at age 25–29. The cancers were less advanced in pill users and thus potentially more treatable (see Hemminki, 1996). Oral contraceptives may decrease the incidence of ovarian and endometrial cancer and do not cause cervical cancer. An association between liver cancer and oral contraceptive use has been reported; but this cancer is rare in Europe and the USA in the absence of some other cause of chronic liver disease such as chronic hepatitis.

Does the pill increase blood pressure? A marked increase in arterial blood pressure occurs in a small percentage of women shortly after starting the combined oral contraceptive pill. This is associated with increased circulating angiotensinogen and disappears when treatment is stopped. Blood pressure is, therefore, monitored carefully when oral contraceptive treatment is started, and an alternative method substituted if necessary.

Is there an impairment in glucose tolerance? Older progestogen preparations could impair glucose tolerance, but this is not a problem with the newer compounds.

Beneficial effects

The combined pill markedly decreases menstrual symptoms such as irregular periods and intermenstrual bleeding. Iron deficiency anaemia and premenstrual tension are reduced, as are benign breast disease, uterine fibroids and functional cysts of the ovaries. Unwanted pregnancy, carrying a maternal mortality ranging from 1 in 10 000 in developed countries to 1 in 150 in Africa, is avoided.

The progestogen-only pill

The drugs used in progestogen-only pills include **norethisterone**, **levonorgestrel** or **ethynodiol**. The pill is taken daily without interruption. The mode of action is primarily on the cervical mucus, which is made inhospitable to sperm. The progestogen probably also hinders implantation through its effect on the endometrium and on the motility and secretions of the fallopian tubes (see above).

Potential beneficial and unwanted effects of the progestogen-only pill

Progestogen-only contraceptives offer a suitable alternative to the combined pill for some women in whom oestrogen is contraindicated, (e.g. because of venous thrombosis, smoking or older age) and are also suitable for women whose blood pressure increases unacceptably during treatment with oestrogen. However, their contraceptive effect is less reliable than that of the combination pill, and missing a dose may result in conception. Disturbances of menstruation (especially irregular bleeding) are common. Only a small proportion of women use this form of contraception, so long-term safety data are less reliable than for the combined pill.

Pharmacokinetics of oral contraceptives: drug interactions

Combined and progestogen-only oral contraceptives are metabolised by hepatic cytochrome P450 enzymes. Since the minimum effective dose of oestrogen is used (in order to avoid excess risk of thromboembolism), any increase in its clearance

Oral contraceptives

The combined pill

- The combined pill contains an oestrogen and a progestogen. It is taken for 21 consecutive days out of 28.
- Mode of action: the oestrogen inhibits follicle-stimulating hormone (FSH) release and, therefore, follicle development; the progestogen inhibits luteinising hormone (LH) release and, therefore, ovulation, and makes cervical mucus inhospitable for sperm; together they render the endometrium unsuitable for implantation.
- Drawbacks: weight gain, nausea, mood changes and skin pigmentation can occur.
- Serious unwanted effects are rare. A small proportion of women develop reversible hypertension; there is evidence both for and against an increased risk of breast cancer; there is a small increased risk of thromboembolism with third-generation pills.
- There are several beneficial effects, not least the avoidance of unwanted pregnancy, which itself carries a not insignificant risk.

The progestogen-only pill

- The progestogen-only pill is taken continuously. It differs from the combined pill in that the contraceptive effect is less reliable and is mainly a result of the alteration of cervical mucus. Irregular bleeding is common.

may result in contraceptive failure, and indeed enzyme-inducing drugs can have this effect not only for combined but also for progesterone-only pills. Such drugs include (par excellence) **rifampicin** and **rifabutin**, as well as **carbamazepine**, **phenytoin**, **griseofulvin** and others. Enterohepatic recycling of oestrogen is mentioned above (p. 433). Broad-spectrum antibiotics such as amoxicillin can disturb this by altering the intestinal flora and cause failure of the combined pill. This does not occur with progesterone-only pills.

OTHER DRUG REGIMENS USED FOR CONTRACEPTION

POSTCOITAL (EMERGENCY) CONTRACEPTION

Oral administration of **levonorgestrel**, alone or combined with oestrogen, is effective if taken within within 72 hours of unprotected intercourse, repeated 12 hours later. Nausea and vomiting are common (and the pills may then be lost: replacement tablets can be taken with an antiemetic such as **domperidone**). Insertion of an intrauterine device is more effective than hormonal methods and works up to 5 days after intercourse.

LONG-ACTING PROGESTOGEN-ONLY CONTRACEPTION

Medroxyprogesterone can be given intramuscularly as a contraceptive. This is effective and safe. However, menstrual irregularities are common, and infertility may persist for many months after cessation of treatment.

Levonorgestrel implanted subcutaneously in non-biodegradable capsules is being used by approximately 3 million women worldwide. This route of administration bypasses the liver, thus avoiding first-pass metabolism. The tubes slowly release their progestogen content over 5 years. Common unwanted effects are irregular bleeding and headache.

A levonorgestrel-impregnated intrauterine device has contraceptive action for 3–5 years.

CONTRACEPTIVES FOR MALES

Oral contraceptives for men remain elusive, but authorities remain optimistic (see, for example, Baird and Glasier, 1999).

THE UTERUS

The physiological and pharmacological responses of the uterus vary at different stages of the menstrual cycle and during pregnancy.

THE MOTILITY OF THE UTERUS

Uterine muscle contracts rhythmically both in vitro and in vivo, the contractions originating in the muscle itself. Myometrial cells in the fundus act as pacemakers and give rise to conducted action potentials. The electrophysiological activity of these pacemaker cells is regulated by the sex hormones.

The non-pregnant human uterus contracts spontaneously but weakly during the first part of the cycle, and more strongly during the luteal phase and during menstruation. Uterine movements are depressed in early pregnancy because oestrogen, potentiated by progesterone, hyperpolarises myometrial cells. This suppresses spontaneous contractions. Towards the end of gestation, however, contractions recommence; these increase in force and frequency and become fully coordinated during parturition. The nerve supply to the uterus includes both excitatory and inhibitory sympathetic components: adrenaline, acting on β_2-adrenoceptors, inhibits uterine contraction, whereas noradrenaline, acting on α-adrenoceptors, stimulates contraction.

DRUGS THAT STIMULATE THE UTERUS

Drugs that stimulate the pregnant uterus and are important in obstetrics include oxytocin, ergometrine and the E and F type prostaglandins.

OXYTOCIN

As explained in Chapter 27, the neurohypophyseal hormone oxytocin (an octapeptide) regulates myometrial activity. Oxytocin release is stimulated by cervical dilatation, and by suckling, but its role in parturition is incompletely understood. Oxytocin for clinical use is prepared synthetically.

Actions

On the uterus Oxytocin contracts the uterus. Oestrogen induces oxytocin receptor synthesis and, consequently, the uterus at term is highly sensitive to this hormone. Given by slow intravenous infusion to induce labour, oxytocin causes regular coordinated contractions that travel from fundus to cervix. Both amplitude and frequency of these contractions are related to dose, the uterus relaxing completely between contractions during low-dose infusion. Larger doses further increase the frequency of the contractions and there is incomplete relaxation between them. Still higher doses cause sustained contractions that interfere with blood flow through the placenta and cause fetal distress or death.

Other actions* Oxytocin contracts myoepithelial cells in the mammary gland, which causes 'milk let-down'—the expression of milk from the alveoli and ducts. It also has a vasodilator action. A weak antidiuretic action, which can result in water retention, occurs if large doses are infused; this may constitute an unwanted effect if oxytocin is used in patients with cardiac or renal disease, or pre-eclampsia.**

*Oxytocin receptors are found not only in the uterus but also in the brain, particularly in the limbic system. Animal experiments have shown that oxytocin is important in mating and parenting behaviour.

**Eclampsia is a pathological condition (involving, among other things, high blood pressure, swelling and seizures) that occurs in pregnant women.

Clinical use

The clinical use of oxytocin is given in the box on page 443.

Pharmacokinetic aspects

Oxytocin can be given by intravenous injection or intramuscularly but is most often given by intravenous infusion. It is inactivated in the liver and kidneys and by circulating placental oxytocinase.

Unwanted effects of oxytocin

Unwanted effects of oxytocin include dose-related hypotension (arising from its vasodilator action), with associated reflex tachycardia. Its antidiuretic hormone-like effect on water excretion by the kidney causes water retention and, unless water intake is curtailed, consequent hyponatraemia.

ERGOMETRINE

Ergot (*Claviceps purpurea*) is a fungus that grows on rye and contains a surprising variety of pharmacologically active substances (see Ch. 12). Ergot poisoning, which was once common, was often associated with abortion. In 1935, **ergometrine** was isolated and was recognised as the oxytocic principle in ergot.

Actions

Ergometrine contracts the human uterus. This action depends partly on the contractile state of the organ. On a contracted uterus (the normal state following delivery), ergometrine has relatively little effect. However, if the uterus is inappropriately relaxed, ergometrine initiates strong contractions, thus reducing bleeding from the placental bed (the raw surface from which the placenta has detached). Ergometrine also has a moderate degree of vasoconstrictor action per se.

The mechanism of action of ergometrine on smooth muscle is not understood. It is possible that it acts partly on α-adrenoceptors, like the related alkaloid ergotamine (see Ch. 8), and partly on 5-hydroxytryptamine (5-HT) receptors.

The clinical use of ergometrine is given in the box on page 443.

Pharmacokinetic aspects and unwanted effects

Ergometrine can be given orally, intramuscularly or intravenously. It has a very rapid onset of action and its effect lasts for 3–6 hours.

Ergometrine can produce vomiting, probably by an effect on dopamine D_2-receptors in the chemoreceptor trigger zone (see Fig. 24.6). Vasoconstriction with an increase in blood pressure associated with nausea, blurred vision and headache can occur, as can vasospasm of the coronary arteries resulting in angina.

PROSTAGLANDINS

Endogenous prostaglandins

Prostaglandins are discussed in detail in Chapter 15. The endometrium and myometrium have substantial prostaglandin-synthesising capacity, particularly in the second, proliferative phase of the menstrual cycle. Prostaglandin (PG) $F_{2\alpha}$ is generated in large amounts and has been implicated in the ischaemic necrosis of the endometrium that precedes menstruation (though it has relatively little vasoconstrictor action on many human blood vessels in contrast to some other mammalian species). Vasodilator prostaglandins, PGE_2 and PGI_2 (prostacyclin), are also generated by the uterus.

In addition to their vasoactive properties, the E- and F-prostaglandins contract the non-pregnant as well as the pregnant uterus. The sensitivity of uterine muscle to prostaglandins increases during gestation. Their role in parturition (if any) is not fully understood, but the finding that cyclooxygenase inhibitors can delay labour (see below) suggests that they do play some part in this.

Prostaglandins also play a part in two of the main disorders of menstruation: dysmenorrhoea (painful menstruation) and menorrhagia (excessive blood loss). Dysmenorrhoea is associated with increased production of PGE_2 and $PGF_{2\alpha}$, both of which cause uterine contractions; *non-steroidal anti-inflammatory drugs*, which inhibit prostaglandin biosynthesis (see Ch. 16), are used to treat spasmodic dysmenorrhoea. Menorrhagia, in the absence of uterine pathology, appears to be caused by a combination of increased vasodilatation and reduced haemostasis, the increased vasodilatation being associated with an increased production of PGE_2 and PGI_2 compared with $PGF_{2\alpha}$. Haemostasis depends on platelet aggregation and fibrin formation, the former providing a surface for the latter (Fig. 20.1) There are fewer platelets in menstrual blood than in circulating blood, and they have a reduced capacity to aggregate and synthesise thromboxane A_2. Increased generation by the uterus of PGI_2 (which inhibits platelet aggregation) could impair haemostasis as well as causing vasodilatation. Cyclooxygenase inhibitors can be of value in treating menorrhagia.

Exogenous prostaglandins

Prostaglandins of the E and F series promote coordinated contractions of the body of the pregnant uterus, while relaxing the cervix. E- and F-prostaglandins reliably cause abortion in early and middle pregnancy, unlike oxytocin, which generally does not cause expulsion of the uterine contents at this stage. The prostaglandins used in obstetrics are **dinoprostone** (PGE_2), **carboprost** (15-methyl $PGF_{2\alpha}$) and **gemeprost** or **misoprostol** (PGE_1 analogues). Dinoprostone can be given intravaginally as a gel or as tablets, or by the extra-amniotic route as a solution. Carboprost is given by deep intramuscular injection. Gemeprost or misoprostol are given intravaginally.

Unwanted effects

Unwanted effects include uterine pain, nausea and vomiting, which occur in about 50% of patients when the drugs are used as abortifacients. Dinoprost may cause cardiovascular collapse if it escapes into the circulation after intra-amniotic injection. Phlebitis can occur at the site of intravenous infusion. When combined with mifepristone, a progestogen antagonist (see p. 434) that sensitises the uterus to prostaglandins, lower doses of

Drugs acting on the uterus

- At parturition, oxytocin causes regular coordinated uterine contractions, each followed by relaxation; ergometrine, an ergot alkaloid, causes uterine contractions with an increase in basal tone. Atosiban, an antagonist of oxytocin, delays labour.
- Prostaglandin (PG) analogues, e.g. dinoprostone (PGE_2) and dinoprost ($PGF_{2\alpha}$), contract the pregnant uterus but relax the cervix. Cyclooxygenase inhibitors inhibit PG synthesis and delay labour. They also alleviate syptoms of dysmenorrhoea and menorrhagia.
- The β_2-adrenoceptor agonists (e.g. ritodrine) inhibit both spontaneous and oxytocin-induced contractions of the pregnant uterus.

Clinical uses of drugs acting on the uterus

Myometrial stimulants (oxytocics)

- Oxytocin is used to induce or augment labour when the uterine muscle is not functioning adequately. It can also be used to treat postpartum haemorrhage.
- Ergometrine can be used to treat postpartum haemorrhage. Carboprost can be used if patients do not respond to ergometrine.
- A preparation containing both oxytocin and ergometrine is used for the management of the third stage of labour; the two agents together can also be used, prior to surgery, to control bleeding owing to incomplete abortion.
- Dinoprostone given by the extra-amniotic route is used for late (second trimester) therapeutic abortion; given as vaginal gel, it is used for cervical ripening and induction of labour.
- Gemeprost, given as vaginal pessary following mifepristone, is used as a medical alternative to surgical termination of pregnancy (up to 63 days of gestation).

Myometrial relaxants

- The β-adrenoceptor agonists (e.g. ritodrine) are used to delay preterm labour.
- Atosiban (oxytocin antagonist) also delays preterm labour.

the prostaglandins (e.g. misoprostol) can be used to terminate pregnancy, and side-effects are reduced.

Clinical use

The clinical use of prostaglandin analogues is given on page 435.

DRUGS THAT INHIBIT UTERINE CONTRACTION

Selective β_2-adrenoceptor agonists, such as **ritodrine** or **salbutamol**, inhibit spontaneous or oxytocin-induced contractions of the pregnant uterus. These uterine relaxants are used in selected patients to prevent premature labour occurring between 22 and 33 weeks of gestation in otherwise uncomplicated pregnancies. They can delay delivery by 48 hours, time that can be used to administer glucocorticoid therapy to the mother so as to mature the lungs of the baby and reduce neonatal respiratory distress, and to optimise logistics such as making sure the baby is born in a facility with neonatal intensive care. It has been difficult to demonstrate that any of the drugs used to delay labour improve the outcome for the baby. Risks to the mother, especially pulmonary oedema, increase after 48 hours and myometrial response is reduced, so prolonged treatment is avoided. Cyclooxygenase inhibitors (e.g. indometacin) inhibit labour, but their use could cause problems in the baby including renal dysfunction and delayed closure of the ductus arteriosus, both of which are influenced by endogenous prostaglandins (see Ch. 23 and 18, respectively).

An oxytocin receptor antagonist, **atosiban**, was recently marketed to inhibit uncomplicated premature labour, and it provides an alternative to a β_2-adrenoceptor agonist. It is given as an intravenous bolus followed by an intravenous infusion for not more than 48 hours. Adverse effects include symptoms of vasodilation, nausea, vomiting, hyperglycaemia and rash.

ERECTILE DYSFUNCTION

Erectile function depends on complex interactions between physiological and psychological factors. Erection is caused by vasorelaxation in the arteries and arterioles supplying the erectile tissue. This increases penile blood flow. Relaxation of trabecular smooth muscle causes filling of the sinusoids. This compresses the plexuses of subtunical venules between the trabeculae and the tunica albuginea, occluding venous outflow and causing erection. During sexual intercourse, reflex contraction of the ischio-cavernosus muscles compresses the base of the corpora cavernosa, and the intracavernosal pressure can reach several hundred millimetres of mercury during this phase of rigid erection. Innervation of the penis includes autonomic and somatic nerves. Nitric oxide is probably the main mediator of erection and is released both from nitrergic nerves and from endothelium (Ch. 14; Fig. 14.5).

Erectile function is adversely affected by several therapeutic drugs (including many antipsychotic, antidepressant and antihypertensive agents), but in long-term randomised controlled trials an appreciable percentage of men who discontinue treatment because of erectile dysfunction had been receiving placebo, and psychiatric and vascular disease can themselves cause sexual dysfunction. Furthermore, erectile dysfunction is common in middle-aged and older men, even if they have no psychiatric or cardiovascular problems. There are several organic causes, including hypogonadism (see above), hyperprolactinaemia (see Ch. 27), pelvic arterial disease and various causes of neuropathy (most commonly diabetes), but often no organic cause is identified, or the problem is a result of a combination of organic and psychological factors, notably anxiety relating to sexual performance, which can establish a vicious circle.

Over the centuries, there has been a huge trade in parts of various creatures that have the misfortune to bear some fancied resemblance to human genitalia, in the pathetic belief that consuming these will restore virility or act as an aphrodisiac (i.e. a drug that stimulates libido). Alcohol (Ch. 42) "provokes the desire but…takes away the performance', and cannabis can also release inhibitions and probably does the same. **Yohimbine** (α_2-antagonist, Ch. 10) may have some positive effect in this regard, but even with meta-analysis the number of subjects randomised is not very impressive and efficacy somewhat unconvincing. **Apomorphine** (dopamine agonist, Ch. 34) causes erections in humans as well as in rodents when injected subcutaneously, but it is a powerful emetic, an effect that is usually regarded as socially unacceptable in this context. Despite this rather obvious disadvantage, a sublingual preparation is licensed for erectile dysfunction.* Nausea is said to subside with continued drug use.

The generally negative picture changed when it was found that injecting vasodilator drugs directly into the corpora cavernosa causes penile erection. **Papaverine** (Ch. 18), if necessary with the addition of **phentolamine**, was used in this way. The route of administration is not acceptable to most men, but diabetics in particular are often not needle-shy and this approach was a real boon to many such patients. **PGE_1** (**alprostadil**) is often combined with other vasodilators when given intracavernosally. It can also be given transurethrally as an alternative (albeit still a somewhat unromantic one) to injection. Adverse effects of all these drugs include priapism, which is no joke! Treatment consists of aspiration of blood (using sterile technique) and, if necessary, cautious intracavernosal administration of a vasoconstrictor such as **phenylephrine**. Intracavernosal and transurethral preparations are still available, but **sildenafil**, which is orally active, is now the drug of choice for most men.

PHOSPHODIESTERASE TYPE V INHIBITORS

Sildenafil, the first selective phosphodiesterase type V inhibitor (see also Chs 14, 18), was being developed for another possible indication and was found incidentally to influence erectile function. In contrast to intracavernosal vasodilators, it is not sufficient of itself to cause erection independent of sexual desire, but it enhances the erectile response to sexual stimulation. It has transformed the treatment of erectile dysfunction.

Mechanism of action

Phosphodiesterase V is the isoform that inactivates cGMP. Nitrergic nerves release nitric oxide (or a related nitrosothiol), which diffuses into smooth muscle cells where it activates guanylate cyclase. The resulting increase in cytoplasmic cGMP mediates vasodilation via activation of protein kinase G (Ch. 14). Consequently, inhibition of phosphodiesterase V potentiates the effect on penile vascular smooth muscle of endothelium-derived nitric oxide and of nitrergic nerves that are activated by sexual stimulation. Other vascular beds are also affected, suggesting other possible uses.**

Pharmacokinetic aspects and drug interactions

Peak plasma concentrations occur approximately 30–120 minutes after an oral dose and are delayed by eating, so it is taken an hour or more before sexual activity. It is given as a single dose as needed. (For possible long-term indications requiring 24 hour enzyme inhibition, it needs to be given three times daily.) It is metabolised by the 3A4 isoenzyme of cytochrome P450, which is induced by **carbamazepine**, **rifampicin** and barbiturates and inhibited by **cimetidine**, macrolide antibiotics, antifungal imidazolines, some antiviral drugs (such as **ritonavir**) and also by grapefruit juice (Ch. 8). These drugs can potentially interact with sildenafil in consequence. A dramatic pharmacodynamic interaction occurs with organic nitrates, which work through increasing cGMP (Ch. 17) and are, therefore, markedly potentiated by sildenafil. Consequenty, concurrent nitrate use contraindicates sildenafil.

Unwanted effects

Many of the unwanted effects of sildenafil are caused by vasodilation in other vascular beds: these include hypotension, flushing and headache. Visual disturbances have occasionally been reported and are of concern since sildenafil has some action on phosphodiesterase VI, which is present in retina and important in vision. The manufacturers advise that sildenafil should not be used in patients with hereditary retinal degenerative diseases (such as retinitis pigmentosa) because of the theoretical risk posed by this.

*Ironically so, since apomorphine was used as 'aversion therapy' in a misguided attempt to 'cure' homosexuality by conditioning individuals to associate homoerotic stimuli with nausea and vomiting, during the not-so-very far off time when homosexuality was classified as a psychiatric disease.

**In particular, pulmonary vasoconstriction in response to hypoxia is almost completely abolished by sildenafil, and it has therapeutic potential in pulmonary hypertension (a serious and poorly treated complication of diseases that cause hypoxaemia).

REFERENCES AND FURTHER READING

Endocrine aspects

Bagatelle C J, Bremner W J 1996 Androgens in men—uses and abuses. N Engl J Med 334: 707–714 (*A review of the biology, pharmacology and use of androgens*)

Baird D T, Glasier A F 1993 Editorial: hormonal contraception. N Engl J Med 328: 1543–1549 (*Pros and cons of hormonal contraception*)

Baird D T, Glasier A F 1999 Science, medicine and the future: contraception. Br Med J 319: 969–972 (*Predicts that antiprogestins will replace progestogen-only pills, and lead to 'once-a-month' pills, and that pills for men will become available in 10–15 years, orally active non-peptide GnRH antagonists*)

Brinton L A, Schairer C 1997 Postmenopausal hormone replacement therapy—time for a reappraisal? N Engl J Med 336: 1821–1822 (*Editorial comment on 20-year retrospective study of 34 000 women*)

Chen Z et al. 1999 Estrogen receptor α mediates the nongenomic activation of endothelial nitric oxide synthase by estrogen. J Clin Invest 103: 401–406 (*Acute vasodilator action of oestrogen may involve membrane ERα rather than the classical intracellular receptor pathway*)

Cummings S R et al. 1999 The effect of raloxifene on risk of breast cancer in postmenopausal women: results of the MORE randomized trial. JAMA 281: 2189–2197 (*7705 postmenopausal women with osteoporosis randomised to raloxifene or placebo and followed for a median of 40 months. Raloxifene reduced the incidence of oestrogen receptor-positive breast cancer by 90%*)

Davidson N E 1995 Breast versus heart versus bone. N Engl J Med 332: 1638–1639

Djerassi C 2001 This man's pill: reflections on the 50th birthday of the pill. Oxford University Press, New York (*Scientific and autobiographical memoir by polymath steroid chemist who worked on 'the pill' at its inception under Syntex in Mexico and has continued thinking about human reproduction in a broad biological and biosocial sense ever since*)

Eastell R 1998 Treatment of postmenopausal osteoporosis. N Engl J Med 338: 736–746 (*Excellent, comprehensive review of pathophysiology and drug treatment of postmenopausal osteoporosis with review of clinical trials of drugs used and future therapies*)

Fuleihan G E-H 1997 Tissue-specific estrogens—the promise for the future. N Engl J Med 337: 1686–1687 (*Editorial on potential use of 'designer oestrogens'*)

Ginsberg J (ed) 1996 Drug therapy in reproductive endocrinology. Arnold, London, pp. 372 (*An excellent, multiauthor textbook on the reproductive system, covering pathophysiology, pharmacology and clinical aspects*)

Grainger D J, Metcalf J C 1996 Tamoxifen: teaching an old drug new tricks. Nat Med 2: 381–385 (*An outline of the actions and mechanisms of action of tamoxifen, namely the anticancer, anti-osteoporotic effects, etc.*)

Gruber C J, Tschugguel W, Schneeberger C, Huber J C 2002 Production and actions of estrogens. N Engl J Med 346: 340–352 (*Review focussing on the new biochemical aspects of the action of oestrogen—including phytoestrogens and selective oestrogen receptor modulators—as well as physiological and clinical aspects*)

Guillebaud J 1998 Time for emergency contraception with levonorgestrol alone. Lancet 352: 46 (*A commentary that expands on the title*)

Hemminki E 1996 Oral contraceptives and breast cancer. Br Med J 313: 63–64 (*An editorial summarising the results of a study that analysed the data from 150 000 women*)

Hotchkiss J, Knobil E 1994 The menstrual cycle and its control. In: Knobil E, Neil J D (eds) The physiology of reproduction. Raven Press, New York, ch. 48, pp. 711–749

Huirne J A F, Lambalk C B 2001 Gonadotrophin-releasing hormone receptor antagonists Lancet 358: 1793–1803 (*Review discussing clinical potential of this relatively new class of drugs*)

Hulley S et al. 1998 Randomized trial of estrogen plus progestin for secondary prevention of coronary heart disease in postmenopausal women. JAMA 280: 605–613 (*2763 postmenopausal women who had suffered a previous coronary event randomised to active or placebo and followed for a mean of 4.1 years. The incidence of fatal myocardial infarction was similar in the two groups despite favourable changes in low and high density lipoproteins cholesterol in the HRT group. Venous thromboembolism was increased by a factor of 2.89 in the active group*)

Jacobs J 1996 Not for everybody. Br Med J 313: 351–352 (*One side of a debate on the desirability of prescribing HRT, the opposite point of view being given by Toozs-Hobson & Cardozo, 1996*)

Khaw K-T 1998 Hormone replacement therapy again: risk–benefit relation differs between population and individuals. Br Med J 316: 1842–1843 (*Emphasises concerns over the risk–benefit balance of long-term use of HRT in healthy women*)

LaCroix A Z, Burke W 1997 Breast cancer and hormone replacement therapy. Lancet 350: 1042–1043

Landers J P, Spelsberg T C 1992 New concepts in steroid hormone expression: transcription factors, proto-oncogenes, and the cascade model for steroid regulation of gene expression. Crit Rev Eukaryotic Gene Express 2: 19–63 (*The molecular biology of steroid hormones*)

Mascarenhas L 1994 Long-acting methods of contraception: much to offer. Br Med J 308: 991–992 (*Editorial*)

McCarthy M, Altemus M 1997 Central nervous system actions of oxytocin and modulation of behaviour in humans. Mol Med Today 3: 269–275 (*Review*)

McPherson K 1996 Third generation oral contraception and venous thromboembolism. Br Med J 312: 68–69 (*Editorial analysing the problem in the title and quoting three other papers on the subject in the same issue*)

Olive D L, Pritts E A 2001 Treatment of endometriosis. N Engl J Med 34: 266–275 (*Critical review of existing evidence—which is thin—forms the basis for sensible recommendations regarding treatment of pelvic pain or infertility from endometriosis using oral ontraceptives and GnRH agonist therapy with oestrogen–progestin add-back*)

Pedersen A T, Lidegaard Ø et al. 1997 Hormone replacement therapy and risk of non-fatal stroke. Lancet 350: 1277–1283

Pritchard K I 1998 Is tamoxifen effective in prevention of breast cancer? Lancet 352: 80–81 (*A large trial in 13 388 women has shown 45% reduction in breast cancer; two smaller trials had not. This is discussed*)

Rosing J, Tans G et al. 1997 Oral contraceptives and venous thromboembolism: different sensitivities to activated protein C in women using second- and third-generation oral contraceptives. Br J Haematol 97: 233–238 (*A proposed explanation for the thrombogenic potential of third-generation pills*)

Toozs-Hobson P, Cardozo L 1996 Hormone replacement therapy for all? Universal prescription is desirable. Br Med J 313: 350–351 (*One side of a debate on the desirability of prescribing HRT, the opposite point of view being given by Jacobs,1996*)

WHO Collaborative Study of Cardiovascular Disease and Steroid Hormone Contraception 1996 Results of international multicentre case-control study on ischaemic stroke and combined oral contraceptives. Lancet 348: 498–510

WHO Collaborative Study of Cardiovascular Disease and Steroid Hormone Contraception 1997 Results of international multicentre case-control study on acute myocardial infarction and combined oral contraceptives Lancet 1997 349: 1202–1209

Uterus

Norwitz E R, Robinson J N, Challis J R 1999 The control of labor. N Engl J Med 341:660-666 (*Review*)

Thornton S, Vatish M, Slater D 2001 Oxytocin antagonists: clinical and scientific considerations. Exp Physiol 86:297–302 (*Reviews rationale for uterine relaxants in preterm labour, evidence for administering atosiban and the role of oxytocin, vasopressin and their receptors in the onset of labour*)

Wray S 1993 Uterine contraction and physiological mechanisms of modulation. Am J Physiol 264 (Cell Physiol 33): C1–C18 (*A review on uterine function*)

Erectile dysfunction

Andersson K-E 2001 Pharmacology of penile erection. Pharmacol Rev 53: 417–450 (*Scholarly review covering cenral and peripheral regulation, and a very wide ranging coverage of the pharmacology of possible future as well as of current therapies*)

Edwards G (ed) 2002 The pharmacokinetics and pharmacodynamics of sildenafil citrate. Br J Clin Pharmacol 53: Suppl 1 (*Articles on this totally novel selective phosphodiesterase type 5 inhibitor, which has revolutionised treatment of erective dysfunction*)

Lue T F 2000 Drug therapy: erectile dysfunction. N Engl J Med 342: 1802–1813 (*Excellent review succinctly covering the physiology of penile erection, pathophysiology and diagnosis of erectile dysfunction, and drug therapy*)

30 Bone metabolism

Overview 446

Bone structure and composition 446

Bone remodelling 446
- The action of cells and cytokines 446
- The turnover of bone minerals 448
- Hormones involved in bone metabolism and remodelling 449

Disorders of bone 451
- Drugs used in bone disorders 451

OVERVIEW

The human skeleton undergoes a continuous process of remodelling throughout life—some bone being resorbed and new bone being laid down. With advancing age, there is an increasing possibility of structural deterioration and decreased bone mineral density (osteoporosis); this constitutes a major health problem throughout the world. Various other conditions can also lead to pathological changes in bone. In this chapter, we consider first the processes involved in bone remodelling and then go on to describe the pharmacological agents used to treat disorders of bone.

BONE STRUCTURE AND COMPOSITION

The human skeleton consists of 80% cortical bone and 20% trabecular bone. Cortical bone is the dense, compact outer part and trabecular bone the inner meshwork. The former predominates in the shafts of long bones, the latter in the vertebrae, the epiphyses of long bones and the iliac crest. Trabecular bone, having a large surface area, is metabolically more active and more affected by factors that lead to bone loss (see below).

The main minerals in bone are calcium salts and phosphates. More than 99% of the calcium in the body is in the skeleton, mostly as crystalline hydroxyapatite but some as non-crystalline phosphates and carbonates; together, these make up half the bone mass.

The organic matrix of bone is *osteoid*, the principal component of which is collagen; but there are also other components such as proteoglycans, osteocalcin and various phosphoproteins, one of which, osteonectin, binds to both calcium and collagen and thus links these two major constituents of bone matrix. Calcium phosphate crystals in the form of hydroxyapatite ($Ca_{10}(PO_4)_6(OH)_2$) are deposited in the osteoid, converting it into hard bone matrix.

Bone plays a major role in calcium homeostasis (see below).

BONE REMODELLING

The process of remodelling involves the following:

- the activity of two main cell types: osteoblasts, which secrete new bone matrix and osteoclasts, which break it down (Fig. 30.1)
- working together these two cell types form the basic multicellular unit (BMU): close cooperation between osteoblasts and osteoclasts is required, the osteoblast being the prime mover in the process in that it controls osteoclast differentiation during cell-to-cell contact. (Fig. 30.2)
- the actions of a variety of cytokines (Figs 30.1 and 30.2)
- the turnover of bone minerals: particularly calcium and phosphate
- the actions of several hormones: parathormone hormone (PTH, parathyroid hormone), the vitamin D family, growth hormone, steroids and calcitonin.

Diet, drugs and physical factors (exercise, loading) also affect remodelling. Bone loss—of 0.5–1% per year—starts in the 35–40 age group in both sexes. The rate accelerates by as much as 10-fold during the menopause in women (or with castration in men) and then gradually settles at 1–3% per year. The loss during the menopause results from increased osteoclast activity (see below) and affects mainly trabecular bone; the later loss in both sexes with increasing age is caused by decreased osteoblast numbers (see below) and affects mainly cortical bone.

THE ACTION OF CELLS AND CYTOKINES

A cycle of remodelling starts with recruitment of osteoclast precursors by cytokines (Fig. 30.1). Osteoblast action regulates the differentiation of these to mature osteoclasts, which adhere to

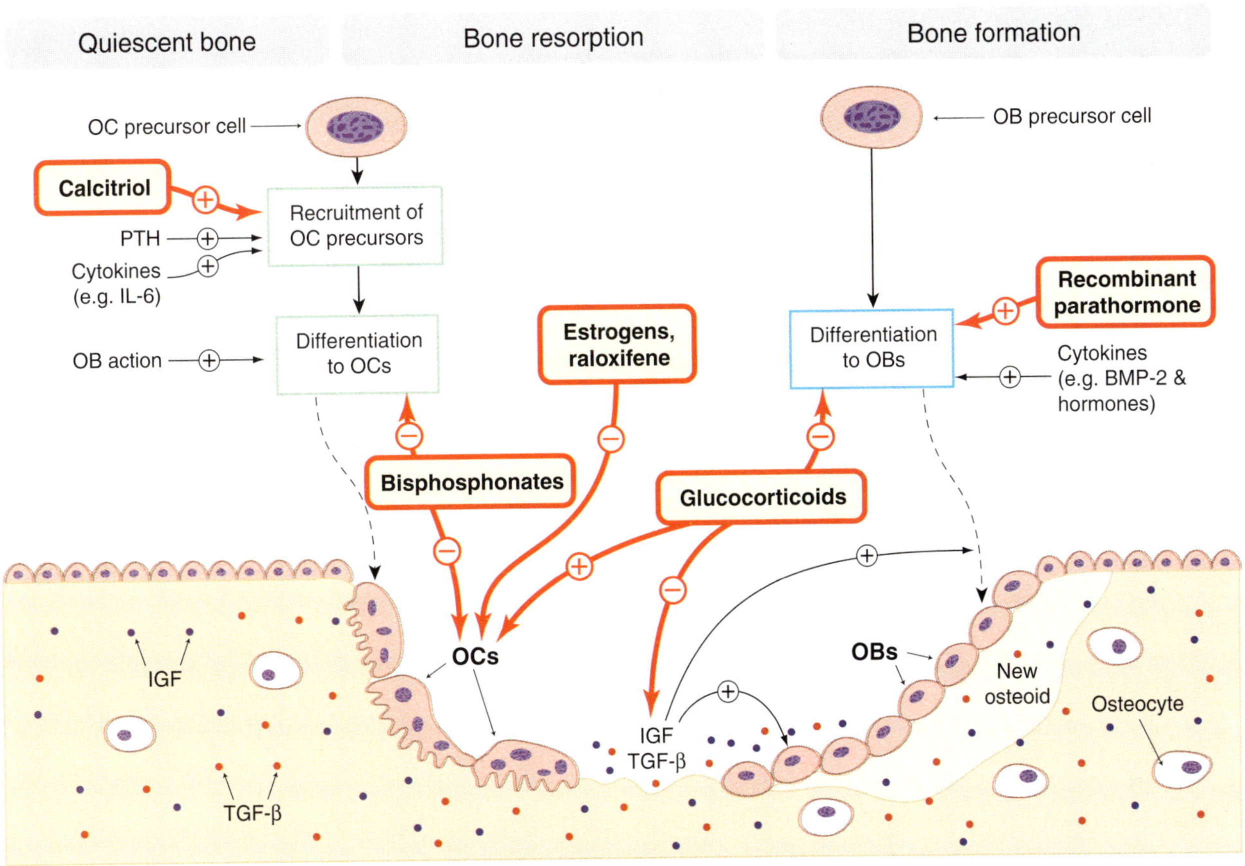

Fig. 30.1 The bone-remodelling cycle and the action of hormones, cytokines and drugs. In quiescent trabecular bone, cytokines such as insulin-like growth factor (IGF) and transforming growth factor-β (TGF-β), shown as dots, are embedded in the bone matrix. During bone resorption, osteoclast (OC) precursor cells, recruited by cytokines and hormones, are activated by osteoblasts (OB) to form mobile multinuclear osteoclasts (see Fig. 30.2), which then move along the bone surface resorbing bone and releasing the embedded cytokines. During bone formation, the released cytokines recruit osteoblasts, which lay down osteoid and embed cytokines IGF and TGF-β in it. Some OBs also become embedded, forming terminal osteocytes. The osteoid then becomes mineralised and lining cells cover the area (not shown). Oestrogens cause apoptosis (programmed cell death) of osteoclasts. Note that pharmacological concentration of glucocorticoids has the effects specified above, but physiological concentrations are required for osteoblast differentiation. (BMP-2, bone morphogenic protein-2; PTH, parathormone (endogenous); rPTH, recombinant PTH; IL-6, interleukin-6.)

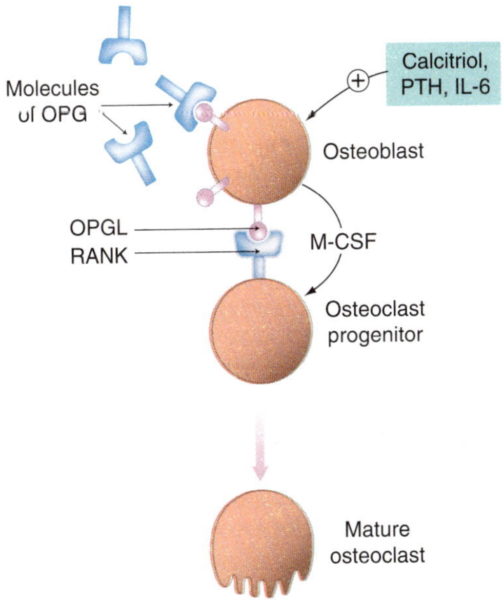

Fig. 30.2 Schematic diagram of the role of the osteoblast in the differentiation and activation of the osteoclast. The osteoblast is stimulated by calcitriol, parathormone (PTH) and interleukin-6 (IL-6) to express a surface ligand, the osteoprotegerin ligand (OPGL). This ligand interacts with a receptor on the osteoclast—an osteoclast differentiation and activation receptor termed RANK (receptor activator of NF-κB). This, with macrophage colony-stimulating factor (M-CSF) released by the osteoblast causes differentiation and activation of the osteoclast progenitors to form mature osteoclasts, which are polarised with a ruffled border on the bone-resorbing side. Fusion of osteoclasts occurs to give giant multinucleated bone-resorbing cells (not shown). The osteoblast also releases 'decoy' molecules of osteoprotegerin (OPG), which can bind OPGL and prevent activation of the RANK.

an area of trabecular bone and move along it digging a pit by secreting H^+ and proteolytic enzymes. This process gradually liberates cytokines such as insulin growth factor (IGF-1) and transforming growth factor-β (TGF-β) that have been embedded in the osteoid (Fig. 30.1) and these in turn recruit and activate successive teams of osteoblasts that have been stimulated to develop from precursor cells, and are awaiting the call to duty (see Fig. 30.1 and below). The osteoblasts invade the site, synthesising and secreting the organic matrix of bone, the osteoid, and secreting IGF-1 and TGF-β (which become embedded in the osteoid; see above). Some osteoblasts become embedded in the osteoid, forming terminal osteocytes; others interact with and activate osteoclast precursors—and we are back to the beginning of the cycle.

Cytokines involved in bone remodelling other than IGF-1 and TGF-β include the bone morphogenic protein-2 (a member of a family of cytokines related to the TGF-β superfamily; Fig. 30.1) — fibroblast growth factor (Fig. 30.1), macrophage colony-stimulating factor (Fig. 30.2), various interleukins (ILs; Fig. 30.1) and two newly discovered factors involved in the osteoblast–osteoclast interaction. These are shown in Figure 30.2. Osteoprotegerin ligand (OPGL) is expressed by the osteoblast and, during cell-to-cell contact, it binds to a receptor on the osteoclast. The receptor is termed (wait for it; biological terminology has fallen over its own feet here) RANK, which stands for receptor activator of NF-κB—NF-κB being the principal transcription factor involved in osteoclast differentiation and activation. The osteoblast also synthesises and releases a molecule termed osteoprotegerin (OPG), identical with RANK, which functions as a decoy receptor. In a sibling-undermining process by the two osteoblast progeny, OPG can bind to OPGL (generated by the very cell that OPG itself is generated by) and inhibit OPGL's binding to its intended partner, RANK (Fig. 30.2).

THE TURNOVER OF BONE MINERALS

The main bone minerals are calcium and phosphorus.

CALCIUM METABOLISM

The daily turnover of bone minerals during remodelling involves about 700 mg calcium. Calcium has numerous roles in physiological functioning. Intracellular Ca^{2+} constitutes only a small proportion of body calcium, but it has a major role in cellular function (see Ch. 3). An influx of Ca^{2+} with increase of Ca^{2+} in the cytosol is part of the signal transduction mechanism of many cells, so the concentration of Ca^{2+} in the extracellular fluid and the plasma needs to be controlled with great precision. The concentration of Ca^{2+} in the cytoplasm of cells is about 100 nmol/l, whereas in the plasma it is about 2.5 mmol/l (i.e. 2.5×10^6 nmol/l). The plasma Ca^{2+} concentration is regulated by complex interactions between PTH and various forms of vitamin D (Figs 30.3 and 30.4). Calcitonin also plays a part.

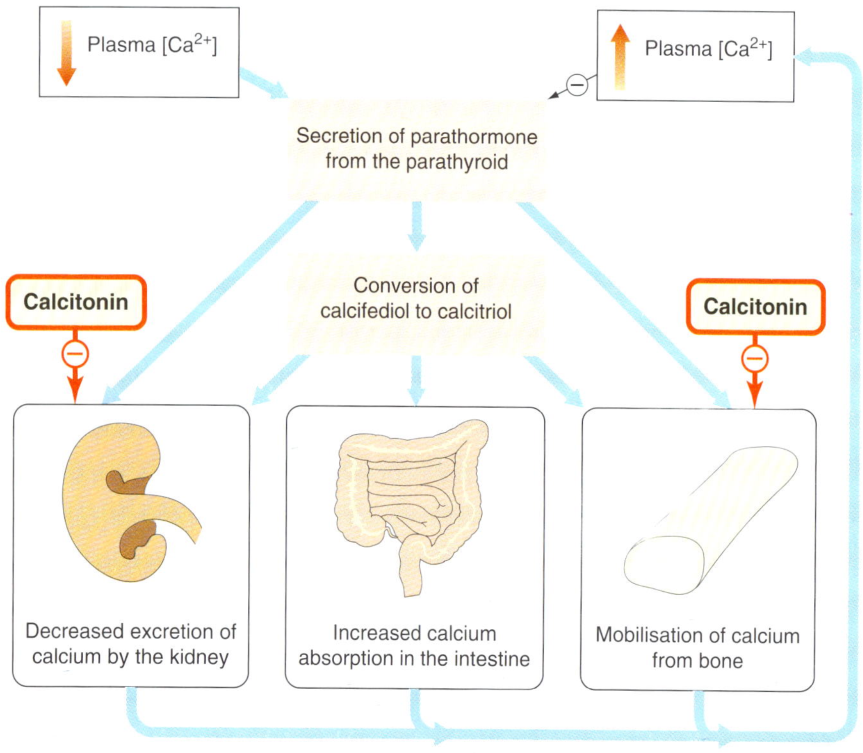

Fig. 30.3 The main factors involved in maintaining the concentration of calcium in the plasma. Calcifediol and calcitriol are metabolites of vitamin D_3 and constitute the 'hormones' 25-hydroxyvitamin D_3 and 1,25-hydroxyvitamin D_3, respectively. Endogenous calcitonin, secreted by the thyroid, inhibits Ca^{2+} mobilisation from bone and decreases its resorption in the kidney, thus reducing blood Ca^{2+} concentrations. Calcitonin is also used therapeutically in osteoporosis.

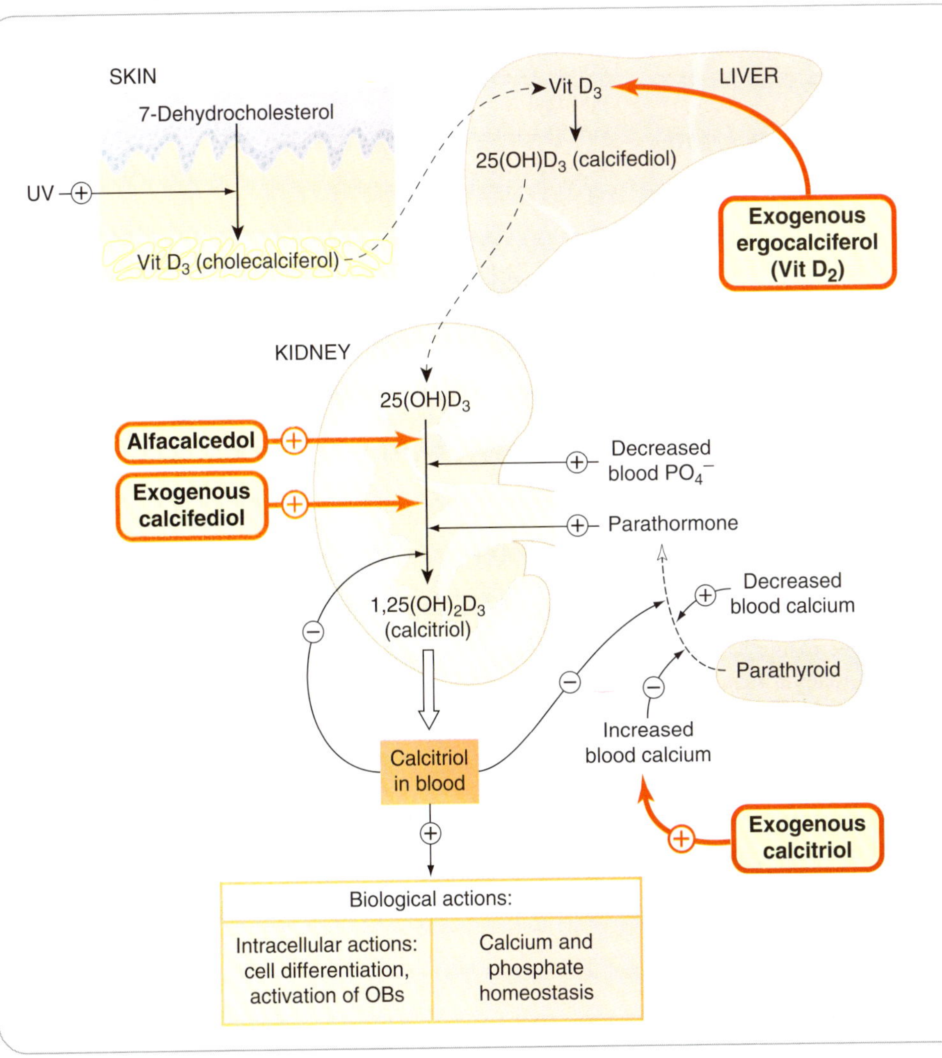

Fig. 30.4 Summary of the actions of the vitamin D endocrine system. Drugs that affect the system are shown in red-bordered boxes. Exogenous ergocalciferol, vitamin D_2 (formed in plants under the influence of ultraviolet (UV)), is converted to the corresponding D_2 metabolites in liver and kidney, as in the D_2 analogue dihydrotachysterol (not shown). Alfacalcidol (1α-hydroxycholecalciferol) is 25-hydroxylated to calcitriol in the liver. (OBs, osteoblasts.)

Calcium absorption in the intestine involves a Ca^{2+}-binding protein, the synthesis of which is regulated by calcitriol (see Fig. 30.3 and below). It is probable that the overall calcium content of the body is regulated largely by this absorption mechanism since normally, urinary Ca^{2+} excretion remains more or less constant. However, with high blood Ca^{2+} concentrations, urinary excretion increases, and with low blood concentrations, urinary excretion can be reduced by PTH and calcitriol, both of which enhance Ca^{2+} reabsorption in the renal tubules (Fig. 30.3).

PHOSPHATE METABOLISM

Phosphates are important constituents of bone and are also critically important in the structure and function of all the cells of the body. They play a significant part in enzymic reactions in the cell; they have roles as intracellular buffers and in the excretion of H^+ in the kidney.

Phosphate absorption is an energy-requiring process regulated by calcitriol (see below). Phosphate deposition in bone, as hydroxyapatite, depends on the plasma concentration of PTH, which, with calcitriol, tends to mobilise both Ca^{2+} and phosphate from the bone matrix. Phosphate is excreted by the kidney; here PTH inhibits reabsorption and thus increases excretion.

HORMONES INVOLVED IN BONE METABOLISM AND REMODELLING

The main hormones involved in bone metabolism and remodelling are PTH, the vitamin D family and calcitonin. Glucocorticoids also affect bone.

PARATHORMONE

PTH is an important physiological regulator of Ca^{2+} metabolism. It maintains the plasma Ca^{2+} concentration by mobilising Ca^{2+} from bone, by promoting its reabsorption by the kidney and, in particular, by stimulating the synthesis of calcitriol, which, in turn, increases Ca^{2+} absorption from the intestine and synergises with PTH in mobilising bone Ca^{2+} (Figs 30.3 and 30.4). PTH promotes phosphate excretion, and thus its net effect is to increase the concentration of Ca^{2+} in the plasma and lower that of phosphate.

The mobilisation of Ca^{2+} from bone by PTH is mediated, at least in part, by stimulation of the recruitment and activation of osteoclasts. In some circumstances, osteoblast activity is also inhibited (not shown in Fig. 30.1).

However, given therapeutically in low intermittent dose, PTH and fragments of PTH paradoxically stimulate osteoblast activity and enhance bone formation (see below).

PTH is synthesised in the cells of the parathyroid glands and stored in vesicles. The principal factor controlling secretion is the concentration of free Ca^{2+} in the plasma, low plasma Ca^{2+} stimulating secretion. The parathyroid cell has a Ca^{2+} sensor in its membrane and Ca^{2+} binding leads to inhibition of PTH secretion.

VITAMIN D

Vitamin D is a prehormone that is converted in the body into a number of biologically active metabolites that function as true hormones, circulating in the blood and regulating the activities of various cell types (see Reichel et al., 1989). Their main action is the maintenance of plasma Ca^{2+} by increasing Ca^{2+} absorption in the intestine, mobilising Ca^{2+} from bone and decreasing its renal excretion (see Fig. 30.3). Vitamin D itself is really a family of hormones belonging to the steroid family of super-hormones. In humans, there are two sources of vitamin D:

- dietary ergocalciferol (D_2), derived from ergosterol in plants
- cholecalciferol (D_3) generated in the skin from 7-dehydrocholesterol by the action of ultraviolet irradiation, the 7-dehydrocholesterol having been formed from cholesterol in the wall of the intestine.

Cholecalciferol (vitamin D_3) is converted to 25-hydroxyvitamin D_3 (calcifediol) in the liver, and this is converted to a series of other metabolites of varying activity in the kidney, the most potent of which is 1,25-dihydroxyvitamin D_3 (*calcitriol*) (see Fig. 30.4). The synthesis of calcitriol from calcifediol is regulated by PTH and is also influenced by the phosphate concentration in the plasma and by the calcitriol concentration itself through a negative feedback mechanism (Fig. 30.4). Receptors for calcitriol have been identified in virtually every tissue except liver and it is now considered that calcitriol may be important in the functioning of many cell types.

The main actions of calcitriol are the stimulation of absorption of Ca^{2+} and phosphate in the intestine and the mobilisation of Ca^{2+} from bone, but it also increases Ca^{2+} reabsorption in the kidney tubules (Fig. 30.3). Its effect on bone involves promotion of maturation of osteoclasts and indirect stimulation of their activity (Figs 30.1 and 30.3). It decreases collagen synthesis by osteoblasts, and its effect on these cells is by the classical steroid pathway, involving intracellular receptors and an effect on the DNA. However, the effect on bone is complex and is clearly not confined to mobilising Ca^{2+}, since in clinical vitamin D deficiency (see below), in which the mineralisation of bone is impaired, administration of vitamin D restores bone formation. One explanation may lie in the fact that calcitriol stimulates synthesis of osteocalcin, the vitamin-K-dependent, Ca^{2+}-binding protein of bone matrix.

OESTROGENS

During reproductive life in the female, oestrogens have an important role in maintenance of bone integrity. They inhibit the cytokines that recruit osteoclasts and oppose the bone-resorbing, Ca^{2+}-mobilising action of PTH. Withdrawal of oestrogen as happens at the menopause can lead to osteoporosis.

CALCITONIN

Calcitonin is a hormone secreted by the specialised 'C' cells found in the thyroid follicles.

The main action of calcitonin is on bone; it inhibits bone resorption by binding to a specific receptor on osteoclasts inhibiting their action. In the kidney it decreases the reabsorption of both Ca^{2+} and phosphate in the proximal tubules. Its overall effect is to decrease the plasma Ca^{2+} concentration. See Figures 33.3 and 33.4.

Secretion is determined mainly by the plasma Ca^{2+} concentration.

GLUCOCORTICOIDS

Physiological concentrations of glucocorticoids are required for osteoblast differentiation. Excessive pharmacological concentrations inhibit bone formation by inhibiting osteoblast differentiation and activity and may stimulate osteoclast action — leading to osteoporosis. This latter effect is also evident when pathological concentrations of endogenous glucocorticoids are present, as in Cushing's syndrome (see Fig. 27.7).

Bone remodelling

- Bone is continuously remodelled throughout life. The events of the remodelling cycle are as follows:
  - —osteoclasts, having been activated by osteoblasts, resorb bone by digging pits in trabecular bone
  - —into these pits the bone-forming osteoblasts secrete osteoid (bone matrix), which consists mainly of collagen but also contains osteocalcin, osteonectin, phosphoproteins and the cytokines insulin growth factor (IGF) and transforming growth factor-β (TGF-β)
  - —the osteoid is then mineralised, i.e. complex calcium phosphate crystals (hydroxyapatites) are deposited.
- Bone metabolism and mineralisation involves the action of parathormone, the vitamin D family, various cytokines (e.g. IGF, TGF-β, interleukin-6, bone morphogenic protein 2) and calcitonin. Declining physiological levels of oestrogens and therapeutic levels of glucocorticoids can result in bone resorption not balanced by bone formation—leading to osteoporosis.

DISORDERS OF BONE

DISORDERS OF THE STRUCTURE OF BONE

The reduction of bone mass with distortion of the microarchitecture is termed *osteoporosis*; a reduction in the mineral content is termed *osteopenia*. Osteoporotic bone can fracture easily after minimal trauma—and frequently does. The commonest causes of osteoporosis are postmenopausal deficiency of oestrogen and age-related deterioration in bone homeostasis, but it can also result from other factors such as excessive glucocorticoid or thyroxine administration and can occur secondary to conditions such as rheumatoid arthritis. Since life expectancy has increased significantly, osteoporosis has become an important public health problem and drugs that prevent its development are being sought actively. Other diseases of bone requiring drug therapy are *osteomalacia* and *rickets* (the juvenile form of osteomalacia) in which there are defects in bone mineralisation owing to vitamin D deficiency, and *Paget's disease*, in which there is distortion of the processes of bone resorption and remodelling.

DISORDERS OF BONE MINERAL METABOLISM

Hypocalcaemia occurs with hypoparathyroidism, vitamin D deficiencies, congenital rickets and some kidney diseases; hypercalcaemia occurs with hyperparathyroidism and some malignancies.

Phosphate deficiency and hypophosphataemia can occur in nutritional deficiency states (e.g. in alcoholics and patients receiving parenteral nutrition).

Hyperphosphataemia is a common problem in patients with renal failure and is treated with Ca^{2+}- or aluminium-containing antacids (Ch. 24) that bind phosphate and prevent its absorption from the gut.

DRUGS USED IN BONE DISORDERS

BISPHOSPHONATES

Bisphosphonates are enzyme-resistant analogues of pyrophosphate—which normally inhibits mineralisation in bone. In bisphosphonates, the P–O–P structure of pyrophosphate is replaced by P–C–P. They reduce the resorption of bone in a dose-dependent manner—mainly by inhibiting recruitment and promoting apoptosis (cell suicide see Ch. 5) of osteoclasts (Fig. 30.1). They also indirectly stimulate osteoblast activity. It is thought that they may be incorporated into the bone matrix and ingested by osteoclasts when these resorb bone.

The main bisphosphonates available for clinical use are **alendronate** and **risedronate**. Others are disodium etidronate, disodium pamidronate and sodium clodronate.

Bisphosphonates are given orally and are poorly absorbed. About 50% of a dose accumulates at sites of bone mineralisation, where it remains, potentially for months or years, until the bone is resorbed. The free drug is excreted unchanged by the kidney.

Clinical uses of bisphosphonates (e.g. alendronate, pamidronate)

- Paget's disease of bone.
- Hypercalcaemia caused by malignant disease.
- Prevention or treatment of postmenopausal osteoporosis (as an alternative or addition to oestrogens).
- Prevention or treatment of glucocorticoid-induced osteoporosis.
- They are under investigation for the treatment of cancer metastases in bone.

Absorption is impaired by food, particularly milk, so the drugs must be taken on an empty stomach.

Unwanted effects

Unwanted effects include gastrointestinal disturbances, which can be severe, and occasionally bone pain. Peptic ulcers have occurred. Alendronate can cause oesophagitis.

Disodium etidronate can increase the risk of fractures owing to reduced calcification of bone; this is less likely if it is given cyclically.

COMPOUNDS RELATED TO OESTROGEN

The decline in natural oestrogen levels is a major factor in postmenopausal osteoporosis and there is evidence that giving hormone replacement therapy (HRT; see Ch. 29) can ameliorate this condition. But HRT has actions on many systems and newer non-hormonal agents have now been developed that exhibit agonist actions on some tissues and antagonist actions on others. These are termed *selective estrogen receptor modulators* (SERMS). **Raloxifene** is a SERM that has agonist activity on oestrogen receptors in bone and the cardiovascular system and antagonist activity on oetrogen receptors in mammary tissue and the uterus.

Raloxifene

Actions and mechanism of action

Raloxifene produces a dose-dependent increase in osteoblast activity and reduction in osteoclast action.

It is well absorbed in the gastrointestinal tract and undergoes extensive first-pass metabolism in the liver to give the glucuronide. Thus bioavailability is only about 2%. It is widely distributed in the tissues and is converted to an active metabolite in liver, lungs, bone, spleen, uterus and kidneys. Its half-life averages 32 hours. It is excreted mainly in the faeces.

Unwanted effects

Hot flushes and leg cramps are common. A more serious effect is venous thromboembolism, which in a recent clinical trial occurred three times more frequently in subjects on raloxifene than in those taking placebo.

When warfarin is given with raloxifene, there is a 10% decrease in prothrombin time; colestyramine reduces the enterohepatic cycling of raloxifene by 60%.

VITAMIN D AND PARATHORMONE

Until recently, there had been little or no clinical use for PTH as such; however, as PTH and fragments of PTH paradoxically stimulate osteoblast activity and enhance bone formation, they are in clinical trial for the treatment of osteoporosis (see below).

Hypoparathyroidism is treated by vitamin D—acute hypoparathyroidism necessitating the use of intravenous Ca^{2+} and injectable vitamin D preparations.

The main vitamin D preparation used clinically is ergocalciferol (vitamin D_2); also available for clinical use are alfacalcidol and calcitriol. All can be given orally and are well absorbed from the intestine. Vitamin D preparations are fat soluble and bile salts are necessary for absorption. Injectable forms of calciferol are available.

Pharmacokinetic aspects

Given orally, vitamin D is bound to a specific α-globulin in the blood. The plasma half-life is about 22 hours but vitamin D can be found in the fat for many months. The main route of elimination is in the faeces.

The clinical use of vitamin D preparations is given in the box.

Unwanted effects

Excessive intake of vitamin D causes hypercalcaemia, the manifestations of which include constipation, depression, weakness and fatigue. There is a reduced ability to concentrate the urine, resulting in polyuria and polydipsia. If hypercalcaemia persists, calcium salts are deposited in the kidney and urine causing renal failure and kidney stones.

Some anticonvulsant drugs (e.g. phenytoin; see Ch. 39) increase the requirement for vitamin D.

Clinical uses of vitamin D

- Deficiency states: prevention and treatment of various forms of rickets, osteomalacia and vitamin D deficiency owing to malabsorption and liver disease (ergocalciferol).
- Hypocalcaemia caused by hypoparathyroidism (ergocalciferol).
- Osteodystrophy of chronic renal failure, which is the consequence of decreased calcitriol generation (calcitriol or alphacalcidol).

Plasma Ca^{2+} levels should be monitored during therapy with vitamin D.

Clinical uses of calcitonin/salcatonin

- Hypercalcaemia (e.g. associated with neoplasia).
- Paget's disease of bone (it relieves the pain and reduces some of the neurological complications).
- Postmenopausal and corticosteroid-induced osteoporosis (with other agents).

CALCITONIN

The preparations available for clinical use (see the clinical box) are porcine (natural) **calcitonin** and **salcatonin** (synthetic salmon calcitonin). Synthetic human calcitonin is now also available. Porcine calcitonin may contain traces of thyroid hormones and can lead to the production of antibodies. Calcitonin is given by subcutaneous or intramuscular injection, and there may be a local inflammatory action at the injection site. It can also be given intranasally. Its plasma half-life is 4–12 minutes, but its action lasts for several hours.

Unwanted effects

Unwanted effects include nausea and vomiting. Facial flushing may occur, as may a tingling sensation in the hands and an unpleasant taste in the mouth.

CALCIUM SALTS

Calcium salts used therapeutically include calcium gluconate and calcium lactate, given orally. Calcium gluconate is also used for intravenous injection; intramuscular injection is not used because it causes local necrosis. An oral preparation of hydroxyapatite is available.

Unwanted effects

Oral calcium salts can cause gastrointestinal disturbance. Intravenous administration requires care, especially in patients taking cardiac glycosides (see Ch. 17).

The clinical use of the calcium salts is given in the box on page 453.

POTENTIAL NEW THERAPIES FOR OSTEOPOROSIS

All current drugs used in osteoporosis *inhibit bone resorption*. They can increase bone mineral density and decrease the risk of fractures. But they do not generally produce a marked increase in bone mass and the reduction of fracture risk is not usually more than 50% of the risk in untreated subjects. Consequently there is now growing interest in the possible value of compounds that *stimulate bone formation* — for use alone or in combination with the resorptive drugs (see Rosen and Bilezekian, 2001). Some contenders are PTH, IGF-1 and growth hormone (see Fig. 30.1). PTH is the most promising of these. When given intermittently in low doses it potently stimulates both trabecular and cortical bone

Clinical uses of calcium salts

- Dietary deficiency.
- Hypocalcaemia caused by hypoparathyroidism or malabsorption (intravenous for acute tetany).
- Calcium carbonate is an antacid; it is poorly absorbed and binds phosphate in the gut. It is used to treat patients with hyperphosphataemia caused by renal failure.
- Prevention and treatment of osteoporosis (often with oestrogen, bisphosphonate, vitamin D or calcitonin).
- Cardiac dysrhythmias caused by severe hyperkalaemia (intravenous; see Ch. 17).

growth. Both recombinant PTH itself and the recombinant peptide fragment (1–34) are in phase III trial.

Potential anabolic agents being considered for future development are fluoride and the statins. These last, commonly given to reduce blood cholesterol (Ch. 19) have been shown to increase the gene expression of bone morphogenic protein 2, and to increase bone formation in vitro.

Possible new antiresorptive agents include osteoprotegerin—a physiological inhibitor of bone resorption—which has shown promise in early clinical trials, and thiazides (Ch. 23), which have a small effect in slowing bone loss and might be of value in combination therapy.

It seems that there is likely to be a significant break-through in fracture prevention in the reasonably near future.

Parathyroid, vitamin D and bone mineral homeostasis

- The vitamin D family are true hormones; precursors are converted to calcifediol in the liver, then to the main hormone, calcitriol, in kidney.
- Calcitriol increases plasma Ca^{2+} by mobilising it from bone, increasing its absorption in the intestine and decreasing its excretion by the kidney.
- Parathormone (PTH) increases blood Ca^{2+} by increasing calcitriol synthesis, mobilising Ca^{2+} from bone and reducing renal Ca^{2+} excretion. (But paradoxically, small doses of PTH given intermittently increase bone formation.)
- Calcitonin (secreted from the thyroid) reduces Ca^{2+} resorption from bone by inhibiting osteoclast activity.

REFERENCES AND FURTHER READING

Allison T, Derynck R 2002 Interfering with bone remodelling. Nature 416: 686–687 (*Short comment on the proposal that osteoclasts can activate the production of their own 'off-switch'—interferon-β protein—which prevents runaway bone loss. The targeted use of interferon-β could have a role in the therapy of osteoporosis*)

Bouillon R 1998 The many faces of rickets. N Engl J Med 338: 681–682 (*Editorial: A succinct account of recent information about the metabolic activation of the vitamin D family and its relation to rickets*)

Bushinskey D A, Monk R D 1998 Calcium. Lancet 352: 306–311 (*Calcium homeostasis, its disorders and the treatment thereof*)

Clemett D, Spenser C M 2000 Raloxifene: a review of its use in postmenopausal osteoporosis. Drugs 60: 379–411 (*Comprehensive review covering the mechanism of action, pharmacology, pharmacokinetic aspects, therapeutic use and adverse effects of raloxifene*)

Compston J E 2001 Sex steroids and bone. Physiol Rev 81: 419–447 (*Excellent, comprehensive review of steroid actions and mechanisms of action on bone, starting with bone structure; clear coverage of remodelling*)

Delmas P 2002 Treatment of postmenopausal osteoporosis. Lancet 359; 2018–20026 (*Excellent up-to-date review*)

Eastell R 1998 Treatment of postmenopausal osteoporosis. N Engl J Med 338: 736–746 (*Excellent, comprehensive review of pathophysiology and drug treatment of postmenopausal osteoporosis with review of clinical trials of drugs used and future therapies*)

Gonzalez E A 2000 The role of cytokines in skeletal remodelling: possible consequences for renal dystrophy. Nephrol Dial Transplant 15: 945–950 (*Succinct article on the role of the osteoprotegerin/RANK/OPGK system in osteoporosis. Excellent figures*)

Groeneveld E H J, Burger E H 2000 Bone morphogenic proteins in human bone regeneration. Eur J Endocrinol 142: 9–21 (*Detailed review describing clinical studies with recombinant bone morphogenic protein (BMP)2 (rhBMP-2), BMP carriers and the potential role of BMP in bone grafts*)

Hill P A 1998 Bone remodelling. Br J Orthodontics 25: 101–107 (*Succinct description of bone turnover with good diagrams*)

Horowitz M C, Xi Y et al. 2001 Control of osteoclastogenesis and bone resorption by members of the TNF family of receptors and ligands. Cytokine Growth Factor Rev 12: 9–18 (*Worthwhile minireview, good diagram*)

Kleerekoper M, Schein J R 2001 Comparative safety of bone remodeling agents with a focus on osteoporosis therapies. J Clin Pharmacol 41: 239–250 (*Covers briefly the epidemiology of osteoporosis. Outlines the various bone remodelling agents available and gives a good summary table of their benefits*)

Kostenuik P J, Shalhoub V 2001 Osteoprotegerin: a physiological and pharmacological inhibitor of bone resorption. Curr Pharmaceut Design 7: 613–635 (*Detailed coverage of the role of OPG/RANK/OPGK in bone remodelling with structure of OPG and its regulation and results of* in vitro *experiments, animal experiments and one clinical trial. States that the OPG pathway 'represents a potential goldmine of therapeutic targets'*)

Lopez F J 2000 New approaches to the treatment of osteoporosis. Curr Opin Chem Biol 4: 383–393 (*Crisp outline of estrogens, SERMs, androgens, bisphosphonates, PTH preparations, calcitonin and potential new agents such as the statins, leptin, osteoprotegerin and oxytocin*)

Lufkin E G, Wong M, Deal C 2001 The role of selective oestrogen receptor modulators in the prevention and treatment of osteoporosis. Rheum Dis Clin North Am 27: 163–184 (*Good description of the pathogenesis of osteoporosis with outline of main current therapies. Gives details of clinical trials with raloxifene and considers combination therapies*)

Manolagas S C 2000 Birth and death of bone cells: basic regulatory mechanisms and implications for the pathogenesis and treatment of osteoporosis. Endocrin Rev 21: 115–137 (*Outstanding, comprehensive review*)

Masi L, Brandi M L 2001 Physiopathological basis of bone turnover. Q J Nucl Med 45: 2–6 (*Crisp article on bone remodelling with useful table of factors that control it*)

Morley P, Whitfield J F, Willick G E 2001 Parathyroid hormone: an anabolic treatment for osteoporosis. Curr Pharmaceut Design 7: 671–687 (*Very worthwhile review. Delineates the anabolic actions of parathyroid*

hormone and cites the results of animal and clinical studies)
Reeve J 2002 Recombinant human parathyroid hormone: osteoporosis is proving amenable to treatment. Br Med J 324: 435–436 (*Editorial on the significance of recombinant human parathyroid hormone for osteoporosis therapy*)
Reichel H, Koeftler H P, Norman A W 1989 The role of the vitamin D endocrine system in health and disease. N Engl J Med 320: 980–991 (*Good comprehensive early review*)
Reid I R, Ames R W et al. 2000 Hydrochlorothiazide reduces loss of cortical bone in normal postmenopausal women: a randomized controlled trial. Am J Med 109: 362–370 (*The results suggest that thiazides may possibly be useful in prevention but not treatment of postmenopausal osteoporosis. See also in the same issue: Sebastien A, pp. 429–430*)
Rodan G A 1998 Mechanism of action of the bisphosphonates. Annu Rev Pharmacol Toxicol 38: 375–388 (*Short lucid review*)
Rosen C J, Bilezekian J P 2001 Anabolic therapy for osteoporosis. J Clin Endocrinol Metab 86: 957–964 (*Well written article clarifying the potential role of non-resorptive agents in the therapy of osteoporosis. Neat figure of the interaction between osteoblasts and osteoclasts*)
Rosen C J, Rackoff P J 2001 Emerging anabolic treatments for osteoporosis. Rheum Dis Clin North Am 27: 215–232 (*Clear account of the potential value of anabolic agents, describing preclinical studies with insulin-like growth factor-1, recombinant growth hormone, recombinant PTH and various combination therapies*)
Watts N B 1999 Postmenopausal osteoporosis. Obstet Gynecol Surv 54: 532–537 (*Short clinical review covering the epidemiology of osteoporosis, delineating the techniques for identifying it and describing briefly the main drugs used in treatment. Useful table of all the main causes of osteoporosis*)
Whitfield J F, Morley P 1995 Small bone-building fragments of parathyroid hormone: new therapeutic agents for osteoporosis. Trends Pharmacol Sci 16: 382–385 (*Useful review with cheerful diagram of bone remodelling*)

SECTION

4

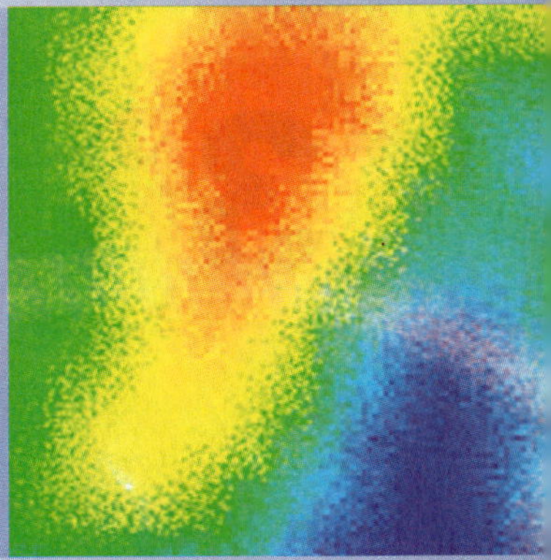

THE NERVOUS SYSTEM

31 Chemical transmission and drug action in the central nervous system

Overview 456

Introduction 456

Chemical signalling in the nervous system 457

Targets for drug action 458

Drug action in the central nervous system 459

The classification of psychotropic drugs 460

OVERVIEW

Brain function is the single most important aspect of physiology that defines the difference between humans and other species. Disorders of brain function, whether primary or secondary to malfunction of other systems, are a major concern of human society, and a field in which pharmacological intervention plays a key role. In this chapter, we introduce some basic principles of neuropharmacology that underly much of the material in the rest of this section.

INTRODUCTION

There are two reasons why understanding the action of drugs on the central nervous system (CNS) presents a particularly challenging problem. The first is that centrally acting drugs are of special significance to mankind. Not only are they of major therapeutic importance,* but they are also the drugs that humans most commonly administer to themselves for non-medical reasons (e.g. alcohol, tea and coffee, cannabis, nicotine, opiates, amphetamines and so on). The second reason is that the CNS is functionally far more complex than any other system in the body, and this makes the understanding of drug effects very much more difficult. The relationship between the behaviour of individual cells and that of the organ as a whole is far less direct in the brain than, for example, in the heart or kidney. In these latter organs, a detailed understanding of how a drug affects the cells gives us a fairly clear idea of what effect it will produce on the organ (and on the animal) as a whole. In the brain, this is simply not true. For example, we may know that a drug mimics the action of 5-hydroxytryptamine (5-HT, serotonin) in its effect on nerve cells, and we know empirically that this type of action is often associated with drugs that cause hallucinations, but the link between these two events remains wholly mysterious. In spite of sustained progress in understanding the cellular and biochemical effects produced by centrally acting drugs, the gulf between the description of drug action at this level and the description of drug action at the functional and behavioural level remains, for the most part, very wide. Attempts to bridge it seem, at times, like throwing candy floss into the Grand Canyon.

A few bridgeheads have none the less been established, some more firmly than others. Thus the relationship between dopaminergic pathways in the extrapyramidal system and the effects of drugs in alleviating or exacerbating the symptoms of Parkinson's disease (see Ch. 34) is clear cut. Also reasonably firm is the link between the functions of noradrenaline (norepinephrine) and 5-HT in certain parts of the brain and the symptoms of depression (see Ch. 38), and that between gamma-aminobutyric acid (GABA) and anxiety (Ch. 36). Less well established is the connection between hyperactivity in dopaminergic pathways and schizophrenia (see Ch. 37). At the other end of the spectrum, attempts to relate the condition of epilepsy to an identifiable cellular disturbance (see Ch. 39) have been very disappointing, even though the abnormal neuronal discharge pattern in epilepsy seems, on the face of it, a much simpler kind of disturbance than, for example, the altered mood of a depressed patient. In this chapter, we outline the general principles governing the action of drugs on the CNS and include a look into the (possible) future. Most neuroactive drugs work by interfering with the chemical signals that underlie brain function, and the next two chapters discuss the major CNS transmitter systems, and the ways in which drugs affect them. In Chapter 34 we focus on neurodegenerative diseases, and the remaining chapters in this section deal with the main classes of neuroactive drug that are currently in use.

Background information will be found in neurobiology textbooks such as Kandel et al. (2000), and in texts on

*In England in 2000, 103 million prescriptions (about 20% of all prescriptions) were for CNS drugs, as defined by the British National Formulary. This amounted to nearly two per person across the whole population.

neuropharmacology such as Cooper et al. (1996), Nestler et al. (2001). For exhaustive coverage, see Bloom & Kupfer (1995).

CHEMICAL SIGNALLING IN THE NERVOUS SYSTEM

The brain (like every other organ in the body!) is basically a chemical machine; it controls the main functions of a higher animal across timescales ranging from milliseconds (e.g. returning a 100 mph tennis serve) to years (e.g. remembering how to ride a bicycle).* The chemical signalling mechanisms cover a correspondingly wide dynamic range, as summarised, in a very general way, in Figure 31.1. Currently, we understand much about drug effects on events at the fast end of the spectrum—synaptic transmission and neuromodulation—but much less about long-term adaptive processes, though it is quite evident that the latter are of great importance for the neurological and psychiatric disorders that are susceptible to drug treatment.

The original concept of neurotransmission envisaged a substance released by one neuron and acting rapidly, briefly, and at short range on the membrane of an adjacent (postsynaptic) neuron, causing excitation or inhibition. The principles outlined in Chapter 9 apply to the central as well as the peripheral nervous system. It is now clear that chemical mediators within the brain can produce slow and long-lasting effects; that they can act rather diffusely, at a considerable distance from their site of release; and that they can produce diverse effects, for example on transmitter synthesis and on the expression of neurotransmitter receptors, in

*Memory of the basic facts of pharmacology seems to come somewhere in the middle of this range (skewed towards the short end).

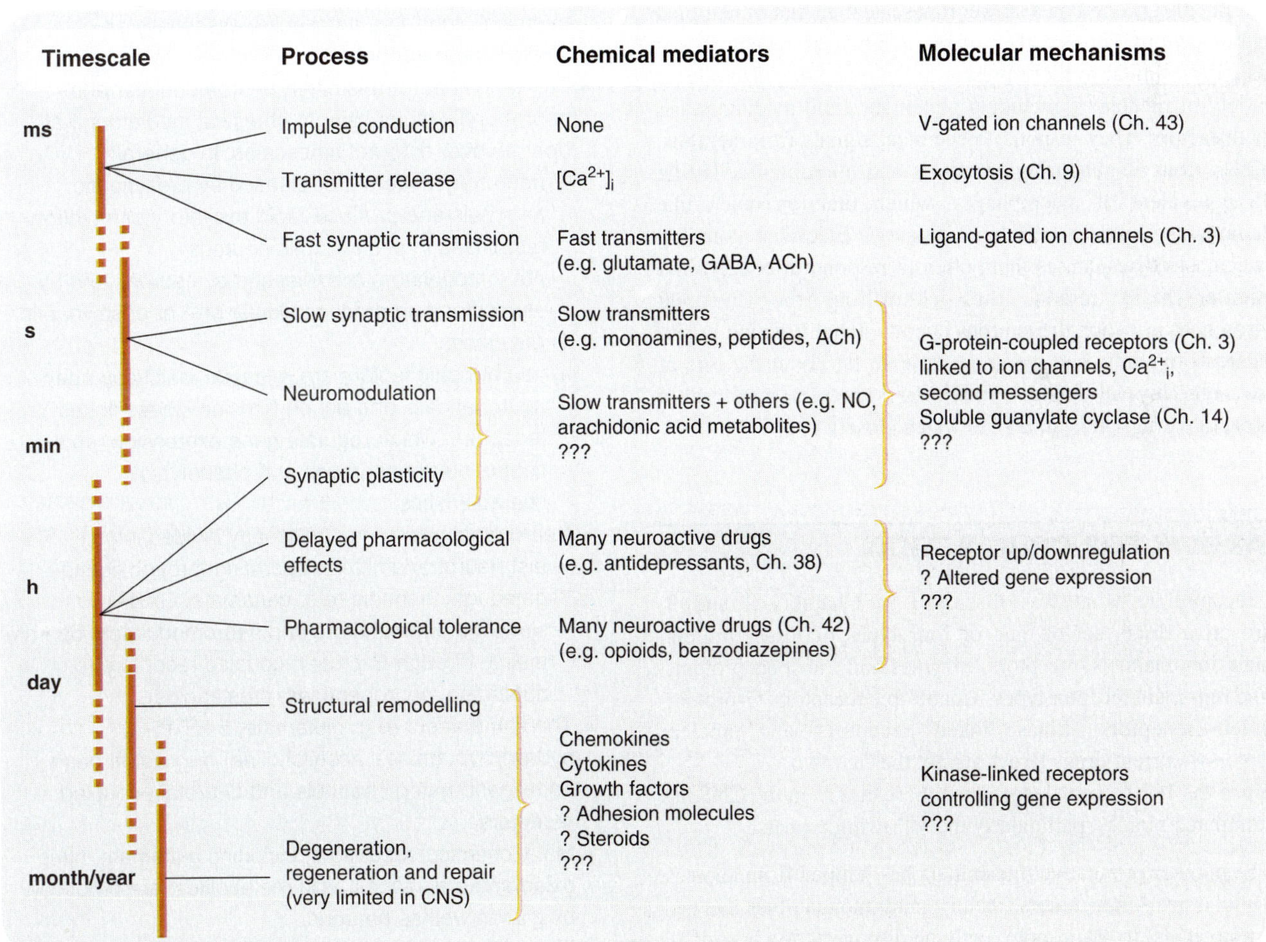

Fig. 31.1 Chemical signalling in the nervous system. Knowledge of the mediators and mechanisms becomes sparser as we move from the rapid events of synaptic transmission to the slower ones involving remodelling and alterations of gene expression. (ACh, acetylcholine' GABA, gamma-aminobutyric acid; NO, nitric oxide; ???, areas of uncertainty.)

addition to affecting the ionic conductance of the postsynaptic cells. The term *neuromodulator* was coined to denote a neuronally released mediator, the actions of which do not conform to the original neurotransmitter concept. The term is not clearly defined, and it covers not only the diffusely acting neuropeptide mediators, but also mediators such as nitric oxide (NO) and arachidonic acid metabolites, which are not stored and released like conventional neurotransmitters and may come from non-neuronal cells as well as neurons. In general, neuromodulation relates to *synaptic plasticity*, including short-term events, such as the regulation of presynaptic transmitter release or postsynaptic excitability, and longer-term events such as neuronal gene regulation.

Neurotrophic factors act over even longer timescales to regulate the growth and morphology of neurons, as well as their functional properties.

Glial cells, particularly astrocytes, which are the main non-neuronal cells in the CNS and outnumber neurons by ten-to-one, also play an important signalling role. Once thought of mainly as housekeeping cells, whose function was merely to look after the fastidious neurons, they are increasingly seen as 'inexcitable neurons' with a major communications role to play (see Bezzi & Volterra, 2001), albeit on a slower timescale than that of neuronal communication. These cells express a range of receptors and transporters similar to those present in neurons; they also release a variety of mediators, including glutamate, lipid mediators and growth factors. They respond to chemical signals from neurons, and also from neighbouring astrocytes and microglial cells (the CNS equivalent of macrophages, which function much like inflammatory cells in peripheral tissues). Electrical coupling between astrocytes causes them often to respond in concert in a particular brain region, thus controlling the chemical environment in which the neurons operate. Glial function in situ is difficult to study, and we know little so far about the role of these cells in pathological conditions, or their response to neuroactive drugs. It is an area to watch closely.

TARGETS FOR DRUG ACTION

To recapitulate what was discussed in Chapters 2 and 3, neuroactive drugs act on one of four types of target protein, namely ion channels, receptors, enzymes and transport proteins. Of the four main receptor types—ionotropic receptors, G-protein-coupled receptors, kinase-linked receptors and nuclear receptors—current drugs target mainly the first two.

Since the 1970s, knowledge about these targets in the CNS has accumulated rapidly, particularly the following aspects.

- The number of putative transmitters has jumped from about 10 'classical' transmitters (mainly small monoamines and amino acids) to 40 or more, with the discovery of a host of neuropeptides (see Ch. 13). At the same time, the importance of other 'non-classical' mediators—NO, eicosanoids, growth factors, etc.—has become apparent (see Barañano et al., 2001).
- Cloning of genes for a wide variety of receptors, ion channels and other functional proteins has revealed a much greater diversity than had been evident from pharmacological studies alone (see Ch. 3). All of the known receptor molecules and ion channels appear to be expressed in at least three or four (often more) subtypes, with quite characteristic distributions in different brain areas. In some cases (e.g. dopamine receptor subtypes, Ch. 33) we are beginning to understand what the diversity means at a functional level, but in many cases (e.g. NMDA (*N*-methyl-D-aspartate) receptors, Ch. 32; sodium channels, Ch. 42), we have no real idea. From the pharmacological standpoint, the molecular diversity of such targets raises the possibility that drugs with improved

Chemical transmission in the central nervous system

- The basic processes of synaptic transmission in the CNS are essentially similar to those operating in the periphery (Ch. 9).
- Glial cells, particularly astrocytes, participate actively in chemical signalling, functioning essentially as 'inexcitable neurons'.
- The terms neurotransmitter, neuromodulator and neurotrophic factor refer to chemical mediators that operate over different timescales. In general:
  - neurotransmitters are released by presynaptic terminals and produce rapid excitatory or inhibitory responses in postsynaptic neurons
  - neuromodulators are released by neurons and by astrocytes and produce slower pre- or postsynaptic responses
  - neurotrophic factors are released mainly by non-neuronal cells and act on tyrosine-kinase-linked receptors, which regulate gene expression, and control neuronal growth and phenotypic characteristics.
- Neurotransmitters may be broady divided into:
  - fast neurotransmitters, operating through ligand-gated ion channels (e.g. glutamate, GABA)
  - slow neurotransmitters and neuromodulators operate mainly through G-protein-coupled receptors (e.g. dopamine, neuropeptides, prostanoids).
- The same agent (e.g. glutamate, 5-HT (5-hydroxytryptamine), acetylcholine) may act through both ligand-gated channels and G-protein-coupled receptors.
- Many chemical mediators, including glutamate, nitric oxide and arachidonic acid metabolites, are produced by glia as well as neurons.
- Many other mediators (e.g. cytokines, chemokines, growth factors, steroids) control long-term changes in the brain (e.g. synaptic plasticity, remodelling, etc.), mainly by affecting gene transcription.

selectivity of action—blocking one kind of sodium channel without affecting others, for example—may be discovered, and these may provide tools with which to study the functional importance of the different isoforms. Other approaches to elucidating the function of specific isoforms include the use of transgenic animals that either lack or overexpress specific isoforms (see Ch. 6), or the use of antisense oligonucleotides (Ch. 53) to block their expression. Great efforts are currently going into studies of this sort, and some successes are described in later chapters. So far, however, the potential of these new approaches in terms of improved drugs for neurological and psychiatric diseases remains largely unrealised. Hope, however (and certainly hype), springs eternal.
- The pathophysiology of neurodegeneration in conditions such as Alzheimer's disease and stroke is beginning to be understood (see Ch. 34), and progress is being made in understanding the mechanisms underlying drug dependence (see Ch. 42). These advances are suggesting new strategies for treating these disabling conditions. Other areas of brain research (e.g. the neurobiology of epilepsy, schizophrenia, depressive illnesses) are advancing less rapidly, but there is still progress to report.

DRUG ACTION IN THE CENTRAL NERVOUS SYSTEM

As we have already emphasised, the molecular and cellular mechanisms underlying drug action in the CNS and in the periphery are essentially similar. Understanding how drugs affect brain function is, however, made difficult by several factors. One is the complexity of neuronal interconnections in the brain—the wiring diagram. Figure 31.2 illustrates in a schematic way the kind of interconnections that typically exist for, say, a noradrenergic neuron in the locus ceruleus (see Ch. 33), shown as *neuron 1* in the diagram, releasing *transmitter a* at its terminals. Release of *a* affects *neuron 2* (which releases *transmitter b*) and also affects neuron 1 by direct feedback and indirectly by affecting presynaptic inputs impinging on neuron 1. The firing pattern of neuron 2 also affects the system, partly through interneuronal connections (*neuron 3*, releasing *transmitter c*). It is clear that the effects on the system of blocking or enhancing the release or actions of one or other of the transmitters will be difficult to predict and will depend greatly on the relative strength of the various excitatory and inhibitory synaptic connections, and on external inputs (*x* and *y* in the diagram). Added to this complexity at the level of neuronal interconnections is the influence of the glial cells, mentioned above. A further important complicating factor is that a range of secondary, adaptive responses is generally set in train by any drug-induced perturbation of the system. Typically, an increase in transmitter release, or interference with transmitter reuptake, is countered by inhibition of transmitter synthesis, enhanced transporter expression or decreased receptor expression. These changes, which involve altered gene expression, generally take time (hours, days or weeks) to develop and are not evident when drug effects are studied in acute experiments.

In the clinical situation, the effects of psychotropic drugs often take weeks to develop, so it is likely that they reflect the adaptive responses rather than the immediate pharmacodynamic effects of the drug. This is well documented for antidepressant drugs (Ch. 38) and some antipsychotic drugs (Ch. 37). The development of dependence on drugs such as opiates, benzodiazepines and psychostimulants is similarly gradual (Ch. 42). Therefore, one has to take into account not only the primary interaction of the drug with its target but also the secondary response of the brain to this primary effect; it is often the secondary response, rather than the primary effect, which leads to clinical benefit.

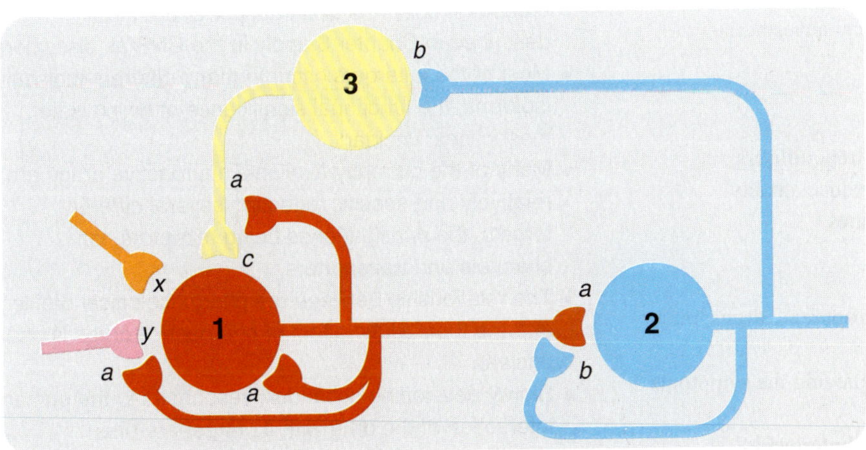

Fig. 31.2 Simplified scheme of neuronal interconnections in the CNS. Neurons 1, 2 and 3 are shown releasing transmitters a, b and c, respectively, which may be excitatory or inhibitory. Boutons of neuron 1 terminate on neuron 2, but also on neuron 1 itself, and on presynaptic terminals of other neurons that make synaptic connections with neuron 1. Neuron 2 also feeds back on neuron 1 via interneuron 3. Transmitters (x and y), released by other neurons are also shown impinging on neuron 1. Even with a such a simple network, the effects of drug-induced interference with specific transmitter systems can be difficult to predict.

A further important factor in CNS pharmacology is the existence of the blood–brain barrier (see Ch. 4), penetration of which requires molecules to *traverse* the vascular endothelial cells, rather than going between them. In general, only small non-polar molecules can diffuse passively across cell membranes. Some neuroactive drugs penetrate the blood–brain barrier in this way, but many do so via transporters, which can act either to facilitate entry into the brain or to diminish it by pumping the compound from the endothelial cell interior back into the bloodstream. Drugs that gain entry in this way include **levodopa** (Ch. 34), **valproate** (Ch. 39) and various sedative histamine antagonists (Ch. 16). Drugs that are excluded include many antibacterial and anticancer drugs that are substrates for the P-glycoprotein transporter (see Chs 4 and 44). Several such transporters have been identified, and their importance in relation to drug action in the brain is becoming increasingly apparent (see review by Tamai & Tsuji, 2000).

THE CLASSIFICATION OF PSYCHOTROPIC DRUGS

Psychotropic drugs are defined as those that affect mood and behaviour. Because these indices of brain function are difficult to define and measure, there is no consistent basis for classifying psychotropic drugs. Instead, we find a confusing melée of terms reating to chemical structure (*benzodiazepines, butyrophenones*, etc.), biochemical target (*monoamine oxidase inhibitors, serotonin reuptake inhibitors*, *opiates*, etc.), behavioural effect (*hallucinogens, psychomotor stimulants*) or clinical use (*antidepressants, antipsychotic agents, antiepileptic drugs*, etc.), together with a number of undefinable rogue categories (*atypical antipsychotic drugs, nootropic drugs*) thrown in for good measure.

However, grumbling about terminology is fruitless. The following classification is based on that suggested in 1967 by the World Health Organization; although flawed, it provides a basis for the material presented later (Chs 36–42).

- Anaesthetic agents
  Definition: drugs used to produce surgical anaesthesia
  Examples: **halothane**, **propofol**
  See Chapter 35.
- Anxiolytics and sedatives
  Synonyms: hypnotics, sedatives, minor tranquillisers
  Definition: drugs that cause sleep and reduce anxiety
  Examples: **barbiturates**, **benzodiazepines**
  See Chapter 36.
- Antipsychotic drugs
  Synonyms: neuroleptic* drugs, antischizophrenic drugs, major tranquillisers
  Definition: drugs that are effective in relieving the symptoms of schizophrenic illness
  Examples: **clozapine**, **chlorpromazine**, **haloperidol**
  See Chapter 37.
- Antidepressant drugs
  Synonym: thymoleptics*
  Definition: drugs that alleviate the symptoms of depressive illness
  Examples: monoamine oxidase inhibitors and tricyclic antidepressants
  See Chapter 38.
- Analgesic drugs
  Definition: drugs used clinically for controlling pain
  Examples: **opiates**, **carbamazepine**
  See Chapter 40.
- Psychomotor stimulants
  Synonym: psychostimulants
  Definition: drugs that cause wakefulness and euphoria
  Examples: **amphetamine**, **cocaine** and **caffeine**
  See Chapter 41.
- Psychotomimetic drugs
  Synonyms: hallucinogens, psychodysleptics*
  Definition: drugs that cause disturbance of perception (particularly visual hallucinations) and of behaviour in ways that cannot be simply characterised as sedative or stimulant effects
  Examples: **lysergic acid diethylamide** (LSD), **mescaline** and **phencyclidine**
  See Chapter 41.

*These strange terms are the remnants of a classification proposed by Javet in 1903, who distinguished psycholeptics (depressants of mental function), psychoanaleptics (stimulants of mental function) and psychodysleptics (drugs that produce disturbed mental function). The term neuroleptic (literally 'nerve-seizing') was coined 50 years later to describe chlorpromazine-like drugs (see Ch. 37). It gained favour, presumably by virtue of its brevity rather than its literal meaning.

Drug action in the central nervous system

- The basic types of drug target (ion channels, receptors, enzymes and transporter proteins) described in Chapter 3 apply in the CNS as elsewhere.
- Most of these targets occur in many different molecular isoforms, the functional significance of which is, in most cases, unclear.
- Many of the currently available neuroactive drugs are relatively non-specific, affecting several different targets, the principal ones being receptors, ion channels and transporters.
- The relationship between the pharmacological profile and the therapeutic effect of neuroactive drugs is often unclear.
- Slowly developing secondary responses to the primary interaction of the drug with its target are often important (e.g. the delayed efficacy of antidepressant drugs, tolerance and dependence with opiates, etc.).

- Cognition enhancers: perhaps this is more of a wishful than a real category
  Synonyms: nootropic drugs
  Definition: drugs that improve memory and cognitive performance
  Examples: **tacrine**, **donepezil**, ?**piracetam**
  See Chapter 31.

Some drugs defy classification in this scheme; for example, **lithium** (see Ch. 38), which is used in the treatment of manic-depressive psychosis, and **ketamine** (see Ch. 35), which is classed as a dissociative anaesthetic but produces psychotropic effects rather similar to those produced by phencyclidine.

USE OF DRUGS IN PSYCHIATRIC ILLNESS

In practice, the use of drugs in psychiatric illness frequently cuts across the specific therapeutic categories listed above. For example, it is common for antipsychotic drugs to be used as 'tranquillisers' to control extremely anxious or unruly patients, or to treat severe depression. Antidepressant drugs are often used to treat intractable pain, and certain psychostimulants are of proven efficacy for treating hyperactive children. The simple-minded pharmacologist, confronted with the realities of clinical practice, may find this confusing. Here we will adhere to the conventional pharmacological categories, but it needs to be emphasised that in clinical use these distinctions are often disregarded.

REFERENCES AND FURTHER READING

Barañano D E, Ferris C D, Snyder S H 2001 Atypical neural messengers. Trends Neurosci 24: 99–106 (*Short trendy review on some established mediators, such as NO, and some speculative ones, such as carbon monoxide and D-serine*)

Bezzi P, Volterra A 2001 A neuron-glia signalling network in the active brain. Curr Opin Neurobiol 11: 387–394 (*Good short review, emphasising the intercommunication between glial cells and neurons—a topic still poorly understood but of growing importance*)

Bloom F E, Kupfer D J (eds) 1995 Psychopharmacology: a fourth generation of progress. Raven Press, New York (*A 2000-page monster with excellent and authoritative articles on basic and clinical aspects*)

Cooper J R, Bloom F E, Roth R H 1996 Biochemical basis of neuropharmacology. Oxford University Press, New York (*Excellent and readable account focussing on basic rather than clinical aspects*)

Kandel E, Schwartz J H, Jessell T M 2000 Principles of neural science, 4th edn. Elsevier, New York (*Excellent and detailed standard text on neurobiology—little emphasis on pharmacology*)

Nestler E J, Hyman S E, Malenka R C 2001 Molecular neuropharmacology. McGraw Hill, New York (*Good modern textbook*)

Tamai I, Tsuji A 2000 Transporter-mediated permeation of drugs across the blood–brain barrier. J Pharm Sci 89: 1372–1388 (*Good review of the role of transport mechanisms in determining transfer of drugs and endogenous molecules into and out of the brain*)

32 Amino acid transmitters

Overview 462

Excitatory amino acids 462
- Role as central transmitters 462
- Metabolism and release of amino acids 462

Glutamate 463
- Glutamate receptor subtypes 463
- Functional role of glutamate receptors 466
- Drugs acting on glutamate receptors 468

Gamma-aminobutyric acid 470
- Synthesis, storage and function 470
- GABA receptors: structure and pharmacology 471
- Drugs acting on GABA receptors 471

Glycine 473

OVERVIEW

In this chapter, we discuss the major neurotransmitters in the central nervous system, namely the excitatory transmitter, glutamate, and the inhibitory transmitters gamma-aminobutyric acid (GABA) and glycine. It is an area in which scientific discoveries have come thick and fast since the 1980s, producing a prolific literature and, for many of us, a measure of information overload. Here we avoid going into great detail but include recent references for those seeking more.

EXCITATORY AMINO ACIDS

ROLE AS CENTRAL TRANSMITTERS

L-Glutamate is the principal and ubiquitous excitatory transmitter in the central nervous system (CNS) (see Cotman et al. 1995 for general review). *Aspartate* plays a similar role in certain brain regions, as possibly does *homocysteate*, but this is controversial. The realisation of glutamate's importance came slowly. By the 1950s (in the words of Krnjevic, one of the glutamate pioneers, 'the era of Prehistory'), work on the peripheral nervous system had highlighted the transmitter roles of acetylcholine and catecholamines, and as the brain also contained these substances, there seemed little reason to look further. The presence of *gamma-aminobutyric acid* (GABA; see below) in the brain and its powerful inhibitory effect on neurons were discovered in the 1950s, and its transmitter role was postulated. At the same time, work by Curtis' group in Canberra showed that glutamate and various other acidic amino acids produced a strong excitatory effect, but it seemed inconceivable that such workaday metabolites could actually be transmitters. Through the 1960s ('the Dark Ages'), GABA and excitatory amino acids (EAAs) were thought, even by their discoverers, to be mere pharmacological curiosities. In the 1970s ('the Renaissance'), the humblest amino acid, glycine, was established as an inhibitory transmitter in the spinal cord, giving the lie to the idea that the transmitters had to be exotic molecules, too beautiful for any role but to sink into the arms of a receptor. Once glycine had been accepted, the rest quickly followed (the 'Baroque era', an apt phrase to describe the intricate detail that has since been added to the basic discovery). A major advance was the discovery of EAA antagonists, based on the work of Watkins in Bristol, which enabled the physiological role of glutamate to be established unequivocally and also led to the realisation that EAA receptors are heterogeneous.

To do justice to the wealth of discovery in this field in just two decades is beyond the range of this book; for recent reviews giving more detail, see Dingledine et al. (1999), Conn & Pin (1997). Here we will concentrate on pharmacological aspects. Disappointingly, no therapeutic drugs have yet been introduced on the basis of EAA mechanisms, in spite of the many potential applications that exist. The 'Industrial revolution' seems to be running late.

METABOLISM AND RELEASE OF AMINO ACIDS

Glutamate is widely and fairly uniformly distributed in the CNS, and its concentration there is much higher than it is in other tissues. It has an important metabolic role, the metabolic and neurotransmitter pools being linked by *transaminase* enzymes that catalyse the interconversion of glutamate and α-oxoglutarate (Fig. 32.1). Glutamate in the CNS comes mainly from either *glucose*, via the tricarboxylic acid (Krebs) cycle, or *glutamine*, which is synthesised by glial cells and taken up by the neurons;

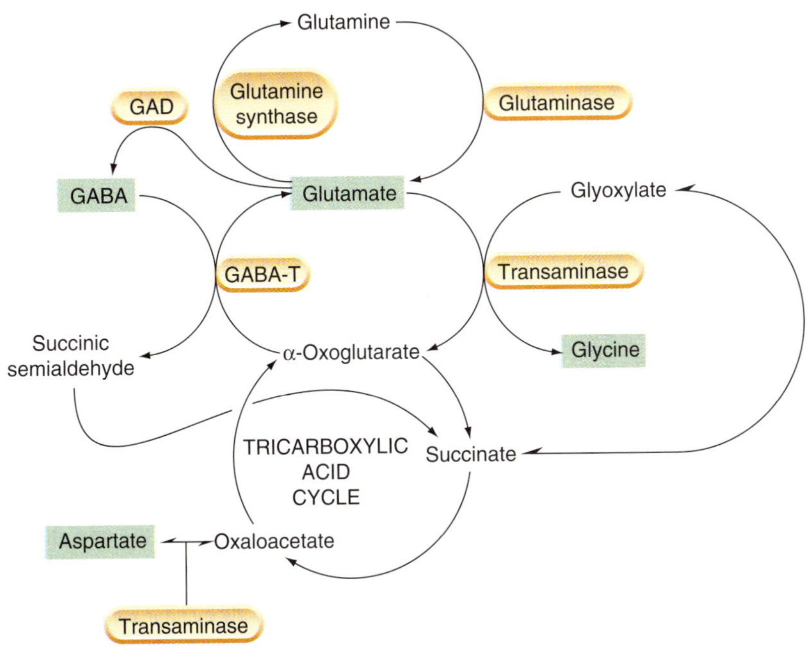

Fig. 32.1 Metabolism of transmitter amino acids in the brain. Transmitter substances are marked with green boxes. (GABA, gamma-aminobutyric acid; GAD, glutamic acid decarboxylase; GABA-T, GABA transaminase.)

very little comes from the periphery. The interconnection between the pathways for the synthesis of EAAs and inhibitory amino acids (GABA and glycine), shown in Figure 32.1, makes it difficult to use experimental manipulations of transmitter synthesis to study the functional role of individual amino acids, since disturbance of any one step will affect both excitatory and inhibitory mediators.

In common with other transmitters, glutamate is stored in synaptic vesicles and released by calcium-dependent exocytosis; specific transporter proteins account for its uptake by neurons and other cells, and for its accumulation by synaptic vesicles (see Ch. 9). In contrast to the situation with monoamine synthesis and transport (Chs 10 and 33), few drugs (none in clinical use) are known that interfere specifically with glutamate metabolism.

The action of glutamate is terminated mainly by carrier-mediated reuptake into the nerve terminals and neighbouring astrocytes (Fig. 32.2). This transport can, under some circumstances (e.g. depolarisation by increased extracellular K^+), operate in reverse and constitute a source of glutamate release (see Takahashi et al., 1997), a process that may occur under pathological conditions such as brain ischaemia (see Ch. 34). Glutamate taken up by astrocytes is converted to *glutamine* and recycled, via transporters, back to the neurons, which convert the glutamine back to glutamate. Glutamine, which lacks the pharmacological activity of glutamate, thus serves as a pool of inactive transmitter under the regulatory control of the astrocytes, which act as ball-boys, returning the ammunition in harmless form in order to rearm the neurons.

Glutamate uptake is coupled to Na^+ entry, and several transporters have been cloned and characterised in detail (see Seal & Amara, 1999).

GLUTAMATE

GLUTAMATE RECEPTOR SUBTYPES

On the basis of studies with selective agonists and antagonists (Fig. 32.3), four main subtypes of EAA receptors can be distinguished, namely *NMDA*,* *AMPA*,* *kainate** and *metabotropic* receptors (Table 32.1), all of which have been cloned and studied in great detail (see Dingledine et al., 1999; Conn & Pin, 1997). The first three are *ionotropic receptors*, named according to their specific agonists (Fig. 32.3). The channel consists of five subunits, each with the 'pore-loop' structure shown in Figure 3.16. NMDA-receptors are assembled from two types of subunit, NR1 and NR2, each of which can exist in different isoforms and splice variants, giving rise to many different receptor isoforms in the brain, the significance of which is not yet understood—a scenario by now familiar to our readers. The subunits constituting AMPA and kainate receptors, termed $GluR_{1-7}$ and $KA_{1,2}$, are closely related, but distinct from NR subunits. AMPA-receptors consist of combinations of $GluR_{1-4}$.** AMPA-receptors lacking the $GluR_2$ subunit have much higher permeability to Ca^{2+} than the others, which has important functional consequences (see Ch. 4). The metabotropic receptors are monomeric G-protein-coupled receptors, linked to

*NMDA is *N*-methyl-D-aspartate; AMPA is α-amino-3-hydroxy-5-hydroxy-5-methyl-4-isoxazoleproprionate; kainate is isolated from seaweed.

**AMPA-receptor subunits are also subject to other kinds of variation, namely *alternative splicing*, giving rise to the engagingly named 'flip' and 'flop' variants, and *RNA editing* at the single amino acid level, both of which contribute yet more functional diversity to this motley family.

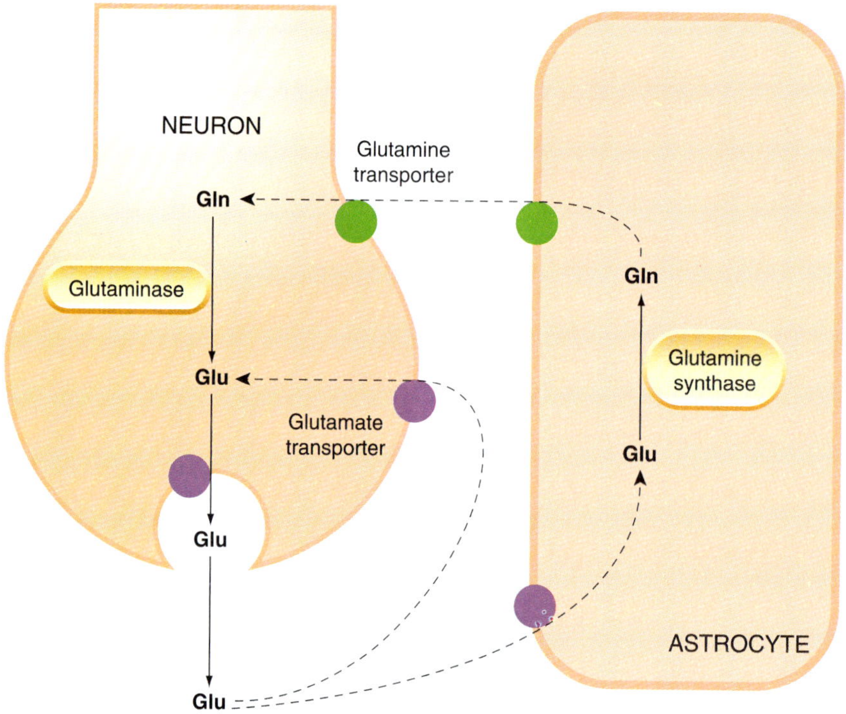

Fig. 32.2 Transport of glutamate (Glu) and glutamine (Gln) by neurons and astrocytes. Released glutamate is captured partly by neurons and partly by astrocytes, which convert it to glutamine. Astrocytes release glutamine via a transporter, and neurons take it up and synthesise glutamate.

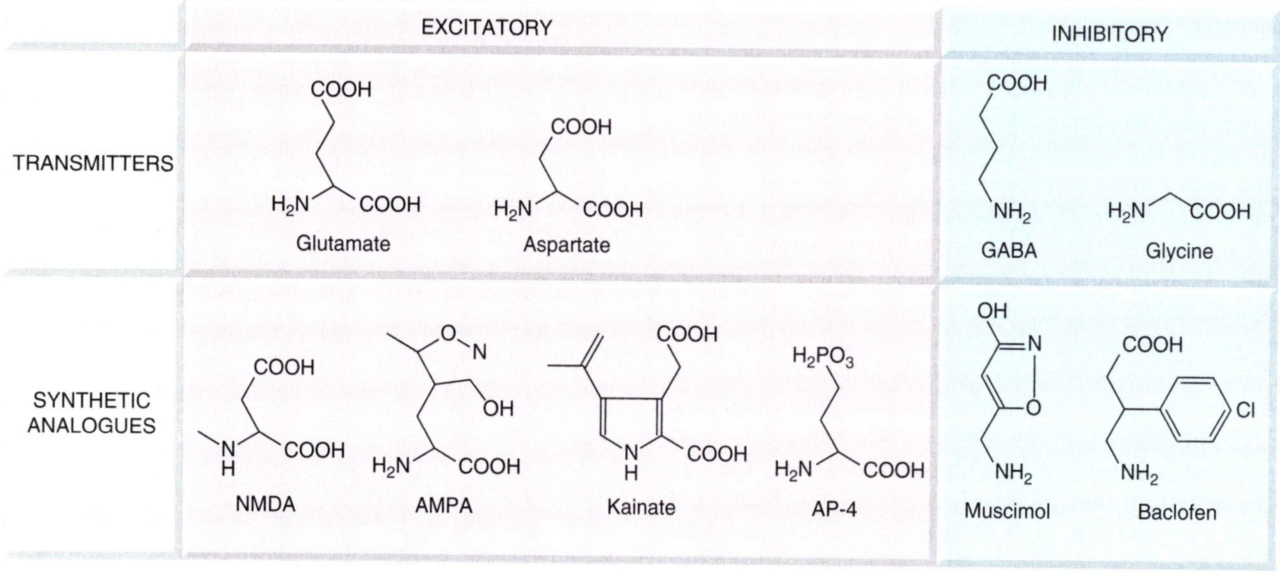

Fig. 32.3 Structures of agonists acting on glutamate, gamma-aminobutyric acid (GABA) and glycine receptors. The receptor specificity of these compounds is shown in Tables 32.1 and 32.2. (NMDA, *N*-methyl-D-aspartate; AMPA, α-amino-3-hydroxy=5=methylisoxazole; AP-4, 3-amino-4-phosphonopentanoic acid.)

Table 32.1 Properties of excitatory amino acid receptors

	NMDA		AMPA	Kainate	Metabotropic
Subunit composition	Pentamers consisting of NR1 & NR2 subunits		Pentamers consisting of $GluR_{1-4}$ subunits (variants associated with alternative splicing and RNA editing)	Pentamers consisting of $GluR_{5-7}$ subunits, plus KA 1–2	Monomeric GPCRs
	Receptor site	**Modulatory site (glycine)**			
Endogenous agonists	Glutamate Aspartate	Glycine, ?D-serine	Glutamate	Glutamate	Glutamate
Other agonists	NMDA	Cycloserine	AMPA Quisqualate	Kainate Domoate	D-AP4, ACPD
Antagonists[a]	AP-5, AP-7 CGS 19755 (selfotel) CPP LY 235959	7-Chlorokynurenic acid ACEA 1021 HA-466	NBQX CNQX LY293558	NBQX LY 377770	MCPG
Other modulators	Polyamines (e.g. spermine, spermidine) Mg^{2+}, Zn^{2+}		Cyclothiazide, Aniracetam, Ampakines[b]	–	–
Channel blockers	Dizocilpine (MK801) Phencyclidine Ketamine Dextromethorphan Mg^{2+}		–	–	Not applicable
Effector mechanisms	Ligand-gated cation channel (slow kinetics, high Ca^{2+} permeability)		Ligand-gated cation channel (fast kinetics; channels possessing $GluR_2$ subunits show low Ca^{2+} permeability)	Ligand-gated cation channel (fast kinetics, low Ca^{2+} permeability)	G-protein-coupled (IP_3 formation and release of Ca^{2+})
Location	Postsynaptic (also glial) Wide distribution		Postsynaptic	Pre- and postsynaptic	Pre- and postsynaptic
Function	Slow EPSP Synaptic plasticity (LTP, LTD) Excitotoxicity		Fast EPSP Wide distribution	Fast EPSP ?presynaptic inhibition Limited distribution	Synaptic modulation Excitotoxicity

ACPD, 1-aminocyclopentane-1,3-dicarboxylic acid; AMPA, α-amino-3-hydroxy-5-methylisoxazole, AP-5, 2-amino-5-phosphonopentanoic acid; AP-7, 2-amino-7-phosphonoheptanoic acid; CNQX, 6-cyano-7-nitroquinoxaline-2,3-dione; CPP, 3-(2-carboxypirazin-4-yl)-propyl-1-phosphonic acid; NMDA, *N*-methyl-D-aspartic acid, NBQX, 2,3-dihydro-6-nitro-7-sulfamoyl-benzoquinoxaline; MCPG, α-methyl-4-carboxyphenylglycine; EPSP, excitatory postsynaptic potential; LTP, long-term potentiation; LTD, long-term depression; IP_3, inositol trisphosphate. (Other structures are shown in Figure 32.3.)

[a]Structures of experimental compounds can be found in review by Brauner-Osborne et al. (2000, J Med Chem 43 2609–2645, 2000)

[b]Ampakine is a term invented to describe a number of compounds that appear to enhance the action of AMPA-receptor agonists.

intracellular second messenger systems (see Ch. 3; Conn & Pin, 1997), and comprise eight subtypes in three main classes (Table 32.1). They are unusual in showing no sequence homology with other G-protein-coupled receptors, and in having a very large extracellular N-terminal tail that contains the glutamate-binding site, in contrast to most amine receptors in which the agonist binding site is buried amongst the transmembrane helices (Ch. 3).

Binding studies show that glutamate receptors are most abundant in the cortex, basal ganglia and sensory pathways. NMDA- and AMPA-receptors are generally colocalised, but kainate receptors have a much more restricted distribution. Expression of the many different receptor subtypes in the brain also shows distinct regional differences, but we have hardly begun to understand the significance of this extreme organisational complexity.

SPECIAL FEATURES OF NMDA-RECEPTORS

NMDA-receptors and their associated channels have been studied in more detail than the other types and show special pharmacological properties, summarised in Figure 32.4, which are postulated to play a role in pathophysiological mechanisms.

- They are highly permeable to Ca^{2+}, as well as to other cations, so activation of NMDA-receptors is particularly effective in promoting Ca^{2+} entry.
- They are readily blocked by Mg^{2+}, and this block shows marked voltage dependence. It occurs at physiological Mg^{2+} concentrations when the cell is normally polarised, but is overcome if the cell is depolarised.
- Activation of NMDA-receptors requires *glycine* as well as glutamate (Fig. 32.5). The binding site for glycine is distinct from the glutamate-binding site, and both have to be occupied for the channel to open. This discovery caused a stir, because glycine had hitherto been recognised as an inhibitory transmitter (see below), so to find it facilitating excitation ran counter to the prevailing doctrine. The concentration of glycine required is low in relation to the concentration of glycine normally present in the brain, suggesting that it may serve as a constant enabling factor for NMDA-receptor-mediated effects of glutamate, rather than as a regulatory mechanism. Competitive antagonists at the glycine site (see Table 32.1) indirectly inhibit the action of glutamate. It has recently been suggested (see Barañano et al., 2001) that a very surprising molecule, namely *D-serine* (surprising, since it is the 'wrong' enantiomer for higher organisms), also activates the NMDA-receptor via the glycine site and can be released from astrocytes.
- Certain well-known anaesthetic and psychotomimetic agents, such as **ketamine** (Ch. 32) and **phencyclidine** (Ch. 38), are selective blocking agents for NMDA-operated channels. The experimental compound **dizocilpine** (codename MK801) shares this property.
- Certain endogenous polyamines (e.g. *spermine*, *spermidine*) act on a different accessory site to facilitate channel opening. The experimental drugs **ifenprodil** and **eliprodil** block their action.

FUNCTIONAL ROLE OF GLUTAMATE RECEPTORS

AMPA-receptors and, in certain brain regions, kainate receptors (see Bleakman & Lodge, 1998) serve to mediate fast excitatory

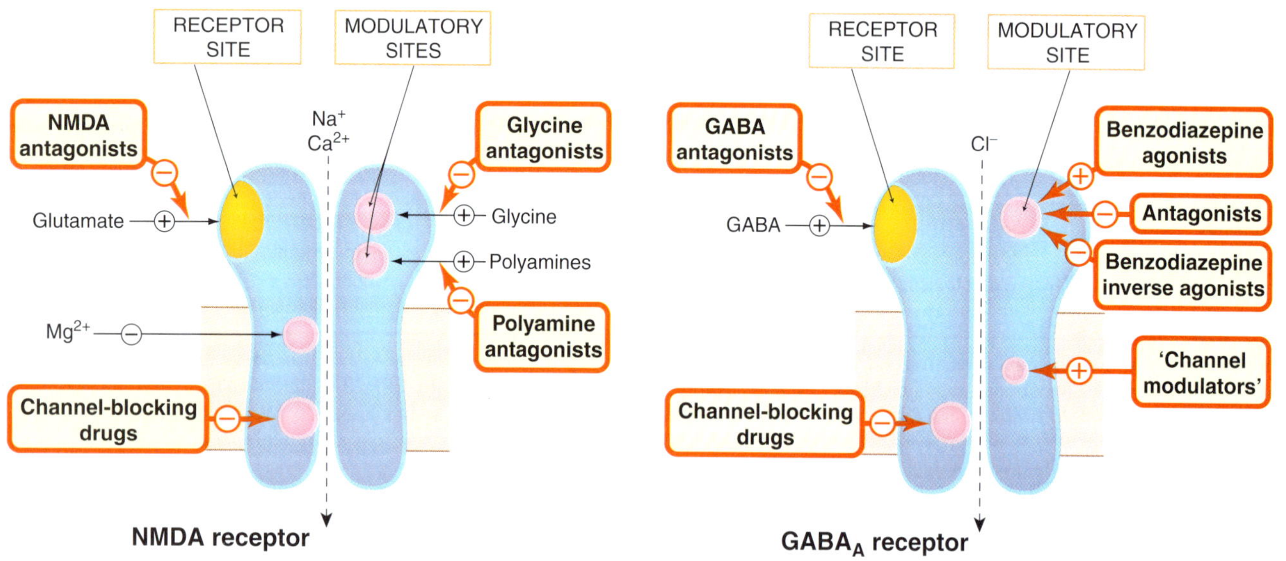

Fig. 32.4 Main sites of drug action on NMDA and $GABA_A$-receptors. Both receptors are multimeric ligand-gated ion channels. Drugs can act as agonists or antagonists at the neurotransmitter receptor site, or at modulatory sites associated with the receptor. They can also act to block the ion channel at one or more distinct sites. In the case of the $GABA_A$-receptor, the mechanism by which 'channel modulators' (e.g. ethanol, anaesthetic agents) facilitate channel opening is uncertain; they may affect both ligand binding and channel sites. The location of the different binding sites shown in the figure is largely imaginary, though study of mutated receptors is beginning to reveal where they actually reside. Examples of the different drug classes are given in Tables 32.1 and 32.2.

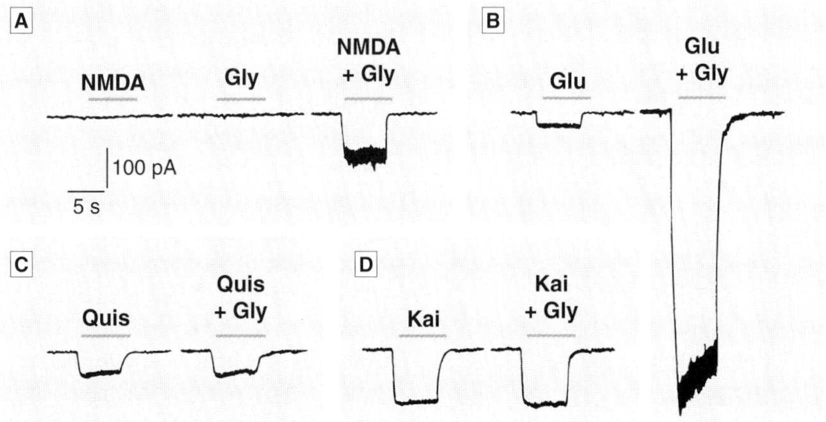

Fig. 32.5 Facilitation of NMDA response by glycine. Voltage-clamp recordings from mouse brain neurons in culture. Downward deflections represent inward current through EAA-activated ion channels. [A] NMDA (10 μmol/l) or glycine (1 μmol/l) applied separately had little or no effect, but together produced a response. [B] The response to glutamate (10 μmol/l, Glu) was strongly potentiated by glycine (1 μmol/l, Gly). [C] and [D] Responses of AMPA and kainate receptors to quisqualate (Quis) and kainate (Kai) were unaffected by glycine. (From: Johnson J W, Ascher P 1987 Nature 325: 529–531.)

synaptic transmission in the CNS—absolutely essential for our brains to function. Kainate receptors also have a presynaptic role (see Frerking & Nicoll, 2000). AMPA-receptors also occur on astrocytes, which (Ch. 31) seem to play a communicative, as well as a merely supportive, role in the brain. NMDA-receptors (which often coexist with AMPA-receptors) contribute a slow component to the excitatory synaptic potential (Fig. 32.6), the magnitude of which varies in different pathways. Metabotropic glutamate receptors are linked either to inositol trisphophate production and release of intracellular Ca^{2+} or to inhibition of adenylate cyclase (see Ch. 3). They are located both pre- and postsynaptically and, like other glutamate receptors, also occur on astrocytes. Their effects on transmission are modulatory, rather than direct, comprising mainly postsynaptic excitatory effects (by inhibition of potassium channels) and presynaptic inhibition (by inhibition of calcium channels).

In general, it appears that NMDA and metabotropic receptors play a role in long-term adaptive and pathological changes in the brain and are of particular interest as potential drug targets.

Two aspects of special importance are *synaptic plasticity*, discussed here, and *excitotoxicity* (discussed in Ch. 34).

SYNAPTIC PLASTICITY

Synaptic plasticity is a general term to describe long-term changes in synaptic connectivity and efficacy, either following physiological alterations in neuronal activity (as in learning and memory) or resulting from pathological disturbances (as in epilepsy, chronic pain or drug dependence). Broadly speaking, synaptic plasticity underlies much of what we call 'brain function', and understanding how it happens has been a holy grail for neurobiologists for decades. Needless to say, no single mechanism is responsible for the many phenomena that fall within the term; however, the discovery of *long-term potentation* (LTP), and the central role of glutamate and NMDA-receptors, represents a big step forward.

LTP (Bliss & Collingridge, 1993; Bennett, 2000) is the term used to describe a long-lasting (hours in vitro, days or weeks in vivo) enhancement of synaptic transmission that occurs at various CNS synapses following a short (conditioning) burst of presynaptic stimulation, typically at about 100 Hz for 1 second. Its counterpart is *long-term depression* (LTD), which is produced by a longer train of stimuli at lower frequency. These phenomena have been studied in great detail in the hippocampus (Fig. 32.6), which plays a central role in learning and memory. It has been argued that 'learning', in the synaptic sense, can occur if synaptic strength is enhanced following *simultaneous* activity in both pre- and postsynaptic neurons. LTP shows this characteristic; it does not occur if presynaptic activity fails to excite the postsynaptic neuron, or if the latter is activated independently, for instance by different presynaptic input. Thus LTP initiation involves both the presynaptic and postsynaptic components, and it results from enhanced activation of AMPA-receptors at EAA synapses. The facilitatory process also appears to involve both pre- and postsynaptic elements (though the small-print argument on this point rumbles on); the release of glutamate is increased, and so is the response of postsynaptic AMPA-receptors to glutamate. Increased expression and trafficking of AMPA-receptors to synaptic sites also occurs. The following experimental results have led to the model shown in Figure 32.7, in which activation

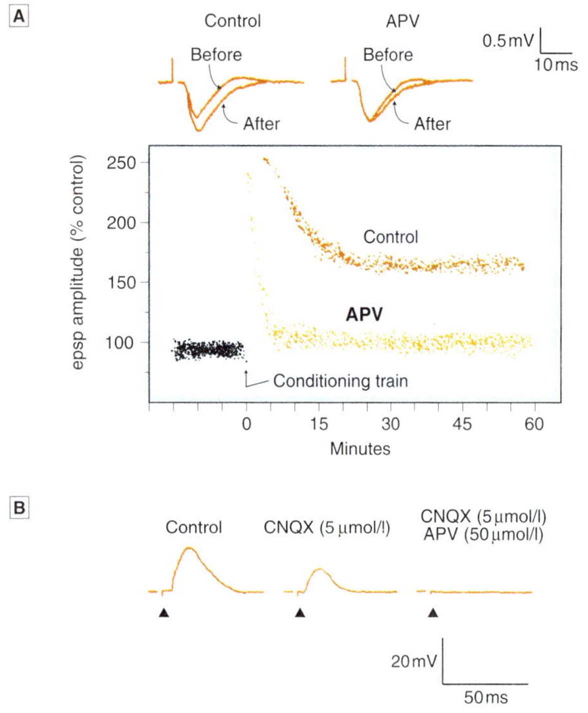

Fig. 32.6 Effects of excitatory amino acid (EAA) receptor antagonists on synaptic transmission. A APV (NMDA antagonist) prevents long-term potentiation (LTP) in the rat hippocampus without affecting the fast excitatory postsynaptic potential (epsp). Top records show the extracellularly recorded fast epsp (downward deflection) before, and 50 minutes after, a conditioning train of stimuli (100 Hz for 2 s). The presence of LTP in the control preparation is indicated by the increase in epsp amplitude. In the presence of APV (50 μmol/l), the normal epsp is unchanged, but LTP does not occur. Lower trace shows epsp amplitude as a function of time. The conditioning train produces a short-lasting increase in epsp amplitude, which still occurs in the presence of APV, but the long-lasting effect is prevented. B Block of fast and slow components of epsp by CNQX (AMPA-receptor antagonist) and APV (NMDA-receptor antagonist). The epsp (upward deflection) in hippocampal neuron recorded with an intracellular electrode is partly blocked by CNQX (5 μmol/l), leaving behind a slow component, which is blocked by APV (50 μmol/l). (From: (A) Malinow R, Madison D, Tsien R W 1988 Nature 335: 821; (B) Andreasen M, Lambert J D, Jensen M S 1989 J Physiol 414: 317–336.)

of NMDA-receptors and metabotropic glutamate receptors indirectly leads to sensitisation of AMPA-receptors.

- NMDA antagonists prevent LTP, without affecting normal, non-potentiated transmission (which depends on AMPA-receptors). Disruption of the gene for the NMDA-receptor has the same effect.
- LTP occurs only if the postsynaptic cell is depolarised at the time when the conditioning burst of stimulation is delivered. Blocking AMPA-receptors prevents this and prevents LTP.
- Antagonists at metabotropic glutamate receptors reduce the duration of LTP; LTP is also impaired in transgenic mice lacking the mGluR1 receptor.
- Calcium entry into the postsynaptic cell is required, and there is evidence that activation of protein kinase C (see Ch. 3), resulting in phosphorylation of AMPA-receptors, is involved in the mechanism of potentiation.
- LTP is reduced by agents that block the synthesis or effects of nitric oxide or arachidonic acid. One or both of these mediators may be the hitherto elusive 'retrograde messenger' through which events in the postsynaptic cell are able to influence the presynaptic nerve terminal.

▼ Two special properties of the NMDA-receptor and channel underlie its involvement in LTP, namely voltage-dependent channel block by Mg^{2+} and its high Ca^{2+} permeability. At normal membrane potentials, the NMDA channel is blocked by Mg^{2+}; a sustained postsynaptic depolarisation produced by glutamate acting repeatedly on AMPA-receptors, however, removes the Mg^{2+} block, and NMDA-receptor activation then allows Ca^{2+} to enter the cell. The metabotropic EAA receptor also contributes to the increase in $[Ca^{2+}]_i$. This rise in $[Ca^{2+}]_i$ in the postsynaptic cell activates protein kinases, phospholipases and nitric oxide synthase, which act jointly (by mechanisms that are not yet fully understood) to facilitate transmission via AMPA-receptors. Initially, during the *induction phase* of LTP, phosphorylation of AMPA-receptors increases their responsiveness to glutamate. Later, during the *maintenance phase*, more AMPA-receptors are recruited to the postsynaptic membrane as a result of altered receptor trafficking; later still, various other mediators and signalling pathways are activated, causing structural changes and leading to a permanent increase in the number of synaptic contacts.

Though LTP is well established as a synaptic phenomenon, its relationship to learning and memory remains controversial, though the evidence is suggestive. For example, NMDA-receptor antagonists applied to the hippocampus impair learning in rats; also, 'saturation' of LTP by electrical stimulation of the hippocampus has been found to impair the ability of rats to learn a maze. Furthermore, LTP-like changes have been detected after learning has taken place. Thus there is hope that drugs capable of enhancing LTP may improve learning and memory.

LTP is just one manifestation of synaptic plasticity whereby neuronal connections respond to changes in the activity of the nervous system. Other phenomena, including short-term potentiation and LTD also occur, and they too appear to involve glutamate receptors (see Malenka & Nicoll, 1993).

DRUGS ACTING ON GLUTAMATE RECEPTORS

ANTAGONISTS

Much effort, particularly by Watkins and his colleagues, has gone into the search for selective glutamate antagonists, partly to provide tools for better understanding the physiological roles of the different types of EAA receptor and partly as potential therapeutic agents with which to treat, for example, epilepsy and neurodegenerative disorders.

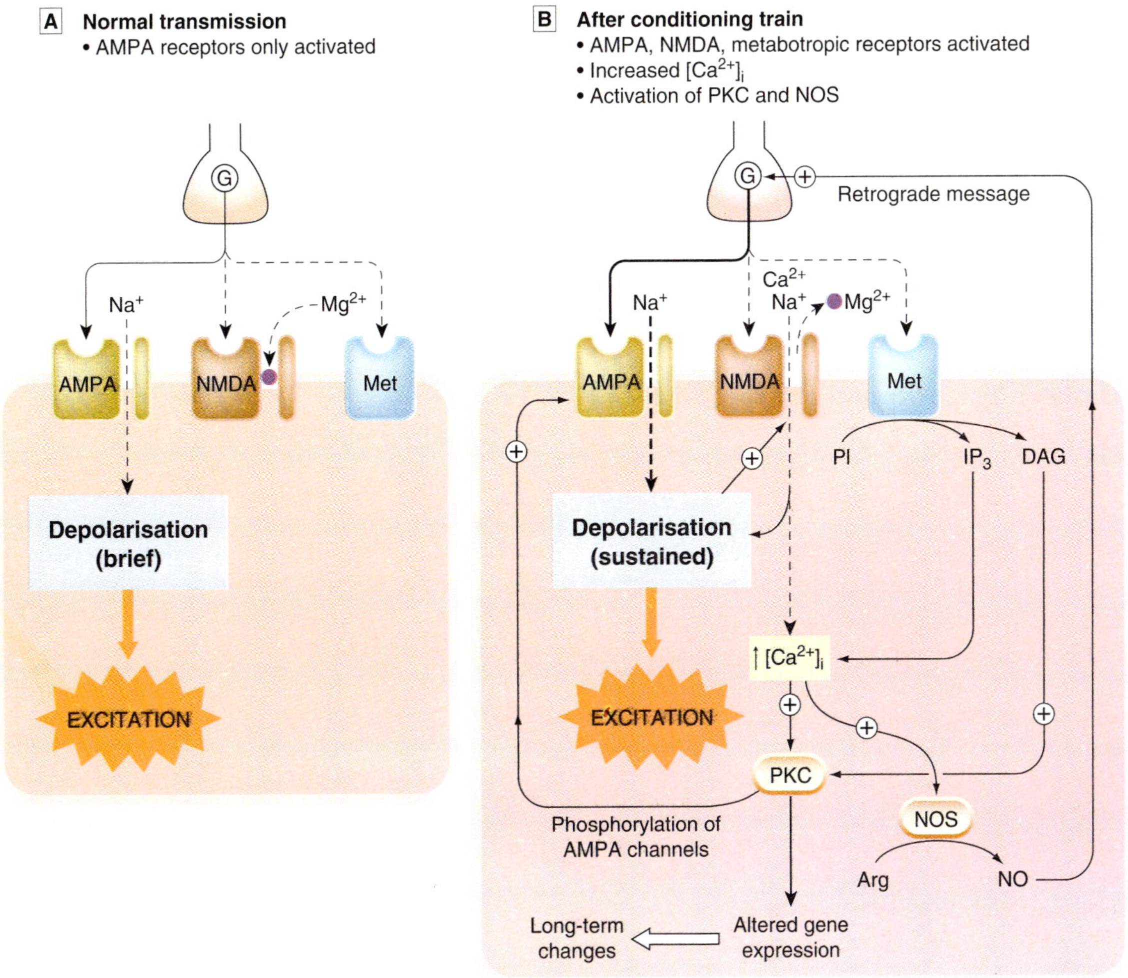

Fig. 32.7 Mechanisms of long-term potentiation (LTP). A With infrequent synaptic activity, glutamate activates mainly AMPA-receptors. There is insufficient glutamate to activate metabotropic (met) receptors, and NMDA-receptor channels are blocked by Mg^{2+}. B After a conditioning train of stimuli, enough glutamate is released to activate metabotropic receptors, and NMDA channels are unblocked by the sustained depolarisation. The resulting increase in $[Ca^{2+}]_i$ activates PKC and NOS. PKC phosphorylates various proteins, including AMPA-receptors (causing facilitation of transmitter action) and other signal transduction molecules controlling gene transcription (not shown) in the postsynaptic cell. Release of NO facilitates glutamate release (retrograde signalling, otherwise known as NO turning back). (G, glutamate; NMDA, *N*-methyl-D-aspartate; AMPA, α-amino-3-hydroxy-5-methylisoxazole; PI, phosphatidylinositol; IP_3, inositol 1,4,5-trisphosphate; DAG, diacylglycerol; PKC, protein kinase; NO, nitric oxide; NOS, nitric oxide synthase.)

The main types of EAA antagonists are shown in Table 32.1. They are selective for the main receptor types, but generally not for specific subtypes. Many of these compounds, though very useful as experimental tools in vitro, are unable to penetrate the blood–brain barrier, so they are not effective when given systemically.

NMDA-receptors, as discussed above, require glycine as well as NMDA to activate them, so blocking of the glycine site is an alternative way to produce antagonism. **Kynurenic acid**, and its more potent analogue **7-chloro-kynurenic acid** act in this way, as do various compounds currently in development

Another site of block is the channel itself, where various substances act, for example **ketamine** and **phencyclidine**. **Dizocilpine**, **remacemide** and **memantine** are more recent examples. These agents are lipid soluble and, therefore, able to cross the blood–brain barrier.

The potential therapeutic interest in glutamate antagonists lies mainly in the reduction of brain damage following strokes and head injury (Ch. 34), in the treatment of epilepsy (Ch. 39) and for various other indications, such as drug dependence (Ch. 42) and schizophrenia (Ch. 37), where the rationale is less clear. Trials with NMDA antagonists and channel blockers have so far proved disappointing, and a serious drawback of these agents is their tendency to cause hallucinatory and other disturbances (also a feature of phencyclidine; Ch. 41), so their usefulness remains to be assessed (see Trist, 2000). Glycine site antagonists may be better in this regard but none is yet registered for clinical use. AMPA-receptor antagonists seem unpromising as therapeutic agents, since the available agents (as might be expected) produce overall CNS depression, including respiratory depression and motor incoordination, with little margin of safety. Only if subtype selectivity can be achieved is this approach likely to succeed. Against this unpromising background, antagonists at metabotropic receptors may offer the best hope (see Nicoletti et al., 1996), but such compounds are not yet available for clinical use. As in other areas, the profusion of molecular subtypes of glutamate receptors is held to be the shining path leading to the discovery of more selective drugs.

Excitatory amino acids (EAAs)

- EAAs, namely glutamate, aspartate, and possibly homocysteate, are the main fast excitatory transmitters in the CNS.
- Glutamate is formed mainly from the tricarboxylic acid cycle intermediate α-oxoglutarate, by the action of GABA aminotransferase
- There are four main EAA receptor subtypes (Table 24.3):
  —NMDA
  —AMPA
  —kainate
  —metabotropic.
- NMDA-, AMPA- and kainate-receptors are ionotropic receptors regulating cation channels; metabotropic receptors are G-protein-coupled receptors and act through intracellular second messengers. There are many molecular subtypes within each class.
- The channels controlled by NMDA-receptors are highly permeable to Ca^{2+} and are blocked by Mg^{2+}.
- AMPA- and kainate-receptors are involved in fast excitatory transmission; NMDA-receptors mediate slower excitatory responses and, through their effect in controlling Ca^{2+} entry, play a more complex role in controlling synaptic plasticity (e.g. long-term potentiation).
- Competitive NMDA-receptor antagonists include AP5 and other experimental compounds; the NMDA-operated ion channel is blocked by dizocilpine, as well as by the psychotomimetic drugs ketamine and phencyclidine.
- CNQX is a selective AMPA receptor antagonist.
- NMDA-receptors require low concentrations of glycine as a co-agonist, in addition to glutamate; 7-chlorokynurenate blocks this action of glycine.
- NMDA-receptor activation is increased by endogenous polyamines, such as spermine, acting on a modulatory site that is blocked by ifenprodil.
- The entry of excessive amounts of Ca^{2+} produced by NMDA-receptor activation can result in cell death: excitotoxicity (see Ch. 34).
- Metabotropic receptors are G-protein-coupled receptors, linked to inositol trisphosphate formation and intracellular Ca^{2+} release. They play a part in glutamate-mediated synaptic plasticity and excitotoxicity. Specific agonists and antagonists are known.
- EAA receptor antagonists have yet to be developed for clinical use.

AGONISTS AND POSITIVE MODULATORS

Various agonists at EAA-receptors that are used experimentally are shown in Table 32.1. From the clinical perspective, interest centres on the theory that positive AMPA-receptor modulators, which act by reducing receptor desensitisation, may improve memory and cognitive performance. **Cyclothiazide** acts in this way but is toxic; drugs such as **piracetam** and **aniracetam,** which are used in dementia (Ch. 34), also sensitise AMPA-receptors, though it is not certain that this accounts for their psychotropic effects.

GAMMA-AMINOBUTYRIC ACID

GABA is the main inhibitory transmitter in the brain. In the spinal cord and brainstem, glycine is also important.

SYNTHESIS, STORAGE AND FUNCTION

GABA occurs in brain tissue, but not in other mammalian tissues, except in trace amounts. In the brain it is particularly abundant (about 10 μmol/g tissue) in the nigrostriatal system and occurs at lower concentrations (2–5 μmol/g) throughout the grey matter.

GABA is formed from glutamate (Fig. 32.1) by the action of *glutamic acid decarboxylase* (GAD), an enzyme found only in GABA-synthesising neurons in the brain. Immunohistochemical labelling of GAD is used to map the GABA pathways in the brain. GABA is destroyed by a transamination reaction, in which the amino group is transferred to α-oxoglutaric acid (to yield glutamate), with the production of succinic semialdehyde, and then succinic acid. This reaction is catalysed by *GABA transaminase*, which is inhibited by **vigabatrine**, a compound used to treat epilepsy (Ch. 39). GABA-ergic neurons and astrocytes take up GABA via specific transporters, and it is this, rather than GABA transaminase, that removes the GABA after it has been released. GABA transport is inhibited by **guvacine** and **nipecotic acid.**

GABA functions as an inhibitory transmitter in many different CNS pathways. It is released mainly from short interneurons, but also from long GABA-ergic tracts running to the cerebellum and striatum. The widespread distribution of GABA, and the fact that virtually all neurons are sensitive to its inhibitory effect, suggest that its function is ubiquitous in the brain. It has been estimated that GABA serves as a transmitter at about 30% of all the synapses in the CNS.

GABA RECEPTORS: STRUCTURE AND PHARMACOLOGY

In common with glutamate, and several other CNS transmitters, GABA acts on two distinct types of receptor, one (the *$GABA_A$-receptor*) being a ligand-gated channel, the other (*$GABA_B$*) being a G-protein-coupled receptor.* $GABA_A$-receptors (see Mehta & Ticku, 1999) belong to the same structural class as nicotinic acetylcholine receptors (see Fig. 3.16). They are pentamers, most of them composed of three different subunits (α, β, γ), each of which can exist in three to six molecular subtypes, so the possible permutations are countless—a familiar pattern of heterogeneity (as yet unlinked to function) typical of neurotransmitter receptors.

$GABA_A$-receptors, located postsynaptically, mediate fast postsynaptic inhibition, the channel being selectively permeable to Cl^-. Because the equilibrium membrane potential for Cl^- is usually negative to the resting potential of the cell, increasing Cl^- permeability hyperpolarises the cell, thereby reducing its excitability.

$GABA_B$-receptors are located pre- and postsynaptically, and they closely resemble metabotropic glutamate receptors. They were cloned in 1997 and were later shown to be unusual in that the functional receptor is a dimer consisting of two different subunits (see Ch. 3). They exert their effects by inhibiting voltage-gated calcium channels (thus reducing transmitter release), and by opening potassium channels (thus reducing postsynaptic excitability), these actions resulting from inhibition of adenylate cyclase.

It is believed that glutamate and GABA, and their receptors, evolved very early, so these receptors probably represent the venerable aristocrats from which upstarts such as the neuropeptide receptors evolved much later.

DRUGS ACTING ON GABA RECEPTORS

$GABA_A$-RECEPTORS

$GABA_A$-receptors resemble NMDA-receptors in that drugs may act at several different sites (Fig. 32.4; see Johnston 1996). These include:

- the GABA-binding site
- one or more modulatory sites
- the ion channel.

$GABA_A$-receptors are the target for several important centrally acting drugs, notably *benzodiazepines*, *barbiturates* and *neurosteroids* (see below). The main agonists, antagonists and modulatory substances that act on GABA receptors are shown in Table 32.2.

Muscimol, derived from a hallucinogenic mushroom, is a powerful $GABA_A$-receptor agonist that hyperpolarises GABA-sensitive neurons. **Bicuculline**, a naturally occurring convulsant compound, is a specific antagonist that blocks the fast inhibitory synaptic potential in most CNS synapses. These compounds are useful experimental tools but have no therapeutic uses.

Benzodiazepines, which have powerful sedative and anxiolytic effects (see Ch. 36), selectively potentiate the effects of GABA on $GABA_A$-receptors. They bind with high affinity to an accessory site (the 'benzodiazepine receptor') on the $GABA_A$-receptor, in such a way that the binding of GABA is facilitated and its agonist effect is enhanced. Studies on recombinant $GABA_A$-receptors have shown that a small region of the γ-subunit confers benzodiazepine sensitivity, and mutations in this region affect the level of constitutive activity (see Ch. 2) at this site, and its sensitivity to benzodiazepines.* Sedative benzodiazepines, such as **diazepam**, are agonists (enhancing the action of GABA), whereas convulsant analogues, such as **flumazenil** (Ch. 36), are antagonists.

Modulators that also enhance the action of GABA, but with a site of action which is less well defined than that of benzodiazepines (shown as 'channel modulators' in Fig. 32.4), include other CNS depressants such as *barbiturates* (see Ch. 36) and neurosteroids. *Neurosteroids* (see Lambert et al., 1995) are compounds that are related to steroid hormones but do not act on conventional intracellular steroid receptors. Interestingly, they include metabolites of progesterone and androgens that are formed in the nervous system and may have a physiological role. Synthetic neurosteroids include **alphaxolone**, developed as an anaesthetic agent (Ch. 35). Another putative endogenous modulator of GABA-mediated transmission is a peptide, *diazepam-binding inhibitor* (DBI), which occurs in the brain and elsewhere, but whose physiological role is unclear.

Picrotoxin (Ch. 41) is a convulsant that acts by blocking the chloride channel associated with the $GABA_A$-receptor, thus blocking the postsynaptic inhibitory effect of GABA. It has no therapeutic uses.

$GABA_B$-RECEPTORS

When the importance of GABA as an inhibitory transmitter was recognised, it was thought that a GABA-like substance might prove to be effective in controlling epilepsy and other convulsive states; since GABA itself fails to penetrate the blood–brain barrier, more lipophilic GABA analogues were sought, one of

*A third class, *$GABA_C$*, has recently been proposed (see Bormann, 2000). Closely resembling $GABA_A$-receptors in their structure and function, $GABA_C$-receptors are constructed from a different family of subunits (termed ρ), and have slightly different pharmacological properties. Their functional significance remains unknown.

*Interestingly, there is evidence from transgenic animals, in which specific $GABA_A$-receptor subunits were knocked out, that the anxiolytic and sedative effects of benzodiazepines are separable in terms of their molecular targets (see Rudolph et al., 2001), a discovery with important implications for the development of improved anxiolytic drugs.

Table 32.2 Properties of inhibitory amino acid receptors

	$GABA_A$			$GABA_B$	Glycine
	Receptor site	**Modulatory site (benzodiazepine)**	**Modulatory site (others)**		
Endogenous agonists	GABA	?DBI	Various neurosteroids (e.g. progesterone metabolites)	GABA	Glycine, β-alanine, taurine
Other agonists	Muscimol	Anxiolytic benzodiazepines (e.g. diazepam)	Barbiturates, steroid anaesthetics (e.g. alphaxolone)	Baclofen	–
Antagonists	Bicuculline	Flumazenil	–	Phaclofen, CGP 35348 & others	Strychnine
Channel blockers	Picrotoxin	Picrotoxin	Picrotoxin	Not applicable	–
Effector mechanisms	Ligand-gated chloride channel	Ligand-gated chloride channel	Ligand-gated chloride channel	G-protein-coupled receptor; inhibition of adenylate cyclase	Ligand-gated chloride channel
Location	Widespread; mainly GABA-ergic interneurons	Widespread; mainly GABA-ergic interneurons	Widespread; mainly GABA-ergic interneurons	Pre- and postsynaptic; widespread	Postsynaptic; mainly in brainstem and spinal cord
Function	Postsynaptic inhibition (fast ipsp)	Postsynaptic inhibition (fast ipsp)	Postsynaptic inhibition (fast ipsp)	Presynaptic inhibition (decreases Ca^{2+} entry Postsynaptic inhibition (increases K^+ permeability)	Postsynaptic inhibition (fast ipsp)

GABA, gamma-aminobutyric acid; DBI, diazepam-binding inhibitor; ipsp, inhibitory postsynaptic potential.

Inhibitory amino acids: GABA and glycine

- GABA is the main inhibitory transmitter in the brain.
- It is present fairly uniformly throughout the brain; there is very little in peripheral tissues.
- GABA is formed from glutamate, by the action of GAD (glutamic acid decarboxylase). Its action is terminated mainly by reuptake, but also by deamination, catalysed by GABA transaminase.
- There are two types of GABA receptor, $GABA_A$ and $GABA_B$.
- $GABA_A$-receptors, which occur mainly postsynaptically, are directly coupled to chloride channels, opening of which reduces membrane excitability. Muscimol is a specific GABA agonist, and the convulsant bicuculline is an antagonist.
- Other drugs that interact with $GABA_A$-receptors and channels include:
  - —benzodiazepine tranquillisers, which act at an accessory binding site to facilitate the action of GABA
  - —convulsants such as picrotoxin, which block the anion channel
  - —neurosteroids, including endogenous progesterone metabolites, and other CNS depressants, such as barbiturates, which facilitate the action of GABA.
- $GABA_B$ receptors are G-protein-coupled receptors, linked to inhibition of cAMP formation. They cause pre- and postsynaptic inhibition by inhibiting calcium channel opening and increasing K^+ conductance. Baclofen is a $GABA_B$-receptor agonist used to treat spasticity. $GABA_B$ antagonists are not yet in clinical use.
- Glycine is an inhibitory transmitter mainly in the spinal cord, acting on its own receptor, structurally and functionally similar to the $GABA_A$-receptor.
- The convulsant drug **strychnine** is a competitive glycine antagonist. **Tetanus toxin** acts mainly by interfering with glycine release.

which, **baclofen**, was introduced in 1972. Unlike GABA, baclofen has little postsynaptic inhibitory effect, and its actions are not blocked by bicuculline. These findings led to the recognition of the $GABA_B$-receptor, for which baclofen is a selective agonist (see Bowery, 1993). Baclofen is used to treat spasticity and related motor disorders (Ch. 36).

Competitive antagonists for the $GABA_B$-receptor include a number of experimental compounds (e.g. **saclofen**) and more potent compounds with improved brain penetration (such as *CGP 35348*). Tests in animals have shown that these compounds produce only slight effects on CNS function (in contrast to the powerful convulsant effects of $GABA_A$ antagonists). The main effect observed, paradoxically, was an antiepileptic action, specifically in an animal model of absence seizures (see Ch. 36) together with enhanced cognitive performance. Whether such compounds will prove to have therapeutic uses remains to be seen.

GLYCINE

Glycine is present in particularly high concentration (5 μmol/g) in the grey matter of the spinal cord. Applied ionophoretically to motoneurons or interneurons, it produces an inhibitory hyperpolarisation that is indistinguishable from the inhibitory synaptic response. **Strychnine** (see Ch. 41), a convulsant poison that acts mainly on the spinal cord, blocks both the synaptic inhibitory response and the response to glycine. This, together with direct measurements of glycine release in response to nerve stimulation, provides strong evidence for its physiological transmitter role. **Beta-alanine** has pharmacological effects and a pattern of distribution very similar to glycine, but its action is not blocked by strychnine.

The inhibitory effect of glycine is quite distinct from its role in facilitating activation of NMDA-receptors (see p. 466).

The glycine receptor resembles the $GABA_A$-receptor; it is a multimeric ligand-gated chloride channel, of which a number of subtypes have been identified by cloning, and mutations of the receptor have been identified in some inherited neurological disorders associated with muscle spasm and reflex hyperexcitability. There are no therapeutic drugs that act by modifying glycinergic transmission. **Tetanus toxin**, a bacterial toxin resembling **botulinum toxin** (Ch. 10), acts selectively to prevent glycine release from inhibitory interneurons in the spinal cord, causing excessive reflex hyperexcitability and violent muscle spasms ('lockjaw').

REFERENCES AND FURTHER READING

Barañano D E, Ferris C D, Snyder S H 2001 Atypical neural messengers. Trends Neurosci 24: 99–106 (*Short trendy review on some established mediators, such as NO, and some speculative ones, such as carbon monoxide and D-serine*)

Bennett M R 2000 The concept of long term potentiation of transmission at synapses. Prog Neurobiol 60: 109–137 (*An excellent and not overly long review of this complex phenomenon*)

Bleakman D, Lodge D 1998 Neuropharmacology of AMPA and kainate receptors. Neuropharmacol 37: 187–204 (*Review giving molecular and functional information on these receptors*)

Bliss T V P, Collingridge G L 1993 A synaptic model of memory: long-term potentiation in the hippocampus. Nature 361: 31–38

Bormann J 2000 The ABC of GABA receptors. Trends Pharmacol Sci 21: 16–19 (*Discussion about the putative $GABA_C$ receptor, mainly a taxonomic dispute at this stage*)

Bowery N G 1993 $GABA_B$ receptor pharmacology. Annu Rev Pharmacol Toxicol 33: 109–147

Conn P J, Pin J-P 1997 Pharmacology and functions of metabotropic glutamate receptors. Annu Rev Pharmacol 37: 205–237

Cotman C W, Kahle J S, Miller S E, Ulas J, Bridges R J 1995 Excitatory amino acid transmission. In: Bloom F E, Kupfer D J (eds) Psychopharmacology: a fourth generation of progress. Raven Press, New York, pp. 75–85

Danysz W, Parsons C G 1998 Glycine and *N*-methyl-D-aspartate receptors: physiological significance and possible therapeutic applications. Pharmacol Rev 80: 598–659 (*Heavyweight review focusing mainly on glycine modulation of NMDA-receptors*)

Dingledine R, Borges K, Bowie D, Traynelis S F 1999 The glutamate receptor ion channels. Pharmacol Rev 51: 8–61 (*Comprehensive review focussing on molecular aspects with section on potential therapeutic applications*)

Frerking M, Nicoll R A 2000 Synaptic kainate receptors. Curr Opin Neurobiol 10: 342–351 (*Review of recent evidence showing that kainate receptors have a synaptic role similar to that of AMPA-receptors*)

Johnston G A R 1996 $GABA_A$-receptor pharmacology. Pharmacol Ther 69: 173–198

Lambert J J, Belelli D, Hill-Venning C, Peters J A 1995 Neurosteroids and $GABA_A$-receptor function. Trends Pharmacol Sci 16: 295–303

Malenka R C, Nicoll R A 1993 NMDA-receptor-dependent synaptic plasticity: multiple forms and mechanisms. Trends Neurosci 16: 521–527

Mehta A K, Ticku M K 1999 An update on $GABA_A$ receptors. Brain Res Rev 29: 196–217 (*Useful review of molecular and pharmacological properties of $GABA_A$-receptors*)

Myers S J, Dingledine R, Borges K 1999 Genetic regulation of glutamate receptor channels. Annu Rev Pharmacol Toxicol 39: 221–241 (*Review of findings with transgenic mice with disordered glutamate receptors*)

Nicoletti F, Bruno V, Copani A, Caasabona G, Knopfel T 1996 Metabotropic glutamate receptors: a new target for the therapy of neurodegenerative disorders? Trends Neurosci 19: 267–271

Rudolph U, Crestani F, Möhler H 2001 $GABA_A$ receptor subtypes—dissecting their pharmacological functions. Trends Pharmacol Sci 22: 188–194 (*Recent data on transgenic mice with altered $GABA_A$-receptors giving rise to changes in benzodiazepine effects*)

Seal R P, Amara S G 1999 Excitatory amino acid transporters: a family in flux. Annu Rev Pharmacol Toxicol 39: 431–456 (*Review covering molecular and physiological aspects of glutamate transporters*)

Takahashi M, Billups B, Rossi D, Sarantis M, Hamann M, Attwell D 1997 The role of glutamate transporters in glutamate homeostasis in the brain. J Exp Biol 200: 401–409

Trist D G 2000 Excitatory amino acid agonists and antagonists: pharmacology and therapeutic applications. Pharm Acta Helv 74: 221–229.

33 Other transmitters and modulators

Overview 474

Introduction 474

Noradrenaline 475
— Noradrenergic pathways in the CNS 475
— Functional aspects 475

Dopamine 476
— Dopaminergic pathways in the CNS 476
— Dopamine receptors 477
— Functional aspects 478

5-Hydroxytryptamine 480
— 5-HT pathways in the CNS 481
— 5-HT receptors in the CNS 481
— Functional aspects 481

Acetylcholine 483
— Cholinergic pathways in the CNS 483
— Acetylcholine receptors 483
— Functional aspects 483

Purines 485

Histamine 485

Other CNS mediators 485
— Melatonin 485
— Nitric oxide 487
— Lipid mediators 488

A final message 488

OVERVIEW

In this chapter we discuss various transmitters, the pathways they are involved in and the receptors. The functional aspects are also outlined. The principal 'amine' transmitters in the central nervous system, namely dopamine, 5-hydroxytryptamine (5-HT) and acetylcholine, are described in this chapter, with briefer coverage of other mediators, including histamine, melatonin and purines. More recently, some 'atypical' chemical mediators, such as nitric oxide (Ch. 14) and lipid metabolites (Ch. 15) have come on the scene, and they are discussed at the end of the chapter. Many of the currently used psychotropic drugs that are discussed in later chapters owe their effects to mechanisms that are related to these mediators.

INTRODUCTION

The monoamines were the first central nervous system (CNS) transmitters to be identified. In the mid-1960s, during the 'monoamine years', a combination of neurochemistry and neuropharmacology led to many important discoveries about the role of CNS transmitters, and about the ability of drugs to influence these systems. The monamines differ from the amino acid transmitters discussed in Chapter 32 in being localised to small populations of neurons with cell bodies in the brainstem and basal forebrain, which project diffusely to cortical and other areas. These amine-containing neurons function as 'modulatory aerosols' and they are broadly associated with high-level behaviours (for example the stereotypic behaviour associated with enhanced dopamine activity; see below), rather than with localised synaptic excitation or inhibition. The other major class of CNS mediators, the neuropeptides, are described in Chapter 13, and information on specific neuropeptides appears in Chapters 26, 27, 29, and 40.

Though we know much about the many different mediators, their cognate receptors, and the effector mechanisms that they control at the cellular level, when describing their effects on brain function, we fall back on relatively crude terms—psychopharmacologists will be at our throats for so underrating the sophistication of their measurements—such as 'motor coordination', 'arousal', 'cognitive impairment', 'exploratory behaviour', etc. The gap between these two levels of understanding (the Grand Canyon referred to in Ch. 31) still frustrates the best efforts to link drug action at the molecular level to drug action at the therapeutic level. The use of antisense oligonucleotides and transgenic animal models to silence particular genes is increasingly being used as a guide to the 'function' of individual receptors and transporters in terms of overall behaviour (see Wei, 1997; Sibley, 1999).* More detail on the content of this chapter can be found in Cooper et al. (1996) and Nestler et al. (2001).

NORADRENALINE

The basic processes responsible for the synthesis, storage, release and reuptake of noradrenaline are the same in the brain as in the periphery (Ch. 11), and the same types of adrenoceptor are also found in pre- and postsynaptic locations in the brain.

NORADRENERGIC PATHWAYS IN THE CNS

Though the transmitter role of noradrenaline in the brain was suspected in the 1950s, detailed analysis of its neuronal distribution only became possible when the fluorescence technique, based on the formation of a fluorescent derivative of catecholamines when tissues are exposed to formaldehyde, was devised by Falck & Hillarp. Detailed maps of the pathways of noradrenergic, dopaminergic and serotonergic neurons in laboratory animals were produced, and the same basic features have since been confirmed in human brains. The cell bodies of noradrenergic neurons occur in small clusters in the pons and medulla, and they send extensively branching axons to many other parts of the brain and spinal cord (Fig. 33.1). The most prominent cluster is the *locus ceruleus* (LC), which is found in the grey matter of the pons. Although it contains only about 10 000 neurons in humans, the axons, running in a discrete medial forebrain bundle, give rise to many millions of noradrenergic nerve terminals throughout the cortex, hippocampus and cerebellum. These nerve terminals do not form distinct synaptic contacts but appear to release transmitter diffusely—justifying the aerosol analogy.

Other noradrenergic neurons lie close to the LC in the pons and medulla. Axons from these cells innervate the hypothalamus, hippocampus and other parts of the forebrain, and they also project to the cerebellum and spinal cord. There is also a smaller group of adrenergic neurons, with cell bodies lying more ventrally in the brainstem. Their fibres run mainly to the pons and medulla and hypothalamus, and they release adrenaline rather than noradrenaline. Rather little is known about them, but they are believed to be important in cardiovascular control.

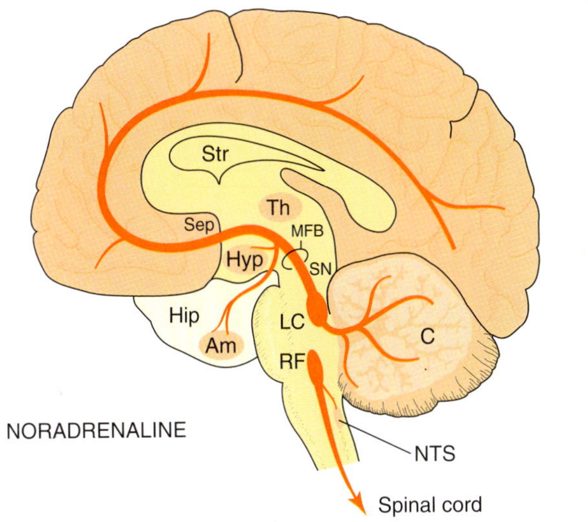

Fig. 33.1 Noradrenaline pathways in the brain. The location of the main groups of cell bodies and fibre tracts is shown in red. Pink areas show the location of noradrenergic terminals. (Am, amygdaloid nucleus; C, cerebellum; LC, locus ceruleus; Hip, hippocampus; Hyp, hypothalamus; MFB, medial forebrain bundle; NTS, nucleus of the tractus solitarius (vagal sensory nucleus); RF, brainstem reticular formation; Sep, septum; SN, substantia nigra; Str, corpus striatum; Th, thalamus.)

FUNCTIONAL ASPECTS

Noradrenaline applied to individual neurons usually causes inhibition, and in most cases this is produced by activation of β-adrenoceptors, linked to cAMP accumulation. In some situations, however, noradrenaline has an excitatory effect, which is mediated by either α- or β-adrenoceptors.

Arousal and mood

Attention has focussed mainly on the LC, which is the source of most of the noradrenaline released in the brain, and from which neuronal activity can be measured by implanted electrodes. LC neurons are silent during sleep and their activity increases with behavioural arousal. 'Wake-up' stimuli of an unfamiliar or threatening kind excite these neurons much more effectively than familiar stimuli. Amphetamine-like drugs, which release catecholamines in the brain, increase wakefulness, alertness and exploratory activity (though, in this case, firing of LC neurons is actually reduced, by feedback mechanisms; see Ch. 41).

There is a close relationship between mood and state of arousal; depressed individuals are usually lethargic and unresponsive to external stimuli. The catecholamine hypothesis of affective disorders (see Ch. 38) suggested that depression results from a functional deficiency of noradrenaline in certain parts of the brain, while mania results from an excess. This remains controversial, and subsequent findings suggest that 5-hydroxytryptamine (5-HT) may be more important than noradrenaline in relation to mood.

Blood pressure regulation

The role of central, as well as peripheral, noradrenergic synapses in blood pressure control is shown by the action of hypotensive drugs such as **clonidine** and **methyldopa** (see Chs 11 and 18), which decrease the discharge of sympathetic nerves emerging from the CNS. They cause hypotension when injected locally into

*Often, 'knockout' animals either fail to survive or appear surprisingly normal, presumably because compensatory mechanisms are able to make up for the deficit; neither outcome is informative with respect to gene function. However, the use of new techniques such as 'conditional transgenesis' (see Rudolph & Möhler, 1999) whereby genes can be switched on and off during the life of the animal, should overcome some of the problems.

Noradrenaline in the CNS

- Mechanisms for synthesis, storage, release and reuptake of noradrenaline in the CNS are essentially the same as in the periphery, as are the receptors (Ch.11).
- Noradrenergic cell bodies occur in discrete clusters, mainly in the pons and medulla, one important such cell group being the locus ceruleus.
- Noradrenergic pathways, running mainly in the medial forebrain bundle, and descending spinal tracts, terminate diffusely in the cortex, hippocampus, hypothalamus, cerebellum and spinal cord.
- The actions of noradrenaline are mainly inhibitory (β-adrenoceptors), but some are excitatory (α- or β-adrenoceptors).
- Noradrenergic transmission is believed to be important in
  - —the 'arousal' system, controlling wakefulness and alertness
  - —blood pressure regulation
  - —control of mood (functional deficiency contributing to depression).
- Psychotropic drugs that act partly or mainly on noradrenergic transmission in the CNS include antidepressants, cocaine, amphetamine. Some antihypertensive drugs (e.g. clonidine, methyldopa) act mainly on noradrenergic transmission in the CNS.

the medulla or fourth ventricle, in much smaller amounts than are required when the drugs are given systemically. Noradrenaline, and other α_2-adrenoceptor agonists, have the same effect when injected locally. Noradrenergic synapses in the medulla probably form part of the baroreceptor reflex pathway, since stimulation or antagonism of α_2-adrenoceptors in this part of the brain has a powerful effect on the activity of baroreceptor reflexes.

Ascending noradrenergic fibres run to the hypothalamus, and descending fibres run to the lateral horn region of the spinal cord, acting to increase sympathetic discharge in the periphery. It has been suggested that these regulatory neurons may release adrenaline, rather than noradrenaline. Some catecholamine-containing cells in the brainstem contain PNMT (phenyl-ethanolamine-*N*-methyltransferase: the enzyme that converts noradrenaline to adrenaline; see Ch. 11) and inhibition of this enzyme interferes with the baroreceptor reflex.

DOPAMINE

Dopamine is particularly important in relation to neuropharmacology, since it is involved in several common disorders of brain function, notably Parkinson's disease, schizophrenia and attention deficit disorder, as well as in drug dependence and certain endocrine disorders. Many of the drugs used clinically to treat these conditions work by influencing dopamine transmission.

The distribution of dopamine in the brain is more restricted than that of noradrenaline. Dopamine is most abundant in the *corpus striatum*, a part of the extrapyramidal motor system concerned with the coordination of movement (see Ch. 34), and high concentrations also occur in certain parts of the *limbic system* and *hypothalamus*.

The synthesis of dopamine follows the same route as that of noradrenaline (see Ch. 11), namely conversion of tyrosine to dopa (the rate-limiting step) followed by decarboxylation to form dopamine (Fig. 33.2). Dopaminergic neurons lack dopamine β-hydroxylase and, therefore, do not produce noradrenaline.

Dopamine is largely recaptured, following its release from nerve terminals, by a specific dopamine transporter, one of the large family monoamine transporters (see Ch. 4). It is metabolised by monoamine oxidase (MAO) and catecholamine *O*-methyltransferase (COMT; see Ch. 11), the main products being dihydroxyphenylacetic acid (DOPAC) and homovanillic acid (HVA, the methoxy derivative of DOPAC). The brain content of HVA is often used as an index of dopamine turnover. Drugs that cause the release of dopamine increase HVA, often without changing the concentration of dopamine. DOPAC and HVA, and their sulfate conjugates, are excreted in the urine, which provides an index of dopamine release in human subjects.

6-Hydroxydopamine, which selectively destroys dopaminergic nerve terminals, is commonly used as a research tool. It is taken up by the dopamine transporter and converted to a reactive metabolite that causes oxidative cytotoxicity.

DOPAMINERGIC PATHWAYS IN THE CNS

Dopaminergic neurons form three main systems (Fig. 33.3).

- *The nigrostriatal pathway* This pathway, which accounts for about 75% of the dopamine in the brain, consists of cell bodies in the *substantia nigra* (forming the A9 cell group in rats) with axons that terminate in the *corpus striatum*. These fibres run in the *medial forebrain bundle* along with other monoamine-containing fibres. The abundance of dopamine-containing neurons in the human striatum can be appreciated from the image shown in Figure 33.4, which was obtained by injecting a dopa derivative containing radioactive fluorine, and scanning for radioactivity 3 hours later by positron emission tomography (PET).
- *The mesolimbic/mesocortical pathways* The cell bodies of these pathways occur in groups in the midbrain (mainly the A10 cell group) and the fibres project, also via the medial forebrain bundle, to parts of the limbic system, especially the *nucleus accumbens* and the *amygdaloid nucleus* and to the frontal cortex.
- *The tuberohypophyseal system* This group of short neurons runs from the ventral hypothalamus to the *median eminence* and *pituitary gland*, the secretions of which they regulate.

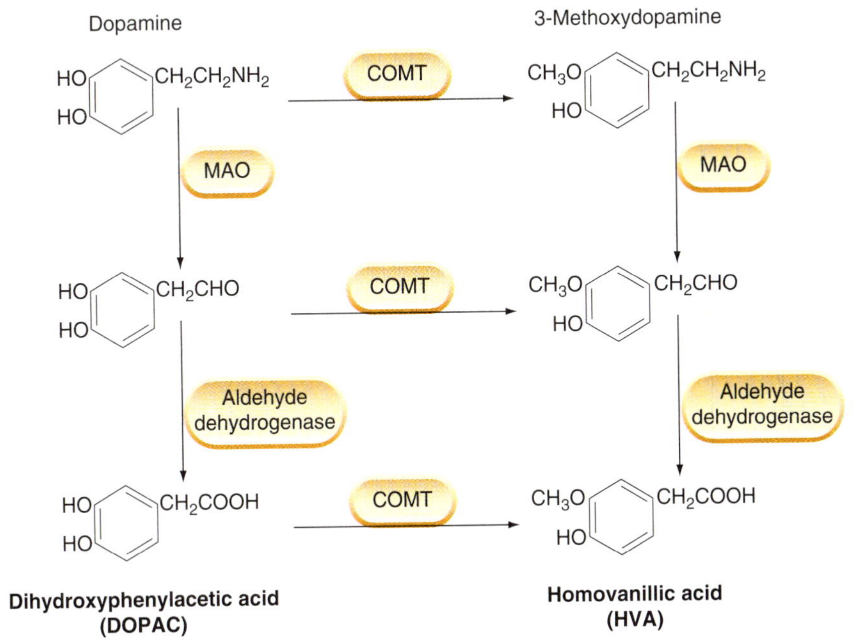

Fig. 33.2 The main pathways for dopamine metabolism in the brain. (MAO, monoamine oxidase; COMT, catechol-*O*-methyl-transferase.)

The functions of these systems are discussed below. There are also many local dopaminergic interneurons in other brain regions, and in the retina.

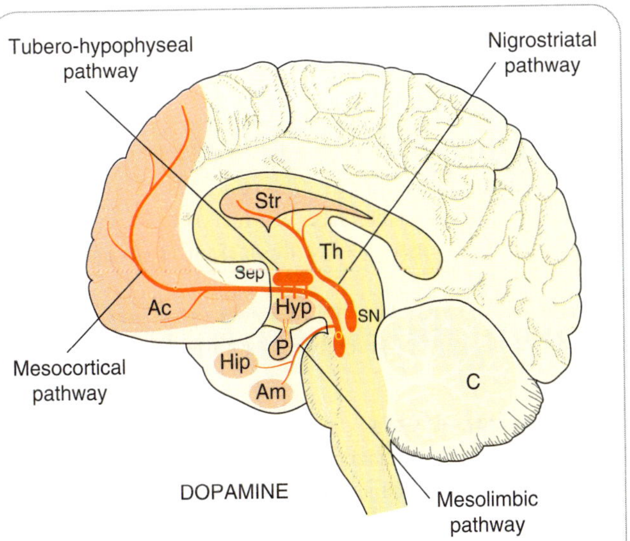

Fig. 33.3 Dopamine pathways in the brain (drawn as in Fig. 33.1). The pituitary gland (P) is shown, innervated with dopaminergic fibres from the hypothalamus. (Ac, nucleus accumbens; other abbreviations as in Fig. 33.1.)

DOPAMINE RECEPTORS

Two types of receptor, D_1 and D_2 (linked, respectively, to activation and inhibition of adenylate cyclase), were originally distinguished on pharmacological and biochemical grounds. Gene cloning revealed further subgroups, D_1 to D_5 (for review, see Jaber et al., 1994; Seeman & van Tol, 1996). The original D_1 family now includes D_1 and D_5, while the D_2 family consists of D_2, D_3 and D_4 (see Table 33.1). Splice variants, leading to long and short forms of D_2, and genetic polymorphisms, particularly of D_4 (see below), have subsequently been identified. All belong to the family of G-protein-coupled transmembrane receptors described in Chapter 3, and their signal transduction mechanisms, linked via adenylate cyclase and/or phospholipid hydrolysis to the control of potassium and calcium channels, arachidonic acid release etc., are similar to those of other such receptors. They are expressed in the brain in distinct but overlapping areas. D_1-receptors are most abundant and widespread in areas receiving a dopaminergic innervation (namely the striatum, the limbic system, thalamus and hypothalamus: Fig. 33.3), as are D_2-receptors, which also occur in the pituitary gland. D_3-receptors occur in the limbic system, but not in the striatum. Since dopamine antagonists used as antipsychotic drugs (Ch. 37) owe their actions to effects in the mesolimbic system, but often cause motor side-effects by blocking receptors in the striatum, there is interest in targeting the D_3- and D_4-receptors as a means of avoiding these side-effects. The D_4-receptor is much more

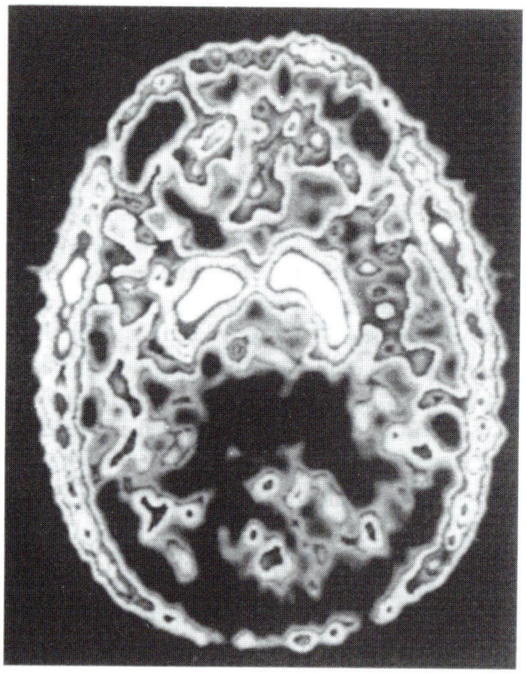

Fig. 33.4 Dopamine in the basal ganglia of a human subject. The subject was injected with 5-fluorodopa labelled with the positron-emitting isotope ^{18}F, which was localised 3 hours later by the technique of positron emission tomography. The isotope is accumulated (white areas) by the dopa-uptake system of the neurons of the basal ganglia, and to a smaller extent in the frontal cortex. It is also seen in the scalp and temporalis muscles. (From: Garnett E S et al. Nature 305: 137.)

weakly expressed, mainly in the cortex and limbic systems, but is a focus of interest because of its possible relationship to the mechanism of schizophrenia (Ch. 37) and drug dependence (Ch. 32).

The D_4-receptor displays an unexpected polymorphism in humans, with a varying number (from 2 to 10) of 16 amino acid repeat sequences being expressed in the third intracellular loop, which participates in G-protein coupling (Ch. 3). However, neither this polymorphism nor the long/short splice variants in the D_2-receptor are associated with significant changes in receptor function. Expectations that D_4-receptor polymorphism might be related to the occurrence of schizophrenia or attention deficit disorder in humans were disappointed after several studies failed to find any correlation. The possible connection with drug dependence is discussed in Chapter 42.

Dopamine, like many other transmitters and modulators, acts presynaptically as well as postsynaptically. Presynaptic D_3-receptors occur mainly on dopaminergic neurons, for example those in the striatum and limbic system, where they act to inhibit dopamine synthesis and release. Dopamine antagonists, by blocking these receptors, increase dopamine synthesis and release and cause accumulation of dopamine metabolites in these parts of the brain. They also cause an increase in the rate of firing of dopaminergic neurons (see Cooper et al., 1996), probably by blocking a neuronal feedback pathway.

Dopamine receptors also mediate various effects in the periphery (mediated by D_1-receptors), notably renal vasodilatation and increased myocardial contractility. Dopamine itself is used clinically in the treatment of circulatory shock (see Ch. 18).

FUNCTIONAL ASPECTS

The functions of dopaminergic pathways divide broadly into:

- motor control (nigrostriatal system)
- behavioural effects (mesolimbic and mesocortical systems)
- endocrine control (tuberohypophyseal system).

Dopamine and motor systems

▼ Ungerstedt showed, in 1968, that bilateral ablation of the substantia nigra in rats, which destroys the nigrostriatal neurons, causes profound catalepsy, the animals becoming so inactive that they die of starvation unless artificially fed. Unilateral lesions produced by 6-hydroxydopamine injection caused the animal to turn in circles *towards* the lesioned side, because of an imbalance of dopamine action in the corpus striatum between the two sides of the brain. Conversely, unilateral injection of **apomorphine** (a dopamine-like agonist) into the striatum causes circling *away* from the injected side. If apomorphine is given systemically to normal rats it causes, as one would expect, no asymmetrical pattern of locomotion, but if given systemically to animals with unilateral lesions of the substantia nigra made days or weeks earlier, apomorphine causes circling away from the lesioned side. This is because denervation supersensitivity (see Ch. 9) one one side, following the destruction of dopaminergic terminals, results in an asymmetric response to apomorphine. In these animals, administration of drugs that act by releasing dopamine (e.g. **amphetamine**) cause turning *towards* the lesioned side, since the dopaminergic nerve terminals are only present on the normal side. This 'turning model' has been extremely useful in investigating the action of drugs on dopaminergic neurons and dopamine receptors.

Parkinson's disease (Ch. 34) is a disorder of motor control, associated with a deficiency of dopamine in the nigrostriatal pathway.

Many antipsychotic drugs (see Ch. 37) are D_2-receptor antagonists, the major side-effect of which is to cause movement disorders, probably associated with block of D_2-receptors in the nigrostriatal pathway.

Transgenic mice lacking D_2-receptors show greatly reduced spontaneous movement, resembling Parkinson's disease.

Behavioural effects

Administration of amphetamine to rats, which releases both dopamine and noradrenaline, causes a cessation of normal 'ratty' behaviour (exploration and grooming) and the appearance of repeated 'stereotyped' behaviour (rearing, gnawing and so on) unrelated to external stimuli. These effects are prevented by dopamine antagonists, and by destruction of dopamine-containing cell bodies in the midbrain, but not by drugs that inhibit the noradrenergic system. These amphetamine-induced

Table 33.1 Dopamine receptors

	Functional role	D_1 type		D_2 type		
		D_1	D_5	D_2	D_3	D_4
Distribution						
Cortex	Arousal, mood	+++	–	++	–	+
Limbic system	Emotion, stereotypic behaviour	+++	+	++	+	
Striatum	Motor control	+++	+	++	+	+
Ventral hypothalamus and anterior pituitary	Prolactin secretion	–	–	++	+	–
Agonists						
Dopamine		+ (low potency)	+ (low potency)	+ (high potency)	+ (high potency)	+ (high potency)
Apomorphine		PA (low potency)	PA (low potency)	+ (high potency)	+ (high potency)	+ (high potency)
Bromocriptine		PA (low potency)	PA (low potency)	+ (high potency)	+ (high potency)	+ (high potency)
Antagonists						
Chlorpromazine		+	+	+++	+++	+
Haloperidol		++	+	+++	+++	+++
Spiperone		–	–	+++	+++	+++
Sulpiride		–	–	+++	++	–
Clozapine		+	+	+	+	++
Signal transduction		Increase cAMP	Increase cAMP	Decrease cAMP and/or increase IP_3	Decrease cAMP and/or increase IP_3	Decrease cAMP and/or increase IP_3
Effect		Mainly postsynaptic inhibition	Mainly postsynaptic inhibition	Pre- and postsynaptic inhibition Stimulation/ inhibition of hormone release	Pre- and postsynaptic inhibition Stimulation/ inhibition of hormone release	Pre- and postsynaptic inhibition Stimulation/ inhibition of hormone release

PA, partial agonist; IP_3, inositol trisphosphate.

motor disturbances in rats probably reflect hyperactivity in the nigrostriatal dopaminergic system.

Amphetamine also causes a general increase in motor activity, which can be measured, for example, by counting electronically the frequency at which a rat crosses from one part of its enclosure to another. This effect, in contrast to stereotypy, appears to be related to the mesolimbic and mesocortical dopaminergic pathways. There is some evidence (see Ch. 37) that schizophrenia in humans is associated with dopaminergic hyperactivity, but attempts to detect behavioural effects of dopamine in animals that might be related to the symptoms of human schizophrenia have been generally unsuccessful. Chronic administration of amphetamine to a few rats in a large colony produces various types of abnormal social interaction, including withdrawal and aggressive behaviour, but it is difficult to quantify such effects or to establish their relationship to schizophrenia in humans.

Amphetamine, cocaine (which acts by inhibiting the dopamine transporter; (Ch. 9) and other addictive drugs (Ch. 42) activate mesocortical dopaminergic 'reward' pathways, which play a key role in drug dependence. The main receptor involved appears to be D_1, and transgenic mice lacking D_1-receptors behave as though generally demotivated, with reduced food intake and insensitivity to amphetamine and cocaine (see Sibley, 1999).

Neuroendocrine function

The tuberohypophyseal dopaminergic pathway (see Fig. 33.3) is involved in the control of prolactin secretion. The hypothalamus secretes various mediators (mostly small peptides; see Ch. 27) that control the secretion of different hormones from the pituitary gland. One of these, which has an inhibitory effect on prolactin release, is dopamine. This system is of clinical importance. Many antipsychotic drugs (see Ch. 37), by blocking D_2-receptors, increase prolactin secretion and can cause breast development and lactation, even in males. **Bromocriptine**, a dopamine receptor agonist derived from ergot, is used clinically to suppress prolactin secretion by tumours of the pituitary gland.

Growth hormone release is increased in normal subjects by dopamine, but bromocriptine paradoxically inhibits the excessive secretion responsible for acromegaly, and it has a useful therapeutic effect provided it is given before excessive growth has taken place (see Ch. 27).

Dopamine in the CNS

- Dopamine is a neurotransmitter as well as being the precursor for noradrenaline. It is degraded in a similar fashion to noradrenaline, giving rise mainly to DOPAC and HVA (see text), which are excreted in the urine.
- There are three main dopaminergic pathways:
  - —nigrostriatal pathway, important in motor control
  - —mesolimbic/mesocortical pathways, running from groups of cells in the midbrain to parts of the limbic system, especially the nucleus accumbens, and to the cortex; they are involved in emotion and drug-induced reward systems
  - —tuberohypophyseal neurons running from the hypothalamus to the pituitary gland, the secretions of which they regulate.
- There are five dopamine receptor subtypes. D_1- and D_5-receptors are linked to stimulation of adenylate cyclase. D_2-, D_3- and D_4-receptors are linked to inhibition of adenylate cyclase. Most known functions of dopamine appear to be mediated mainly by receptors of the D_2 family.
- Receptors of the D_2 family may be implicated in schizophrenia. The D_4-receptor shows marked polymorphism in humans.
- Parkinson's disease is associated with a deficiency of nigrostriatal dopaminergic neurons.
- Behavioural effects of an excess of dopamine activity consist of stereotyped behaviour patterns and can be produced by dopamine-releasing agents (e.g. amphetamine) and dopamine agonists (e.g. apomorphine).
- Hormone release from the anterior pituitary gland is regulated by dopamine, especially prolactin release (inhibited) and growth hormone release (stimulated).
- Dopamine acts on the chemoreceptor trigger zone to cause nausea and vomiting.

Vomiting

Pharmacological evidence strongly suggests that dopaminergic neurons have a role in the production of nausea and vomiting. Thus, nearly all dopamine receptor agonists (e.g. bromocriptine) and other drugs that increase dopamine release in the brain (e.g. **levodopa**; Ch. 34) cause nausea and vomiting as side-effects, while many dopamine antagonists (e.g. *phenothiazines*, **metoclopramide**; Ch. 24) have antiemetic activity. D_2-receptors occur in the area of the medulla (chemoreceptor trigger zone) associated with the initiation of vomiting (Ch. 24) and are assumed to mediate this effect.

5-HYDROXYTRYPTAMINE

The occurrence and functions of 5-HT in the periphery are described in Chapter 12. Interest in 5-HT as a possible CNS transmitter dates from 1953, when Gaddum found that **lysergic acid diethylamide** (LSD), a drug known to be a powerful hallucinogen, acted as a 5-HT antagonist on peripheral tissues and suggested that its central effects might also be related to this action. The presence of 5-HT in the brain was demonstrated a few years later. Even though brain accounts for only about 1% of the total body content, 5-HT is an important CNS transmitter (see Cooper et al., 1996).

In its formation, storage and release, 5-HT resembles noradrenaline (see Fig. 12.1). Its precursor is tryptophan, an amino acid derived from dietary protein, the plasma content of which varies considerably according to food intake and time of day. Tryptophan is actively taken up into neurons, converted by tryptophan hydroxylase to 5-hydroxytryptophan and then decarboxylated by a non-specific amino acid decarboxylase to 5-HT. Tryptophan hydroxylase can be selectively and irreversibly inhibited by ***p*-chlorophenylalanine** (PCPA). Availability of tryptophan, and the activity of tryptophan hydroxylase are thought to be the main processes that regulate 5-HT synthesis. The decarboxylase is very similar, if not identical, to dopa decarboxylase and does not play any role in regulating 5-HT synthesis. Following release, 5-HT is largely recovered by neuronal uptake, this mechanism being inhibited by many of the same drugs (e.g. *tricyclic antidepressants*) that inhibit catecholamine uptake. The carrier is not identical, however, and inhibitors show varying degrees of specificity between the two. *Specific serotonin reuptake inhibitors* (SSRIs; see Ch. 38) constitute an important group of antidepressant drugs. 5-HT is degraded almost entirely by MAO (Fig. 12.1), which converts it to 5-hydroxyindole acetaldehyde, most of which is dehydrogenated to form 5-hydroxyindole acetic acid (5-HIAA), which is excreted in the urine.

5-HT PATHWAYS IN THE CNS

The distribution of 5-HT-containing neurons (Fig. 33.5), resembles that of noradrenergic neurons. The cell bodies are grouped in the pons and upper medulla, close to the midline (raphe) and are often referred to as *raphe nuclei*. The rostrally situated nuclei project, via the medial forebrain bundle, to many parts of the cortex, hippocampus, basal ganglia, limbic system and hypothalamus. The caudally situated cells project to the cerebellum, medulla and spinal cord.

5-HT RECEPTORS IN THE CNS

The main 5-HT receptor types are shown in Table 12.1. All are G-protein-coupled receptors except for 5-HT_3, which is a ligand-gated cation channel. All are expressed in the CNS, and their functional roles have been extensively analysed. With 14 identified subtypes, and a large number of pharmacological tools of relatively low specificity, assigning clear-cut functions to 5-HT receptors is not simple. A detailed account of our present state of knowledge is given by Barnes & Sharp (1999). Knowledge about the newer members of the family (5-HT_{5-7} receptors) is very limited.

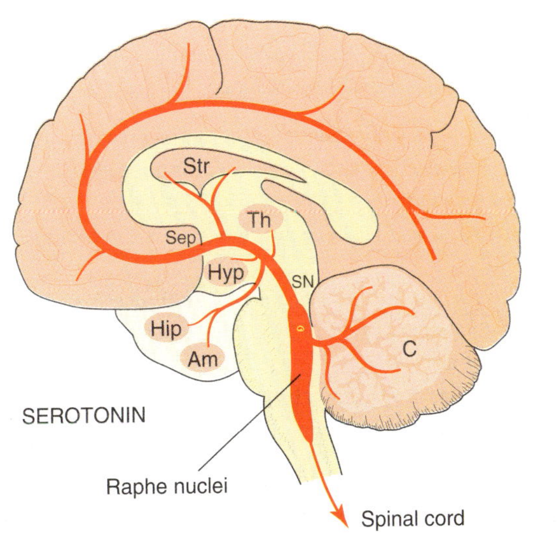

Fig. 33.5 5-Hydroxytryptamine (serotonergic) pathways in the brain. (Abbreviations and drawn as in Fig. 33.1.)

Certain generalisations can be made.

- 5-HT_1-receptors are predominantly inhibitory in their effects. 5-HT_{1A}-receptors are expressed as autoreceptors by the 5-HT neurons in the raphe nuclei, and their autoinhibitory effect tends to limit the rate of firing of these cells. They are also widely distributed in the limbic system and are believed to be the main target of drugs used to treat anxiety and depression (see Chs 36 and 38). 5-HT_{1B}- and 5-HT_{1D}-receptors are found mainly as presynaptic inhibitory receptors in the basal ganglia. Agonists acting on peripheral 5-HT_{1D}-receptors are used to treat migraine (see Ch. 12).
- 5-HT_2-receptors (mostly 5-HT_{2A} in the brain) exert an excitatory postsynaptic effect and are abundant in the cortex and limbic system. They are believed to be the target of various hallucinogenic drugs (see Ch. 41). The use of 5-HT_2-receptor antagonists such as **methysergide** in treating migraine is discussed in Chapter 12.
- 5-HT_3-receptors are found chiefly in the *area postrema* (a region of the medulla involved in vomiting; see Ch. 21) and other parts of the brainstem, extending to the dorsal horn of the spinal cord. They are also widely, but more sparsely, present in certain parts of the cortex. They are excitatory ionotropic receptors, and specific antagonists (e.g. **ondansetron**, see Chs 12 and 24) are used to treat nausea and vomiting. They may also have anxiolytic effects, but this is less clear.
- 5-HT_4-receptors are important in the gastrointestinal tract (see Chs 12, 24) and are also expressed in the brain, particularly in the striatum. They exert an presynaptic facilitatory effect, particularly on acetylcholine release, thus enhancing cognitive performance.

Although the remaining members of the 5-HT receptor family are known to be expressed in discrete areas of the brain, little is known so far about their function. Specific agonists and antagonists at these receptors are being investigated, but none is currently in clinical use.

FUNCTIONAL ASPECTS

The precise localisation of 5-HT neurons in the brainstem has allowed their electrical activity to be studied in detail and correlated with behavioural and other effects produced by drugs thought to affect 5-HT-mediated transmission. 5-HT cells show an unusual, highly regular slow discharge pattern and are strongly inhibited by 5-HT_1-receptor agonists, suggesting a local inhibitory feedback mechanism.

In vertebrates, certain physiological and behavioural functions relate particularly to 5-HT pathways (see Barnes & Sharp, 1999), namely:

- hallucinations and behavioural changes
- sleep, wakefulness and mood
- feeding behaviour
- control of sensory transmission.

Hallucinatory effects

Many hallucinogenic drugs (e.g. LSD, Ch. 41) are agonists at 5-HT_{2A}-receptors and depress the firing of brainstem 5-HT neurons. These neurons exert an inhibitory influence on cortical neurons, and it is suggested that a loss of cortical inhibition underlies the hallucinogenic effect, as well as certain behavioural effects in experimental animals, such as the 'wet-dog shakes' that occur in rats when the 5-HT precursor 5-HTP is administered. Many antipsychotic drugs (Ch. 37) are antagonists at 5-HT_{2A}-receptors, in addition to blocking dopamine D_2-receptors.

Sleep, wakefulness and mood

Lesions of the raphe nuclei or depletion of 5-HT by PCPA administration abolishes sleep in experimental animals, whereas micro-injection of 5-HT at specific points in the brainstem induces sleep. Attempts to cure insomnia in humans by giving 5-HT precursors (tryptophan or 5-hydroxytryptophan) have, however, proved unsuccessful. There is evidence that 5-HT, as well as noradrenaline, may be involved in the control of mood (see Ch. 38), and the use of tryptophan to enhance 5-HT synthesis has been tried in depression, with equivocal results.

Feeding and appetite

In experimental animals, 5-HT_{1A} agonists, such as 8-OH-DPAT (8-hydroxy-2-(di-n-propylamino)tetralin), cause hyperphagia, leading to obesity. Antagonists acting on 5-HT_2-receptors, including several antipsychotic drugs used clinically, also increase appetite and cause weight gain. Conversely, antidepressant drugs that inhibit 5-HT uptake (SSRI; see Ch. 38) cause loss of appetite.

Sensory transmission

After lesions of the raphe nuclei or administration of PCPA, animals show exaggerated responses to many forms of sensory stimulus. They are startled much more easily and also quickly develop avoidance responses to stimuli that would not normally produce this effect. It appears that the normal ability to disregard irrelevant forms of sensory input requires intact 5-HT pathways. The 'sensory enhancement' produced by hallucinogenic drugs may be partly a result of antagonism of 5-HT. 5-HT also exerts an inhibitory effect on transmission in the pain pathway, both in the spinal cord and in the brain, and there is a synergistic effect between 5-HT and analgesics such as morphine (see Ch. 40). Thus depletion of 5-HT by PCPA, or selective lesions of the descending 5-HT-containing neurons that run to the dorsal horn, antagonise the analgesic effect of morphine, while inhibitors of 5-HT uptake have the opposite effect.

Other possible roles

Other putative roles of 5-HT include various autonomic and endocrine functions, such as the regulation of body temperature, blood pressure and sexual function. Further information can be found in Azmitia & Whitaker-Azmitia (1995) and Cooper et al. (1996).

5-Hydroxytryptamine (5-HT) in the CNS

- The processes of synthesis, storage, release, reuptake and degradation of 5-HT in the brain are very similar to events in the periphery (Ch. 9).
- Availability of tryptophan is the main factor regulating synthesis.
- Urinary excretion of 5-HIAA (see text) provides a measure of 5-HT turnover.
- 5-HT neurons are concentrated in the midline raphe nuclei in the pons and medulla, projecting diffusely to the cortex, limbic system, hypothalamus and spinal cord, similar to the noradrenergic projections.
- Functions associated with 5-HT pathways include:
  - —various behavioural responses (e.g. hallucinatory behaviour, 'wet-dog shakes')
  - —feeding behaviour
  - —control of mood and emotion
  - —control of sleep/wakefulness
  - —control of sensory pathways, including nociception
  - —vomiting.
- 5-HT can exert inhibitory or excitatory effects on individual neurons, acting either presynaptically or postsynaptically.
- The main receptor subtypes (see Table 12.1) in the CNS are 5-HT_{1A}, 5-HT_{1B}, 5-HT_{1D}, 5-HT_2, 5-HT_3. Associations of behavioural and physiological functions with these receptors have been partly worked out. Other receptor types (5-HT_{4-7}) also occur in the CNS, but less is known about their function.

Several classes of drug used clinically influence 5-HT-mediated transmission. They include:

- SSRIs, such as **fluoxetine**, used as antidepressants (Ch. 38)
- $5HT_{1D}$-receptor agonists, such as **sumatriptan** (Ch. 12), used to treat migraine
- **buspirone**, a 5-HT_{1A}-receptor agonist used in treating anxiety (Ch. 36)
- 5-HT_3-receptor antagonists, such as **ondansetron,** used as antiemetic agents (see Ch. 24); these are also active in animal models of anxiety
- antipsychotic drugs (e.g. **clozapine**, Ch. 37), which owe their efficacy partly to an action on 5-HT receptors.

Efforts are being made to identify drugs that selectively target other 5-HT receptor subtypes in the hope of discovering improved drugs for use in different CNS indications. As a result, many code-named compounds have been described and characterised experimentally, but very few have been registered for clinical use in recent years.

ACETYLCHOLINE

There are numerous cholinergic neurons in the CNS, and the basic processes by which acetylcholine is synthesised, stored and released are the same as in the periphery (see Ch. 10). Various biochemical markers have been used to locate cholinergic neurons in the brain, the most useful being choline acetyltransferase, the enzyme responsible for acetylcholine synthesis, and the transporters that capture choline and package acetylcholine, which can be labelled by immunofluorescence. Biochemical studies on acetylcholine precursors and metabolites are generally more difficult than corresponding studies on other amine transmitters, because the relevant substances, choline and acetate, are involved in many processes other than acetylcholine metabolism.

CHOLINERGIC PATHWAYS IN THE CNS

Acetylcholine is very widely distributed in the brain, occurring in all parts of the forebrain (including the cortex), midbrain and brainstem, though there is little in the cerebellum. Some of the main cholinergic pathways in the brain are shown in Figure 33.6. Cholinergic neurons in the forebrain and brainstem send diffuse projections to many parts of the cortex and hippocampus – a pattern similar to that of the amine pathways described above. These neurons lie in a small area of the basal forebrain, forming the *magnocellular forebrain nuclei* (so-called because the cell bodies are conspicuously large). Degeneration of one of these, the *nucleus basalis of Meynert,* which projects mainly to the cortex, is associated with Alzheimer's disease (Ch. 34). Another cluster, the *septohippocampal nucleus*, provides the main cholinergic input to the hippocampus and is involved in memory. In addition, there are—in contrast to the monoamine pathways—many local cholinergic interneurons, particularly in the corpus striatum, these being important in relation to Parkinson's disease and Huntington's chorea (Ch. 34).

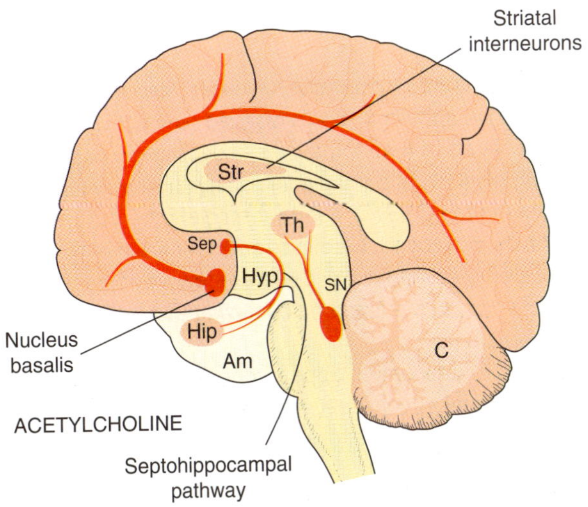

Fig 33.6 Acetylcholine pathways in the brain. (Abbreviations and drawn as in Fig. 33.1.)

ACETYLCHOLINE RECEPTORS

Acetylcholine has mainly excitatory effects, which are mediated by various subtypes of either nicotinic (ionotropic) or muscarinic (G-protein-coupled) receptors (see Ch. 10). Some muscarinic receptors are inhibitory.

The muscarinic receptors in the brain are predominantly of the M_1 class (i.e. M_1-, M_3- and M_5-subtypes; see Ch. 10), and the central actions of muscarinic antagonists and anticholinesterases depend on block and stimulation of these receptors, respectively. Muscarinic receptors act presynaptically to inhibit acetylcholine release from cholinergic neurons; muscarinic antagonists, by blocking this inhibition, markedly increase acetylcholine release. Many of the behavioural effects associated with cholinergic pathways seem to be produced by acetylcholine acting on muscarinic receptors.

Nicotinic receptors, are also widespread in the brain but are much sparser than muscarinic receptors. They are typical pentameric ionotropic receptors (Ch. 3; Jones et al., 1999; Dani, 2000), assembled from α- and β-subunits, each of which come in several isoforms. The main ones occurring in the brain are the heteropentameric α4β2 subtype (occurring mainly in the cortex) and the homomeric α7 subtype (mainly in the hippocampus). Other isoforms occur at lower densities in many brain regions. For the most part, nicotinic acetylcholine receptors are located presynaptically and act to facilitate the release of other transmitters, such as glutamate and dopamine, though in a few situations they function postsynaptically to mediate fast excitatory transmission as in the periphery. Nicotine (see Ch. 42) exerts its central effects by agonist action on nicotinic receptors of the α4β2 subtype.

Many of the drugs that block nicotinic receptors (e.g. **tubocurarine**; see Ch. 10) do not cross the blood–brain barrier, and even those that do (e.g. **mecamylamine**) produce no major CNS side-effects.

FUNCTIONAL ASPECTS

The functional roles of cholinergic pathways have been deduced mainly from studies of the action of drugs that mimic, accentuate or block the actions of acetylcholine, and recently from studies of transgenic animals in which particular nicotinic receptors were deleted or mutated (see Cordero-Erausquin et al., 2000) .

The main functions ascribed to cholinergic pathways are related to arousal, learning and memory, and motor control. Electroencephalographic (EEG) recording can be used to monitor the state of arousal in humans or in experimental animals. A drowsy, inattentive state is associated with a large amplitude, low-frequency EEG record, which switches to a low-amplitude, high-frequency pattern on arousal by any sensory stimulus. Administration of **physostigmine** (an anticholinesterase that crosses the blood–brain barrier) produces EEG arousal, whereas

atropine has the opposite effect. It is presumed that the cholinergic projection from the ventral forebrain to the cortex mediates this response. The relationship of this response to behaviour is confusing, however, for physostigmine in humans causes a state of lethargy and anxiety, and in rats it depresses exploratory activity, whereas atropine causes excitement and agitation in humans, and increases exploratory activity in rats, effects opposite to what one might expect.

▼ There is evidence that cholinergic pathways, in particular the septohippocampal pathway, are involved in learning and short-term memory (see Hagan & Morris, 1988). For example (Fig. 33.7), mice may be trained to execute a maze-running manoeuvre in response to a buzzer, and many will remember the correct response when retested 7 days later. Intracerebral injection of a muscarinic agonist, **arecoline**, immediately after the training session reduces the percentage of animals that forget the correct response when retested, whereas an injection of the muscarinic antagonist **hyoscine** (scopolamine) has the opposite effect. In the experiment shown in Figure 33.7, a deliberate bias was introduced in that the mice selected for the arecoline test were particularly dim (the fast-learners having been excluded), and the training was brief, so that the forgetting rate in the control group was about 70%; an optimal dose of arecoline reduced this to about 15%. The hyoscine test was done on the cleverest mice (the no-hopers being excluded), and the training was more thorough, so the forgetting rate in the control group was only about 20%, and this was increased by hyoscine. More recently, synthetic muscarinic agonists have been shown partially to restore learning and memory deficits induced in experimental animals by lesions of the septohippocampal cholinergic pathway. Hyoscine also impairs memory in human subjects and causes amnesia when used as preanaesthetic medication. Nicotine increases alertness and can also enhance learning and memory, as can various synthetic agonists at neuronal nicotinic receptors. Nevertheless, transgenic mice with disruption of brain nicotinic receptors perform normally in a simple spatial learning task. In conclusion, both nicotinic and muscarinic receptors may play a role in learning and memory, while nicotinic receptors also mediate behavioural arousal.

Transgenic mice that overexpress acetylcholinesterase (and hence show impaired cholinergic transmission) behave normally but develop a learning deficit after a few months (Beeri et al., 1995). The interpretation is not simple, however, since these mice also respond poorly to muscarinic and nicotinic agonists, suggesting that more complex secondary effects were produced.

Involvement of neuronal nicotinic receptors in pain transmission is suggested by the recent finding that **epibatidine**, a compound extracted from frog skin and is a selective agonist at these receptors, has powerful analgesic properties in animals (Ch. 40), as does nicotine itself..

The significance of cholinergic neurons in neurodegenerative conditions such as dementia and Parkinson's disease is discussed in Chapter 34.

SECRETED ACETYLCHOLINESTERASE

▼ In addition to its well-established role as a membrane enzyme responsible for the rapid hydrolysis of acetylcholine (see Ch. 10), there is evidence that acetylcholinesterase may itself be released by neuronal activity, particularly in the substantia nigra, and can modulate various processes (see Appleyard, 1992; Greenfield, 1996). This view, somewhat controversial, is supported by evidence suggesting that injection of

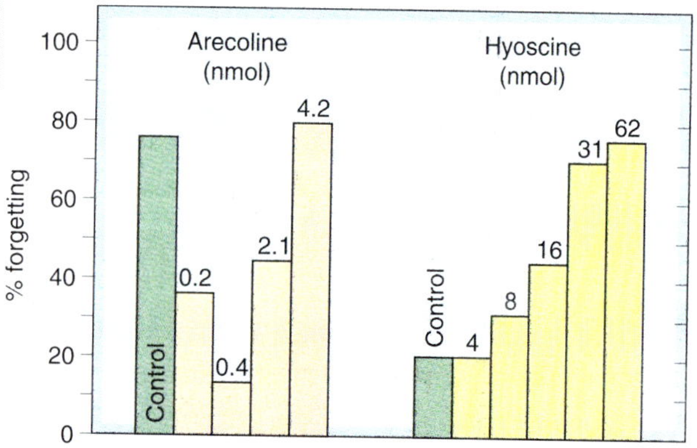

Fig 33.7 Effect of arecoline and hyoscine on learning. Mice were trained to perform a behavioural feat in order to avoid an electric shock and tested for their ability to remember it 7 days later. The group that performed least well (left) were given the cholinergic agonist arecoline by intracerebroventricular injection; at low doses, their performance improved markedly, but at higher doses, their performance declined. The group that performed best in the initial test were given the muscarinic-receptor antagonist hyoscine, which caused a deterioration of their performance. (From Flood et al. 1981 Brain Res 215: 177–185.)

Acetylcholine in the CNS

- Synthesis, storage and release of acetylcholine in the CNS are essentially the same as in the periphery (Ch.10).
- Acetylcholine is widely distributed in the CNS, important pathways being:
  —basal forebrain (magnocellular) nuclei, which send a diffuse projection to most forebrain structures, including the cortex
  —septohippocampal projection
  —short interneurons in the striatum and nucleus accumbens.
- Certain neurodegenerative diseases, especially dementia and Parkinson's disease (see Ch. 34), are associated with abnormalities in cholinergic pathways.
- Both nicotinic and muscarinic acetylcholine receptors occur in the CNS. The former mediate the central effects of nicotine. Nicotinic receptors are mainly located presynaptically; there are few examples of transmission mediated by postsynaptic nicotinic receptors.
- Muscarinic receptors appear to mediate the main behavioural effects associated with acetylcholine, namely effects on arousal, and on learning and short-term memory.
- Muscarinic antagonists (e.g. hyoscine) cause amnesia.
- Acetylcholinesterase released from neurons may have functional effects distinct from cholinergic transmission.

purified acetylcholinesterase into regions of the brain devoid of cholinergic synapses can cause various behavioural effects. One possibility is that acetylcholinesterase possesses some protease activity, and that its effects are secondary to the production of peptide fragments from local protein substrates. Whatever the mechanism, the concept of an enzyme functioning as a released neural mediator is a novel one, the implications of which remain to be explored.

PURINES

Both adenosine and ATP act as transmitters and/or modulators in the CNS (for review, see Dunwiddie & Masino, 2001; Robertson et al., 2001) as they do in the periphery (Ch. 12). Mapping the pathways is difficult, because purinergic neurons are not easily identifiable histochemically, but it is likely that adenosine serves as a very widespread neuromodulator, while ATP has more specific synaptic functions, as a fast transmitter and as a local modulator.

Adenosine is produced intracellularly from ATP (see Fig. 12.4). It is not packaged into vesicles but is released mainly by carrier-mediated transport. Since the intracellular concentration of ATP (several millimoles per litre) greatly exceeds that of adenosine, conversion of a small proportion of ATP results in a large increase in adenosine. ATP is packaged into vesicles and released by exocytosis as a conventional transmitter, but it can also leak out of cells under conditions of tissue damage, the released ATP being quickly converted to adenosine (Fig. 12.4). These special characteristics of adenosine metabolism suggest that it serves mainly as safety mechanism, protecting the neurons from damage when their viability is threatened, for example by ischaemia or seizure activity.

As discussed in Chapter 12, adenosine produces its effects through G-protein-coupled receptors (with receptor subtypes A_1, A_2 and A_3) while ATP acts on P_2-receptors, P_{2X} being ligand-gated cation channels, P_{2Y} being G-protein-coupled. P_{2Y}-receptors produce mainly inhibitory effects, while the P_{2X}-receptors are excitatory, producing both pre- and postsynaptic effects in much the same way as nicotinic receptors. All of these receptors are more or less widely distributed in the brain.

The overall effect of adenosine and of various adenosine receptor agonists is inhibitory, leading to effects such as drowsiness, motor incoordination, analgesia and anticonvulsant activity. Xanthines, such as **caffeine** (Ch. 41), which are antagonists at A_2-receptors, produce arousal and alertness. Many synthetic adenosine agonists have been developed, since such drugs could be useful in treating conditions such as epilepsy, pain and sleep disorders. A further possible use is in neuroprotection, since the inhibitory effect of adenosine on neuronal excitability and glutamate release is able, in experimental models, to protect the brain against ischaemic damage (see Ch. 34).

Little is known about the function of ATP as a chemical mediator in the brain. Because it is quickly metabolised to ADP and adenosine, its pharmacological actions are difficult to unravel, and there are few selective agonists or antagonists for ATP receptors. It may play a role in nociception, since ATP is released by tissue damage and causes pain by stimulating unmyelinated afferent nerve terminals, which express P_{2X}-receptors.

HISTAMINE

Histamine is present in the brain in much smaller amounts than in other tissues, such as skin and lung, but undoubtedly serves a neurotransmitter role (see Brown et al., 2001). Histaminergic neurons are restricted to a small part of the hypothalamus, and their axons run to virtually all parts of the brain—an 'aerosol' arrangement similar to other monoamines. Unusually, no uptake mechanism for histamine is present, its action being terminated instead by enzymic methylation.

Histamine acts on three types of receptor (H_{1-3}; Ch. 15), all of which are G-protein-coupled receptors and occur in most brain regions. H_1-receptors are mainly located postsynaptically and cause excitation; H_2- and H_3-receptors are inhibitory, respectively post- and presynaptic, H_3-receptors being inhibitory autoreceptors on histamine-releasing neurons.

▼ Like other monoamine transmitters, histamine is involved in many different CNS functions. Histamine release follows a distinct circadian pattern, the neurons being active by day and silent by night. H_1-receptors in the cortex and reticular activating system contribute to arousal and wakefulness, and H_1-receptor antagonists produce sedation (see Ch. 15). Other functions ascribed to histamine include control of food and water intake, thermoregulation, etc., but these are less well characterised.

OTHER CNS MEDIATORS

We now move from the comfortable neuropharmacological territory of the 'classical' monoamines to some of the frontier towns, bordering on the Wild West. Useful drugs are still few and far between in this area, and if applied pharmacology is your main concern, you can safely skip the next part and wait a few years for law and order to be established.

MELATONIN

▼ Melatonin (reviewed by Brzezinski, 1997) is something of a mystery. It is synthesised exclusively in the pineal, an endocrine gland that plays a role in establishing circadian rhythms. The gland contains two enzymes, not found elsewhere, which convert 5-HT by acetylation and O-methylation to melatonin, its hormonal product. Melatonin secretion (in all animals, whether diurnal or nocturnal in their habits) is high at night, and low by day. This rhythm is controlled by input from the retina, via a noradrenergic retinohypothalamic tract that terminates in the suprachiasmatic nucleus in the hypothalamus, a structure often termed the 'biological clock', which generates the circadian rhythm. This area controls the pineal, not directly, but via sympathetic fibres supplying the gland. This retinal control system serves to inhibit melatonin secretion when the light intensity is high. It does not itself generate the circadian rhythm but rather 'entrains' it to the light–dark cycle. Circadian rhythms, including the rhythmic secretion of melatonin, continue even in the absence of light–dark cues, but usually with a periodicity rather longer than 24 hours.

Melatonin receptors (as you will have guessed) are widespread and come in different types. The main ones are typical G-protein-coupled receptors, found mainly in the brain and retina but also in peripheral tissues. Another type has been identified as one of the previous 'orphan receptors' (see Ch. 3), a member of the retinoic acid intracellular receptor family which regulates gene transcription. We currently know very little about the physiological processes that are controlled by melatonin, though there is intense research activity in this area.

The use of melatonin for medicinal purposes has become something of an 'alternative medicine' fad, though there are few properly controlled trials of its efficacy. Given orally, melatonin is well absorbed, but quickly metabolised, its plasma half-life being a few minutes. It has been promoted as a means of controlling jet-lag, or of improving the performance of night-shift workers, based on its ability to reset the circadian clock, and controlled studies have confirmed that melatonin given in the evening can alleviate the effects of jet-lag. A single dose appears to have the effect of resynchronising the physiological secretory cycle, though it is not clear how this occurs. It causes sleepiness, and there is some disagreement about whether its actions are distinguishable from those of conventional hypnotic drugs (see Ch. 36). Claims that melatonin produces other effects (e.g. on mood and immune function) have yet to be confirmed.

Other transmitters and modulators

Histamine

- Histamine fulfils the criteria for a neurotransmitter. Histaminergic neurons originate in a small area of the hypothalamus and have a widespread distribution.
- H_1-, H_2- and H_3-receptors are widespread in the brain. H_1- and H_3-receptors are mainly excitatory; H_2-receptors are inhibitory.
- The functions of histamine are not well understood, the main clues being that histaminergic neurons are active during waking hours, and H_1-receptor antagonists are strongly sedative.
- H_1-receptor antagonists are antiemetic.

Purines

- ATP functions as a neurotransmitter, being stored in vesicles and released by exocytosis. It acts, via ionotropic receptors, as a fast excitatory transmitter in certain pathways and, via metabotropic receptors, as a neuromodulator.
- Cytosolic ATP is present at relatively high concentration and can be released directly if neuronal viability is compromised (e.g. in stroke).
- Released ATP is rapidly converted to ADP, AMP and adenosine.
- Adenosine Is not stored in vesicles but is released by carrier mechanisms or generated from released ATP, mainly under pathological conditions.
- Adenosine exerts mainly inhibitory effects, through A_1- and A_2-receptors, resulting in sedative, anticonvulsant and neuroprotective effects, and acting as a safety mechanism.
- Methylxanthines (e.g. caffeine) are antagonists at A_2-receptors and increase wakefulness.

Melatonin

- Melatonin is synthesised from 5-HT, mainly in the pineal gland, from which it is released as a circulating hormone.
- Secretion is controlled by light intensity, being low by day and high by night. Fibres from the retina run to the suprachiasmatic nucleus ('biological clock'), which controls the pineal gland via its sympathetic innervation.
- Melatonin acts on several types of receptor in the brain and periphery. Given orally, it causes sedation and also 'resets' the biological clock, being used for this purpose to counter jet-lag.
- Other claimed actions of melatonin (e.g. on mood and immune function) are controversial.

Nitric oxide (NO; see Ch.14)

- Neuronal nitric oxide synthetase (nNOS) is present in many CNS neurons, and NO production is increased by mechanisms (e.g. transmitter action) that raise intracellular Ca^{2+}.
- NO affects neuronal function by increasing cGMP formation, producing both inhibitory and excitatory effects on neurons.
- In larger amounts, NO forms peroxynitrite, which contributes to neurotoxicity.
- Inhibition of nNOS reduces long-term potentiation and depression, probably because NO functions as a retrograde messenger. Inhibition of nNOS also protects against ischaemic brain damage in animal models.
- Carbon monoxide shares many properties with NO and may also be a neural mediator.

Lipid mediators

- Arachidonic acid is produced in neurons by receptor-mediated hydrolysis of phospholipid. It is converted to various eicosanoids and to anandamide.
- Arachioline acid itself, as well as its active products, can produce rapid and slow effects by regulation of ion channels and protein kinase cascades. Such effects can occur in the donor cell, or in adjacent cells and nerve terminals.
- Anandamide is an endogenous activator of cannabinoid receptors (Ch 51) and also of the vanilloid receptor (Ch. 40).
- The functional role of lipid mediators in the CNS is still poorly understood.

NITRIC OXIDE

Nitric oxide (NO) as a peripheral mediator is discussed in Chapter 14. Its significance as an important chemical mediator in the nervous system became apparent only in the 1990s and demanded a considerable readjustment of our views about neurotransmission and neuromodulation (for review, see Dawson & Snyder, 1994). The main defining criteria for transmitter substances—namely that neurons should possess machinery for synthesising and storing the substance, that it should be released from neurons by exocytosis, that it should interact with specific membrane receptors, and that there should be mechanisms for its inactivation—do not apply to NO. Moreover, it is an inorganic toxic gas, not at all the kind of molecule we are used to. The mediator function of NO, and probably also carbon monoxide (CO), is now well established, however (see Bredt & Snyder, 1992; Vincent, 1995; Barañano et al., 2001). NO diffuses rapidly through cell membranes, and its action is not highly localised. Its half-life depends greatly on the chemical environment, ranging from seconds in blood to several minutes in normal tissues. The presence of superoxide, with which NO reacts (see below), shortens its half-life considerably.

NO in the nervous system is produced mainly by the constitutive neuronal form of *nitric oxide synthase* (nNOS; see Ch. 14), which can be detected either histochemically or by immunolabelling. It is present in roughly 2% of neurons, both short interneurons and long-tract neurons, in virtually all brain areas, with particular concentrations in the cerebellum and hippocampus. It occurs in cell bodies and dendrites, as well as in axon terminals, suggesting (since NO is not stored but released as it is made) that the release of NO is not restricted to conventional neurotransmitter release sites. nNOS is calmodulin dependent and is activated by a rise in intracellular Ca^{2+} concentration, which can occur by many mechanisms, including action potential conduction and neurotransmitter action. Many studies have shown that NO production is increased by activation of synaptic pathways, or by other events such as brain ischaemia (see Ch. 34).

NO exerts its effects in two main ways:

- by activation of soluble guanylate cyclase, leading to the production of cGMP and various phosphorylation cascades (Ch. 3); this 'physiological' control mechanism operates at low NO concentrations of about 0.1 μmol/l
- by reacting with the superoxide free radical to generate peroxynitrite, a highly toxic anion, which acts by oxidising various intracellular proteins; this requires concentrations of 1–10 μmol/l, which are achieved in brain ischaemia.

There is good evidence that NO plays a role in long-term potentiation and depression (see Ch. 32), since these phenomena are reduced or prevented by NOS inhibitors, and are absent in transgenic mice in which the nNOS gene has been disrupted.

Based on the same kind of evidence, NO is also believed to play an important part in the mechanisms by which ischaemia causes neuronal death (see Ch. 34). There is also speculation that it may be involved in other processes, including neurodegeneration in Parkinson's disease, senile dementia and amyotrophic lateral sclerosis, and the local control of blood flow linked to neuronal activity. If substantiated, these theories will open up major new therapeutic possibilities in some hitherto intractable disease areas.

CARBON MONOXIDE

▼ CO is best known as a poisonous gas present in vehicle exhaust; it binds strongly to haemoglobin, causing tissue anoxia. However, it is also formed endogenously and has many features in common with NO (see Verma et al., 1993; Barañano et al., 2001). Neurons and other cells contain a CO-generating enzyme, *haem oxygenase*, and CO also activates guanylate cyclase.

The role of CO as a CNS mediator is less well established, but there is some evidence that it plays a role in the cerebellum, and also in olfactory neurons, where cGMP-sensitive ion channels are involved in the transduction process.

Undoubtedly, further functions of NO and CO in the brain remain to be identified, and novel therapeutic approaches may come from targeting the different steps in the synthetic and signal transduction pathways for these surprising mediators. We may have to endure the ponderous whimsy of many 'NO' puns, but it should be worth it in the end.

LIPID MEDIATORS

▼ The formation of arachidonic acid and its conversion to *eicosanoids* (mainly prostaglandins, leukotrienes and HETEs (hydroxy-eicosatetraenoic acids); see Ch. 15) and to the endogenous cannabinoid receptor ligand **anandamide** (see Ch. 42) are known to take place in the CNS. They doubtless play an important role, though our knowledge in this area is still fragmentary (for reviews, see Piomelli, 1995; Piomelli et al., 2000), partly because there are few selective inhibitors that can be used to probe the various steps in the rather lengthy biochemical pathways through which the mediators are formed and exert their effects. Figure 33.8 shows a schematic view of the different possibilities, but it should be realised that evidence as to the functional importance of these pathways is still very limited.

Phospholipid cleavage, leading to arachidonic acid production, occurs in neurons in response to receptor activation by many different mediators, including neurotransmitters. The arachidonic acid so formed can act directly as an intracellular messenger, controlling both ion channels and various parts of the protein kinase cascade (see Ch. 3) and producing both rapid and delayed effects on neuronal function. Arachiolonic acid can also be metabolised to anandamide and to eicosanoids, some of which (principally the HETEs) can also act as intracellular messengers acting in the same cell. Eicosanoids can also exert an *autocrine* effect via membrane receptors expressed by the cell. Both arachidonic acid itself and its products escape readily from the cell of origin and can affect neighbouring structures, including presynaptic terminals (retrograde signalling) and adjacent cells (*paracrine* signalling), by acting on receptors or by acting directly as intracellular messengers. Theoretically, the possibilities are endless, but there are so far only a few instances where this system is known to play a significant role. These include our old friend long-term potentiation (Ch. 32), one component of which is prevented by inhibition of phospholipase A_2, where arachidonic acid is believed to serve as a retrograde messenger causing facilitation of transmitter release by the presynaptic nerve terminal. A second well-studied system is the *Aplysia* sensory neuron, where the effects of various inhibitory mediators, acting on membrane receptors, are exerted through the intracellular actions of arachidonic acid and its products.

One surprise in this field has been the discovery that anandamide, besides being an agonist at cannabinoid receptors, also activates vanilloid

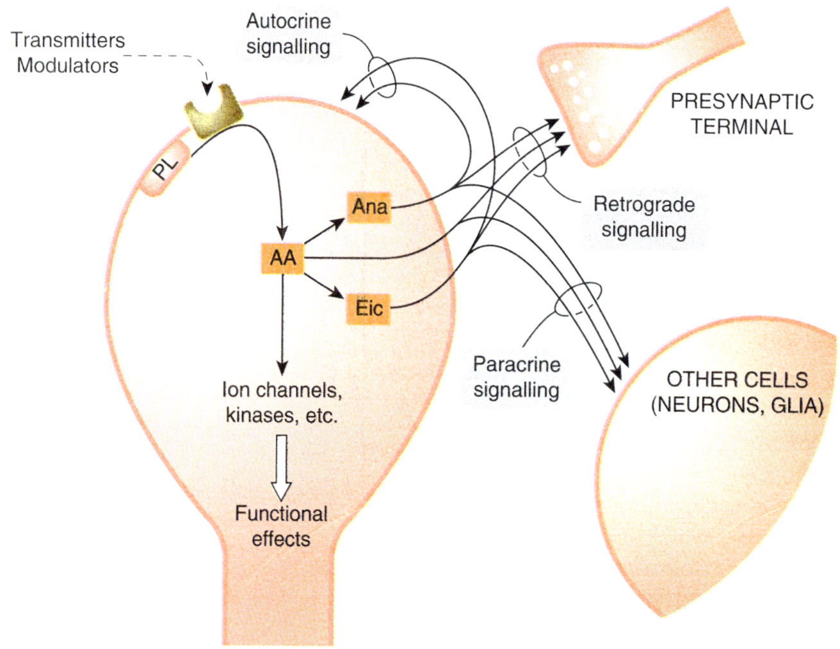

Fig. 33.8 Postulated modes of signalling by lipid mediators. Arachidonic acid is formed by receptor-mediated cleavage of membrane phospholipid. It can act directly as an intracellular messenger, on ion channels or components of different kinase cascades, producing various long- and short-term effects. It can also be converted to eicosanoids (prostaglandins, leukotrienes or HETEs) or to anandamide. HETEs can also act directly as intracellular messengers. All of these mediators diffuse out of the cell, and exert effects on presynaptic terminals and neighbouring cells, acting either on extracellular receptors, or intracellularly. There are examples of most of these modes of signalling, but only limited information about their functional significance in the nervous system. (AA, arachidonic acid; Ana, anandamide; Eic, eicosanoids; PL, membrane phospholipid; HETEs, hydroxyeicosatetraenoic acids.)

receptors (see Ch. 40), which are involved in the response of peripheral sensory nerve terminals to painful stimuli. What role, if any, anandamide has in pain transmission remains to be seen.

A FINAL MESSAGE

In the last two chapters, we have taken a long and tortuous tour through the brain and its chemistry, with two questions at the back of our minds. What mediators and what receptors play a key role in what brain functions? How does the information relate to existing and future drugs that aim to correct malfunctions? Despite the efforts of a huge army of researchers deploying an arsenal of powerful new techniques, the answers to these questions seem to remain as elusive as ever. Though transgenic techniques allow specific gene products (i.e. proteins) to be modified in a much more precise and controllable way than can be achieved pharmacologically, behavioural analysis of transgenic animals has failed to clear the air very much. The array of potential CNS targets—comprising multiple receptor subtypes, many with the added complexity of heteromeric assemblies, splice variants, etc., along with regulatory mechanisms that control their expression and localisation—continues to grow in complexity. Speculation about the best target to aim at in order to ameliorate the effect of a particular brain malfunction, such as stroke or schizophrenia, has become less focussed, even if better informed, than it was two decades ago. In the ensuing chapters in this section, we shall find that most of the therapeutic successes have come from chance discoveries that were followed up empirically; few have followed a logical, mechanism-based route to success. Optimists believe that this is changing and advise: Hang in there—good things will come out of all this sooner than you might suppose.

REFERENCES AND FURTHER READING

Appleyard M E 1992 Secreted acetylcholinesterase: non-classical aspects of a classical enzyme. Trends Neurosci 15: 485–490 (*Review of the controversial function of acetylcholinesterase as a secreted mediator*)

Azmitia E C, Whitaker-Azmitia P M 1995 Anatomy, cell biology and plasticity of the serotonergic system. In: Bloom F E, Kupfer D J (eds) Psychopharmacology: a fourth generation of progress. Raven Press, New York (*General review article*)

Barañano D E, Ferris C D, Snyder S H 2001. Atypical neural messengers. Trends Neurosci 24: 99–106 (*Short trendy review on some established mediators, such as NO, and some speculative ones, such as CO and D-serine*)

Barnes N M, Sharp T 1999 A review of central 5-HT receptors and their function. Neuropharmacology 38: 1083--152 (*Detailed compilation of data relating to distribution, pharmacology and function of 5-HT receptors in the CNS. Useful information source but not particularly illuminating*)

Beeri R, Andres C, Lev-Lehman E et al. 1995 Transgenic expression of human acetylcholinesterase induces progressive cognitive deterioration in mice. Curr Biol 5: 1063–1071 (*Describes a transgenic mouse model with impaired cholinergic transmission, leading to cognitive changes*)

Bredt D S, Snyder S H 1992 Nitric oxide, a novel neuronal messenger. Neuron 8: 3–11 (*Widely quoted review article which anticipates many later discoveries*)

Brown R E, Stevens D R, Haas H L 2001 The physiology of brain histamine. Prog Neurobiol 63: 637–672 (*Useful review article*)

Brzezinski A 1997 Melatonin in humans. N Engl J Med 336: 186–195 (*Clear and well referenced review article. Recommended as an introduction*)

Cooper J R, Bloom F E, Roth R H 1996 Biochemical basis of neuropharmacology. Oxford University Press, New York (*Clear and well written textbook giving more detailed information on many topics covered in this chapter*)

Cordero-Erausquin M, Marubio L M, Klink R, Changeux J-P 2000 Nicotinic receptor function: new perspectives from knockout mice. Trends Pharmacol Sci 21: 211–217 (*Short review article*)

Dani J A 2000 Overview of nicotinic receptors and their roles in the central nervous system. Biol Psychiatry 49: 166–174 (*Useful review article*)

Dawson T M, Snyder S H 1994 Gases as biological messengers: nitric oxide and carbon monoxide in the brain. J Neurosci 14: 5147–5159 (*Excellent introductory review, summarising ideas in a new area*)

Dunwiddie T V, Masino S A 2001 The role and regulation of adenosine in the central nervous system. Annu Rev Neurosci 24: 31–55 (*Good short review emphasising the protective role of adenosine*)

Greenfield S A 1996 Non-classical actions of cholinesterases; role in cellular differentiation, tumorigenesis and Alzheimer's disease. Neurochem Int 28: 485–490 (*Review of possible functions of secreted acetylcholinesterase*)

Hagan J J, Morris R G M 1988 The cholinergic hypothesis of memory: a review of animal experiments. In: Iversen L L, Iversen S, Snyder S H (eds) Handbook of psychopharmacology, vol. 20, pp. 237–323 Plenum, New York (*Useful summary, now rather dated, of evidence implicating acetylcholine in learning and memory*)

Jones S, Sudweeks S, Yakel J L 1999 Nicotinic receptors in the brain: correlating physiology with function. Trends Neurosci 12: 555–561 (*Review focussing on role of nicotinic acetylcholine receptors in cognitive functions*)

Jaber M, Robinson S W, Missale C, Caron M G 1996 Dopamine receptors and brain function. Neuropharmacology 35: 1503–1519 (*Useful general review*)

Nestler E J, Hyman S E, Malenka R C 2001 Molecular neuropharmacology. McGraw Hill, New York (*Good modern textbook*)

Piomelli D 1995 Arachidonic acid. In: Bloom F E, Kupfer D J (eds) Psychopharmacology: a fourth generation of progress. Raven Press, New York (*Excellent review article*)

Piomelli D, Giuffrida A, Calignano A, Fonseca F R 2000 The endocannabinoid system as a target for therapeutic drugs. Trends Pharmacol Sci 21: 218–224 (*Short review article on role of anandamide in CNS*)

Robertson S J, Ennion S J, Evans R J, Edwards F A 2001 Synaptic P_{2X} receptors. Curr Opin Neurobiol 11: 378–386 (*Review on transmitter role of ATP focussing on receptor pharmacology*)

Rudolph U, Möhler H 1999 Genetically modified animals in pharmacological research: future trends. Eur J Pharmacol 375: 327–337

Seeman P, van Tol H H M 1994 Dopamine receptor pharmacology. Trends Pharmacol Sci 15: 264–270 (*Introductory review article*)

Sibley D R 1999 New insights into dopaminergic receptor function using antisense and genetically altered animals. Annu Rev Pharmacol Toxicol 39: 313–341

Verma A, Hirsch D J, Glatt C E, Ronnett G V, Snyder S H 1993 Carbon monoxide: a putative neural messenger. Science 259: 381–384 (*Speculative review, which points out similarities with NO*)

Vincent S R (ed) 1995 Nitric oxide in the nervous system. Academic Press, London (*Useful compendium of review articles on all aspects of NO in the nervous system*)

Wei L-N 1997 Transgenic animals as new approaches in pharmacological studies. Annu Rev Pharmacol Toxicol 27: 119–141

34 Neurodegenerative disorders

Overview 490

Mechanisms of neuronal death 490
- Excitotoxicity 491
- Apoptosis 491
- Oxidative stress 493

Ischaemic brain damage 493

Alzheimer's disease 494
- Pathogenesis 494
- Therapeutic approaches 496

Parkinson's disease 497
- Features of Parkinson's disease 497
- Pathogenesis 497
- Drug treatment of Parkinson's disease 499

Huntington's disease 501

Neurodegenerative prion diseases 501

OVERVIEW

As a rule, dead neurons in the adult CNS are not replaced,* nor can their terminals regenerate when their axons are interrupted. Therefore, any pathological process causing neuronal death generally has irreversible consequences. At first sight, this appears to be very unpromising territory for pharmacological intervention, and indeed drug therapy currently has rather little to offer, except in the case of Parkinson's disease (see below). Nevertheless, the incidence and social impact of neurodegenerative brain disorders in ageing populations has resulted in a massive research effort in recent years, and the improved understanding of the molecular basis of these disorders now offers real hope for therapeutic progress in the not-too-distant future. In this chapter, we discuss:

- **mechanisms responsible for neuronal death, focussing on protein deposition (amyloidosis), excitotoxicity, oxidative stress and apoptosis**
- **pharmacological approaches (so far hypothetical) to preventing neuronal loss**
- **pharmacological approaches to compensation for neuronal loss.**

The discussion focuses mainly on three common neurodegenerative conditions, namely *dementia (Alzheimer's disease)*, *ischaemic brain damage (stroke)* and *Parkinson's disease.* The hurried reader may safely skip straight to page 497 without missing anything of current therapeutic importance.

*It is recognised that new neurons are formed from progenitor cells in certain regions of the adult brain, even in primates. Whether this occurs in the cortex, and whether it plays any role in learning and memory, is a matter of dispute (see Gross, 2000; Rakic, 2002). Certainly, it plays little if any role in brain repair. However, learning how to harness the inherent ability of neuronal progenitors (stem cells) to form new neurons is seen as an obvious approach to treating neurodegenerative disorders.

MECHANISMS OF NEURONAL DEATH

Acute injury to cells causes them to undergo *necrosis*, recognised pathologically by cell swelling, vacuolisation and lysis, and associated with Ca^{2+} overload of the cells and membrane damage (see below). Necrotic cells typically spill their contents into the surrounding tissue, evoking an inflammatory response. Cells can also die by *apoptosis* or programmed cell death (see Raff, 1998), a slower process that occurs normally during development and is essential for many processes throughout life, for example development, immune regulation and tissue remodelling. Apoptosis, as well as necrosis, occurs in many neurodegenerative disorders (including acute conditions such as stroke and head injury; for review, see Bredesen (1995)). The distinction between necrosis and apoptosis as processes leading to neurodegeneration is not absolute, for challenges such as excitotoxicity and oxidative stress may be enough to kill cells directly by necrosis, or, if less intense, may induce them to undergo apoptosis. Both processes, therefore, represent possible targets for putative neuroprotective drug therapy. Pharmacological interference with the apoptotic pathway may become possible in the future, but for the present, most efforts are directed at the processes involved in cell necrosis, and at compensating pharmacologically for the neuronal loss.

EXCITOTOXICITY

In spite of its ubiquitous role as a neurotransmitter (Ch. 32), *glutamate* is highly toxic to neurons, a phenomenon dubbed *excitotoxicity* (see Choi, 1988). A low concentration of glutamate applied to neurons in culture kills the cells, and the finding in the 1970s that glutamate given orally produces neurodegeneration in vivo caused considerable alarm, because of the widespread use of glutamate as a 'taste-enhancing' food additive. The 'Chinese restaurant syndrome'—an acute attack of neck stiffness and chest pain—is well known, but so far the possibility of more serious neurotoxicity from dietary glutamate is only hypothetical.

Local injection of **kainic acid** is used experimentally to produce neurotoxic lesions. It acts by excitation of local glutamate-releasing neurons, and the release of glutamate, acting on NMDA (*N*-methyl-D-aspartate) and also metabotropic receptors (Ch. 32) leads to neuronal death.

Calcium overload is the essential factor in excitotoxicity. The mechanisms by which this occurs and leads to cell death are as follows (Fig. 34.1).

- Glutamate activates NMDA, AMPA (α-amino-3-hydroxy-5-methyl-4-isoxazolepropionate) and metabotropic receptors (sites 1, 2 and 3 in Fig. 34.1). Activation of AMPA receptors depolarises the cell, which unblocks the NMDA-channels (see Ch. 32), permitting Ca^{2+} entry. Depolarisation also opens voltage-activated calcium channels (site 4), releasing more glutamate. Metabotropic receptors cause the release of intracellular Ca^{2+} from the endoplasmic reticulum. Sodium entry further contributes to Ca^{2+} entry by stimulating Ca^{2+}/Na^+ exchange (site 5). Depolarisation inhibits or reverses glutamate uptake (site 6), thus increasing the extracellular glutamate concentration.
- The mechanisms that normally operate to counteract the rise in $[Ca^{2+}]_i$ include the Ca^{2+} efflux pump (site 7) and, indirectly, the Na^+ pump (site 8).
- `The mitochondria and endoplasmic reticulum act as capacious sinks for Ca^{2+} and normally keep $[Ca^{2+}]_i$ under control. Loading of the mitochondrial stores beyond a certain point, however, disrupts mitochondrial function, reducing ATP synthesis, thus reducing the energy available for the membrane pumps and for Ca^{2+} accumulation by the endoplasmic reticulum. Formation of reactive oxygen species (ROS) is also enhanced. This represents the danger point at which positive feedback exaggerates the process.
- Raised $[Ca^{2+}]_i$ affects many processes, the chief ones relevant to neurotoxicity being:
  —increased glutamate release
  —activation of proteases (calpains) and lipases, causing membrane damage
  —activation of nitric oxide (NO) synthase (NOS); while low concentrations of NO are neuroprotective, high concentrations, in the presence of ROS, generate peroxynitrite and hydroxyl free radicals, which damage many important biomolecules, including membrane lipids, proteins and DNA
  —increased arachidonic acid release, which increases free radical production and also inhibits glutamate uptake (site 6).

Glutamate and Ca^{2+} are arguably the two most ubiquitous chemical signals, extracellular and intracellular respectively, underlying brain function, so it is disconcerting that such cytotoxic mayhem can be unleashed when they get out of control. Both are stored in dangerous amounts in subcellular organelles, like hand-grenades in an ammunition store. Defence against excitotoxicity is clearly essential if our brains are to have any chance of staying alive. Mitochondrial energy metabolism provides one line of defence (see above), and impaired mitochondrial function, by rendering neurons vulnerable to excitotoxic damage, may be a factor in various neurodegenerative conditions, including Parkinson's disease (PD).

The role of excitotoxicity in ischaemic brain damage is well established (see below), and it is also believed to be a factor in other neurodegenerative diseases, such as those discussed below (see Lipton & Rosenberg, 1994).

▼ There are several examples of neurodegenerative conditions caused by environmental toxins, acting as agonists on glutamate receptors (see Olney, 1990). *Domoic acid* is a glutamate analogue produced by mussels, which was identified as the cause of an epidemic of severe mental and neurological deterioration in a group of Newfoundlanders in 1987. On the island of Guam, a syndrome combining the features of dementia, paralysis and PD was traced to an excitotoxic amino acid, β-methylaminoalanine, in the seeds of a local plant. Discouraging the consumption of these seeds has largely eliminated the disease.

APOPTOSIS

Apoptosis (Ch. 5) can be initiated by various cell surface signals (see review by Steller, 1995). The cell is systematically dismantled and the shrunken remnants are removed by macrophages without causing inflammation. Apoptotic cells can be identified by a staining technique that detects the characteristic DNA breaks. In general, neural apoptosis is initiated by the absence of particular growth factors, resulting in altered gene transcription and the activation of specific 'cell death' proteins. Apoptosis is often associated with excitotoxicity, even in acute neurodegenerative conditions in humans, though the link is not well understood. Many different signalling pathways can result in apoptosis (see Raff, 1998), but in all cases the final pathway resulting in cell death is the activation of a family of proteases (*caspases*) that inactivate various intracellular proteins. Neural apoptosis is normally prevented by neuronal growth factors, including nerve growth factor and brain-derived neurotrophic factor, secreted proteins that are required for the survival of different populations of neurons in the central nervous system (CNS). These growth factors regulate the expression of the two gene products Bax and Bcl-2, Bax being pro-apoptotic and Bcl-2 being anti-apoptotic (see Raff 1998; also Fig. 5.5). Blocking apoptosis by interfering at specific points on these pathways

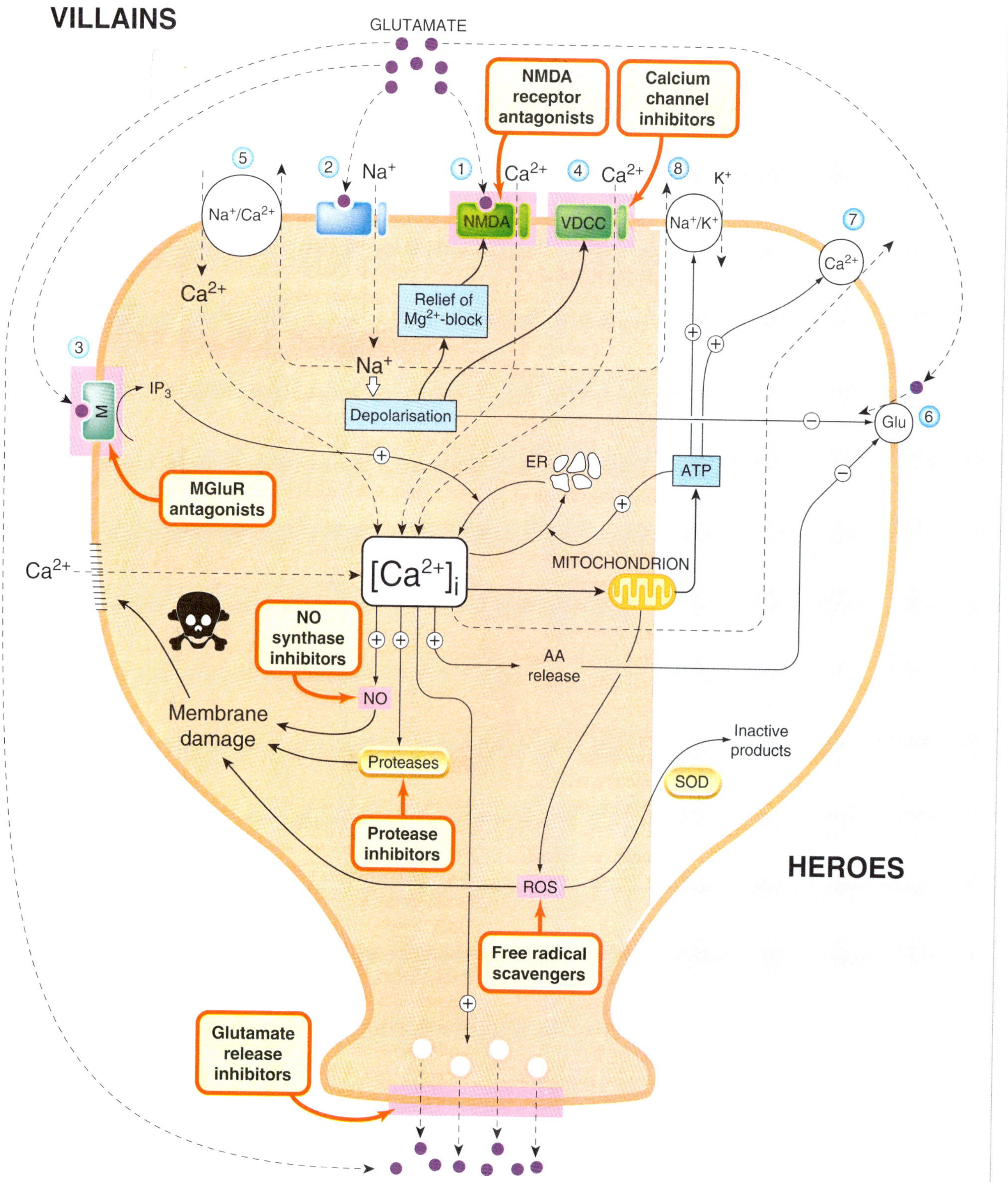

Fig. 34.1 Mechanisms of excitotoxicity. Membrane receptors, ion channels and transporters, identified by numbers 1–8, are discussed in the text. Possible sites of action of neuroprotective drugs (not yet of proven clinical value) are highlighted. Mechanisms on the left (villains) are those that favour cell death, while those on the right (heroes) are protective. See text for details. (ER, endoplasmic reticulum; AA, arachidonic acid; ROS, reactive oxygen species; SOD, superoxide dismutase; NMDA, *N*-methyl-D-aspartate; VDCC, coltage-controlled calcium channel; IP_3, inositol trisphosphate; NO, nitric oxide.)

represents an attractive strategy for developing neuroprotective drugs, but one which has yet to bear fruit.

OXIDATIVE STRESS

The brain derives nearly all its energy from mitochondrial oxidative phosphorylation, which generates ATP at the same time as reducing molecular oxygen to water. Under certain conditions, ROS, for example oxygen and hydroxyl free radicals, and hydrogen peroxide may be generated as side-products of this process (see Coyle & Puttfarken, 1993). Oxidative stress is the result of excessive production of these reactive species. They can also be produced as a by-product of other biochemical pathways, including NO synthesis and arachidonic acid metabolism (which are implicated in excitotoxicity; see above), as well as the mixed function oxidase system (see Ch. 8). Unchecked, ROS attack many key molecules, including enzymes, membrane lipids and DNA. Not surprisingly, defence mechanisms are provided, in the form of enzymes such as *superoxide dismutase* (SOD) and *catalase*, as well as antioxidants, such as *ascorbic acid*, *glutathione* and *α-tocopherol* (vitamin E), which normally keep these reactive species in check. Some cytokines, especially tumour necrosis factor (TNF-α), which is produced in conditions of brain ischaemia or inflammation (Ch. 15), exert a protective effect, partly by increasing the expression of SOD (see Rothwell et al., 1996). Transgenic animals lacking TNF receptors show enhanced susceptibility to brain ischaemia. Mutations of the gene encoding SOD (Fig. 34.1) are associated with a progressive form of motor neuron disease known as *amyotrophic lateral sclerosis*, a fatal paralytic disease resulting from progressive degeneration of motoneurons; transgenic mice expressing mutated SOD develop a similar condition (see Louvel et al., 1997). It is possible that accumulated or inherited mutations in enzymes such as those of the mitochondrial respiratory chain lead to a congenital or age-related increase in susceptibility to oxidative stress, which is manifest in different kinds of inherited neurodegenerative disorder (such as Huntington's disease), and in age-related neurodegeneration (see Beal et al., 1993).

Several possible targets for therapeutic intervention with neuroprotective drugs are shown in Figure 34.1. Activity in this area is intense, but with little practical outcome so far. One recent, though modest, success is **riluzole**, a compound that inhibits both the release and the postsynaptic action of glutamate; this drug retards to some degree the deterioration of patients with amyotrophic lateral sclerosis. For reviews of hopes and achievements in various neurodegenerative diseases, see Lipton & Rosenberg (1994), Green & Cross (1997) and Wyss-Coray & Mucke (2002).

Excitotoxicity and oxidative stress

- Excitatory amino acids (EAA, e.g. glutamate) can cause neuronal death.
- Excitotoxicity is associated mainly with activation of NMDA-receptors, but other types of EAA receptors also contribute.
- Excitotoxicity results from a sustained rise in intracellular Ca^{2+} concentration (Ca^{2+} overload).
- Excitotoxicity can occur under pathological conditions (e.g. cerebral ischaemia, epilepsy) in which excessive glutamate release occurs. It can also occur when chemicals such as kainic acid are administered.
- Raised intracellular Ca^{2+} causes cell death by various mechanisms, including activation of proteases, formation of free radicals, and lipid peroxidation. Formation of nitric oxide and arachidonic acid are also involved.
- Various mechanisms act normally to protect neurons against excitotoxicity, the main ones being Ca^{2+} transport systems, mitochondrial function and the production of free radical scavengers.
- Oxidative stress refers to conditions (e.g. hypoxia) in which the protective mechanisms are compromised, reactive oxygen species (ROS) accumulate and neurons become more susceptible to excitotoxic damage.
- Excitotoxicity caused by environmental chemicals may contribute to some neurodegenerative disorders.
- Measures designed to reduce excitotoxicity include the use of glutamate antagonists, calcium channel blocking drugs (calcium antagonists) and free radical scavengers; none is yet proven for clinical use.

ISCHAEMIC BRAIN DAMAGE

After heart disease and cancer, strokes are the commonest cause of death in Europe and North America, and the 70% that are non-fatal are the commonest cause of disability.

PATHOPHYSIOLOGY

Interruption of blood supply to the brain initiates the cascade of neuronal events shown in Figure 34.1; these lead. in turn, to later consequences, including cerebral oedema and inflammation, which can also contribute to brain damage (see Dirnagl et al., 1999). Further damage can occur following reperfusion, because of the production of ROS when the oxygenation is restored. Reperfusion injury may be an important component in stroke patients. These secondary processes often take hours to develop and may offer hope for therapeutic intervention. The lesion produced by occlusion of a major cerebral artery consists of a central core in which the neurons quickly undergo irreversible necrosis, surrounded by a *penumbra* of compromised tissue in which inflammation and apoptotic cell death develop over a period of several hours. It is assumed that neuroprotective therapies, given within a few hours, might inhibit this secondary penumbral damage.

Glutamate excitotoxicity plays a critical role in brain ischaemia. Ischaemia causes depolarisation of neurons, and the release of large amounts of glutamate. Calcium ion accumulation occurs, partly as a result of glutamate acting on NMDA-receptors, for both Ca^{2+} entry and cell death following cerebral ischaemia are inhibited by drugs that block NMDA-receptors or channels (see Ch. 32). NO also builds up, to levels much higher than can be produced by normal neuronal activity (i.e. to levels that are toxic, rather than modulatory).

THERAPEUTIC APPROACHES

In animal models involving cerebral artery occlusion, a long list of drugs targeted at the mechanisms shown in Figure 34.1 can reduce the size of the infarct. These include glutamate antagonists, calcium and sodium channel inhibitors, free radical scavengers, anti-inflammatory drugs, protease inhibitors, and others. It seems that almost anything works.

However, attempts to develop drugs for therapeutic use have so far been disappointing (see de Keyser et al., 1999). Controlled clinical trials on stroke patients are problematic and very expensive, partly because of the large variability of outcome in terms of spontaneous functional recovery, which means that large groups of patients (typically several hundred) need to be followed for several months. The need to start therapy within hours of the attack is an additional problem. Nonetheless, many trials have been completed (see de Keyser et al., 1999), with few if any signs of efficacy.* The dispiriting list of failures includes calcium and sodium channel blockers (e.g. **nimodipine**, **fosphenytoin**), NMDA-receptor antagonists (**selfotel**, **eliprodil**, **dextromethorphan**), drugs that inhibit glutamate release (**adenosine analogues**, **lobeluzole**), drugs that enhance GABA effects (e.g. **clormethiazole**), and various free radical scavengers (e.g. **tirilazad**).

Ischoaemic brain damage: stroke

- Stroke is associated with intracerebral thrombosis or haemorrhage (less common), resulting in rapid death of neurons by necrosis in the centre of the lesion, followed by more gradual (hours) degeneration of cells in penumbra from excitotoxicity and inflammation.
- Spontaneous functional recovery occurs to a highly variable degree.
- Though many types of drug that interfere with excitotoxicity (see text) are able to reduce infarct size in experimental animals, none of these has so far proved efficacious in humans.
- Tissue plasminogen activator, which disperses blood clots, is beneficial if it is given within 3 hours.

ALZHEIMER'S DISEASE

Loss of intellectual ability with age is considered to be a normal process, rate and extent of which is very variable. Alzheimer's disease (AD) was originally defined as presenile dementia, but it now appears that the same pathology underlies the dementia irrespective of the age of onset. AD refers to dementia that does not have an antecedent cause, such as stroke, brain trauma or alcohol. Its prevalence rises sharply with age, from about 5% at 65 to 90% or more at 95. Until recently, age-related dementia was considered to result from the steady loss of neurons that normally goes on throughout life, possibly accelerated by a failing blood supply associated with atherosclerosis. Studies since the mid-1980s have, however, revealed specific genetic and molecular mechanisms underlying AD (reviewed by Selkoe, 1993, 1997), which have opened new therapeutic opportunities (see Yamada & Nabeshima, 2000; Hardy & Selkoe, 2002).

PATHOGENESIS

AD is associated with brain shrinkage, and localised loss of neurons, mainly in the hippocampus and basal forebrain. Two microscopic features are characteristic of the disease, namely extracellular *amyloid plaques*, consisting of amorphous extracellular deposits of β-amyloid protein (known as Aβ), and intraneuronal *neurofibrillary tangles*, comprising filaments of a phosphorylated form of a microtuble-associated protein (Tau). These appear also in normal brains, though in smaller numbers. The early appearance of amyloid deposits presages the development of AD, though symptoms may not develop for many years. Altered processing of amyloid protein from its precursor (APP; see below) is now recognised as the key to the pathogenesis of AD. This conclusion is based on several lines of evidence, particularly the genetic analysis of certain, relatively rare, types of familial AD, in which mutations of the APP gene, or of other genes that control amyloid processing, have been discovered. The APP gene resides on chromosome 21, which is duplicated in Down's syndrome, in which early AD-like dementia occurs in association with overexpression of APP.

▼ Amyloid deposits consist of aggregates of Aβ (Fig. 34.2) containing 40 or 42 residues. Aβ40 is produced normally in small amounts, whereas Aβ42 is overproduced as a result of the genetic mutations mentioned above. Both proteins aggregate to form amyloid plaques, but Aβ42 shows a stronger tendency than Aβ40 to do so and appears to be the main culprit in amyloid formation. Aβ40 and Aβ42 are produced by proteolytic cleavage of a much larger APP, a membrane protein normally expressed by many cells, including CNS neurons. The proteases that cut out the Aβ sequence are known as *secretases*. Normally *α-secretase* acts to release the large extracellular domain as soluble APP, which serves various poorly understood trophic functions. Formation of Aβ involves cleavage at two different points, including one in the intramembrane domain of APP, by *β- and γ- secretases* (Fig. 34.2). Gamma-secretase is a clumsy enzyme that lacks precision and cuts APP at different points in the same vicinity, generating Aβ fragments of different lengths, including Aβ40

*The one drug that shows significant efficacy so far discovered is the biopharmaceutical 'clot-buster' tissue plasminogen activator (tPA, see Ch. 20). It has to be given within 3 hours of the thrombosis and gives only slight benefit, at the risk of making matters worse if the stroke is haemorrhagic rather than thrombotic.

and Aβ42. Mutations in this region of the APP gene affect the preferred cleavage point, tending to favour formation of Aβ42. Mutations of the unrelated *presenilin* genes result in increased activity of γ-secretase, because the presenilin proteins are involved in regulating the activity of this enzyme. These different AD-related mutations increase the ratio of Aβ42 to Aβ40, which can be detected in plasma, serving as a marker for familial AD. Mutations in another gene, that for the lipid transport protein apoprotein E4, also predispose to AD, probably because expression of abnormal ApoE4 proteins facilitates the aggregation of Aβ.

It is uncertain exactly how Aβ accumulation causes neurodegeneration (see Yankner, 1996). There is some evidence that the cells die by apoptosis, though an inflammatory response is also evident. Expression of mutations related to AD in transgenic animals causes plaque formation and neurodegeneration and also increases the susceptibility of CNS neurons to other challenges, such as ischaemia, excitotoxicity and oxidative stress; this increased vulnerability may be the cause of the progressive neurodegeneration in AD. These transgenic models will be of great value in testing potential drug therapies aimed at retarding the neurodegenerative process.

The other main player on the biochemical stage is Tau, the protein of which the neurofibrillary tangles are composed (Fig. 34.2). Their role in neurodegeneration is unclear, though similar 'tauopathies' occur in many neurodegenerative conditions (see Lee et al., 2001). Tau is a normal constituent of neurons, being associated with intracellular microtubules. In AD and other tauopathies, it becomes abnormally phosphorylated and is deposited intracellularly as *paired helical filaments* with a characteristic microscopic appearance. When the cells die, these filaments aggregate as extracellular neurofibrillary tangles. It is possible, but not proven, that Tau phosphorylation is enhanced by the presence of Aβ plaques. Whether hyperphosphorylation and intracellular deposition of Tau harms the cell is not certain, though it is known that Tau phosphorylation impairs fast axonal transport, a process that depends on microtubules.

Loss of cholinergic neurons

Though changes in many transmitter systems have been observed, mainly from measurements on postmortem AD brain tissue, a relatively selective loss of cholinergic neurons in the

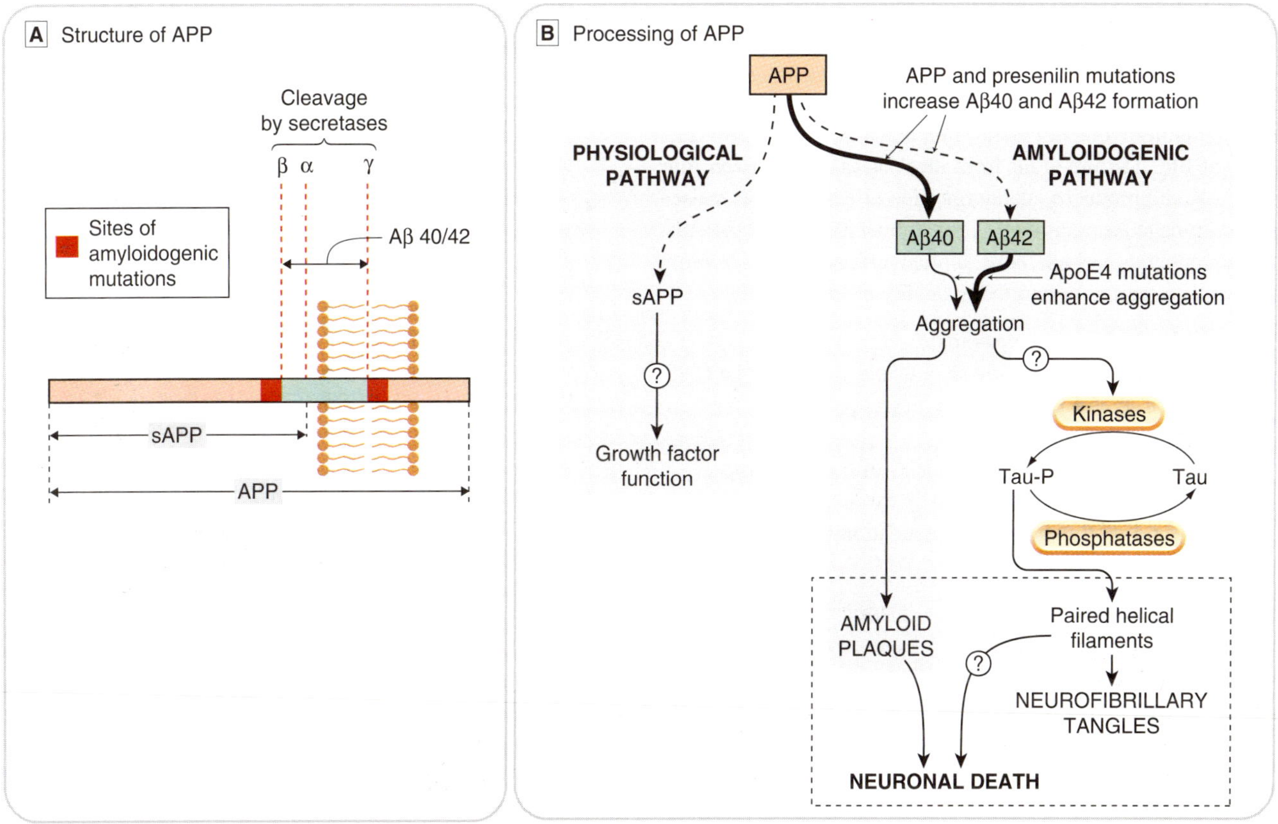

Fig. 34.2 Pathogenesis of Alzheimer's disease. A Structure of amyloid precursor protein (APP), showing origin of secreted APP (sAPP) and Aβ amyloid protein. The regions involved in amyloidogenic mutations discovered in some cases of familial Alzheimer's disease are shown flanking the Aβ sequence. APP cleavage involves three proteases: secretases α, β and γ. Alpha-secretase produces soluble APP, whereas β- and γ-secretases generate amyloid β-protein (Aβ). Gamma-secretase can cut at different points, generating Aβ peptides of varying lengths, including Aβ40 and Aβ42, the latter having a high tendency to aggregate as amyloid plaques. B Processing of APP. The main 'physiological' pathway gives rise to sAPP, which exerts a number of trophic functions. Cleavage of APP at different sites gives rise to Aβ amyloid, the predominant form normally being Aβ40, which is weakly amyloidogenic. Mutations in APP or presenilins increase the proportion of APP that is degraded via the amyloidogenic pathway and also increase the proportion converted to the much more strongly amyloidogenic form Aβ42. Aggregation of Aβ is favoured by mutations in the *apoE4* gene. (Tau, microtubule-associated protein.)

basal forebrain nuclei (Ch. 33) is characteristic. This discovery, made in 1976, implied that pharmacological approaches to restoring cholinergic function might be feasible, leading to the use of cholinesterase inhibitors to treat AD (see below).

Choline acetyltransferase (CAT) activity in the cortex and hippocampus is reduced considerably (30–70%) in AD but not in other disorders such as depression or schizophrenia; acetylcholinesterase activity is also greatly reduced. Muscarinic receptor density, determined by binding studies, is not affected, but nicotinic receptors, particularly in the cortex, are reduced.

THERAPEUTIC APPROACHES

Recent advances in understanding the process of neurodegeneration in AD have yet to result in therapies able to retard it. Currently, cholinesterase inhibitors (see Ch. 10) are the only drugs approved for treating AD, though many drugs have have been claimed to improve cognitive performance, and several new approaches are being explored (see Aisen & Davis, 1997).

Cholinesterase inhibitors

Tacrine was the first drug approved for treating AD, on the basis that enhancement of cholinergic transmission might compensate for the cholinergic deficit. Trials showed modest improvements in tests of memory and cognition in about 40% of patients with AD, but no improvement in other functional measures that affect quality of life. Tacrine is far from ideal; it has to be given four times daily and produces cholinergic side-effects, such as nausea and abdominal cramps, as well as hepatotoxicity in some patients. Later compounds, which have limited efficacy but are more effective than tacrine in improving quality of life, include:

- **donepezil**, which is not hepatotoxic
- **rivastigmine,** a longer-lasting drug that is claimed to be CNS selective and, therefore, to produce fewer peripheral cholinergic side-effects
- **galanthamine**, an alkaloid from plants of the snowdrop family, which is claimed to act partly by cholinesterase inhibition and partly by allosteric activation of brain nicotinic acetylcholine receptors.

Other drugs aimed at improving cholinergic function that are being investigated include a variety of muscarinic and nicotinic receptor agonists, none of which look promising on the basis of early clinical results.

Other drugs

▼ **Dihydroergotamine** was used for many years to treat dementia. It acts as a cerebral vasodilator, but trials showed it to produce little if any cognitive improvement. 'Nootropic' drugs, such as **piracetam** and **aniracetam,** improve memory in animal tests, possibly by enhancing glutamate release, but are probably ineffective in AD.

Inhibiting neurodegeneration

▼ For most of the disorders discussed in this chapter, including AD, the holy grail, which so far eludes us, would be a drug that retards neurodegeneration. Now that we have several well-characterised targets, such as Aβ formation by the β- and γ-secretases, Aβ neurotoxicity, etc., together with a range of transgenic animal models of AD on which compounds can be tested, the prospects certainly look brighter than they did a decade ago (see Hardy & Selkoe, 2002). Particular developments are worth mentioning.

- Inhibitors of β- and γ-secretase are undergoing clinical trials.
- An ingenious new approach was taken by Schenk et al. (1999), who immunised AD transgenic mice with Aβ protein and found that this not only prevented plaque formation but actually reversed it, suggesting an immunological approach that might be used in humans. However, clinical trials with an antibody directed against Aβ showed that it tended to cause CNS inflammation, so the project was abandoned.
- Epidemiological studies reveal that some non-steroidal anti-inflammatory drugs (NSAIDs; see Ch. 15), used routinely to treat arthritis, reduce the likelihood of developing AD. **Ibuprofen** and **indometacin** have this effect, though other NSAIDs, such as **aspirin**, do not, nor do anti-inflammatory steroids such as **prednisolone.** Recent work (see de Strooper & König, 2001) suggests that NSAIDs may reduce Aβ42 formation by regulating γ-secretase, an effect unrelated to cyclooxygenase inhibition by which NSAIDs reduce inflammation. It may, therefore, be possible to find compounds that target γ-secretase selectively, without inhibiting cyclooxygenase, thus avoiding the side-effects associated with current NSAIDs.

Dementia and Alzheimer's disease

- Alzheimer's disease (AD) is a common age-related dementia, distinct from vascular dementia associated with brain infarction.
- The main pathological features of AD comprise amyloid plaques, neurofibrillary tangles and a loss of neurons (particularly cholinergic neurons of the basal forebrain).
- Amyloid plaques consist of the Aβ fragment of amyloid precursor protein (APP), a normal neuronal membrane protein, produced by the action of β- and γ-secretases. AD is associated with excessive Aβ formation, resulting in neurotoxicity.
- Familial AD (rare) results from mutations in the genes for APP, or the unrelated presenilin, both of which cause increased Aβ formation.
- Neurofibrillary tangles comprise aggregates of a highly phosphorylated form of a normal neuronal protein (Tau). The relationship of these structures to neurodegeneration is not known.
- Loss of cholinergic neurons is believed to account for much of the learning and memory deficit in AD.
- Anticholinesterases (tacrine, donepezil, rivastigmine) give proven, though limited, benefit in AD.
- Many other drugs, including putative vasodilators (dihydroergotamine), muscarinic agonists (arecoline, pilocarpine) and cognition enhancers (piracetam, aniracetam), give no demonstrable benefit and are not officially approved.
- Certain anti-inflammatory drugs, and also clioquinol (a metal chelating agent), may retard neurodegeneration and are undergoing clinical evaluation.

- Aβ plaques bind copper and zinc, and removal of these metal ions promotes dissolution of the plaques. The amoebicidal drug **clioquinol** is a metal chelating agent that causes regression of amyloid deposits in animal models of AD and is currently undergoing clinical trials.
- Shortage of growth factors (particularly **nerve growth factor**) may contribute to the loss of forebrain cholinergic neurons in AD. Administering growth factors into the brain is not realistic for routine therapy, but alternative approaches, such as implanting cells engineered to secrete nerve growth factor, are under investigation.

PARKINSON'S DISEASE

FEATURES OF PARKINSON'S DISEASE

PD is a progressive disorder of movement that occurs mainly in the elderly. The chief symptoms are:

- tremor at rest, usually starting in the hands ('pill-rolling' tremor), which tend to diminish during voluntary activity
- muscle rigidity, detectable as an increased resistance in passive limb movement
- suppression of voluntary movements (hypokinesis), caused partly by muscle rigidity and partly by an inherent inertia of the motor system, which means that motor activity is difficult to stop as well as to initiate.

Parkinsonian patients walk with a characteristic shuffling gait. They find it hard to start, and once in progress they cannot quickly stop or change direction. PD is commonly associated with dementia, probably because the degenerative process is not confined to the basal ganglia but also affects other parts of the brain.

PD often occurs with no obvious underlying cause, but it may be the result of cerebral ischaemia, viral encephalitis or other types of pathological damage. The symptoms can also be drug induced, the main drugs involved being those that reduce the amount of dopamine in the brain (e.g. reserpine; see Ch. 11) or block dopamine receptors (e.g. antipsychotic drugs, such as **chlorpromazine**; see Ch. 37). There are rare instances of early-onset PD, which runs in families, and two specific gene mutations have been identified (*synuclein* and *parkin*). Study of these gene mutations has given some clues about the mechanism underlying the neurodegenerative process (see below).

NEUROCHEMICAL CHANGES

PD affects the basal ganglia, and its neurochemical origin was discovered in 1960 by Hornykiewicz, who showed that the dopamine content of the substantia nigra and corpus striatum (see Ch. 33) in postmortem brains of patients with PD was extremely low (usually less than 10% of normal), associated with a loss of dopaminergic neurons in the substantia nigra and degeneration of nerve terminals in the striatum. Other monoamines, such as noradrenaline and 5-hydroxytryptamine (5-HT) were much less affected than dopamine. Later studies (e.g. with positron emission tomography to reveal dopamine transport in the striatum; see Fig. 33.3) have shown a loss of dopamine over several years, with symptoms of PD appearing only when the striatal dopamine content has fallen to 20–40% of normal. Lesions of the nigrostriatal tract or chemically induced depletion of dopamine in experimental animals also produce symptoms of PD. The symptom most clearly related to dopamine deficiency is *hypokinesia*, which occurs immediately and invariably in lesioned animals. Rigidity and tremor involve more complex neurochemical disturbances of other transmitters (particularly acetylcholine, noradrenaline, 5-HT and GABA (gamma-aminobutyric acid)) as well as dopamine. In experimental lesions, two secondary consequences follow damage to the nigrostriatal tract, namely a hyperactivity of the remaining dopaminergic neurons, which show an increased rate of transmitter turnover, and an increase in the number of dopamine receptors, which produces a state of denervation hypersensitivity (see Ch. 9). The striatum expresses mainly D_1- (excitatory) and D_2- (inhibitory) receptors (see Ch. 33), but fewer D_3- and D_4-receptors.

The intrinsic cholinergic neurons of the corpus striatum (which has the highest content of acetylcholine, CAT and acetylcholinesterase in the brain) are also involved in PD (as well as Huntington's disease; see Fig. 34.3). Acetylcholine release from the striatum is strongly inhibited by dopamine, and it is suggested that hyperactivity of these cholinergic neurons (associated with the lack of dopamine) leads to the symptoms of PD, whereas hypoactivity (associated with a surfeit of dopamine, secondary to a deficiency of GABA) results in the hyperkinetic movements and hypotonia characteristic of Huntington's disease (Fig. 34.3). In both conditions, therapies aimed at redressing the balance between the dopaminergic and cholinergic neurons are, up to a point, beneficial.

PATHOGENESIS

PD is believed to be caused mainly by environmental factors, though the rare types of hereditary PD have provided some valuable clues about the mechanism. As with other neurodegenerative disorders, the damage is caused by three familiar villains, namely excitotoxicity, oxidative stress and apoptosis (see Olanow & Tatton, 1999). Aspects of the pathogenesis and animal models of PD are described by Beal (2001).

Neurotoxins

New light was thrown on the possible aetiology of PD by a chance event. In 1982 a group of young drug addicts in California suddenly developed an exceptionally severe form of PD (known as the 'frozen addict' syndrome), and the cause was traced to the compound *1-methyl-4-phenyl-1,2,3,6-tetrahydropyridine (MPTP)*, which was a contaminant in a preparation used as a heroin substitute (see Langston, 1985). MPTP causes irreversible destruction of nigrostriatal dopaminergic neurons in various species and produces a PD-like state in primates. MPTP acts by being converted to a toxic metabolite, MPP^+, by the enzyme *monoamine oxidase* (MAO: specifically by the MAO-B subtype; see Ch. 38). MPP^+ is taken up by the dopamine transport system and thus acts selectively on dopaminergic neurons; it inhibits

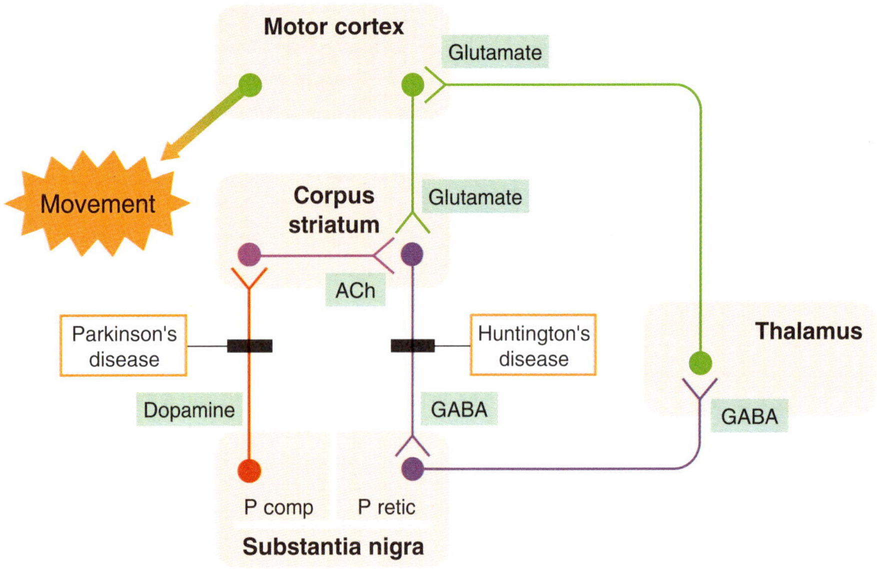

Fig. 34.3 Simplified diagram of the organisation of the extrapyramidal motor system, and the defects that occur in Parkinson's disease and Huntington's disease. In the former, the inhibitory dopaminergic pathway from the substantia nigra (pars compacta) to the striatum is impaired, increasing the activity of GABAergic cells in the striatum, which in turn inhibit GABAergic cells in the substantia nigra (pars reticulata), thus reducing the restraint on the thalamus and cortex, causing rigidity. The dopaminergic inhibition of the striatal cells is opposed by excitatory cholinergic interneurons, The defect can be counteracted by dopamine (D_2 or D_3) agonists or by acetylcholine (muscarinic) antagonists. In Huntington's disease, the GABAergic striatonigral pathway is impaired, producing effects opposite to the changes in Parkinson's disease. (P comp, pars compacta; P ret, pars reticulata; GABA, gamma-aminobutyric acid; ACh, acetylcholine.)

mitochondrial oxidation reactions, producing oxidative stress (see above). MPTP appears to be selective in destroying nigrostriatal neurons and does not affect dopaminergic neurons elsewhere—the reason for this is unknown. **Selegiline**, a selective MAO-B inhibitor (see below), prevents MPTP-induced neurotoxicity by blocking its conversion to MPP^+. Selegiline is also used in treating PD (see below); as well as inhibiting dopamine breakdown, it might also work by blocking the metabolic activation of a putative endogenous, or environmental, MPTP-like substance* that is involved in the causation of PD. Whether or not its action reflects the natural pathogenesis of PD, MPTP is a very useful experimental tool for testing possible therapies.

Various herbicides, such as *rotenone*, that selectively inhibit mitochondrial function cause a PD-like syndrome in animals, suggesting that environmental toxins could be a factor in human PD, since impaired mitochondrial function is a feature of the disease in humans.

Molecular aspects

▼ PD, as well as several other neurodegenerative disorders, is associated with the development of protein aggregates known as *Lewy bodies* in various parts of the brain. They consist largely of *α-synuclein*, a synaptic protein of unknown function which is present in large amounts in normal brains. Mutations affecting α-synuclein occur in rare types of hereditary PD (see above), and it is believed that such mutations render the protein resistant to degradation within cells, causing it to pile up in Lewy bodies. Consistent with this hypothesis, the other mutation associated with PD (*parkin*) also affects a protein that participates in intracellular protein degradation. Though many questions remain, the picture that begins to emerge is that PD is associated with defective disposal of α-synuclein, allowing it to accumulate in Lewy bodies. By unknown mechanisms, the presence of Lewy bodies renders neurons particularly susceptible to

*It is possible that dopamine itself could be the culprit, since oxidation of dopamine gives rise to potentially toxic metabolites.

Parkinson's disease

- Parkinson's disease (PD) is a degenerative disease of the basal ganglia causing tremor at rest, muscle rigidity and hypokinesia, often with dementia.
- PD is often idiopathic, but it may follow stroke, virus infection or can be drug-induced (antipsychotic drugs).
- PD is associated with early degeneration of dopaminergic nigrostriatal neurons, followed by more general neurodegeneration.
- PD can be induced by MPTP (see text), a neurotoxin affecting dopamine neurons. Similar environmental neurotoxins, as well as genetic factors, may be involved in human PD.

oxidative stress. In PD, such oxidative stress, targeted to dopaminergic neurons, could result from the action of MPTP-like environmental toxins.

DRUG TREATMENT OF PARKINSON'S DISEASE

Despite past optimism, none of the drugs used to treat PD affect the progression of the disease. For general reviews of current and future approaches, see Hagan et al. (1997) and Stern (1997). The drugs used fall into the following categories:

- drugs that replace dopamine (e.g. **levodopa**, usually used concomitantly with peripherally acting dopa decarboxylase inhibitors, e.g. **carbidopa**, **benserazide**). **Entacapone**, an inhibitor of catechol-*O*-methyl transferase (COMT), is also used to inhibit dopamine inactivation.
- drugs that mimic the action of dopamine at D_2- or D_3-receptors (e.g. **bromocriptine**, **pergolide**, **lisuride**, **pramipexole**)
- MAO-B inhibitors (e.g. **selegiline**)
- drugs that release dopamine (e.g. **amantadine**)
- muscarinic acetylcholine receptor antagonists (e.g. **benzatropine**).

LEVODOPA

Levodopa is the first-line treatment for PD; it is nearly always combined with a peripheral dopa decarboxylase inhibitor, either **carbidopa** or **benserazide**, which reduces the dose needed by about 10-fold and diminishes the peripheral side-effects. It is well absorbed from the small intestine, a process which relies on active transport, though much of it is inactivated by MAO in the wall of the intestine. The plasma half-life is short (about 2 hours). Conversion to dopamine in the periphery, which would otherwise account for about 95% of the levodopa dose, and cause troublesome side-effects, is largely prevented by the decarboxylase inhibitor. Decarboxylation occurs rapidly within the brain, since the decarboxylase inhibitors do not penetrate the blood–brain barrier. It is not certain whether the effect depends on an increased release of dopamine from the few surviving dopaminergic neurons or on a 'flooding' of the striatum with exogenous dopamine. Animal studies suggest that levodopa can act even when no dopaminergic nerve terminals are present. However, the therapeutic effectiveness of levodopa decreases as the disease advances, so part of its action may rely on the presence of functional dopaminergic neurons. Combination of levodopa with an inhibitor of COMT (see Ch. 11), such as **entacapone**, in order to inhibit its degradation has been shown to improve clinical response.

Therapeutic effectiveness

About 80% of patients show initial improvement with levodopa, particularly of rigidity and hypokinesia, and about 20% are restored virtually to normal motor function. As time progresses, the effectiveness of levodopa gradually declines (Fig. 34.4). In a typical study of 100 patients treated with levodopa for 5 years, only 34 were better than they had been at the beginning of the trial, 32 patients having died and 21 having withdrawn from the trial. It is likely that the loss of effectiveness of levodopa mainly reflects the natural progression of the disease, but receptor downregulation and other compensatory mechanisms may also contribute. There is no evidence that levodopa can actually accelerate the neurodegenerative process through overproduction of dopamine, as was suspected on theoretical grounds (see above). Overall, levodopa increases the life expectancy of patients with PD, probably as a result of improved motor function, though some symptoms (e.g. dysphagia, cognitive decline) are not improved.

Unwanted effects

There are two main types of unwanted effect: dyskinesia and 'on–off' effects.

Dyskinesia

Involuntary writhing movements (dyskinesia) develop in the majority of patients within 2 years of starting levodopa therapy. These movements usually affect the face and limbs and can become very severe. They disappear if the dose of levodopa is reduced, but this causes rigidity to return. Consquently, the margin between the beneficial and the unwanted effect becomes

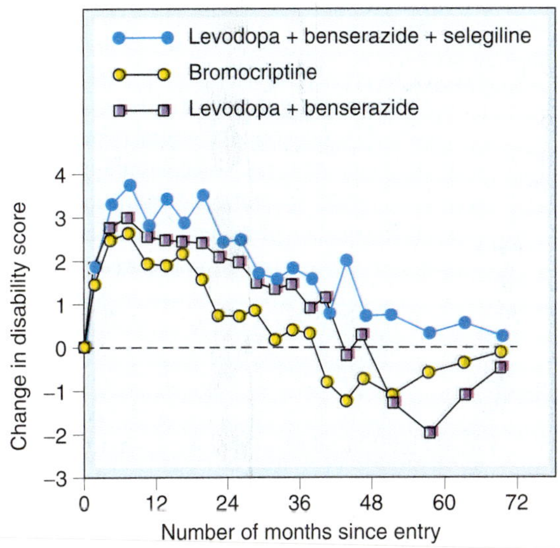

Fig. 34.4 Comparison of levodopa/benserazide, levodopa/ benserazide/ selegiline and bromocriptine on progression of Parkinson's disease symptoms. Patients (249–271 in each treatment group) were assessed on a standard disability rating score. Before treatment, the average rate of decline was 0.7 units/year. All three treatments produced improvement over the initial rating for 2–3 years, but the effect declined, either because of refractoriness to the drugs, or because of disease progression. Bromocriptine appeared slightly less effective than levodopa regimens, and there was a higher drop-out rate because of side-effects in this group. (Parkinson's Disease Research Group 1993 Br Med J 307 469-472, 1993.)

progressively narrower, an effect that appears to be related to the duration of levodopa treatment.

'On–off' effect

Rapid fluctuations in clinical state can occur where hypokinesia and rigidity may suddenly worsen, for anything from a few minutes to a few hours, and then improve again. This on–off effect is not seen in untreated patients with or without other anti-PD drugs. The 'off effect' can be so sudden that patients stop while walking and feel rooted to the spot or are unable to rise from a chair in which they had sat down normally a few moments earlier. The mechanism of this remarkable effect is not understood. In some patients, the fluctuations reflect the changing plasma levodopa concentration, and it is suggested that, as the disease advances, the ability of neurons to store dopamine is lost, so the therapeutic benefit of levodopa depends increasingly on the continuous formation of extraneuronal dopamine, which is dependent on a continuous supply of levodopa. The use of sustained-release preparations, or co-administration of COMT inhibitors such as **entacapone** (see above), may be used to counteract the fluctuations in plasma concentration of levodopa.

Acute effects

In addition to these slowly developing side-effects, levodopa produces several acute effects, which are experienced by most patients at first but tend to disappear after a few weeks. The main ones are:

- nausea and anorexia: **domperidone**, a peripherally acting dopamine antagonist, may be useful in preventing this effect
- hypotension, usually of minor importance, but may cause postural hypotension in patients on antihypertensive drugs
- psychological effects: levodopa, by increasing dopamine activity in the brain, can produce a schizophrenia-like syndrome (see Ch. 37) with delusions and hallucinations; more commonly, in about 20% of patients, it causes confusion, disorientation, insomnia or nightmares.

SELEGILINE

Selegiline is a MAO inhibitor that is selective for MAO-B, which predominates in dopamine-containing regions of the CNS. It, therefore, lacks the unwanted peripheral effects of non-selective MAO inhibitors used to treat depression (Ch. 36), and, in contrast to them, does not provoke the 'cheese reaction' or interact so frequently with other drugs. Inhibition of MAO-B protects dopamine from intraneuronal degradation, and this was initially used as an adjunct to levodopa. Long-term trials showed that the combination of selegiline and levodopa was more effective than levodopa alone in relieving symptoms and prolonging life. Recognition of the role of MAO-B in neurotoxicity (see above) suggested that selegiline might be neuroprotective, rather than merely enhancing the action of levodopa, but clinical studies do not support this A large-scale trial (Fig. 34.4) showed no difference when selegiline was added to levodopa/benserazide treatment.

OTHER DRUGS USED IN PARKINSON'S DISEASE

Dopamine receptor agonists

Bromocriptine, derived from the ergot alkaloids (see Ch. 12), is a potent agonist at dopamine (D_2) receptors in the CNS. It inhibits the anterior pituitary gland and was first introduced for the treatment of galactorrhoea and gynaecomastia (Ch. 27), but it is effective also in PD (Fig. 34.4). Its duration of action is longer (plasma half-life 6–8 hours) than that of levodopa, so it does not need to be given so frequently. It was hoped that bromocriptine might be effective in patients who had become refractory to levodopa through loss of dopaminergic neurons, but this has not been clearly established. **Apomorphine**, given subcutaneously, sometimes with a continuous pump, is also used. Other dopamine-receptor agonists, such as **lisuride**, **pergolide** and **pramipexole**, are also used. Pramipexole, recently introduced, may have antioxidant effects, as well as a protective effect on mitochondria. Whether these potentially neuroprotective properties are significant clinically remains to be discovered.

Amantadine

Amantadine was introduced as an antiviral drug, and it was discovered by accident in 1969 to be beneficial in PD. Many possible mechanisms for its action have been suggested, based on neurochemical evidence of increased dopamine release, inhibition of amine uptake or a direct action on dopamine receptors. Most authors now suggest, although not with much conviction, that increased dopamine release is primarily responsible for the clinical effects.

Amantadine is less effective than levodopa or bromocriptine, and its action declines with time. Its side-effects are considerably less severe, though qualitatively similar to those of levodopa.

Acetylcholine antagonists

For more than a century, until levodopa was discovered, **atropine** and related drugs were the main form of treatment for PD. Muscarinic acetylcholine receptors exert an excitatory effect, opposite to that of dopamine, on striatal neurons (see Fig. 34.3) and also exert a presynaptic inhibitory effect on dopaminergic nerve terminals. Suppression of these effects thus makes up, in part, for a lack of dopamine. The action of muscarinic antagonists is more limited than that of levodopa, and they diminish tremor more than rigidity or hypokinesia (which are more disabling in their effects). Furthermore, their side-effects—dry mouth, constipation, impaired vision, urinary retention—are often troublesome. They are used mainly to treat PD in patients receiving antipsychotic drugs (which are dopamine antagonists and thus nullify the effect of levodopa; see Ch. 37). The drugs used for this purpose (e.g. **benzatropine**) have less peripheral effect in relation to their central effect than does atropine. Drowsiness and confusion are the main unwanted effects.

NEURAL TRANSPLANTATION

▼ PD is the first neurodegenerative disease for which neural transplantation was attempted in 1982, amid much publicity. Various

Drugs used in Parkinson's disease

- Drugs act by counteracting deficiency of dopamine in basal ganglia or by blocking muscarinic receptors. None of the available drugs affects the underlying neurodegeneration.
- The most effective drug is **levodopa**, a dopamine precursor that passes the blood–brain barrier; it is given with an inhibitor of peripheral dopa decarboxylase (e.g. **carbidopa**) to minimise side-effects. Sometimes a COMT (catechol *O*-methyltransferase) inhibitor (e.g. **entacapone**) is also given, to retard dopamine metabolism.
- Levodopa is effective in most patients initially but often loses efficacy after about 2 years.
- Main unwanted effects of levodopa are involuntary movements, which occur in most patients within 2 years, and unpredictable 'on–off effect'. Others are nausea, postural hypotension and occasionally psychotic symptoms.
- Other useful drugs include bromocriptine (dopamine agonist), selegiline (monoamine oxidase-B inhibitor), amantadine (? enhances dopamine release) and benztropine (muscarinic receptor antagonist, used for parkinsonism caused by antipsychotic drugs).
- Neurotransplantation, still in an experimental phase, may be effective, but results are variable.

transplantation approaches have been tried, based on the injection of dissociated fetal cells directly into the striatum. Trials in patients with PD (see Bjorklund & Lindvall, 2000; Barker & Rosser, 2001) have mainly involved injection of midbrain neurons from aborted human fetuses. The success rate has been very variable, but reasonably encouraging, and postmortem studies have shown that such transplants are able to survive and establish synaptic connections. Some patients have gone on to develop serious dyskinesias, possibly as a result of dopamine overproduction. The use of fetal material is, of course, fraught with difficulties (usually cells from five or more fetuses are needed for one transplant). Hopes for the future rest mainly on the possibility of developing preparations of immortalised neuronal precursor cells, which can be multiplied in culture, and which will differentiate into functional postmitotic neurons after transplantation. Efforts are continuing to develop transplantation as a means of treating other conditions, such as Huntington's disease, stroke and epilepsy, as well as PD, but the field remains highly controversial (Bjorklund & Lindvall, 2000; Barker & Rosser, 2001).

HUNTINGTON'S DISEASE

▼ Huntington's disease is an inherited (autosomal dominant) disorder resulting in progressive brain degeneration, starting in adulthood and causing rapid deterioration and death. It is the commonest of a group of so-called 'trinucleotide-repeat' neurodegenerative diseases, associated with the expansion of the number of repeats of the CAG sequence in specific genes, and hence the number (50 or more) of consecutive glutamine (Gln) residues in the expressed protein (see Gusella & MacDonald, 2000). The larger the number of repeats, the earlier the appearance of symptoms. The protein coded by the Huntington's disease gene, *huntingtin*, interacts with various regulatory proteins, including one of the caspases (see above) that participates in excitotoxicity and apoptosis. Some of these interactions are enhanced by the poly-Gln repeat in the mutant protein, and this may account for the neuronal loss, which affects mainly the cortex and the striatum, resulting in progressive dementia and severe involuntary jerky (choreiform) movements. Studies on postmortem brains showed that the dopamine content of the striatum was normal or slightly increased, while there was a 75% reduction in the activity of glutamic acid decarboxylase, the enzyme responsible for GABA synthesis (Ch. 33). It is believed that the loss of GABA-mediated inhibition in the basal ganglia produces a hyperactivity of dopaminergic synapses, so the syndrome is in some senses a mirror image of PD (Fig. 34.3). The effects of drugs that influence dopaminergic transmission are correspondingly the opposite of those that are observed in PD, dopamine antagonists being effective in reducing the involuntary movements, while drugs such as levodopa and bromocriptine make them worse. Drugs used to alleviate the symptoms include dopamine antagonists, such as **chlorpromazine** (Ch. 37), and the GABA agonist **baclofen** (Ch. 32). These do not affect the course of the disease, and it is possible that drugs which inhibit excitotoxicity, or possibly neural transplantation procedures, when these become available (see above) may prove useful.

NEURODEGENERATIVE PRION DISEASES

▼ A group of human and animal diseases associated with a characteristic type of neurodegeneration, known as *spongiform encephalopathy* because of the vacuolated appearance of the affected brain, has recently been the focus of intense research activity (see Collinge, 2001; Prusiner, 2001). A key feature of these diseases is that they are transmissible through an infective agent, though not, in general, across species. The recent upsurge of interest has been spurred mainly by the discovery that the bovine form of the disease, bovine spongiform encephalopathy (BSE), is transmissible to humans. Different human forms of the disease include Creutzfeldt–Jakob disease (CJD, which is unrelated to BSE) and the new variant form (nvCJD), as yet very rare, which results from eating, or close contact with, infected beef or human tissue. Another human form is *kuru*, a neurodegenerative disease affecting cannibalistic tribes in Papua New Guinea. These diseases cause a progressive, and sometimes rapid, dementia and loss of motor coordination, for which no therapies currently exist. *Scrapie*, a common disease of domestic sheep, is another example, and it may have been the practice of feeding sheep offal to domestic cattle that initiated an epidemic of BSE in Britain during the 1980s, leading to the appearance of nvCJD in humans in the mid-1990s. Although the BSE epidemic has been controlled, there is concern that many more human cases may develop in its wake, since the incubation period—known to be long—is uncertain. The infectious agent responsible for spongiform encephalopathies is, unusually, a protein, known as a prion The protein involved (PrP^{C}) is a normal cytosolic constituent of the brain and other tissues, with uncertain functions. As a result of altered glycosylation, the protein can become misfolded, forming the insoluble PrP^{Sc} form, which has the ability to recruit normal PrP^{C} molecules to the misfolded PrP^{Sc}, thus starting a chain reaction. PrP^{Sc}—the infective agent—accumulates and aggregates as insoluble fibrils and is responsible for the progressive neurodegeneration. In support of this unusual form of infectivity, it has been shown that injection of PrP^{Sc} into normal mice causes spongiform encephalopathy, whereas PrP knockout mice, which are otherwise fairly normal, are resistant, since they lack the substrate for the autocatalytic generation of PrP^{Sc}. Fortunately the infection does not easily cross between species, since there are differences between the PrP genes of different species. It is possible that a mutation of the PrP gene in either sheep or cattle produced the variant form that became infective in humans.

This chain of events bears some similarity to that of AD, in that the brain accumulates an abnormal form of a normally expressed protein.

There is as yet no known treatment for this type of encephalopathy, but laboratory experiments suggest that two very familiar drugs, namely **clioquinol** (an antimalarial drug, mentioned above as a possible therapy for AD) and **chlorpromazine** (a widely used antipsychotic drug, Ch. 37), can inhibit PrP^{Sc} aggregation. Both are under investigation for treating human CJD.

REFERENCES AND FURTHER READING

Aisen P S, Davis K L 1997 The search for disease-modifying treatment of Alzheimer's disease. Neurology 48: S35–S41 (*Good review article on current and prospective therapies*)

Barker R A, Rosser A E 2001 Neural transplantation therapies for Parkinson's and Huntington's diseases. Drug Discov Today 6: 575–582 (*Informative and balanced review article on a controversial topic*)

Beal M F, Hyman B T, Koroshetz W 1993 Do defects in mitochondrial energy metabolism underlie the pathology of neurodegenerative diseases? Trends Neurosci 16: 125–131

Beal F W 2001 Experimental models of Parkinson's disease. Nat Rev Neurosci 2: 325–332 (*Useful review article covering many aspects of PD pathogenesis*)

Bjorklund A, Lindvall O 2000 Cell replacement therapies for central nervous system disorders. Nat Neurosci 3: 537–544 (*Upbeat review by pioneers in the field of neural transplantation*)

Bredesen D E 1995 Neural apoptosis. Ann Neurol 38: 839–851 (*Useful review with discussion of relevance to clinical disorders*)

Choi D W 1988 Calcium-mediated neurotoxicity: relationship to specific channel types and role in ischaemic damage. Trends Neurosci 11: 465–469

Collinge J 2001 Prion diseases of humans and animals: their causes and molecular basis. Annu Rev Neurosci 24: 519–550 (*Useful review article*)

Coyle J T, Puttfarken P 1993 Oxidative stress, glutamate and neurodegenerative disorders. Science 262: 689–695 (*Good review article*)

de Keyser J, Sulter G, Luiten P G 1999 Clinical trials with neuroprotective drugs in ischaemic stroke: are we doing the right thing? Trends Neurosci 22: 535–540 (*Short summary of the largely unsuccessful clinical trials of drugs targeting a wide variety of mechanisms thought to be important in stroke*)

de Strooper B, König G 2001 An inflammatory drug prospect. Nature 414: 159–160 (*Informative commentary on publication by Weggen et al. in the same issue, describing effects of NSAIDs on APP cleavage*)

Dirnagl U, Iadecola C, Moskowitz M A 1999 Pathobiology of ischaemic stroke: an integrated view. Trends Neurosci 22: 391–397 (*Useful review of mechanisms underlying neuronal damage in stroke*)

Green R A, Cross A J (eds) 1997 Neuroprotective agents in cerebral ischaemia. Int Rev Neurobiol 40 (*Compendium of articles summarising preclinical and clinical data*)

Gross C G 2000 Neurogenesis in the adult brain: death of a dogma. Nat Rev Neurosci 1: 67–73 (*Reviews evidence for the formation of new neurons in the adult brain, a process with important therapeutic implications if we could discover how to enlist it for brain repair. See Rakic (2002) for a more sceptical assessment*)

Gusella J F, MacDonald M E 2000 Molecular genetics: unmasking polyglutamine triggers in neurodegenerative disease. Nat Rev Neurosci 1: 109–115 (*General review on trinucleotide repeat disorders, and how the brain damage is produced*)

Hagan J J, Middlemiss D N, Sharpe PC, Poste G H 1997 Parkinson's disease: prospects for improved therapy. Trends Pharmacol Sci 18: 156–163 (*Excellent review of current trends*)

Hardy J, Selkoe D J 2002 The amyloid hypothesis of Alzheimer's disease: progress and problems on the road to therapeutics. Science 297: 353–356 (*Good short review summing up the current status of the amyloid hypothesis, with a realistic assessment of therapeutic prospects*)

Langston W J 1985 MPTP and Parkinson's disease. Trends Neurosci 8: 79–83 (*Readable account of the MPTP story by its discoverer*)

Lee V M-Y, Goedert M, Trojanowski J Q 2001 Neurodegenerative tauopathies. Annu Rev Neurosci 24: 1121–1159 (*Detailed review of the uncertain role of Tau proteins in neurodegeneration*)

Lipton S A, Rosenberg P A 1994 Excitatory amino acids as a final common pathway for neurologic disorders. N Engl J Med 330: 613–622 (*Review emphasising central role of glutamate in neurodegeneration*)

Louvel E, Hugon J, Doble A 1997 Therapeutic advances in amyotrophic lateral sclerosis. Trends Pharmacol Sci 18: 196–203 (*Recent summary of research and clinical trials data—mostly negative—on neuroprotective strategies in a progressive neurodegenerative disease*)

Olanow C W, Tatton W G 1999 Etiology and pathogenesis of Parkinson's disease. Annu Rev Neurosci 22: 123–144 (*Useful review of environmental and genetic factors in PD*)

Olney J W 1990 Excitotoxic amino acids and neuropsychiatric disorders. Annu Rev Pharmacol Toxicol 30: 47–71 (*Dated, but comprehensive review, covering psychiatric as well as neurological diseases*)

Prusiner S B 2001 Neurodegenerative disease and prions. N Engl J Med 344: 1544–1551 (*General review article by the discoverer of prions*)

Raff M 1998. Cell suicide for beginners. Nature 396: 119–122 (*An excellent short review on apoptosis*)

Rakic P 2002 Neurogenesis in the adult primate cortex: an evaluation of the evidence. Nat Rev Neurosci 3: 65–71 (*Critical review suggesting that neurogenesis in adult primates is probably very limited, contrary to recent accounts—see Gross (2000)*)

Rothwell N J, Luheshi G, Toulmond S 1996 Cytokines and their receptors in the central nervous system: physiology, pharmacology and pathology. Pharmacol Ther 69: 85–95 (*Useful short review of an emerging area*)

Schenk D et al. 1999 Immunization with amyloid-beta attenuates Alzheimer-disease-like pathology in the PDAPP mouse, Nature 400: 173–7 (*Report of an ingenious experiment that could have implications for treatment of AD in humans*)

Selkoe D J 1993 Physiological production of the β-amyloid protein and the mechanism of Alzheimer's disease. Trends Neurosci 16: 403–409 (*Introductory review by one of the pioneers of the amyloid theory*)

Selkoe D J 1997 Alzheimer's disease: genotypes, phenotype and treatments. Science 275: 630–631 (*Short but informative summary of recent advances in Alzheimer genetics*)

Steller H 1995 Mechanisms and genes of cellular suicide. Science 267: 1445–1449 (*Review on apoptosis, not only neuronal*)

Stern M B 1997 Contemporary approaches to the pharmacotherapeutic management of Parkinson's disease. Neurol 49(suppl 1): S2–S9 (*Good review of current and future approaches*)

Wyss-Coray T, Mucke L 2002 Inflammation in neurodegenerative disease—a double-edged sword. Neuron 35: 419–432 (*Detailed review emphasising balance between harmful and protective roles of inflammation, and implications for therapeutics*)

Yamada K, Nabeshima T 2000 Animal models of Alzheimer's disease and evaluation of anti-dementia drugs (*Describes pathology of AD, transgenic and other animal models and therapeutic approaches*)

Yankner B A 1996 Mechanisms of neuronal degeneration in Alzheimer's disease. Neuron 16: 921–932 (*Review focussing on reasons why neurons are damaged by amyloid deposition*)

General anaesthetic agents

35

Overview 503

Introduction 503

Mechanism of action of anaesthetic drugs 504
- Lipid theory 504
- Effects on ion channels 504

The effects of anaesthetics on the nervous system 505
- Stages of anaesthesia 505

Effects on the cardiovascular and respiratory systems 506

Inhalation anaesthetics 506
- Pharmacokinetic aspects 506
- The solubility of anaesthetics 507
- Induction and recovery 507
- Metabolism and toxicity of inhalation anaesthetics 508

Individual inhalation anaesthetics 509
- Halothane 510
- Nitrous oxide 510
- Enflurane 510
- Isoflurane 510
- Other inhalation anaesthetics 511

Intravenous anaesthetic agents 511
- Thiopental 512
- Etomidate 513
- Propofol 513
- Other induction agents 513

OVERVIEW

General anaesthetics are used as an adjunct to surgical procedures in order to render the patient unaware of, and unresponsive to, painful stimulation. They are given systemically and exert their main effects on the central nervous system, in contrast to local anaesthetics (see Ch. 42), which work by blocking conduction of impulses in peripheral sensory nerves. Though we now take them for granted, general anaesthetics are the drugs that paved the way for modern surgery.

In this chapter, we describe the pharmacology of the main agents in current use, which fall into two main groups, inhalation agents and intravenous agents. Information on the clinical pharmacology and use of anaesthetic agents can be found in textbooks of anaesthesia (e.g. Miller, 1999).

INTRODUCTION

Many drugs, including, for example, ethanol and morphine, can produce a state of insensibility and obliviousness to pain but are not used as anaesthetics. For a drug to be useful as an anaesthetic it must be readily controllable, so that induction and recovery are rapid, allowing the level of anaesthesia to be adjusted as required during the course of the operation. For this reason it was only when inhalation anaesthetics were first discovered, in 1846, that surgical operations under controlled anaesthesia became a practical possibility. Until that time, surgeons relied on being able to operate at lightning speed, and most operations were amputations. Inhalation is still the commonest route of administration for anaesthetics, though induction is usually carried out with intravenous agents.

▼ The use of **nitrous oxide** to relieve the pain of surgery was suggested by Humphrey Davy in 1800. He was the first person to make nitrous oxide and he tested its effects on several people, including himself and the Prime Minister, noting that it caused euphoria, analgesia and loss of consciousness. The use of nitrous oxide, billed as 'laughing gas', became a popular fairground entertainment and came to the notice of an American dentist Horace Wells, who had a tooth extracted under its influence while he himself squeezed the inhalation bag. **Ether** also first gained publicity in a disreputable way, through the spread of 'ether frolics' at which it was used to produce euphoria among the guests (explosions, too, one might have thought). William Morton, also a dentist and a student at Harvard Medical School, used it successfully to extract a tooth in 1846 and then suggested to Warren, the chief surgeon at Massachusetts General Hospital, that he should administer it for one of Warren's operations. Warren grudgingly agreed, and on 16 October 1846 a large audience was gathered in the main operating theatre; after some preliminary fumbling, Morton's demonstration was a spectacular success. 'Gentlemen, this is no humbug' was the most gracious comment that Warren could bring himself to make to the assembled audience. A more wordy appreciation came later from Oliver Wendell Holmes (1847), the neurologist–poet–philosopher who first coined the word 'anaesthesia'. 'The knife is searching for disease, the pulleys are dragging back dislocated limbs—Nature herself is working out the primal curse which doomed the tenderest of her creatures to the sharpest of her trials, but the fierce extremity of suffering has been steeped in the waters of forgetfulness, and the deepest furrow in the knotted brow of agony has been smoothed forever'. Morton subsequently sank into an endless and bitter dispute over the patent rights and contributed nothing more to medical science. In the same year James Simpson, professor of obstetrics in Glasgow, used chloroform to relieve the pain of childbirth, bringing on himself fierce denunciation from the clergy, one of whom wrote: 'Chloroform is a decoy of Satan, apparently offering itself to bless women; but in the end it will harden society and rob God of the deep, earnest cries which arise in time of trouble, for help'. Opposition was effectively silenced in 1853 when Queen Victoria gave birth to her seventh child under the influence of chloroform, and the procedure became known as *anaesthésie à la reine*.

MECHANISM OF ACTION OF ANAESTHETIC DRUGS

Unlike most drugs, inhalation anaesthetics, which include substances as diverse as halothane, nitrous oxide and xenon, belong to no recognisable chemical class. The shape and electronic configuration of the molecule is evidently unimportant, and the pharmacological action seems to require only that the molecule has certain physicochemical properties. Early theories, particularly the lipid theory (see below), were, therefore, based on rather general physicochemical ideas. Since we now know much more about the functional components of cell membranes—the principal structures affected by anaesthetic drugs—the emphasis has shifted towards identifying specific protein targets.

Accounts of the different theories of anaesthesia are given by Halsey (1989), Franks & Lieb (1994) and Little (1996).

LIPID THEORY

Overton & Meyer, at the turn of the 20th century, showed a close correlation between anaesthetic potency and lipid solubility in a diverse group of simple and unreactive organic compounds that were tested for their ability to immobilise tadpoles (see Franks & Lieb, 1994) This led to a bold theory, formulated by Meyer in 1937: 'Narcosis commences when any chemically indifferent substance has attained a certain molar concentration in the lipids of the cell'.

The relationship between anaesthetic activity and lipid solubility has been repeatedly confirmed. Figure 35.1 shows results obtained in humans where the minimal alveolar concentration (MAC; inversely proportional to potency) required to produce a lack of response to painful stimulation is plotted against lipid solubility, expressed as oil:water partition coefficient, for a wide range of inhalation anaesthetics. The Overton–Meyer studies did not suggest any particular mechanism but revealed an impressive correlation that any theory of anaesthesia needs to take into account. Oil:water partition should predict partition into membrane lipids, in agreement with abundant evidence that anaesthesia is caused by an alteration of membrane function.

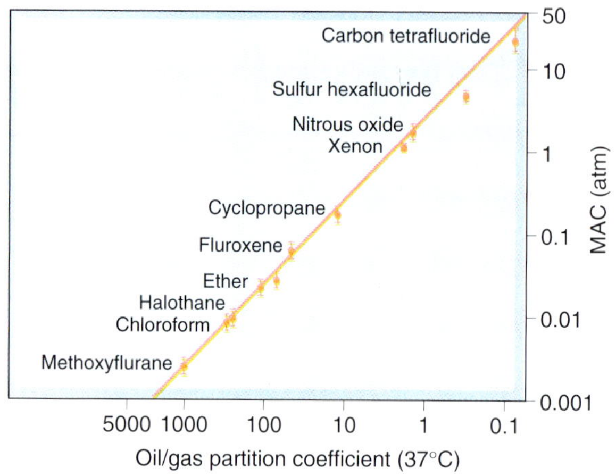

Fig. 35.1 Correlation of anaesthetic potency with oil:gas partition coefficient. Anaesthetic potency in humans is expressed as minimum alveolar partial pressure (MAC) required to produce surgical anaesthesia. There is a close correlation with lipid solubility, expressed as the oil:gas partition coeffecient. (From: Halsey 1989.)

How the simple introduction of inert foreign molecules into the cell membrane could cause a functional disturbance is not explained. Two possible mechanisms, namely *volume expansion* and *increased membrane fluidity,* have been suggested and tested experimentally, but both are now largely discredited (see Halsey, 1989; Little, 1996), and attention has swung from lipids to proteins.

EFFECTS ON ION CHANNELS

Anaesthetics can bind to proteins, as well as lipids, first demonstrated in experiments on luciferase (the enzyme responsible for the luminescent reaction of fireflies). Luciferase itself has no relevance to anaesthesia, but later work showed that anaesthetics also interact with functional membrane proteins, particularly a wide range of ligand-gated ion channels (see Franks & Lieb, 1994; Krasowski & Harrison, 1999). Many anaesthetic agents are able, at concentrations reached during anaesthesia, to inhibit the function of excitatory receptors, such as the ionotropic glutamate, acetylcholine or 5-hydroxytryptamine (5-HT) receptors, as well as enhancing the function of inhibitory receptors, such as gamma-aminobutyric acid (GABA)-A and glycine. Studies with genetically engineered receptors show that these effects depend on the presence of particular domains in the receptor protein, which appear to consist of specific 'modulatory sites' through which the anaesthetic drugs exert their effects on channel function. Another type of channel that appears to be specifically anaesthetic sensitive is one of the 'two-pore-domain' potassium channels, known as TREK (see Ch. 4), which is activated, thus reducing membrane excitability, in the presence of low concentrations of several volatile anaesthetics (see Franks & Lieb, 1999). It is now clear that anaesthetics affect the function of

Theories of anaesthesia

- Many simple, unreactive compounds produce narcotic effects, the extreme example being the inert gas xenon.
- Anaesthetic potency is closely correlated with lipid solubility (Overton–Meyer correlation), not with chemical structure.
- Earlier theories of anaesthesia postulate interaction with the lipid membrane bilayer. Recent work favours interaction with ligand-gated membrane ion channels.
- Most anaesthetics enhance the activity of inhibitory $GABA_A$-receptors and many inhibit activation of excitatory receptors, such as glutamate and nicotinic acetylcholine receptors.

many ion channels, and it is likely that these effects account for their overall effects on the central nervous system (CNS).

The current emphasis on protein targets leaves the very striking correlation between anaesthetic potency and lipid solubility described above somewhat dangling in the wind with no satisfactory explanation. One possibility is that anaesthetics concentrate at the lipid–protein interface within the membrane and thereby affect the functioning of membrane proteins. As Little (1996) emphasises, individual anaesthetics differ in their actions and affect cellular function in several different ways, so a simple unitary theory is unlikely to be sufficient.

THE EFFECTS OF ANAESTHETICS ON THE NERVOUS SYSTEM

At the cellular level, the effect of anaesthetics is mainly to inhibit synaptic transmission, any effects on axonal conduction probably being unimportant in practice (see Pocock & Richards, 1993).

Inhibition of synaptic transmission could be the result of reduction of transmitter release, inhibition of the action of the transmitter, or reduction of the excitability of the postsynaptic cell. Though all three effects have been described, most studies suggest that reduced transmitter release and reduced postsynaptic response are the main factors. A reduction of acetylcholine release has been shown in studies on peripheral synapses, and reduced sensitivity to excitatory transmitters (through inhibition of ligand-gated ion channels; see above) occurs at both peripheral and central synapses.

The action of inhibitory synapses may be enhanced or reduced by anaesthetics. Enhancement of inhibitory synaptic action occurs particularly with barbiturates (p. 471), though similar effects also occur with volatile anaesthetics (see Little, 1996).

Much effort has gone into identifying a particular brain region on which anaesthetics act to produce their effect (see Angel, 1993). The most sensitive region appears to be the thalamic sensory relay nuclei and the deep layer of the cortex to which these nuclei project. This constitutes the route taken by sensory impulses reaching the cortex, so inhibition can result in a lack of awareness of sensory input.

Anaesthetics, even in low concentrations, cause short-term amnesia, i.e. experiences occurring during the influence of the drug are not recalled later even though the subject was responsive at the time.* It is likely that interference with hippocampal function produces this effect, for it is known that the hippocampus is involved in short-term memory and that certain hippocampal synapses are highly susceptible to inhibition by anaesthetics.

As the anaesthetic concentration is increased, all brain functions are affected, including motor control and reflex activity, respiration and autonomic regulation. Therefore, it is not possible to identify a critical 'target site' in the brain responsible for all the phenomena of anaesthesia.

STAGES OF ANAESTHESIA

When a slowly acting anaesthetic, such as ether, is given on its own, certain well-defined stages are passed through as its concentration in the blood increases.

- *Stage I—Analgesia* The subject is conscious but drowsy. Responses to painful stimuli are reduced. The degree of analgesia actually varies greatly with different agents; it is pronounced with ether and nitrous oxide, but not with halothane.
- *Stage II—Excitement* The subject loses consciousness and no longer responds to non-painful stimuli but responds in a reflex fashion to painful stimuli. Other reflexes, for example the cough reflex and gagging in response to pharyngeal stimulation, are present and often exaggerated. The subject may move, talk incoherently, hold his breath, choke or vomit. Irregular ventilation may affect the absorption of the anaesthetic agent. It is a dangerous state, and modern anaesthetic procedures are designed to eliminate it.
- *Stage III—Surgical anaesthesia* Spontaneous movement ceases and respiration becomes regular. If anaesthesia is light, some reflexes (e.g. responses to pharyngeal and peritoneal stimulation) are still present, and muscles show appreciable tone. With deepening anaesthesia, these reflexes disappear, and the muscles relax fully. Respiration becomes progressively shallower, with the intercostal muscles failing before the diaphragm.
- *Stage IV—Medullary paralysis* Respiration and vasomotor control cease, and death occurs within a few minutes.

Single anaesthetic agents are rarely used on their own, and progression through these stages is seldom observed in practice. The anaesthetic state, for clinical purposes, consists of three main

*The benzodiazepine **flunitrazepam** recently achieved a nasty notoriety, since its amnesia-producing and tranquillising effect led to its use as a rapists' aid.

components, namely loss of consciousness, analgesia, and muscle relaxation; in practice these effects are produced with a combination of drugs rather than with a single anaesthetic agent. For example, a common procedure would be to produce unconsciousness rapidly with an intravenous induction agent (e.g. **propofol**), to maintain unconsciousness and produce analgesia with one or more inhalation agents (e.g. **nitrous oxide** and **halothane**), which might be supplemented with an intravenous analgesic agent (e.g. an *opiate*; see Ch. 40), and to produce muscle paralysis with a neuromuscular blocking drug (e.g. **atracurium**; see Ch. 10). Such a procedure results in much faster induction and recovery, avoiding long (and hazardous) periods of semiconsciousness, and it enables surgery to be carried out with relatively little impairment of homeostatic reflexes.

Pharmacological effects of anaesthetic agents

- Anaesthesia involves three main neurophysiological changes: unconsciousness, loss of response to painful stimulation and loss of reflexes.
- At supra-anaesthetic doses, all anaesthetic agents can cause death by loss of cardiovascular reflexes and respiratory paralysis.
- At the cellular level, anaesthetic agents affect synaptic transmission rather than axonal conduction. The release of excitatory transmitters and the response of the postsynaptic receptors are both inhibited. GABA-mediated inhibitory transmission is enhanced by most anaesthetics.
- Though all parts of the nervous system are affected by anaesthetic agents, the main targets appear to be the thalamus, cortex and hippocampus.
- Most anaesthetic agents (with exceptions, such as ketamine and benzodiazepines) produce similar neurophysiological effects and differ mainly in respect of their pharmacokinetic properties and toxicity.
- Most anaesthetic agents cause cardiovascular depression, by effects on the myocardium and blood vessels as well as on the nervous system. Halogenated anaesthetic agents are likely to cause cardiac dysrhythmias, accentuated by circulating catecholamines.

EFFECTS ON THE CARDIOVASCULAR AND RESPIRATORY SYSTEMS

Though all anaesthetics decrease the contractility of isolated heart preparations, their effects on cardiac output and blood pressure in humans vary, mainly because of concomitant actions on the sympathetic nervous system. Some agents (e.g. nitrous oxide) cause an increased sympathetic discharge and increased plasma noradrenaline concentration and tend to increase blood pressure, whereas others (e.g. halothane and other halogenated anaesthetics) have the opposite effect.

Many anaesthetics, especially halogenated agents, cause cardiac dysrhythmias, particularly ventricular extrasystoles. The mechanism is not well understood but involves sensitisation to adrenaline. The usual manifestation is the appearance of ventricular ectopic beats; careful electrocardiographic monitoring shows that these occur very commonly in patients under halothane anaesthesia without producing any harmful effect. If catecholamine secretion is excessive, however, there is a risk of precipitating ventricular fibrillation, which is a particular hazard if stage II of the induction process is unduly prolonged.

With the exception of nitrous oxide and ketamine, all anaesthetics depress respiration markedly, and increase arterial partial pressure of carbon dioxide. Nitrous oxide has much less effect, mainly because its low potency prevents very deep anaesthesia from being produced with this drug (see below).

INHALATION ANAESTHETICS

PHARMACOKINETIC ASPECTS

An important characteristic of an inhalation anaesthetic is the speed at which the arterial blood concentration, which governs the pharmacological effect, follows changes in the concentration of the drug in the inspired air. Ideally, the blood concentration should follow as quickly as possible, so that the depth of anaesthesia can be controlled rapidly. In particular, the blood concentration should fall to a subanaesthetic level rapidly when administration is stopped, so that the patient recovers consciousness with minimal delay. A prolonged semicomatose state, in which respiratory reflexes are weak or absent, is hazardous to life.

The only quantitatively important route by which inhalation anaesthetics enter and leave the body is via the lungs. Metabolic degradation of anaesthetics (see below), though important in relation to their toxicity, is generally insignificant in determining their duration of action. Anaesthetics are all small, lipid-soluble molecules, which cross the alveolar membrane with great ease. It is, therefore, the rate of delivery of drug to and from the lungs, via the inspired air and the bloodstream, that determines the overall kinetic behaviour of an anaesthetic. The reason that anaesthetics vary in their kinetic behaviour is that their relative solubilities in blood, and in body fat, vary between one drug and another.

The main factors that determine the speed of induction and recovery can be summarised as:

- properties of the anaesthetic
  —blood:gas partition coefficient (i.e. solubility in blood)
  —oil:gas partition coefficient (i.e. solubility in fat)
- Physiological factors
  —alveolar ventilation rate
  —cardiac output.

THE SOLUBILITY OF ANAESTHETICS

For practical purposes, anaesthetics can be regarded physicochemically as ideal gases: their solubility in different media is expressed as *partition coefficients*, defined as the ratio of the concentration of the agent in two phases at equilibrium.

The *blood:gas partition coefficient* is the main factor that determines the rate of induction and recovery of an inhalation anaesthetic, and the lower the blood:gas partition coefficient the faster the induction and recovery.

The *oil:gas partition coefficient*, a measure of fat solubility, determines the potency of an anaesthetic (as already discussed) and also influences the kinetics of its distribution in the body, the main effect being that high lipid solubility tends to delay recovery from the effects of anaesthesia. Values of blood:gas and oil:gas partition coefficients for some anaesthetics are given in Table 35.1.

INDUCTION AND RECOVERY

The brain has a large blood flow, and the blood–brain barrier is freely permeable to anaesthetics, so the concentration of anaesthetic in the brain closely tracks that in the arterial blood. The kinetics of transfer of anaesthetic between the inspired air and the arterial blood, therefore, determine the kinetics of the pharmacological effect.

If an anaesthetic is added to the inspired air at a concentration that, at equilibrium, will produce surgical anaesthesia, the rate at which this equilibrium is approached depends mainly on the blood:gas partition coefficient. Contrary to what one might intuitively suppose, the *lower* the solubility in blood, the *faster* is the process of equilibration. This is because less drug has to be transferred via the lungs to the blood in order to achieve a given partial pressure. Therefore, a single lungful of air containing a

Table 35.1 Characteristics of inhalation anaesthetics

Drug	Partition coefficients: Blood:gas	Partition coefficients: Oil:gas	MAC (% v/v)	Induction/ recovery	Main adverse effects	Notes
Ether	12.0	65	1.9	Slow	Respiratory irritation Nausea and vomiting Explosion risk	Now obsolete, except where facilities are minimal
Halothane	2.4	220	0.8	Medium	Hypotension Cardiac arrhythmias Hepatotoxicity (with repeated use) Malignant hyperthermia (rare)	In common use, but declining in favor of newer agents Significant metabolism to trifluoracetate
Nitrous oxide	0.5	1.4	100[a]	Fast	Few adverse effects Risk of anemia (with prolonged or repeated use)	Good analgesic effect Low potency precludes use as sole anaesthetic agent—normally combined with other inhalation agents
Enflurane	1.9	98	0.7	Medium	Risk of convulsions (slight) Malignant hyperthermia (rare)	Widely used Similar characteristics to halothane, with less risk of hepatic toxicity
Isoflurane	1.4	91	1.2	Medium	Few adverse effects Possible risk of coronary ischemia in susceptible patients	Widely used as alternative to halothane
Desflurane	0.4	23	6.1	Fast	Respiratory tract irritation, cough, bronchospasm	Used for day-case surgery, because of fast onset and recovery (comparable to nitrous oxide)
Sevoflurane	0.6	53	2.1	Fast	Few reported Theoretical risk of renal toxicity owing to fluoride	Recently introduced Similar to desflurane

MAC, minimum alveolar concentration.
[a]Theoretical value, based on experiments under hyperbaric conditions.

low-solubility agent will bring the partial pressure in the blood closer to that of the inspired air than is the case for a high-solubility agent, and a smaller number of breaths (i.e. a shorter time) will be needed to reach equilibrium. The same principle applies in reverse for washout of the drug, recovery being faster with a low-solubility agent. Figure 35.2 shows the much faster equilibration for nitrous oxide—a low-solubility agent—than for ether—a high solubility agent (now obsolete)

The transfer of anaesthetic between blood and tissues also affects the kinetics of equilibration. Figure 35.3 shows a very simple model of the circulation in which two tissue compartments are included. Body fat has a low blood flow and often a high anaesthetic solubility (see Table 35.1); it constitutes about 20% of the volume of a normal male. Consequently, for a drug such as halothane, which is about 100 times more soluble in fat than in water, the amount present in fat after complete equilibration would be roughly 95% of the total amount in the body. Because of the low blood flow it takes many hours for the drug to enter and leave the fat, which results in a pronounced slow phase of equilibration following the rapid phase associated with the blood–gas exchanges (Fig. 35.2). The more fat soluble the anaesthetic and the fatter the patient, the more pronounced this slow phase becomes.

Of the physiological factors affecting the rate of equilibration of inhalation anaesthetics, alveolar ventilation is the most important. The greater the ventilation rate, the faster is the process of equilibration, particularly for drugs that have high blood:gas partition coefficients. The use of respiratory depressant drugs, such as morphine (see Ch. 40), can thus retard recovery from anaesthesia. Changes in cardiac output produce complex effects. Increasing the cardiac output tends to slow down the early phase of induction but speed up the later phase of equilibration.

Recovery from anaesthesia involves the same processes as induction but in reverse (Fig. 35.2), the rapid phase of recovery being followed by a slow 'hangover'. If anaesthesia with a highly fat-soluble drug has been maintained for a long time, so that the fat has had time to accumulate a substantial amount of the anaesthetic, this hangover can become very pronounced and the patient may remain drowsy for some hours. Because of these kinetic factors, the search for improved inhalation anaesthetics has focussed on agents with low blood and tissue solubility. Newer drugs, which show kinetic properties similar to those of nitrous oxide but have higher potency, include **sevoflurane** and **desflurane** (Table 35.1).

METABOLISM AND TOXICITY OF INHALATION ANAESTHETICS

Metabolism, though not generally important as a route of elimination of inhalation anaesthetics, can generate toxic

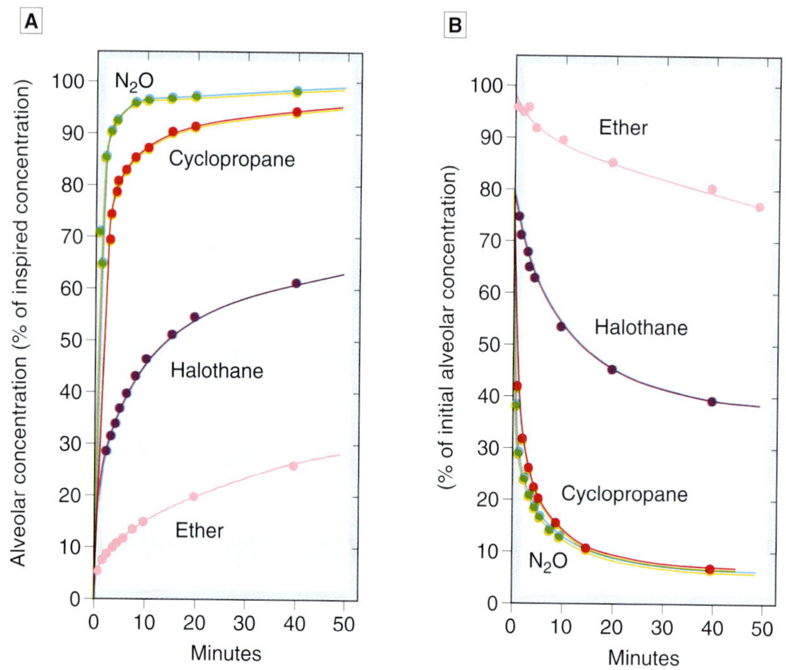

Fig. 35.2 Rate of equilibration of inhalation anaesthetics in humans. The curves show alveolar concentration (which closely reflects arterial blood cencentration) as a function of time during induction and recovery. The overall rate of equilibration varies with water solubility. There is also a slow phase of equilibration, most marked with highly lipid-soluble drugs (ether and halothane), owing to the slow transfer between blood and fat (Fig. 35.3). A Induction. B Recovery. (From: Papper E M, Kitz R (eds) 1963 Uptake and distribution of anaesthetic agents. McGraw-Hill, New York.)

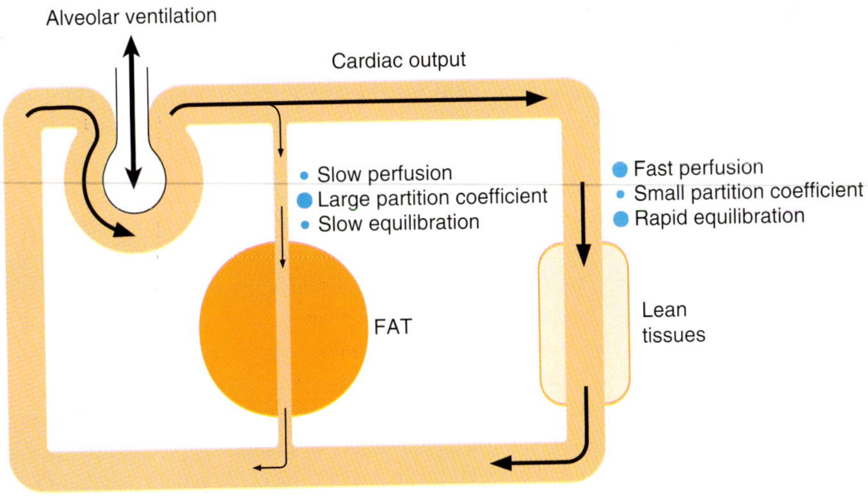

Fig. 35.3 Factors affecting the rate of equilibration of inhalation anaesthetics in the body. The body is represented as two compartments. Lean tissues, including the brain, have a large blood flow and low partition coefficient for anaesthetics and, therefore, equilibrate rapidly with the blood. Fat tissues have a small blood flow and large partition coefficient and, therefore, equilibrate slowly, acting as a reservoir of drug during the recovery phase.

metabolites. **Chloroform** (now obsolete) causes hepatotoxicity associated with free radical formation in liver cells. **Methoxyflurane**, a halogenated ether, is now very rarely used because about 50% is metabolised, generating fluoride and oxalate, which cause renal toxicity. **Enflurane** and **sevoflurane** also generate fluoride, but at much lower (non-toxic) levels (Table 35.1). **Halothane** is the only volatile anaesthetic in current use that undergoes substantial metabolism, about 30% being converted to bromide, trifluoroacetic acid and other metabolites, which may be responsible for the rare occurrence of liver toxicity (see below).

The problem of toxicity of low concentrations of anaesthetics inhaled over long periods by operating theatre staff causes much concern, following the demonstration that such chronic low-level exposure leads to liver toxicity (associated with metabolite formation) in experimental animals. Epidemiological studies of operating theatre staff, compared with similar groups of subjects not exposed to anaesthetic agents, have shown increased incidence of liver disease and of certain types of leukaemia, and of spontaneous abortion and congenital malformations, Though causation has not been clearly established, strict measures are used to minimise the escape of anaesthetics into the air of operating theatres.

Pharmacokinetic properties of inhalation anaesthetics

- Rapid induction and recovery are important properties of an anaesthetic agent, allowing flexible control over the depth of anaesthesia.
- Speed of induction and recovery are determined by two properties of the anaesthetic: solubility in blood (blood:gas partition coefficient) and solubility in fat (lipid solubility).
- Agents with low blood:gas partition coefficients produce rapid induction and recovery (e.g. nitrous oxide, desflurane); agents with high blood:gas partition coefficients show slow induction and recovery (e.g. halothane).
- Agents with high lipid solubility (e.g. halothane) accumulate gradually in body fat and may produce a prolonged hangover if used for a long operation.
- Some halogenated anaesthetics (especially halothane and methoxyflurane) are metabolised. This is not very important in determining their duration of action but contributes to toxicity (e.g. renal toxicity associated with fluoride production with methoxyflurane—no longer used).

INDIVIDUAL INHALATION ANAESTHETICS

The inhalation anaesthetics currently used in developed countries are **halothane**, **nitrous oxide**, **enflurane** and **isoflurane**. **Ether**, now largely obsolete, is still used in some parts of the world. It is explosive, and highly irritant, and commonly causes postoperative nausea and respiratory complications. **Methoxyflurane** (see above) is rarely used because of its renal toxicity. **Desflurane** and **sevoflurane** have gained popularity since they overcome many of the problems of the earlier drugs. The newer compounds are all halogen-substituted hydrocarbons of very similar 'spot-the difference' structure. After 50 years of this kind of musical-chairs chemistry, there is a sense that we may have reached the end of the line with sevoflurane. **Xenon,** an inert gas shown many years ago to have anaesthetic properties, is making something of a comeback in the clinic, since—not being metabolised—it lacks toxicity, but its relatively low potency and high cost are disadvantages.

HALOTHANE

Halothane is a widely used inhalation anaesthetic, but its use is now declining in favour of isoflurane and other drugs (see below). It is non-explosive and non-irritant; induction and recovery are relatively fast; it is highly potent and can easily produce respiratory and cardiovascular failure, so the concentration administered needs to be controlled accurately. Even in normal anaesthetic concentrations, halothane causes a fall in blood pressure, partly because of myocardial depression and partly because of vasodilatation. Halothane is not analgesic and has a relaxant effect on the uterus, which limits its usefulness for obstetric purposes.

Adverse effects

In common with many halogenated anaesthetics, halothane sensitises the heart to adrenaline, and it tends to cause cardiac dysrhythmias, particularly ventricular extra-systoles. Though this does not normally matter, it can be important in special circumstances, e.g. in operations for phaeochromocytoma (see Ch. 11), where there is a risk of precipitating ventricular fibrillation.

Two rare, but serious, adverse reactions are associated with halothane, namely *hepatotoxicity* and *malignant hyperthermia*. In a major study in 1986 of 850 000 cases involving anaesthesia with different agents, nine deaths from liver failure not attributable to any other recognisable cause were reported, seven of which had received halothane. Subsequent reports suggest that the risk is associated with repeated administration of halothane. In the UK, a study of 62 cases of unexplained serious liver disease showed that 66% were associated with repeated halothane administration. Halothane undergoes metabolism (see above), partly by oxidation to trifluoroacetic acid, which reacts covalently with many proteins. This happens particularly in liver cells, where halothane metabolism takes place, and the mechanism of hepatotoxicity is thought to involve an immune response to certain fluoroacetylated liver enzymes.

Malignant hyperthermia results from excessive metabolic heat production in skeletal muscle, as a result of excessive release of Ca^{2+} from the sarcoplasmic reticulum. The result is a dramatic rise in body temperature, associated with muscle contractures and acidosis, which can be fatal unless treated promptly. Malignant hyperthermia can be triggered by a number of drugs, including other halogenated anaesthetics and neuromuscular-blocking drugs (see Ch. 10). Susceptibility to it has a genetic basis, being associated with mutations in the gene encoding the *ryanodine receptor*, which controls Ca^{2+} release from the sarcoplasmic reticulum (Ch. 4). Why such mutations induce sensitivity of the channel to anaesthetics and other drugs is not clear. Malignant hyperthermia is treated with **dantrolene**, a muscle relaxant drug that blocks these calcium channels.

NITROUS OXIDE

Nitrous oxide (N_2O, not to be confused with nitric oxide, NO) is an odourless gas with many advantageous features for anaesthesia; it is in widespread use. It is rapid in action, because of its low blood:gas partition coefficient (Table 35.1), and is also an effective analgesic agent in concentrations too low to cause unconsciousness. It is used in this way to reduce pain during childbirth. The potency of nitrous oxide is low; even at a concentration of 80% in the inspired gas mixture (the maximum possible without reducing the oxygen content), nitrous oxide does not produce surgical anaesthesia. It is not, therefore, used on its own as an anaesthetic, but it is very often used (as 70% nitrous oxide in oxygen) as an adjunct to volatile anaesthetics, allowing them to be used at lower concentrations. During recovery from nitrous oxide anaesthesia, the transfer of the gas from the blood into the alveoli can be sufficient to reduce, by dilution, the alveolar partial pressure of oxygen, producing a transient hypoxia (known as the second gas effect), but this is only important in patients with respiratory disease.

Given for brief periods, nitrous oxide is devoid of any serious toxic effects, but prolonged exposure (over 6 hours) causes inactivation of methionine synthase, an enzyme required for DNA and protein synthesis, resulting in bone marrow depression, which may cause anaemia and leucopenia. This does not normally occur with brief exposure to nitrous oxide, but prolonged or repeated use needs to be avoided. It should also be avoided in patients with anaemia related to vitamin B_{12} deficiency. Prolonged exposure to very low concentrations of nitrous oxide, far below the level causing anaesthesia, may affect protein and DNA synthesis very markedly, and nitrous oxide has been suspected to be a cause of the increased frequency of abortion and fetal abnormality among operating theatre staff.

ENFLURANE

Enflurane is a halogenated ether, similar to halothane in its potency and moderate speed of induction. It was introduced as an alternative to methoxyflurane, its advantages being that it causes little production of fluoride (and, therefore, lacks renal toxicity) and is less fat soluble than methoxyflurane so that recovery is faster. The main drawback to enflurane, which otherwise has many favourable characteristics, is that it can cause seizures, either during induction or following recovery from anaesthesia. In this connection, it is interesting that a related substance, a fluorine-substituted diethyl ether, hexafluoroether, is a powerful convulsant agent, though the mechanism is not understood. Enflurane, in common with other halogenated anaesthetics, can induce malignant hyperthermia.

ISOFLURANE

Isoflurane, which is now the most widely used volatile anaesthetic, is similar to enflurane in many respects. It is not appreciably metabolised and shows little sign of toxicity; it also lacks the proconvulsive property of enflurane. It is an expensive drug, because of the difficulty in separating isomers formed during synthesis. It tends to cause hypotension and is a powerful coronary vasodilator. Paradoxically, this can exacerbate cardiac ischaemia in patients with coronary disease, because of the 'steal' phenomenon (see Ch. 17).

Individual inhalation anaesthetics

- The main agents in current use in developed countries are halothane, nitrous oxide, isoflurane, enflurane, desflurane and sevoflurane. Ether is largely obsolete.
- **Halothane**:
  - —widely used agent
  - —potent, non-explosive and non-irritant, hypotensive; may cause dysrhythmias; about 30% metabolised
  - —hangover likely, because of high lipid solubility
  - —risk of liver damage if used repeatedly.
- **Nitrous oxide**:
  - —low potency, therefore must be combined with other agents
  - —rapid induction and recovery
  - —good analgesic properties
  - —risk of bone marrow depression with prolonged administration.
- **Enflurane**:
  - —halogenated anaesthetic similar to halothane
  - —less metabolism than halothane; therefore, there is less risk of toxicity
  - —faster induction and recovery than halothane (less accumulation in fat)
  - —some risk of epilepsy-like seizures.
- **Isoflurane**:
  - —similar to enflurane but lacks epileptogenic property
  - —may precipitate myocardial ischaemia in patients with coronary disease.
  - —Irritant to respiratory tract
- **Desflurane** and **sevoflurane** are similar to isoflurane but have faster onset and recovery and lack of respiratory irritation.
- **Ether**:
  - —obsolete except where modern facilities are not available
  - —easy to administer and control
  - —slow onset and recovery, with postoperative nausea and vomiting
  - —analgesic and muscle relaxant properties
  - —highly explosive
  - —irritant to respiratory tract.

OTHER INHALATION ANAESTHETICS

Desflurane, introduced recently, is chemically similar to isoflurane, but its lower solubility in blood and fat means that induction and recovery are faster, so it is gaining in use as an anaesthetic for day-case surgery. It is not appreciably metabolised. Its potency is lower than that of the drugs described above, the MAC being about 6%. At the concentrations used for induction (about 10%), desflurane causes some respiratory tract irritation, which can lead to coughing and bronchospasm.

Sevoflurane, another recent introduction, resembles desflurane but is more potent and does not cause respiratory irritation. It is partially (about 3%) metabolised, and detectable levels of fluoride are produced, though this does not appear to be sufficient to cause toxicity. Like other halogenated anaesthetics, sevoflurane can cause malignant hyperthermia in genetically susceptible individuals.

Many inhalation anaesthetics have been introduced and gradually superseded, mainly because of their inflammable nature or because of toxicity. They include chloroform (hepatotoxicity and cardiac dysrhythmias), diethyl ether (explosive and highly irritant to the respiratory tract, leading to postoperative complications), vinyl ether (explosive), cyclopropane (explosive, strongly depressant to respiration, and hypotensive), trichloroethylene (chemically unstable, no special advantages), methoxyflurane (slow recovery and renal toxicity).

Further information is available in many excellent textbooks of anaesthesia (e.g. Bowdle et al., 1994; Miller, 1999).

INTRAVENOUS ANAESTHETIC AGENTS

Even the fastest-acting inhalation anaesthetics, such as nitrous oxide, take a few minutes to act and cause a period of excitement before anaesthesia is produced. Intravenous anaesthetics act much more rapidly, producing unconsciousness in about 20 seconds, as soon as the drug reaches the brain from its site of injection. These drugs (e.g. **thiopental**, **etomidate**, **propofol**; see below) are normally used for induction of anaesthesia. They are preferred by patients, since injection generally lacks the menacing quality associated with a face-mask in an apprehensive individual.

Other drugs used as intravenous induction agents include certain benzodiazepines (see Ch. 36), such as **diazepam** and **midazolam**, which act rather less rapidly than the drugs listed above. Though intravenous anaesthetics on their own are generally unsatisfactory for producing maintained anaesthesia because their elimination from the body is relatively slow compared with that of inhalation agents, **propofol** can be used in this way, and the duration of action of **ketamine** is sufficient that it can be used for short operations without the need for an inhalation agent.

The combined use of **droperidol**, a dopamine antagonist related to antipsychotic drugs (Ch. 34), and an opiate analgesic, such as **fentanyl** (Ch. 40), can be used to produce a state of deep sedation and analgesia (known as *neuroleptanalgesia*) in which the patient remains responsive to simple commands and questions but does not respond to painful stimuli or retain any memory of the procedure. This is used for minor surgical procedures, such as endoscopy.

The properties of the main intravenous anaesthetics are summarised in Table 35.2. Agents now withdrawn because of a high incidence of acute allergic reactions, producing hypotension and bronchoconstriction, include propanidid and althesin.

THIOPENTAL

Thiopental belongs to the barbiturate class of CNS depressants (Ch. 36) and is the only one of importance in anaesthesia. It has very high lipid solubility, and this accounts for the speed and transience of its effect when it is injected intravenously (see below). The free acid is insoluble in water, so thiopental is given as the sodium salt. This solution is strongly alkaline and is unstable, so the drug must be dissolved immediately before it is used.

Pharmacokinetic aspects

On intravenous injection, thiopental causes unconsciousness within about 20 seconds, and this lasts for 5–10 minutes. The anaesthetic effect closely parallels the concentration of thiopental in the blood reaching the brain, because its high lipid solubility allows it to cross the blood–brain barrier without noticeable delay.

The blood concentration of thiopental declines rapidly, by about 80% within 1–2 minutes, following the initial peak after intravenous injection, because the drug is redistributed, first to tissues with a large blood flow (liver, kidneys, brain, etc.) and more slowly to muscle. Uptake into body fat, though favoured by the high lipid solubility of thiopental, occurs only slowly because of the low blood flow to this tissue. After several hours, however, most of the thiopental present in the body will have accumulated in body fat, the rest having been metabolised. Recovery from the anaesthetic effect occurs within about 5 minutes, governed entirely by redistribution of the drug to well-perfused tissues; very little is metabolised in this time. After the initial rapid decline, the blood concentration drops more slowly, over several hours, as the drug is taken up by body fat and metabolised. Consequently, thiopental produces a long-lasting 'hangover'; furthermore, repeated intravenous doses cause progressively longer periods of anaesthesia, since the plateau in blood concentration becomes progressively more elevated as more drug accumulates in the body. For this reason, thiopental cannot be used to maintain surgical anaesthesia, but only as an induction agent.

Thiopental binds to plasma albumin (roughly 70% of the blood content normally being bound). The fraction bound is less in states of malnutrition, liver disease or renal disease, which affect the concentration and drug-binding properties of plasma albumin; this can appreciably reduce the dose needed for induction of anaesthesia.

Actions and side-effects

The actions of thiopental on the nervous system are very similar to those of inhalation anaesthetics, though it has no analgesic effect and can cause profound respiratory depression even in amounts that fail to abolish reflex responses to painful stimuli.

Its long after-effect, associated with a slowly declining plasma concentration, means that drowsiness and some degree of respiratory depression persist for some hours.

Table 35.2 Properties of intravenous anesthetic agents

Drug	Speed of induction and recovery	Main unwanted effects	Notes
Thiopental	Fast (cumulation occurs, giving slow recovery) Hangover	Cardiovascular and respiratory depression	Widely used as induction agent for routine purposes
Etomidate	Fast onset, fairly fast recovery	Excitatory effects during induction and recovery Adrenocortical suppression	Less cardiovascular and respiratory depression than with thiopental Causes pain at injection site
Propofol	Fast onset, very fast recovery	Cardiovascular and respiratory depression	Rapidly metabolised Possible to use as continuous infusion Causes pain at injection site
Ketamine	Slow onset, after-effects common during recovery	Psychotomimetic effects following recovery Postoperative nausea, vomiting and salivation	Produces good analgesia and amnesia
Midazolam	Slower than other agents		Little respiratory or cardiovascular depression

Accidental injection of thiopental around, rather than into, the vein or into an artery can cause local tissue necrosis and ulceration or severe arterial spasm, which can result in gangrene. Immediate injection of procaine, through the same needle, is the recommended procedure if this accident occurs. The risk is small, now that lower concentrations of thiopental are used for intravenous injection. Thiopental, like other barbiturates, can precipitate an attack of porphyria in susceptible individuals (see Ch. 52).

Intravenous anaesthetic agents

- Most commonly used for induction of anaesthesia, followed by inhalation agent.
- Thiopental, etomidate and propofol are most commonly used; all act within 20–30 seconds if given intravenously.
- **Thiopental**:
  - —barbiturate with very high lipid solubility
  - —rapid action because of rapid transfer across blood–brain barrier; short duration (about 5 minutes) becaue of redistribution, mainly to muscle
  - —slowly metabolised and liable to accumulate in body fat; therefore, may cause prolonged effect if given repeatedly
  - —no analgesic effect
  - —narrow margin between anaesthetic dose and dose causing cardiovascular depression
  - —risk of severe vasospasm if accidentally injected into artery.
- **Etomidate**:
  - —similar to thiopental but more quickly metabolised
  - —less risk of cardiovascular depression
  - —may cause involuntary movements during induction
  - —possible risk of adrenocortical suppression.
- **Propofol**:
  - —rapidly metabolised
  - —very rapid recovery; no cumulative effect
  - —useful for day-case surgery
- **Ketamine**:
  - —analogue of phencyclidine, with similar properties
  - —action differs from other agents; probably related to effect on NMDA-type glutamate receptors
  - —onset of effect is relatively slow (2–5 minutes)
  - —produces 'dissociative' anaesthesia, in which patient may remain conscious, though amnesic and insensitive to pain
  - —high incidence of dysphoria, hallucinations, etc. during recovery; used mainly for minor procedures in children.

ETOMIDATE

Etomidate has gained favour over thiopental on account of the larger margin between the anaesthetic dose and the dose needed to produce respiratory and cardiovascular depression. It is also more rapidly metabolised than thiopental and, therefore, less likely to cause a prolonged hangover. In other respects, etomidate is very similar to thiopental, though it appears more likely to cause involuntary movements during induction, and to cause postoperative nausea and vomiting. With prolonged use, etomidate appears to suppress the adrenal cortex, which has been associated with an increase in mortality in severely ill patients. It is, therefore, only used as an induction agent, and is preferable to thiopental in patients at risk of circulatory failure.

PROPOFOL

Propofol, introduced in 1983, is also similar in its properties to thiopental but has the advantage of being very rapidly metabolised and, therefore, giving rapid recovery without any hangover effect. This enables it to be used as a continuous infusion to maintain surgical anaesthesia without the need for any inhalation agent. Propofol lacks the tendency to cause involuntary movement and adrenocortical suppression seen with etomidate. It is particularly useful for the growing practice of day-case surgery.

OTHER INDUCTION AGENTS

KETAMINE

▼ Ketamine closely resembles, both chemically and pharmacologically, **phencyclidine**, which is a 'street-drug' with a pronounced effect on sensory perception (see Ch. 42). Both drugs produce a similar anaesthesia-like state and profound analgesia, but ketamine produces considerably less euphoria and sensory distortion than phencyclidine and is thus more useful in anaesthesia. Both drugs are believed to act by blocking activation of one type of excitatory amino acid receptor (the NMDA-receptor; see Ch. 32).

Given intravenously, ketamine takes effect more slowly (2–5 minutes) than thiopental and produces a different effect, known as 'dissociative anaesthesia' in which there is a marked sensory loss and analgesia, as well as amnesia and paralysis of movement, without actual loss of consciousness. During induction and recovery, involuntary movements and peculiar sensory experiences often occur. Ketamine does not act simply as a depressant, and it produces cardiovascular and respiratory effects quite different from those of most anaesthetics. Blood pressure and heart rate are usually increased, and respiration is unaffected by effective anaesthetic doses. The main drawback of ketamine, in spite of the safety associated with a lack of overall depressant activity, is that hallucinations, and sometimes delirium and irrational behaviour, are common during recovery. These after-effects limit the usefulness of ketamine but are said to be less marked in children;* therefore, ketamine, often in conjunction with a benzodiazepine, is often used for minor procedures in paediatrics.

*A cautionary note: many adverse effects are claimed to be less marked in children, perhaps because they cannot verbalise their experiences. Until recently, muscle relaxants alone were used without anaesthesia during cardiac surgery in neonates. The babies did not complain of pain, but their circulating catecholamine levels were astronomical.

MIDAZOLAM

Midazolam, a benzodiazepine (Ch. 36), is appreciably slower in the onset and offset of its action than the drugs discussed above, but it lacks the tendency to cause respiratory and cardiovascular depression, which can be an advantage in some patients. It is often used as a preoperative sedative for procedures such as endoscopy where full anaesthesia is not required.

REFERENCES AND FURTHER READING

Angel A 1993 Central neuronal pathways and the process of anaesthesia. Br J Anaesth 71: 148–163 (*Review of effects of anaesthetics at the neurophysiological level*)

Bowdle T A, Horita A, Kharasch E D 1994 The pharmacologic basis of anesthesiology. Churchill Livingstone, New York (*Comprehensive textbook*)

Franks N P, Lieb W R 1994 Molecular and cellular mechanisms of general anaesthesia. Nature 367: 607–614 (*Good discussion of the opposing 'lipid' and 'protein' theories by pioneers from the protein camp*)

Franks N P, Lieb W J, 1999 Background K^+ channels: an important target for volatile anesthetics? Nat Neurosci 2: 395–396 (*Short commentary on recent evidence suggesting that anaesthetics can activate TREK channels*)

Halsey M J 1989 Physicochemical properties of inhalation anaesthetics. In: Nunn J F, Utting J E, Brown B R (eds) General anaesthesia. Butterworth, London (*Good summary of evidence supporting lipid theories of anaesthesia*)

Little H J 1996 How has molecular pharmacology contributed to our understanding of the molecular mechanism(s) of general anaesthesia? Pharmacol Ther 69: 37–58 (*Balanced account of the strengths and shortcomings of current theories*)

Krasowski M D, Harrison N L 1999 General anaesthetic actions on ligand-gated ion channels. Cell Mol Life Sci 55: 1278–1303 (*Reviews recent evidence for specific effects on ion channels as cause on anaesthesia*)

Miller R D (ed) 1999 Anaesthesia. Churchill Livingstone, New York (*Comprehensive textbook*)

Pocock G, Richards C D 1993 Excitatory and inhibitory synaptic mechanisms in anaesthesia. Br J Anaesth 71: 134–147 (*Summary of evidence showing that anaesthetics can enhance as well as inhibit synaptic function*)

36 Anxiolytic and hypnotic drugs

Overview 515

The nature of anxiety and measurement of anxiolytic activity 515
- Animal models of anxiety 516
- Tests on humans 516

Classification of anxiolytic and hypnotic drugs 516

Benzodiazepines 517
- Chemistry and structure–activity relationships 517
- Mechanism of action 518
- Pharmacological effects and uses 518
- Pharmacokinetic aspects 518
- Unwanted effects 521

Benzodiazepine antagonists 523

Buspirone 523

Barbiturates 523

Other potential anxiolytic drugs 524

OVERVIEW

In this chapter, we discuss the nature of anxiety and the drugs used to treat it (anxiolytic drugs), as well as drugs used to treat insomnia (hypnotic drugs). Though the clinical objectives are different, there is some overlap between these two groups, reflecting the fact that anxiolytic drugs commonly cause a degree of sedation and drowsiness. There are, however, many sedative and hypnotic drugs that lack specific anxiolytic effects. In high doses, all of these drugs cause unconsciousness and, eventually, death from respiratory and cardiovascular depression. Benzodiazepines form the most important group, though anxiolytic and hypnotic drugs from an earlier era are still in use. In recent years, a number of drugs acting on 5-hydroxytryptamine (5-HT) receptors in the brain, which do not have strong sedative activity, have been introduced as anxiolytic agents. Possible new approaches, based on neuropeptide mediators, are also discussed briefly.

THE NATURE OF ANXIETY AND MEASUREMENT OF ANXIOLYTIC ACTIVITY

The normal *fear response* to threatening stimuli comprises several components, including defensive behaviours, autonomic reflexes, arousal and alertness, corticosteroid secretion and negative emotions. In *anxiety states*, these reactions occur in an anticipatory manner, independently of external events. The distinction between a 'pathological' and a 'normal' state of anxiety is not clear-cut but represents the point at which the symptoms interfere with normal productive activities. Despite (or perhaps because of) this loose distinction, anxiolytic drugs are among the most frequently prescribed substances, used regularly by upwards of 10% of the population in most developed countries.

Anxiety disorders as recognised clinically include:

- *generalised anxiety disorder* (an ongoing state of excessive anxiety lacking any clear reason or focus)
- *panic disorder* (attacks of overwhelming fear occurring in association with marked somatic symptoms, such as sweating, tachycardia, chest pains, trembling, choking, etc): such attacks can be induced even in normal individuals by infusion of sodium lactate, and the condition appears to have a genetic component
- *phobias* (strong fears of specific things or situations, e.g. snakes, open spaces, flying, social interactions)
- *Post-traumatic stress disorder* (anxiety triggered by insistent recall of past stressful experiences).

It should be stressed that the treatment of such disorders generally involves psychological approaches rather than, or in addition to, drug treatment. Furthermore, other types of drug, particularly antidepressants (Ch. 38) and sometimes antipsychotic drugs (Ch. 37), are often used to treat anxiety disorders, in addition to the anxiolytic drugs described here.

ANIMAL MODELS OF ANXIETY

▼ In addition to the subjective (emotional) component of human anxiety, there are measurable behavioural and physiological effects, which also occur in exerimental animals. In biological terms, anxiety induces a particular form of behavioural inhibition, which occurs in response to environmental events that are novel, non-rewarding (under conditions where reward is expected) or punishing. In animals, this behavioural inhibition may take the form of immobility, or suppression of a behavioural response such as bar-pressing to obtain food (see below). To develop new anxiolytic drugs, it is important to have animal tests that give a good guide to activity in humans, and much ingenuity has gone into developing and validating such tests.

For example, a rat placed in an unfamiliar environment normally responds by remaining immobile, though alert ('behavioural suppression'), for a time, which may represent 'anxiety' produced by the strange environment. This immobility is reduced if anxiolytic drugs are administered. The 'elevated cross-maze' is a widely used test model. Two arms of the raised horizontal cross are closed in, and the others are open. Normally rats spend most of their time in the closed arms and avoid the open arms (afraid, possibly, of falling off). Administration of anxiolytic drugs increases the time spent in the open arms and also increases the mobility of the rats, as judged by the frequency of crossing the intersection.

Conflict tests can also be used. For example, a rat trained to press a bar repeatedly to obtain a food pellet normally achieves a high and consistent response rate. A conflict element is then introduced: at intervals, indicated by an auditory signal, bar pressing results in an occasional 'punishment' in the form of an electric shock in addition to the reward of a food pellet. Normally, the rat ceases pressing the bar (behavioural inhibition), and thus avoids the shock, while the signal is sounding. The effect of an anxiolytic drug is to relieve this suppressive effect, so that the rats continue bar-pressing for reward in spite of the 'punishment'. Other types of psychotropic drug are not effective, nor are analgesic drugs. Other evidence confirms that anxiolytic drugs affect the level of behavioural inhibition produced by the conflict situation, rather than simply raising the pain threshold.

In other tests, aggressive behaviour is produced experimentally by lesions of the midbrain septum, or by housing mice in individual cages and then introducing a stranger. Anxiolytic drugs reduce the amount of aggressive behaviour displayed. They also increase the amount of 'social' interaction occurring between pairs of rats placed in an unfamiliar environment, this being a situation in which social interaction is greatly decreased in control animals. In many of these tests, the response is an increase in behavioural activity, so it is clear that the anxiolytic drugs are producing something more than a non-specific sedation.

TESTS ON HUMANS

Various 'anxiety scale' tests have been devised, based on standard patient questionnaires. These have confirmed the efficacy of many anxiolytic drugs, though placebo treatment often also produces highly significant responses.

Other tests rely on measurement of the somatic and autonomic effects associated with anxiety. An example is the galvanic skin response (GSR) in which the electrical conductivity of the skin is used as a measure of sweat production. Any novel stimulus, whether pleasant or unpleasant, causes a response. This forms the basis of the lie-detector test. If an innocuous stimulus is repeated at intervals, the magnitude of the response decreases (habituation). The rate of habituation is less in anxious patients than in normal subjects, and it is increased by anxiolytic drugs.

Measurement of anxiolytic activity

- Behavioural tests in animals are based on measurements of the behavioural inhibition (considered to reflect 'anxiety') in response to conflict or novelty.
- Human tests for anxiolytic drugs employ psychiatric rating scales or measures of autonomic responses, such as the galvanic skin response.
- Tests such as these can distinguish between anxiolytic drugs (benzodiazepines, buspirone, etc.) and sedatives (e.g. barbiturates).

A human version of the conflict test described above involves the substitution of money for food pellets, and the use of graded electric shocks as punishment. As with rats, administration of diazepam increases the rate of button-pressing for money during the periods when the punishment was in operation, though the subjects reported no change in the painfulness of the electric shock. Subtler forms of torment and reward are not hard to imagine.

CLASSIFICATION OF ANXIOLYTIC AND HYPNOTIC DRUGS

The main groups of drug (see review by Argyropoulos et al., 2000) are as follows.

- **Benzodiazepines** This is the most important group, used as anxiolytic and hypnotic agents.

Classes of anxiolytic and hypnotic drug

- Benzodiazepines, the most important class, are used for treating both anxiety states and insomnia.
- 5-HT_{1A}-receptor agonists have been recently introduced and show anxiolytic activity with little sedation.
- The β-adrenoceptor antagonists are used mainly to reduce physical symptoms of anxiety (tremor, palpitations, etc.); they have no effect on the affective component.
- Miscellaneous other agents (e.g. methaqualone, chloral hydrate) are still used occasionally to treat insomnia (benzodiazepines are preferable in most cases).
- Barbiturates are now largely obsolete as anxiolytic/sedative agents.

- **Buspirone** This 5-HT_{1A}-receptor agonist is anxiolytic but not appreciably sedative.
- The β-adrenoceptor antagonists (e.g. **propranolol**; Ch. 11) These are used to treat some forms of anxiety, particularly where physical symptoms, such as sweating, tremor and tachycardia, are troublesome. Their effectiveness depends on block of peripheral sympathetic responses rather than on any central effects. They are sometimes used by actors and musicians to reduce the symptoms of stage fright, but their use by snooker players to minimise tremor is banned as unsportsmanlike.
- **Barbiturates** These are now largely obsolete, superseded by benzodiazepines. Their use is now confined to anaesthesia (Ch. 35) and the treatment of epilepsy (Ch. 39).
- Miscellaneous other drugs (e.g. **chloral hydrate, meprobamate** and **methaqualone**). They are no longer recommended, but therapeutic habits die hard, and they are occasionally used. Sedative antihistamines (see Ch. 13), such as **diphenhydramine**, are sometimes used as sleeping pills, particularly for wakeful children.

BENZODIAZEPINES

The first benzodiazepine, **chlordiazepoxide**, was synthesised by accident in 1961, the unusual seven-membered ring having been produced as a result of an unplanned reaction in the laboratories of Hoffman la Roche. Its unexpected pharmacological activity was recognised in a routine screening procedure, and benzodiazepines quite soon became the most widely prescribed drugs in the pharmacopoeia.

CHEMISTRY AND STRUCTURE–ACTIVITY RELATIONSHIPS

The basic chemical structure of benzodiazepines consists of a seven-membered ring fused to an aromatic ring, with four main substituent groups that can be modified without loss of activity. Thousands of compounds have been made and tested, and about 20 are available for clinical use, the most important ones being listed in Table 36.1. They are basically similar in their pharmacological actions, though some degree of selectivity has

Table 36.1 Characteristics of benzodiazepines in humans

Drug	Half-life of parent compound (h)	Active metabolite	Half-life of metabolite (h)	Overall duration of action	Main uses
Triazolam,[a] midazolam	2–4	Hydroxylated derivative	2	Ultra-short (<6 h)	Hypnotic* Midazolam used as intravenous anaesthetic
Zolpidem[b]	2	No		Ultra-short (~ 4 h)	Hypnotic
Lorazepam, oxazepam, temazepam, lormetazepam	8–12	No		Short (12–18 h)	Anxiolytic, hypnotic
Alprazolam	6–12	Hydroxylated derivative	6	Medium (24 h)	Anxiolytic, antidepressant
Nitrazepam	16–40	No		Medium	Hypnotic, anxiolytic
Diazepam, chlordiazepoxide	20–40	Nordazepam	60	Long (24–48 h)	Anxiolytic, muscle relaxant Diazepam used intravenously as anticonvulsant
Flurazepam	1	Desmethyl-flurazepam	60	Long	Anxiolytic
Clonazepam	50	No		Long	Anticonvulsant, anxiolytic (especially mania)

[a]Triazolam has been withdrawn from use in UK on account of side-effects.
[b]Zolpidem is not a benzodiazepine but acts at the same site.

been reported. For example, some, such as **clonazepam,** show anticonvulsant activity with less-marked sedative effects.From a clinical point of view, differences in pharmacokinetic behaviour among different benzodiazepines (see below) are more important than differences in profile of activity. Drugs with a similar structure have been discovered that specifically antagonise the effects of the benzodiazepines, e.g. **flumazenil** (see below).

MECHANISM OF ACTION

Benzodiazepines (once thought, in the absence of evidence to the contrary, to be acting as 'non-specific depressants') act selectively on gamma-aminobutyric acid A ($GABA_A$) receptors (Ch. 32), which mediate fast inhibitory synaptic transmission throughout the central nervous system (CNS). Benzodiazepines enhance the response to GABA, by facilitating the opening of GABA-activated chloride channels (Fig. 36.1). They bind specifically to a regulatory site of the receptor, distinct from the GABA binding site, and act allosterically to increase the affinity of GABA for the receptor. Single channel recordings show an increase in the frequency of channel opening by a given concentration of GABA, but no change in the conductance or mean open time, consistent with an effect on GABA binding rather than the channel-gating mechanism. Benzodiazepines do not affect receptors for other amino acids, such as glycine or glutamate (Fig. 36.1).

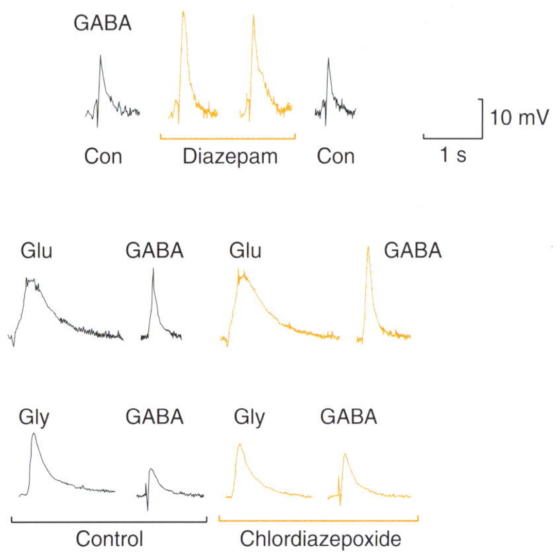

Fig. 36.1 Potentiating effect of benzodiazepines and chlordiazepoxide on the action of gamma-aminobutyric acid (GABA). Drugs were applied by ionophoresis to mouse spinal cord neurons grown in tissue culture, from micropipettes placed close to the cells. The membrane was hyperpolarised to −90 mV, and the cells were loaded with Cl^- from the recording microelectrode, so inhibitory amino acids (GABA and glycine), as well as excitatory ones (glutamate), caused depolarising responses. The potentiating effect of diazepam is restricted to GABA responses, glutamate and glycine responses being unaffected.

▼ The $GABA_A$-receptor is a ligand-gated ion channel (see Ch. 3) consisting of a pentameric assembly built from a collection of 18 or more different subunits. Many different combinations occur in different parts of the brain, and linking this diversity with physiological function and pharmacological specificity presents a difficult, though familiar, problem. Progress has recently been made, however, in understanding the effects of benzodiazepines at the molecular level (see Rudolph et al., 2001), which may point the way to novel drugs with more specific actions. The α-subunit of the pentameric complex occur in six isoforms (α_1–α_6) Mutation of a single amino acid (histidine 101) in the α-subunit eliminates benzodiazepine sensitivity. This has been used in an ingenious series of experiments on transgenic mice in which this residue has been mutated in four of the different α-subunits. The animals were then tested to determine which benzodiazepine effects were eliminated in these different mutants, with the interesting result that mutation of the α_1-subunit (the most widely expressed variant) eliminated the sedative and amnesia-producing actions of benzodiazepines, as well as diminishing the anticonvulsant effect, whereas mutation of α_2 (expressed mainly in the limbic system) eliminated the anxiolytic effect but left the sedative effect unaltered. Different benzodiazepine effects can thus be linked to different GABA receptor subtypes, raising the possibility of developing novel drugs with more selective effects than existing benzodiazepines, An important advance would be an α_2-selective compound with anxiolytic but not sedative actions.

Peripheral benzodiazepine binding sites, not associated with GABA receptors, are known to exist in many tissues, but their function and pharmacological significance are unknown.

PHARMACOLOGICAL EFFECTS AND USES

The main effects of benzodiazepines are:

- reduction of anxiety and aggression
- sedation and induction of sleep
- reduction of muscle tone and coordination
- anticonvulsant effect
- anterograde amnesia.

Reduction of anxiety and aggression

Benzodiazepines show anxiolytic effects in animal tests, as described above, and also exert a marked 'taming' effect, allowing animals to be handled more easily.* If given to the dominant member of a pair of animals (e.g. mice or monkeys) housed in the same cage, benzodiazepines reduce the number of attacks by the dominant individual and increase the number of attacks made upon him. With the possible exception of **alprazolam** (Table 36.1), benzodiazepines do not have antidepressant effects. Benzodiazepines may paradoxically produce an increase in irritability and aggression in some individuals. This appears to be particularly pronounced with the ultra-short-acting drug **triazolam** (and led to its withdrawal in the UK and some other countries) and is generally more common with short-acting compounds. It is probably a manifestation of the benzodiazepine withdrawal syndrome, which occurs with all of

*This depends on the species. Cats actually become more excitable, as a colleague of one of the authors discovered to his cost when attempting to sedate a tiger in the Baltimore zoo.

these drugs (see below) but is more acute with drugs that have an action that wears off rapidly.

Benzodiazepines are used mainly for treating acute anxiety states, but their use is declining in favour of antidepressants (Ch. 38), coupled with behavioural therapies in more severe cases.

The use of benzodiazepines as anxiolytic agents is reviewed by Shader & Greenblatt (1993).

Sedation and induction of sleep

Benzodiazepines decrease the time taken to get to sleep and increase the total duration of sleep, though the latter effect occurs only in subjects who normally sleep for less than about 6 hours each night. Both effects tend to decline when benzodiazepines are taken regularly for 1–2 weeks.

On the basis of electroencephalography measurements, several levels of sleep can be recognised. Of particular psychological importance is 'rapid eye movement' (REM) sleep, which is associated with dreaming, and 'slow wave' (SW) sleep, which corresponds to the deepest level of sleep when the metabolic rate and adrenal steroid secretion are at their lowest and the secretion of growth hormone is at its highest (see Ch. 27). All hypnotic drugs reduce the proportion of REM sleep, though benzodiazepines affect it less than other hypnotics. Artificial interruption of REM sleep causes irritability and anxiety, even if the total amount of sleep is not reduced, and the lost REM sleep is made up for at the end of such an experiment by a rebound increase. The same rebound in REM sleep is seen at the end of a period of administration of benzodiazepines or other hypnotics. It is, therefore, assumed that REM sleep has a beneficial function, and that the relatively slight reduction of REM sleep by benzodiazepines is a point in their favour.

The proportion of SW sleep is significantly reduced by benzodiazepines, though growth hormone secretion is unaffected.

Figure 36.2 shows the improvement of subjective ratings of sleep quality produced by a benzodiazepine, and the rebound decrease at the end of a 32-week period of drug treatment. It is notable that, though tolerance to objective effects such as reduced sleep latency occurs within a few days, this is not obvious in the subjective ratings.

Sedation appears to be a function of activity on $GABA_A$-receptors containing α_2-subunits (see above), so in theory it may be possible to develop non-sedating benzodiazepines that retain anxiolytic and/or anticonvulsant effects, but this has not yet been achieved.

Though long-term use of benzodiazepines as sleeping pills is undesirable, owing to tolerance, dependence and hangover effects, occasional use (e.g. by shift-workers, plane travellers, etc.) is effective.

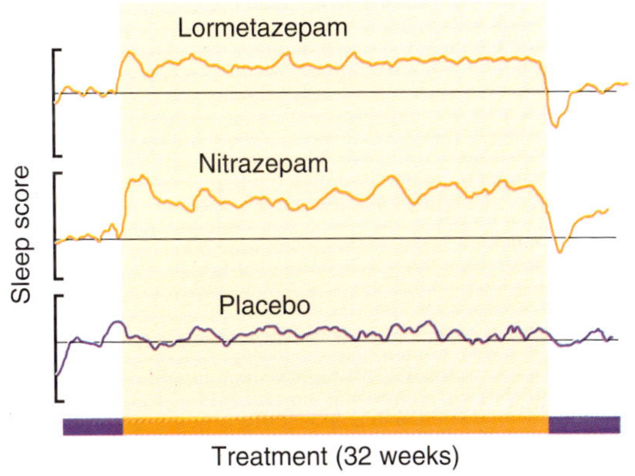

Fig. 36.2 Effects of long-term benzodiazepine treatment on sleep quality. A group of 100 poor sleepers were given, under double-blind conditions, lormetazepam 5 mg, nitrazepam 2 mg, or placebo nightly for 24 weeks, the test period being preceded and followed by 4 weeks of placebo treatment. They were asked to assess, on a subjective rating scale, the quality of sleep during each night and the results are expressed as a 5-day rolling average of these scores. The improvement in sleep quality was maintained during the 24-week test period, and was followed by a 'rebound' worsening of sleep when the test period ended. (From: Oswald I et al. 1982 Br Med J 284: 860–864.)

Reduction of muscle tone and coordination

Benzodiazepines reduce muscle tone by a central action that is independent of their sedative effect. Cats are particularly sensitive to this action, and some benzodiazepines (e.g. **clonazepam**, **flunitrazepam**) reduce decerebrate rigidity in doses that are much smaller than those needed to produce behavioural effects. In other species, the effect is less clear. Coordination can be tested by measuring the length of time for which mice can stay on a slowly rotating horizontal plastic rod, or the time taken for them to escape from confinement by climbing up the inside of a tubular chimney. Performance in these acrobatic tricks is impaired by benzodiazepines and other sedatives, but it is not clear that particular drugs show selectivity in this respect in species other than the cat. Studies in humans have failed to show differences between benzodiazepines.

Increased muscle tone is a common feature of anxiety states in humans and may contribute to the aches and pains, including headache, that often trouble anxious patients. The relaxant effect of benzodiazepines may, therefore, be clinically useful. A reduction of muscle tone appears to be possible without appreciable loss of coordination. Other clinical uses of muscle relaxants are discussed in Chapter 39.

Anticonvulsant effects

All of the benzodiazepines have anticonvulsant activity in experimental animal tests. They are highly effective against chemically induced convulsions caused by **leptazol**, **bicuculline** and similar drugs (see Chs 39 and 41) but less so against electrically induced convulsions. Benzodiazepines do not affect strychnine-induced convulsions in experimental animals. Both bicuculline and strychnine are believed to act by blocking the action of inhibitory transmitters in the CNS; strychnine exerts its effect on glycine receptors (see Ch. 38), whereas bicuculline and several other chemical convulsant agents act on $GABA_A$-receptors (Ch. 29). Since benzodiazepines enhance the action of GABA but not glycine, the selectivity of their anticonvulsant action is explicable. **Clonazepam** (see above), because of its selective anticonvulsant action, is used to treat epilepsy (Ch. 39), as is **diazepam**, which is given intravenously to control life-threatening seizures in *status epilepticus*.

Anterograde amnesia

Benzodiazepines obliterate memory of events experienced while under their influence, an effect not seen with other CNS depressants. Minor surgical procedures can thus be performed without leaving unpleasant memories.

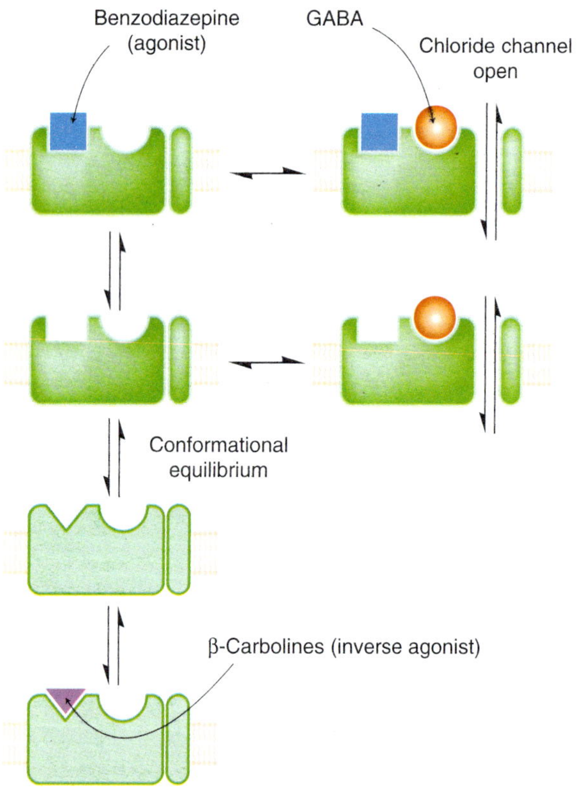

Fig 36.3 Model of benzodiazepine/gamma-aminobutyric acid (GABA) receptor interaction. Benzodiazepine agonists (e.g. diazepam) and antagonists (e.g. flumazenil) are believed to bind to a site on the GABA receptor distinct from the GABA-binding site. A conformational equilibrium exists between states in which the benzodiazepine receptor exists in its agonist-binding conformation (above) and in its antagonist-binding conformation (below). In the latter state, the GABA receptor has a much reduced affinity for GABA; consequently, the chloride channel remains closed.

IS THERE AN ENDOGENOUS BENZODIAZEPINE-LIKE MEDIATOR?

▼ Whether there is an endogenous ligand for the benzodiazepine receptors, whose function is to regulate the action of GABA, is still uncertain. The main candidate is a 10 kDa peptide, *diazepam-binding inhibitor* (DBI), isolated from rat brain. This peptide binds strongly to the benzodiazepine binding site of the $GABA_A$-receptor and has the opposite effect to benzodiazepines, i.e. it inhibits chloride channel opening by GABA and, when injected into the brain, has an anxiogenic and proconvulsant effect. Other possible endogenous modulators of $GABA_A$-receptors include steroid metabolites (see Ch. 32). There is also evidence that benzodiazepines themselves may occur naturally in the brain. At present, there is no general agreement on the identity and function of an endogenous ligand.

BENZODIAZEPINE INVERSE AGONISTS AND ANTAGONISTS

▼ The term 'inverse agonist' (Ch. 2) is applied to drugs that bind to benzodiazepine receptors and exert the opposite effect to that of conventional benzodiazepines, producing signs of increased anxiety and convulsions. DBI is an example, and some benzodiazepine analogues act similarly. It is possible (see Fig. 36.3) to explain these complexities in terms of the two-state model discussed in Chapter 2, by postulating that the benzodiazepine receptor exists in two distinct conformations, only one of which (A) can bind a GABA molecule and open the chloride channel. The other conformation (B) cannot bind GABA. Normally, with no benzodiazepine receptor ligand present, there is an equilibrium between these two conformations; sensitivity to GABA is present, but submaximal. Benzodiazepine agonists (e.g. diazepam) are postulated to bind preferentially to conformation A, thus shifting the equilibrium in favour of A and enhancing GABA sensitivity. Inverse agonists bind selectively to B and have the opposite effect. Competitive antagonists, such as **flumazenil** (see below), bind equally to A and B and consequently do not disturb the conformational equilibrium but antagonise the effect of both agonists and inverse agonists. Some of the molecular variants of the $GABA_A$-receptor (see above) seem to show different relative affinities for agonists, antagonists and inverse agonists, and it is possible that this reflects differences in the equilibrium between the A and B states as a function of the subunit composition of the receptor.

PHARMACOKINETIC ASPECTS

Benzodiazepines are well absorbed when given orally, usually giving a peak plasma concentration in about 1 hour. Some (e.g. **oxazepam**, **lorazepam**) are absorbed more slowly. They bind strongly to plasma protein, and their high lipid solubility causes many of them to accumulate gradually in body fat. These two factors result in distribution volumes not far from 1 l/kg body weight for most benzodiazepines. They are normally given by mouth but can be given intravenously (e.g. **diazepam** in status epilepticus, **midazolam** in anaesthesia). Intramuscular injection often results in slow absorption.

Benzodiazepines are all metabolised, and they are eventually excreted as glucuronide conjugates in the urine. They vary greatly in duration of action, and can be roughly divided into short-, medium- and long-acting compounds (Table 36.1). Several are converted to active metabolites, such as *N*-desmethyldiazepam (nordazepam), which has a half-life of about 60 hours, and which accounts for the tendency of many benzodiazepines to produce cumulative effects and long hangovers when they are given at regular intervals. The short-acting compounds are those that are metabolised directly by conjugation with glucuronide. The main pathways are shown in Figure 36.4. Figure 36.5 shows the gradual build-up and slow disappearance of nordazepam from the plasma of a human subject given diazepam daily for 15 days.

Advancing age affects the rate of oxidative reactions more than that of conjugation reactions. Thus the effect of the long-acting benzodiazepines, which may be used regularly as hypnotics or anxiolytic agents for many years, tends to increase with age, and it is common for drowsiness and confusion to develop insidiously for this reason.*

*At the age of 91, the grandmother of one of the authors was growing increasingly forgetful and mildly dotty, having been taking nitrazepam for insomnia regularly for years. To the author's lasting shame, it took a canny general practitioner to diagnose the problem. Cancellation of the nitrazepam prescription produced a dramatic improvement.

UNWANTED EFFECTS

Unwanted effects may be divided into:

- toxic effects resulting from acute overdosage
- unwanted effects occurring during normal therapeutic use
- tolerance and dependence.

Acute toxicity

Benzodiazepines in acute overdose are considerably less dangerous than most other anxiolytic/hypnotic drugs. Since such agents are often used in attempted suicide, this is an important advantage. In overdose, benzodiazepines cause prolonged sleep, without serious depression of respiration or cardiovascular function. However, in the presence of other CNS depressants, particularly alcohol, benzodiazepines can cause severe, even life-threatening, respiratory depression. The availability of an

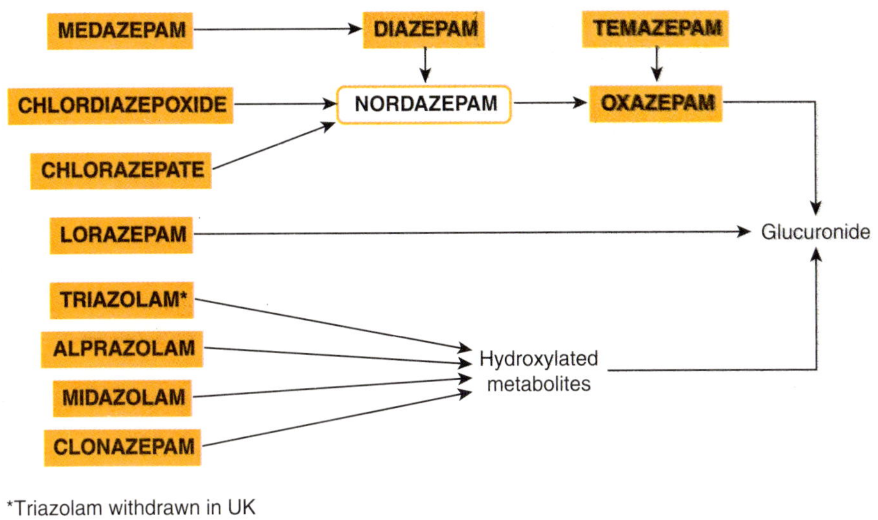

Fig. 36.4 The metabolism of benzodiazepines. The N-demethylated metabolite nordazepam is formed from a number of benzodiazepines and is important because it is biologically active and has a very long half-life. Compounds with pharmacological activity are shown in blue. Drugs available for clinical use are shown in shaded boxes.

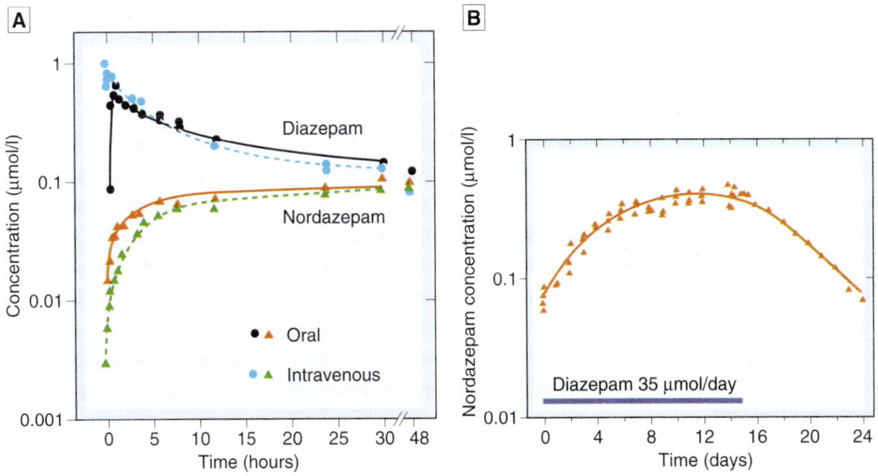

Fig. 36.5 Pharmacokinetics of diazepam in humans. [A] Concentrations of diazepam and nordazepam following a single oral or intravenous dose. Note the very slow disappearance of both substances after the first 20 hours. [B] Accumulation of nordazepam during 2 weeks' daily administration of diazepam, and slow decline (half-life about 3 days) after cessation of diazepam administration. (Data from: Kaplan S A et al. 1973 J Pharmacol Sci 62: 1789.)

effective antagonist, **flumazenil**, means that the effects of an acute overdose can be counteracted,* which is not possible for most CNS depressants.

Side-effects during therapeutic use

The main side-effects of benzodiazepines are drowsiness, confusion, amnesia and impaired coordination, which considerably affects manual skills such as driving performance. Benzodiazepines enhance the depressant effect of other drugs, including alcohol, in a more than additive way. The long and unpredictable duration of action of many benzodiazepines is important in relation to side-effects. Long-acting drugs such as nitrazepam are no longer used as hypnotics, and even shorter-acting compounds such as lorazepam can produce a substantial day-after impairment of job performance and driving skill.

Tolerance and dependence

Tolerance (i.e. a gradual escalation of dose needed to produce the required effect) occurs with all benzodiazepines, as does *dependence*, which is their main drawback. They share these properties with other hypnotics and sedatives. Tolerance is less marked than it is with barbiturates, which produce pharmacokinetic tolerance because of induction of hepatic drug-metabolising enzymes—this does not occur with benzodiazepines. Such tolerance as does occur appears to represent a change at the receptor level, but the mechanism is not well understood.

The sleep-inducing effect shows relatively little tolerance (Fig. 36.2). In a study with intravenous diazepam given to normal subjects, its euphoric effect was not present in those taking oral diazepam daily. It is not clear whether tolerance to the anxiolytic effect is significant.

Benzodiazepines produce dependence, and this is a major problem. In human subjects and patients, stopping benzodiazepine treatment after weeks or months causes an increase in symptoms of anxiety, together with tremor and dizziness. Though animals show only a weak tendency to self-administration of benzodiazepines, withdrawal after chronic administration causes physical symptoms similar to those that follow opiate withdrawal (see Ch. 42), namely nervousness, tremor, loss of appetite and sometimes convulsions.** The withdrawal syndrome, in both animals and humans, is slower in onset than with barbiturates, probably because of the long plasma half-life of most benzodiazepines. Short-acting benzodiazepines cause more abrupt withdrawal effects. With **triazolam**, a very short-acting drug and no longer in use, the withdrawal effect occurred within a few hours, even after a single dose, producing early-morning insomnia and daytime anxiety when the drug was used as a hypnotic.

The physical and psychological withdrawal symptoms make it difficult for patients to give up taking benzodiazepines, but *addiction* (i.e. severe psychological dependence which outlasts the physical withdrawal syndrome), which occurs with many drugs of abuse (Ch. 42), is not a major problem.

*In practice, patients are usually left to sleep it off, since there is a risk of seizures with flumazenil; however, flumazenil may be useful diagnostically to exclude coma of other causes.

**Withdrawal symptoms can be more severe. A relative of one of the authors, advised to stop taking benzodiazepines after 20 years, suffered hallucinations, and one day tore down all the curtains, convinced that they were on fire.

Benzodiazepines

- Act by binding to a specific regulatory site on the $GABA_A$-receptor, thus enhancing the inhibitory effect of GABA. Subtypes of the $GABA_A$-receptor exist in different regions of the brain and differ in their sensitivity to benzodiazepines.
- Anxiolytic benzodiazepines are agonists at this regulatory site. Other benzodiazepines (e.g. flumazenil) are antagonists and prevent the actions of the anxiolytic benzodiazepines. A further class of inverse agonists is recognised, which reduce the effectiveness of GABA and are anxiogenic; they are not used clinically.
- Endogenous ligands for the benzodiazepine-binding site are believed to exist. They include peptide and steroid molecules, but their physiological function is not yet understood.
- Benzodiazepines cause:
  —reduction of anxiety and aggression
  —sedation, leading to improvement of insomnia
  —muscle relaxation and loss of motor coordination
  —suppression of convulsions (antiepileptic effect)
  —anterograde amnesia.
- Differences in the pharmacological profile of different benzodiazepines are minor; clonazepam appears to have more anticonvulsant action in relation to its other effects. Different $GABA_A$-receptor isoforms are believed to mediate sedative and anxiolytic effects.
- Benzodiazepines are active orally and differ mainly in respect of their duration of action. Short-acting agents (e.g. lorazepam and temazepam, half-lives 8–12 hours) are metabolised to inactive compounds and are used mainly as sleeping pills. Some long-acting agents (e.g. diazepam and chlordiazepoxide) are converted to a long-lasting active metabolite (nordazepam).
- Some are used intravenously, e.g. diazepam in status epilepticus; midazolam in anaesthesia.
- Zolpidem is a short-acting drug that is not a benzodiazepine but acts similarly.
- Benzodiazepines are relatively safe in overdose. Their main disadvantages are interaction with alcohol, long-lasting hangover effects, withdrawal symptoms and the development of dependence.

BENZODIAZEPINE ANTAGONISTS

Competitive antagonists of benzodiazepines were first discovered in 1981. The best-known compound is **flumazenil**. This compound was originally reported to lack effects on behaviour or on drug-induced convulsions when given on its own, though it was later found to possess some 'anxiogenic' and proconvulsant activity. Flumazenil can be used to reverse the effect of benzodiazepine overdosage (normally used only if respiration is severely depressed) or to reverse the effect of benzodiazepines such as midazolam used for minor surgical procedures. Flumazenil acts quickly and effectively when given by injection, but its action lasts for only about 2 hours, so drowsiness tends to return. It is often used in treating comatose patients suspected of having overdosed with benzodiazepines even before the diagnosis is confirmed on the basis of a blood sample. Convulsions may rarely occur in patients treated with flumazenil, and this is more common in patients receiving tricyclic antidepressants (Ch. 38). Reports that flumazenil improves the mental state of patients with severe liver disease (hepatic encephalopathy) and alcohol intoxication have not been confirmed in controlled trials.

BUSPIRONE

Buspirone is a partial agonist at 5-HT_{1A}-receptors (Ch. 12) used to treat various anxiety disorders. It also binds to dopamine receptors, but it is likely that its 5-HT-related actions are important in relation to anxiety suppression, since related anxiolytic compounds (e.g. **ipsapirone** and **gepirone**; see Traber & Glaser, 1987) show high specificity for 5-HT_{1A}-receptors, which are inhibitory autoreceptors that reduce the release of 5-HT and other mediators. They also inhibit the activity of noradrenergic locus ceruleus neurons (Ch. 33) and, thus, interfere with arousal reactions. However, buspirone takes days or weeks to produce its effect in humans, suggesting a more complex indirect mechanism of action. Buspirone is ineffective in controlling panic attacks.

Buspirone, ipsapirone and gepirone have side-effects quite different from those of benzodiazepines. They do not cause sedation or motor incoordination, nor have withdrawal effects been reported. Their main side-effects are nausea, dizziness, headache and restlessness, which generally seem to be less troublesome than the side-effects of benzodiazepines.

5-HT_{1A} agonists as anxiolytic drugs

- Buspirone is a potent (though non-selective) agonist at 5-HT_{1A}-receptors.
- Ipsapirone and gepirone are similar.
- Anxiolytic effects take days or weeks to develop.
- Side-effects appear less troublesome than with benzodiazepines; they include dizziness, nausea, headache, but not sedation or loss of coordination.

BARBITURATES

The sleep-inducing properties of barbiturates were discovered early in the 20th century, and hundreds of compounds were made and tested. Until the 1960s, they formed the largest group of hypnotics and sedatives in clinical use. Barbiturates all have depressant activity on the CNS, producing effects similar to those of inhalation anaesthetics. They cause death from respiratory and cardiovascular depression if given in large doses, which is one of the main reasons that they are now little used as anxiolytic and hypnotic agents. **Pentobarbital** and similar typical barbiturates with a duration of action of 6–12 hours are still very occasionally used as sleeping pills and anxiolytic drugs, but they are less safe than benzodiazepines. Pentobarbital is often used as an anaesthetic for laboratory animals.

Barbiturates that remain in widespread use are those which have specific properties, such as **phenobarbital**, used for its anticonvulsant activity (see Ch. 39), and **thiopental**, which is widely used as an intravenous anaesthetic agent (see Ch. 35).

Barbiturates share with benzodiazepines the ability to enhance the action of GABA, but they bind to a different site on the GABA_A-receptor/chloride channel, and their action is less specific.

Apart from the risk of dangerous overdose, the main disadvantages of barbiturates are that they induce a high degree of tolerance and dependence, and that they strongly induce the synthesis of hepatic cytochrome P450 and conjugating enzymes, thus increasing the rate of metabolic degradation of many other drugs and giving rise to a number of potentially troublesome drug interactions (Ch. 51). Because of enzyme induction, barbiturates are also dangerous to patients suffering from the metabolic disease porphyria.

Barbiturates

- Barbiturates are non-selective CNS depressants that produce effects ranging from sedation and reduction of anxiety to unconsciousness and death from respiratory and cardiovascular failure. Therefore, they are dangerous in overdose.
- They act partly by enhancing action of GABA but are less specific than benzodiazepines.
- Barbiturates are mainly used in anaesthesia and treatment of epilepsy; use as sedative/hypnotic agents is no longer recommended.
- They are potent inducers of hepatic drug-metabolising enzymes, especially cytochrome P450 system, so are liable to cause drug interactions. They also precipitate attacks of acute porphyria in susceptible individuals.
- Tolerance and dependence occur.

OTHER POTENTIAL ANXIOLYTIC DRUGS

▼ Besides the $GABA_A$- and $5\text{-}HT_{1A}$-receptor mechanisms discussed above, many other transmitters and receptors have been implicated in anxiety and panic disorders (see Sandford et al., 2000), particularly noradrenaline, and neuropeptides such as cholecystokinin (CCK) and substance P. Anxiolytic drugs aimed at these targets are in development, but none is so far available for clinical use.

$5\text{-}HT_3$-receptor antagonists, such as **ondansetron** (Ch. 15), show anxiolytic activity in animal models but have not proved efficacious in controlled human trials. As mentioned earlier, 5-HT uptake inhibitors, such as **fluoxetine**, and mixed 5-HT/noradrenaline uptake inhibitors, which are used as antidepressant drugs (Ch. 38), also show efficacy in anxiety disorders.

Antagonists to the neuropeptide CCK (see Ch. 13) have been tested as anxiolytic drugs. CCK, which is expressed in many areas of the brainstem and midbrain that are involved in arousal, mood and emotion, has been considered as a possible mediator of panic attacks, but non-peptide CCK antagonists have proved ineffective in clinical trials.

REFERENCES AND FURTHER READING

Argyropoulos S V, Sandford J J, Nutt D J 2000 The psychobiology of anxiolytic drugs. Part 2: pharmacological treatments of anxiety. Pharmacol Therapeu 88: 213–227 (*General review article on clinically used anxiolytic drugs*)

Rudolph U, Crestani F, Möhler H 2001 $GABA_A$ receptor subtypes: dissecting their pharmacological functions. Trends Pharmacol Sci 22: 188–194 (*Describes recent work with transgenic mice expressing mutated $GABA_A$-receptors, suggesting that anxiolytic and sedative actions of benzodiazepines may be separable*)

Sandford J J, Argyropoulos S V, Nutt D J 2000 The psychobiology of anxiolytic drugs. Part 1: basic neurobiology. Pharmacol Ther 88: 197–212 (*Explains brain mechanisms thought to underly actions of anxiolytic drugs*)

Shader R I, Greenblatt D J 1993 Use of benzodiazepines in anxiety disorders. N Engl J Med 328: 1398–1405

Traber J, Glaser T 1987 $5\text{-}HT_{1A}$ receptor-related anxiolytics. Trends Pharmacol Sci 8: 432–437

Antipsychotic drugs

37

Overview 525

The nature of schizophrenia 525
— Aetiology and pathogenesis of schizophrenia 526

Antipsychotic drugs 528
— Classification of antipsychotic drugs 528
— General properties 528
— Mechanism of action 528
— Pharmacological effects 530
— Pharmacokinetic aspects 533
— Clinical use and clinical efficacy 533

OVERVIEW

In this chapter, we focus on schizophrenia and the drugs used to treat it. We start by describing the illness and what is known of its pathogenesis, including the various neurochemical hypotheses and their relation to the actions of the main types of antipsychotic drug that are in use or in development.

Psychotic illnesses include various disorders, but the term antipsychotic drugs—also known as neuroleptic drugs, antischizophrenic drugs, or major tranquillisers—conventionally refers to those used to treat schizophrenia, one of the most common and debilitating forms of florid mental illness. Pharmacologically, they are characterised as dopamine receptor antagonists, though many of them also act on other targets, particularly 5-hydroxytryptamine (5-HT) receptors, which may contribute to their clinical efficacy. Existing drugs have many drawbacks in terms of their efficacy and side-effects. Gradual improvements are being achieved as new drugs are developed, but radical new approaches will probably have to wait until we have a better understanding of the biological nature of the disease, which is still poorly understood.*

THE NATURE OF SCHIZOPHRENIA

Schizophrenia (see Lewis & Lieberman, 2000) affects about 1% of the population. It is one of the most important forms of psychiatric illness, because it affects young people, is often chronic and usually highly disabling. There is a strong hereditary factor in its aetiology, and evidence suggestive of a fundamental biological disorder (see below). The main clinical features of the disease are:

- **positive symptoms**:
  —delusions (often paranoid in nature)
  —hallucinations, usually in the form of voices, and often exhortatory in their message
  —thought disorder, comprising wild trains of thought, garbled sentences and irrational conclusions, sometimes associated with the feeling that thoughts are inserted or withdrawn by an outside agency
  —abnormal behaviours, such as stereotyped or occasionally aggressive behaviours.
- **negative symptoms**:
  —withdrawal from social contacts
  —flattening of emotional responses.

In addition, deficits in cognitive function (e.g. attention, memory) are often present, together with anxiety and depression, leading to suicide in about 10% of cases. The clinical phenotype varies greatly, particularly with respect to the balance between negative and positive symptoms, and this may have a bearing on the efficacy of antipsychotic drugs in individual cases.

▼ A characteristic feature of schizophrenia is a defect in 'selective attention'. Whereas a normal individual quickly accommodates to stimuli of a familiar or inconsequential nature and responds only to stimuli that are unexpected or significant, the ability of schizophrenic patients to discriminate between significant and insignificant stimuli seems to be impaired. For example, the ticking of a clock may command as much attention as the words of a companion; a chance thought, which a normal person would dismiss as inconsequential, may become an irresistible

*In this respect, it is interesting that the study of schizophrenia lags some years behind that of Alzheimer's disease (Ch. 34), where understanding of the pathogenesis has progressed rapidly to the point where promising new drug targets can be identified. In spite of this, pragmatists can argue that drugs against Alzheimer's disease are so far only marginally effective, whereas current antipsychotic drugs deliver great benefits, even though we do not quite know how they work.

imperative. 'Latent inhibition' is a form of behavioural testing in animals that can be used as a model for this type of sensory habituation. If a rat is exposed to a 'conditioned' stimulus (such as a bell), followed by an 'unconditioned' stimulus (e.g. a foot shock), which it can avoid (e.g. by pressing a bar), it will quickly learn to press the bar as soon as it hears the bell—the conditioned response. However, if it has previously heard the bell several times without any ensuing foot shock, it will learn the conditioned response less quickly, having learned to disregard the bell. Latent inhibition is a measure of the inhibitory effect of pre-exposure to the conditioned stimulus on acquisition of the conditioned response. It is often impaired in schizophrenic subjects and in animals treated with amphetamine, or psychotomimetic drugs such as lysergic acid diethylamide (LSD), and is restored by many antipsychotic drugs.

Schizophrenia often begins in adolescence or young adult life; it can follow a relapsing and remitting course, or be chronic and progressive, particularly in cases with a later onset. Chronic schizophrenia used to account for most of the patients in long-stay psychiatric hospitals; following the closure of many of these in the UK, it now accounts for many of society's outcasts.

AETIOLOGY AND PATHOGENESIS OF SCHIZOPHRENIA

GENETIC AND ENVIRONMENTAL FACTORS

The cause of schizophrenia remains unclear, but it involves a combination of genetic and environmental factors (see Lewis & Lieberman, 2000). The disease shows a strong, but incomplete, hereditary tendency. In first-degree relatives, the risk is about 10%; even in monozygotic twins, one of whom has schizophrenia, the probability of the other being affected is only about 50%. Genetic linkage studies aimed at identifying schizophrenia susceptibility genes have identified likely chromosomes, but not yet any specific genes. Some environmental influences early in development have been identified as possible predisposing factors, including maternal virus infections and high blood pressure during pregnancy. This and other evidence suggests that schizophrenia is associated with a neurodevelopmental disorder, affecting mainly the cerebral cortex, and occurring in the first few months of prenatal development (see Harrison, 1997). This view is supported by brain imaging studies showing cortical atrophy, with enlargement of the cerebral ventricles. These structural changes are present in schizophrenic patients presenting for the first time and are probably not progressive, suggesting that they represent an early irreversible aberration in brain development rather than a gradual neurodegeneration. Studies of postmortem schizophrenic brains show evidence of misplaced cortical neurons with abnormal morphology. Psychological factors, such as stress, may precipitate acute episodes but are not the underlying cause.

NEUROCHEMICAL THEORIES

Current ideas about the neurochemical mechanisms in schizophrenia came from analysing the effects of antipsychotic and propsychotic drugs—from pharmacology rather than from neurochemistry. Instead of neurochemical theory providing the basis for rational drug treatment, the opposite occurred: drugs found by chance to be effective have provided the main clues about the nature of the disorder. Indeed, an intensive search for neurochemical abnormalities in schizophrenia proved frustrating for many years, no biochemical markers being found either in postmortem brain material or in other samples from living patients. Only recently (see below) have imaging studies proved more successful in detecting neurochemical abnormalities.

The main neurochemical theories centre on dopamine and glutamate, though other mediators, particularly 5-HT, are also receiving attention.

Dopamine theory

The dopamine theory was proposed by Carlsson—awarded a Nobel prize in 2000—on the basis of indirect pharmacological evidence in humans and experimental animals. **Amphetamine** releases dopamine in the brain and can produce in humans a behavioural syndrome indistinguishable from an acute schizophrenic episode—very familiar to doctors who treat drug users. In animals, dopamine release causes a specific pattern of stereotyped behaviour, which resembles the repetitive behaviours sometimes seen in schizophrenic patients. Potent D_2-receptor agonists (e.g. **apomorphine** and **bromocriptine**; Ch. 33) produce similar effects in animals, and these drugs, like amphetamine, exacerbate the symptoms of schizophrenic patients. Furthermore, dopamine antagonists and drugs that block neuronal dopamine storage (e.g. **reserpine**) are effective in controlling the positive symptoms of schizophrenia, and in preventing amphetamine-induced behavioural changes. There is a strong correlation between clinical antipsychotic potency and activity in blocking D_2-receptors (Fig. 37.1), and receptor imaging studies have shown that clinical efficacy of antipsychotic drugs is consistently achieved when D_2-receptor occupancy reaches about 80%.

▼ There is no consistent biochemical evidence for excessive dopamine synthesis or release in schizophrenia. Furthermore, the production of prolactin, which might be expected to be abnormally low if dopaminergic transmission was facilitated, is normal in schizophrenic patients. One difficulty in interpreting such studies is that nearly all schizophrenic patients are treated with drugs that are known to affect dopamine metabolism, whereas the non-schizophrenic control group are not. Even where it has been possible to allow for this factor, however, the results are still generally negative. A well-controlled study by Reynolds (1983), however, showed a raised dopamine content postmortem in the amygdala of schizophrenic subjects, the noradrenaline content being normal. The best evidence for increased dopamine release in schizophrenic patients comes from imaging studies (Laruelle et al., 1999). A radioligand imaging technique was used to measure binding of a specific antagonist (**raclopride**) to D_2-receptors in the striatum. Injection of amphetamine caused dopamine release, and thus displacement of raclopride, measured as a reduction of the signal intensity. This reduction was greater by a factor of two or more in schizophrenic compared with control subjects, implying a greater amphetamine-induced release of dopamine. The effect was greatest in schizophrenics during acute attacks, and absent during spontaneous remissions—clear evidence linking dopamine release to the symptomatology.

An increase in dopamine receptor density in schizophrenia has been reported in some studies, but not consistently, and the interpretation is complicated by the fact that antipsychotic drug treatment is known to increase dopamine receptor expression.

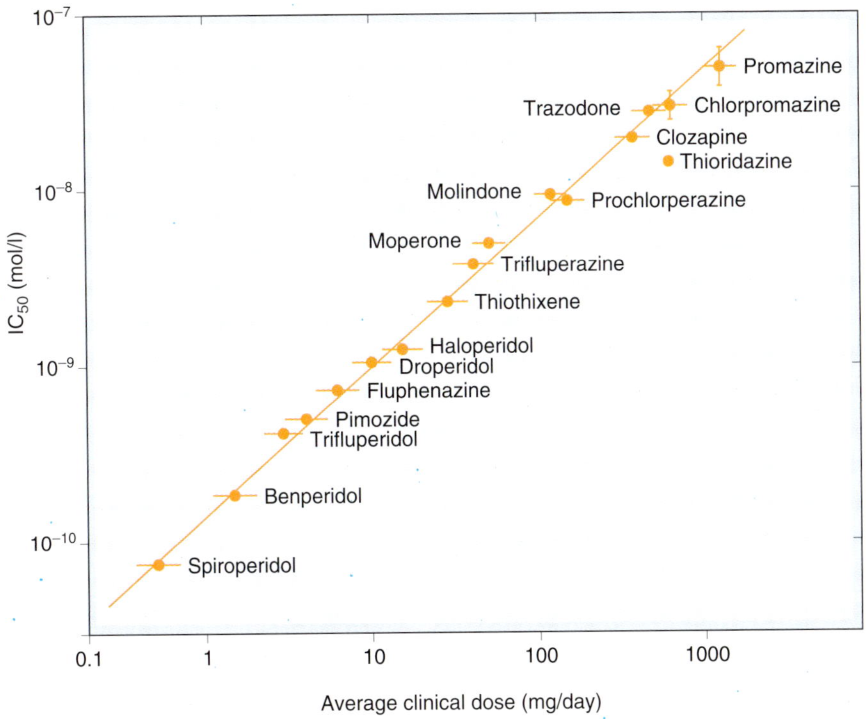

Fig. 37.1 Correlation between the clinical potency and affinity for dopamine D_2-receptors among neuroleptic drugs. Clinical potency is expressed as the daily dose used in treating schizophrenia, and binding activity is expressed as the concentration needed to produce 50% inhibition of haloperidol binding. (From: Seeman P et al. 1976 Nature 361:717.)

The D_4-receptor has also attracted attention on account of the high degree of genetic polymorphism that it shows in human subjects, and because some of the newer antipsychotic drugs (e.g. **clozapine**; see below) turn out to have a high affinity for this receptor subtype. Genetic studies have, however, failed to show any relationship between schizophrenia and D_4-receptor polymorphism. Moreover, a specific D_4-receptor antagonist proved ineffective in clinical trials.

Glutamate theory

Another transmitter implicated in the pathophysiology of schizophrenia is—you will not be surprised to learn—glutamate (see Goff & Coyle, 2001). The glutamate NMDA (N-methyl-D-asparate) receptor antagonists, such as **phencyclidine**, **ketamine** and **dizocilpine** (Ch. 32), produce psychotic symptoms (e.g. hallucinations, thought disorder) in humans, and reduced glutamate concentrations and glutamate receptor densities have been reported in postmortem brains of schizophrenics—one of the few fairly consistent findings.

▼ Though schizophrenia is difficult to diagnose in a mouse, transgenic mice in which NMDA receptor expression is reduced (not abolished, since this is fatal) show stereotypic behaviours and reduced social interaction that are suggestive of schizophrenia, and which respond to antipsychotic drugs—evidence which supports the glutamate hypothesis. According to this view, glutamate and dopamine exert excitatory and inhibitory effects, respectively, on GABA-ergic striatal neurons, which project to the thalamus and constitute a sensory 'gate' (see below). Too little glutamate, or too much dopamine, disables the gate, allowing uninhibited sensory input to reach the cortex.

Other theories

Other transmitters that may be important include 5-HT and noradrenaline. The idea that 5-HT dysfunction could be involved in schizophrenia was based on the fact that LSD (see Ch. 41) produces schizophrenia-like symptoms, and this idea has drifted in and out of favour many times (see Busatto & Kerwin, 1997).

Many effective antipsychotic drugs, in addition to blocking dopamine receptors (see below), also act as 5-HT receptor antagonists. 5-HT has a modulatory effect on dopamine pathways, so the two theories are not incompatible. Affinity for $5\text{-}HT_{2A}$-receptors is a feature of many of the recently developed 'atypical' antipsychotic drugs (see below), which produce fewer extrapyramidal side-effects than the earlier dopamine-selective compounds, Controversy exists as to whether the $5\text{-}HT_2$-receptor block contributes to the antipsychotic effect or merely reduces the undesirable side-effects associated with D_2-receptor antagonists.

Summary

In conclusion, the dopamine hyperactivity theory of schizophrenia is supported by considerable evidence. Though it is undoubtedly an oversimplification, and relates only to the positive symptoms, it provides the best framework for understanding the action of antipsychotic drugs, though effects on 5-HT and other receptors may contribute significantly to the clinical profile of some of the newer drugs. (See Jones & Pilowski (2002) and Strange (1999) for current status.)

The nature of schizophrenia

- Schizophrenia psychotic illness is characterised by delusions, hallucinations and thought disorder (positive symptoms), together with social withdrawal, flattening of emotional responses and cognitive impairment (negative symptoms).
- Acute episodes (mainly positive symptoms) frequently recur and develop into chronic schizophrenia, with predominantly negative symptoms.
- Incidence is about 1% of population, with a strong, but not invariable, hereditary component.
- Pharmacological evidence is generally consistent with dopamine overactivity hypothesis, supported by biochemical findings and imaging studies.
- There is also evidence for involvement of glutamate and 5-HT.

Classification of antipsychotic drugs

- Main categories are:
  - —classical *'typical' antipsychotics* (e.g. chlorpromazine, haloperidol, fluphenazine, thioridazine, flupenthixol, clopenthixol)
  - —recent 'atypical' antipsychotics (e.g. clozapine, risperidone, sertindole, quetiapine)
- Distinction between typical and atypical groups is not clearly defined, but rests on:
  - —receptor profile
  - —incidence of extrapyramidal side-effects (less in atypical group)
  - —efficacy in treatment-resistant group of patients
  - —efficacy against negative symptoms.

ANTIPSYCHOTIC DRUGS

CLASSIFICATION OF ANTIPSYCHOTIC DRUGS

More than 20 different antipsychotic drugs are available for clinical use, but with certain exceptions the differences between them are minor.

A distinction is drawn between the drugs that were originally developed (e.g. **chlorpromazine**, **haloperidol** and many similar compounds), often referred to as *classical* or *typical* antipsychotic drugs, and more recently developed agents (e.g. **clozapine**, **risperidone**), which are termed *atypical* antipsychotic drugs. These terms are widely used, but not clearly defined, and experts argue endlessly about what 'atypical' actually means. It often refers to the diminished tendency of some newer compounds to cause unwanted motor side-effects (see below), but it is also used to describe compounds with a pharmacological profile somewhat different from that of 'classical' compounds, or to describe compounds which improve the negative as well as the positive symptoms. In practice, it merely serves—not very usefully—to distinguish the large group of ('classical') pre-1980 drugs (phenothiazines, thioxanthenes and butyrophenones), which are very similar in their properties, from a more diverse group of newer compounds described below.

Table 37.1 summarises the main drugs that are in clinical use.

GENERAL PROPERTIES

The therapeutic activity of the prototype drug, chlorpromazine, in schizophrenic patients was discovered through the acute observations of a French surgeon, Laborit, in 1947. He tested various substances, including promethazine, for their ability to alleviate signs of stress in patients undergoing surgery and concluded that promethazine had a calming effect that was different from mere sedation. Elaboration of the phenothiazine structure produced chlorpromazine, the antipsychotic effect of which was demonstrated, at Laborit's instigation, by Delay & Deniker in 1953. This drug was unique in controlling the symptoms of psychotic patients without excessively sedating them. The clinical efficacy of phenothiazines was discovered long before their mechanism of action was understood.

Pharmacological investigation showed that phenothiazines blocked the actions of many different mediators, including histamine, catecholamines, acetylcholine and 5-HT, and this multiplicity of actions led to the trade name Largactil for chlorpromazine. It is now clear (see Fig. 37.1) that antagonism at dopamine receptors is the main determinant of antipsychotic action.

MECHANISM OF ACTION

DOPAMINE RECEPTORS AND DOPAMINERGIC NEURONS

The classification of dopamine receptors in the central nervous system (CNS) is discussed in Chapter 33 (see Table 33.1). There are five subtypes, which fall into two functional classes: the D_1 type, comprising D_1 and D_5 and the D_2 type, comprising D_2, D_3 and D_4. The antipsychotic drugs owe their therapeutic effects mainly to blockade of D_2-receptors. As stated above, antipsychotic effects require about 80% block of D_2-receptors. Antagonism at D_2-receptors can be measured in experimental animals by various tests, such as inhibition of amphetamine-induced stereotypic behaviour, or of apomorphine-induced turning behaviour in animals with unilateral striatal lesions (see Ch. 33), and in vitro by the ability to inhibit the binding of a radioactive D_2 antagonist (e.g. spiroperidol) to brain membrane fragments. The earlier compounds, phenothiazines, thioxanthenes and butyrophenones, show some preference for D_2- over D_1-receptors; some of the newer agents (e.g. sulpiride, remoxipride)

Table 37.1 Characteristics of antipsychotic drugs

Drug	Receptor affinity						Main side-effects				Notes
	D_1	D_2	α-adr	H_1	mACh	5-HT_2	EPS	Sed.	Hypo.	Other	
Classical											
Chlorpromazine	++	+++	+++	++	++	++	++	++	++	Increased prolactin (gynaecomastia) Hypothermia Anticholinergic effects Hypersensitivity reactions Obstructive jaundice	Phenothiazine class **Fluphenazine, trifluperazine** are similar, but: • do not cause jaundice • less hypotension • more EPS Fluphenazine available as depot preparation
Thioridazine	+	++	+++	+	++	++	+	++	++	As chlorpromazine, but does not cause jaundice	Phenothiazine class First drug with lower EPS tendency
Haloperidol	+	+++	++	–	±	+	+++	—	++	As chlorpromazine, but does not cause jaundice Fewer anticholinergic side-effects	Butyrophenone class Widely used antipsychotic drug Strong EPS tendency
Flupenthixol	++	+++	++	++	–	+++	++	+	+	Increased prolactin (gynaecomastia) Restlessness	**Clopenthixol** is similar Available as depot preparations
Atypical											
Sulpiride	—	+++	—	—	—	—	+	+	—	Increased prolactin (gynaecomastia)	Benzamide class Selective D_2/D_3 antagonist Less EPS than haloperidol Poorly absorbed. **Remoxipride and pimozide** (long acting) are similar
Clozapine	++	++	++	++	++	+++	—	++	+	Risk of agranulocytosis (~1%): regular blood counts required Seizures Sedation Salivation Anticholinergic side-effects Weight gain	Dibenzodiazepine class Potent antagonist at D_4-receptors No EPS Shows efficacy in "treatment-resistant" patients Effective against negative and positive symptoms **Olanzapine** is similar, without risk of agranulocytosis
Risperidone	—	++	++	++	++	+++	+	++	+	Weight gain EPS at high doses Hypotension	Significant risk of EPS ? Effective against negative symptoms Potent on D_4-receptors
Sertindole	—	++	++	—	—	+++	+	+	++	Ventricular arrhythmias (ECG checks advisable) Weight gain Nasal congestion	Long plasma half-life (~3 days) ? Effective against negative symptoms
Quetiapine	—	+	+++	—	+	+	+	++	++	Tachycardia Agitation Dry mouth Weight gain	Novel type, acting mainly on α-adrenoceptors Not yet fully evaluated

$D_{1/2}$, types of dopamine receptor; EPS, extrapyramidal side-effects; Sed., sedation; Hypo., hypotension; adr, adrenoceptor; mACh, muscarine acetylcholine; ECG, electrocardiograph.

are highly selective for D_2-receptors, whereas clozapine is relatively non-selective between D_1 and D_2 but has high affinity for D_4.

In animal tests, all antipsychotic drugs initially *increase* and later *decrease* the electrical activity of midbrain dopaminergic neurons in the substantia nigra and ventral tegmentum and also the release of dopamine in regions containing dopaminergic nerve terminals (see O'Donnell & Grace, 1996). These changes are possibly associated with changes in dopamine receptor expression (see below). Effects on the mesolimbic/mesocortical dopamine pathways are believed to correlate with antipsychotic effects, whereas effects on the nigrostriatal pathways are responsible for the unwanted motor effects produced by antipsychotic drugs (see below). For example, haloperidol, a classical drug with pronounced motor effects, acts on both sets of dopamine neurons, whereas clozapine, an atypical drug which lacks motor effects, affects only the ventral tegmental neurons.

Antipsychotic drugs, like many neuroactive compounds, take several weeks to take effect, even though their receptor-blocking action is immediate.* When antipsychotic drugs are administered chronically, the increase in activity of dopaminergic neurons is transient and gives way after about 3 weeks to inhibition (Fig. 37.2), at which time both the biochemical and electrophysiological markers of activity decline.

Another delayed effect seen with chronic administration of antipsychotic drugs is proliferation of dopamine receptors, detectable as an increase in haloperidol binding (see Seeman, 1987); there is also a pharmacological supersensitivity to dopamine, somewhat akin to the phenomenon of denervation supersensitivity. At present neither the mechanism of the delayed effects nor their relationship to the clinical response is at all well understood.

Antipsychotic drugs show varying patterns of selectivity in their receptor-blocking effects (Table 37.1), some having high affinity for 5-HT and/or D_4-receptors. The connection between their receptor specificity and their functional and therapeutic effects, despite a wealth of fine argument, remains hidden. Were it understood, we might not have to resort in desperation to words like 'atypical' to hide our uncertainty.

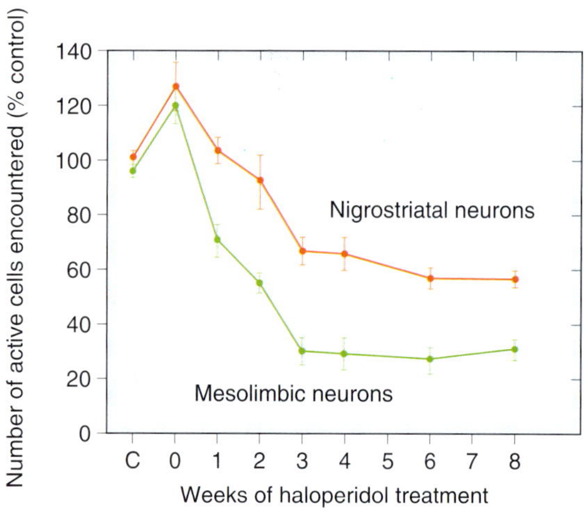

Fig. 37.2 Effect of chronic haloperidol treatment on the activity of dopaminergic neurons in the rat brain. In both regions the activity of dopaminergic neurons, recorded with microelectrodes from anaesthetised animals, initially increases and then declines, reaching a steady level after 3 weeks. (From: White F J, Wang R Y 1983 Life Sci 32: 983.)

Mechanism of action of antipsychotic drugs

- All antipsychotic drugs are antagonists at dopamine D_2 receptors but most also block other monoamine receptors, especially 5-HT_2. Clozapine also blocks D_4-receptors.
- Antipsychotic potency generally runs parallel to activity on D_2-receptors, but other activities may determine side-effect profile.
- Antipsychotics take days or weeks to work, suggesting that secondary effects (e.g. increase in number of D_2-receptors in limbic structure) may be more important than direct effect of D_2-receptor block.

PHARMACOLOGICAL EFFECTS

BEHAVIOURAL EFFECTS

Antipsychotic drugs produce many behavioural effects in experimental animals (see Ögren 1996), but no single test is known that distinguishes them clearly from other types of psychotropic drug. Antipsychotic drugs reduce spontaneous motor activity and in larger doses cause *catalepsy*, a state in which the animal remains immobile even when placed in an unnatural position. Inhibition of the locomotor hyperactivity induced by amphetamine is used as an indicator of the required antipsychotic action of these drugs, whereas ability to cause catalepsy is used as an indicator of their tendency to cause unwanted extrapyramidal symptoms in clinical use (see below). These effects probably reflect D_2-receptor antagonism in the mesocortical/mesolimbic and the striatonigral pathways, respectively. Other tests reveal effects that are not associated with motor inhibition. For example, in a conditioned avoidance model, a rat may be trained to respond to a conditioned stimulus, such as a buzzer, by remaining immobile and thereby avoiding a painful shock; chlorpromazine impairs performance in this test, as well as

*Their sedating effect is also immediate, allowing them to be used in acute behavioural emergencies.

in tests that demand active motor responses. In doses too small to reduce spontaneous motor activity, chlorpromazine reduces social interactions (grooming, mating, fighting, etc.) and also impairs performance in discriminant tests (e.g. requiring the animal to respond differently to red and green lights).

Inhibition of amphetamine-induced behavioural changes occurs with all of the 'classical' antipsychotic drugs, reflecting their action on D_2-receptors. Some of the atypical drugs, which have less activity on D_2-receptors, are less active in such models, and also in the catalepsy model, but are equally efficacious in conditioned avoidance tests. Both classical and atypical drugs, moreover, reduce the hyperactivity caused by phencyclidine (a glutamate antagonist; Ch. 32), which causes a schizophrenia-like syndrome in humans. Conditioned avoidance and phencyclidine tests in animals are, therefore, used as guides to antipsychotic activity in humans.

In humans, the effect of antipsychotic drugs is to produce a state of apathy and reduced initiative. The subject displays few emotions, is slow to respond to external stimuli and tends to drowse off. The patient is, however, easily aroused and can respond to questions accurately, with no marked loss of intellectual function. Aggressive tendencies are strongly inhibited. The effects in humans differ from those of hypnotic and anxiolytic drugs, which cause drowsiness and confusion, with euphoria rather than apathy.

Many antipsychotic drugs show antiemetic activity (see Ch. 24), reflecting antagonism at dopamine receptors. The antihistamine activity of many phenothiazines is also important.

UNWANTED EFFECTS

Extrapyramidal motor disturbances and tardive dyskinesia

Antipsychotic drugs produce two main kinds of motor disturbance in humans, *acute dystonias* and *tardive dyskinesia*, collectively termed extrapyramidal side-effects, which result directly or indirectly from D_2-receptor blockade. These effects constitute one of the main disadvantages of all of the 'classical' antipsychotic drugs. The term 'atypical' was originally applied to some of the newer compounds that show much less tendency to produce extrapyramidal effects.

Acute dystonias

Acute dystonias are involuntary movements (muscle spasms, protruding tongue, torticollis, etc.), and often a Parkinson-type syndrome (Ch. 34). They occur commonly in the first few weeks, often declining with time, and they are reversible on stopping drug treatment. The occurrence of acute dystonias is consistent with block of the dopaminergic nigrostriatal pathway, and there is evidence that the relative selectivity of atypical antipsychotic drugs for the mesolimbic/mesocortical pathway accounts for the diminished risk of acute dystonias. Concomitant block of muscarinic acetylcholine receptors may also mitigate the motor effects of dopamine receptor block, since the two receptor systems act in opposite ways (Ch. 34).

Tardive dyskinesia

Tardive dyskinesia (see Klawans et al., 1988) develops after months or years (hence 'tardive') in 20–40% of patients treated with classical antipsychotic drugs and is one of the main problems of antipsychotic therapy. Its seriousness lies in the fact that it is a disabling and often irreversible condition, which often gets worse when antipsychotic therapy is stopped, and is resistant to treatment. The syndrome consists of involuntary movements, often of the face and tongue, but also of the trunk and limbs, which can be severely disabling. It resembles that seen after prolonged treatment of Parkinson's disease with levodopa. The incidence depends greatly on the drug dosage, the age of the patient (commonest in patients over 50) and on the drug used.

There are several theories about the mechanism of tardive dyskinesia (see Casey, 1995). One is that it is associated with a gradual increase in the number of D_2-receptor sites in the striatum, which is less marked with the atypical antipsychotic drugs. Another possibility is that chronic block of inhibitory dopamine receptors enhances catecholamine and/or glutamate release in the striatum, leading to excitotoxic neurodegeneration (Ch. 34). The reason why atypical antipsychotic drugs (e.g. clozapine, olanzapine, sertindole) are better in this regard is not clear. A possible explanation (see Kapur & Seeman, 2001) lies in differences in the *rate* at which compounds dissociate from D_2-receptors. With a rapidly dissociating compound, a brief surge of dopamine can effectively overcome the block by competition

Antipsychotic-induced motor disturbances

- Major problem of antipsychotic drug treatment.
- Two main types of disturbance occur:
  - —acute, reversible dystonias and Parkinson-like symptoms
  - —slowly developing tardive dyskinesia, often irreversible.
- Acute symptoms comprise involuntary movements, of tremor and rigidity, and are probably the direct consequence of block of nigrostriatal dopamine receptors.
- Tardive dyskinesia comprises mainly involuntary movements of face and limbs, appearing after months or years of antipsychotic treatment. It may be associated with proliferation of dopamine receptors (possibly presynaptic) in corpus striatum. Treatment is generally unsuccessful.
- Incidence of acute dystonias and tardive dyskinesia is less with atypical antipsychotics, and particularly low with clozapine. This may reflect relatively strong muscarinic receptor block with these drugs, or a degree of selectivity for the mesolimbic, as opposed to the nigrostriatal, dopamine pathways.

(Ch. 2), whereas with a slowly dissociating compound, the level of block takes a long time to respond to the presence of endogenous dopamine and is in practice non-competitive. It could, therefore, be that motor effects are avoided if the level of receptor block can give way readily to competition from physiological surges of dopamine, whereas this is not a factor of importance for the psychotropic effects. Whether this kinetic explanation will prove more sustainable than the many attempts to relate the tendency to cause motor side-effects to the receptor profile of different compounds remains to be seen. Clozapine has relatively high affinity for D_1- and D_4-receptors, compared with D_2-receptors, and also has marked antimuscarinic activity, as do some other antipsychotic drugs, such as thioridazine, which may counteract its effects on the motor system.

Endocrine effects

Dopamine, released in the median eminence by neurons of the tuberohypophyseal pathway (see Chs 27 and 33) acts physiologically via D_2-receptors as an inhibitor of prolactin secretion. The result of blocking D_2-receptors by antipsychotic drugs is thus to increase the plasma prolactin concentration (Fig. 37.3), resulting in breast swelling, pain and lactation, which can occur in men as well as women. As can be seen from Figure 37.3, the effect is maintained during chronic antipsychotic administration, without any habituation. Other less-pronounced endocrine changes have also been reported, including a decrease of growth hormone secretion, but these, unlike the prolactin response, are unimportant clinically.

Other unwanted effects

Sedation, which tends to decrease with continued use, occurs with many antipsychotic drugs. Antihistamine (H_1) activity is a property of phenothiazines and contributes to their sedative and antiemetic properties (Ch. 24), but not to their antipsychotic action.

Phenothiazines and, to a variable extent, other antipsychotic drugs, block a variety of receptors, particularly acetylcholine (muscarinic), histamine (H_1), noradrenaline (α) and 5-HT (Table 37.1).

Blocking muscarinic receptors produces a variety of peripheral effects, including blurring of vision and increased intraocular pressure, dry mouth and eyes, constipation and urinary retention (see Ch. 10). It may, however, also be beneficial in relation to extrapyramidal side-effects. Acetylcholine acts in opposition to dopamine in the basal ganglia (see Ch. 31) and it is possible that the relative lack of extrapyramidal side-effects with clozapine and thioridazine is a consequence of their high antimuscarinic potency (see above).

Blocking α-adrenoceptors results in the important side-effect in humans of orthostatic hypotension (see Ch. 18), but it does not seem to be important for the antipsychotic action.

Weight gain is a common and troublesome side-effect, particularly associated with some of the 'atypical' drugs, and probably related to 5-HT antagonism.

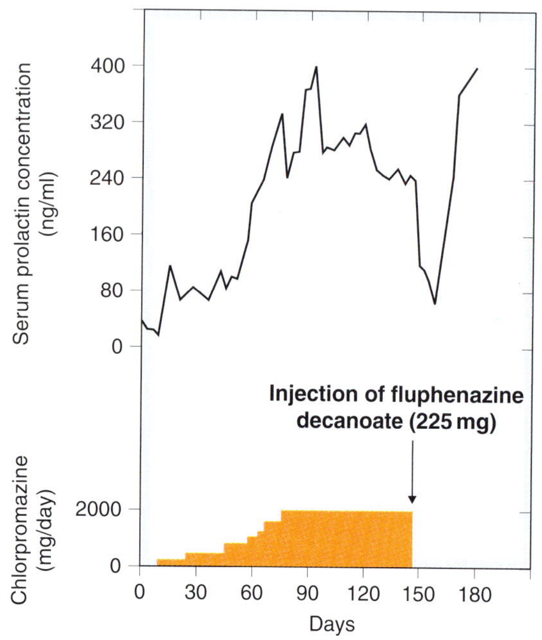

Fig. 37.3 Effects of antipsychotic drugs on prolactin secretion in a schizophrenic patient. When daily dosage with chlorpromazine was replaced with a depot injection of fluphenazine, the plasma prolactin initally dropped, because of the delay in absorption, and then returned to a high level. (From: Meltzer H Y et al. 1978 In: Lipton et al. (eds) Psychopharmacology. A generation in progress. Raven Press, New York.)

Unwanted effects of antipsychotic drugs

- Important side-effects common to most drugs are extrapyramidal motor disturbances (see separate box) and endocrine disturbances (increased prolactin release); these are secondary to dopamine receptor block. Sedation, hypotension and weight gain are also common.
- Other side-effects (dry mouth, blurred vision, hypotension, etc.) result from blockade of other receptors, particularly α-adrenoceptors and muscarinic acetylcholine receptors.
- Obstructive jaundice sometimes occurs with phenothiazines.
- Some antipsychotics cause agranulocytosis as a rare and serious idiosyncratic reaction. With clozapine, leucopenia is common and requires routine monitoring.
- Antipsychotic malignant syndrome is a rare but potentially dangerous idiosyncratic reaction.

Various idiosyncratic and hypersensitivity reactions can occur, the most important being:

- Jaundice, which occurs with older phenothiazines, such as chlorpromazine. The jaundice is usually mild, and of obstructive origin, and disappears quickly when the drug is stopped or substituted by an antipsychotic drug of a different class.
- Leucopenia and agranulocytosis are rare, but potentially fatal, and occur in the first few weeks of treatment. The incidence of leucopenia (usually reversible) is less than 1 in 10 000 for most antipsychotics, but much higher (1–2%) with clozapine, the use of which, therefore, requires regular monitoring of blood cell counts. Provided the drug is stopped at the first sign of leucopenia or anaemia, the effect is reversible. Olanzapine appears to be free of this disadvantage.
- Urticarial skin reactions are common but usually mild. Excessive sensitivity to ultraviolet light may also occur.
- Antipsychotic malignant syndrome is a rare but serious complication, similar to the malignant hyperthermia syndrome seen with certain anaesthetics (see Ch. 35). Muscle rigidity is accompanied by a rapid rise in body temperature and mental confusion. It is usually reversible, but death from renal or cardiovascular failure occurs in 10–20%.

PHARMACOKINETIC ASPECTS

Chlorpromazine, which is typical of many phenothiazines, is erratically absorbed into the bloodstream after oral administration. Figure 34.4 shows the wide range of variation of the peak plasma concentration as a function of dose in 14 patients. Among four patients treated at the high dosage level of 6–8 mg/kg, the variation in peak plasma concentration was nearly 90-fold; two showed marked side-effects, one was correctly controlled and one showed no clinical response.

The relationship between the plasma concentration and the clinical effect of antipsychotic drugs is also highly variable, and the dosage has to be adjusted on a trial-and-error basis. This is made even more difficult by the fact that at least 40% of schizophrenic patients fail to take drugs as prescribed. It is remarkably fortunate that the acute toxicity of antipsychotic drugs is slight, given the unpredictability of the clinical response.

The plasma half-life of most antipsychotic drugs is 15–30 hours, clearance depending entirely on hepatic transformation by a combination of oxidative and conjugative reactions.

Most antipsychotic drugs can be given orally or by intramuscular injection, once or twice a day. Slow-release (depot) preparations of many are available, in which the active drug is esterified with heptanoic or decanoic acid and dissolved in oil. Given as an intramuscular injection, the drug acts for 2–4 weeks but initially may produce acute side-effects. These preparations are widely used as a means of overcoming compliance problems.

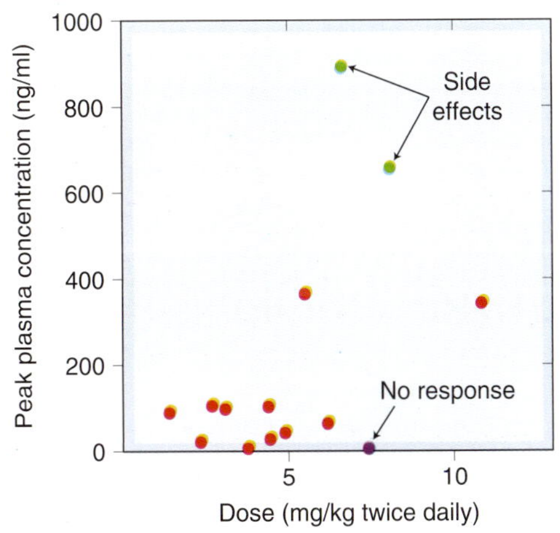

Fig. 37.4 Individual variation in the relation between dose and plasma concentration of chlorpromazine in a group of schizophrenic patients. (Date: Curry S H et al. 1970 Arch Gen Psychiat 22: 289.)

CLINICAL USE AND CLINICAL EFFICACY

The major use of antipsychotic drugs is in the treatment of schizophrenia and acute behavioural emergencies, but they are also widely used as adjunct therapy in the treatment of other illnesses, such as psychotic depression and mania. Some of the newer antipsychotics (e.g. **sulpiride**) have been claimed to have specific antidepressant actions. Phenothiazines are also useful as antiemetics (see Ch. 24). Minor uses include the treatment of Huntington's chorea (mainly haloperidol; see Ch. 34).

The clinical efficacy of antipsychotic drugs in enabling schizophrenic patients to lead more normal lives has been

Clinical efficacy of antipsychotic drugs

- Antipsychotic drugs are effective in controlling symptoms of acute schizophrenia, when large doses may be needed.
- Long-term antipsychotic treatment is often effective in preventing recurrence of schizophrenic attacks, and this is a major factor in allowing schizophrenic patients to lead normal lives.
- Depot preparations are often used for maintenance therapy.
- Antipsychotic drugs are not generally effective in improving negative schizophrenic symptoms, though newer drugs are claimed to relieve these symptoms.
- Approximately 40% of chronic schizophrenic patients are poorly controlled by antipsychotic drugs; clozapine may be effective in some of these 'antipsychotic-resistant' patients.
- There are small, if any, overall differences in efficacy between different antipsychotic drugs, though side-effects differ significantly.

demonstrated in many controlled trials. The inpatient population (mainly chronic schizophrenics) of mental hospitals declined sharply in the 1950s and 1960s. The efficacy of the newly introduced antipsychotic drugs was a significant enabling factor, as well as the changing public and professional attitudes towards hospitalisation of the mentally ill.

Antipsychotic drugs, apart from their side-effects, have two main shortcomings.

- They are effective in only about 70% of schizophrenic patients; for any single drug the success rate is lower. The remaining 30% are classed as 'treatment-resistant', and present a major therapeutic problem. The reason for the difference between responsive and unresponsive patients is unknown at present.*
- While they control the positive symptoms (thought disorder, hallucinations, delusions, etc.) effectively, they are ineffective in relieving the negative symptoms (emotional flattening, social isolation).

The newer atypical antipsychotic drugs, particularly clozapine, may overcome these shortcomings to some degree, showing efficacy in treatment-resistant patients and improving negative, as well as positive, symptoms. However, a recent meta-analysis (Geddes et al., 2000) suggests that these newer drugs, while clearly reducing the risk of motor side-effects, are not significantly better in terms of efficacy or other side-effects. The older drugs, Geddes et al. suggest, may have gained a bad name for causing troublesome side-effects because of the common practice of overdosing beyond the useful therapeutic range.

In current practice, the increasing use of atypical antipsychotic drugs—despite their high cost—is fully justified by the low level of motor side-effects that they produce, but whether they are better in other respects remains uncertain.

*Recent evidence suggests that responsiveness to clozapine is related to polymorphisms of the gene encoding the 5-HT_{2A}-receptor. Determination of a patient's individual genotype with respect to six polymorphisms gave 77% success in predicting his or her response to clozapine.

REFERENCES AND FURTHER READING

Busatto G F, Kerwin R W 1997 Perspectives on the role of serotonergic mechanisms in the pharmacology of schizophrenia. J Psychopharmacol 11: 3–12 (*Assesses the evidence implicating 5-HT as well as dopamine in the action of antipsychotic drugs*)

Casey D E 1995 Tardive dyskinesia: pathophysiology. In: Bloom F E, Kupfer D J (eds) Psychopharmacology: a fourth generation of progress. Raven Press, New York

Geddes J, Freemantle N, Harrison P, Bebbington P 2000 Atypical antipsychotics in the treatment of schizophrenia: systematic overview and meta-regression analysis. Br Med J 321: 1371–1376 (*Survey of trials comparing atypical and classical drugs showing few clearcut differences apart from motor side-effects*)

Goff D C, Coyle J T 2001 The emerging role of glutamate in the pathophysiology and treatment of schizophrenia. Am J Psychiatry 158: 1367–1377 (*Good review article on pathophysiology, though referring to role in treatment is premature*)

Harrison P J 1997 Schizophrenia: a disorder of development. Curr Opin Neurobiol 7: 285–289 (*Reviews persuasively the evidence favouring abnormal early brain development as the basis of schizophrenia*)

Jones H M, Pilowsky L S 2002 Dopamine and antipsychotic drug action revisited. Br J Psychiatry 181: 271–275 (*Useful update reviewing recent clinical imaging data supporting the dopamine hypothesis*)

Kapur S, Seeman P 2001 Does fast dissociation from the dopamine D_2 receptor explain the action of atypical antipsychotics? A new hypothesis. Am J Psychiatry 158: 360–369 (*Suggests that differences in dissociation rates, rather than receptor selectivity profiles, may account for differing tendency of drugs to cause motor side-effects*)

Klawans H L, Tanner C M, Goetz C G 1988 Epidemiology and pathophysiology of tardive dyskinesias. Adv Neurol 49: 185–197

Laruelle M, Abi-Dargham A, Gil R, Kegeles L, Innis R 1999 Increased dopamine transmission in schizophrenia: relationship to illness phases. Biol Psych 46: 56–72 (*The first direct evidence for increased dopamine function as a cause of symptoms in schizophrenia*)

Lewis D A, Lieberman J A 2000 Catching up on schizophrenia: natural history and neurobiology. Neuron 28: 325–334 (*Useful review summarising present understanding of the nature of schizophrenia*)

O'Donnell P, Grace A A 1996 Basic neurophysiology of antipsychotic drug action. In: Chernansky J G (ed) Antipsychotics. Handbook of experimental pharmacology, Springer, Berlin, vol. 120 (*Review of effects of antipsychotic drugs at the neurophysiological level, emphasising distinction between acute and chronic effects*)

Ögren S O1996 The behavioural pharmacology of typical and atypical antipsychotic drugs. In: Csernasky J G (ed) Antipsychotics. Handbook of experimental pharmacology. Springer, Berlin, vol. 120

Reynolds G P 1983 Increased concentrations and lateral asymmetry of amygdala dopamine in schizophrenia. Nature 305: 527–529 (*Demonstrates unilateral increase of brain dopamine in postmortem schizophrenic brains—one of the few positive neurochemical findings*)

Seeman P 1987 Dopamine receptors and the dopamine hypothesis of schizophrenia. Synapse 1: 133–152 (*Convincing, and widely quoted, review of role of dopamine receptors in schizophrenia*)

Strange P G 2001 Antipsychotic drugs: importance of dopamine receptors for mechanisms of therapeutic actions and side effects. Pharmacol Rev 53: 119–133 (*Good review favouring dopamine hypothesis*)

Drugs used in affective disorders

38

Overview 535

The nature of depression 535

The theories of depression 536
- The monoamine theory 536
- Animal models of depression 538

Antidepressant drugs 538
- Types of antidepressant drug 538
- Measurement of antidepressant activity 538
- Mechanism of action of antidepressant drugs 539
- Tricyclic antidepressant drugs 539
- Selective 5-HT uptake inhibitors 544
- Monoamine axidase inhibitors 545
- Other antidepressant drugs 547

Electroconvulsive therapy 547

Clinical effectiveness of antidepressant treatments 548

Mood-stabilising drugs 548
- Lithium 548

OVERVIEW

Depression is an extremely common psychiatric condition, about which a variety of neurochemical theories exist and for which a corresponding variety of different types of drug is used in treatment. It is a field in which therapeutic empiricism has led the way, with mechanistic understanding tending to lag behind, part of the difficulty being that animal models cannot address the mood change that defines the human condition. In this chapter, we discuss the current understanding of the nature of the disorder and describe the major drugs that are used to treat it. A good summary of our present state of knowledge is given by Wong & Licinio (2001).

THE NATURE OF DEPRESSION

Depression is the most common of the affective disorders (disorders of mood rather than disturbances of thought or cognition); it may range from a very mild condition, bordering on normality, to severe (psychotic) depression accompanied by hallucinations and delusions. Worldwide, depression is a major cause of disability and premature death.

The symptoms of depression include emotional and biological components:

- emotional symptoms:
  —misery, apathy and pessimism
  —low self-esteem: feelings of guilt, inadequacy and ugliness
  —indecisiveness, loss of motivation.
- biological symptoms:
  —retardation of thought and action
  —loss of libido
  —sleep disturbance and loss of appetite.

There are two distinct types of depressive syndrome, namely *unipolar depression*, in which the mood swings are always in the same direction, and *bipolar affective disorder*, in which depression alternates with mania. Mania is in most respects exactly the opposite, with excessive exuberance, enthusiasm and self-confidence, accompanied by impulsive actions, these signs often being combined with irritability, impatience and aggression, and sometimes with grandiose delusions of the Napoleonic kind. As with depression, the mood and actions are inappropriate to the circumstances.

Unipolar depression is commonly (about 75% of cases) non-familial, clearly associated with stressful life-events and accompanied by symptoms of anxiety and agitation; this type is sometimes termed *reactive depression*. Other patients (about 25%, sometimes termed *endogenous depression*) show a familial pattern, unrelated to external stresses, and with a somewhat different symptomatology. This distinction is made clinically, but there is little evidence that antidepressant drugs show significant selectivity between these conditions.

Bipolar depression, which usually appears in early adult life, is less common and results in oscillating depression and mania over a period of a few weeks. There is a strong hereditary tendency, but no specific gene or genes have been identified either by genetic linkage studies of affected families, or by comparison of affected and non-affected individuals..

THEORIES OF DEPRESSION

THE MONOAMINE THEORY

The main biochemical theory of depression is the monoamine hypothesis, proposed by Schildkraut in 1965, which states that depression is caused by a functional deficit of monoamine transmitters at certain sites in the brain, while mania results from a functional excess. For reviews of the evolving status of the theory, see Baker & Dewhurst (1985), Maes & Meltzer (1995), Manji et al. (2001).

The monoamine hypothesis grew originally out of associations between the clinical effects of various drugs that cause or alleviate symptoms of depression and their known neurochemical effects on monoaminergic transmission in the brain. Initially the hypothesis was formulated in terms of noradrenaline, but subsequent work showed that most of the observations were equally consistent with 5-hydroxytryptamine (5-HT) being the key substance. This pharmacological evidence, which is summarised below, gives general support to the monoamine hypothesis, though there are several anomalies. Attempts to obtain more direct evidence, by studying monoamine metabolism in depressed patients or by measuring changes in the number of monoamine receptors in postmortem brain tissue, have tended to give inconsistent and equivocal results, and the interpretation of these studies is often problematic, since the changes described are not specific to depression. Similarly, investigation by functional tests of the activity of known monoaminergic pathways (e.g. those controlling pituitary hormone release) in depressed patients have also given equivocal results.

PHARMACOLOGICAL EVIDENCE

Table 38.1 summarises the main pharmacological evidence supporting the monoamine hypothesis. Though it provides reasonable support for the theory, there are several examples of drugs that might have been predicted to improve or worsen depressive symptoms but fail to do so convincingly. It has to be recognised that the basis for predicting the effects of drugs on mood is, at best, very simple-minded. For example, supplying a transmitter precursor will not necessarily increase the release of transmitter unless availability of the precursor is rate limiting. Similarly, a drug that releases monoamines from normal nerve terminals may fail to do so if the nerve terminals are functionally defective. The pharmacological evidence does not enable a clear distinction to be drawn between the noradrenaline and 5-HT theories of depression. Clinically, it seems that inhibitors of noradrenaline reuptake and of 5-HT reuptake are equally effective as antidepressants (see below) though individual patients may respond better to one or the other.

Any theory of depression has to take account of the fact that the direct biochemical effects of antidepressant drugs appear very rapidly, whereas their antidepressant effects take weeks to develop. A similar situation exists in relation to antipsychotic drugs (Ch. 37) and some anxiolytic drugs (Ch. 36), suggesting that the secondary, adaptive changes in the brain, rather than the primary drug effect, are responsible for the clinical improvement. With our increasing understanding of the link between membrane receptors and long-term changes in cell function (Ch. 3), the dilemma may largely disappear. A rapid change in the concentration of, say, 5-HT, as well as producing immediate effects on cell function, can, if sustained, also produce slowly developing trophic changes associated with changes in gene expression. Rather than thinking of the monoamine deficiency as causing direct changes in the activity of putative 'happy' or 'sad' neurons in the brain, we should perhaps think of the monoamines as regulators of gradual adaptive responses, the time course of which is paralleled by mood changes. Evidence for such adaptive changes in monoamine receptor function is discussed below (p. 539).

Table 38.1 Pharmacological evidence supporting the monoamine hypothesis of depression

Drug	Principal action	Effect in depressed patients
Tricyclic antidepressants	Block NA and 5-HT reuptake	Mood ↑
MAO inhibitors	Increase stores of NA and 5-HT	Mood ↑
Reserpine	Inhibits NA and 5-HT storage	Mood ↓
α-Methyltyrosine	Inhibits NA synthesis	Mood ↓ Calming of manic patients
Methyldopa	Inhibits NA synthesis	Mood ↓
Electroconvulsive therapy	?Increases CNS responses to NA and 5-HT	Mood ↑
Tryptophan (5-hydroxytryptophan)	Increases 5-HT synthesis	Mood? ↑ in some studies

MAO, monoamine oxidase; NA, noradrenaline; 5-HT; 5-hydroxytryptamine.

BIOCHEMICAL STUDIES

Many studies have sought to test the amine hypothesis by looking for biochemical abnormalities in cerebrospinal fluid (CSF), blood or urine, or in postmortem brain tissue, from depressed or manic patients. They have included studies of monoamine metabolites, receptors, enzymes and transporters, largely with negative results. The major metabolites of noradrenaline and 5-HT, respectively, are 3-methoxy-4-hydroxyphenylglycol (MHPG) and 5-hydroxyindoleacetic acid (5-HIAA). These appear in the CSF, blood and urine (see Chs 11, 12 and 33). There are two fundamental problems in relating changes in the concentration of these metabolites in body fluids to changes in transmitter function in the brain. One is that many secondary factors can affect their concentration, such as diet; transport between CSF, blood and urine; or release of monoamines from non-cerebral sites. The second is that many patients receive drug treatment, which affects the metabolite concentrations markedly.

Studies of urinary MHPG excretion in normal and depressed subjects have shown convincingly that the level is reduced in bipolar depressive patients and is lower during the depressive than during the manic phase. In unipolar depression, however, MHPG excretion, though highly variable between patients, is not significantly lower than in controls, so support for the monoamine theory is at best equivocal. Plasma noradrenaline actually tends to be higher in depressed than in normal subjects, possibly because it reflects peripheral sympathetic activity, which increases with the anxiety that often accompanies depression. It too shows a cyclic variation in bipolar depressive patients.

Results pertaining to altered 5-HT metabolism are also highly variable (see Maes & Meltzer, 1995). Studies of 5-HIAA in CSF and urine have generally failed to find any clear correlation with depression. Low levels of 5-HIAA occur in the brain and CSF of suicide victims but could be associated with violent behaviour rather than with depression. More consistent changes have been reported in the plasma concentration of L-tryptophan (TRP, the precursor of 5-HT). Though the resting levels are not significantly different in depressed patients, the rise in plasma TRP following an intravenous or oral dose is reduced, implying lower 'TRP availability'.

Other evidence in support of the monoamine theory is that agents known to block either noradrenaline or 5-HT synthesis consistently reverse the therapeutic effects of antidepressant drugs that act selectively on the two transmitter systems (see below).

NEUROENDOCRINE STUDIES

Various attempts have been made to test for a functional deficit of monoamine pathways in depression. Hypothalamic neurons controlling pituitary function receive noradrenergic and 5-HT inputs, which control the discharge of these cells. Hypothalamic cells release *corticotrophin-releasing hormone* (CRH), which stimulates pituitary cells to secrete adrenocorticotrophic hormone, leading, in turn, to cortisol secretion. The plasma cortisol concentration is usually high in depressed patients and it fails to respond with the normal fall when a synthetic steroid, such as dexamethasone, is given. This formed the basis of a clinical test, the *dexamethasone suppression test* (also used in the diagnosis of Cushing's syndrome; see p. 416). Other hormones in plasma are also affected; For example, growth hormone concentration is reduced and prolactin is increased. In general, these changes are consistent with deficient monoamine transmission, but they are not specific to depressive illness.

CRH is widely distributed in the brain and has behavioural effects that are distinct from its endocrine functions. Injected into the brain of experimental animals, CRH mimics some effects of depression in humans, such as diminished activity, loss of appetite, and increased signs of anxiety. Furthermore, CRH concentrations in the brain and CSF of depressed patients are increased. Consequently, CRH hyperfunction, as well as monoamine hypofunction, may be associated with depression (see Holsboer, 1999).

In summary, there is considerable circumstantial evidence to suggest that Schildkraut's monoamine theory is basically correct, though it requires a good deal of special pleading to accommodate many of the clinical observations. There are, however, some inconsistencies, of which the most obvious are the following:

- neither amphetamine nor cocaine have antidepressant actions, despite their ability to enhance monoamine transmission.

Monoamine theory of depression

- The monoamine theory, proposed in 1965, suggests that depression results from functionally deficient monoaminergic (noradrenaline and/or 5-HT) transmission in the CNS.
- The theory was based on the ability of known antidepressant drugs (tricyclic antidepressants and monoamine oxidase inhibitors) to facilitate monoaminergic transmission, and of drugs such as reserpine to cause depression.
- Biochemical studies on depressed patients do not clearly support the monoamine hypothesis in its simple form.
- An abnormally weak response of plasma cortisol to exogenous steroid (dexamethasone suppression test) is common in depression and may reflect defective monoamine transmission in the hypothalamus.
- Though the monoamine hypothesis in its simple form is insufficient as an explanation of depression, pharmacological manipulation of monoamine transmission remains the most successful therapeutic approach.
- Current approaches focus on other mediators (e.g. corticotrophin-releasing hormone), signal transduction pathways, growth factors, etc., but theories remain imprecise.

- antidepressant drugs have a delayed therapeutic effect, which coincides in time with an apparent inhibition rather than facilitation of monoaminergic transmission
- some clinically effective antidepressants seem to lack any actions that could enhance monoamine transmission
- the biochemical changes associated with depression have, in several studies, been identical with changes observed in manic patients.

Recognising these inconsistencies, many authors (see Ashton, 1992; Manji et al, 2001) have suggested more complicated mechanisms than a simple transmitter deficit, and have invoked dopamine, acetylcholine and peptides in delicately balanced arrays in attempts to account for all the facts. The focus has shifted to the long-term effects of agents that enhance or inhibit transmitter function, mediated through foot-soldiers of neuroplasticity such as growth factors and changes in gene expression. Receptor downregulation and its counterpart, supersensitivity, are examples of such long-term effects that may be associated with depression. The complexities of these models currently go beyond the experimental data, and, despite its shortcomings, Schildkraut's basic hypothesis remains the best basis for understanding the actions of antidepressant drugs. It clearly needs to be modified and elaborated, but clinical and experimental studies in the last few years may have generated more prose than progress in this direction, possibly because the methodology for studying transmitter function in humans lacks sufficient precision.

ANIMAL MODELS OF DEPRESSION

▼ Progress in unravelling the neurochemical mechanisms is, as in so many areas of psychopharmacology, limited by the lack of good animal models of the clinical condition. There is no known animal condition corresponding to the inherited condition of depression in humans, but various procedures have been described that produce in animals behavioural states (withdrawal from social interaction, loss of appetite, reduced motor activity, etc.) typical of human depression (see review by Porsolt, 1985). For example, the delivery of repeated inescapable painful stimuli leads to a state of 'learned helplessness', in which even when the animal is free to escape it fails to do so. Mother–infant separation in monkeys, and administration of amine-depleting drugs such as reserpine, also produce states that superficially resemble human depression. As well as being inherently distasteful, these experiments often require elaborate and expensive experimental protocols, and the similarity of these states to human depression is questionable. However, the learned helplessness state and the effect of mother–infant separation can be reversed by tricyclic antidepressants and increased by small doses of α-methyl-*p*-tyrosine (which inhibits noradrenaline synthesis), suggesting a basic similarity to the human state.

ANTIDEPRESSANT DRUGS

TYPES OF ANTIDEPRESSANT DRUG

Antidepressant drugs fall into the following categories:

- inhibitors of monoamine uptake:
  - —tricyclic antidepressants (TCA), e.g. **imipramine**, **amitriptyline**: these are non-selective (or in some cases noradrenaline-selective) inhibitors of monoamine uptake
  - —selective 5-HT (serotonin) uptake inhibitors (SSRI), e.g. **fluoxetine**, **fluvoxamine**, **paroxetine**, **sertraline**
  - —other inhibitors that are chemically unrelated to TCA but similar pharmacologically, e.g. **maprotiline, reboxetine.**
- monoamine oxidase (MAO) inhibitors (MAOI), e.g. **phenelzine, tranylcypromine**, which are non-selective with respect to the MAO-A and B subtypes (see below); **moclobemide**, which is MAO-A-selective
- miscellaneous antidepressants: these are compounds with non-selective receptor-blocking effects and their antidepressant actions are poorly understood (e.g. **mianserin, bupropion, trazodone**).

Table 38.2 summarises the main features of these types of drug. A recent update is provided by Frazer (1997).

Mention should also be made of electroconvulsive therapy (ECT) which is effective and usually acts more rapidly than antidepressant drugs (see later section).

MEASUREMENT OF ANTIDEPRESSANT ACTIVITY

▼ The clinical effectiveness of the first MAOI and TCA drugs was discovered by chance when these drugs were given to patients for other reasons. **Iproniazid**, the first MAOI, was originally used to treat tuberculosis, being chemically related to **isoniazid** (see Ch. 45); **imipramine**, the first TCA, resembles **chlorpromazine** (see Ch. 37) and was first tried as an antipsychotic drug. Later, the monoamine hypothesis of depression produced a biochemical rationale for their antidepressant actions and, hence, ways of testing new compounds as a preliminary to clinical trials. The results of such biochemical tests are successful in predicting clinical efficacy for conventional TCA and MAOI but fail to predict efficacy with many newer antidepressant drugs. Various behavioural tests have also been used (see above), though there is no animal model that satisfactorily resembles depressive illness in humans. Some of the most useful tests are the following.

- *Potentiation of noradrenaline effects in the periphery* Stimulation of sympathetic nerves or administration of noradrenaline causes contraction of smooth muscle, which is enhanced if the noradrenaline reuptake mechanism of the nerve terminal is blocked (see Ch. 11). This test gives positive results with monoamine uptake inhibitors but does not reveal MAOI or atypical antidepressant activity.
- *Potentiation of the central effects of amphetamine* Amphetamine works partly by releasing noradrenaline in the brain, and its actions are enhanced both by MAOI and by uptake inhibitors. Some atypical antidepressants also give a positive response, making it a useful test for predicting activity in humans.
- *Antagonism of reserpine-induced depression* Reserpine depletes the brain of both noradrenaline and 5-HT, causing various measurable effects (hypothermia, bradycardia, reduced motor activity, etc.), which are reduced by antidepressant drugs. This test also reveals activity among the atypical antidepressants.
- *Block of amine uptake in vitro* Among TCA there is a fairly good correlation between antidepressant activity and potency in inhibiting noradrenaline or 5-HT uptake, but MAOI and many other antidepressants have no effect.

A general point that has to be borne in mind when using in vitro tests to assess potential antidepressants is that many drugs (particularly TCA) are metabolised to pharmacologically active

Types of antidepressant drugs

- Main types are:
  - —monoamine uptake inhibitors (tricyclic antidepressants (TCA), selective 5-HT reuptake inhibitors (SSRI) and others)
  - —monoamine oxidase inhibitors (MAOI)
  - —miscellaneous ('atypical') antidepressants, mainly non-selective receptor antagonists (e.g. bupropion, trazodone, mirtazepine).
- TCA and SSRI act by inhibiting uptake of noradrenaline and/or 5-HT by monoaminergic nerve terminals, thus acutely facilitating transmission.
- MAOIs inhibit one or both forms of brain MAO, thus increasing the cytosolic stores of noradrenaline and 5-HT in nerve terminals. Inhibition of MAO-A correlates with antidepressant activity. Most are non-selective; moclobemide is specific for MAO-A.
- Mode of action of 'atypical' antidepressants is poorly understood.
- All types of antidepressant drug take at least 2 weeks to produce any beneficial effects, even though their pharmacological effects are produced immediately, indicating that secondary adaptive changes are important.
- The most consistent adaptive change seen with different types of antidepressant drug is downregulation of β- and α_2-adrenoceptors, as well as 5-HT_2-receptors. How this is related to therapeutic effect is not clear.

substances in vivo, and it is often unclear whether the parent drug or the metabolite is actually responsible for the clinical effect.

MECHANISM OF ACTION OF ANTIDEPRESSANT DRUGS

In the absence of a simple mechanistic theory to account for antidepressant action (see above), it is useful to look for pharmacological effects that the various drugs have in common, concentrating mainly on the slow adaptive changes that follow a similar time course to the therapeutic effect. This approach has led to the discovery that certain monoamine receptors, in particular β_1- and β_2-adrenoceptors, are consistently downregulated following chronic antidepressant treatment. This can be demonstrated in experimental animals as a reduction in the number of binding sites, as well as by a reduction in the functional response to agonists (e.g. stimulation of cAMP formation by β-adrenoceptor agonists). Receptor downregulation probably also occurs in humans, since endocrine responses to clonidine, an α_2-adrenoceptor agonist, are reduced by long-term antidepressant treatment. Other receptors have also been studied; α_1-adrenoceptors are not consistently affected, but 5-HT_2-receptors are also downregulated.

How these findings relate to the monoamine theory is unclear at present. Loss of β-adrenoceptors as a factor in alleviating depression does not fit comfortably with theory, since β-adrenoceptor antagonists are not antidepressant, though it is the most consistent change reported. Impaired presynaptic inhibition, secondary to downregulation of α_2-adrenoceptors might, it is argued, facilitate monoamine release and thus facilitate transmission. Consistent with this possibility is the fact that some newer antidepressant drugs, such as **mirtazapine** (Table 38.2), are antagonists at various inhibitory presynaptic receptors, including α_2-adrenoceptors.

As already stressed, the delayed effect of antidepressants suggests that events downstream from the direct cellular effects of monoamines are probably important. Consequently, effects on signal transduction mechanisms, including kinases, transcription factors and growth factors, are being actively investigated (see Manji et al., 2001), but it is too early to say whether this will lead to new therapeutic agents.*

In the following sections, we describe the main classes of antidepressant drug in more detail. Drugs not covered here are summarised in Table 38.2.

TRICYCLIC ANTIDEPRESSANT DRUGS

Tricyclic antidepressants are an important group of antidepressants in clinical use. They are, however, far from ideal in practice, and it was the need for drugs that act more quickly and reliably and produce fewer side-effects that led to the introduction of newer SSRI drugs and other antidepressants (see below).

Testing of antidepressant drugs

- Animal models of depression include,
  - —learned helplessness model
  - —reversal of reserpine-induced behavioural syndrome
  - —mother–infant separation in primates.
- None is a good model for human depressive illness, but they are the best available for testing new drugs.
- Biochemical and pharmacological measures include inhibition of monoamine uptake, receptor-blocking activity, enhancement of peripheral noradrenergic transmission.
- Clinical testing of antidepressant drugs necessitates allowance for large placebo effects.

*In a study by Malberg et al. (2000), several antidepressant drugs given to rats were found to increase neurogenesis in the hippocampus, raising the interesting possibility that actual brain remodelling may be involved in their therapeutic effects.

Table 38.2 Types of antidepreassant drugs and their characteristics

Type and examples	Action	Unwanted effects	Risk of overdose	Pharmacokinetics	Notes
Monoamine uptake inhibitors					
1. Tricyclic (TCA)	Inhibition of NA/5-HT reuptake	Sedation Anticholinergic effects (dry mouth, constipation, blurred vision, urinary retention, etc.) Postural hypotension Seizures Impotence Interaction with CNS depressants (esp. alcohol, MAOIs)	Ventricular dysrhythmias High risk in combination with CNS depressants		'First-generation' antidepressants, still very widely used, though newer compounds generally have fewer side-effects and lower risk with overdose
Imipramine	Non-selective	As above	As above	$t_{1/2}$ 4–18 h; converted to desipramine	
Desipramine	NA-selective	As above	As above	$t_{1/2}$ 12–24 h	
Amitriptyline	Non-selective	As above	As above	$t_{1/2}$ 12–24 h; converted to nortriptyline	Widely used, also for neuropathic pain (Ch. 40)
Nortriptyline	NA-selective (slight)	As above	As above	Long $t_{1/2}$ 24–96 h	Long duration Less sedative
Clomipramine	Non-selective	As above	As above	$t_{1/2}$ 18–24 h	Also used for anxiety disorders
2. Selective serotonin (5-HT) reuptake inhibitors (SSRI)	All highly selective for 5-HT	Nausea, Diarrhoea Agitation Insomnia Anorgasmia Inhibit metabolism of other drugs, so risk of interactions	Low risk in overdose, but must not be used in combination with MAOIs		
Fluoxetine				Long $t_{1/2}$ 24–96 h	
Fluvoxamine				$t_{1/2}$ 18–24 h	Less nausea than other SSRIs
Paroxetine				$t_{1/2}$ 18–24 h	Withdrawal reaction
Citalopram				$t_{1/2}$ 24–36 h	
Sertraline				$t_{1/2}$ 24–36 h	
3. Miscellaneous					
Maprotiline	Selective NA uptake inhibitor	As TCA, no significant advantages	As TCA	Long $t_{1/2}$ ~40 h	No significant advantages over TCAs
Reboxetine	Selective NA uptake inhibitor	Dizziness Insomnia Anticholinergic effects	Safe in overdose. (low risk of cardiac dysrhythmia)	$t_{1/2}$ ~12 h	Safer and fewer side-effects than TCA
Venlafaxine	Weak non-selective NA/5-HT uptake inhibitor. Also non-selective receptor-blocking effects	As SSRIs Withdrawal effects common and troublesome if doses are missed	Safe in overdose	Short $t_{1/2}$ ~5 h	Claimed to act more rapidly than other antidepressants, and to work better in 'treatment-resistant' patients

Table 38.2 *Continued*

Type and examples	Action	Unwanted effects	Risk of overdose	Pharmacokinetics	Notes
St John's wort (active principle: hyperforin)	Weak non-selective NA/5-HT uptake inhibitor. Also non-selective receptor blocking effects	Few side-effects reported	Risk of drug interactions through enhanced drug metabolism (e.g. loss of efficacy of ciclosporin, antidiabetic drugs)	$t_{1/2}$ ~12 h	Freely available as crude herbal preparation. Effective in clinical trials. Similar to other antidepressants, but fewer acute side-effects. Risk of serious drug interactions
Monoamine oxidase inhibitors (MAOIs)	Inhibit MAO-A and/or MAO-B Earlier compounds have long duration of action because of covalent binding to enzyme				
Phenelzine	Non-selective	'Cheese reaction' to tyramine-containing foods (see text) Anticholinergic side-effects Hypotension Insomnia Weight gain Liver damage (rare)	Many interactions (TCAs, opioids, sympathomimetic drugs)—risk of severe hypertension due to cheese reaction	$t_{1/2}$ 1–2 h Duration of action long because of irreversible binding	
Tranylcypromine	Non-selective	As phenelzine	As phenelzine	$t_{1/2}$ 1–2 h Duration of action long because of irreversible binding	
Isocarboxazid	Non-selective	As phenelzine	As phenelzine	Long $t_{1/2}$ ~36 h	
Moclobemide	MAO-A selective Short-acting	Nausea Insomnia, Agitation	Interactions less severe than other MAOIs; no cheese reactions reported	$t_{1/2}$ 1–2 h	Safer alternative to earlier MAOIs
Miscellaneous antidepressants					
Bupropion	Not known. Weak dopamine uptake inhibitor	Dizziness Anxiety Seizures	Safe in overdose	$t_{1/2}$ ~12 h	Used mainly in depression associated with anxiety
Trazodone	Weak 5-HT uptake inhibitor. Also blocks 5-HT_2- and H_1-receptors (enhances NA/5-HT release)	Sedation Hypotension Cardiac dysrhythmias	Safe in overdose	$t_{1/2}$ 6–12 h	Nefazodone and mianserin are similar
Mirtazapine	Blocks $\alpha 2$, 5-HT_2- and 5-HT_3-receptors	Dry mouth Sedation Weight gain	No serious drug interactions	$t_{1/2}$ 20–40 h	Claimed to have faster onset of action than other antidepressants

NA, noradrenaline; 5-HT, 5-hydroxytryptamine

Chemical aspects

TCA are closely related in structure to the phenothiazines (Ch. 37) and were initially produced (in 1949) as potential antipsychotic drugs. **Imipramine** was found to be of no use in schizophrenia, but effective in depression, so other compounds, such as **clomipramine**, were synthesised. They differ from phenothiazines principally in the incorporation of an extra atom into the central ring (Fig. 38.1), which twists the structure so that the molecule is no longer planar as in phenothiazines.

Similar changes to the structure of thioxanthene-type antipsychotic drugs resulted in drugs such as **amitriptyline**. All of these compounds are tertiary amines, with two methyl groups attached to the basic nitrogen atom. They are quite rapidly demethylated in vivo (Fig. 38.2) to the corresponding secondary amines (**desipramine**, **nortriptyline**, etc.), which are themselves active and may be administered as drugs in their own right. Other tricyclic derivatives with slightly modified bridge structures include **doxepin**. The pharmacological differences between these drugs are not very great and relate mainly to their side-effects, which are discussed below.

Mechanism of action

As discussed above, the main effect of TCA is to block the uptake of amines by nerve terminals by competition for the binding site of the transport protein (Ch. 11). Synthesis of amines, storage in synaptic vesicles and release are not directly affected, though some TCA appear to increase transmitter release indirectly by blocking presynaptic α_2-adrenoceptors. Most TCA inhibit noradrenaline and 5-HT uptake by brain synaptosomes to a similar degree (Fig. 38.3) but have much less effect on dopamine uptake. It has been suggested that improvement of emotional symptoms reflects mainly an enhancement of 5-HT-mediated transmission, whereas relief of biological symptoms results from facilitation of noradrenergic transmission. Interpretation is made difficult by the fact that the major metabolites of TCA have considerable pharmacological activity (in some cases greater than that of the parent drug) and often differ from the parent drug in respect of their noradrenaline/5-HT selectivity (Table 38.3).

In addition to their effects on amine uptake, most TCA affect one or more types of neurotransmitter receptor, including muscarinic acetylcholine receptors, histamine receptors and 5-HT receptors (see Frazer, 1997). The antimuscarinic effects of TCA do not contribute to their antidepressant effects but are responsible for various troublesome side-effects (see below).

Actions and unwanted effects

In non-depressed human subjects, TCA cause sedation, confusion and motor incoordination. These effects occur also in depressed patients in the first few days of treatment but tend to wear off in 1–2 weeks as the antidepressant effect develops. In experimental animals, TCA produce sedation, but they are able to reverse the depressant effect of reserpine treatment.

Dibenzazepines

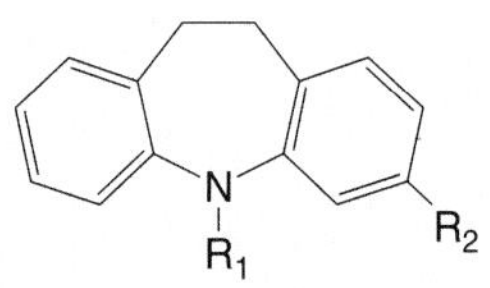

Drug	R_1	R_2
Imipramine	$-CH_2CH_2CH_2N(CH_3)_2$	H
Desipramine	$-CH_2CH_2CH_2NHCH_3$	H
Clomipramine	$-CH_2CH_2CH_2N(CH_3)_2$	Cl

Dibenzcycloheptenes

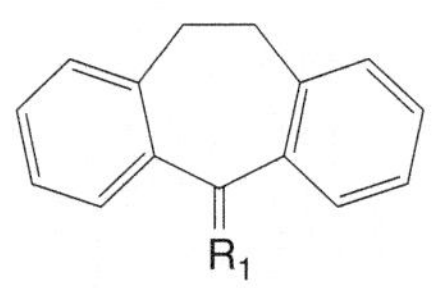

Drug	R_1
Amitriptyline	$=CHCH_2CH_2N(CH_3)_2$
Nortriptyline	$=CHCH_2CH_2NHCH_3$

Fig. 38.1 Chemical structures of tricyclic antidepressants.

Table 38.3 Inhibition of neuronal noradrenaline and 5-HT uptake by tricyclic antidepressants and their metabolites

Drug/metabolite	NA uptake	5-HT uptake
Imipramine	+++	++
Desmethylimipramine (DMI)	++++	+
Hydroxy-DMI	+++	–
Clomipramine (CMI)	++	+++
Desmethyl-CMI	+++	+
Amitriptyline (AMI)	++	++
Nortriptyline (desmethyl-AMI)	+++	++
Hydroxynortriptyline	++	++

NA, noradrenaline; 5-HT, 5-hydroxytryptamine.

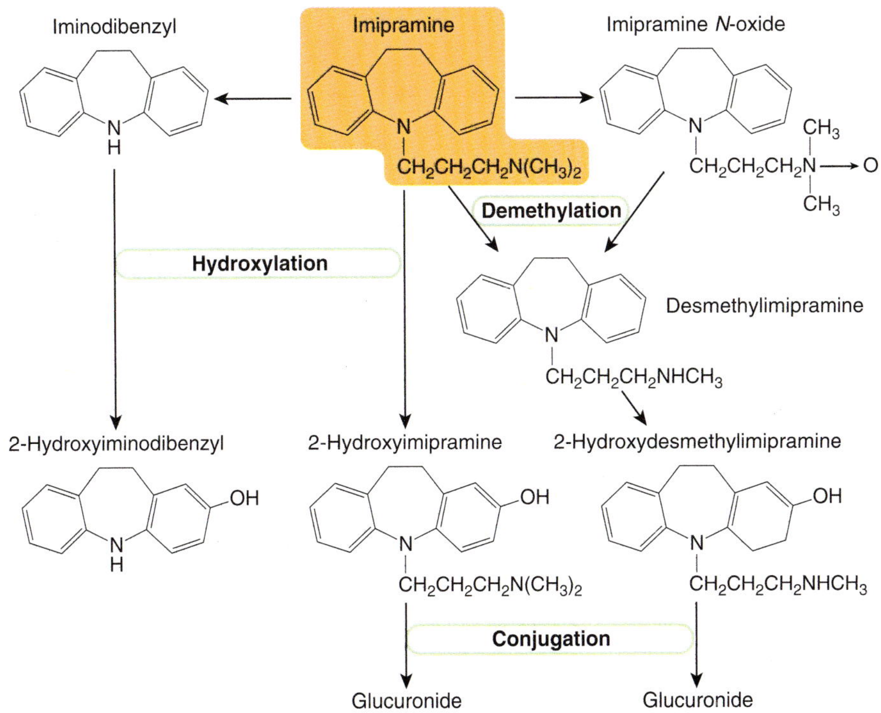

Fig. 38.2 Metabolism of imipramine, which is typical of that of other tricyclic antidepressants.

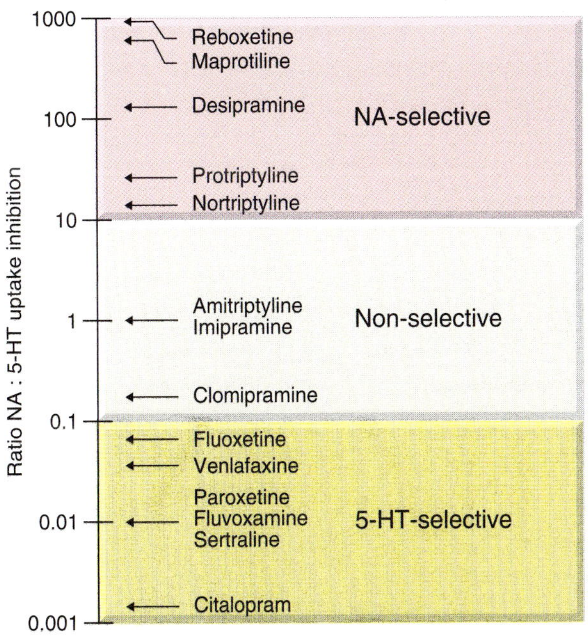

Fig. 38.3 Selectivity of inhibition of noradrenaline (NA) and 5-hydroxytryptamine (5-HT) uptake by various antidepressants.

Unwanted effects with normal clinical dosage

TCA produce a number of troublesome side-effects, mainly because of interference with autonomic control.

Atropine-like effects include dry mouth, blurred vision, constipation and urinary retention. These effects are strong with amitriptyline, and much weaker with desipramine. Postural hypotension occurs with TCA. This may seem anomalous for drugs that enhance noradrenergic transmission, and it possibly results from an effect on adrenergic transmission in the medullary vasomotor centre. The other common side-effect is sedation (see above), and the long duration of action means that daytime performance is often affected by drowsiness and difficulty in concentrating.

TCA, particularly in overdose, may cause ventricular dysrhythmias associated with prolongation of the Q–T interval (see Ch. 17). This is thought to result from blocking of a particular type of cardiac potassium channel known as the HERG channel (Ch. 4). TCA used in normal doses increase slightly, but significantly, the risk of sudden cardiac death.

Interactions with other drugs

TCA are particularly likely to cause adverse effects when given in conjunction with other drugs (see Ch. 51). They are strongly bound to plasma protein, so their effects tend to be enhanced by competing drugs (e.g. **aspirin** and **phenylbutazone**). They rely on hepatic microsomal metabolism for elimination from the body, and this may be inhibited by competing drugs (e.g. antipsychotic drugs and some steroids).

TCA cause a strong potentiation of the effects of alcohol, for reasons that are not well understood, and deaths have occurred as a result of this, when severe respiratory depression has followed a bout of drinking. TCA also interact with various antihypertensive drugs (see Ch. 18) with potentially dangerous consequences, so their use in hypertensive patients requires close monitoring.

Acute toxicity

Antidepressant drugs (most commonly TCA) are often used for attempted suicide, so their acute toxic effects are a matter of some practical importance. In the UK, TCA overdose is estimated to cause about 400 deaths annually. The main effects are on the central nervous system (CNS) and the heart. The initial effect of TCA overdosage is to cause excitement and delirium, which may be accompanied by convulsions. This is followed by coma and respiratory depression lasting for some days before a gradual recovery. Pronounced atropine-like effects are produced, with flushing, dry mouth and skin, and inhibition of gut and bladder.

Cardiac dysrhythmias (see above) are common with TCA overdose, and sudden death may occur from ventricular fibrillation.

One form of treatment that has been reported to control the main CNS effects is the use of the anticholinesterase **physostigmine** (see Ch. 10), though this is not recommended routinely. This suggests that the antimuscarinic effects of TCA may be partly responsible, and indeed the symptoms produced closely resemble those of atropine poisoning.

Pharmacokinetic aspects

TCA are all rapidly absorbed when given orally and bind strongly to plasma albumin, most being 90–95% bound at therapeutic plasma concentrations. They bind to extravascular tissues, which accounts for their generally large distribution volumes (usually 10–50 l/kg; see Ch. 7) and low rates of elimination. This extravascular sequestration means that extracorporeal dialysis is ineffective in acute overdosage.

TCA are metabolised in the liver by two main routes (Fig. 38.2), namely *N-demethylation*, whereby tertiary amines are converted to secondary amines (e.g. imipramine to desmethylimipramine, amitriptyline to nortriptyline), and *ring hydroxylation*. Both the desmethyl and the hydroxylated metabolites commonly retain biological activity (see Table 38.3). During prolonged treatment with TCA, the plasma concentration of these metabolites is usually comparable to that of the parent drug, though there is wide variation between individuals. Inactivation of the drugs occurs by glucuronide conjugation of the hydroxylated metabolites, the glucuronides being excreted in the urine.

The overall half-times for elimination of TCA are generally long, ranging from 10 to 20 hours for imipramine and desipramine to about 80 hours for protriptyline. They are even longer in elderly patients. Therefore, gradual accumulation is possible, leading to slowly developing side-effects. The relationship between plasma concentrations and the therapeutic effect may not be simple, according to a study on nortriptyline (Fig. 38.4) which showed that too high a plasma concentration actually reduced the antidepressant effect, and there is quite a narrow 'therapeutic window'. Whether this is true for other antidepressant drugs is not known.

Tricyclic antidepressants (TCA)

- TCA are chemically related to phenothiazine, and some have similar non-selective receptor-blocking actions.
- Important examples are imipramine, amitriptyline and clomipramine.
- Widely used as antidepressants.
- Most are long acting, and they are often converted to active metabolites.
- Important side-effects: sedation (H_1-block), postural hypotension (α-adrenoceptor block), dry mouth, blurred vision, constipation (muscarinic block), occasionally mania and convulsions. Risk of ventricular dysrhythmias through potassium HERG channel block.
- TCAs are dangerous in acute overdose, causing confusion and mania, and cardiac dysrhythmias.
- They are liable to interact with other drugs, e.g. alcohol, anaesthetics, hypotensive drugs and non-steroidal anti-inflammatory drugs; TCA should not be given with monoamine oxidase inhibitors (MAOI).

SELECTIVE 5-HT UPTAKE INHIBITORS

Drugs that inhibit 5-HT uptake (termed SSRI) include **fluoxetine**, **fluvoxamine**, **paroxetine**, **citalopram** and **sertraline** (see Table 38.2). Fluoxetine is currently the most prescribed antidepressant. As well as showing selectivity with respect to 5-HT over noradrenaline uptake, they are less likely than TCA to cause

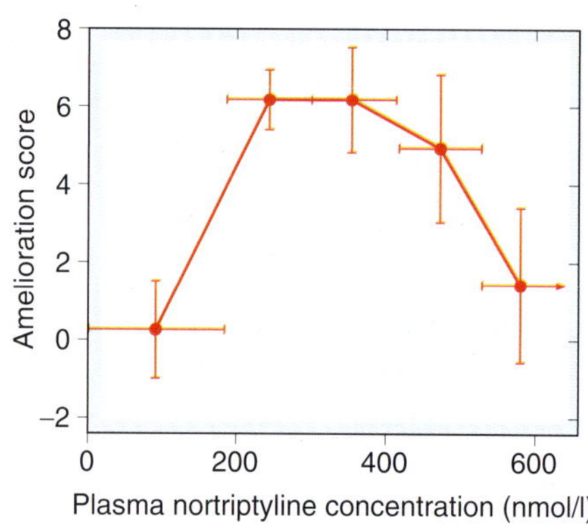

Fig. 38.4 'Therapeutic window' for nortriptyline. The antidepressant effect, determined from subjective rating scales, is optimal at plasma concentrations between 200 and 400 nmol/l and declines at higher levels.

anticholinergic side-effects and are less dangerous in overdose. In contrast to MAOI (see below), they do not cause 'cheese reactions'. They are as effective as TCA and MAOI in treating depression of moderate degree but probably less effective than TCA in treating severe depression.

Pharmacokinetic aspects

SSRIs are well absorbed orally and have plasma half-lives of 15–24 hours, fluoxetine being longer-acting (24–96 hours). The delay of 2–4 weeks before the therapeutic effect develops is similar to that seen with other antidepressants. Paroxetine and fluoxetine are not used in combination with TCA because they may inhibit TCA hepatic metabolism, and hence increase TCA toxicity.

Unwanted effects

Common side-effects are nausea, anorexia, insomnia, loss of libido and failure of orgasm.

In combination with MAOI, SSRIs can result in 'serotonin syndrome' associated with tremor, hyperthermia and cardiovascular collapse, from which deaths have occurred. There have been reports of increased aggression, and occasionally violence, in patients treated with fluoxetine, but these have not been confirmed by controlled studies.

In spite of the apparent advantages of SSRI over TCA in terms of side-effects, the combined results of many trials show no overall difference in terms of patient acceptability (Song et al., 1993).

The SSRIs are used in a variety of psychiatric disorders, as well as in depression, including anxiety disorders, panic attacks, and obsessive–compulsive disorder.

MONOAMINE OXIDASE INHIBITORS

Drugs of the MAOI type were among the first to be introduced clinically as antidepressants but were largely superseded by TCA and other types of antidepressant with clinical efficacies that were considered better and with generally less side-effects. The main examples are **phenelzine**, **tranylcypromine** and **iproniazid**. These drugs cause irreversible inhibition of the enzyme and do not distinguish between the two main isozymes (see below). Recently, the discovery of reversible inhibitors that show isozyme selectivity has rekindled interest in this class of drug. Though several studies have shown a reduction in platelet MAO activity in certain groups of depressed patients, there is no clear evidence that abnormal MAO activity is involved in the pathogenesis of depression.

MAO (see Ch. 11) is found in nearly all tissues and exists in two similar molecular forms, coded by separate genes (see Table 38.4). MAO-A has a substrate preference for 5-HT and is the main target for the antidepressant MAOI. MAO-B has a substrate preference for phenylethylamine, and both enzymes act on noradrenaline and dopamine. Type B is selectively inhibited by **selegiline**, which is used in the treatment of parkinsonism (see Ch. 34). Disruption of the gene for MAO-A in mice causes increased brain accumulation of 5-HT and, to a lesser extent, noradrenaline, along with aggressive behaviour (Shih et al., 1999). A family has been reported with an inherited mutation leading to loss of MAO-A activity; family members showed mental retardation and violent behaviour patterns. Most antidepressant MAOI act on

Other monoamine uptake inhibitors

- Inhibit monoaine uptake by a noradrenaline-selective (e.g. maprotiline, reboxetine) or non-selective (e.g. venlafaxine) mechanism.
- Generally similar to tricyclic antidepressants pharmacologically but have fewer side-effects, especially with respect to cardiac effects, so safer in overdose.

Selective 5-HT uptake inhibitors (SSRI)

- Examples include fluoxetine, fluvoxamine, paroxetine, sertraline, citalopram.
- Antidepressant actions are similar in efficacy and time course to those of tricyclic antidepressants (TCA).
- Acute toxicity is less than that of monoamine oxidase inhibitors (MAOI) or TCA, so overdose risk is reduced.
- Side-effects include nausea, insomnia. and sexual dysfunction.
- No food reactions but dangerous 'serotonin reaction' (hyperthermia, muscle rigidity, cardiovascular collapse) can occur if given with MAOI.
- Currently the most commonly prescribed antidepressants; also used for some other psychiatric indications.

Table 38.4 Substrates and inhibitors for type A and type B monoamine oxidase

	Type A	Type B
Preferred substrates	Noradrenaline 5-HT	Phenylethylamine Benzylamine
Non-specific substrates	Dopamine Tyramine	Dopamine Tyramine
Specific inhibitors	Clorgiline Moclobemide	Selegiline
Non-specific inhibitors	Pargyline Tranylcypromine Isocarboxazid	Pargyline Tranylcypromine Isocarboxazid

both forms of MAO, but clinical studies with subtype-specific inhibitors have shown clearly that antidepressant activity, as well as the main side-effects of MAOI, is associated with MAO-A inhibition. MAO is located intracellularly, mostly associated with mitochondria, and has two main functions.

- Within nerve terminals, MAO regulates the free intraneuronal concentration of noradrenaline or 5-HT and hence the releasable stores of these transmitters. It is not involved in the inactivation of released transmitter. The biochemical role of MAO in noradrenergic nerves and the effect of MAOI on transmitter metabolism are discussed in Chapter 11.
- MAO is important in the inactivation of endogenous and ingested amines, which would otherwise produce unwanted effects. An example is tyramine, an ingested amine which is a substrate for both MAO-A and MAO-B, and is important in producing some of the side-effects of MAOI (see below).

Chemical aspects

MAOI are substrate analogues with a phenylethylamine-like structure and most contain a reactive group (e.g. hydrazine, propargylamine, cyclopropylamine) that enables the inhibitor to bind covalently to the enzyme, resulting in a non-competitive and long-lasting inhibition. Recovery of MAO activity after inhibition takes several weeks with most drugs but is quicker after tranylcypromine, which forms a less stable bond with the enzyme. **Moclobemide** acts as a reversible competitive inhibitor.

MAOI are not particularly specific in their actions and inhibit a variety of other enzymes as well as MAO, including many enzymes involved in the metabolism of other drugs. This is responsible for some of the many clinically important drug interactions associated with MAOI.

Pharmacological effects

MAOI cause a rapid and sustained increase in the 5-HT, noradrenaline and dopamine content of the brain, 5-HT being affected most and dopamine least. Similar changes occur in peripheral tissues such as heart, liver and intestine, and increases in the plasma concentrations of these amines are also detectable. Although these increases in tissue amine content are largely the result of accumulation within neurons, transmitter release in response to nerve activity is not increased. In contrast to the effect of TCA, MAOI do not increase the response of peripheral organs, such as the heart and blood vessels, to sympathetic nerve stimulation. The main effect of MAOI is to increase the cytoplasmic concentration of monoamines in nerve terminals, without greatly affecting the vesicular stores which form the pool that is releasable by nerve stimulation. The increased cytoplasmic pool results in an increased rate of spontaneous leakage of monoamines, and also an increased release by indirectly acting sympathomimetic amines such as amphetamine and tyramine (see Ch. 11). This occurs because these amines work by displacing noradrenaline from the vesicles into the nerve terminal cytoplasm, from which it may either leak out and produce a response or be degraded by MAO (see Fig. 11.9). Inhibition of MAO increases the proportion that escapes and thus enhances the response. Tyramine thus causes a much greater rise in blood pressure in MAOI-treated animals than in controls. This mechanism is important in relation to the 'cheese reaction' produced by MAOI in humans (see later section).

In normal human subjects, MAOI cause an immediate increase in motor activity, and euphoria and excitement develop over the course of a few days. This is in contrast to TCA, which cause only sedation and confusion when given to non-depressed subjects. MAOI (like TCA) are also effective in reversing the behavioural effects of reserpine treatment. The effects of MAOI on amine metabolism develop rapidly, and the effect of a single dose lasts for several days. There is a clear discrepancy, as with TCA, between the rapid biochemical response and the delayed antidepressant effect.

The mechanisms underlying the antidepressant effects of MAOI are not well understood, but MAOI cause a delayed downregulation of β-adrenoceptors and $5\text{-}HT_2$-receptors similar to that produced by TCA.

Unwanted effects and toxicity

Many of the unwanted effects of MAOI result directly from MAO inhibition, but some are produced by other mechanisms.

Hypotension is a common side-effect; indeed pargyline was at one time used as an antihypertensive drug. One possible explanation for this effect—the opposite of what might have been expected—is that amines such as dopamine or octopamine are able to accumulate within peripheral sympathetic nerve terminals and displace noradrenaline from the storage vesicles, thus reducing noradrenaline release associated with sympathetic activity.

Excessive central stimulation may cause tremors, excitement, insomnia and, in overdose, convulsions.

Weight gain, associated with increased appetite, occurs in a proportion of patients and can be so extreme as to require the drug to be discontinued.

Atropine-like side-effects (dry mouth, blurred vision, urinary retention, etc.) are common with MAOI, though they are less of a problem than with TCA.

MAOI of the hydrazine type (e.g. phenelzine and iproniazid) produce, very rarely (less than 1 in 10 000), severe hepatotoxicity, which seems to be caused by the hydrazine moiety of the molecule. Their use in patients with liver disease is, therefore, unwise.

Interaction with other drugs and foods

Interaction with other drugs and foods is the most serious problem with MAOI and is the main factor that caused their clinical use to decline. The special advantage claimed for the new reversible MAOI, such as **moclobemide**, is that these interactions are reduced.

The *'cheese reaction'* is a direct consequence of MAO inhibition and occurs when normally innocuous amines produced during fermentation (mainly tyramine) are ingested. Tyramine is normally metabolised by MAO in the gut wall and liver and so little dietary

Monoamine oxidase inhibitors (MAOI)

- Main examples are phenelzine, tranylcypromine, isocarboxazid and moclobemide.
- For many years superseded by tricyclic antidepressants (TCA), mainly because of drug and food interactions; currently undergoing a revival.
- Action is long lasting (weeks) because of irreversible inhibition of MAO. Moclobemide has a short duration of action.
- Main side-effects: postural hypotension (sympathetic block); atropine-like effects (as with TCA); weight gain; CNS stimulation, causing restlessness, insomnia; liver damage (rare).
- Acute overdose causes CNS stimulation, sometimes convulsions.
- May cause severe hypertensive response to tyramine-containing foods ('cheese reaction'); this does not occur with moclobemide.
- MAOI should not be given simultaneously with TCA or 5-HT reuptake inhibitors (SSRI).
- Interact with many drugs (e.g. pethidine, causing hyperpyrexia and hypotension.)

tyramine reaches the systemic circulation. MAO inhibition allows tyramine to be absorbed and also enhances its sympathomimetic effect, as discussed above. The result is acute hypertension, giving rise to a severe throbbing headache, and occasionally even to intracranial haemorrhage. Though many foods contain some tyramine, it appears that at least 10 mg tyramine needs to be ingested to produce such a response and the main danger is from ripe cheeses and from concentrated yeast products such as Marmite. Administration of indirectly acting sympathomimetic amines (e.g. **ephedrine, amphetamine**) is also likely to cause severe hypertension in patients receiving MAOI; directly acting agents, such as noradrenaline (norepinephrine) used in conjunction with local anaesthetic injection (see Ch. 43), are not hazardous.

Hypertensive episodes have also been reported in patients given TCA and MAOI simultaneously. The probable explanation is that inhibition of noradrenaline reuptake further enhances the cardiovascular response to dietary tyramine, thus accentuating the cheese reaction. This combination of drugs can also produce excitement and hyperactivity.

MAOIs interact with some drugs to cause not merely an enhancement of their action but an abnormal syndrome. An important example is the opioid analgesic **pethidine** (see Ch. 40), which may cause severe hyperpyrexia, with restlessness, coma and hypotension when given in combination with MAOI. The mechanism is not known for certain, but it is likely that an abnormal pethidine metabolite is produced because of inhibition of the normal demethylation pathway.

A comparison of the main characteristics of MAOI and other antidepressant drugs is given in Table 38.2.

Other antidepressant drugs

- Heterogeneous group, including, trazodone, mirtazapine and bupropion.
- No common mechanism of action. Act mainly as non-selective antagonists at presynaptic receptors, possibly enhancing amine release.
- Delay in therapeutic response is similar to tricyclic antidepressants (TCA) and monoamine oxidase inhibitors. Mirtazapine may act more rapidly.
- Unwanted effects and acute toxicity vary but are generally less than with TCA.

OTHER ANTIDEPRESSANT DRUGS

Uncertainty about the exact biochemical mode of action of antidepressants has meant that the development of new drugs has often been empirical. The main claims made for these newer agents are:

- fewer side-effects (e.g. sedation and anticholinergic effects)
- lower acute toxicity in overdose
- action with less delay
- efficacy in patients non-responsive to TCA or MAOI.

In practice, the newer drugs, though no more efficacious than TCA, generally have fewer side-effects and less acute toxicity, but only **mirtazapine** appears to be more rapid in action.

▼ Two substances have been touted as 'natural' antidepressants, namely **L-tryptophan** (TRP) and **St John's wort.** Because of their origins, they are freely available and are not subject to normal regulatory controls relating to purity, safety or efficacy. TRP is the amino acid precursor of 5-HT. Given as a dietary supplement, it produces very limited antidepressant effects. In pure form, it has no adverse effects, but there have been several outbreaks of a sometimes fatal muscle disorder caused by a manufacturing impurity. St John's wort contains many active substances, one of which, **hyperforin,** is a monomine transport inhibitor. Its antidepressant activity has been confirmed in many trials and it has few acute side-effects, so is better tolerated than many conventional antidepressants. It does, however, interact with other drugs, by inducing drug-metabolising enzymes (Ch. 8). There have been cases of delayed transplant rejection because of this interaction in patients who took St. John's wort while receiving the immunosuppressant ciclosporin.

ELECTROCONVULSIVE THERAPY

A faulty line of reasoning, namely that schizophrenia and epilepsy were considered to be mutually exclusive, led to the use of induced convulsions as therapy for psychological disorders in the 1930s; though useless in schizophrenia, its efficacy in treating severe depression has been repeatedly confirmed. ECT in humans involves stimulation through electrodes placed on either side of the head, with the patient lightly anaesthetised, paralysed with a neuromuscular-blocking drug so as to avoid physical injury, and artificially ventilated. More recently, a technique involving transcranial magnetic stimulation, which does not require these precautions, has been introduced. Controlled trials have shown ECT to be at least as effective as antidepressant drugs, with response rates ranging between 60 and 80%; it appears to be the most effective treatment for severe suicidal depression. The main disadvantage of ECT is that it often causes confusion and memory loss lasting for days or weeks.

The effect of ECT on experimental animals has been carefully analysed to see if it provides clues as to the mode of action of antidepressant drugs, but the clues it gives are enigmatic. 5-HT synthesis and uptake are unaltered, and noradrenaline uptake is somewhat increased (in contrast to the effect of TCA). Decreased β-adrenoceptor responsiveness, both biochemical and behavioural, occurs with both ECT and long-term administration of antidepressant drugs, but changes in 5-HT-mediated responses tend to go in opposite directions (see Maes & Meltzer, 1995).

CLINICAL EFFECTIVENESS OF ANTIDEPRESSANT TREATMENTS

The overall clinical efficacy of antidepressants has been established in many well-controlled clinical trials. However, it is clear that a substantial proportion of patients recover spontaneously, and that placebo responders are very common;* moreover, 30–40% of patients fail to improve with drug treatments. Controlled trials show there is little to choose in terms of overall efficacy between any of the drugs currently in use, but clinical experience suggests that individual patients may respond better to one drug than to another. Attempts to identify which patients will respond on the basis of behavioural or biochemical measurements (e.g. platelet MAO activity, MHPG excretion) have not been successful.

MOOD-STABILISING DRUGS

Mood-stablising drugs are used to control the mood swings characteristic of manic-depressive (bipolar) illness. **Lithium** is most commonly used, but recently antiepileptic drugs such as **carbamazepine**, **valproate** and **gabapentin** (Ch. 39), which have fewer side-effects and problems than lithium, have also proved efficacious.

Used prophylactically in bipolar depression, mood-stabilising drugs prevent the swings of mood and thus reduce both the depressive and the manic phases of the illness. They are given over long periods, and their beneficial effects take 3–4 weeks to develop. Given in an acute attack, they are effective only in reducing mania, not during the depressive phase (though lithium is sometimes used as an adjunct to antidepressants in severe cases of unipolar depression).

*Placebo responses are particularly evident in antidepressant trials, patients being influenced by the attitude of the prescriber, who is, in turn, influenced by claims for the latest in a long line of drugs. A nightmare for hospital formulary committees!

LITHIUM

Other drugs (e.g. antipsychotics) are equally effective in treating acute mania; they act more quickly and are considerably safer, so the clinical use of lithium is mainly confined to prophylactic control of manic-depressive illness.

The psychotropic effect of lithium was discovered in 1949 by Cade, who had predicted that urate salts should prevent the induction by uraemia of a hyperexcitability state in guinea-pigs. He found lithium urate to produce an effect, quickly discovered that it was caused by lithium rather than urate, and went on to show that lithium produced a rapid improvement in a group of manic patients.

Pharmacological effects and mechanism of action

Lithium is clinically effective at a plasma concentration of 0.5–1 mmol/l; above 1.5 mmol/l it produces a variety of toxic effects. Consequently, the therapeutic window is narrow. In normal subjects, 1 mmol/l lithium in plasma has no appreciable psychotropic effects. It does, however, produce many detectable biochemical changes, and it is still extremely unclear how these may be related to its therapeutic effect.

Lithium is a monovalent cation that can mimic the role of Na^+ in excitable tissues, being able to permeate the fast voltage-sensitive channels that are responsible for action potential generation (see Ch. 4). It is, however, not pumped out by the Na^+/K^+-ATPase and, therefore, tends to accumulate inside excitable cells, leading to a partial loss of intracellular K^+, and depolarisation of the cell.

The biochemical effects of lithium are complex, but its therapeutic actions are generally ascribed to two mechanisms (see Nahorski et al., 1991; Atack et al., 1995).

- The phosphatidylinositol (PI) pathway (see Ch. 3) is blocked at the point where inositol phosphate is hydrolysed to free inositol. This step is required for the regeneration of PI in the membrane after it has been hydrolysed by agonist action, as described in Chapter 3. Lithium thus causes a depletion of membrane PI and accumulation of intracellular inositol phosphate. The result is inhibition of agonist-stimulated inositol trisphosphate formation through various PI-linked receptors and, therefore, block of many receptor-mediated effects.
- Hormone-induced cAMP production is usually reduced (e.g. the response of renal tubular cells to antidiuretic hormone, and of the thyroid to thyroid-stimulating hormone; see Chs 23 and 28). This is not, however, a pronounced effect in the brain.

It is believed that the effects of lithium on these two important second messenger systems account for its therapeutic effect, and that its cellular selectivity depends on the uptake of lithium in varying amounts, reflecting the activity of sodium channels in different cells. This could explain its relatively selective action in the brain and kidney, even though many other tissues use the same second messengers. Lacking knowledge of the the nature of the disturbance underlying the mood swings in bipolar

Lithium

- Inorganic ion taken orally as lithium carbonate.
- Mechanism of action is not understood. The main biochemical possibilities are:
  —interference with inositol trisphosphate formation.
  —interference with cAMP formation.
- Acts to control mania as well as depression. Lithium is mainly used prophylactically in bipolar depression.
- Long plasma half-life and narrow therapeutic window.
- Hence, side-effects are common, and monitoring of plasma concentration essential, especially in presence of renal disease. Action enhanced by diuretic drugs.
- Main unwanted effects: nausea, thirst and polyuria, hypothyroidism, tremor, weakness, mental confusion, teratogenesis. Acute overdose causes confusion, convulsions and cardiac dysrhythmias.
- Alternative mood-stabilising drugs (e.g. carbamazepine, valproate, gabapentin) are gaining favour because of better side-effect and safety profile.

depression, we remain ignorant of the link between the biochemical and the prophylactic effects of lithium.

Pharmacokinetic aspects and toxicity

Lithium is given by mouth as the carbonate salt and is excreted by the kidney. About half of an oral dose is excreted within about 12 hours—the remainder, which presumably represents lithium taken up by cells, is excreted over the next 1–2 weeks. This very slow phase means that, with regular dosage, lithium accumulates slowly over approximately 2 weeks before a steady state is reached. The narrow therapeutic limit for the plasma concentration (approximately 0.5–1.5 mmol/l) means that monitoring is essential. Sodium depletion reduces the rate of excretion by increasing the reabsorption of lithium by the proximal tubule, and thus increases the likelihood of toxicity. Diuretics that act distal to the proximal tubule (Ch. 23) also have this effect, and renal disease also predisposes to lithium toxicity.

The main toxic effects that may occur during treatment are:

- nausea, vomiting and diarrhoea
- tremor
- renal effects:
  —polyuria (with resulting thirst) resulting from inhibition of the action of antidiuretic hormone; Na^+ retention associated with increased aldosterone secretion
  —serious renal tubular damage may occur with prolonged treatment, making it essential to monitor renal function regularly in lithium-treated patients
- thyroid enlargement, sometimes associated with hypothyroidism
- weight gain.

Acute lithium toxicity results in various neurological effects, progressing from confusion and motor impairment, to coma, convulsions and death if the plasma concentration reaches 3–5 mmol/l.

REFERENCES AND FURTHER READING

Ashton H 1992 Brain systems, disorders and psychotropic drugs. Blackwell Science, Oxford (*Comprehensive monograph*)

Atack J R, Broughton H B, Pollack S J 1995 Inositol monophosphatase—a putative target for Li^+ in the treatment of bipolar disorder. Trends Neurosci 18: 343–349 (*Review of evidence suggesting that lithium action depends on interference with inositol recycling, and hence role of IP in intracellular signalling*)

Baker G B, Dewhurst W G 1985 Biochemical theories of affective disorders. In: Dewhurst W G, Baker G B (eds) Pharmacotherapy of affective disorders. Croom Helm, Beckenham (*Useful review of earlier hypotheses relating monoamine disturbances to mood disorders*)

Frazer A 1997 Pharmacology of antidepressants. J Clin Psychopharmacol 17: 2S–18S (*Good general review*)

Holsboer F 1999 The rationale for corticotrophin-releasing hormone receptor (CRH-R) antagonists to treat depression and anxiety. J Psychiatr Res 33: 181–214 (*Reviews the evidence linking CRH with depressive illness*)

Maes M, Meltzer H Y 1995 The serotonin hypothesis of major depression. In: Bloom F E, Kupfer D J (eds) Psychopharmacology: the fourth generation of progress. Raven Press, New York (*Review showing how emphasis has shifted towards the involvement of 5-HT, rather than noradrenaline, in the aetiology of depression*)

Malberg J E, Eisch A J, Nestler E, Duman R S 2000 Chronic antidepressant treatment increases neurogensis in the rat hippocampus. J Neurosci 20: 9104–9110 (*New idea relating to the mechnism of action of antidepressant drugs*)

Manji H K, Drevets W C, Charney D S 2001 The cellular neurobiology of depression. Nat Med 7: 541–547 (*Speculative review of the possible mechanisms and role of neurodegeneration and neuroplasticity in depressive disorders, attempting to move beyond the monoamine theory*)

Nahorski S R, Ragan C I, Challiss R A J 1991 Lithium and the phosphoinositide cycle: an example of uncompetitive inhibition and its pharmacological consequences. Trends Pharmacol Sci 12: 297–303 (*Short review article; see also Atack et al. 1995*)

Porsolt R D 1985 Animal models of affective disorders. In: Dewhurst W G, Baker G B (eds) Pharmacotherapy of affective disorders. Croom Helm, Beckenham (*Useful review of animal models, still mainly valid despite date*)

Shih J C, Chen K, Ridd M J 1999 Monoamine oxidase: from genes to behaviour. Annu Rev Neurosci XX: 197–217 (*Review of recent work on transgenic mice with MAO mutation or deletion*)

Song F, Freemantle N, Sheldon T A et al. 1993 Selective serotonin reuptake inhibitors: meta-analysis of efficacy and acceptability. Br Med J 306: 683–687 (*Summary of clinical trials data showing limitations as well as advantages of SSRIs*)

Wong M-L, Licinio J 2001 Research and treatment approaches to depression. Nat Rev Neurosci 2: 343–351 (*Excellent summary of the current—somewhat patchy—state of knowledge about the biochemical and genetic basis of depression, and the mechanism of action of antidepressant drugs*)

39 Antiepileptic drugs

Overview 550

The nature of epilepsy 550
— Types of epilepsy 550
— Neural mechanisms and animal models of epilepsy 552

Mechanism of action of antiepileptic drugs 553

Antiepileptic drugs 554
— Phenytoin 555
— Carbamazepine 555
— Valproate 556
— Ethosuximide 557
— Phenobarbital 557
— Benzodiazepines 558
— Newer antiepileptic drugs 558

Muscle spasm and centrally acting muscle relaxants 559

OVERVIEW

Epilepsy is a very common disorder, characterised by *seizures*, which take various forms and result from episodic neuronal discharges, the form of the seizure depending on the part of the brain affected. Epilepsy affects 0.5–1% of the population. Often there is no recognisable cause, although it may develop after brain damage, such as trauma, infection or tumour growth, or other kinds of neurological disease, including various inherited neurological syndromes. Epilepsy is treated mainly with drugs, though brain surgery may be used for severe cases. Current antiepileptic drugs are effective in controlling seizures in about 70% of patients, but their use is often limited by side-effects. In attempting to improve the efficacy and side-effect profile, many new antiepileptic drugs have been developed since the mid-1990s—one of the most active areas of drug development. Improvements have been steady rather than spectacular, and epilepsy remains a difficult problem, despite the fact that controlling reverberative neuronal discharges would seem, on the face of it, to be a much simpler problem than controlling those aspects of brain function that determine emotions, mood and cognitive function.

In this chapter we describe the nature of epilepsy, the neurobiological mechanisms underlying it and the animal models that can be used to study it. We then proceed to describe the various classes of drug that are used to treat it, the mechanisms by which they work and their pharmacological characteristics. More information on the topics covered here is given by Eadie & Vajda (2000).

Centrally acting muscle relaxants are discussed briefly at the end of the chapter.

THE NATURE OF EPILEPSY

The characteristic event in epilepsy is the *seizure*, which is associated with the episodic high-frequency discharge of impulses by a group of neurons in the brain. What starts as a local abnormal discharge may then spread to other areas of the brain. The site of the primary discharge and the extent of its spread determines the symptoms that are produced, which range from a brief lapse of attention to a full-blown convulsive fit lasting for several minutes. The particular symptoms produced depend on the function of the region of the brain that is affected. Thus involvement of the motor cortex causes convulsions; involvement of the hypothalamus causes peripheral autonomic discharge, and involvement of the reticular formation in the upper brainstem leads to loss of consciousness.

Abnormal electrical activity during a seizure can be detected by electroencephalograph (EEG) recording from electrodes distributed over the surface of the scalp. Various types of seizure can be recognised on the basis of the nature and distribution of the abnormal discharge (Fig. 39.1).

TYPES OF EPILEPSY

The clinical classification of epilepsy defines two major seizure categories, namely *partial* and *generalised*, though there is some overlap and many varieties of each. Either form is classified as

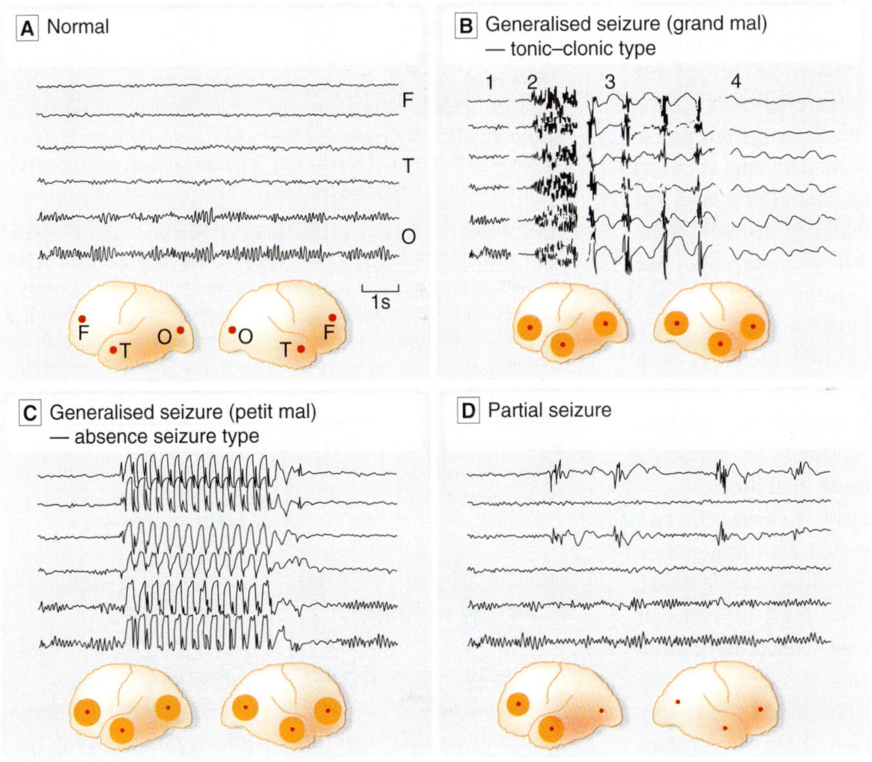

Fig. 39.1 Electroencephalograph (EEG) records in epilepsy. [A] Normal EEG recorded from frontal (F), temporal (T) and occipital (O) sites on both sides, as shown in the inset diagram. The α-rhythm (10/s) can be seen in the occipital region. [B] Sections of EEG recorded during a generalised tonic–clonic (grand mal) seizure. 1. Normal record. 2. Onset of tonic phase. 3. Clonic phase. 4. Postconvulsive coma. [C] Generalised absence seizure (petit mal) showing sudden brief episode of 3/s 'spike and wave' discharge. [D] Partial seizure with synchronous abnormal discharges in left frontal and temporal regions. (From: Eliasson S G et al. 1978 Neurological pathophysiology, 2nd edn. Oxford University Press, New York.)

simple (if consciousness is not lost) or *complex* (if consciousness is lost).

PARTIAL SEIZURES

Partial seizures are those in which the discharge begins locally, and often remains localised. The symptoms depend on the brain region or regions involved, and include involuntary muscle contractions, abnormal sensory experiences or autonomic discharge, or effects on mood and behaviour, often termed psychomotor epilepsy. The EEG discharge in this type of epilepsy is normally confined to one hemisphere (Fig 39.1D). Partial seizures can often be attributed to local cerebral lesions, and their incidence increases with age. In complex partial seizures, loss of consciousness may occur at the outset of the attack, or somewhat later, when the discharge has spread from its site of origin to regions of the brainstem reticular formation

An epileptic focus in the motor cortex results in attacks, sometimes called Jacksonian epilepsy, consisting of repetitive jerking of a particular muscle group, which spreads and may involve much of the body within about 2 minutes before dying out. The patient loses voluntary control of the affected parts of the body but does not necessarily lose consciousness. In psychomotor epilepsy, which is often associated with a focus in the temporal lobe, the attack may consist of stereotyped purposive movements such as rubbing or patting movements, or much more complex behaviour such as dressing or walking or hair-combing. The seizure usually lasts for a few minutes, after which the patient recovers with no recollection of the event. The behaviour during the seizure can be bizarre and accompanied by a strong emotional response.

Complex partial seizures are among the commonest types of epilepsy.

GENERALISED SEIZURES

Generalised seizures involve the whole brain, including the reticular system, thus producing abnormal electrical activity throughout both hemispheres. Immediate loss of consciousness is characteristic of generalised seizures. Two important categories are *tonic–clonic seizures* (grand mal, Fig. 39.1B) and *absence seizures* (petit mal, Fig. 39.1C). A tonic–clonic seizure consists of an initial strong contraction of the whole musculature, causing a rigid extensor spasm. Respiration stops and defaecation, micturition and salivation often occur. This tonic phase lasts for about 1 minute and is followed by a series of violent, synchronous jerks, which gradually dies out in 2–4 minutes. The patient stays unconscious for a few more minutes and then gradually recovers, feeling ill and confused. Injury may occur during the convulsive episode. The EEG shows generalised continuous high-frequency activity in the tonic phase, and an intermittent discharge in the clonic phase.

Absence seizures occur in children; they are much less dramatic but may occur more frequently (many seizures each day), than tonic–clonic seizures. The patient abruptly ceases whatever he or she was doing, sometimes stopping speaking in mid-sentence, and stares vacantly for a few seconds, with little or no motor disturbance. The patient is unaware of his or her surroundings and recovers abruptly with no after-effects. The EEG pattern shows a characteristic rhythmic discharge during the period of the seizure (Fig. 36.1C). The rhythmicity appears to be caused by oscillatory feedback between the cortex and the thalamus, the special properties of the thalamic neurons being dependent on the calcium channels that they express (see Willoughby, 1999). The pattern differs from that of partial seizures, where a high-frequency asynchronous discharge spreads out from a local focus. Accordingly (see below), the drugs used specifically to treat absence seizures act mainly by blocking calcium channels, whereas drugs effective against other types of epilepsy act mainly by blocking sodium channels or enhancing gamma-aminobutyric acid (GABA) -mediated inhibition.

A particularly severe kind of epilepsy, *Lennox–Gastaut syndrome*, occurs in children and is associated with progressive mental retardation, possibly a reflection of excitotoxic neurodegeneration (see Ch. 34). About one third of cases of epilepsy are familial, but few specific gene defects have been identified.*

With optimal drug therapy, epilepsy is controlled completely in about 75% of patients, but about 10% (50 000 in Britain) continue to have seizures at intervals of 1 month or less, which severely disrupts their life and work. There is, therefore, a need to improve the efficacy of therapy.

NEURAL MECHANISMS AND ANIMAL MODELS OF EPILEPSY

▼ The underlying neuronal abnormality in epilepsy is poorly understood. In general, excitation will naturally tend to spread throughout a network of interconnected neurons but is normally prevented from doing so by inhibitory mechanisms. Thus epileptogenesis can arise if excitatory transmission is facilitated or inhibitory transmission is reduced. In certain respects epileptogenesis resembles long-term potentiation (Ch. 32), and similar types of use-dependent synaptic plasticity may be involved (see Kulmann et al., 2000). Because detailed studies are difficult to carry out on epileptic patients, many different animal models of epilepsy have been investigated (see Löscher, 1999). These include a variety of genetic strains that show epilepsy-like characteristics (e.g. mice that convulse briefly in response to certain sounds, baboons that show photically induced seizures, and beagles with an inherited abnormality that closely resembles human epilepsy). Recently, several transgenic mouse strains have been reported that show spontaneous seizures. They include knockout mutations of various ion channels, receptors and other synaptic proteins. It is too early to say whether these will be useful as models of human epilepsy. Local cortical damage (e.g. by applying aluminium oxide paste or crystals of a cobalt salt) results in focal epilepsy. Local application of penicillin crystals has a similar effect, probably by interfering with inhibitory synaptic transmission. Convulsant drugs, such as **pentylenetetrazol** (PTZ, see Ch. 41), are often used, particularly in the testing of antiepileptic agents, and seizures caused by electrical stimulation of the whole brain are used for the same purpose. It has been found empirically that drugs which inhibit PTZ-induced convulsions and raise the threshold for production of electrically induced seizures are generally effective against absence seizures, whereas those that reduce the duration and spread of electrically induced convulsions are effective in focal types of epilepsy, such as tonic–clonic seizures.

The *kindling model* may approximate the human condition more closely than directly evoked seizure models. Low-intensity electrical stimulation of certain regions of the limbic system such as the amygdala with implanted electrodes normally produces no seizure response. If a brief period of stimulation is repeated daily for several days, however, the response gradually increases until very low levels of stimulation will evoke a full seizure, and eventually seizures begin to occur spontaneously. Once produced, the kindled state persists indefinitely. This change is prevented by glutamate (*N*-methyl-D-aspartate (NMDA)) subtype receptor antagonists and may involve processes similar to those that cause long-term potentiation of synaptic transmission in the hippocampus (see Ch.

*Some rare hereditary forms of epilepsy have been linked to mutations in potassium or sodium channels In one type, the mutation turned out to be in a ubiquitous endogenous protease inhibitor, cystatin B, previously unsuspected of any connection with neuronal function. Comment of an expert in epilepsy genetics, quoted in Science: 'Boy, what a surprising thing!'

Nature of epilepsy

- Epilepsy affects about 0.5% of the population.
- The characteristic event is the seizure, which is often associated with convulsions but may occur in many other forms.
- The seizure is caused by an asynchronous high-frequency discharge of a group of neurons, starting locally and spreading to a varying extent to affect other parts of the brain. In absence seizures, the discharge is regular and oscillatory.
- Partial sizures affect localised brain regions, and the attack may involve mainly motor, sensory or behavioural phenomena. Unconsciousness occurs when the reticular formation is involved. Generalised seizures affect the whole brain.
- Two common forms of epilepsy are the tonic–clonic fit (grand mal) and the absence seizure (petit mal). Status epilepticus is a life-threatening condition in which seizure activity is uninterrupted.
- Many animal models have been devised, including electrically and chemically induced generalised seizures, production of local chemical damage and kindling. These provide good prediction of antiepileptic drug effects in humans.
- The neurochemical basis of the abnormal discharge is not well understood. It may be associated with enhanced excitatory amino acid transmission, impaired inhibitory transmission, or abnormal electrical properties of the affected cells. The glutamate content in areas surrounding an epileptic focus may be increased.
- Repeated epileptic discharge can cause neuronal death (excitotoxicity).
- Current drug therapy is effective in 70–80% of patients.

32). In human focal epilepsies, surgical removal of a damaged region of cortex fails to cure the condition, as though the abnormal discharge from the region of primary damage had somehow produced a secondary hyperexcitability elsewhere in the brain. Furthermore, prophylactic treatment with antiepileptic drugs for 2 years following severe head injury reduces the subsequent incidence of post-traumatic epilepsy, which suggests that a phenomenon similar to kindling may underlie this form of epilepsy.

The *kainate model* entails a single injection of the glutamate receptor agonist kainic acid into the amygdaloid nucleus of a rat. After transient intense stimulation, spontaneous seizures begin to occur 2–4 weeks later, and again continue indefinitely. It is believed that excitotoxic damage to inhibitory neurons is responsible, associated with structural remodelling of excitatory synaptic connections, changes that may also be a factor in human epilepsies.

By intracellular recording techniques it is known that neurons from which the epileptic discharge originates display an unusual type of electrical behaviour, termed the paroxysmal depolarising shift (PDS), during which the membrane potential suddenly decreases by about 30 mV and remains depolarised for up to a few seconds before returning to normal. A burst of action potentials often accompanies this depolarisation (Fig. 39.2). This event probably results from the abnormally exaggerated and prolonged action of an excitatory transmitter. Activation of NMDA-receptors (see Ch. 32) produces 'plateau-shaped' depolarising responses very similar to the PDS, as well as initiating seizure activity. This membrane response occurs because of the voltage-dependent blocking action of Mg^{2+} on channels operated by NMDA-receptors (see Ch. 32). Glutamate must undoubtedly participate in the epileptic discharge, but efforts to develop glutamate antagonists as antiepileptic drugs have so far been unsuccessful. It is known that repeated seizure activity can lead to neuronal degeneration, possibly as a result of excitotoxicity (Ch. 34).

Studies on experimental epilepsy in the kindling or kainate models have revealed a deficit in various markers of GABA-mediated inhibitory transmission, and an increase of markers associated with glutamate-mediated excitation (see Jarrott, 1999). Human studies have shown less-consistent changes, though studies on brain samples removed at operation suggest that the epileptic focus contains more glutamate than normal, though the GABA content is not affected. Potassium-stimulated glutamate release is also increased in the epileptic focus compared with normal tissue.

Recent studies (see Binder et al., 2001) suggest that *neurotrophins*, particularly *brain-derived neurotrophic factor* (BDNF), may play a role in epileptogenesis. BDNF, which acts on a membrane receptor tyrosine kinase (Ch. 3), enhances membrane excitability and also stimulates synapse formation. Production and release of BDNF is increased in the kindling models, and there is also evidence for its involvement in human epilepsy. Specific blocking agents represent a possible future strategy for treating epilepsy, but remain to be identified.

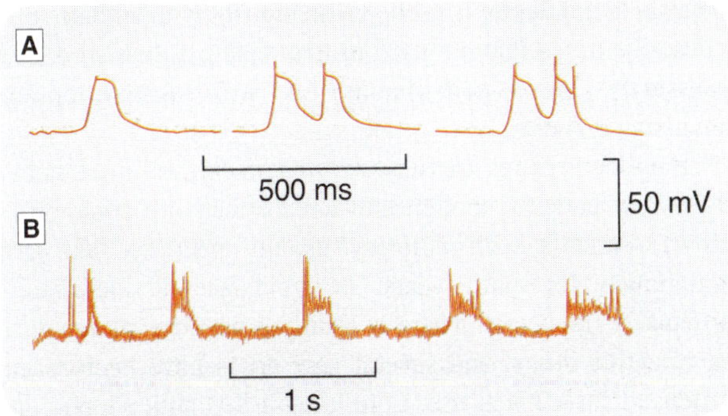

Fig. 39.2 'Paroxysmal depolarising shift' (PDS) compared with experimental activation of glutamate receptors of the NMDA type. A PDS recorded with an intracellular microelectrode from cortical neurons of anaesthetised cats. Seizure activity was induced by topical application of penicillin. **B** Intracellular recording from caudate nucleus of anaesthetised cat. NMDA was applied by ionophoresis from a nearby micropipette. Note the periodic waves of depolarisation, associated with a burst of action potentials, which closely resemble the PDS. (NMDA, *N*-methyl D-aspartate.) (From: (A) Matsumoto H, Marsan C A 1964 Exp Neurol 9: 286; (B) Herrling P L et al. 1983 J Physiol 339: 207.)

MECHANISM OF ACTION OF ANTIEPILEPTIC DRUGS

Three main mechanisms appear to be important in the action of antiepileptic drugs (see Meldrum 1996):

- enhancement of GABA action
- inhibition of sodium channel function
- inhibition of calcium channel function.

Other mechanisms that may operate with some drugs are inhibition of glutamate release and block of glutamate receptors. Many of the current antiepileptic drugs were developed empirically on the basis of activity in animal models, such as the electroshock seizure test. Their mechanism of action at the cellular level is not fully understood. As with drugs used to treat cardiac dysrhythmias (Ch. 17), the aim is to prevent the paroxysmal discharge without affecting normal transmission. It is clear that properties such as use-dependence and voltage-dependence of channel-blocking drugs (see Ch. 4) are important in achieving this selectivity, but our understanding remains fragmentary.

Enhancement of GABA action

Several antiepileptic drugs (e.g. **phenobarbital** and **benzodiazepines**) enhance the activation of $GABA_A$-receptors, thus facilitating the GABA-mediated opening of chloride channels (see Chs 32 and 36). A recently introduced drug **vigabatrin** (see below) acts by inhibiting the enzyme GABA transaminase, which is responsible for inactivating GABA, and **tiagabine** inhibits GABA uptake; both thereby enhance the action of GABA as an inhibitory transmitter. **Gabapentin** (see below) was designed as an agonist at $GABA_A$-receptors but ironically was found to be an effective antiepileptic drug in spite of having little or no effect on GABA receptors or on the transporter; its mechanism of action remains uncertain (see Macdonald, 1999).

Inhibition of sodium channel function

Several of the most important antiepileptic drugs (e.g. **phenytoin**, **carbamazepine**, **valproate**, **lamotrigine**) affect membrane excitability by an action on voltage-dependent sodium channels (see Ch. 4), which carry the inward membrane current necessary for the generation of an action potential. Their blocking action shows the property of use-dependence (see Ch 4); in other words, they block preferentially the excitation of cells that are firing repetitively, and the higher the frequency of firing, the greater the block produced. This characteristic, which is relevant to the ability of drugs to block the high-frequency discharge that occurs in an epileptic fit without unduly interfering with the low-frequency firing of neurons in the normal state, arises from the ability of blocking drugs to discriminate between sodium channels in their resting, open and inactivated states. Depolarisation of a neuron (such as occurs in the PDS described above) increases the proportion of the sodium channels in the inactivated state. Antiepileptic drugs bind preferentially to channels in this state, preventing them from returning to the resting state, and thus reducing the number of functional channels available to generate action potentials.

Inhibition of calcium channels

Several antiepileptic drugs have minor effects on calcium channels (see Table 39.1), but only **ethosuximide** specifically blocks the T-type calcium channel, activation of which is believed to play a role in the rhythmic discharge associated with absence seizures. **Gabapentin** may act on L-type calcium channels, but whether this is important for its antiepileptic properties is uncertain.

Other mechanisms

The action of many antiepileptic drugs remains poorly understood (see Levy et al., 1995; Meldrum 1996; MacDonald, 1999). **Phenobarbital** is a barbiturate (see Ch. 36) that has a greater antiepileptic effect and relatively less sedative action than other barbiturates, though its GABA-potentiating action is similar. However, phenobarbital is as effective against electrically induced convulsions as it is against PTZ-induced convulsions in rats or mice, whereas benzodiazepines, which act similarly on GABA-mediated transmission, are without effect on electrically induced convulsions. Phenobarbital reduces the electrical activity of neurons within a chemically induced epileptic focus in the cortex, whereas diazepam (a benzodiazepine) does not suppress the focal activity but prevents it from spreading. The action of phenobarbital cannot, therefore, be solely a result of its interaction with GABA, and it is likely that it also acts by inhibiting excitatory synaptic responses, though little is known about the mechanism.

Phenytoin has been studied in great detail. It not only causes use-dependent block of sodium channels (see above) but also affects other aspects of membrane function, including calcium channels, and post-tetanic potentiation, as well as intracellular protein phosphorylation by calmodulin-activated kinases, which could also interfere with membrane excitability and synaptic function.*

Obvious targets for potential antiepileptic drugs are the receptors for excitatory amino acids (see Ch. 32), and antagonists acting on NMDA, AMPA (α-amino-3-hydroxy-5-methyl-4-isoxazolepropionate) or metabotropic glutamate receptors all show anticonvulsant activity in various animal models. Few of these drugs have yet been tested in humans, but in general they show a narrow margin between the desired anticonvulsant effect and unacceptable side-effects, such as loss of motor coordination.

Mechanism of action of antiepileptic drugs

- Current antiepileptic drugs are thought to act mainly by three main mechanisms:
  - —reducing electrical excitablity of cell membranes, mainly through use-dependent block of sodium channels
  - —enhancing GABA-mediated synaptic inhibition: this may be achieved by an enhanced postsynaptic action of GABA, by inhibiting GABA transaminase or by drugs with direct GABA-agonist properties
  - —inhibiting T-type calcium channels (important in controlling absence siezures).
- Newer drugs act by other mechanisms, yet to be elucidated.
- Drugs that block glutamate receptors are effective in animal models but are not yet developed for clinical use.

ANTIEPILEPTIC DRUGS

The term antiepileptic is used synonymously with anticonvulsant to describe drugs that are used to treat epilepsy (which does not necessarily cause convulsions) as well as non-epileptic convulsive disorders.

Antiepileptic drugs are fully effective in controlling seizures in 50–80% of patients, though unwanted effects are common (see below). Patients with epilepsy usually need to take drugs continuously for many years, so avoidance of side-effects is particularly important. There is clearly a need for more specific and effective drugs, and several new drugs have been recently introduced for clinical use. Long-established antiepileptic drugs (see Table 39.1) include **phenytoin, carbamazepine, valproate, ethosuximide** and **phenobarbital**, together with various benzodiazepines, such as **diazepam, clonazepam** and **clobazam**. The newer drugs, the place of which in therapy is still being evaluated, include **vigabatrin, gabapentin, lamotrigine, felbamate, tiagabine** and **topiramate.**

*The highly complex actions of established antiepileptic drugs are apt to make discouraging reading for those engaged in trying to develop new drugs on simple rational principles. Serendipity, not science, appears to be the path to therapeutic success.

PHENYTOIN

Phenytoin is the most important member of the hydantoin group of compounds, which are structurally related to the barbiturates. It is highly effective in reducing the intensity and duration of electrically induced convulsions in mice, though ineffective against PTZ-induced convulsions. Despite its many side-effects and unpredictable pharmacokinetic behaviour, phenytoin is widely used, being effective against various forms of partial and generalised seizures, though not against absence seizures, which may even get worse.

Pharmacokinetic aspects

Phenytoin has certain pharmacokinetic peculiarities that need to be taken into account when it is used clinically. It is well absorbed when given orally, and about 80–90% of the plasma content is bound to albumin. Other drugs, such as salicylates, phenylbutazone and valproate, inhibit this binding competitively (see Ch. 51). This increases the free phenytoin concentration but also increases hepatic clearance of phenytoin, so it may enhance or reduce the effect of the phenytoin in an unpredictable way. Phenytoin is metabolised by the hepatic mixed function oxidase system and excreted mainly as the glucuronide. It causes enzyme induction and thus increases the rate of metabolism of other drugs (e.g. oral anticoagulants). The metabolism of phenytoin itself can be either enhanced or competitively inhibited by various other drugs that share the same hepatic enzymes. Phenobarbital produces both effects, and since competitive inhibition is immediate whereas induction takes time, it initially enhances and later reduces the pharmacological activity of phenytoin. Ethanol has a similar dual effect.

The metabolism of phenytoin shows the characteristic of saturation (see Ch. 4), which means that over the therapeutic plasma concentration range the rate of inactivation does not increase in proportion to the plasma concentration. The consequences of this are:

- the plasma half-life (approximately 20 hours) increases as the dose is increased
- the steady-state mean plasma concentration, achieved when a patient is given a constant daily dose, varies disproportionately with the dose. (Figure 39.3 shows that in one patient increasing the dose by 50% caused the steady-state plasma concentration to increase more than fourfold.)

The range of plasma concentration over which phenytoin is effective without causing excessive unwanted effects is quite narrow (approximately 40–100 μmol/l). The very steep relationship between dose and plasma concentration, and the many interacting factors, mean that there is considerable individual variation in the plasma concentration achieved with a given dose. A radioimmunoassay for phenytoin in plasma is available, and its use has helped considerably in achieving an optimal therapeutic effect. The past tendency was to add further drugs for patients where a single drug failed to give adequate control. It is now recognised that much of the unpredictability can be ascribed to pharmacokinetic variability, and regular plasma monitoring has reduced the use of polypharmacy.

Unwanted effects

Side-effects of phenytoin begin to appear at plasma concentrations exceeding 100 μmol/l and may be severe above about 150 μmol/l. The milder side-effects include vertigo, ataxia, headache and nystagmus, but not sedation. At higher plasma concentrations, marked confusion with intellectual deterioration occurs; these effects occur acutely and are quickly reversible. Hyperplasia of the gums, which is disfiguring rather than harmful, often develops gradually, as does hirsutism, which probably results from increased androgen secretion. Megaloblastic anaemia, associated with a disorder of folate metabolism, sometimes occurs and can be corrected by giving folic acid (Ch. 21). Hypersensitivity reactions, mainly rashes, are quite common. Phenytoin has also been implicated as a cause of the increased incidence of fetal malformations in children born to epileptic mothers, particularly the occurrence of cleft palate, associated with the formation of an epoxide metabolite. Severe idiosyncratic reactions, including hepatitis and skin reactions, occur in a small proportion of patients.

CARBAMAZEPINE

Carbamazepine is chemically derived from the tricyclic antidepressant drugs (see Ch. 38) and was found in a routine screening test to inhibit electrically evoked seizures in mice. Pharmacologically and clinically its actions resemble those of

Clinical uses of antiepileptic drugs

- Tonic–clonic (grand mal) seizures:
  - —carbamazepine (preferred because of low incidence of side-effects), phenytoin, valproate
  - —use of a single drug is preferred when possible to avoid pharmacokinetic interactions
  - —newer agents (not yet fully assessed) include vigabatrin, lamotrigine, felbamate, gabapentin.
- Partial (focal) seizures: carbamazepine, valproate; clonazepam or phenytoin are alternatives.
- Absence seizures (petit mal): ethosuximide or valproate
  - —valproate is used when absence seizures coexist with tonic–clonic seizures, since most other drugs used for tonic–clonic seizures can worsen absence seizures.
- Myoclonic seizures: diazepam intravenously or (in absence of accessible veins) rectally.
- Neuropathic pain, e.g. carbamazepine, gabapentin (see Ch. 40).
- To stabilise mood (as an alternative to lithium), e.g. carbamazepine, valproate (see Ch. 38).

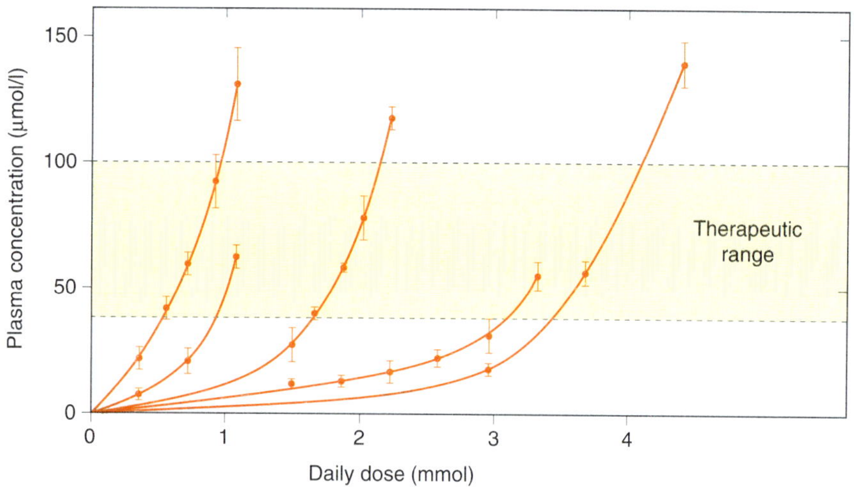

Fig. 39.3 Non-linear relationship between daily dose of phenytoin and steady-state plasma concentration in five individual human subjects. Although the therapeutic range is quite broad (40–100 µmol/l), the daily dose required varies greatly between individuals; for any one individual, the dose has to be adjusted rather precisely to keep within the acceptable plasma concentration range. (Redrawn from: Richens A, Dunlop A 1975 Lancet ii: 247.)

phenytoin, though it appears to be particularly effective in treating complex partial seizures (e.g. psychomotor epilepsy). It is also used to treat various types of neuropathic pain (see Ch. 40), including trigeminal neuralgia, an exceedingly painful condition that is probably associated with a paroxysmal discharge of neurons associated with the trigeminal sensory pathway. Though not obviously associated with epilepsy, this condition probably involves similar neuronal mechanisms. Carbamazepine is now one of the most widely used antiepileptic drugs and is occasionally used in treating manic-depressive illness (see Ch. 38).

Pharmacokinetic aspects

Carbamazepine is well absorbed. Its plasma half-life is about 30 hours when it is given as a single dose, but it is a strong inducing agent, and the plasma half-life shortens to about 15 hours when it is given repeatedly. A slow-release preparation is used for patients who experience dose-related side-effects (see below).

Unwanted effects

Carbamazepine produces a variety of unwanted effects, ranging from drowsiness, dizziness and ataxia to more severe mental and motor disturbances. It can also cause water retention and a variety of gastrointestinal and cardiovascular side-effects. The incidence and severity of these effects is relatively low, however, compared with other drugs. Treatment is usually started with a low dose, which is built up gradually to avoid dose-related toxicity. Severe bone marrow depression, causing neutropenia, and other severe forms of hypersensitivity reaction have occurred but are very rare.

Carbamazepine is a powerful inducer of hepatic microsomal enzymes and thus accelerates the metabolism of many other drugs, such as phenytoin, oral contraceptives, warfarin, corticosteroids, etc. In general it is inadvisable to combine it with other antiepileptic drugs. **Ozcarbazepine,** introduced recently, is a pro-drug that is metabolised to a compound closely resembling carbamazepine, and its actions are very similar.

VALPROATE

Valproate is a simple monocarboxylic acid, chemically unrelated to any other class of antiepileptic drug, and in 1963 it was discovered quite accidentally to have anticonvulsant properties in mice. It inhibits most kinds of experimentally induced convulsion and is effective in many kinds of epilepsy, being particularly useful in certain types of infantile epilepsy, where its low toxicity and lack of sedative action are important, and in adolescents in whom grand mal and petit mal coexist, since valproate (unlike most antiepileptic drugs) is effective against both. Like carbamazepine, valproate is sometimes used as a mood stabiliser, for example in bipolar depressive illness (Ch. 38).

Mechanism of action

Valproate has many effects and probably works by several mechanisms—a familiar refrain in many areas of neuropharmacology—of which the details remain uncertain (see Macdonald, 1999).

Valproate causes a significant increase in the GABA content of the brain and is a weak inhibitor of two enzyme systems that inactivate GABA, namely GABA transaminase and succinic semialdehyde dehydrogenase, but in vitro studies suggest that these effects would be very slight at clinical dosage. Other more potent inhibitors of these enzymes (e.g. **vigabatrin**; see below) also increase GABA content and have an anticonvulsant effect in experimental animals. There is some evidence that valproate enhances the action of GABA by a postsynaptic action, but no clear evidence that it affects inhibitory synaptic responses. It also has effects on sodium channels, weaker than those of phenytoin.

Valproate is well absorbed orally and is excreted, mainly as the glucuronide, in the urine, the plasma half-life being about 15 hours.

Unwanted effects

Compared with most antiepileptic drugs, valproate is relatively free of unwanted effects. It causes thinning and curling of the hair in about 10% of patients. The most serious side-effect is hepatotoxicity. An increase in serum glutamic oxaloacetic transaminase, which signals liver damage of some degree, commonly occurs, but proven cases of valproate-induced hepatitis are rare. The few cases of fatal hepatitis in valproate-treated patients may well have been caused by other factors. Valproate is teratogenic, causing spina bifida and other neural tube defects so should not be given to pregnant women.

The major antiepileptic drugs

- The main drugs in current use are: phenytoin, carbamazepine, valproate and ethosuximide.
- **Phenytoin**:
  - —acts mainly by use-dependent block of sodium channels
  - —effective in many forms of epilepsy, but not absence seizures
  - —metabolism shows saturation kinetics; therefore, plasma concentration can vary widely and monitoring is needed
  - —drug interactions are common
  - —main unwanted effects are confusion, gum hyperplasia, skin rashes, anaemia, teratogenesis
  - —widely used in treatment of epilepsy; also used as antidysrhythmic agent.
- **Carbamazepine**:
  - —derivative of tricyclic antidepressants
  - —similar profile of that of phenytoin, but with fewer unwanted effects
  - —effective in most forms of epilepsy (except absence seizures); particularly effective in psychomotor epilepsy; also useful in trigenimal neuralgia
  - —strong enzyme-inducing agent; therefore, many drug interactions
  - —low incidence of unwanted effects; principally sedation, ataxia, mental disturbances, water retention.
- **Valproate**:
  - —chemically unrelated to other antiepileptic drugs
  - —mechanism of action not clear; weak inhibition of GABA transaminase; some effect on sodium channels
  - —related few unwanted effects: baldness, teratogenicity, liver damage (rare, but serious).
- **Ethosuximide**:
  - —the main drug used to treat absence seizures, may exacerbate other forms
  - —acts by blocking T-type calcium channels
  - —relatively few unwanted effects, mainly nausea and anorexia.
- Secondary drugs include:
  - —phenobarbital: highly sedative
  - —various benzodiazepines (e.g. clonazepam); diazepam used in treating status epilepticus.

ETHOSUXIMIDE

Ethosuximide, which belongs to the succinimide class, is another drug developed empirically by modifying the barbituric acid ring structure. Pharmacologically and clinically, however, it is different from the drugs so far discussed in that it is active against PTZ-induced convulsions in animals and against absence seizures in humans, with little or no effect on other types of epilepsy. It supplanted **trimethadione**, the first drug found to be effective in absence seizures, which had major side-effects. Ethosuximide is used clinically for its selective effect on absence seizures,

The mechanism of action of ethosuximide and trimethadione appears to differ from that of other antiepileptic drugs. The main effect described is inhibition of T-type calcium channels, which may play a role in generating the 3/second firing rhythm in thalamic relay neurons which is characteristic of absence seizures.

Ethosuximide is well absorbed, and it is metabolised and excreted much like phenobarbital, with a plasma half-life of about 50 hours. Its main side-effects are nausea and anorexia, sometimes lethargy and dizziness, and it is said to precipitate tonic–clonic seizures in susceptible patients. Very rarely it can cause severe hypersensitivity reactions.

PHENOBARBITAL

Phenobarbital was one of the first barbiturates to be developed and its antiepileptic properties were recognised in 1912. In its action against experimentally induced convulsions and clinical forms of epilepsy it closely resembles phenytoin; it affects the duration and intensity of artificially induced seizures, rather than the seizure threshold, and is (like phenytoin) ineffective in treating absence seizures. **Primidone**, now rarely used, acts by being metabolised to phenobarbital. It often causes hypersensitivity reactions. The clinical uses of phenobarbital are virtually the same as those of phenytoin, though phenytoin is preferred because of the absence of sedation.

Pharmacokinetic aspects

The pharmacokinetic behaviour of phenobarbital is straightforward. It is well absorbed and about 50% of the drug in the blood is bound to plasma albumin. It is eliminated slowly from the plasma (half-life, 50–140 hours). About 25% is excreted unchanged in the urine. Since phenobarbital is a weak acid, its ionisation and hence renal elimination are increased if the urine is made alkaline (see Ch. 8). The remaining 75% is metabolised, mainly by oxidation and conjugation, by the hepatic microsomal enzymes. Phenobarbital is a powerful inducer of liver enzymes, and it lowers the plasma concentration of several other drugs (e.g. steroids, oral contraceptive, warfarin, tricyclic antidepressants) to an extent that is clinically important.

Unwanted effects

The main unwanted effect of phenobarbital is sedation, which often occurs at plasma concentrations within the therapeutic range for seizure control. This is a serious drawback, since the drug may have to be used for years on end. Some degree of tolerance to the sedative effect seems to occur, but objective tests of cognition and motor performance show impairment even after long-term treatment. Other unwanted effects that may occur with clinical dosage include megaloblastic anaemia (similar to that caused by phenytoin), mild hypersensitivity reactions and osteomalacia. Like other barbiturates (see Ch. 51) it must not be given to patients with porphyria. In overdose, phenobarbital produces coma and respiratory and circulatory failure, as do all barbiturates.

BENZODIAZEPINES

Diazepam, given intravenously, is used to treat *status epilepticus*, a life-threatening condition in which epileptic seizures occur almost without a break. Its advantage in this situation is that it acts very rapidly compared with other antiepileptic drugs. With most benzodiazepines (see Ch. 36), the sedative effect is too pronounced for them to be used for maintenance therapy. **Clonazepam**, and the related compound **clobazam**, are claimed to be relatively selective as antiepileptic drugs. Sedation is the main side-effect of these compounds, and an added problem may be the withdrawal syndrome, which results in an exacerbation of seizures if the drug is stopped.

NEWER ANTIEPILEPTIC DRUGS

For about 25 years, from the mid-1960s, the inventiveness of the pharmaceutical industry in producing improved antiepileptic drugs dried up. Around 1985, the muse returned, and a spate of new drugs were developed over the next 10–15 years, several of which are now in use, and more are under evaluation (see Eadie & Vajda, 1999).

VIGABATRIN

Vigabatrin, the first 'designer drug' in the epilepsy field, is a vinyl-substituted analogue of GABA that was designed as an inhibitor of the GABA-metabolising enzyme GABA transaminase. Vigabatrin is extremely specific for this enzyme and works by forming an irreversible covalent bond. In animal studies, vigabatrin increases the GABA content of the brain and also increases the stimulation-evoked release of GABA, implying that GABA transaminase inhibition can increase the releasable pool of GABA and effectively enhance inhibitory transmission. In humans, vigabatrin increases the content of GABA in the cerebrospinal fluid. Although its plasma half-life is short, it produces a long-lasting effect because the enzyme is blocked irreversibly, and the drug can be given by mouth once daily. Evidence of neurotoxicity was found in animals but has not been found in humans, removing one of the main question marks hanging over this drug.

The main drawback of vigabatrin is the occurrence of depression, and occasionally psychotic disturbances, in a minority of patients; otherwise it is relatively free from side-effects.

Vigabatrin has been reported to be effective in a substantial proportion of patients resistant to the established drugs, and it may represent an important therapeutic advance.

LAMOTRIGINE

Lamotrigine, though chemically unrelated, resembles phenytoin and carbamazepine in its pharmacological effects, acting on sodium channels and inhibiting the release of excitatory amino acids. It appears that, despite its similar mechanism of action, lamotrigine has a broader therapeutic profile than the earlier drugs, with significant efficacy against absence seizures. Its main side-effects are nausea, dizziness and ataxia, and hypersensitivity reactions (mainly mild rashes, but occasionally more severe). Its plasma half-life is about 24 hours, with no particular pharmacokinetic anomalies, and it is taken orally.

FELBAMATE

Felbamate is an analogue of an obsolete anxiolytic drug, **meprobamate**. It is active in many animal seizure models and has a broader clinical spectrum than earlier antiepileptic drugs, but its mechanism of action at the cellular level is uncertain. It has only a weak effect on sodium channels, little effect on GABA but causes some block of the NMDA-receptor channel (Ch. 32). Its acute side-effects are mild, mainly nausea, irritability and insomnia, but it occasionally causes severe reactions, resulting in aplastic anaemia or hepatitis. For this reason, its recommended use is limited to a form of intractable epilepsy in children (Lennox–Gastaut syndrome) that is unresponsive to other drugs. Its plasma half-life is about 24 hours, and it can enhance the plasma concentration of other antiepileptic drugs given concomitantly.

GABAPENTIN

Gabapentin was designed as a simple analogue of GABA that would be sufficiently lipid soluble to penetrate the blood–brain barrier. It turned out to be an effective anticonvulsant in several animal models, but, surprisingly, not by acting on GABA receptors. It has no effect on sodium channels. It may inhibit calcium channels, and also binds with high affinity to a specific site in the brain, which appears to be the amino acid transporter system that occurs in many neurons and other cells. The mechanistic implications of this are unknown, and its mode of action remains an intriguing mystery. The side-effects of gabapentin (mainly sedation and ataxia) are less severe than with many antiepileptic drugs. The absorption of gabapentin from the intestine depends on the amino acid carrier system and shows the property of saturability, which means that increasing the dose does not proportionately increase the amount absorbed. This makes gabapentin relatively safe and free of side-effects associated with overdosing. Its plasma half-life is about 6 hours, requiring dosing two to three times daily. It is excreted unchanged in the urine and is free of interactions with other drugs. It has limited efficacy when used on its own, so it is used mainly as add-on therapy. It is also used as an analgesic to treat neuropathic pain (Ch. 40). A pro-drug, **pregabalin,** which is more potent than gabapentin, is in development.

TIAGABINE

Tiagabine, an analogue of GABA that is able to penetrate the blood–brain barrier, acts by inhibiting the reuptake of GABA by neurons and glia and was the product of rational drug design. It enhances the extracellular GABA concentration, as measured in microdialysis experiments, and also potentiates and prolongs GABA-mediated synaptic responses in the brain. It has a short plasma half-life, and its main side-effects are drowsiness and confusion. The clinical usefulness of tiagabine has not yet been fully assessed.

New antiepileptic drugs

- **Vigabatrin**:
  - —acts by inhibitng GABA transaminase
  - —effectve in patients unresponsive to conventional drugs
  - —main side-effects: drowsiness, behavioural and mood changes.
- **Lamotrigine**:
  - —acts by inhibiting sodium channels
  - —broad therapeutic profile
  - —main side-effects are hypersensitivity reactions (especially skin rashes).
- **Felbamate**:
  - —mechanisms of action unknown
  - —broad therapeutic profile
  - —use limited to intractable disease because of the risk of severe hypersensitivity reactions.
- **Gabapentin**:
  - —mechanism of action not known
  - —saturable absorption; therefore, it is safe in overdose
  - —relatively free of side-effects.
- **Tiagabine**:
  - —GABA-uptake inhibitor
  - —side-effects are dizziness and confusion
  - —not yet fully evaluated.
- **Topiramate**:
  - —complex actions, not fully understood
  - —similar to phenytoin with fewer side-effects and simpler pharnacokinetics
  - —risk of teratogenesis.

TOPIRAMATE

Topiramate is a recently introduced drug that, mechanistically, appears to do a little of everything, blocking sodium channels, enhancing the action of GABA, blocking AMPA-receptors and, for good measure, weakly inhibiting carbonic anhydrase. Its therapeutic spectrum resembles that of phenytoin, and it is claimed to produce less-severe side-effects, as well as being devoid of the pharmacokinetic properties that cause trouble with phenytoin. Its main drawback is that (like many antiepileptic drugs) it is teratogenic in animals, so it should not be used in women of child-bearing age. Currently, it is recommended for use as add-on therapy in refractory cases of epilepsy.

MUSCLE SPASM AND CENTRALLY ACTING MUSCLE RELAXANTS

Many diseases of the brain and spinal cord produce an increase in muscle tone, which can be painful and disabling. Spasticity, resulting from birth injury or cerebral vascular disease, and the paralysis produced by spinal cord lesions are examples. Local injury or inflammation, as in arthritis, can have the same effect, and chronic back pain is also often associated with local muscle spasm.

Certain centrally acting drugs are available that have the effect of reducing the background tone of the muscle without seriously affecting its ability to contract transiently under voluntary control. The distinction between voluntary movements and 'background tone' is not clear cut, and the selectivity of those drugs is not complete. Postural control, for example, is usually jeopardised by centrally acting muscle relaxants. Furthermore, drugs that affect motor control generally produce rather widespread effects on the central nervous system, and drowsiness and confusion turn out to be very common side-effects of these agents. The main groups of drug that have been used to control muscle tone are:

- **mephenesin** and related drugs
- **baclofen**
- **benzodiazepines** (see Ch. 36)
- **botulinum toxin** (see Ch. 10): injected into a muscle, this neurotoxin causes long-lasting paralysis confined to the site of injection. Its use to treat local muscle spasm is increasing.

MEPHENESIN

Mephenesin is an aromatic ether that acts mainly on the spinal cord, causing a selective inhibition of polysynaptic excitation of motor neurons. Thus it strongly inhibits the flexor reflex without affecting the tendon jerk reflex, which is monosynaptic, and it abolishes decerebrate rigidity. Its mechanism of action at the cellular level is unknown. Mephenesin is little used clinically, though it is sometimes given as an intravenous injection to reduce acute muscle spasm resulting from injury.

Table 39.1 Properties of the main antiepileptic drugs

Drug	Sites of action: Sodium channel	GABA$_A$-receptor	Calcium channel	Other	Main uses	Main unwanted effects	Pharmacokinetics
Phenytoin	++				All types *except* absence seizures	Ataxia, vertigo Gum hypertrophy Hirsutism Megaloblastic anaemia Fetal malformation Hypersensitivity reactions	Half-life ~ 24 h Saturation kinetics; therefore unpredictable plasma levels Plasma monitoring often required
Carbamazepine[a]	++				All types *except* absence seizures Especially temporal lobe epilepsy (Also used in trigeminal neuralgia) Most widely used antiepileptic drug	Sedation, ataxia Blurred vision Water retention Hypersensitivity reactions Leucopenia, liver failure (rare)	Half-life 12–18 h (longer initially) Strong induction of microsomal enzymes; therefore, risk of drug interactions
Valproate	+	?+		GABA transaminase inhibition	Most types, including absence seizures	Generally less than with other drugs Nausea Hair loss Weight gain Fetal malformations	Half-life 12–15 h
Ethosuximide[b]			++		Absence seizures May exacerbate tonic/clonic seizures	Nausea, anorexia Mood changes Headache	Long plasma half-life (~ 60 h)
Phenobarbital[c]	?+	+			All types *except* absence seizures	Sedation, depression Contraindicated in porphyria (as are other barbituates; Ch. 36)	Long plasma half-life (>60 h) Strong induction of microsomal enzymes; therefore, risk of drug interactions (e.g. with phenytoin)
Benzodiazepines: e.g. clonazepam, clobazam, diazepam		++			All types Diazepam used intravenously to control *status epilepticus*	Sedation Withdrawal syndrome (see Ch. 36)	See Ch. 36
Vigabatrin				GABA transaminase inhibition	All types Appears to be effective in patients resistant to other drugs.	Sedation Behavioural and mood changes (occasionally psychosis) Visual field defects	Short plasma half-life, but enzyme inhibition is long lasting
Lamotrigine	++		?+	Inhibits glutamate release	All types	Dizziness Sedation Skin rashes	Plasma half-life 24–36 h
Gabapentin			?+		Not yet fully assessed	Few side effects, mainly sedation	Plasma half-life 6–9 h

[a]**Oxcarbazepine**, recently introduced, is similar. Claimed to have fewer side-effects.
[b]**Trimethadione** is similar to ethosuximide in that it acts selectively against absence seizures. Its greater toxicity (especially the risk of severe hypersensitivity reactions, means that ethosuximide has largely replaced it in clinical use.
[c]**Primidone** is pharmacologically similar to phenobarbital and is converted to phenobarbital in the body. It has no clear advantages and is more liable to produce hypersensitivity reactions, so it is now rarely used.
See text for details of newer antiepileptic drugs (**felbamate, tiagabine, topiramate**), not yet fully evaluated.

BACLOFEN

Baclofen (see Ch. 32) is a chlorophenyl derivative of GABA, originally prepared as a lipophilic GABA-like agent in order to assist penetration of the blood–brain barrier, which GABA itself does not do. Baclofen is a selective agonist at presynaptic $GABA_B$-receptors (see Ch. 32). The antispastic action of baclofen is exerted mainly on the spinal cord, where it inhibits both monosynaptic and polysynaptic activation of motor neurons.

It is effective when given by mouth and is used in the treatment of spasticity associated with multiple sclerosis or spinal injury. However, it is ineffective in cerebral spasticity caused by birth injury.

Baclofen produces various unwanted effects, particularly drowsiness, motor incoordination and nausea, and it may also have behavioural effects. It is not useful in epilepsy.

CANNABIS

Anecdotal evidence suggests that smoking cannabis (Ch. 41) relieves the painful muscle spasms occurring in multiple sclerosis. A controlled trial is under way to assess this, with a view to legalising the prescription of cannabis for this purpose.

REFERENCES AND FURTHER READING

Binder D K, Croll S D, Gall C M, Scharfman H E 2001 BDNF and epilepsy: too much of a good thing? Trends Neurosci 24: 47–53 (*Recent ideas on possible role of BDNF in epileptogenesis*)

Eadie M J, Vajda F J (eds) 1999 Handbook of experimental pharmacology, vol. 138: Antiepileptic drugs: pharmacology and therapeutics. Springer, Berlin (*Useful collection of articles covering all aspects of antiepileptic drugs*)

Hopkins A, Shorvon S, Cascino G 1995 Epilepsy, 2nd edn. Chapman & Hall, London (*Comprehensive general textbook*)

Jarrott B 1999 Epileptogenesis: biochemical aspects. In: Eadie M J, Vajda F J (eds) Antiepileptic drugs: pharmacology and therapeutics. Handbook of experimental pharmacology, Springer, Berlin, vol. 138, pp. 87–121 (*Review article describing possible neurochemical mechanisms underlying epilepsy—mostly speculative*)

Kulmann D M, Asztely F, Walker M C 2000 The role of mammalian ionotropic receptors in synaptic plasticity: LTP, LTD and epilepsy. Cell Mol Life Sci 57: 1551–1561 (*Draws parallels between epileptogensis and other well-studied forms of synaptic plasticity*)

Levy R H, Mattson R H, Meldrum B S, Dreifuss F E, Penry J K (eds) 1995 Antiepileptic drugs, 4th edn. Raven Press, New York (*Comprehensive general textbook*)

Löscher W 1999 Animal models of epilepsy and epileptic seizures. In: Eadie M J, Vajda F J (eds) Antiepileptic drugs: pharmacology and therapeutics. Handbook of experimental pharmacology, Springer, Berlin, vol. 138, pp 19–62 (*Comprehensive review article*)

Macdonald R L 1999 Cellular actions of antiepileptic drugs. In: Eadie M J, Vajda F J (eds) Antiepileptic drugs: pharmacology and therapeutics. Handbook of experimental pharmacology, Springer, Berlin, vol. 138, pp 123–150 (*Good review article including information on new drugs*)

Meldrum B S 1996 Update on the mechanism of action of antiepileptic drugs. Epilepsia 37: S4–S11 (*Excellent review article summarising current knowledge on mechanisms*)

Willoughby J O 1999 Epileptogenesis: electrophysiology. In: Eadie M J, Vajda F J (eds) Antiepileptic drugs: pharmacology and therapeutics. Handbook of experimental pharmacology, Springer, Berlin, vol. 138, pp 63–85 (*Review article*)

40 Analgesic drugs

Overview 562

Neural mechanisms of pain 562
- Nociceptive afferent neurons 562
- Modulation in the nociceptive pathway 563
- Neuropathic pain 566
- Pain and nociception 567
- Chemical mediators in the nociceptive pathway 567
- Transmitters and modulators in the nociceptive pathway 570

Analgesic drugs 572
- Morphine-like drugs 572
- Other opioid analgesics 581
- Opioid antagonists 582
- Other analgesic drugs 583

New approaches 583

OVERVIEW

Pain is a disabling accompaniment of many medical conditions, and pain control is one of the most important therapeutic priorities.

In this chapter, we discuss the neural mechanisms responsible for different types of pain, and the various drugs that are used to reduce it. The 'classical' analgesic drugs, notably opiates and non-steroidal anti-inflammatory drugs (described in Ch. 16), have their origins in natural products that have been used for centuries. The original compounds, typified by morphine and aspirin are still in widespread use, but many synthetic compounds that act by the same mechanisms have been developed. Opiate analgesics are described in this chapter. Next, we consider various other drug classes, such as antidepressants (e.g. amitriptyline) and antiepileptic drugs (e.g. carbamazepine), which clinical experience has shown to be effective in certain types of pain. Finally, looking into the future, many potential new drug targets have emerged during the 1990s as our knowledge of the neural mechanisms underlying pain has advanced. We describe briefly some of these new approaches at the end of the chapter.

NEURAL MECHANISMS OF PAIN

Pain is a subjective experience, hard to define exactly, even though we all know what we mean by it. Typically, it is a direct response to an untoward event associated with tissue damage, such as injury, inflammation or cancer, but severe pain can arise independently of any obvious predisposing cause (e.g. trigeminal neuralgia), or persist long after the precipitating injury has healed (e.g. phantom limb pain). It can also occur as a consequence of brain or nerve injury (e.g. following a stroke or herpes infection). Pain conditions of the latter kind, not directly linked to tissue injury, are very common, and a major cause of disability and distress; in general they respond less well to conventional analgesic drugs than do conditions where the immediate cause is clear. In these cases, we need to think of pain in terms of disordered neural function, comparable to schizophrenia or epilepsy, rather than simply as a 'normal' response to tissue injury. Therefore, it is useful to distinguish two components, either or both of which may be involved in pathological pain states: (i) the peripheral nociceptive afferent neuron, which is activated by noxious stimuli; (ii) the central mechanisms by which the afferent input generates a pain sensation.

Good accounts of the neural basis of pain can be found in Besson & Chaouch (1987) and Wall & Melzack (1999).

NOCICEPTIVE AFFERENT NEURONS

Under normal conditions, pain is associated with electrical activity in small diameter primary afferent fibres of peripheral nerves (see Raja et al., 1999). These nerves have sensory endings in peripheral tissues and are activated by stimuli of various kinds (mechanical, thermal, chemical; Cesare & McNaughton, 1997; Julius & Basbaum, 2001). They are distinguished from other sorts of mechanical and thermal receptors by their higher threshold, since they are normally activated only by stimuli of noxious intensity—sufficient to cause some degree of tissue damage. Recordings of activity in single afferent fibres in human subjects have shown that stimuli sufficient to excite these small afferent fibres also evoke a painful sensation. Many of these fibres are non-myelinated C-fibres with low conduction velocities (<1 m/s); this group is known as *C-polymodal nociceptors*. Others are fine myelinated (Aδ) fibres, which conduct more rapidly but respond to similar peripheral stimuli. Though there are some species differences, the majority of the C-fibres in peripheral nerves are associated with polymodal nociceptive endings. Afferents from muscle and viscera also convey nociceptive information. In the nerves from these tissues, the Aδ-fibres are connected to high-threshold mechanoreceptors, while the unmyelinated fibres are connected to C-polymodal nociceptors, as in the skin.

Experiments on human subjects, in which recording or stimulating electrodes are applied to cutaneous sensory nerves, have shown that activity in the Aδ-fibres causes a sensation of sharp, well-localised pain, whereas C-fibre activity causes a dull burning pain.

With many pathological conditions, tissue injury is the immediate cause of the pain, and this results in the local release of a variety of chemical agents, which are assumed to act on the nerve terminals, either activating them directly or enhancing their sensitivity to other forms of stimulation. The pharmacological properties of nociceptive nerve terminals are discussed in more detail below.

The cell bodies of spinal nociceptive afferent fibres lie in dorsal root ganglia; fibres enter the spinal cord via the dorsal roots, ending in the grey matter of the dorsal horn (Fig. 40.1). Most of the nociceptive afferents terminate in the superficial region of the dorsal horn, the C-fibres and some Aδ-fibres innervating cell bodies in laminae I and II, while other A-fibres penetrate deeper into the dorsal horn (lamina V). Cells in laminae I and V give rise to the main projection pathways from the dorsal horn to the thalamus.

The non-myelinated afferent neurons contain several neuropeptides (see Ch. 13), particularly substance P and calcitonin gene-related peptide (CGRP). These are released as mediators at both the central and peripheral terminals and play an important role in the pathology of pain.

MODULATION IN THE NOCICEPTIVE PATHWAY

Acute pain is generally well accounted for in terms of *nociception*—an excessive noxious stimulus giving rise to an intense and unpleasant sensation. In contrast, most chronic pain states* are associated with aberrations of the normal physiological pathway, giving rise to *hyperalgesia* (an increased amount of pain associated with a mild noxious stimulus), *allodynia* (pain evoked by a non-noxious stimulus), or *spontaneous pain* without any precipitating stimulus. An analogy is with an old radio set that plays uncontrollably loudly (hyperalgesia), receives two stations at once (allodynia) or produces random shrieks and whistles (spontaneous pain spasms). These distortions in the transmission line are beginning to be understood in terms of various types of positive and negative modulation in the nociceptive pathway, discussed in more detail below. Some of the main mechanisms are summarised in Figure 40.2.

HYPERALGESIA AND ALLODYNIA

▼ Anyone who has suffered a burn or sprained ankle has experienced hyperalgesia and allodynia. Hyperalgesia involves both sensitisation of peripheral nociceptive nerve terminals and central facilitation of transmission at the level of the dorsal horn and thalamus—changes embraced by the term neuroplasticity. The peripheral component results

*Defined as pain which outlasts the precipitating tissue injury. Many clinical pain states fall into this category. The dissociation of pain from noxious input is most evident in 'phantom limb' pain, which occurs after amputations and may be very severe. The pain is usually not relieved by local anaesthetic injections, implying that electrical activity in afferent fibres is not an essential component. At the other extreme, noxious input with no pain, there are many well-documented reports of mystics and showmen who subject themselves to horrifying ordeals with knives, burning embers, nails and hooks (undoubtedly causing massive afferent input) without apparently suffering pain.

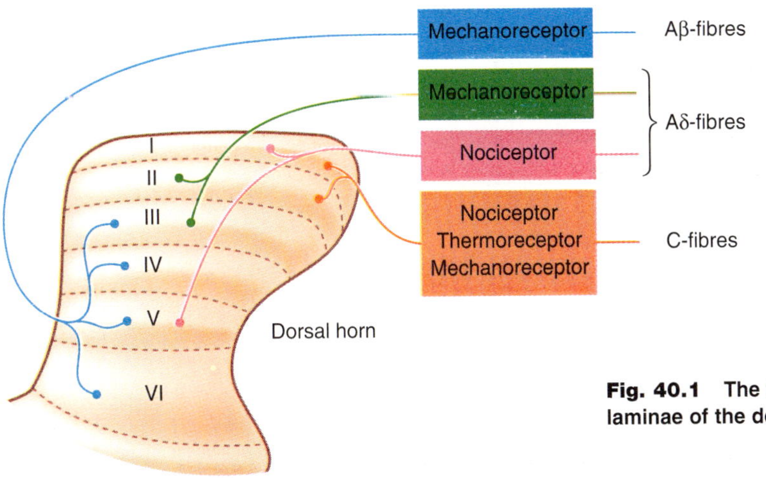

Fig. 40.1 The termination of afferent fibres in the six laminae of the dorsal horn of the spinal cord.

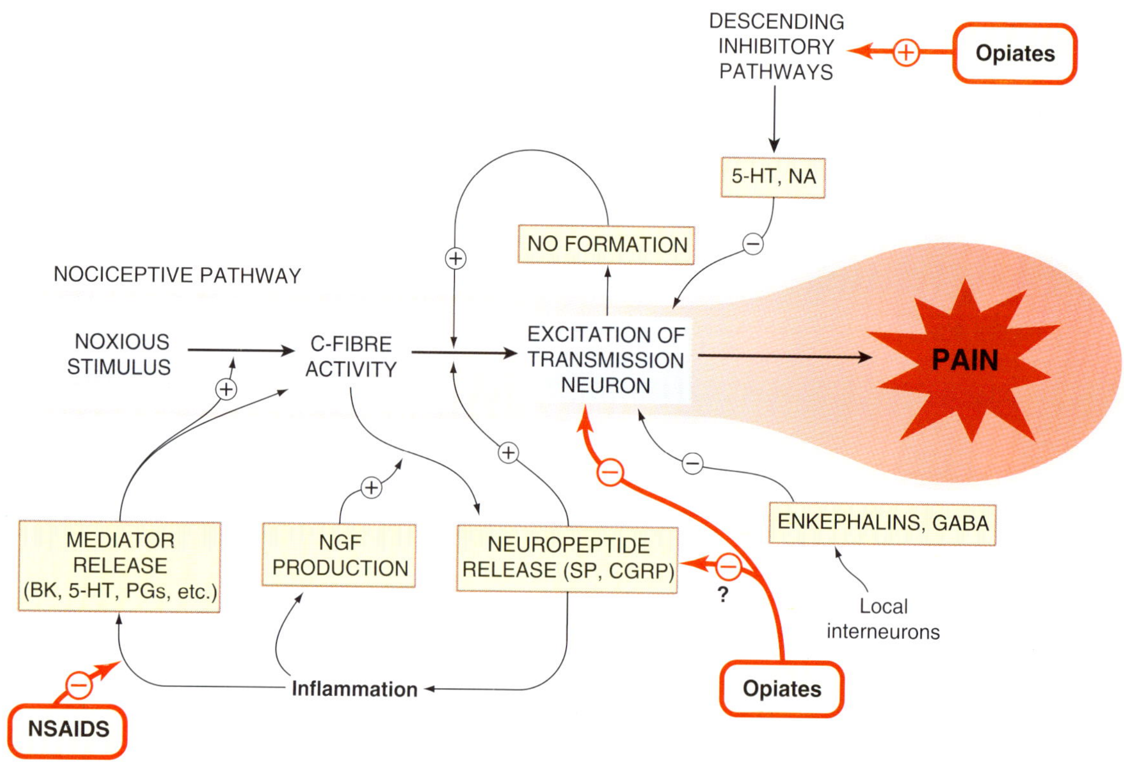

Fig. 40.2 Summary of modulatory mechanisms in the nociceptive pathway. (5-HT, 5-hydroxytyptamine; NA, noradrenaline; BK, bradykinin; PGs, prostalgandins; NGF, nerve growth factor; SP, substance P; CGRP, calcitonin gene-related peptide; GABA, gamma-aminobutyric acid; NSAIDs, non-steroidal anti-inflammatory drugs; NO, nitric oxide.)

from the action of mediators such as bradykinin, prostaglandins, etc. acting on the nerve terminals (see below). The central component reflects facilitation of synaptic transmission. This has been well studied in the dorsal horn (see Yaksh, 1999). The synaptic responses of dorsal horn neurons to nociceptive inputs display the phenomenon of 'wind-up'—i.e. the synaptic potentials steadily increase in amplitude with each stimulus—when repeated stimuli are delivered at physiological frequencies (see Fig. 40.3). This activity-dependent facilitation of transmission has many features in common with the phenomenon of long-term potentiation in the hippocampus, described in Chapter 32, and the chemical mechanisms underlying it also appear to be similar (see McMahon et al., 1993; Fig. 40.3). In the dorsal horn, the facilitation is blocked by NMDA (*N*-methyl-D-asparate) receptor antagonists, also by antagonists of substance P, a slow excitatory transmitter released by nociceptive afferent neurons (see above), and by inhibitors of nitric oxide (NO) synthesis. Substance P produces a slow depolarising response in the postsynaptic cell, which builds up during repetitive stimulation, and (as with long-term potentiation; see Fig. 32.6) is believed to enhance NMDA-receptor-mediated transmission. This results in Ca^{2+} influx and activation of NO synthase (see Ch. 14), the released NO acting to facilitate transmission by mechanisms that have yet to be elucidated. Substance P and CGRP released from primary afferent neurons also act in the periphery, promoting inflammation by their effects on blood vessels and cells of the immune system (Ch. 15). This mechanism, known as *neurogenic inflammation*, acts to amplify and sustain the inflammatory reaction, and the accompanying activation of nociceptive afferent fibres. There is evidence that these processes (summarised in Fig. 40.2) are also involved in pathological hyperalgesia (e.g. that associated with inflammatory responses), in which central facilitation is known to occur (see Coderre et al., 1993). Other mechanisms can also contribute to central facilitation. *Nerve growth factor* (NGF) a cytokine-like mediator produced by peripheral tissues, particularly in inflammation, acts specifically on nociceptive afferent neurons, increasing their electrical excitability, chemosensitivity and peptide content, and also promoting the formation of synaptic contacts. Increased NGF production may be an important mechanism by which nociceptive transmission becomes facilitated by tissue damage, leading to hyperalgesia (see McMahon, 1996). Increased gene expression in sensory neurons is induced by NGF and other inflammatory mediators; the upregulated genes include those encoding vatious neuropeptide precursors, receptors and channels and have the overall effect of facilitating transmission at the first synaptic relay in the dorsal horn.

THE SUBSTANTIA GELATINOSA AND THE GATE CONTROL THEORY

Cells of lamina II of the dorsal horn (the *substantia gelatinosa*, SG) are mainly short inhibitory interneurons projecting to lamina I and lamina V, and they regulate transmission at the first synapse of the nociceptive pathway, between the primary afferent fibres and the spinothalamic tract transmission neurons. This

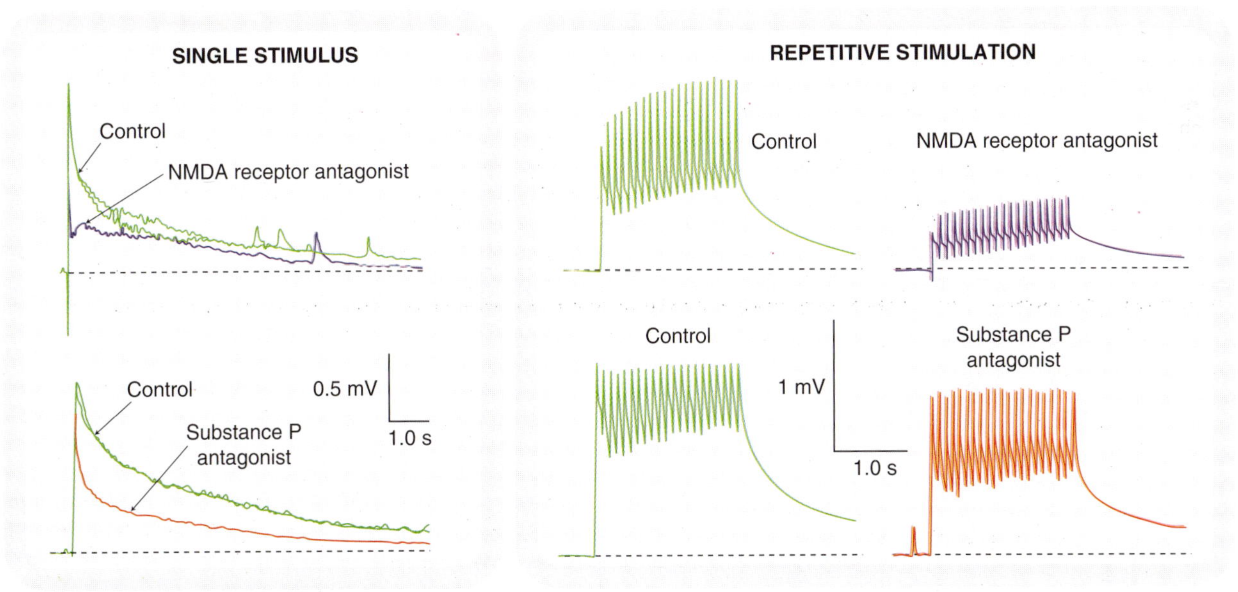

Fig. 40.3 Effect of glutamate and substance P antagonist on nociceptive transmission in the rat spinal cord. The rat paw was inflamed by ultraviolet irradiation 2 days before the experiment, a procedure that induces hyperalgesia and spinal cord facilitation. The synaptic response was recorded from the ventral root, in response to stimulation of C-fibres in the dorsal root with single stimuli (left) or repetitive stimuli (right). The effect of the NMDA-receptor antagonist D-AP5 (see Ch. 32) and the substance P antagonist RP 67580 (selective for the tachykinin NK_2-receptor) are shown. The slow component of the synaptic response is reduced by both antagonists (left-hand traces), as is the 'wind-up' in response to repetitive stimulation (right-hand traces). These effects are much less pronounced in the normal animal. Therefore, both glutamate, acting on NMDA receptors, and substance P, acting on NK_2-receptors, are involved in nociceptive transmission, and their contribution increases as a result of inflammatory hyperalgesia. (Records kindly provided by L Urban and S W Thompson.)

gatekeeper function gave rise to the term 'gate control theory', proposed by Wall & Melzack in 1965. According to this view (summarised in Fig. 40.4) the SG cells respond both to the activity of afferent fibres entering the cord (thus allowing the arrival of impulses via one group of afferent fibres to regulate the transmission of impulses via another pathway) and to the activity of descending pathways (see below). The SG is rich in both opioid peptides and opioid receptors and may be an important site of action for morphine-like drugs (see below). Further studies have added extra detail to the dorsal horn circuitry shown schematically in Figure 40.4 (see Fields & Basbaum, 1994), and it is evident that similar 'gate' mechanisms also operate in the thalamus.

From the spinothalamic tracts, the projection fibres form synapses mainly in the ventral and medial parts of the thalamus with cells having axons projecting to the somatosensory cortex. In the medial thalamus in particular, many cells respond specifically to noxious stimuli in the periphery and lesions in this area cause analgesia. Functional imaging studies in conscious subjects (see Rainville et al., 1997) suggest that the affective component of pain sensation involves a specific region of the cingulate cortex, distinct from the somatosensory cortex (lesions of which do not prevent the sensation of pain, though they can alter its quality).

DESCENDING INHIBITORY CONTROLS

As mentioned above, descending pathways constitute one of the gating mechanisms that control impulse transmission in the dorsal horn (see Fields & Basbaum, 1994). A key part of this descending system is the *periaqueductal grey* (PAG) area of the midbrain, a small area of grey matter surrounding the central canal. In 1969, Reynolds found that electrical stimulation of this brain area in the rat caused analgesia sufficiently intense that abdominal surgery could be performed without anaesthesia and without eliciting any marked response. Non-painful sensations were unaffected. The PAG receives inputs from many other brain regions, including the hypothalamus, cortex and thalamus, and it is thought to represent the mechanism whereby cortical and other inputs act to control the nociceptive 'gate' in the dorsal horn.

The main neuronal pathway activated by PAG stimulation runs first to an area of the medulla close to the midline, known as the *nucleus raphe magnus* (NRM), and thence via fibres running in the dorsolateral funiculus of the spinal cord, which form synaptic connections on dorsal horn interneurons. The major transmitter at these synapses is 5-hydroxytryptamine (5-HT), and the interneurons in turn act to inhibit the discharge of spinothalamic neurons (Fig. 40.5). The NRM itself receives an input from spinothalamic neurons, via the adjacent *nucleus reticularis*

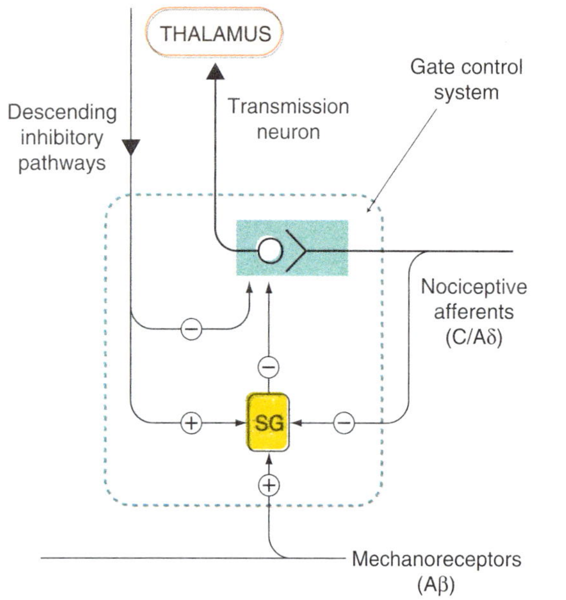

Fig. 40.4 Schematic diagram of the gate control system. This system regulates the passage of impulses from the peripheral afferent fibres to the thalamus via transmission neurons originating in the dorsal horn. Neurons in the substantia gelatinosa (SG) of the dorsal horn act to inhibit the transmission pathway. Inhibitory interneurons are activated by descending inhibitory neurons or by non-nociceptive afferent input. They are inhibited by nociceptive C-fibre input, so the persistent C-fibre activity facilitates excitation of the transmission cells by either nociceptive or non-nociceptive inputs. This autofacilitation causes successive bursts of activity in the nociceptive afferents to become increasingly effective in activating transmission neurons. Details of the interneuronal pathways are not shown. (From: Melzack R, Wall P D 1982 The challenge of pain. Penguin, Harmondsworth.)

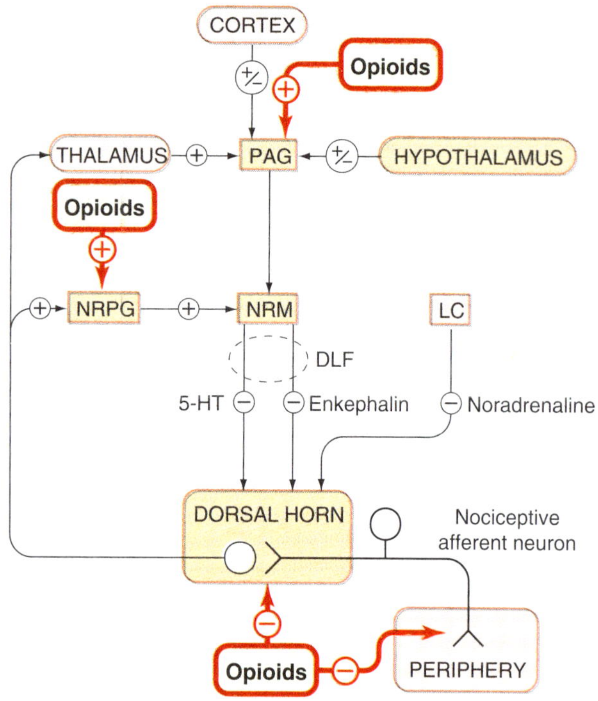

Fig. 40.5 The descending control system, showing the main sites of action of opioids on pain transmission. Opioids excite neurons in the periaqueductal grey matter (PAG) and in the nucleus reticularis paragigantocellularis (NRPG), which in turn project to the rostroventral medulla, which includes the nucleus raphe magnus (NRM). From the NRM, 5-HT- and enkephalin-containing neurons run to the substantia gelatinosa of the dorsal horn, and exert an inhibitory influence on transmission. Opioids also act directly on the dorsal horn, as well as on the peripheral terminals of nociceptive afferent neurons. The *locus ceruleus* (LC) sends noradrenergic neurons to the dorsal horn, which also inhibit transmission. The pathways shown in this diagram represent a considerable oversimplification but depict the general organisation of the supraspinal control mechanisms. Blue shaded boxes represent areas rich in opioid peptides. DLF, dorsolateral funiculus; 5-HT, 5-hydroxytryptamine. (For more detailed information, see Fields & Basbaum 1994.)

paragigantocellularis (NRPG), so this descending inhibitory system may form part of a regulatory feedback loop whereby transmission through the dorsal horn is controlled according to the amount of activity reaching the thalamus.

The descending inhibitory pathway is probably an important site of action for opioid analgesics (see below). Both PAG and SG are particularly rich in enkephalin-containing neurons, and opioid antagonists, such as **naloxone** (see later section), can prevent electrically induced analgesia, which would suggest that opioid peptides may function as transmitters in this system. The physiological role of opioid peptides in regulating pain transmission has been controversial, mainly because under normal conditions naloxone has relatively little effect on pain threshold. Under pathological conditions, however, when stress is present, naloxone causes hyperalgesia, implying that the opioid system is active.

There is also a noradrenergic pathway from the locus ceruleus (see Ch. 33), which has a similar inhibitory effect on transmission in the dorsal horn (Fig. 40.5).

NEUROPATHIC PAIN

Neurological disease affecting the sensory pathway can produce severe chronic pain—termed neuropathic pain—unrelated to any peripheral tissue injury. This occurs with CNS disorders, such as stroke and multiple sclerosis, or with conditions associated with peripheral nerve damage, such as mechanical injury, diabetic neuropathy or herpes zoster infection (shingles). The pathophysiological mechanisms underlying this kind of pain are poorly understood, though spontaneous activity in damaged sensory neurons is thought to be a factor. The sympathetic nervous system also plays a part, since damaged sensory neurons can express α-adrenoceptors and develop a sensitivity to noradrenaline that they do not possess under normal conditions.

Modulation of pain transmission

- Transmission in the dorsal horn is subject to various modulatory influences, constituting the 'gate control' mechanism.
- Descending pathways from the midbrain and brainstem exert a strong inhibitory effect on dorsal horn transmission. Electrical stimulation of the midbrain periaqueductal grey area causes analgesia through this mechanism.
- The descending inhibition is mediated mainly by enkephalins, 5-HT, noradrenaline and adenosine. Opioids cause analgesia partly by activating these descending pathways, partly by inhibiting transmission in the dorsal horn, and partly by inhibiting excitation of sensory nerve terminals in the periphery.
- Repetitive C-fibre activity facilitates transmission through the dorsal horn ('wind-up') by mechanisms involving activation of NMDA and substance P receptors.

Thus physiological stimuli that evoke sympathetic responses can produce severe pain, a phenomenon described clinically as *sympathetically mediated pain*. Neuropathic pain, which appears to be a component of many types of clinical pain (including common conditions such as back pain, cancer pain, as well as amputation pain), is generally difficult to control with conventional analgesic drugs. Potential new drug targets are discussed below.

PAIN AND NOCICEPTION

▼ As emphasised above, the perception of noxious stimuli (termed 'nociception' by Sherrington) is not the same thing as pain, which is a subjective experience and includes a strong emotional (affective) component. The amount of pain that a particular stimulus produces depends on many factors other than the stimulus itself. A stabbing sensation in the chest will cause much more pain if it occurs spontaneously in a middle-aged man than if it is caused by a 2-year-old poking him in the ribs with a sharp stick. The nociceptive component may be much the same, but the affective component is quite different. Animal tests of analgesic drugs commonly measure nociception and involve testing the reaction of an animal to a mildly painful stimulus, often mechanical or thermal. Such measures include the tail-flick test (measuring the time taken for a rat to withdraw its tail when a standard radiant heat stimulus is applied) or the paw pressure test (measuring the withdrawal threshold when a normal or inflamed paw is pinched with increasing force). Similar tests can be used on human subjects, who simply indicate when a stimulus begins to feel painful, but the pain in these circumstances lacks the affective component. Clinically, spontaneous pain of neuropathic origin is coming to be recognised as particularly important, but this is difficult to model in animal studies for both technical and ethical reasons. It is recognised clinically that many analgesics, particularly those of the morphine-type, can greatly reduce the distress associated with pain even though the patient reports no great change in the intensity of the actual sensation. It is much more difficult to devise tests that measure this affective component, and it is important to realise that it may be at least as significant as the antinociceptive component in the action of these drugs. There is often a poor correlation between the activity of analgesic drugs in animal tests (which mainly assess antinociceptive activity) and their clinical effectiveness.

CHEMICAL MEDIATORS IN THE NOCICEPTIVE PATHWAY

CHEMOSENSITIVITY OF NOCICEPTIVE NERVE ENDINGS

In most cases, stimulation of nociceptive endings in the periphery is chemical in origin. Excessive mechanical or thermal stimuli can obviously cause acute pain, but the persistence of such pain after the stimulus has been removed, or the pain resulting from inflammatory or ischaemic changes in tissues, generally reflects an altered chemical environment of the pain afferents. The field was opened up in the 1960s by Keele & Armstrong, who developed a simple method for measuring the pain-producing effect of various substances that act on cutaneous nerve endings. They produced small blisters on the forearm of human subjects and applied chemicals to the blister base, recording the degree of pain that the subjects reported. Techniques of electrical recording from sensory nerves, more recently studies of the membrane responses of neurons in culture, and the application of molecular biology techniques to identify receptors and signal transduction pathways in nociceptive neurons have produced a wealth of new information, and the humble nociceptive neuron has bathed in a limelight that more aristocratic neurons might envy. The current state of knowledge is reviewed by Bevan (1999) and Julius & Basbaum (2001) and summarised in Fig. 40.6.

The main groups of substances that stimulate pain endings in the skin (see Rang et al., 1994) are discussed below.

The vanilloid receptor

▼ **Capsaicin**, the substance in chilli peppers that gives them their pungency, selectively excites nociceptive nerve terminals, causing intense pain if injected into the skin or applied to sensitive structures such as the cornea.* It produces this effect by binding to a receptor expressed by nociceptive afferent neurons. The receptor, known as the vanilloid receptor because many capsaicin-like compounds are based on the structure of vanillic acid, is a typical ligand-gated cation channel (Ch. 3); it was cloned in 1997 and named VR1, in anticipation of further members of the vanilloid receptor family being discovered.** Agonists such as capsaicin open the channel, which is permeable to Na^+, Ca^{2+} and other cations, causing depolarisation and initiation of action potentials. The vanilloid receptor responds not only to capsaicin-like agonists but also to other stimuli, including temperatures in excess of about 45°C (the threshold for pain) and H^+ concentrations in the micromolar range (pH 5.5 and below), which also cause pain. The receptor thus has unusual 'polymodal' characteristics that closely match those of nociceptive neurons, and it is believed to play a central role in nociception. VR1 is, like many other ionotropic receptors, modulated by phosphorylation, and several of the pain-producing substances that act through G-protein-coupled receptors (e.g. *bradykinin*, see below) work by sensitising VR1.

*Anyone who has rubbed their eyes after cutting up strong peppers will know this.

**In the event, the further family members have proved not to be sensitive to vanilloids, so the terminology is confusing.

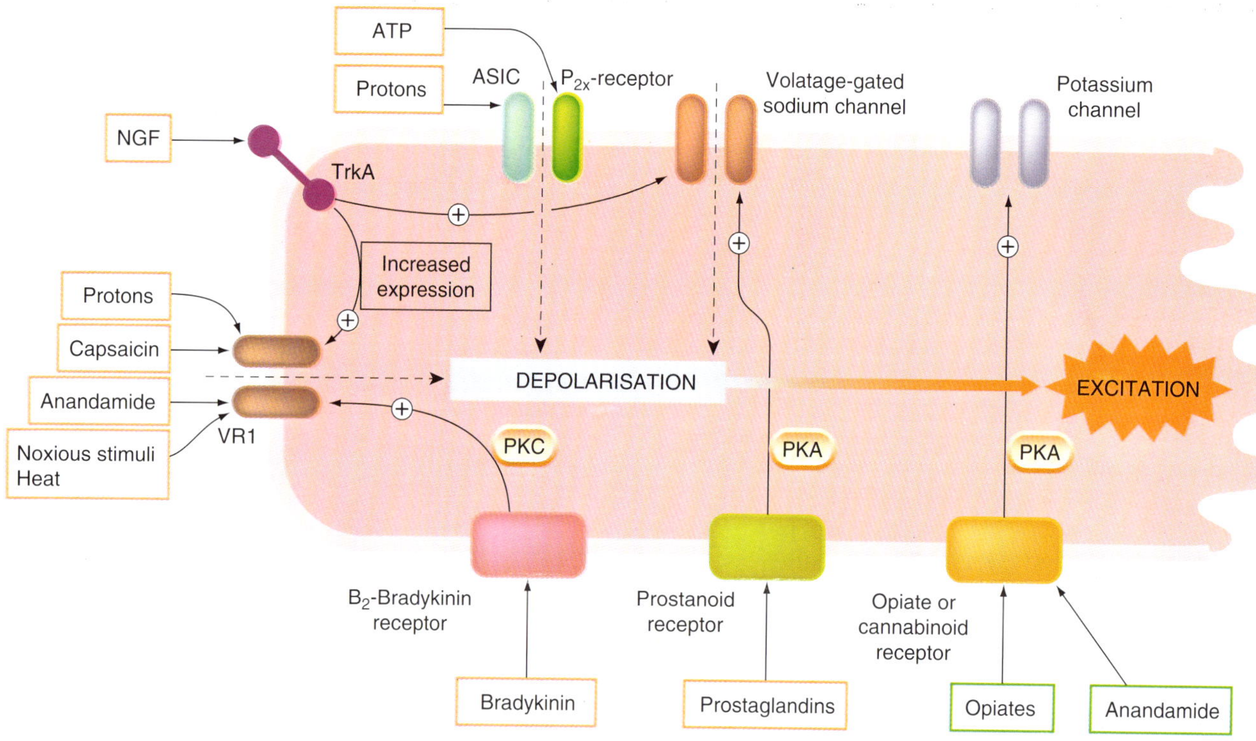

Fig. 40.6 Channels, receptors and transduction mechanisms of nociceptive afferent terminals. Only the main channels and receptors are shown. Ligand-gated channels include acid-sensitive channels (ASIC), ATP-sensitive channels (P_{2X}-receptors) and the capsaicin-sensitive channel (VR1), which is also sensitive to protons and to temperature. Various facilitatory and inhibitory G-protein-coupled receptors are shown, which regulate channel function through various second messenger systems. Growth factor such as nerve growth factor (NGF) act via kinase-linked receptors (TrkA) to control ion channel function and gene expression. (PKC, protein kinase C; PKA, protein kinase A; orange boxes, excitatory mediates; green boxes, inhibitory mediators.)

A search for endogenous ligands for VR1 revealed surprisingly that **anandamide** (a lipid mediator previously identified as an agonist at cannabinoid receptors; see Ch. 42) is also a VR1 agonist, though less potent than capsaicin. Whether this has physiological significance is not currently known. Confirming the role of VR1 in nociception, it has been found that VR1 knockout mice show reduced responsiveness to noxious heat and also fail to show thermal hyperalgesia in response to inflammation.

The latter observation is interesting, since VR1 expression is known to be increased by inflammation, and this may be a key mechanism by which primary hyperalgesia is produced.

Capsaicin and related irritant substances

Capsaicin is a potent vanilloid receptor agonist that selectively stimulates nociceptive nerve endings, as described above. Similar substances exist in other pungent plants (ginger, black pepper, etc.) but none is as potent as capsaicin. **Resiniferatoxin**, a compound produced by some plants of the *Euphorbia* family, whose sap causes painful skin irritation, is so far the most potent agonist known.

There are several interesting features of the action of capsaicin:

- The large influx of Ca^{2+} into nerve terminals that it produces results in peptide release (mainly substance P and CGRP), causing intense vascular and other physiological responses. The Ca^{2+} influx may be enough to cause nerve terminal degeneration, which takes days or weeks to recover. Attempts to use topically applied capsaicin to relieve painful skin conditions have had some success, but the initial strong irritant effect is a major disadvantage.
- Capsaicin applied to the bladder causes degeneration of primary afferent nerve terminals and has been used to treat incontinence associated with bladder hyper-reactivity in patients with stroke or spinal injury. C-fibre afferents in the bladder serve a local reflex function, which promotes emptying when the bladder is distended, the reflex being exaggerated when central control is lost.
- Given to neonatal animals, capsaicin causes an irreversible loss of polymodal nociceptors, since the cell bodies (not just the terminals) are killed. The animals grow up with greatly reduced responses to painful stimuli. This has been used as an experimental procedure for investigating the role of these neurons.

- Unlike mammals, birds do not respond to capsaicin, because avian VR1 differs from mammalian VR1. Consequently, birds eat chilli peppers and distribute their seeds, while mammals (other than humans—the only masochistic mammal) avoid them.

Kinins

The most active kinins are *bradykinin* and *kallidin* (see Ch. 15), two closely related peptides produced under conditions of tissue injury by the proteolytic cleavage of the active kinins from a precursor protein contained in the plasma (reviewed by Dray & Perkins, 1993). Bradykinin is a potent pain-producing substance, acting partly by release of prostaglandins, which strongly enhance the direct action of bradykinin on the nerve terminals (Fig. 40.7). Bradykinin acts by combining with specific G-protein-coupled receptors (Ch. 3) and produces its cellular effects through production of various intracellular messengers (see Cesare & McNaughton, 1997). Specific competitive antagonists, based on the peptide structure of bradykinin, such as **icatibant** (Ch. 15), have recently been developed, and these show analgesic and anti-inflammatory properties. Such peptides are not suitable for clinical use as analgesics but may provide a new principle on which to base future analgesic drugs.

Bradykinin receptors are coupled to activation of a specific isoform of protein kinase C (PKCε), which phosphorylates VR1 and facilitates opening of the VR1 channel.

Prostaglandins

Prostaglandins do not themselves cause pain, but they strongly enhance the pain-producing effect of other agents such as 5-HT or bradykinin (Fig. 40.7). Prostaglandins of the E and F series are released in inflammation (Ch. 15) and also during tissue ischaemia. They sensitise nerve terminals to other agents partly

Mechanisms of pain and nociception

- *Nociception* is the mechanism whereby noxious peripheral stimuli are transmitted to the central nervous system. *Pain* is a subjective experience, not always associated with nociception.
- Polymodal nociceptors (PMN) are the main type of peripheral sensory neuron that responds to noxious stimuli. The majority are non-myelinated C-fibres with endings that respond to thermal, mechanical and chemical stimuli.
- Chemical stimuli acting on PMN to cause pain include bradykinin, protons, ATP and vanilloids (e.g. capsaicin). PMN are sensitised by prostaglandins, which explains the analgesic effect of aspirin-like drugs, particularly in the presence of inflammation.
- The vanilloid receptor VR1 responds to noxious heat as well as capsaicin-like agonists. The lipid mediator anandamide is an agonist at vanilloid receptors, as well as being an endogenous cannabinoid receptor agonist.
- Nociceptive fibres terminate in the superficial layers of the dorsal horn, forming synaptic connections with transmission neurons running to the thalamus.
- PMN neurons release glutamate (fast transmitter) and various peptides (especially substance P), which act as slow transmitters. Peptides are also released peripherally and contribute to neurogenic inflammation.
- Neuropathic pain, associated with damage to neurons of the nociceptive pathway rather than an excessive peripheral stimulus, is frequently a component of chronic pain states and may respond poorly to opioid analgesics.

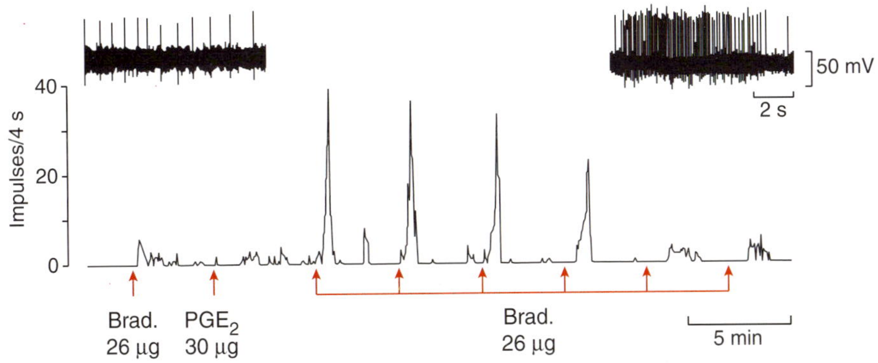

Fig. 40.7 Response of a nociceptive afferent neuron to bradykinin and prostaglandin. Recordings were made from a nociceptive afferent fibre supplying a muscle, and drugs were injected into the arterial supply. **Upper records**: single fibre recordings showing discharge caused by bradykinin (Brad.) alone (left), and by bradykinin following injection of prostaglandin E_2 (PGE_2, right). **Lower trace**: ratemeter recording of single fibre discharge showing long-lasting enhancement of response to bradykinin after an injection of PGE_2. Prostaglandin itself did not evoke a discharge. (From: Mense S 1981 Brain Res 225: 95.)

by inhibiting potassium channels and partly by facilitating—through second-messenger-mediated phosphorylation reactions (see Ch. 3)—the cation channels opened by noxious agents. It is of interest that bradykinin itself causes prostaglandin release, and thus has a powerful 'self-sensitising' effect on nociceptive afferents. Other eicosanoids, including prostaglandin I_2 (PGI_2), leukotrienes and the unstable HETE (hydroxy-eicosatetraenoic acid) derivatives (Ch. 15), may also be important, but information is sparse (see Rang et al., 1998). The analgesic effects of non-steroidal anti-inflammatory drugs (NSAIDs; Ch. 15) result from inhibition of prostaglandin synthesis.

Other peripheral mediators

Various metabolites and substances are released from damaged or ischaemic cells, or inflamed tissues, including 5-HT, histamine, lactic acid, ATP and K^+, many of which affect nociceptive nerve terminals (Fig. 40.6).

5-HT causes excitation, but studies with antagonists suggest that it plays at most a minor role. Histamine is also active but causes itching rather than actual pain. Both of these substances are known to be released locally in inflammation (see Ch. 15).

Low pH excites nociceptive afferent neurons partly by opening proton-activated cation channels (acid-sensitive ion channels or ASICs), and partly by facilitation of VR1 (see above). ATP acts similarly. A type of ATP receptor restricted to sensory neurons, termed P_{2X3} (see Ch. 12), mediates this excitatory response (see Burnstock & Wood 1996). However, P_{2X3}-receptor knockout mice show fairly normal pain responses, so the physiological role of ATP in nociception may be limited.

Opioid peptides released peripherally have an inhibitory effect on nociceptor excitability, as do cannabinoids. These agents act through G-protein-coupled receptors (GPCR) that are negatively coupled to adenylate cyclase, and hence their effects oppose those of prostaglandins. The physiological significance of these medaitors in the periphery is uncertain.

TRANSMITTERS AND MODULATORS IN THE NOCICEPTIVE PATHWAY

TACHYKININS

▼ **Substance P**, discovered in 1931 by von Euler & Gaddum, was the first neuropeptide to be discovered, and it still enjoys prima donna status. In 1931, there was no simple way to purify or determine the structure of a peptide, and it remained a pharmacological curiosity. Nearly 20 years later, Erspamer found another peptide, **eledoisin**, in a Mediterranean octopus, that had very similar actions to substance P. He purified this from nearly 2 tons of octopus and elucidated its sequence (Fig. 40.8). Encouraged, he did the same for some amphibian peptides, which turned out to have very similar sequences. He called them tachykinins (fast-acting) to distinguish them from bradykinin, which has a much slower action on smooth muscle. In 1970, substance P was purified from hypothalamus and shown to belong to the tachykinin family, which are characterised by the terminal sequence Phe–X–Gly–Leu–Met–NH_2 (unblushingly referred to as the 'canonical sequence' by peptide pundits).

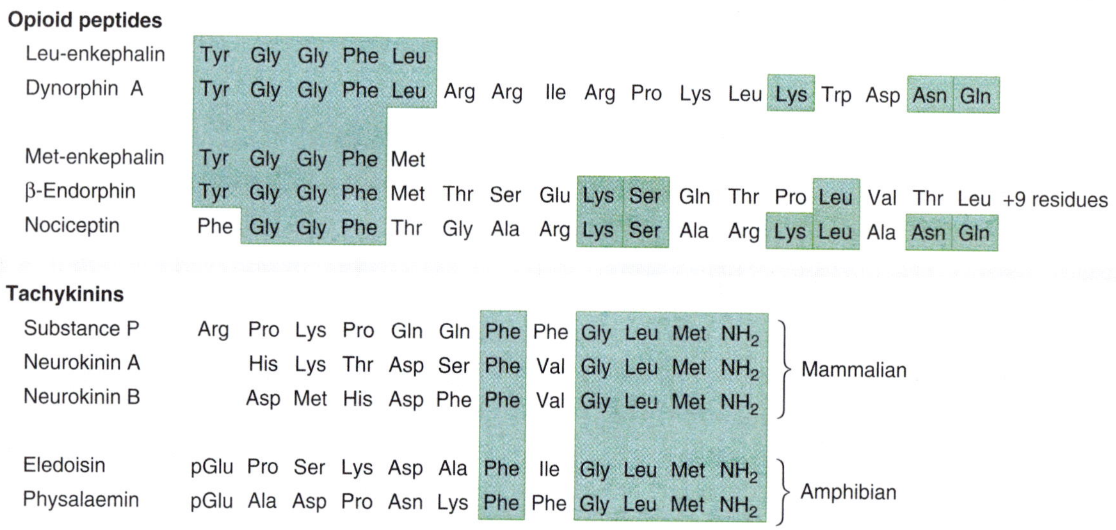
Opioid peptides
Leu-enkephalin Tyr Gly Gly Phe Leu
Dynorphin A Tyr Gly Gly Phe Leu Arg Arg Ile Arg Pro Lys Leu Lys Trp Asp Asn Gln
Met-enkephalin Tyr Gly Gly Phe Met
β-Endorphin Tyr Gly Gly Phe Met Thr Ser Glu Lys Ser Gln Thr Pro Leu Val Thr Leu +9 residues
Nociceptin Phe Gly Gly Phe Thr Gly Ala Arg Lys Ser Ala Arg Lys Leu Ala Asn Gln
Tachykinins
Substance P Arg Pro Lys Pro Gln Gln Phe Phe Gly Leu Met NH2
Neurokinin A His Lys Thr Asp Ser Phe Val Gly Leu Met NH2
Neurokinin B Asp Met His Asp Phe Phe Val Gly Leu Met NH2
Mammalian
Eledoisin pGlu Pro Ser Lys Asp Ala Phe Ile Gly Leu Met NH2
Physalaemin pGlu Ala Asp Pro Asn Lys Phe Phe Gly Leu Met NH2
Amphibian

Fig. 40.8 Structure of opioid and tachykinin peptides, with common amino acids highlighted.

Subsequently, two less-abundant mammalian tachykinins, *neurokinin* (NK) *A* and *B*, were identified. As often happens in the peptide field, several groups converged on these substances and called them by different names, causing a merry confusion. The tachykinins, like other neuropeptides (Ch. 13), are formed by cleavage of larger protein precursors, preprotachykinins. Substance P and NKA are represented in the same preprotachykinin gene, and tissue-specific splicing patterns allow either substance P alone, or both peptides, to be formed in different situations. Detailed information on the tachykinins can be found in various reviews (e.g. Maggio, 1988; Maggi et al., 1993).

Distribution

▼ Substance P and NKA, which are derived from the same gene, are distributed widely in the nervous system, but especially in nociceptive primary afferent neurons and the dorsal horn. Nociceptive sensory neurons express several neuropeptides, which are released at both the central and the peripheral terminals when the neurons are activated. Release of peptides at the peripheral terminals of these neurons is thought to play a part in 'neurogenic inflammation' (see Holzer, 1988). Substance P-containing terminals are abundant in the walls of many blood vessels, and also in the gastrointestinal tract, airways and skin.

Tachykinin receptors

▼ Three tachykinin receptor subtypes exist, NK_1, NK_2 and NK_3, the preferred agonists being substance P, NKA and NKB, respectively. All are typical GPCR acting through various signal transduction pathways (Ch. 3). Most of the known effects of tachykinins are mediated by NK_1- or NK_2-receptors, with much interspecies variation. Less is known about NK_3-receptors, and their role seems to be more limited. Substance P, acting on NK_1-receptors, and NKA, acting on NK_2-receptors, elicit very slow excitatory synaptic potentials in dorsal horn neurons, which are insufficient on their own to excite the postsynaptic neuron but may build up during repetitive activity to produce a burst of action potentials lasting for a few seconds in response to each stimulus. Inflammation, through the action of NGF, increases the substance P content of nociceptive neurons and enhances these slow excitatory responses in the spinal cord, an adaptive change that may be an important factor in hyperalgesia (Fig. 40.3). The presence of abundant NK_1-receptors in the superficial layers of the dorsal horn can be revealed by immunofluorescent labelling. Using this technique, Mantyh et al. (1995) showed that a noxious stimulus to the rat's paw, which releases substance P from primary afferent terminals, causes internalisation of these surface receptors, through agonist-induced endocytosis (see Ch. 3). The physiological significance of this remains uncertain, but the result confirms the postulated modulatory role of substance P in the nociceptive pathway.

Tachykinins elicit a wide range of responses from cells of many types, including neurons, smooth muscle, vascular endothelium, exocrine gland cells, mast cells and cells of the immune system (see review by Maggi et al., 1993), the overall pattern of effects being similar to that seen with agents such as bradykinin (Ch. 15) or 5-HT (Ch. 12). Most types of smooth muscle, including that of the gastrointestinal tract and airways, contract in response to tachykinins. Blood vessels show a mixture of constrictor and dilator responses (endothelium-dependent; see Ch. 16), together with increased permeability, leading to oedema formation. Many neurons, including central and autonomic neurons, show a slow excitatory response, as described above. Intrathecal application of substance P causes a scratching response in conscious animals and may produce hyperalgesia, consistent with the postulated transmitter role of SP in the nociceptive pathway. Mast cells are activated, and release histamine, and various exocrine glands, including salivary glands, are also stimulated.

There is evidence to suggest that substance P is involved not only in the nociceptive pathway, but also in inflammatory conditions, such as arthritis, asthma, hay fever, inflammatory bowel disease and migraine (see Maggi et al., 1993).

Tachykinins

- There are three endogenous tachykinins—substance P, neurokinin A (NKA) and neurokinin B (NKB)—which are widely distributed in the central and peripheral nervous systems.
- Nociceptive sensory neurons express substance P and NKA and release them in the periphery and in the dorsal horn. Inflammation increases substance P expression.
- Substance P release in the periphery when nociceptors are activated contributes to neurogenic inflammation. Its release in the dorsal horn contributes to the wind-up phenomenon.
- There are three tachykinin receptors—NK_1, NK_2 and NK_3—which have NKA and NKB, respectively, as their preferred agonists.
- Nociceptive transmission and neurogenic inflammation are mediated mainly through NK_1-receptors.
- Selective NK_1-receptor antagonists have proved ineffective as analgesic agents.

Tachykinin antagonists

▼ Various peptide analogues of substance P with receptor antagonist properties have been described and used in experimental studies. In 1991, the first non-peptide tachykinin antagonist (CP 96345) was developed from a lead obtained by random screening. Others quickly followed, and there are now several peptide and non-peptide tachykinin antagonists that distinguish between the receptor subtypes (see Maggi et al., 1993). Many of these are active in animal models of inflammatory pain, but disappointingly, none is effective in humans, so the high hopes of developing a new class of analgesic for clinical use were quickly dashed. As a consolation prize, NK_1 antagonists are unexpectedly showing promise in clinical trials for the treatment of depression and anxiety (see Longmore et al., 1997).

OPIOID PEPTIDES

In 1975, Hughes & Kosterlitz succeeded in isolating from the brain two pentapeptides that competed strongly with morphine-like drugs for binding to receptors in the brain, and which had pharmacological actions closely resembling those of morphine itself. This outstanding work showed that the hitherto mysterious actions of morphine (see below) stemmed from its ability to mimic the actions of a family of endogenous mediators, the *opioid peptides*. This very satisfying result fuelled the expectation that the discovery of other neuropeptides might similarly illuminate the actions of other types of drug that affect the central nervous system (CNS); to date, however, morphine-like drugs remain the only class known to act by mimicking peptides. For general reviews of opioid peptides, see Cooper et al. (1996) and Nestler et al. (2001). Opioid peptides, defined as peptides with opiate-like pharmacological effects, are coded by three distinct genes, whose products are, respectively, *preproopiomelanocortin* (POMC), *preproenkephalin* and *preprodynorphin* (see Ch. 13).* The mediators about which most is known are β-endorphin, met-enkephalin, leu-enkephalin and dynorphin. In the brain, these peptides are widely distributed. In the spinal cord, dynorphin occurs mainly in interneurons, while the enkephalins are found mainly in long descending pathways from the midbrain to the dorsal horn. Opioid peptides are also produced by many non-neuronal cells, including endocrine and exocrine glands and cells of the immune system, as well as in brain areas distinct from those involved in nociception, and correspondingly, they play a regulatory role in many different physiological systems, as reflected in the rather complex pharmacological properties of opiate drugs (see below).

The receptors through which opioid peptides exert their effects are described below.

OTHER CENTRAL MEDIATORS

Glutamate (see Ch. 32) This excitatory amino acid is released from primary afferent neurons and, acting on AMPA receptors, is responsible for fast synaptic transmission at the first synapse in the dorsal horn. There is also a slower NMDA-receptor-mediated response, which is important in relation to the wind-up phenomenon (see Fig. 40.3).

Gamma-aminobutyric acid (GABA; see Ch. 32) This is released by spinal cord interneurons and inhibits transmitter release by primary afferent terminals in the dorsal horn (see Malcangio & Bowery, 1996).

5-HT This is the transmitter of inhibitory neurons running from the NRM to the dorsal horn.

Noradrenaline This is the transmitter of the inhibitory pathway from the locus ceruleus to the dorsal horn, and possibly also in other antinociceptive pathways.

Adenosine This plays a dual role in regulating nociceptive transmission, activation of A_1-receptors causing analgesia while activation of A_2-receptors does the reverse. There is evidence for descending inhibitory purinergic pathways acting on pain transmission through A_1-receptors (see Sawynok & Sweeney, 1996).

*A fourth class of opioid peptide, *nociceptin*, has also been discovered (see Henderson & McKnight, 1997), the structure of which (Fig. 40.8) derives from a distinct precursor. Nociceptin was identified as the endogenous ligand for a novel opioid receptor-like protein (ORL) that had been detected by screening for homologues of the known opioid receptors. Because none of the then-known opioid peptides recognised ORL, it was classed as an 'orphan receptor' (Ch. 3). The discovery of nociceptin means that it is no longer an orphan, but little is yet known about the function of this system. The name nociceptin was coined because earlier studies showed that it caused hyperalgesia when injected into the brain—the opposite of other opioid peptides. Later studies showed, however, that its effects on nociception are more complex and can go in either direction (see Henderson & McKnight, 1997). To add to the confusion, the nociceptin precursor also contains another active peptide, *nocistatin*, that has actions which oppose those of nociceptin.

ANALGESIC DRUGS

MORPHINE-LIKE DRUGS

The term *opioid* applies to any substance, whether endogenous or synthetic, that produces morphine-like effects that are blocked by antagonists such as naloxone. The older term, *opiate*, is restricted to synthetic morphine-like drugs with non-peptidic structures. The field is reviewed thoroughly by Herz (1993).

Opium is an extract of the juice of the poppy *Papaver somniferum*, which has been used for social and medicinal purposes for thousands of years, as an agent to produce euphoria, analgesia and sleep, and to prevent diarrhoea. It was introduced in Britain at the end of the 17th century, usually taken orally as 'tincture of laudanum', addiction to which acquired a certain social cachet during the next 200 years. The situation changed when the hypodermic syringe and needle were invented in the mid-19th century and opiate dependence began to take on a more sinister significance.

CHEMICAL ASPECTS

Opium contains many alkaloids related to morphine. The structure of morphine (Fig. 40.9) was determined in 1902 and since then many semisynthetic compounds (produced by chemical modification of morphine) and fully synthetic opiates have been studied. In addition to morphine-like compounds, opium also contains **papaverine**, a smooth muscle relaxant (see Ch. 18).

The main drugs that are discussed in this section are:

- morphine analogues: these are compounds closely related in structure to morphine and often synthesised from it: they may be agonists (e.g. **morphine**, **diamorphine** (heroin) and **codeine**), partial agonists (e.g. **nalorphine** and **levallorphan**) or antagonists (e.g. **naloxone**)
- synthetic derivatives with structures unrelated to morphine:
  —phenylpiperidine series, e.g. **pethidine** and **fentanyl**
  —methadone series, e.g. **methadone** and **dextropropoxyphene**
  —benzomorphan series, e.g. **pentazocine** and **cyclazocine**
  —semisynthetic thebaine derivatives, e.g. **etorphine** and **buprenorphine**.

Mention should also be made of **loperamide**, an opiate that does not enter the brain and, therefore, lacks analgesic activity. Like other opiates (see below) it inhibits peristalsis, and it is used to control diarrhoea (see Ch. 24).

Morphine analogues

Morphine is a phenanthrene derivative with two planar rings and two aliphatic ring structures, which occupy a plane roughly at right angles to the rest of the molecule (Fig. 40.9). Variants of the morphine molecule have been produced by substitution at one or both of the hydroxyl groups or at the nitrogen atom.

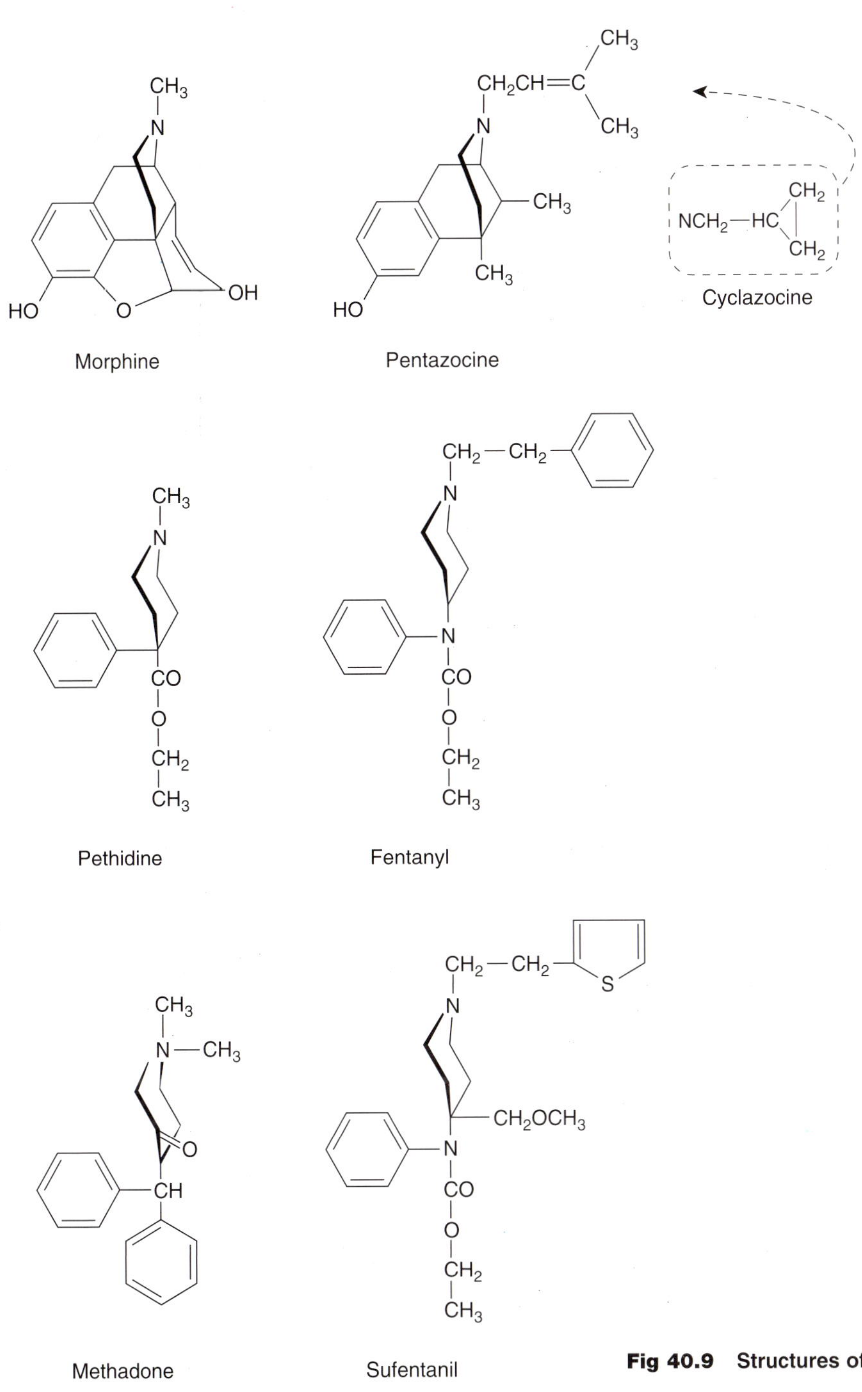

Fig 40.9 **Structures of some opiate analgesics.**

Synthetic derivatives

Phenylpiperidine series The first fully synthetic morphine-like drug, **pethidine** (known as meperidine in USA), was discovered accidentally when new atropine-like drugs were being sought. It is chemically unlike morphine, though its pharmacological actions are very similar. **Fentanyl** and **sufentanil** are more potent and shorter-acting derivatives that are used intravenously to treat severe pain or as an adjunct to anaesthesia.

Methadone series Although the structural formula of **methadone** bears no obvious chemical relationship to that of morphine, assumes a similar conformation in solution and was designed by reference to the common three-dimensional structural features of morphine and pethidine (Fig. 40.9). It is

Opioid analgesics

- There are three main families of endogenous opioid peptides (see Ch. 13); these have analgesic activity and have many physiological functions, but they are not used as drugs.
- Opioid drugs include:
  - —phenanthrene derivatives, structurally related to morphine
  - —synthetic compounds with a variety of dissimilar structures but similar pharmacological effects.
- Important morphine-like agonists include diamorphine and codeine; other structurally related compounds are partial agonists (e.g. nalorphine and levallorphan) or antagonists (e.g. naloxone).
- The main groups of synthetic analogues are the piperidines (e.g. pethidine and fentanyl), the methadone-like drugs, the benzomorphans (e.g. pentazocine) and the thebaine derivatives (e.g. buprenorphine).
- Opioid analgesics may be given orally, by injection, or intrathecally to produce analgesia.

Opioid receptors

- The μ-receptors are thought to be responsible for most of the analgesic effects of opioids, and for some major unwanted effects (e.g. respiratory depression, euphoria, sedation and dependence). Most of the analgesic opioids are μ-receptor agonists.
- The δ-receptors are probably more important in the periphery but may also contribute to analgesia.
- The κ-receptors contribute to analgesia at the spinal level and may elicit sedation and dysphoria; they produce relatively few unwanted effects and do not contribute to dependence. Some analgesics are relatively κ-selective.
- The σ-receptors are not true opioid receptors but are the site of action of certain psychotomimetic drugs, to which some opioids also bind.
- All opioid receptors are linked through G-proteins to inhibition of adenylate cyclase. They also facilitate opening of potassium channels (causing hyperpolarisation), and inhibit opening of calcium channels (inhibiting transmitter release). These membrane effects are not linked to the decrease in cAMP formation.
- Functional heterodimers, formed by combination of different types of opioid receptor, may occur and give rise to further pharmacological diverstity.

longer-acting than morphine but otherwise very similar to it. **Dextropropoxyphene** is very similar and used clinically for treating mild or moderate pain.

Benzomorphan series The most important members of this class are **pentazocine** and **cyclazocine** (Fig. 40.9). These drugs differ from morphine in their receptor-binding profile (see below) and so have somewhat different actions and side-effects.

Thebaine derivatives **Etorphine** is a highly potent morphine-like drug used mainly in veterinary practice. **Buprenorphine** resembles morphine but is a partial agonist (see below); thus, although very potent, its maximal effect is less than that of morphine, and it antagonises the effect of other opioids.

OPIOID RECEPTORS

Direct evidence that opioids are recognised by specific receptors came from binding studies by Snyder and his colleagues in 1973, though the existence of specific antagonists had earlier suggested that such receptors must exist. Various pharmacological observations implied that more than one type of receptor was involved, the original suggestion of multiple receptor types arising from in vivo studies of the spectrum of actions (analgesia, sedation, pupillary constriction, bradycardia, etc.) produced by different drugs. It was also found that some opioids, but not all, were able to relieve withdrawal symptoms in morphine-dependent animals, and this was interpreted in terms of distinct receptor subtypes. The conclusion (see Dhawan et al., 1996) from these and many subsequent pharmacological studies, now confirmed by receptor cloning, is that three types of opioid receptor, termed μ, δ and κ (all of them typical G-protein-coupled receptors), mediate the main pharmacological effects of opiates, as summarised in Table 40.1.* There is pharmacological evidence for further subdivisions of each of these three subtypes; it is possible (see Ch. 3) that their tendency to combine as functional dimers can account for this pharmacological diversity, but this remains to be confirmed. Recent studies on the characteristics of transgenic mouse strains lacking each of the three main subtypes show that the major pharmacological effects of morphine, including analgesia, are mediated by the μ-receptor.

The interaction of various opioid drugs and peptides with the various receptor types is summarised in Table 40.2. In addition to endogenous peptides and drugs in clinical use, some agents that are used as experimental tools for distinguishing the different receptor subtypes are also shown.

*A fourth subtype, σ, was also postulated in order to account for the 'dysphoric' effects (anxiety, hallucinations, bad dreams, etc.) produced by some opiates. The σ-receptors are, however, not true opioid receptors, since many other types of psychotropic drug also interact with them, and their biological role remains unclear (see Walker et al., 1990). Of the opiate drugs, only benzomorphans, such as **pentazocine** and **cyclazocine**, bind appreciably to σ-receptors, which is consistent with their known psychotomimetic properties.

Table 40.1 Functional effects associated with the main types of opioid receptor

	μ	δ	κ
Analgesia			
Supraspinal	+++	–	–
Spinal	++	++	+
Peripheral	++	–	++
Respiratory depression	+++	++	–
Pupil constriction	++	–	+
Reduced GI motility	++	++	+
Euphoria	+++	–	–
Dysphoria	–	–	+++
Sedation	++	–	++
Physical dependence	+++	–	+

Table 40.2 Selectivity of opioid drugs and peptides for receptor subtypes

	μ	δ	κ
Endogenous peptides			
β-Endorphin	+++	+++	+++
Leu-enkephalin	+	+++	–
Met-enkephalin	++	+++	–
Dynorphin	++	+	+++
Opiate drugs			
Pure agonists			
Morphine, codeine, oxymorphone, dextropropoxyphene	+++	+	+
Methadone	+++	–	–
Meperidine	++	+	+
Etorphine, bremazocine	+++	+++	+++
Fentanyl, sufentanil	+++	+	–
Partial mixed agonists			
Pentazocine, ketocyclazocine	+	+	++
Nalbuphine	+	+	(++)
Nalorphine	++	–	(++)
Buprenorphine	(+++)	–	++
Antagonists			
Naloxone	+++	+	++
Naltrexone	+++	+	+++
Research tools (receptor-selective)			
DAMGO[a]	+++	–	–
DPDPE[a]	–	++	–
U50488[a]	–	–	+++
CTOP[a]	+++	–	–
Naltrindole, diprenorphine	–	+++	–
Nor-binaltorphimine	+	+	+++

Note: Blue + symbols represent **agonist** activity; partial agonists in parentheses
Black + symbols denote **antagonist** activity.
– symbols represent weak or no activity.

[a]DAMGO, DPDPE and CTOP are synthetic opioid-like peptides, more receptor-selective than endogenous opioids. U50488 is a synthetic opiate.

AGONISTS AND ANTAGONISTS

Opioids vary not only in their receptor specificity but also in their efficacy at the different types of receptor. Thus some agents act as agonists on one type of receptor and as antagonists or partial agonists at another, producing a very complicated pharmacological picture. Some of this complexity may reflect the existence of receptor heterodimers with functional properties that differ from those of the well-studied monomeric opiate receptors.

Three main categories may be distinguished (Table 40.2):

Pure agonists This group includes most of the typical morphine-like drugs. They all have high affinity for μ-receptors and generally lower affinity for δ- and κ-sites. Some drugs of this type, notably **codeine**, **methadone** and **dextropropoxyphene**, are sometimes referred to as weak agonists, since their maximal effects, both analgesic and unwanted, are less than those of morphine, and they do not cause dependence. Whether they are truly partial agonists is not established.

Partial agonists and mixed agonist–antagonists These drugs are typified by **nalorphine** and **pentazocine** and combine a degree of agonist and antagonist activity on different receptors. Nalorphine, for example, is an agonist when tested on guinea-pig ileum, but it also inhibits competitively the effect of morphine on this tissue (consistent with a partial agonist profile; see Ch. 2). In vivo, it shows a similar mixture of agonist and antagonist actions. Pentazocine and cyclazocine, by comparison, are antagonists at μ-receptors, but partial agonists on δ- and κ-receptors. Most of the drugs in this group tend to cause dysphoria, rather than euphoria, an effect mediated by the κ-receptor or the non-opioid σ-receptor.

Antagonists These drugs produce very little effect when given on their own but block the effects of opioids. The most important examples are **naloxone** and **naltrexone**.

MECHANISM OF ACTION OF OPIOIDS

The opioids have probably been studied more intensively than any other group of drugs in the effort to understand their powerful effects in molecular, biochemical and physiological terms, and to use this understanding to develop opioid drugs as analgesics with significant advantages over morphine. While the receptor biology is well worked out, the physiological pathways that are regulated by opioids, which underlie their analgesic and other actions, are only partly understood. Even so, morphine—described by Osler as 'God's own medicine'—remains the standard against which any new analgesic is assessed. Useful reviews on the neuropharmacology of opiates include Pasternak (1993) and Yaksh (1997).

Cellular actions

Opioid receptors belong to the family of G-protein-coupled receptors and inhibit adenylate cyclase, so reducing the intracellular cAMP content (see Dhawan et al., 1996). All three receptor subtypes exert this effect, and they also exert effects on ion channels through a direct G-protein coupling to the channel. By these means, opioids promote the opening of potassium channels and inhibit the opening of voltage-gated calcium channels, which are the main effects seen at the membrane level. These membrane effects reduce both neuronal excitability (since the increased K^+ conductance causes hyperpolarisation of the membrane) and transmitter release (owing to inhibition of Ca^{2+} entry). The overall effect is, therefore, inhibitory at the cellular level. Nonetheless, opioids increase activity in some neuronal pathways (see below) by suppressing the firing of inhibitory interneurons. At the cellular level, all three receptor subtypes mediate very similar effects, though the heterogeneous distribution of the receptors means that particular neurons and pathways are affected selectively by different agonists.

Effects on the nociceptive pathway

Opioid receptors are widely distributed in the brain, and their relationship to the nociceptive pathway is summarised in Figure 40.5. Opioids are effective as analgesics when given intrathecally in minute doses, implying that a central action can account for their analgesic effect. Injection of morphine into the PAG region causes marked analgesia, which can be prevented by surgical interruption of the descending pathway to NRM or by blocking 5-HT synthesis pharmacologically with *p*-chlorophenylalanine. This latter procedure blocks the 5-HT pathway running from NRM to the dorsal horn. Moreover, systemic morphine is rendered less effective in suppressing nociceptive spinal reflexes by transection of the spinal cord in the neck, and the firing of neurons associated with the descending inhibitory pathways is increased by morphine, confirming that there is a significant supraspinal component of the overall effect.

At the spinal level, morphine inhibits transmission of nociceptive impulses through the dorsal horn and suppresses nociceptive spinal reflexes, even in patients with spinal cord transection. It inhibits release of substance P from dorsal horn neurons in vitro and in vivo (Fig. 40.10), by a presynaptic inhibitory effect on the central terminals of nociceptive afferent neurons. Microinjection of morphine into the dorsal horn also produces this effect. However, direct measurement of substance P release (by an antibody-covered microprobe inserted directly into the dorsal horn) failed to show any inhibition of release when morphine was given systemically in analgesic doses, implying that an action on primary afferent terminals may not be important in producing its therapeutic effect.

There is also evidence (see Stein & Yassouridis, 1997) that opiates inhibit the discharge of nociceptive afferent terminals in the periphery, particularly under conditions of inflammation, in which the expression of opioid receptors by sensory neurons is increased. Injection of morphine into the knee joint following surgery to the joint provides effective analgesia, undermining the age-old belief that opioid analgesia is exclusively a central phenomenon.

PHARMACOLOGICAL ACTIONS

Morphine is typical of many opioid analgesics and will be taken as the reference compound.

The most important effects of morphine are on the CNS and the gastrointestinal tract, though numerous effects of lesser significance on many other systems have been described.

Effects on the central nervous system

Analgesia

Morphine is effective in most kinds of acute and chronic pain, though opioids in general are less useful in neuropathic pain

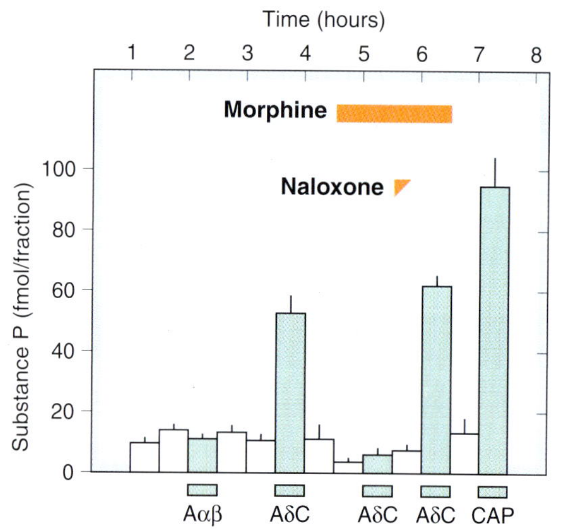

Fig. 40.10 Morphine inhibits the release of substance P from cat spinal cord. Substance P was measured by radioimmunoassay in the fluid superfusing the spinal cord. Stimulation of the sciatic nerve at low intensity stimulates large myelinated fibres (Aα and Aβ) only and evokes no release. Increasing the stimulus strength to recruit Aδ and C fibres causes substance P release. The release is blocked by morphine, this effect being antagonised by naloxone. Capsaicin (CAP) added to the fluid superfusing the spinal cord also releases substance P. (From: Yaksh T L et al. 1980 Nature 286: 155.)

syndromes (such as phantom limb and other types of deafferentation pain, trigeminal neuralgia, etc.) than in pain associated with tissue injury, inflammation or tumour growth.

As well as being antinociceptive, morphine also reduces the affective component of pain. This reflects its supraspinal action, possibly at the level of the limbic system, which is probably involved in the euphoria-producing effect. Drugs such as nalorphine and pentazocine share the antinociceptive actions of morphine but have much less effect on the psychological response to pain.

Euphoria

Morphine causes a powerful sense of contentment and well-being. This is an important component of its analgesic effect, since the agitation and anxiety associated with a painful illness or injury are thereby reduced. If morphine or diamorphine ('heroin') is given intravenously, the result is a sudden 'rush' likened to an 'abdominal orgasm'. The euphoria produced by morphine depends considerably on the circumstances. In patients who are distressed, it is pronounced, but in patients who become accustomed to chronic pain, morphine causes analgesia with little or no euphoria. Some patients report restlessness rather than euphoria under these circumstances.

Euphoria appears to be mediated through μ-receptors and to be balanced by the dysphoria associated with κ-receptor activation (see Table 40.1). Thus, different opioid drugs vary greatly in the amount of euphoria that they produce. It does not occur with codeine or with pentazocine to any marked extent, and nalorphine, in doses sufficient to cause analgesia, produces dysphoria.

Respiratory depression

Respiratory depression, resulting in increased arterial partial pressure of carbon dioxide ($P\text{CO}_2$), occurs with a normal analgesic dose of morphine or related compounds. Analgesia and respiratory depression are both mediated by μ-receptors, and the balance between them is thus the same for most opioids. The depressant effect is associated with a decrease in the sensitivity of the respiratory centre to $P\text{CO}_2$. Neurons in the medullary respiratory centre itself do not appear to be directly depressed, but opioids applied to the ventral surface of the medulla in the region where carbon dioxide chemosensitivity is maximal have a powerful depressant effect on respiration.

Respiratory depression by opioids is not accompanied by depression of the medullary centres controlling cardiovascular function (in contrast to the action of anaesthetics and other general depressants). This means that respiratory depression produced by opioids is much better tolerated than a similar degree of depression caused by, say, a barbiturate. Nonetheless, respiratory depression is the most troublesome unwanted effect of these drugs, and, unlike that caused by general CNS depressant drugs, it occurs at therapeutic doses. It is the commonest cause of death in acute opioid poisoning.

Depression of cough reflex

Cough suppression, surprisingly, does not correlate closely with the analgesic and respiratory depressant actions of opioids, and its mechanism at the receptor level is unclear. In general, increasing substitution on the phenolic hydroxyl group of morphine increases antitussive relative to analgesic activity. Thus codeine suppresses cough in subanalgesic doses and is often used in cough medicines (see Ch. 22). **Pholcodine** is even more selective, though these agents cause constipation as an unwanted effect.

Nausea and vomiting

Nausea and vomiting occur in up to 40% of patients when they first take morphine, and these effects do not seem to be separable from the analgesic effect among a range of opioid analgesics. The site of action is the area postrema (chemoreceptor trigger zone) a region of the medulla where chemical stimuli of many kinds may initiate vomiting (see Ch. 24).* Nausea and vomiting following morphine injection are usually transient and disappear with repeated administration.

Pupillary constriction

Pupillary constriction is a centrally mediated effect, caused by μ- and κ-receptor-mediated stimulation of the oculomotor nucleus. Pinpoint pupils are an important diagnostic feature in overdosage with morphine and related drugs, because most other causes of coma and respiratory depression produce pupillary dilatation.

Effects on the gastrointestinal tract

Morphine increases tone and reduces motility in many parts of the gastrointestinal system, resulting in constipation, which may be severe and very troublesome to the patient. The resulting delay in gastric emptying can considerably retard the absorption of other drugs. Pressure in the biliary tract increases because of contraction of the gall bladder and constriction of the biliary sphincter. Opiates should be avoided in patients suffering from biliary colic caused by gallstones, in whom pain may be increased rather than relieved. The rise in intrabiliary pressure can cause a transient increase in the concentration of amylase and lipase in the plasma.

The action of morphine on visceral smooth muscle is probably mediated mainly through the intramural nerve plexuses, since the increase in tone is reduced or abolished by atropine. It is partly mediated by a central action of morphine, since intraventricular injection of morphine inhibits propulsive gastrointestinal movements. The local effect of morphine and other opioids on neurons of the myenteric plexus is inhibitory, associated with hyperpolarisation resulting from an increased K^+ conductance. The receptors involved in these effects are of the μ, κ and δ type, with much variation between different preparations and different species.

Other actions of opioids

Morphine releases histamine from mast cells, by an action unrelated to opioid receptors. This release of histamine can cause

*The chemically related compound **apomorphine** is more strongly emetic than morphine, through its action as a dopamine agonist; despite its name, it is inactive on opioid receptors. It was at one time used as a conditioned 'aversion therapy' for treating various kinds of unwanted behaviour.

Actions of morphine

- The main pharmacological effects are:
  - —analgesia
  - —euphoria and sedation
  - —respiratory depression and suppression of cough
  - —nausea and vomiting
  - —pupillary constriction
  - —reduced gastrointestinal motility, causing constipation
  - —histamine release, causing bronchoconstriction and hypotension.
- The most troublesome unwanted effects are constipation and respiratory depression.
- Morphine may be given by injection (intravenous or intramuscular) or by mouth, often as slow-release tablets.
- Acute overdosage with morphine produces coma and respiratory depression.
- Morphine is metabolised to morphine 6-glucuronide (M6G), which is more potent as an analgesic.
- Morphine and M6G, are the active metabolites of diamorphine and codeine.

local effects, such as urticaria and itching at the site of the injection, or systemic effects, namely bronchoconstriction and hypotension. The bronchoconstrictor effect can have serious consequences for asthmatic patients, to whom morphine should not be given. Pethidine does not produce this effect.

Hypotension and bradycardia occur with large doses of most opioids, through an action on the medulla. With morphine and similar drugs, histamine release may contribute to the hypotension.

Effects on smooth muscle other than that of the gastrointestinal tract and bronchi are slight, though spasm of the ureters, bladder and uterus sometimes occur. The Straub tail reaction, an improbable phenomena beloved of pharmacologists, consists of a raising and stiffening of the tail of rats or mice given opioid drugs, and is caused by spasm of a muscle at the base of the tail. It was through this effect that the analgesic action of pethidine was discovered.

Opioids also exert complex immunosuppressant effects, which may be important as a link between the nervous system and immune function (see Sibinga & Goldstein, 1988). The pharmacological significance of this is not yet clear, but there is evidence in humans that the immune system is depressed by long-term opioid abuse, leading to increased susceptibility to infections.

TOLERANCE AND DEPENDENCE

Tolerance to opioids (i.e. an increase in the dose needed to produce a given pharmacological effect) develops rapidly and is readily demonstrated. *Dependence* is a different phenomenon, much more difficult to define and measure, which involves two separate components, namely physical and psychological dependence (see Ch. 42). Physical dependence is associated with a physiological withdrawal syndrome (or *abstinence syndrome*), which can be reproduced in experimental animals and appears to be closely related to tolerance. Morphine also produces strong psychological dependence, expressed as craving for the drug, which is probably more important than the physical withdrawal syndrome as a factor causing dependence in humans but is far harder to study.

Tolerance

Tolerance can be detected within 12–24 hours of morphine administration. Figure 40.11 shows the increase in the equianalgesic dose of morphine (measured by the hot-plate test) that occurred when a slow-release pellet of morphine was implanted subcutaneously in mice. The pellet was removed 8 hours before the test to allow its effect to disappear before the test was carried out. Within 3 days the equianalgesic dose increased about fivefold. Sensitivity returned to normal within about 3 days of removing the pellet. Tolerance extends to most of the pharmacological effects of morphine, including analgesia, emesis, euphoria, and respiratory depression, but affects the constipating and pupil-constricting actions much less. Thus, addicts may take 50 times the normal analgesic dose of morphine with relatively little respiratory depression, but marked constipation and pupillary constriction.

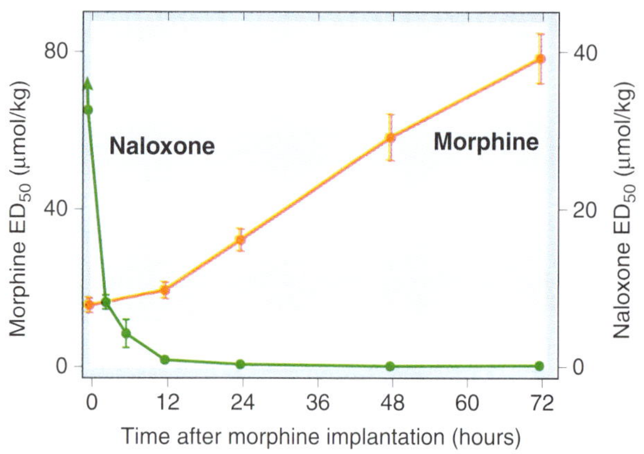

Fig. 40.11 Development of morphine tolerance in mice. The median effective dose (ED_{50}) for analgesia (hot-plate test) produced by subcutaneous injection of a test dose of morphine (orange line) was measured at intervals after implantation of a slow-release pellet of morphine, the pellet being removed 8 hours before the assay in order to allow the circulating morphine concentration to fall to zero before the test dose was given. The ED_{50} increases about fivefold after 72 hours. Simultaneously, the dose of naloxone needed to precipitate withdrawal symptoms (green line) decreases very markedly. (From: Way E L et al. 1969 J Pharmacol Exp Ther 167: 1.)

The cellular mechanisms responsible for tolerance are discussed in Chapter 42. Certain possibilities can be excluded, such as increased metabolic degradation, reduced affinity of opioids for their receptors, downregulation of opioid receptors and inhibition of the release of endogenous opioids. Tolerance is a general phenomenon of opioid receptor ligands, irrespective of which type of receptor they act upon. Cross-tolerance occurs between drugs acting at the same receptor, but not between opioids that act on different receptors. In clinical settings, the opiate dose required for effective pain relief may increase as a result of developing tolerance, but it does not constitute a major problem.

Physical dependence

Physical dependence is characterised by a clear-cut abstinence syndrome. In experimental animals (for example, rats), abrupt withdrawal of morphine after chronic administration for a few days causes an increased irritability, loss of weight and a variety of abnormal behaviour patterns, such as body shakes, writhing, jumping and signs of aggression. These reactions decrease after a few days, but abnormal irritability and aggression persist for many weeks. Human addicts show a similar abstinence syndrome, somewhat resembling severe influenza, with yawning, pupillary dilatation, fever, sweating, piloerection,* nausea, diarrhoea and insomnia.

Tolerance and dependence

- Tolerance develops rapidly, accompanied by physical withdrawal syndrome.
- The mechanism of tolerance is unclear (see Ch. 42). It is not pharmacokinetic in origin and receptor downregulation is not a major factor.
- Dependence is satisfied by μ-receptor agonists, and the withdrawal syndrome is precipitated by μ-receptor antagonists.
- Dependence comprises two components: (i) physical dependence, associated with the withdrawal syndrome, lasting for a few days; (ii) psychological dependence, associated with craving, lasting for months or years. Psychological dependence rarely occurs in patients being given opioids as analgesics.
- Weak, long-acting μ-receptor agonists, such as methadone, may be used to relieve withdrawal symptoms.
- Certain opioid analgesics, such as codeine, pentazocine and buprenorphine, are much less likely to cause physical or psychological dependence.

*Causing goose pimples. This is the origin of the phrase 'cold turkey' used to describe the effect of morphine withdrawal.

Extreme restlessness and distress are accompanied by a strong craving for the drug. The physical symptoms are maximal after 2–3 days and largely disappear in 8–10 days, though some residual symptoms and physiological abnormalities persist for several weeks. Re-administration of morphine rapidly abolishes the abstinence syndrome.

Many physiological changes have been described in relation to the abstinence syndrome. For example, spinal reflex hyperexcitability occurs in morphine-dependent animals, and it can be produced by chronic intrathecal as well as systemic administration of morphine. The noradrenergic pathways emanating from the locus ceruleus (see above) may also play an important role in causing the abstinence syndrome, and the α_2-adrenoceptor agonist clonidine is sometimes used to alleviate it. The rate of firing of locus ceruleus neurons is reduced by opioids, and increased during the abstinence syndrome. Similar changes affect dopaminergic neurons in the ventral tegmental area that project to the nucleus accumbens. These cells receive input from opioid-containing neurons and constitute the 'reward pathway' responsible for the strong reinforcing effect of opioids (see Ch. 42).

PHARMACOKINETIC ASPECTS

Table 40.3 summarises the pharmacokinetic properties of the main opioid analgesics. The absorption of morphine congeners by mouth is variable. Morphine itself is slowly and erratically absorbed and is commonly given by intravenous or intramuscular injection to treat acute severe pain; oral morphine is, however, often used in treating chronic pain, and slow-release preparations are available to increase its duration of action. Codeine is well absorbed and normally given by mouth. Most morphine-like drugs undergo considerable first-pass metabolism and are, therefore, markedly less potent when taken orally than when injected.

The plasma half-life of most morphine analogues is 3–6 hours. Hepatic metabolism is the main mode of inactivation, usually by conjugation with glucuronide. This occurs at the 3- and 6-OH groups, and these glucuronides constitute a considerable fraction of the drug in the bloodstream. Morphine 6-glucuronide is, surprisingly, more active as an analgesic than morphine itself, and it contributes substantially to the pharmacological effect. Morphine 3-glucuronide has been claimed to antagonise the analgesic effect of morphine, but the significance of this experimental finding is uncertain. Morphine glucuronides are excreted in the urine; consequently, the dose needs to be reduced in cases of renal failure. Glucuronides also reach the gut via biliary excretion, where they are hydrolysed, most of the morphine being reabsorbed (enterohepatic circulation). Because of low conjugating capacity in neonates, morphine-like drugs have a much longer duration of action; because even a small degree of respiratory depression can be hazardous, morphine congeners should not be used in the neonatal period, nor used as analgesics during childbirth. Pethidine (see below) is a safer alternative for this purpose.

Table 40.3 Characteristics of the main opioid analgesic drugs

DRUG	Uses	Route of administration	Pharmacokinetic aspects	Main adverse effects	Notes
Morphine	Widely used for acute and chronic pain	Oral, including sustained-release form Injection[a] Intrathecal	Half-life 3–4 h Converted to active metabolite (morphine 6-glucuronide)	Sedation, Respiratory depression Constipation Nausea and vomiting Itching (histamine release) Tolerance and dependence Euphoria	Tolerance and withdrawal effects not common when used for analgesia
Diamorphine	Acute and chronic pain	Oral Injection	Acts more rapidly than morphine because of rapid brain penetration. Metabolised to morphine	As morphine	Not available in all countries Considered (irrationally) to be analgesic of last resort Also known as heroin
Hydromorphone	Acute and chronic pain	Oral Injection	Half-life 2–4 h No active metabolites	As morphine but allegedly less sedative	**Levorphanol** is similar, with longer duration of action
Methadone	Chronic pain Maintenance of addicts	Oral Injection	Long half-life (>24 h) Slow onset	As morphine but little euphoric effect Accumulation may occur because of long half-life	Slow recovery results in attenuated withdrawal syndrome
Pethidine	Acute pain	Oral Intramuscular injection	Half-life 2–4 h Active metabolite (norpethidine) may account for stimulant effects	As morphine, anticholinergic effects Risk of excitement and convulsions	Known as meperidine in USA. Interacts with monoamine oxidase inhibitors (MAOI; Ch. 38)
Buprenorphine	Acute and chronic pain	Sublingual Injection Intrathecal	Half-life about 12 h Slow onset Inactive orally because of first-pass metabolism	As morphine but less pronounced Respiratory depression not reversed by naloxone (therefore not suitable for obstetric use)	Useful in chronic pain with patient-controlled injection systems
Pentazocine	Mainly acute pain	Oral Injection	Half-life 2–4 h	Psychotomimetic effects (dysphoria) Irritation at injection site May precipitate morphine withdrawal syndrome (μ-antagonist effect)	Nalbuphine is similar
Fentanyl	Acute pain Anaesthesia	Intravenous Epidural Transdermal patch	Half-life 1–2 h	As morphine	High potency allows transdermal administration **Sufentanil** is similar
Codeine	Mild pain	Oral	Acts as pro-drug Metabolised to morphine and other active opioids	Mainly constipation No dependence liability	Effective only in mild pain Also used to suppress cough Dihydrocodeine is similar
Dextropropoxyphene	Mild pain	Mainly oral	Half-life ~4 h Active metabolite (norpropoxyphene) with half-life ~24 h	Respitory depression. May cause convulsions (possible by action of norpropoxyphene)	Similar to codeine
Tramadol	Acute (mainly postoperative) and chronic pain	Oral Intravenous	Well absorbed Half-life 4–6 h	Dizziness May cause convulsions No respiratory depression	Metabolite of trazodone Mechanism of action uncertain Weak agonist at opioid receptors Also inhibits noradrenaline uptake

[a]Injections may by given intravenously, intramuscularly or subcutaneously for most drugs.

Analogues that have no free hydroxyl group in the 3-position (i.e. diamorphine, codeine) are metabolised to morphine, which accounts for all or part of their pharmacological activity. Morphine produces very effective analgesia when administered intrathecally and is often used in this way by anaesthetists, the advantage being that the sedative and respiratory depressant effects are reduced, though not completely avoided.

For the treatment of chronic or postoperative pain, opioids are being increasingly used 'on demand' (patient-controlled analgesia). The patients are provided with an infusion pump, which they control, the maximum possible rate of administration being limited to avoid acute toxicity. Contrary to fears, patients show little tendency to use excessively large doses and become dependent; instead the dose is adjusted to achieve analgesia without excessive sedation and is reduced as the pain subsides. Being in control of their own analgesia, the patients' anxiety and distress is reduced, and analgesic consumption actually tends to decrease.

UNWANTED EFFECTS

The main unwanted effects of morphine and related drugs are listed in Table 40.3.

Acute overdosage with morphine results in coma and respiratory depression, with characteristically constricted pupils. It is treated by giving naloxone intravenously. This also serves as a diagnostic test, for failure to respond to **naloxone** indicates a cause other than opioid poisoning for the comatose state. There is a danger of precipitating a severe withdrawal syndrome with naloxone, since opioid poisoning occurs mainly in addicts.

OTHER OPIOID ANALGESICS

Diamorphine (heroin) is the diacetyl derivative of morphine. A strong smell of vinegar commonly provides the lead to illicit heroin producers, at least in fiction. In the body, it is rapidly deacetylated to morphine, and its effects are indistinguishable. However, because of its greater lipid solubility it crosses the blood–brain barrier more rapidly than morphine and gives a greater 'rush' when injected intravenously. It is said to be less emetic than morphine, but the evidence for this is slight. It is still available in the UK for clinical use as an analgesic though it is banned in many countries. Its only advantage over morphine is its greater solubility, which allows smaller volumes to be given orally. It exerts the same respiratory depressant effect as morphine and, if given intravenously, is more likely to cause dependence. Its duration of action (about 2 hours) is shorter than that of morphine.

Codeine (3-methoxymorphine) is more reliably absorbed by mouth than morphine but has only 20% or less of the analgesic potency. Furthermore, its analgesic effect does not increase appreciably at higher dose levels. It is, therefore, used mainly as an oral analgesic for mild types of pain (headache, backache, etc.). Unlike morphine, it causes little or no euphoria and is rarely addictive, so it is available freely without prescription. It is often combined with paracetamol in proprietary analgesic preparations. In relation to its analgesic effect, codeine produces the same degree of respiratory depression as morphine, but the limited response even at high doses means that it is seldom a problem in practice. It does, however, cause constipation. Codeine has marked antitussive activity and is often used in cough mixtures (see Ch. 22). **Dihydrocodeine** is pharmacologically very similar, having no substantial advantages or disadvantages over codeine. About 10% of the population is resistant to the analgesic effect of codeine, because they lack the demethylating enzyme which converts it to morphine.

Dextropropoxyphene is similar to codeine but has a longer duration of action. It was thought to be safe in overdose and free from dependence liability, but experience has shown that neither is the case.

Pethidine (meperidine) is very similar to morphine in its pharmacological effects, except that it tends to cause restlessness rather than sedation, and it has an additional antimuscarinic action, which may cause dry mouth and blurring of vision as side-effects. It produces a very similar euphoric effect and is equally liable to cause dependence. Its duration of action is appreciably shorter than that of morphine, and the route of metabolic degradation is different. Pethidine is partly N-demethylated in the liver to norpethidine, which has a hallucinogenic and convulsant effect. This becomes significant with large oral doses of pethidine, producing an overdose syndrome rather different from that of morphine. Pethidine is preferred to morphine for analgesia during labour, because it is shorter acting. The difference in the duration of action of morphine and pethidine is particularly marked in the neonate. This is because the conjugation reactions, on which the excretion of morphine, but not of pethidine, depends, are deficient in the newborn. Severe reactions, consisting of excitement, hyperthermia and convulsions, have been reported when pethidine is given to patients receiving monoamine oxidase inhibitors. This seems to be caused by inhibition of an alternative metabolic pathway, leading to increased norpethidine formation, but the details are not known.

Fentanyl and **sufentanil** are highly potent phenylpiperidine derivatives, with actions similar to morphine but short lasting, particularly sufentanil. Their main use is in anaesthesia, and they may be given intrathecally. They are also used in patient-controlled infusion systems, where a short duration of action is advantageous.

Etorphine is a morphine analogue of remarkable potency, more than 1000 times that of morphine, but otherwise very similar in its actions. Its high potency confers no particular clinical advantage, but it is used to immobilise wild animals for trapping and research purposes, since the required dose, even for an elephant, is small enough to be incorporated into a dart or pellet.

Methadone is also pharmacologically similar to morphine, the main difference being that its duration of action is considerably longer (plasma half-life >24 hours) and it is claimed to have less sedative action. The increased duration seems to occur because the drug is bound in the extravascular compartment and slowly released. One consequence is that the physical abstinence syndrome is less acute than with morphine or other short-acting drugs, though the psychological dependence is no less pronounced. Methadone is widely used as a means of treating morphine and diamorphine addiction. In the presence of methadone, an injection of morphine does not cause the normal euphoria, and the lack of a physical abstinence syndrome makes it possible to wean addicts from morphine or diamorphine by giving regular oral doses of methadone—an improvement if not a cure.*

Pentazocine is a mixed agonist–antagonist (see earlier section). In low doses, its potency and effects are very similar to those of morphine, but increasing the dose does not cause a corresponding increase in the effects produced. Therefore, at high doses, pentazocine causes only slight respiratory depression, and it causes marked dysphoria, with nightmares and hallucinations, rather than euphoria. It also tends to raise, rather than lower, arterial blood pressure. These differences mean that pentazocine has less tendency to cause dependence, and its acute toxicity is much less than that of morphine. Its antagonist activity is apparent in the fact that, given concurrently with morphine, pentazocine actually reduces the analgesic and other actions of morphine, and it can even precipitate an abstinence syndrome in morphine addicts. Binding studies show that it has a higher affinity for κ- than for μ-receptors, and also acts on non-opioid σ-receptors, this spectrum being somewhat different from that of conventional opioid drugs. Though much less addictive than the conventional opioids, pentazocine still has an appreciable tendency to cause dependence and is far from the ideal morphine substitute that it was originally thought to be.

Buprenorphine is a partial agonist on μ-receptors. It is less liable to cause dysphoria than pentazocine, but it is more liable to cause respiratory depression. It has a long duration of action. Its abuse liability is probably less than that of morphine.

Meptazinol and **dezocine** are recently introduced opiates of unusual chemical structure. Meptazinol can be given orally or by injection and has a short plasma half-life. It seems to be relatively free of morphine-like side-effects, causing neither euphoria nor dysphoria, nor severe respiratory depression. It does, however, produce nausea, sedation and dizziness, and it has atropine-like side-effects. Because of its short duration of action and lack of respiratory depression, it may have advantages for obstetric analgesia. Dezocine is a partial agonist at μ-receptors, with analgesic activity similar to that of morphine, but with respiratory depressant activity that reaches a 'ceiling' at high doses. It has not yet been fully evaluated.

OPIOID ANTAGONISTS

Nalorphine is closely related in structure to morphine and was the first specific antagonist to be discovered. It provided the first clear evidence in favour of a specific receptor for morphine, recognition of which led to the successful search for endogenous mediators. Nalorphine has, in fact, a more complicated action than that of a simple competitive antagonist (Table 40.2). In low doses, it is a competitive antagonist and blocks most actions of morphine in whole animals or isolated tissues. Higher doses, however, are analgesic and mimic the effects of morphine. These effects probably reflect an antagonist action on μ-receptors, coupled with a partial agonist action on δ- and κ-receptors, the latter causing dysphoria, which makes it unsuitable for use as an analgesic. Nalorphine can itself produce physical dependence, but it can also precipitate a withdrawal syndrome in morphine or diamorphine addicts. Nalorphine now has few clinical uses.

Naloxone was the first pure opioid antagonist, with affinity for all three opioid receptors. It blocks the actions of endogenous opioid peptides as well as those of morphine-like drugs, and it has been extensively used as an experimental tool to determine the physiological role of these peptides, particularly in pain transmission.

Given on its own, naloxone produces very little effect in normal subjects, but it produces a rapid reversal of the effects of morphine and other opioids, including partial agonists such as pentazocine and nalorphine. It has little effect on pain threshold under normal conditions but causes hyperalgesia under conditions of stress or inflammation, when endogenous opioids are produced. This occurs, for example, in patients undergoing dental surgery, or in animals subjected to physical stress. Naloxone also inhibits acupuncture analgesia, which is known to be associated with the release of opioid peptides. Analgesia produced by PAG stimulation is also prevented.

The main clinical use of naloxone is to treat respiratory depression caused by opioid overdosage, and occasionally to reverse the effect of opioid analgesics, used during labour, on the respiration of the newborn baby. It is usually given intravenously and its effects are produced immediately. It is rapidly metabolised by the liver and its effect lasts only 2–4 hours, which is

Opioid antagonists

- Pure antagonists include naloxone (short acting) and naltrexone (long acting). They block μ-, δ- and κ-receptors more-or-less equally. Selective antagonists are available as experimental tools.
- Other drugs, such as nalorphine and pentazocine, produce a mixture of agonist and antagonist effects.
- Naloxone does not affect pain threshold normally but blocks stress-induced analgesia and can exacerbate clinical pain.
- Naloxone rapidly reverses opioid-induced analgesia and respiratory depression; it is used mainly to treat opioid overdose or to improve breathing in newborn babies affected by opioids given to the mother.
- Naloxone precipitates withdrawal symptoms in morphine-dependent patients or animals. Pentazocine may also do this.

*The benefits come mainly from removing the risks of self-injection and the need to finance the drug habit through crime.

considerably shorter than that of most morphine-like drugs. Consequently, it may have to be given repeatedly.

Naloxone has no important unwanted effects of its own but precipitates withdrawal symptoms in addicts. It can be used to detect opioid addiction.

Naltrexone is very similar to naloxone but with the advantage of a much longer duration of action (half-life about 10 hours). It may be of value in addicts who have been 'detoxified', since it nullifies the effect of a dose of opiate should the patient's resolve fail. Its use in other conditions, such as alcoholism and septic shock, is being investigated, though the role of opioid peptides in these conditions is controversial.

Specific antagonists at μ-, δ- and κ-receptors are available for experimental use (Table 40.2), but not yet for clinical purposes.

OTHER ANALGESIC DRUGS

▼ Besides opioids and NSAIDs (see Ch. 16), several other drugs are used as analgesics, particularly to treat neuropathic pain states, which respond poorly to conventional analgesic drugs and pose a major clinical problem.

- **Tramadol** (see Table 40.3), a metabolite of the antidepressant **trazodone** (Ch. 38), is widely used as an analgesic for postoperative pain. It is a weak agonist at μ-opioid receptors and also a weak inhibitor of noradrenaline reuptake. It is effective as an analgesic and appears to have a better side-effect profile than most opioids.
- Tricyclic antidepressants, particularly **imipramine** and **amitriptyline** (Ch. 38)**,** act centrally by inhibiting noradrenaline reuptake and are highly effective in relieving neuropathic pain in some, but not all, patients. Their action is independent of their antidepressant effects, and selective serotonin (5-HT) reuptake inhibitors are not effective.
- Antiepileptic drugs (Ch 39) such as **carbamazepine, gabapentin** and occasionally **phenytoin** are sometimes effective in neuropathic pain.
- **Ketamine**, a dissociative anaesthetic (Ch. 33), which works by blocking NMDA-receptor channels, has analgesic properties, probably directed at the 'wind-up' phenomenon in the dorsal horn (Fig. 40.3). Given intrathecally, its effects on memory and cognitive function are largely avoided.
- Intravenous **lidocaine**, a local anaesthetic drug (Ch. 43) with a short plasma half-life, can give long-lasting relief in neuropathic pain states. It probably acts by blocking spontaneous discharges from damaged sensory nerve terminals, but the reason for its persistent analgesic effect is not clear.

Clinical uses of analgesic drugs

- Analgesics are used to treat and prevent pain, e.g.
  - —pre- and postoperatively
  - —common painful conditions including headache, dysmenorrhoea, labour, trauma, burns
  - —many medical and surgical emergencies (e.g. myocardial infarction, renal colic, etc.)
  - —terminal disease (especially metatastic cancer).
- Opioid analgesics are used in some non-painful conditions, e.g. acute heart failure (because of their haemodynamic effects) and terminal chronic heart failure (to relieve distress).
- The choice and route of administration of analgesic drugs depends on the nature and duration of the pain.
- A progressive approach is often used, starting with non-steroidal anti-inflammatory drugs (NSAIDs), supplemented first by weak opioid analgesics and then by strong opioids.
- In general, severe acute pain is treated with strong opioids (e.g. morphine, fentanyl) given by injection. Mild inflammatory pain (e.g. sprains, mild arthralgia) is treated with NSAIDs (e.g. ibuprofen) or by paracetamol supplemented by weak opioids (e.g. codeine, dextropropoxyphene). Severe pain (e.g. cancer pain) is treated with strong opioid given orally, intrathecally, epidurally or by subcutaneous injection. Patient-controlled infusion systems are useful postoperatively.
- Chronic neuropathic pain is often unresponsive to opioids and is treated with tricyclic antidepressants (e.g. amitrityline) or anticonvulsants (e.g. carbamazepine, gabapentin).

NEW APPROACHES

▼ It can be seen from the earlier discussion of the neural mechanisms involved in pain and nociception that there are many potential sites at which drugs might act to inhibit transmission of information from the periphery to the thalamus and cortex. Attempts to develop new types of drug have tended to be dominated by opioid agonists on the one hand and NSAIDs on the other, but other possibilities are now being considered, and may find their way into clinical use. They include:

- Enkephalinase inhibitors, such as **thiorphan**, act by inhibiting the metabolic degradation of endogenous opioid peptides. They have been shown to produce analgesia, together with other morphine-like effects, without causing dependence.
- The various ion channels that play a role in nociceptive nerves (Fig. 40.6) may represent useful drug targets. They include the vanilloid receptor, for which antagonists have been identified, and certain sodium channel subtypes that are specific for these nerve terminals.
- Various neuropeptides, such as *somatostatin* (see Ch. 27) and *calcitonin* (see Ch. 28), produce powerful analgesia when applied intrathecally, and there are clinical reports suggesting that they may have similar effects when used systemically to treat endocrine disorders.
- Glutamate antagonists acting on NMDA- or AMPA-receptors show analgesic activity in animal models, but it has not yet been possible to obtain this effect in humans without unacceptable side-effects. Antagonists at the metabotropic glutamate receptor (mGluR5) are currently in development and have fewer side-effects.
- Adenosine analogues, and adenosine kinase inhibitors, could mimic or enhance the inhibitory effect of adenosine on nociceptive pathways.
- Agonists at nicotinic acetylcholine receptors may be analgesic, based on **epibatidine** (an alkaloid from frog skin, which is a potent nicotinic agonist, and—unexpectedly—a potent analgesic as well). Derivatives with fewer side-effects are under investigation.
- Agonists at cannabinoid receptors, including **tetrahydrocannabinol** (Ch. 42), have strong analgesic effects in animal models, supported by

anecdotal reports from dope-smokers. Cannabinoid receptors have an inhibitory effect on nociceptive afferent terminals and also on dorsal horn transmission. Formal trials are in progress to assess the clinical value of such compounds.

We should recall that analgesia was, for best part of a century, a therapeutic need addressed only by opioids and NSAIDs, and the only new drugs to be developed as analgesics in recent years have been look-alikes in these two families. As often happens, clinical observation rather than pharmacological inventiveness has expanded the range by discovering, for example, the efficacy of tricyclic antidepressants in pain treatment. The long list of new possibilites under investigation suggests that the tide of inventiveness may have resumed after a long gap, but it is too early to say whether it will lead to better therapies. Morphine is, as expected of 'God's own medicine', very hard to beat.

REFERENCES AND FURTHER READING

Besson J-M, Chaouch A 1987 Peripheral and spinal mechanisms of nociception. Physiol Rev 67: 67–186

Bevan S 1999 Nociceptive peripheral neurons: cellular properties. In: Wall P D, Melzack R (eds) Textbook of pain, 5th edn. Churchill Livingstone, Edinburgh, ch. 3 (*Describes receptors, ion channels and signalling mechanisms of nociceptive neurons*)

Burnstock G, Wood J N 1996 Purinergic receptors: their role in nociception and primary afferent neurotransmission. Curr Opin Neurobiol 6: 526–532 (*Review of a novel cloned ATP receptor, which is expressed selectively by nociceptive sensory neurons*)

Cesare P, McNaughton P 1997 Peripheral pain mechanisms. Curr Opin Neurobiol 7: 493–499 (*Review article discussing recent work on sensitisation of heat responses by other agents*)

Coderre T J, Katz J, Vaccarino A L, Melzack R 1993 Contribution of central neuroplasticity to pathological pain: review of clinical and experimental evidence. Pain 52: 259–285

Cooper J R, Bloom F E, Roth R H 1996 The biochemical basis of neuropharmacology. Oxford University Press, New York (*Excellent textbook, with good account of opioid peptides*)

Dhawan B N, Cesselin F, Raghubir R et al. 1996 Classification of opioid receptors. Pharmacol Rev 48: 567–592 (*The last word on opioid receptor classification from the International Union of Pharmacology subcommittee entrusted with the task*)

Dray A, Perkins M 1993 Bradykinin and inflammatory pain. Trends Neurosci 16: 99–104

Fields H L, Basbaum A I 1994 Central nervous system mechanisms of pain modulation. In: Wall P D, Melzack R (eds) Textbook of pain. Churchill Livingstone, Edinburgh

Henderson G, McKnight A T 1997 The orphan opioid receptor and its endogenous ligand—nociceptin/orphanin FQ. Trends Pharmacol Sci 18: 293–300 (*Review article summarising what we know about the newly discovered opioid peptide and its receptor*)

Herz A (ed) 1993 Handbook of experimental pharmacology, vol. 104: Opioids. Springer-Verlag, Berlin (*Definitive compendium of reviews on all aspects of opioid pharmacology*)

Holzer P 1988 Local effector functions of capsaicin-sensitive sensory nerve endings: involvement of tachykinins, calcitonin gene-related peptide and other neuropeptides. Neuroscience 24: 739–768 (*Review of neurogenic inflammation and other peripheral effector roles of peptidergic afferent neurons*)

Julius D, Basbaum A I 2001 Molecular mechanisms of nociception. Nature 413: 203–210 (*Review article focussing mainly on receptors and channels involved in activation of sensory nerves by noxious stimuli*)

Longmore J, Hill R G, Hargreaves R J 1997 Neurokinin-receptor antagonists: pharmacological tool and therapeutic drugs. Can J Physiol Pharmacol 75: 612–621 (*Review article on new tachykinin antagonists*)

Maggi C A, Pattachini R, Rovero P, Giachetti A 1993 Tachykinin receptors and tachykinin receptor antagonists. J Auton Pharmacol 13: 23–93 (*Comprehensive review*)

Maggio J E 1988 Tachykinins. Annu Rev Neurosci 11: 13–28 (*General review*)

Malcangio M, Bowery N 1996 GABA and its receptors in the spinal cord. Trends Pharmacol Sci 17: 457–462 (*Review article on role of GABA in the nociceptive pathway*)

Mantyh P et al. 1995 Receptor endocytosis and dendrite reshaping in spinal neurons after somatosensory stimulation. Science 268: 1629–1632 (*Elegant study with immunofluorescent receptor labelling revealing substance P-mediated receptor plasticity in dorsal horn neurons*)

McMahon S B 1996 NGF as a mediator of inflammatory pain. Philos Trans R Soc Lond 351: 431–440 (*Review of evidence implicating NGF as a mediator of inflammatory pain and hyperalgesia, including studies of a novel type of NGF inhibitor*)

McMahon S B, Lewin G R, Wall P D 1993 Central hyper-excitability triggered by noxious inputs. Curr Opin Neurobiol 3: 602–610 (*Review of mechanisms of dorsal horn plasticity*)

Nestler E J, Hyman S E, Malenka R C 2001 Molecular neuropharmacology. McGraw Hill, New York (*Good modern textbook*)

North R A 1993 Opioid actions on membrane ion channels. In: Herz A (ed) Handbook of experimental pharmacology, vol. 104: Opioids. Springer-Verlag, Berlin

Pasternak G W 1993 Pharmacological mechanisms of opioid analgesics. Clin Neuropharmacol 16: 1–18 (*Review of physiological mechanisms of opiate analgesia*)

Rainville P, Duncan G H, Price D D, Carrier B, Bushnell M C 1997 Pain affect encoded in human anterior cingulate but not somatosensory cortex. Science 277: 968–971 (*Imaging study showing cortical area involved in affective component of pain*)

Raja S N, Meyer R A, Ringkamp M, Campbell J N 1999 Chapter 1 In: Wall P D, Melzack R (eds) Textbook of pain, 4th edn. Churchill Livingstone, Edinburgh, ch. 1, pp. 11–57 (*Good general account of peripheral nociceptor functions*)

Rang H P, Bevan S J, Perkins M N 1998 Peripherally acting analgesic agents. In: Sawynok J, Cowan A (eds) Novel aspects of pain management: opioids and beyond. John Wiley, New York

Rang H P, Bevan S, Dray A 1994 Nociceptive peripheral neurons: cellular properties. In: Wall P D, Melzack R (eds) Textbook of pain. Churchill Livingstone, Edinburgh (*Review of chemosensitivity of primary afferent neurons*)

Sawynok J, Sweeney M I 1996 The role of purines in nociception. Neuroscience 32: 557–569 (*Review article drawing attention to role of adenosine as a modulator in nociceptive transmission*)

Sibinga N E S, Goldstein A 1988 Opioid peptides and opioid receptors in cells of the immune system. Annu Rev Immunol 16: 219–249 (*Summarises evidence implicating opioid peptides in control of immune system*)

Stein C, Yassouridis A 1997 Peripheral morphine analgesia. Pain 71: 119–121 (*Short polemic emphasising that opioid analgesia has a significant peripheral component*)

Walker J M, Bowen W D, Walker F O, Matsumoto R R, De Costa B, Rice K C 1990 Sigma receptors: biology and function. Pharmacol Rev 42: 355–402

Wall P D, Melzack R (eds) 1999 Textbook of pain, 4th edn. Churchill Livingstone, Edinburgh (*Large multiauthor reference book*)

Yaksh T L 1997 Pharmacology and mechanisms of opioid analgesic activity. Acta Anaesthesiol Scand 41: 94–111 (*Review of evidence relating to sites of action and receptor specificity of analgesic effect of opioids*)

Yaksh T L 1999 Spinal systems and pain processing: development of novel analgesic drugs with mechanistically defined models. Trends Pharmacol Sci 20: 329–337 (*Good general review article on spinal cord mechanisms—more general than its title suggests*)

CNS stimulants and psychotomimetic drugs

41

Overview 585

Convulsants and respiratory stimulants 585

Psychomotor stimulants 587
- Amphetamines and related drugs 587
- Cocaine 589
- Methylxanthines 590

Psychotomimetic drugs 591
- LSD, psilocybin and mescaline 591
- Phencyclidine 592

OVERVIEW

In this chapter, we describe drugs that have a predominantly stimulant effect on the central nervous system; these fall into three broad categories:

- **convulsants and respiratory stimulants**
- **psychomotor stimulants**
- **psychotomimetic drugs.**

Drugs in the first category have relatively little effect on mental function and appear to act mainly on the brainstem and spinal cord, producing exaggerated reflex excitability, an increase in activity of the respiratory and vasomotor centres and, with higher dosage, convulsions.

Drugs in the second category have a marked effect on mental function and behaviour, producing excitement and euphoria, reduced sensation of fatigue and an increase in motor activity.

Drugs in the third category mainly affect thought patterns and perception, distorting cognition in a complex way and producing effects that may superficially resemble psychotic illness.

Table 41.1 summarises the classification of the drugs that are discussed in this chapter. Several of these drugs have no clinical uses but are recognised as drugs of abuse on the strength of their tendency to produce dependence. This aspect is discussed in Chapter 42.

CONVULSANTS AND RESPIRATORY STIMULANTS

Convulsants and respiratory stimulants (sometimes called *analeptics*) are a chemically diverse group of substances with mechanisms of action that are, with some exceptions, not well understood. Such drugs were once used to treat patients in terminal coma or with severe respiratory failure. Although temporary restoration of function could sometimes be achieved, mortality was not reduced, and the treatment carried a considerable risk of causing convulsions, which left the patient more deeply comatose than before. They were used mainly to give the impression that something was being done for a patient in extremis. There remains a very limited clinical use for respiratory stimulants in treating acute ventilatory failure (see Ch. 22), **amiphenazole** and **doxapram** (Table 41.1) being most commonly used since these drugs carry less risk of causing convulsions than earlier compounds.

Also included in this group are various compounds, such as **strychnine**, **picrotoxin** and **pentylenetetrazol**, which are of interest as experimental tools, but have no clinical uses.

Strychnine is an alkaloid found in the seeds of an Indian tree; it has been used for centuries as a poison (mainly vermin, but also human; it is much favoured in detective stories of a certain genre). It is a powerful convulsant and acts throughout the central nervous system (CNS) but particularly on the spinal cord, causing violent extensor spasms that are triggered by minor sensory stimuli, the head being thrown back and the face fixed, we are told, in a hideous grin. These effects result from blocking receptors for glycine, which is the main inhibitory transmitter acting on motoneurons. The action of strychnine superficially resembles that of **tetanus toxin**, a protein neurotoxin produced by the anaerobic bacterium *Clostridium tetani*, which blocks the release of glycine from inhibitory interneurons. This is very similar to the action of botulinum toxin (see Ch. 10), which is produced by another bacterium of the *Clostridium* genus and causes paralysis by blocking acetylcholine release. In small doses, strychnine causes a measurable improvement in visual and auditory acuity; it was until quite recently included in various

Table 41.1 Central nervous system stimulants and psychotomimetic drugs

Category	Examples	Mode of action	Clinical significance
Convulsants and respiratory stimulants (analeptics)			
Respiratory stimulants	Amiphenazole	Not known	Occasionally used as respiratory stimulant
	Doxapram	Not known	Short-acting respiratory stimulant sometimes given by intravenous infusion to treat acute respiratory failure
Miscellaneous convulsants	Strychnine	Antagonist of glycine Main action is to increase reflex excitability of spinal cord	No clinical uses
	Bicuculline	Competitive antagonist of GABA	No clinical uses
	Picrotoxin	Non-competitive antagonist of GABA	Clinical use as respiratory stimulant; now obsolete; risk of convulsions
	Nikethamide	Not known	As picrotoxin
	Pentylenetetrazol	Not known	No clinical use. Convulsant activity in experimental animals provides a useful model for testing antiepileptic drugs (see Ch. 39)
Psychomotor stimulants			
	Amphetamine and related compounds, e.g. dexamphetamine, methylamphetamine, methylphenidate, fenfluramine, MDMA	Release of catecholamines Inhibition of catecholamine uptake	Methylphenidate and dexamphetamine used to treat ADHD in children; otherwise very limited clinical use Some agents used occasionally as appetite suppressants Risk of dependence, sympathomimetic side-effects and pulmonary hypertension Mainly important as drugs of abuse
	Cocaine	Inhibition of catecholamine uptake Local anaesthetic	Important as drug of abuse Risk of fetal damage Occasionally used for nasopharyngeal and ophthalmic anesthesia (see Ch. 43)
	Methylxanthines, e.g. caffeine, theophylline	Inhibition of phosphodiesterase Antagonism of adenosine A_2 receptors (relevance of these actions to central effects is not clear)	Clinical uses unrelated to stimulant activity, though caffeine is included in various 'tonics' Theophylline used for action on cardiac and bronchial muscle Constituents of beverages
Psychotomimetic drugs (hallucinogens)	Lysergic acid diethylamide (LSD)	Mixed agonist/antagonist at 5-HT receptors (see Ch. 12)	No clinical use Important as drug of abuse
	Mescaline	Not known. Chemically similar to amphetamine	
	Psilocybin	Chemically related to 5-HT, probably acts on 5-HT receptors	
	Tetrahydrocannabinol (THC)	Acts as CNS depressant with mild psychotomimetic effects	No established clinical use[a] See Chapter 42
	Phencyclidine	Chemically similar to ketamine (see Ch. 35) Acts on σ-receptors (Ch. 40). Also blocks NMDA receptor-operated ion channels (see Ch. 32)	Originally proposed as an anaesthetic, now important as drug of abuse and as a model for schizophrenia

[a]**Nabilone,** a synthetic cannabinoid, is sometimes used as an antiemetic to reduce nausea during cancer chemotherapy.
MDMA, methylenedioxymethamphetamine; ADHD, attention deficit hyperactivity disorder; GABA, gamma-aminobutyric acid; NMDA, *N*-methyl-D-aspartate; 5-HT, 5-hydroxytryptamine.

'tonics', on the basis that CNS stimulation should restore both the weary brain and the debilitated body.

Bicuculline, also a plant alkaloid, resembles strychnine in its effects but acts by blocking receptors for gamma-aminobutyric acid (GABA) rather than glycine. Its action is confined to $GABA_A$-receptors, which control Cl^- permeability, and it does not affect $GABA_B$-receptors (see Ch. 32). Its main effects are on the brain rather than the spinal cord, and it is a useful experimental tool for studying GABA-mediated transmission; it has no clinical uses.

Picrotoxin (obtained from the fishberry) also blocks the action of GABA on chloride channels, though not competitively. The plant's name reflects the native practice of incapacitating fish by throwing berries into the water. Picrotoxin, like bicuculline, causes convulsions and has no clinical uses.

Pentylenetetrazol (PTZ) acts similarly, though its mode of action is unknown. Inhibition of PTZ-induced convulsions by antiepileptic drugs (see Ch. 39) correlates quite well with their effectiveness against absence seizures, and PTZ has occasionally been used diagnostically in humans, since it can precipitate the typical electroencephalograph (EEG) pattern of absence seizures in susceptible patients.

Amiphenazole and **doxapram** are similar to the above drugs but have a bigger margin of safety between respiratory stimulation and convulsions. Doxapram also causes nausea, coughing and restlessness, which limit its usefulness. It is rapidly eliminated, and it is occasionally used as an intravenous infusion in patients with acute respiratory failure.

Convulsants and respiratory stimulants

- This is a diverse group of drugs that have little clinical use, though several are useful as experimental tools.
- Certain short-acting respiratory stimulants (e.g. doxapram, amiphenazole) can be used in acute respiratory failure.
- Strychnine is a convulsant poison that acts mainly on the spinal cord, by blocking receptors for the inhibitory transmitter glycine.
- Picrotoxin and bicuculline act as $GABA_A$-antagonists; bicuculline blocks the $GABA_A$-receptor site, whereas picrotoxin appears to block the ion channel.
- Pentylenetetrazol (PTZ) works by an unknown mechanism. PTZ-induced convulsions provide an animal model for testing antiepileptic drugs, giving good correlation with effectiveness in preventing absence seizures.

PSYCHOMOTOR STIMULANTS

AMPHETAMINES AND RELATED DRUGS

Amphetamine, and its active dextro-isomer **dextroamphetamine**, together with **methamphetamine** and **methylphenidate**, form a group of drugs with very similar pharmacological properties (see Fig. 41.1), which includes 'street drugs' such as **methylenedioxymethamphetamine** (MDMA or 'ecstasy'; see below). **Fenfluramine**, though chemically similar, has slightly different pharmacological effects. All of these drugs act by releasing monoamines from nerve terminals in the brain. Noradrenaline and dopamine are the most important mediators in this connection, but 5-hydroxytryptamine (5-HT) release also occurs, particularly with fenfluramine.

Pharmacological effects

The main central effects of amphetamine-like drugs are:

- locomotor stimulation
- euphoria and excitement
- stereotyped behaviour
- anorexia.

In addition, amphetamines have peripheral sympathomimetic actions, producing a rise in blood pressure and inhibition of gastrointestinal motility.

In experimental animals, amphetamines on the one hand cause increased alertness, locomotor activity and grooming; they also increase aggressive activity. On the other, systematic exploration of novel objects by unrestrained rats is reduced by amphetamine. The animals run around more but appear less attentive to their surroundings. Studies of conditioned responses suggest that amphetamines increase the overall rate of responding without affecting the training process markedly. For example, in a fixed

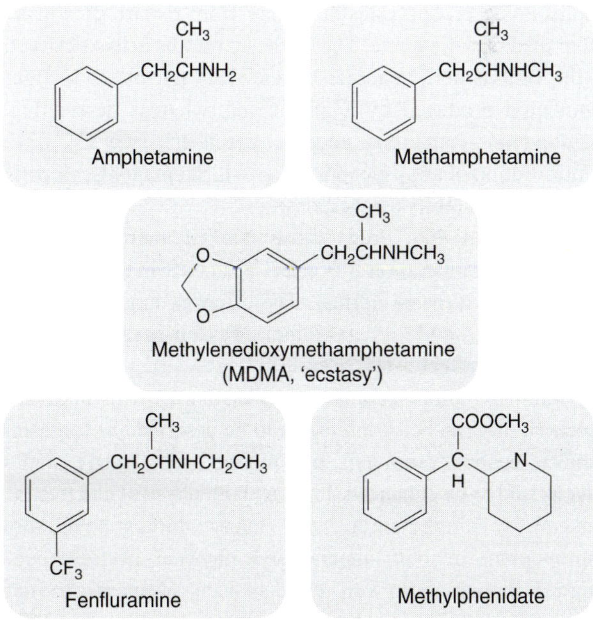

Fig. 41.1 Structures of amphetamine-like drugs.

interval schedule where a reward for lever-pressing is forthcoming only after a fixed interval (say 10 minutes) following the last reward, trained animals normally press the lever very infrequently in the first few minutes after the reward, and increase the rate towards the end of the 10-minute interval when another reward is due. The effect of amphetamine is to increase the rate of unrewarded responses at the beginning of the 10-minute interval without affecting (or even reducing) the rate towards the end of the period. The effects of amphetamine on more sophisticated types of conditioned response, for example those involving discriminative tasks, are not clear cut, and there is no clear evidence that either the rate of learning of such tasks or the final level of performance that can be achieved is affected by the drug. Put crudely, amphetamine makes the animals busier rather than brighter.

With large doses of amphetamines, stereotyped behaviour occurs. This consists of repeated actions, such as licking, gnawing, rearing or repeated movements of the head and limbs. These activities are generally inappropriate to the environment, and with increasing doses of amphetamine they take over more and more of the behaviour of the animal. These behavioural effects are evidently produced by the release of catecholamines in the brain, since pretreatment with 6-hydroxydopamine, which depletes the brain of both noradrenaline and dopamine, abolishes the effect of amphetamine, as does pretreatment with α-methyltyrosine, an inhibitor of catecholamine biosynthesis (see Ch. 11). Similarly, tricyclic antidepressants and monoamine oxidase inhibitors (see Ch. 38) potentiate the effects of amphetamine, presumably by blocking amine reuptake or metabolism. Interestingly, reserpine, which inhibits vesicular storage of catecholamines (see Ch. 11), does not block the behavioural effects of amphetamine. This is probably because amphetamine releases cytosolic rather than vesicular catecholamines (see Ch. 11). The behavioural effects of amphetamine probably result mainly from release of dopamine rather than noradrenaline. The evidence for this is that destruction of the central noradrenergic bundle does not affect locomotor stimulation produced by amphetamine, whereas destruction of the dopamine-containing nucleus accumbens (see Ch. 33), or administration of antipsychotic drugs which antagonise dopamine (see Ch. 37), inhibits this response.

Amphetamine-like drugs cause marked anorexia, but with continued administration this effect wears off in a few days and food intake returns to normal. The effect is most marked with **fenfluramine** and its D-isomer **dexfenfluramine**, which preferentially affect 5-HT release.

In humans, amphetamine causes euphoria; with intravenous injection, this can be so intense as to be described as 'orgasmic'. Subjects become confident, hyperactive and talkative, and sex drive is said to be enhanced. Fatigue, both physical and mental, is reduced by amphetamine, and many studies have shown improvement of both mental and physical performance in fatigued, though not in well-rested subjects. Mental performance is improved for simple tedious tasks much more than for difficult tasks, and amphetamines have been used to improve the performance of soldiers, military pilots and others who need to remain alert under extremely fatiguing conditions. It has also been in vogue as a means of helping students to concentrate before and during examinations, but the improvement caused by reduction of fatigue can be offset by the mistakes of overconfidence.* Amphetamine-like drugs bring about a small but significant improvement of athletic performance, particularly in endurance events. They are banned in sporting events and easily detected in urine.

Tolerance and dependence

If amphetamine is taken repeatedly over the course of a few days, which occurs when users seek to maintain the euphoric 'high' that a single dose produces, a state of 'amphetamine psychosis' can develop, which closely resembles an acute schizophrenic attack (see Ch. 37), with hallucinations, accompanied by paranoid symptoms and aggressive behaviour. At the same time, repetitive stereotyped behaviour may develop (e.g. polishing shoes or stringing beads). The close similarity of this condition to schizophrenia, and the effectiveness of antipsychotic drugs in controlling it, is consistent with the dopamine theory of schizophrenia discussed in Chapter 37. When the drug is stopped after a few days, there is usually a period of deep sleep, and on awakening, the subject feels lethargic, depressed, anxious (sometimes even suicidal) and hungry. Even a single dose of amphetamine, insufficient to cause psychotic symptoms, usually leaves the subject later feeling tired and depressed. These after-effects may be the result of depletion of the normal stores of noradrenaline and dopamine, but the evidence for this is not clear cut. A state of amphetamine dependence can be produced in experimental animals—thus, rats quickly learn to press a lever in order to obtain a dose of amphetamine, and they also become inactive and irritable in the withdrawal phase. These effects do not occur with fenfluramine.

Tolerance develops rapidly to the peripheral sympathomimetic and anorexic effects of amphetamine, but more slowly to the other effects (locomotor stimulation euphoria and stereotyped behaviour). Dependence on amphetamine appears to be a consequence of the unpleasant after-effect that it produces, and the insistent memory of euphoria, which leads to a desire for a repeat dose. There is no clear-cut physical withdrawal syndrome such as occurs with opiates. It is estimated that only about 5% of users progress to full-blown dependence, the usual pattern being that the dose is increased as tolerance develops, and then uncontrolled 'binges' occur in which the user takes the drug repeatedly over a period of a day or more, remaining continuously intoxicated. Large doses may be consumed in such binges, with a high risk of acute toxicity, and the demand for the drug displaces all other considerations.

Experimental animals, given unlimited access to amphetamine, take it in such large amounts that they die from the cardiovascular

*Pay heed to the awful warning of the medical student who, it is said, having taken copious amounts of dextroamphetamine, left the examination hall in confident mood, having spent 3 hours writing his name over and over again.

effects within a few days. Given limited amounts, they too develop a 'binge' pattern of dependence.

Pharmacokinetic aspects

Amphetamine is readily absorbed from the gastrointestinal tract, and freely penetrates the blood–brain barrier. It does this more readily than other indirectly acting sympathomimetic amines, such as ephedrine or tyramine (Ch. 11), which probably explains why it produces more marked central effects than those drugs. It is also readily absorbed from the nasal mucosa, and is often taken by 'snorting'. Amphetamine is mainly excreted unchanged in the urine, and the rate of excretion is increased when the urine is made more acidic (see Ch. 8). The plasma half-life of amphetamine varies from about 5 hours to 20–30 hours, depending on urine flow and urinary pH.

Clinical use and unwanted effects

The main use of amphetamines is in the treatment of *attention deficit/hyperactivity disorder (ADHD)*, particularly in children, **methylphenidate** being the drug most commonly used (although dexamphetamine can also be used), at doses lower than those causing euphoria and other side-effects. ADHD is a common condition in children, whose incessant overactivity and very limited attention span disrupt their education and social development. The efficacy of amphetamines has been confirmed in many controlled trials. Disorders of dopamine pathways are suspected to underly ADHD symptomatology, but the mechanism of action of amphetamines is unclear.

Narcolepsy is a disabling condition, probably a form of epilepsy, in which the patient suddenly and unpredictably falls asleep at frequent intervals during the day. Amphetamine is helpful but not completely effective.

As appetite suppressants in humans, for use in treating obesity, amphetamine derivatives proved relatively ineffective and have been largely abandoned because of their tendency to cause pulmonary hypertension, which can be so severe as to necessitate heart–lung transplantation.

The limited clinical usefulness of amphetamine is offset by its many unwanted effects, including hypertension, insomnia, tremors, risk of exacerbating schizophrenia and risk of dependence.

Sudden deaths have occurred in 'ecstasy' users, even after a single, moderate dose. The drug can induce a condition resembling 'heat-stroke' and associated with muscle damage and renal failure. It also causes inappropriate secretion of antidiuretic hormone, leading to thirst, overhydration and hyponatraemia ('water intoxication').

COCAINE

Cocaine (see reviews by Gawin & Ellinwood, 1988; Johanson & Fischman, 1989) is found in the leaves of a South American shrub, coca. These leaves are used for their stimulant properties by natives of South America, particularly those living at high altitude, who use it to reduce fatigue during work at these altitudes. Considerable mystical significance was attached to the powers of cocaine to boost the flagging human spirit, and Freud tested it extensively on his patients and his family. As a result of Freud's experiments with cocaine, his ophthalmologist colleague, Köller, obtained supplies of the drug and discovered its local anaesthetic action (Ch. 43), but the psychostimulant effects of cocaine have not proved to be clinically useful. However, they led to it becoming at one time the most frequently abused substance in Western countries, though its use has decreased somewhat since 1990. The mechanisms and treatment of cocaine abuse are discussed in Chapter 42.

Pharmacological effects

Cocaine inhibits catecholamine uptake by the noradrenaline and dopamine transporters (see Ch. 11), thereby enhancing the peripheral effects of sympathetic nerve activity and producing a marked psychomotor stimulant effect. The latter produces euphoria, garrulousness, increased motor activity and a magnification of pleasure, similar to the effects of amphetamine. Its effects resemble those of amphetamines, though it has less tendency to produce stereotyped behaviour, delusions, hallucinations and paranoia. With excessive dosage, tremors and convulsions, followed by respiratory and vasomotor depression, may occur. The peripheral sympathomimetic actions lead to tachycardia, vasoconstriction and an increase in blood pressure. Body temperature may increase, owing to the increased motor activity coupled with reduced heat loss. Like amphetamine, cocaine produces no clear-cut physical dependence syndrome but tends to cause depression and dysphoria, coupled with craving for the drug (see Ch. 42), following the initial stimulant effect. Withdrawal of cocaine after administration for a few days causes a marked deterioration of motor performance and learned behaviour, which are restored by resuming dosage with the drug. There is, therefore, a considerable degree of psychological dependence. The pattern of dependence, evolving from occasional use through escalating dosage to compulsive binges, is identical to that seen with amphetamines.

The duration of action of cocaine (about 30 minutes when given intravenously) is much shorter than that of amphetamine.

Pharmacokinetic aspects

Cocaine is readily absorbed by many routes. For many years, illicit supplies consisted of the hydrochloride salt, which could be given by nasal inhalation or intravenously. The latter route produces an intense and immediate euphoria, whereas nasal inhalation produces a less dramatic sensation—and also tends to cause atrophy and necrosis of the nasal mucosa and septum. Cocaine use increased dramatically when the free base form ('crack') became available as a street drug. Unlike the salt, this can be smoked, giving an effect as rapid as that of intravenous administration, with less inconvenience and social stigma. The social, economic and even political consequences of this small change in formulation have been far-reaching.

A cocaine metabolite is deposited in hair, and analysis of its content along the hair shaft allows the pattern of cocaine consumption to be monitored, a technique which has revealed a much higher incidence of cocaine use than was voluntarily reported. Cocaine exposure in utero can be estimated from analysis of the hair of neonates.

Cocaine is still occasionally used topically as a local anaesthetic, mainly in ophthalmology and minor nose and throat surgery, but it has no other clinical uses. It is a valuable pharmacological tool for the study of catecholamine release and reuptake, because of its relatively specific action in blocking uptake 1.

Adverse effects

Toxic effects occur commonly in cocaine abusers. The main acute dangers are cardiac dysrhythmias and coronary or cerebral thrombosis. Slowly developing damage to the myocardium can also occur, leading to heart failure, even in the absence of acute cardiac effects.

Cocaine can severely impair brain development in utero (see Volpe, 1992). The brain size is significantly reduced in babies exposed to cocaine in pregnancy, and the incidence of neurological and limb malformations is also increased. The incidence of ischaemic and haemorrhagic brain lesions, and of sudden infant death, is also higher in cocaine-exposed babies. Interpretation of the data is difficult because many cocaine-abusers also take other illicit drugs that may affect fetal development, but the probability is that cocaine is highly detrimental.

The main adverse effect of amphetamines and cocaine is dependence, with its potentially severe effect on quality of life (Ch. 42).

Effects of amphetamines and cocaine

Amphetamines

- The main effects are:
  - —increased motor activity
  - —euphoria and excitement
  - —anorexia
  - —with prolonged administration, stereotyped and psychotic behaviour.
- Effects result mainly from release of catecholamines, especially noradrenaline and dopamine.
- Stimulant effect lasts for a few hours and is followed by depression and anxiety.
- Tolerance to the stimulant effects develops rapidly, though peripheral sympathomimetic effects may persist.
- Amphetamines may be useful in treating narcolepsy and also (paradoxically) to control hyperkinetic children. They are no longer used as appetite suppressants owing to the risk of pulmonary hypertension..
- Amphetamine psychosis, which closely resembles schizophrenia, can develop after prolonged use.
- Their main importance is in drug abuse.

Cocaine

- Cocaine acts by inhibiting catecholamine uptake (especially dopamine) by nerve terminals.
- Behavioural effects of cocaine are very similar to those of amphetamines, though psychotomimetic effects are rarer. Duration of action is shorter.
- Cocaine used in pregnancy impairs fetal development and may produce fetal malformations.
- As drugs of abuse, amphetamines and cocaine produce strong psychological dependence and carry a high risk of severe adverse reactions.

METHYLXANTHINES

Various beverages, particularly tea, coffee and cocoa, contain methylxanthines to which they owe their mild central stimulant effects. The main compounds responsible are *caffeine* and *theophylline*. The nuts of the cola plant also contain caffeine, which is present in cola-flavoured soft drinks. However, the most important sources, by far, are coffee and tea, which account for more than 90% of caffeine consumption. A cup of instant coffee or strong tea contains 50–70 mg caffeine, while filter coffee contains about twice as much. Among adults in tea- and coffee-drinking countries, the average daily caffeine consumption is about 200 mg. Further information on the pharmacology and toxicology of caffeine is presented by Nehlig et al. (1992) and Fredholm et al. (1999).

Pharmacological effects

Methylxanthines have the following major pharmacological actions:

- CNS stimulation
- diuresis (see Ch. 23)
- stimulation of cardiac muscle (see Ch. 17)
- relaxation of smooth muscle, especially bronchial muscle (see Ch. 22).

The latter two effects resemble those of β-adrenoceptor stimulation (see Ch. 11). This is thought to be because methylxanthines (especially **theophylline**) inhibit phosphodiesterase, which is responsible for the intracellular metabolism of cAMP (Ch. 3). They thus increase intracellular cAMP and produce effects that mimic those of mediators that stimulate adenylate cyclase. Methylxanthines also antagonise many of the effects of adenosine, acting on both A_1- and A_2-receptors (see Ch. 12). Transgenic mice lacking functional A_2-receptors are abnormally active and aggressive, and they fail to show increased motor activity in response to caffeine (Ledent et al., 1997), suggesting that antagonism at A_2-receptors accounts for part, at least, of its CNS stimulant action. The concentration of caffeine reached in plasma and brain after two or three cups of strong coffee—about 100 μmol/l—is sufficient to produce appreciable adenosine receptor block, and a small degree of phosphodiesterase inhibition. The diuretic effect probably results from vasodilatation of the afferent glomerular arteriole, causing an increased glomerular filtration rate.

Methylxanthines

- Caffeine and theophylline produce psychomotor stimulant effects.
- Average caffeine consumption from beverages is about 200 mg/day.
- Main psychological effect is reduced fatigue and improved mental performance, without euphoria. Even large doses do not cause stereotyped behaviour or psychotomimetic effects.
- Methylxanthines act mainly by antagonism at purine A_2-receptors, and partly by inhibiting phosphodiesterase, thus producing effects similar to those of β-adrenoceptor agonists.
- Peripheral actions are exerted mainly on heart, smooth muscle and kidney.
- Theophylline is used clinically as a bronchodilator; caffeine is not used clinically.

Caffeine and theophylline have very similar stimulant effects on the CNS. Human subjects experience a reduction of fatigue, leading to insomnia, with improved concentration and a clearer flow of thought. This is confirmed by objective studies which have shown that caffeine reduces reaction time and produces an increase in the speed at which simple calculations can be performed (though without much improvement in accuracy). Performance at motor tasks, such as typing and simulated driving, is also improved, particularly in fatigued subjects. Mental tasks, such as syllable-learning, association tests and so on, are also facilitated by moderate doses (up to about 200 mg caffeine, or about three cups of coffee) but inhibited by larger doses. By comparison with amphetamines, methylxanthines produce less locomotor stimulation and do not induce euphoria, stereotyped behaviour patterns or a psychotic state, but their effects on fatigue and mental function are similar.

Tolerance and habituation develop to a small extent, but much less than with amphetamines, and withdrawal effects are slight. Caffeine does not lead to self-administration in animals, and it cannot be classified as a dependence-producing drug.

Clinical use and unwanted effects

There are few clinical uses for caffeine. It is included with aspirin in some preparations for treating headaches and other aches and pains, and with ergotamine in some antimigraine preparations, the object being to produce a mildly agreeable sense of alertness. Theophylline is used mainly as a bronchodilator in treating severe asthmatic attacks (see Ch. 22). Caffeine has few unwanted side-effects and is safe even in very large doses. In vitro tests show that it has mutagenic activity, and large doses are teratogenic in animals. However, epidemiological studies have shown no evidence of carcinogenic or teratogenic effects of tea or coffee drinking in humans.

PSYCHOTOMIMETIC DRUGS

Psychotomimetic drugs (also referred to as *psychedelic* or *hallucinogenic* drugs) affect thought, perception and mood, without causing marked psychomotor stimulation or depression. Thoughts and perceptions tend to become distorted and dream-like, rather than being merely sharpened or dulled, and the change in mood is likewise more complex than a simple shift in the direction of euphoria or depression. Not surprisingly, the categorisation of these drugs is very imprecise, and there is no sharp dividing line between the effects of, say, cocaine and those of lysergic acid diethylamide (LSD) or cannabis. Psychotomimetic drugs fall broadly into two groups:

- those with a chemical resemblance to known neurotransmitters (catecholamines or 5-HT): these include LSD and psilocybin, which are related to 5-HT; mescaline and MDMA ('ecstasy'; see above), which are related to amphetamine
- drugs unrelated to monoamine neurotransmitters, e.g. phencyclidine.

LSD, PSILOCYBIN AND MESCALINE

LSD is an exceptionally potent psychotomimetic drug, capable of producing strong effects in humans in doses less than 1 μg/kg. It is a chemical derivative of lysergic acid, which occurs in the cereal fungus ergot (see Ch. 12). It was first synthesised by Hoffman in 1943. Hoffman deliberately swallowed about 250 μg LSD and wrote 30 years later of the experience: 'the faces of those around me appeared as grotesque coloured masks...marked motoric unrest, alternating with paralysis...heavy feeling in the head, limbs and entire body, as if they were filled with lead...clear recognition of my condition, in which state I sometimes observed, in the manner of an independent observer, that I shouted half insanely'. These effects lasted for a few hours, after which Hoffman fell asleep, 'and awoke next morning feeling perfectly well'. Apart from these dramatic psychological effects, LSD has few physiological effects. **Mescaline**, which is derived from a Mexican cactus and has been known as a hallucinogenic agent for many centuries, was made famous by Aldous Huxley in 'The doors of perception'. **Psilocybin** is obtained from a fungus and has very similar properties. Both have basically similar effects to LSD but are much less potent.

Pharmacological effects

The main effects of these drugs are on mental function, most notably an alteration of perception in such a way that sights and sounds appear distorted and fantastic. Hallucinations visual, auditory, tactile or olfactory also occur, and sensory modalities may become confused, so that sounds are perceived as visions. Thought processes tend to become illogical and disconnected, but subjects generally retain insight into the fact that their disturbance is drug induced and generally find the experience exhilarating. Occasionally, LSD produces a syndrome that is extremely disturbing to the subject (the 'bad trip') in which the hallucinatory experience takes on a menacing quality and may be accompanied by paranoid delusions. This sometimes goes so far as to produce homicide or suicide attempts, and in many respects, the state has features in common with acute schizophrenic illness. Furthermore, 'flashbacks' of the hallucinatory experience have been reported weeks or months later.

LSD acts on various 5-HT receptor subtypes (see Ch. 12), and in the CNS it is believed to work mainly as a 5-HT_2-receptor agonist (see Cooper et al., 1996). It inhibits the firing of 5-HT-containing neurons in the raphe nuclei (see Ch. 33), apparently by acting as an agonist on the inhibitory autoreceptors of these cells. The action of mescaline is apparently different, however, and exerted mainly on noradrenergic neurons. It is still quite unclear how changes in cell firing rates might be related to the psychotomimetic action of these drugs.

The main effects of psychotomimetic drugs are subjective, so it is not surprising that animal tests which reliably predict psychotomimetic activity in humans have not been devised. Attempts to measure changes in perception by behavioural conditioning studies have given variable results, but some authors have claimed that effects consistent with increased sensory 'generalisation' (i.e. a tendency to respond similarly to any sensory stimulus) can be detected in this way. One of the more bizarre tests involves spiders, whose normal elegantly symmetrical webs become jumbled and erratic if the animals are treated with LSD.

Dependence and adverse effects

Neither LSD nor other psychotomimetic agents (except for phencyclidine; see below) are self-administered by experimental animals. Indeed, in contrast to most of the drugs that are widely abused by humans, they have aversive rather than reinforcing properties in behavioural tests. Tolerance to the effects of LSD develops quite quickly, and there is cross-tolerance between it and most other psychotomimetics.

There is no physical withdrawal syndrome in animals or humans.

There has been much concern over reports that LSD and other psychotomimetic drugs, as well as causing potentially dangerous 'bad trips', can lead to more persistent mental disorder (see Abraham & Aldridge 1993). There are recorded instances in which altered perception and hallucinations have lasted for up to 3 weeks following a single dose of LSD, and of precipitation of attacks in schizophrenic patients. Furthermore, it is believed that LSD can occasionally initiate long-lasting schizophrenia. This, coupled with the fact that the occasional 'bad trip' can result in severe injury through violent behaviour, means that LSD and other psychotomimetics must be regarded as highly dangerous drugs, far removed from the image of peaceful 'experience enhancers' that the hippy subculture* of the 1960s so enthusiastically espoused.

*You may recall the Beatles' lyric 'Lucy in the Sky with Diamonds', also the phrase 'Drop out; tune in; turn on' coined by Timothy Leary, whose ashes were sent into orbit in 1997.

PHENCYCLIDINE

Phencyclidine was originally intended as an intravenous anaesthetic agent but was found to produce in many patients a period of disorientation and hallucinations following recovery of consciousness. **Ketamine** (see Ch. 35), a close analogue of phencyclidine, is better as an anaesthetic, though it too can cause symptoms of disorientation. Phencyclidine is now of interest mainly as a drug of abuse (now declining in popularity).

Pharmacological effects

The effects of phencyclidine resemble those of other psychotomimetic drugs (see Johnson & Jones, 1990) but also include analgesia, which was one of the reasons for its introduction as an anaesthetic agent. It can also cause stereotyped motor behaviour, like amphetamine. It has the same reported tendency as LSD to cause occasional 'bad trips' and to lead to recurrent psychotic episodes. Its mode of action at a cellular level is not well understood. Specific high-affinity binding sites occur on neuronal membranes, particularly in the frontal cortex and hippocampus, and it appears to have two distinct sites of action. One site is the σ-receptor recognised by various opioids of the

Psychotomimetic drugs

- The main types are:
  - —LSD, psilocybin and mescaline (actions related to 5-HT and catecholamines)
  - —phencyclidine.
- Their main effect is to cause sensory distortion of a fantastic and halluciantory nature.
- LSD is exceptionally potent, producing a long-lasting sense of dissociation and disordered thought, sometimes with frightening hallucinations and delusions, which can lead to violence. Hallucinatory episodes can recur after a long interval.
- LSD and phencyclidine precipitate schizophrenic attacks in susceptible patients, and LSD may cause long-lasting psychopathological changes.
- LSD appears to act as an agonist at 5-HT_2-receptors, and suppresses electrical activity in 5-HT raphe neurons, an action that appears to correlate with psychotomimetic activity.
- They do not cause physical dependence and tend to be aversive, rather than reinforcing, in animal models.
- The mechanism of action of phencyclidine is complex; it binds to the σ-receptor and also blocks the glutamate-activated NMDA-receptor channel, as well as interacting with other neurotransmitter systems.

benzomorphan type (Ch. 40), while the other is the glutamate-operated ion channel (the NMDA (*N*-methyl-D-aspartate) receptor channel; see Ch. 32), which is blocked by phencyclidine as well as by ketamine. The σ-receptor is generally believed to mediate the effects of dysphoria and hallucinations produced by certain opiates, and this may account for the psychotomimetic effects of phencyclidine. At present it is unclear whether the NMDA-receptor channel action is important. However, studies with **dizocilpine**, an NMDA channel blocker (see Ch. 32) that lacks affinity for the σ-receptor, suggest that it has much less psychotomimetic activity than phencyclidine, though other behavioural effects are similar. Which, if either, of the two phencyclidine-binding sites is the key to its behavioural effects remains undecided. One prominent question, however, is whether there may be an endogenous ligand for either of the phencyclidine-binding sites, and, if so, whether such substances might be involved in the causation of schizophrenia (see Debonnel, 1993).

REFERENCES AND FURTHER READING

Abraham H D, Aldridge A M 1993 Adverse consequences of lysergic acid diethylamide. Addiction 88: 1327–1334

Cooper J R, Bloom F E, Roth R H 1996 The biochemical basis of neuropharmacology. Oxford University Press, New York (*Good coverage on mode of action of LSD and amphetamines*)

Debonnel G 1993 Current hypotheses on sigma receptors and their physiological role: possible implications in psychiatry. J Psychiatr Neurosci 18: 157–172

Fredholm B B, Battig K, Holmes J, Nehlig A, Zwartau E E 1999 Actions of caffeine in the brain with special reference to factors that contribute to its widespread use. Pharmacol Rev 51: 83–133 (*Comprehensive review article, covering pharmacological, behavioural and social aspects*)

Gawin F H, Ellinwood E H 1988 Cocaine and other stimulants. N Engl J Med 318: 1173–1182

Johanson C-E, Fischman M W 1989 The pharmacology of cocaine related to its abuse. Pharmacol Rev 41: 3–47

Johnson K M, Jones S M 1990 Neuropharmacology of phencyclidine: basic mechanisms and therapeutic potential. Annu Rev Pharmacol Toxicol 30: 707–750

Ledent C et al. 1997 Aggressiveness, hypoalgesia and high blood pressure in mice lacking the adenosine A_{2a} receptor. Nature 388: 674–678 (*Study of transgenic mice showing loss of stimulant effects of caffeine in mice lacking A_2-receptors*)

Nehlig A, Daval J-L, Debry G 1992 Caffeine and the central nervous system: mechanisms of action, biochemical, metabolic and psychostimulant effects. Brain Res Rev 17: 139–170

Volpe J J 1992 Effect of cocaine on the fetus. N Engl J Med 327: 399–407

42 Drug dependence and drug abuse

Overview 594

Introduction 594

The nature of drug dependence 595
- Reward pathways 596
- Habituation mechanisms 596
- Genetic factors 597
- Pharmacological approaches to treating drug dependence 598

Nicotine and tobacco 598
- Pharmacological effects of smoking 599
- Pharmacokinetic aspects 599
- Tolerance and dependence 600
- Harmful effects of smoking 601

Ethanol 603
- Pharmacological effects of ethanol 603
- Pharmacokinetic aspects 605
- Tolerance and dependence 607

Cannabis 608
- Chemical aspects 608
- Pharmacological effects 609
- Receptors and endogenous ligands 609
- Tolerance and dependence 609
- Pharmacokinetic aspects 609
- Adverse effects 610
- Clinical use of cannabis—a controversial topic 610

OVERVIEW

Drug dependence describes the situation in which drug taking assumes a compulsive quality. All drugs that engender dependence have major central nervous system effects. In this chapter we discuss some general aspects of drug dependence and drug abuse and describe the pharmacology of three important drugs, which have no place in therapy but are consumed in large amounts, namely nicotine, ethanol and cannabis. Other important drugs of abuse, such as opiates, amphetamines and cocaine, are described in other chapters.

INTRODUCTION

There are many drugs that human beings consume because they choose to, and not because they are advised to by doctors. Society in general disapproves, because in most cases there is a social cost; for certain drugs, this is judged to outweigh the individual benefit, and their use is banned in many countries. In Western societies, the three most commonly used non-therapeutic drugs are caffeine, nicotine and ethanol, all of which are legally and freely available. Many more drugs are taken in large quantities, though their manufacture, sale and consumption has been declared illegal in most Western countries, except when it is under the direction of the medical profession. A list of the more important ones is given in Table 42.1. This list does not include drugs that are used illicitly by body-builders and sportsmen to enhance their physical performance. These are covered in other chapters of this book, and a general account is given by Mottram (1988).

The reasons why particular drugs should come to be used in a way that constitutes a problem to society are complex and largely outside the scope of this book. The drug and its pharmacological activity are only the starting point, though drug-taking is clearly seen by society in a quite different light from other forms of addictive self-gratification, such as opera-going, football or sex. At first sight, the 'drugs of abuse' form an extremely heterogeneous pharmacological group; we can find little in common at the molecular and cellular level between say, morphine, cocaine and barbiturates. What links them is that people find their effect pleasurable (hedonic) and tend to want to repeat it, an action which reflects the effect—common to all dependence-producing drugs—of activating mesolimbic dopaminergic neurons (see below). This hedonic effect becomes a problem when:

- the want becomes so insistent that it dominates the lifestyle of the individual and damages his or her quality of life
- the habit itself causes actual harm to the individual or the community.

Examples of the latter are the mental incapacity and liver damage caused by ethanol, the many diseases associated with smoking, the high risk of infection (especially with human immunodeficiency virus (HIV)) and the serious risk of overdosage with most narcotics, plus the criminal behaviour resorted to when an addict needs to finance the habit.

Table 42.1 The main drugs of abuse

Type	Examples	Dependence liability	Discussed in
Narcotic analgesics	Morphine	Very strong	Ch. 40
	Diamorphine	Very strong	Ch. 40
General CNS depressants	Ethanol	Strong	This chapter
	Barbiturates	Strong	Ch. 36
	Methaqualone	Moderate	Ch. 36
	Glutethimide	Moderate	Ch. 36
	Anaesthetics	Moderate	Ch. 35
	Solvents	Strong	–
Anxiolytic drugs	Benzodiazepines	Moderate	Ch. 36
Psychomotor stimulants	Amphetamines	Strong	Ch. 41
	Cocaine	Very strong	Ch. 41
	Caffeine	Weak	Ch. 41
	Nicotine	Very strong	This chapter
Psychotomimetic agents	LSD	Weak or absent	Ch. 41
	Mescaline	Weak or absent	Ch. 41
	Phencyclidine	Moderate	Ch. 41
	Cannabis	Weak or absent	This chapter

LSD, lysergic acid diethylamide

Other drugs with abuse potential are described elsewhere in this book (see Table 39.1). For further information on various aspects of drug abuse, see Shuckit (1995), Friedman et al. (1996), Hyman & Malenka (2001).

THE NATURE OF DRUG DEPENDENCE

Drug dependence describes the state when drug-taking becomes compulsive, taking precedence over other needs. The older term *drug addiction* is not clearly defined but generally implies a state of physical dependence (see below). *Drug abuse* and *substance abuse* are more general terms, meaning any recurrent use of substances that are illegal, or that cause harm to the individual, including drugs in sport. *Tolerance*—the decrease in pharmacological effect on repeated administration of the drug—often accompanies the state of dependence, and it is possible that related mechanisms account for both phenomena (see below). *Withdrawal syndrome* or *abstinence syndrome* describes the adverse effects, both physical and psychological, of stopping taking a drug. Several psychotropic drugs, including antidepressant and antipsychotic agents, produce withdrawal syndromes but are not addictive, so it is important to distinguish this type of commonly observed 'rebound' phenomenon from true dependence.

The common feature of the various types of psychoactive drug that can engender dependence is that all produce a *rewarding* effect. In animal studies, where this cannot be inferred directly, it is manifest as positive reinforcement (i.e. an increase in the probability of occurrence of any behaviour that results in the drug being administered). Thus, with all dependence-producing drugs, spontaneous self-administration can be induced in animal studies. Coupled with the direct rewarding effect of the drug, there is usually also a process of *habituation*, or *adaptation*, when the drug is given repeatedly or continuously, such that cessation of the drug has an *aversive* effect, negative reinforcement, from which the subject will attempt to escape by self-administration of the drug. The physical withdrawal syndrome, associated with the state of physical dependence, is one manifestation of this type of habituation; the intensity and nature of physical withdrawal symptoms varies from one class of drug to another, being particularly marked with opioids. It is less important in sustaining drug-seeking behaviour than psychological habituation, which is associated with a craving that is not related to physical symptoms. A degree of physical dependence is common when patients receive opioid analgesics in hospital for several days, but this almost never leads to addiction. By comparison, addicts who are nursed through and recover fully from the physical abstinence syndrome are still extremely likely to revert to drug-taking later. Consequently, physical dependence is not the major factor in long-term drug dependence. In addition to the positive and negative reinforcement associated with drug administration and withdrawal, *conditioning* plays a significant part in sustaining drug dependence. When a particular environment or location, or the sight of a syringe or cigarette, becomes associated with the pleasurable experience of drug-taking, the antecedent stimulus itself evokes the response, as with Pavlov's dogs. The same happens in reverse, so that the antecedents of not taking the drug become aversive. This kind of conditioning is generally more persistent and less easily extinguished than unconditioned reinforcement, and it probably accounts for the high relapse rate of 'weaned' addicts. The psychological factors in drug dependence are discussed by Koob (1996) and summarised in Figure 42.1.

Animal models provide some insight into the short-term neurobiological basis of reward and habituation, but in humans drug dependence represents a *stable* change in brain function, sustained by processes that are more complex and long lasting than the neurobiological changes so far studied in experimental animals.

REWARD PATHWAYS

▼ Virtually all dependence-producing drugs so far tested, including opioids, nicotine, amphetamines, ethanol and cocaine, activate the *reward pathway*—the mesolimbic dopaminergic pathway (see Ch. 33), which runs, via the medial forebrain bundle, from the ventral tegmental area of the midbrain (A10 cell group in rats) to the nucleus accumbens and limbic region (see Nestler, 2001a). Even though their primary sites of action are generally elsewhere in the brain, all of these drugs increase the release of dopamine in the nucleus accumbens, as shown by microdialysis and other techniques (see Spanagel & Weiss, 1999). Some stimulate firing of A10 cells, whereas others, such as amphetamine and cocaine, release dopamine or prevent its reuptake (see Ch. 11). Their *hedonic* effect results from activation of this pathway, rather than from a subjective appreciation of the diverse other effects (such as alertness or disinhibition) that the drugs produce. Chemical or surgical interruption of this dopaminergic pathway impairs drug-seeking behaviours in many experimental situations. Deletion of D_2-receptors in a transgenic mouse strain eliminated the reward properties of morphine administration, without eliminating other opiate effects, and it did not prevent the occurrence of physical withdrawal symptoms in morphine-dependent animals (Maldonado et al. 1997), suggesting that the dopaminergic pathway is responsible for the positive reward but not for the negative withdrawal effects. There is evidence that other mediators, particularly 5-hydroxytryptamine (5-HT), glutamate and gamma-aminobutyric acid (GABA), influence the mesolimbic dopamine pathway, and possibly other reward pathways. In general, manipulations that increase 5-HT activity (e.g. 5-HT agonists or uptake blockers; see Chs 11 and 38) reduce drug-seeking behaviour. 5-HT-uptake inhibitors (e.g. **zimeldine**) or 5-HT agonists (e.g. **buspirone**) reduce slightly the alcohol consumption in alcoholic patients, as does **acamprosate**, a NMDA (*N*-methyl-D-asparate) glutamate receptor antagonist, recently introduced for treating alcoholism (see below). These therapeutic approaches, based on the neurochemical manipulation of the reward pathway, are yet to be fully evaluated.

HABITUATION MECHANISMS

▼ The cellular mechanisms involved in habituation to the effects of drugs such as opioids and cocaine have been studied in some detail (see Nestler, 2001a). Both classes of drug produce, on chronic administration, an increase in the activity of adenylate cyclase in brain regions such as the nucleus accumbens, which compensates for their acute inhibitory effect on cAMP formation, and produce a rebound increase in cAMP when the drug is terminated (Fig. 42.2). Chronic opioid treatment increases the amount, not only of adenylate cyclase itself but also of other components of the signalling pathway, including the G-proteins and various protein

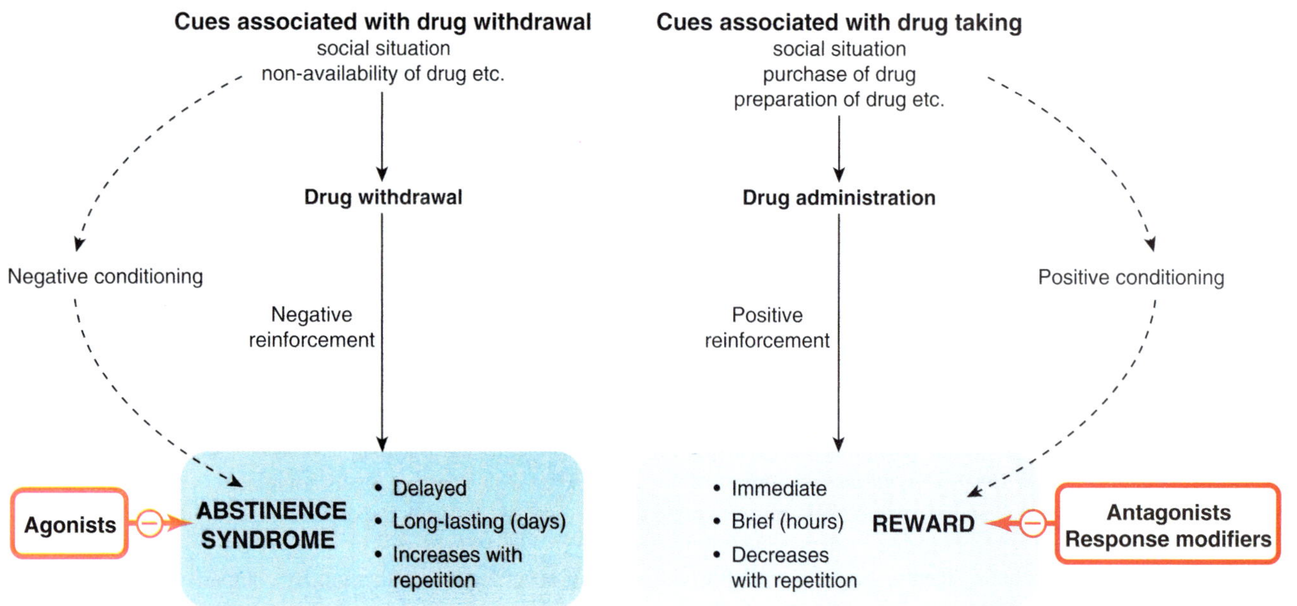

Fig. 42.1 Psychological factors involved in drug dependence.

kinases. This increase in cAMP affects many cellular functions through the increased activity of various cAMP-dependent protein kinases, which control the activity of ion channels (making the cells more excitable), as well as various enzymes and transcription factors.* Similar effects also occur with cocaine, but much less is known about other dependence-producing drugs. These changes (see Fig. 42.3) probably account for the relatively short-term (days to weeks) phenomena of tolerance and dependence, but the long-term processes responsible for craving and relapse—the major issues in human addiction—are very poorly understood at the neurochemical level.

*One particular transcription factor, CREB (cAMP response element-binding protein) may play a central role. It is upregulated in the nucleus accumbens by long-term administration of opiates or cocaine, and transgenic animals lacking CREB show reduced withdrawal symptoms (see Nestler, 2001b).

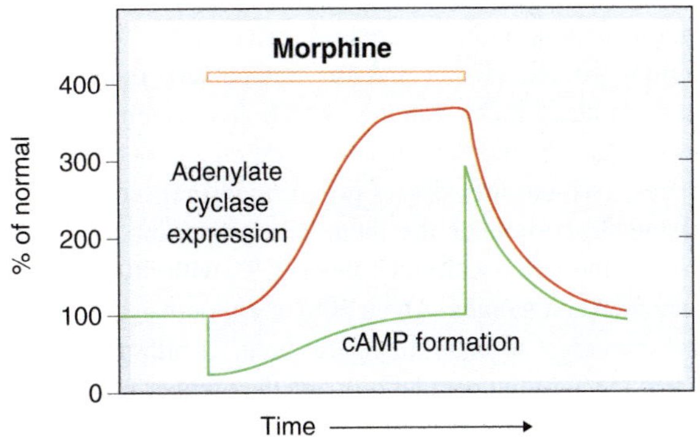

Fig. 42.2 Biochemical mechanism postulated to explain morphine tolerance and dependence. Morphine inhibits adenylate cyclase thus reducing cAMP formation (green line). A secondary rise in adenylate cyclase expression occurs (red line), so cAMP production recovers in the presence of morphine (i.e. tolerance develops). On cessation of morphine treatment, excessive cAMP production occurs, causing withdrawal symptoms, until the high level of adenylate cyclase expression returns to normal. (From: Sharma S K et al. 1975 Proc Natl Acad Sci USA 72: 3092.)

Drug dependence

- Dependence is defined as a compulsive craving that develops as a result of repeated administration of the drug.
- Dependence occurs with a wide range of psychotropic drugs, acting by many different mechanisms.
- The common feature of dependence-producing drugs is that they have a positive reinforcing action ('reward') associated with activation of the mesolimbic dopaminergic pathway.
- Dependence is often associated with (i) tolerance to the drug, which can arise by various biochemical mechanisms; (ii) a physical abstinence syndrome, which varies in type and intensity for different classes of drug; (iii) psychological dependence (craving), which may be associated with the tolerance-producing biochemical changes.
- Psychological dependence, which usually outlasts the physical withdrawal syndrome, is the major factor leading to relapse among treated addicts.
- Though genetic factors contribute to drug-seeking behaviour, no specific genes have yet been identified.

GENETIC FACTORS

Epidemiological studies, particularly in alcoholism, show clear evidence of a genetic component in the pathogenesis of drug abuse. Twin studies suggest that genetic factors contribute up to 60% of an individual's susceptibility to most forms of drug abuse. There are also well-characterised genetic strains of rats and mice—and also humans (see below)—that differ in their tendency to self-administer alcohol, or in the intensity of withdrawal symptoms following chronic opioid administration. However, attempts to find 'drug abuse genes' have not yet succeeded, despite earlier claims that mutations of the gene

	Drug-taking		Drug withdrawal	
State produced:	Acute drugged state	→ *Days–weeks* → Chronic drugged state	Acute abstinence	→ *Months–years* → Chronic abstinence
Effect:	Reward	Tolerance, dependence	Withdrawal syndrome	Craving
Mechanism:	Activation of mesolimbic DA pathway. ? Other reward pathways	Adaptive changes in receptors, transporters, 2nd messengers, etc. (e.g. ↑adenylate cyclase, ↑DA transporter)	Uncompensated adaptive changes (e.g. ↓DA, ↑glutamate)	Not known

Fig. 42.3 Cellular and physiological mechanisms involved in drug dependence. (DA, dopamine.)

encoding the dopamine D_4-receptor* were associated with drug abuse. Transgenic animals lacking or overexpressing many different receptors and other signalling molecules show changes in their susceptibility to dependence-producing drugs (see Nestler, 2000b), but the connection, if any, between such models and genetic factors in humans remains uncertain.

PHARMACOLOGICAL APPROACHES TO TREATING DRUG DEPENDENCE

From the discussion above, it will be clear that drug dependence involves many psychosocial, and some genetic factors, as well as neuropharmacological mechanisms, so drug treatment is only one component of the therapeutic approaches that are used.

The main pharmacological approaches (see O'Brien 1997) are summarised in Table 42.2.

NICOTINE AND TOBACCO

Tobacco growing, chewing and smoking was indigenous throughout the American subcontinent and Australia at the time that European explorers first visited these places. Smoking spread through Europe during the 16th century, coming to England mainly as a result of its enthusiastic espousal by Raleigh at the court of Elizabeth I. James I strongly disapproved of both Raleigh and tobacco, and initiated the first antismoking campaign in the early 17th century with the support of the Royal College of Physicians. Parliament responded by imposing a substantial duty on tobacco, thereby setting up the dilemma (from which we show no sign of being able to escape) of giving the State an economic interest in the continuation of smoking at the same time that its official expert advisers were issuing emphatic warnings about its dangers.

Until the latter half of the 19th century, tobacco was smoked in pipes, and by men. Cigarette manufacture began at the end of the 19th century, and now cigarettes account for more than 90% of tobacco consumption. The trend in cigarette consumption this century is shown in Figure 42.4. From a peak level in the early 1970s, cigarette consumption in the UK dropped by about 50%, the main factors being increased price, adverse publicity, restrictions on advertising and the compulsory publication of health warnings. Filter cigarettes (which give a somewhat lower delivery of tar and nicotine than standard cigarettes) and low-tar cigarettes (which are also low in nicotine) constitute an increasing proportion of the total. The proportion of cigarette smokers in the UK is currently about 25%, with little difference between men and women. About 10% of children aged 10–15 are regular smokers. Currently, there are about 1.1 billion smokers in the world (18% of the population), and the number in third world countries is increasing rapidly. Five trillion (5×10^{12}) cigarettes are sold each year, about 5000 per smoker.

For reviews on nicotine and smoking, see Balfour & Fagerstrom (1996), Benowitz (1996).

Table 42.2 Pharmacological approaches to treating drug dependence

Mechanism	Examples
Substitution, to alleviate withdrawal symptoms	Methadone, used short-term to blunt opiate withdrawal Benzodiazepines, to blunt alcohol withdrawal
Long-term substitution	Methadone substitution for opiate addiction Nicotine patches or chewing gum
Blocking response	Naltrexone to block opiate effects Mecamylamine to block nicotine effects Immunisation against cocaine to produce circulating antibody (not yet proven)
Aversive therapies	Disulfiram to induce unpleasant response to ethanol
Modification of craving	Bupropion (antidepressant) Naltrexone (blocks opiate receptors—also of value in treating other addictions) Clonidine (α-adrenoceptor agonist) Acamprosate (NMDA-receptor antagonist)

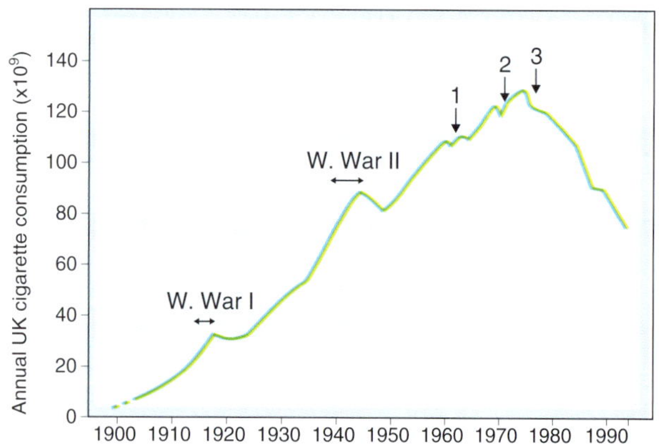

Fig. 42.4 Cigarette consumption in the UK 1900–1994. Numbers 1, 2 and 3 refer to publication of Royal College of Physicians reports on smoking and health. Since 1980, drop in consumption has closely followed price increases. (Data from: Ashton H, Stepney R 1982 Smoking psychology and pharmacology. Tavistock Publications, London; Townsend 1996 Price and consumption of tobacco. Br Med Bull 52: 132–142.)

*Dubbed the 'adventure gene' because mutations appear to be associated with manifestations of a risky lifestyle.

Tobacco smoking

- Cigarette consumption in the UK is now declining, after reaching a peak in the mid-1970s.
- The worldwide prevalence of smoking is now about 18% of the adult population, each smoker using on average 5000 cigarettes per year.
- Nicotine is the only pharmacologically active agent in tobacco, apart from carcinogenic tars and carbon monoxide.
- The amount of nicotine absorbed from an average cigarette is about 0.8–1.5 mg, which causes the plasma nicotine concentration to reach 100–200 nmol/l. These values depend greatly on the type of cigarette, and on the extent of inhalation of the smoke.

PHARMACOLOGICAL EFFECTS OF SMOKING

Nicotine* is the only pharmacologically active substance in tobacco smoke, apart from carcinogenic tars and carbon monoxide (see below). The acute effects of smoking can be mimicked by injection of nicotine and are blocked by mecamylamine, an antagonist at neuronal nicotinic acetylcholine receptors (see Ch. 10).

Effects on the central nervous system

The central effects of nicotine are complex and cannot be summed up overall simply in terms of stimulation or inhibition. At the cellular level, nicotine acts on nicotinic acetylcholine receptors of the $\alpha 4\beta 2$ subtype (see Ch. 33), which are widely expressed in the brain, particularly in the cortex and hippocampus, and are believed to play a role in cognitive function. These receptors are ligand-gated cation channels located both pre- and postsynaptically, causing neuronal excitation and enhanced transmitter release (see Jones et al., 1999). As well as activating the receptors, nicotine also causes desensitisation, which may be an important component of its effects, since the effects of a dose of nicotine are diminished in animals after sustained exposure to the drug. Chronic nicotine administration leads to a substantial increase in the number of nicotinic acetylcholine receptors (an effect opposite to that produced by sustained administration of most receptor agonists), which may represent an adaptive response to prolonged receptor desensitisation. It is likely that the overall effect of nicotine reflects a balance between activation of nicotinic acetylcholine receptors, causing neuronal excitation, and desensitisation, causing synaptic block.

At the spinal level, nicotine inhibits spinal reflexes, causing skeletal muscle relaxation, which can be measured by electromyography. This relaxation may result from stimulation of the inhibitory Renshaw cells in the ventral horn of the spinal cord. The higher level functioning of the brain, as reflected in the subjective sense of alertness or by the electroencephalograph (EEG) pattern, can be affected in either direction by nicotine, according to dose and circumstances. Smokers report that smoking wakes them up when they are drowsy and calms them down when they are tense, and EEG recordings broadly bear this out. It also seems that small doses of nicotine tend to cause arousal, whereas large doses do the reverse. Tests of motor and sensory performance (e.g. reaction time measurements or vigilance tests) in humans generally show improvement after smoking, and nicotine enhances learning in rats. Some elaborate tests have been conducted to see, for example, whether the effect of nicotine on performance and aggression varies according to the amount of stress. In one such test, the subject first has to name the colours of a series of squares (low stress) and then has to name the colours in which the names of other colours are written (high stress). The difference between the scores, reflecting the extent by which performance is affected by stress, was diminished by smoking. Some tests border on nasty-mindedness, such as one in which subjects played a complicated logical game with a computer which initially played fair and then began to cheat randomly, causing stress and aggression in the subjects and a decline in their performance. Smoking, it was reported, did not reduce the anger but did reduce the decline in performance.

Nicotine and other agonists such as **epibatidine** (Ch. 40) have significant analgesic activity.

Peripheral effects

The peripheral effects of small doses of nicotine result from stimulation of autonomic ganglia (see Ch. 10) and of peripheral sensory receptors, mainly in the heart and lungs. Stimulation of these receptors elicits various autonomic reflex responses, causing tachycardia, increased cardiac output and arterial pressure, reduction of gastrointestinal motility, and sweating. When people smoke for the first time, they usually experience nausea and sometimes vomit, probably because of stimulation of sensory receptors in the stomach. All of these effects decline with repeated dosage, though the central effects remain. Secretion of adrenaline and noradrenaline from the adrenal medulla contribute to the cardiovascular effects, and release of antidiuretic hormone from the posterior pituitary causes a decrease in urine flow. The plasma concentration of free fatty acids is increased, probably owing to sympathetic stimulation and adrenaline secretion.

Smokers weigh, on average, about 4 kg less than non-smokers, mainly because of reduced food intake; giving up smoking usually causes weight gain associated with increased food intake.

PHARMACOKINETIC ASPECTS

An average cigarette contains about 0.8 g of tobacco and 9–17 mg nicotine, of which about 10% is normally absorbed by the

*From the plant *Nicotiana*, named after Jean Nicot, French ambassador to Portugal, who presented seeds to the French king, having been persuaded of the medical value of smoking tobacco leaves by natives of South America. Smoking was believed to protect against illness, particularly the plague.

smoker. This fraction varies greatly with the habits of the smoker and the type of cigarette.

Nicotine in cigarette smoke is rapidly absorbed from the lungs, but poorly from the mouth and nasopharynx. Therefore, inhalation is required to give appreciable absorption of nicotine, each puff delivering a distinct bolus of drug to the central nervous system (CNS). Pipe or cigar smoke is less acidic than cigarette smoke, and the nicotine tends to be absorbed from the mouth and nasopharynx, rather than the lungs. Absorption is considerably slower than from inhaled cigarette smoke, resulting in a later and longer-lasting peak in the plasma nicotine concentration (Fig. 42.5). An average cigarette, smoked over 10 minutes, causes the plasma nicotine concentration to rise to 15–30 ng/ml (100–200 nmol/l), falling to about half within 10 minutes and then more slowly over the next 1–2 hours. The rapid decline results mainly from redistribution between the blood and other tissues; the slower decline results from hepatic metabolism, mainly by oxidation to an inactive ketone metabolite, *cotinine*. This has a long plasma half-life, and measurement of plasma cotinine concentration provides a useful measure of smoking behaviour. A nicotine patch applied for 24 hours causes the plasma concentration to rise to 75–150 nmol/l over 6 hours and to remain fairly constant for about 20 hours. Administration by nasal spray or chewing gum results in a time course intermediate between that of smoking and the nicotine patch.

TOLERANCE AND DEPENDENCE

As with other dependence-producing drugs, three separate but related processes—tolerance, physical dependence and psychological dependence—contribute to the overall state of dependence, in which taking the drug becomes compulsive.

The effects of nicotine associated with peripheral ganglionic stimulation show rapid tolerance, perhaps as a result of desensitisation of nicotinic acetylcholine receptors by nicotine. With large doses of nicotine, this desensitisation produces a block of ganglionic transmission rather than stimulation (see Ch. 10). Tolerance to the central effects of nicotine (e.g. in the arousal response) is much less than in the periphery. The increase in the number of nicotinic receptors in the brain produced by chronic nicotine administration in animals (see above) also occurs in heavy smokers. Since the cellular effects of nicotine are diminished, it is possible that the additional binding sites represent desensitised, rather than functional receptors.

The addictiveness of smoking is solely caused by nicotine. Rats choose to drink dilute nicotine solution in preference to water if given a choice, and in a situation in which lever-pressing causes an injection of nicotine to be delivered, they quickly learn to self-administer it. Similarly, monkeys who have been trained to smoke, by providing a reward in response to smoking behaviour, will continue to do so spontaneously (i.e. unrewarded) if the smoking medium contains nicotine, but not if nicotine-free tobacco is offered instead. Like other dependence-producing drugs (see above), nicotine causes excitation of the mesolimbic pathway and increased dopamine release in the nucleus accumbens. Transgenic mice in which expression of the β_2-subunit of the acetylcholine receptor is prevented lose the rewarding effect of nicotine and its dopamine-releasing effect (Picciotto et al., 1998), confirming the role of nicotinic acetylcholine receptors and mesolimbic dopamine release in the response to nicotine. In contrast to normal mice, the mutant mice could not be induced to self-administer nicotine, even though they did so with cocaine. Further evidence implicating brain nicotinic acetylcholine receptors in the addictive property of nicotine comes from experiments with mecamylamine, an antagonist at nicotinic acetylcholine receptors. If monkeys are habituated to tobacco-smoking so that they choose to puff smoke

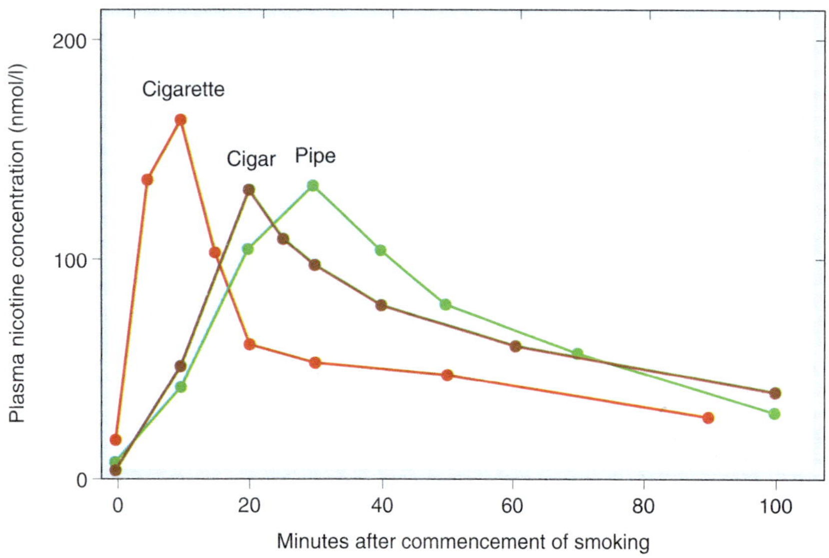

Fig. 42.5 Nicotine concentration in plasma during smoking. The subjects were habitual smokers who smoked a cigarette, cigar or pipe according to their usual habit. (From: Bowman W C, Rand M 1980 Textbook of pharmacology. Blackwell, Oxford, ch. 4.)

in preference to air, administration of mecamylamine causes them to switch to puffing air instead of smoke.

A physical withdrawal syndrome occurs in both humans and experimental animals accustomed to regular nicotine administration. Its main features are increased irritability, impaired performance of psychomotor tasks, aggressiveness and sleep disturbance. The withdrawal syndrome is much less severe than that produced by opiates, and it can be alleviated not only by nicotine but also by amphetamine, a finding consistent with the postulated role of dopamine in the reward pathway. The nicotine withdrawal syndrome lasts for 2–3 weeks, though the craving for cigarettes persists for much longer than this; relapses during attempts to give up cigarette smoking occur most commonly at a time when the physical withdrawal syndrome has long since subsided.

HARMFUL EFFECTS OF SMOKING

The life expectancy of smokers is shorter than that of non-smokers. For example, in a 1971 study of British doctors, the proportion of heavy smokers dying between the ages of 35 and 65 was estimated to be 40% compared with 15% for non-smokers. For a recent analysis, see Peto et al. (1996). Smoking is, by a large margin, the the biggest preventable cause of death, responsible for about 1 in 10 adult deaths worldwide. Apart from the acquired immunodeficiency syndrome (AIDS), smoking is the only major cause of death that is increasing rapidly. In 1990, smoking was responsible for 10% (3 million out of 30 million) of deaths worldwide; by 2030, this is expected to increase to 17% (10 million out of 60 million), mainly because of the growth of smoking in Asia, Africa and Latin America (Peto et al., 1999).

The *main health risks* are as follows.

Cancer This particularly occurs in the lung and upper respiratory tract, but also in the oesophagus, pancreas and bladder. Smoking 20 cigarettes per day is estimated to increase the risk of lung cancer about 10-fold. Approximately 90% of lung cancers are caused by smoking. Pipe and cigar smoking carry much less risk than cigarette smoking, though the risk is still appreciable. Tar, rather than nicotine, is responsible for the cancer risk.

Coronary heart disease and other forms of peripheral vascular disease The mortality among men aged 55–64 from coronary thrombosis is about 60% greater in men who smoke 20 cigarettes per day than in non-smokers. Though the increase in risk is less than it is for lung cancer, the actual number of excess deaths associated with smoking is larger, because coronary heart disease is so common. Other kinds of peripheral vascular disease (e.g. stroke, intermittent claudication and diabetic gangrene) are also strongly smoking related. Many studies have suggested that nicotine is mainly responsible for the adverse effect of smoking on the incidence of cardiovascular disease. Another factor may be carbon monoxide (see below). Surprisingly, there is no clear increase in ischaemic heart disease in pipe and cigar smokers, even though similar blood nicotine and carboxyhaemoglobin concentrations are reached, suggesting that nicotine and carbon monoxide may not be the only causative factors.

Pharmacology of nicotine

- At a cellular level, nicotine acts on nicotinic acetylcholine receptors, mainly of the $\alpha4\beta2$ subtype, to cause neuronal excitation. Its central effects are blocked by receptor antagonists such as mecamylamine.
- At the behavioural level, nicotine produces a mixture of inhibitory and excitatory effects.
- Nicotine shows reinforcing properties, associated with increased activity in the mesolimbic dopaminergic pathway, and self-administration can be elicited in animal studies.
- Electroencephalography changes show an arousal response, and subjects report increased alertness, accompanied by a reduction of anxiety and tension.
- Learning, particularly under stress, is facilitated by nicotine.
- Peripheral effects of nicotine result mainly from ganglionic stimulation: tachycardia, increased blood pressure and reduced gastrointestinal motility. Tolerance develops rapidly to these effects.
- Nicotine is metabolised, mainly in the liver, within 1–2 hours. Its inactive metabolite, cotinine, has a long plasma half-life and can be used as a measure of smoking habits.
- Nicotine gives rise to tolerance, physical dependence and psychological dependence (craving); it is highly addictive. Attempts at long-term cessation succeed in only about 20%.
- Nicotine replacement therapy (chewing gum or skin patch preparations) improves the chances of giving up smoking, but only when combined with active counselling.

Chronic bronchitis Chronic bronchitis is much more common in smokers than non-smokers. Nonetheless, in contrast to lung cancer, chronic bronchitis has declined in prevalence since the 1950s. This is generally attributed to cleaner air and other social changes, and smoking now appears to be the most important remaining cause. Its effect is probably caused by tar and other irritants, rather than nicotine.

Harmful effects in pregnancy Smoking, particularly during the latter half of pregnancy, significantly reduces birth weight (by about 8% in women who smoke 25 or more cigarettes per day during pregnancy) and increases perinatal mortality (by an estimated 28% in babies born to mothers who smoke in the last half of pregnancy). There is evidence that children born to smoking mothers remain behind, in both physical and mental development, for at least 7 years. By 11 years of age, the difference is no longer significant. These effects of smoking, though measurable, are much smaller than the effects of other factors, such as social class and birth order. Various other complications of pregnancy are also more common in women who smoke, including spontaneous abortion (increased 30–70% by smoking), premature delivery (increased about 40%) and placenta praevia (increased 25–90%). Nicotine is excreted in breast milk in sufficient amounts to cause tachycardia in the infant.

Potential protective effects of nicotine Parkinson's disease is approximately twice as common in non-smokers as in smokers. Some studies have found the same to be true of Alzheimer's disease, though this remains very controversial. It is possible that this reflects a protective effect of nicotine, but it could be that common genetic factors underly smoking behaviour and susceptibility to these diseases.

Harmful agents

The agents probably responsible for the harmful effects are:

- *Tar and irritants*, such as nitrogen dioxide, formaldehyde, etc. Cigarette smoke tar contains many known carcinogenic hydrocarbons, as well as tumour promoters, which account for the high cancer risk. It is likely that the various irritant substances are also responsible for the increase in bronchitis and emphysema.
- *Nicotine* probably accounts for retarded fetal development, because of its vasoconstrictor properties, but it is not known whether it also causes the increase in cardiovascular risk.
- *Carbon monoxide*. The average carbon monoxide content of cigarette smoke is about 3%. Carbon monoxide has a high affinity for haemoglobin and the average carboxyhaemoglobin content in the blood of cigarette smokers is about 2.5% (compared with 0.4% for non-smoking urban dwellers). In very heavy smokers, up to 15% of haemoglobin may be carboxylated, a level which affects fetal development in rats. This factor may also contribute to the increased incidence of heart and vascular disease. Fetal haemoglobin has a higher affinity for carbon monoxide than adult haemoglobin, and the proportion of carboxyhaemoglobin is higher in fetal than maternal blood.

'Low tar' cigarettes give a lower yield of both tar and nicotine than standard cigarettes. However, it has been shown that smokers puff harder, inhale more and smoke more cigarettes when low tar brands are substituted for standard brands. The end result may be a slightly reduced intake of tar and nicotine, but an increase in carbon monoxide intake, with no net gain in terms of safety.

Harmful effects of smoking

- Smoking accounts for about 10% of deaths worldwide, mainly through:
  —cancer, especially lung cancer, of which about 90% of cases are smoking-related; carcinogenic tars are responsible
  —ischaemic heart disease; both nicotine and carbon monoxide may be responsible
  —chronic bronchitis; tars are mainly responsible.
- Smoking in pregnancy reduces birth weight and retards childhood development. It also increases abortion rate and perinatal mortality. Nicotine, and possibly carbon monoxide, are responsible.
- However, the incidence of Parkinson's disease is lower in smokers than non-smokers.

PHARMACOLOGICAL APPROACHES TO TREATMENT OF NICOTINE DEPENDENCE

Most smokers would like to quit, but few succeed.* The most successful smoking-cure clinics, using a combination of psychological and pharmacological treatments, achieve a success rate of about 25%, measured as the percentage of patients still abstinent after 1 year. The main pharmacological approach used is *nicotine replacement therapy* (see Benowitz, 1993); adjunct therapies include the antidepressant **bupropion**, **clonidine** and the nicotinic receptor antagonist **mecamylamine**.

Nicotine replacement therapy is used mainly to assist smokers to quit by relieving the psychological and physical withdrawal syndrome. Because nicotine is relatively short acting, and not well absorbed from the gastrointestinal tract, it is given either in the form of chewing gum, used several times daily, or as a transdermal patch, which is replaced daily. These preparations cause various side-effects, particularly nausea and gastrointestinal cramps, cough, insomnia and muscle pains. Because of the risk of coronary spasm, nicotine should not be used in patients with heart disease. Transdermal patches often cause local irritation and itching. The conclusion of many double-blind trials of nicotine against placebo is that these preparations, combined with professional counselling and supportive therapy, roughly double the chances of successfully breaking the smoking habit, but the success rate measured as abstinence 1 year after ceasing treatment is still only about 25%. Nicotine on its own, without counselling and support, is no more effective than placebo, so its use as an over-the-counter smoking remedy has little justification. Though of limited value as an aid to abstinence, the long-term use of nicotine can significantly reduce cigarette consumption by smokers. In Sweden, the use of 'smokeless tobacco' (i.e. nicotine by inhalation) is widespread, and the tobacco consumption and smoking-related death rate is much lower than elsewhere in Europe or North America.

The identification of the $\alpha4\beta2$ nicotinic acetylcholine receptor subtype as the putative 'nicotine receptor' in the brain may allow selective agonists to be developed as nicotine substitutes with fewer side-effects, but this remains theoretical at present.

Bupropion (Ch. 38) appeared to be as effective as nicotine replacement therapy in recent trials, even in non-depressed

*Freud tried unsuccessfully to give up for 45 years before dying of cancer at the age of 83.

patients, and has fewer side-effects. It may act by increasing dopamine activity in the nucleus accumbens.

Clonidine, an α_2-adrenoceptor agonist (see Ch. 11) reduces the withdrawal effects of several dependence-producing drugs, including opioids and cocaine and nicotine.* Clonidine may be given orally or as a transdermal patch and is about as effective as nicotine substitution in assisting abstinence. The side-effects of clonidine (hypotension, dry mouth, drowsiness) are troublesome, however, and it is not widely used.

The use of mecamylamine, which antagonises the effects of nicotine, is not promising. Small doses actually increase smoking, presumably because the antagonism can be overcome by increasing the amount of nicotine. Larger doses of mecamylamine, which abolish the effects of nicotine more effectively, have so many autonomic side-effects (see Ch. 10) that compliance is poor.

ETHANOL

Judged on a molar basis, the consumption of ethanol far exceeds that of any other drug. The ethanol content of various drinks ranges from about 2.5% (weak beer) to about 55% (strong spirits), and the size of the normal measure is such that a single drink usually contains about 8–12 g (0.17–0.26 mole) ethanol. It is by no means unusual to consume 1–2 mole at a sitting, equivalent to about 0.5 kg of most other drugs. Its low pharmacological potency is reflected in the range of plasma concentrations needed to produce pharmacological effects: minimal effects occur at about 10 mmol/l (46 mg/100 ml), and 10 times this concentration may be lethal. The average per capita ethanol consumption in the UK is about 8 litres/year (expressed as pure ethanol) a figure that has changed little since the 1980s, the main change having been a growing consumption of wine in preference to beer.

For practical purposes, ethanol intake is often expressed in terms of units. One unit is equal to 8 g ethanol and is the amount contained in half a pint of normal strength beer, one measure of spirits or one standard glass of wine. Based on the health risks described below, the current official recommendation is a maximum of 21 units/week for men and 14 units/week for women. It is estimated that in the UK, about 25% of men and 7% of women exceed these levels. The annual government revenue from drink (mainly tax) amounts to about £7 billion, whereas the social cost is estimated at £2 billion. Views differ as to whether this represents a good bargain or a moral outrage.

PHARMACOLOGICAL EFFECTS OF ETHANOL

Effects on the central nervous system

The main effects of ethanol are on the CNS (see review by Charness et al., 1989), where its depressant actions resemble those of volatile anaesthetics (Ch. 35). At a cellular level, the effect of ethanol is purely depressant, though it increases impulse activity—presumably by disinhibition—in some parts of the CNS, notably in the mesolimbic dopaminergic neurons that are involved in the reward pathway described above. The main theories of ethanol action (see reviews by Little, 1991; Tabakoff & Hoffman, 1996; Lovinger, 1997) are:

- enhancement of GABA-mediated inhibition, similar to the action of benzodiazepines (see Ch. 36)
- inhibition of Ca^{2+} entry through voltage-gated calcium channels
- inhibition of NMDA-receptor function.

Ethanol enhances the action of GABA acting on $GABA_A$-receptors in a similar way to benzodiazepines (see Ch. 36). Its effect is, however, smaller and less consistent than that of benzodiazepines, and no clear effect on inhibitory synaptic transmission in the CNS has been demonstrated for ethanol. The benzodiazepine antagonist **flumazenil** reverses the central depressant actions of ethanol (see Lister & Nutt, 1987), but this appears to result from physiological antagonism rather than from a direct pharmacological interaction. The use of flumazenil to reverse ethanol intoxication and treat dependence has not found favour for several reasons. It carries a risk of causing seizures and could cause an increase in ethanol consumption and thus increase long-term toxic manifestations.

Ethanol inhibits transmitter release in response to nerve terminal depolarisation, by inhibiting the opening of voltage-sensitive calcium channels in neurons.

The excitatory effects of glutamate are inhibited by ethanol at concentrations that produce CNS depressant effects in vivo. NMDA-receptor activation is inhibited at lower ethanol concentrations than are required to affect AMPA-receptors (see Ch. 33). Other effects produced by ethanol include an enhancement of the excitatory effects produced by activation of nicotinic acetylcholine receptors and $5\text{-}HT_3$-receptors. The relative importance of these various effects in the overall effects of ethanol on CNS function is not clear at present.

The effects of acute ethanol intoxication in humans are well known and include slurred speech, motor incoordination, increased self-confidence and euphoria. The effect on mood varies among individuals, most becoming louder and more outgoing, but some becoming morose and withdrawn. At higher levels of intoxication, the mood tends to become highly labile, with euphoria and melancholy, aggression and submission, often occurring successively. The association between alcohol and violence is well documented.

Intellectual and motor performance and sensory discrimination show uniform impairment by ethanol, but subjects are generally unable to judge this for themselves. For example, bus drivers were asked to drive through a gap which they selected as the minimum for their bus to pass through; ethanol caused them not only to hit the barriers more often at any given gap setting but also to set the gap to a narrower dimension, often narrower than the bus.

Much effort has gone into measuring the effect of ethanol on driving performance in real life, as opposed to artificial tests

*It also reduces postmenopausal flushing, which may represent a physiological oestrogen withdrawal response.

under experimental conditions. In an US study of city drivers, it was found that the probability of being involved in an accident was unaffected at blood ethanol concentrations up to 50 mg/100 ml (10.9 mmol/l); by 80 mg/100 ml (17.4 mmol/l) the probability was increased about fourfold and by 150 mg/100 ml (32.6 mmol/l) about 25-fold. In the UK, driving with a blood ethanol concentration greater than 80 mg/100 ml constitutes a legal offence.

The relationship between plasma ethanol concentration and effect is highly variable. A given concentration produces a larger effect when the concentration is rising than when it is steady or falling. A substantial degree of tissue tolerance develops in habitual drinkers, with the result that a higher plasma ethanol concentration is needed to produce a given effect (see below). In one study, 'gross intoxication' (assessed by a battery of tests that measured speech, gait and so on) occurred in 30% of subjects between 50 and 100 mg/100 ml and in 90% of subjects with more than 150 mg/100 ml. Coma generally occurs at about 300 mg/100 ml and death from respiratory failure is likely at 400–500 mg/100 ml.

In addition to the acute effects of ethanol on the nervous system, chronic administration also causes irreversible neurological effects (see Charness et al., 1989). These may result from ethanol itself, or from metabolites such as acetaldehyde or fatty acid esters. The majority of chronic alcoholics show a degree of dementia associated with ventricular enlargement detectable by brain-imaging techniques. Degeneration in the cerebellum and other specific brain regions can also occur, as well as peripheral neuropathy. Some of these changes are not caused by ethanol itself but by accompanying thiamine deficiency, which is common in alcoholics.

Ethanol significantly enhances—sometimes to a dangerous extent—the CNS depressant effects of many other drugs, including benzodiazepines, antidepressants, antipsychotic drugs and opiates.

Effects on other systems

The main cardiovascular effect of ethanol is to produce cutaneous vasodilatation, central in origin, which causes a warm feeling but actually increases heat loss.

Ethanol increases salivary and gastric secretion. This is partly a reflex effect produced by the taste and irritant action of ethanol. However, heavy consumption of spirits causes damage directly to the gastric mucosa, causing chronic gastritis. Both this and the increased acid secretion are factors in the high incidence of gastric bleeding in alcoholics.

Ethanol produces a variety of endocrine effects. In particular, it increases the output of adrenal steroid hormones, by stimulating the anterior pituitary gland to secrete adrenocorticotrophic hormone. However, the increase in plasma hydrocortisone usually seen in alcoholics (producing a 'pseudo-Cushing's syndrome') is partly a result of inhibition by ethanol of hydrocortisone metabolism in the liver.

Diuresis is a familiar effect of ethanol. It is caused by inhibition of antidiuretic hormone secretion; tolerance develops rapidly, so the diuresis is not sustained. There is a similar inhibition of oxytocin secretion, which can cause delayed parturition at term. Attempts have been made to use this effect in premature labour, but the dose needed is large enough to cause obvious drunkenness in the mother. If the baby is born prematurely in spite of the ethanol, it too may be intoxicated at birth, sufficiently for respiration to be depressed. The procedure evidently has serious disadvantages.

Chronic male alcoholics are often impotent and show signs of feminisation. This is associated with impaired testicular steroid synthesis, but induction of hepatic microsomal enzymes by ethanol, and hence an increased rate of testosterone inactivation, also contributes.

Effects of ethanol on the liver

Together with brain damage, liver damage is the most serious long-term consequence of excessive ethanol consumption (see Lieber, 1995). In the sequence of effects, increased fat accumulation (fatty liver) progresses to hepatitis (i.e. inflammation of the liver) and eventually to irreversible hepatic necrosis and fibrosis. Diversion of portal blood flow around the fibrotic liver often causes oesophageal varices to develop, which can bleed suddenly and catastrophically. Increased fat accumulation in the liver occurs, in rats or in humans, after a single large dose of ethanol. The mechanism is complex, the main factors being:

- increased release of fatty acids from adipose tissue, which is the result of increased stress, causing sympathetic discharge
- impaired fatty acid oxidation, because of the metabolic load imposed by the ethanol itself.

With chronic ethanol consumption, many other factors contribute to the liver damage. One is malnutrition, for an alcoholic may satisfy much of his calorie requirement from ethanol itself as 300 g ethanol (equivalent to one bottle of whisky), provides about 2000 kcal; however, unlike a normal diet, it provides no vitamins, amino acids or fatty acids. Thiamine deficiency is an important factor in causing chronic neurological damage (see above). The hepatic changes occurring in alcoholics are partly caused by chronic malnutrition but mainly result from the cellular toxicity of ethanol, which promotes inflammatory changes in the liver.

The overall incidence of chronic liver disease is a function of cumulative ethanol consumption over many years. Consequently, overall consumption (expressed as g/kg body weight per day multiplied by years of drinking) provides an accurate predictor of the incidence of cirrhosis. An increase in the plasma concentration of the liver enzyme gamma-glutamyl transpeptidase provides an index of liver damage, though not specific to ethanol.

Effects on lipid metabolism, platelet function and atherosclerosis

Moderate drinking reduces mortality associated with coronary heart disease, the maximum effect—about 30% reduction of mortality*—being achieved at a level of 2–3 units/day (see

*The effect is much more pronounced (>50% reduction) in men with high plasma concentrations of low-density lipoprotein cholesterol (see Ch. 19).

Groenbaek et al., 1994). Most evidence suggests that ethanol, rather than any specific beverage such as red wine, is the essential factor. Two mechanisms have been proposed. The first involves the effect of ethanol on the plasma lipoproteins that are the carrier molecules for cholesterol and other lipids in the bloodstream (see Ch. 19). Epidemiological studies, as well as studies on volunteers, have shown that ethanol, in daily doses too small to produce obvious CNS effects, can over the course of a few weeks increase plasma high-density lipoprotein concentration, thus exerting a protective effect against atheroma formation.

Ethanol may also protect against ischaemic heart disease by inhibiting platelet aggregation. This effect occurs at ethanol concentrations in the range achieved by normal drinking in humans (10–20 mmol/l) and probably results from inhibition of arachidonic acid formation from phospholipid. In humans, the magnitude of the effect depends critically on dietary fat intake, and it is not yet clear how important it is clinically.

The effect of ethanol on fetal development

The adverse effect of ethanol consumption during pregnancy on fetal development was demonstrated in the early 1970s, when the term *fetal alcohol syndrome* (FAS) was coined.

The feature of full-blown FAS include:

- abnormal facial development, with wide-set eyes, short palpebral fissures and small cheek bones
- reduced cranial circumference
- retarded growth
- mental retardation and behavioural abnormalities, often taking the form of hyperactivity and difficulty with social integration
- other anatomical abnormalities, which may be major or minor (e.g. congenital cardiac abnormalities, malformation of the eyes and ears).

A lesser degree of impairment, termed *alcohol-related neurolodevelopmental disorder* (ARND), results in behavioural problems and cognitive and motor deficits, often associated with reduced brain size. Full-blown FAS occurs in about 3 per 1000 live births and affects about 30% of children born to alcoholic mothers. It is rare with mothers who drink less than about 5 units/day. ARND is about three times as common. Though there is no clearly defined safe threshold, there is no evidence that amounts less than about 2 units/day are harmful. There is no critical period during pregnancy when ethanol consumption is likely to lead to FAS, though one study suggests that FAS incidence correlates most strongly with ethanol consumption very early in pregnancy, even before pregnancy is recognised, implying that not only pregnant women but also women who are likely to become pregnant must be advised not to drink heavily. Experiments on rats and mice suggest that the effect on facial development may be produced very early in pregnancy (up to 4 weeks in humans), while the effect on brain development is produced rather later (up to 10 weeks).

Other adverse effects of chronic ethanol consumption include gastritis, associated with increased acid secretion and the direct irritant effect of ethanol, immunosuppression, leading to increased incidence of infections such as pneumonia, and increased cancer risk, particularly of the mouth, larynx and oesophagus.

Effects of ethanol

- Ethanol consumption is generally expressed in units of 10 ml (8 g) pure ethanol. Per capita consumption in Britain is about 8 litres/year.
- Ethanol acts as a general CNS depressant, similar to volatile anaesthetic agents, producing the familiar effects of acute intoxication.
- Several cellular mechanisms are postulated: inhibition of calcium channel opening, enhancement of GABA action and inhibitory action at NMDA-type glutamate receptors.
- Effective plasma concentrations:
  —threshold effects: about 40 mg/100 ml (5 mmol/l)
  —severe intoxication: about 150 mg/100 ml
  —death from respiratory failure: about 500 mg/100 ml.
- Main peripheral effects are self-limiting diuresis (reduced antidiuretic hormone secretion), cutaneous vasodilatation and delayed labour (reduced oxytocin secretion).
- Neurological degeneration occurs in heavy drinkers, causing dementia and peripheral neuropathies.
- Long-term ethanol consumption causes liver disease, progressing to cirrhosis and liver failure.
- Moderate ethanol consumption has a protective effect against ischaemic heart disease.
- Excessive consumption in pregnancy causes impaired fetal development, associated with small size, abnormal facial development and other physical abnormalities, and mental retardation.
- Tolerance, physical dependence and psychological dependence all occur with ethanol.
- Drugs used to treat alcohol dependence include disulfiram (aldehyde dehydrogenase inhibitor), naltrexone (opiate antagonist) and acamprosate (NMDA-receptor antagonist).

PHARMACOKINETIC ASPECTS

Metabolism of ethanol

Ethanol is rapidly absorbed, an appreciable amount being absorbed from the stomach. A substantial fraction is cleared by first-pass hepatic metabolism. Hepatic metabolism of ethanol shows saturation kinetics (see Ch. 8) at quite low ethanol concentrations, so the fraction of ethanol removed decreases as the concentration reaching the liver increases. Therefore, if ethanol absorption is rapid and portal vein concentration is high, most of the ethanol escapes into the systemic circulation, whereas with slow absorption, more is removed by first-pass metabolism. This is one reason why drinking ethanol on an empty stomach produces a much greater pharmacological effect. Ethanol is quickly distributed throughout the body water, the rate of its redistribution depending mainly on the blood flow to individual tissues, as with volatile anaesthetics (see Ch. 35).

Ethanol is about 90% metabolised, 5–10% being excreted unchanged in expired air and in urine. This fraction is not pharmacokinetically significant, but it provides the basis for estimating blood ethanol concentration from measurements on breath or urine. The ratio of ethanol concentrations in blood and alveolar air, measured at the end of deep expiration, is relatively constant, 80 mg/100 ml of ethanol in blood producing 35 μg/100 ml in expired air, this being the basis of the breathalyser test. The concentration in urine is more variable and provides a less accurate measure of blood concentration.

Ethanol metabolism occurs almost entirely in the liver, and mainly by a pathway involving successive oxidations, first to acetaldehyde and then to acetic acid (Fig. 42.6). Since ethanol is often consumed in large quantities (compared with most drugs), 1–2 mol daily being by no means unusual, it constitutes a substantial load on the hepatic oxidative systems. The oxidation of 2 mol ethanol consumes about 1.5 kg of the cofactor NAD^+ (nicotine adenine dinucleotide). Availability of NAD^+ limits the rate of ethanol oxidation to about 8 g/hour in a normal adult, independently of ethanol concentration (Fig. 42.7), causing the process to show saturating kinetics (Ch. 8). It also leads to competition between the ethanol and other metabolic substrates for the available NAD^+ supplies, which may be a factor in ethanol-induced liver damage (see Ch. 52). The intermediate metabolite acetaldehyde is a reactive and toxic compound and this may also contribute to the hepatotoxicity. A small degree of esterification of ethanol with various fatty acids also occurs in the tissues, and these esters may also contribute to long-term toxicity.

Alcohol dehydrogenase is a soluble cytoplasmic enzyme, confined mainly to liver cells, which oxidises ethanol at the same time as reducing NAD^+ to NADH (Fig. 42.6). Ethanol metabolism causes the ratio of NAD^+ to NADH to fall, and this has other metabolic consequences (e.g. increased lactate, and slowing down of the tricarboxylic acid cycle). The limitation on ethanol metabolism imposed by the limited rate of NAD^+ regeneration has led to attempts to find a 'sobering-up' agent that works by regenerating NAD^+ from NADH. One such agent is **fructose**, which is reduced by an NADH-requiring enzyme. In large doses, it causes a measurable increase in the rate of ethanol metabolism, but not enough to have a useful effect on the rate of return to sobriety.

Normally, a trivial amount of ethanol is metabolised by the microsomal mixed function oxidase system (see Ch. 8), but induction of this system occurs in alcoholics. Ethanol can affect the metabolism of other drugs that are metabolised by the system (e.g. **phenobarbital**, **warfarin** and **steroids**), with an initial inhibitory effect produced by competition, followed by enhancement owing to enzyme induction.

Nearly all of the acetaldehyde produced is converted to acetate in the liver, by aldehyde dehydrogenase (Fig. 42.6). Normally, only a little acetaldehyde escapes from the liver, giving a blood acetaldehyde concentration of 20–50 μmol/l after an intoxicating dose of ethanol in humans. The circulating acetaldehyde usually has little or no effect, but the concentration may become much larger under certain circumstances and produce toxic effects. This occurs if aldehyde dehydrogenase is inhibited by drugs such as

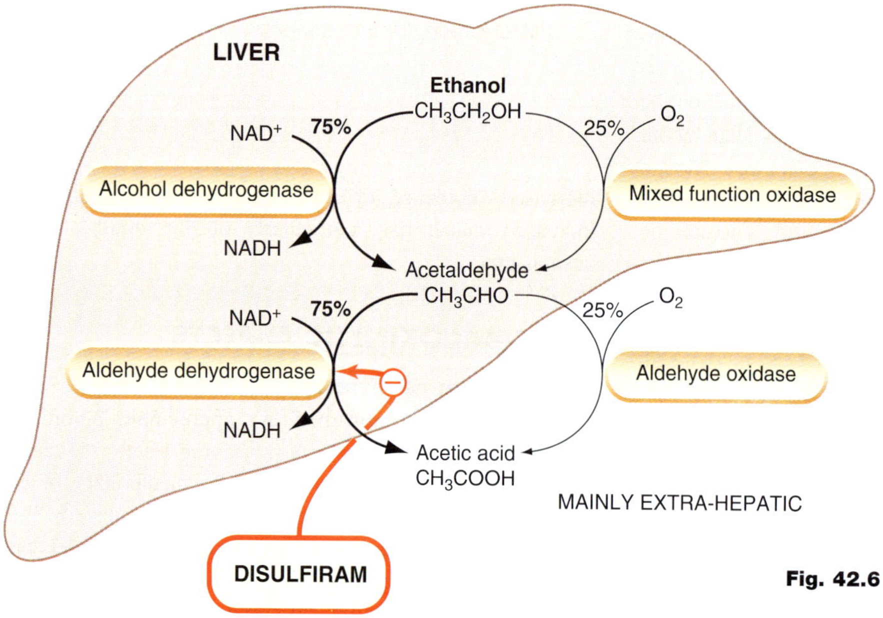

Fig. 42.6 Metabolism of ethanol.

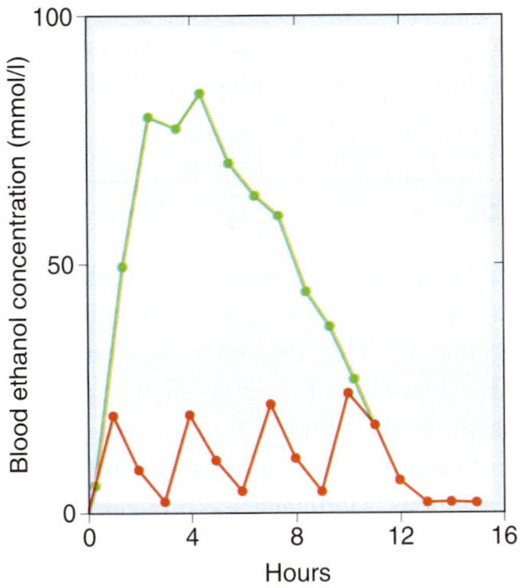

Fig. 42.7 Zero-order kinetics of ethanol elimination in rats. Rats were given ethanol orally (104 mmol/kg) either as a single dose, or as four divided doses. The single dose results in a much higher and more sustained blood ethanol concentration than the same quantity given as divided doses. Note that, after the single dose, ethanol concentration declines linearly, the rate of decline being similar after a small or large dose, because of the saturation phenomenon. (From: Kalant H et al. 1975 Biochem Pharmacol 24: 431.)

disulfiram. In the presence of disulfiram, which produces no marked effect when given alone, ethanol consumption is followed by a severe reaction, comprising flushing, tachycardia, hyperventilation and considerable panic and distress, which is caused by excessive acetaldehyde accumulation in the bloodstream. This reaction is extremely unpleasant, but not harmful, and disulfiram can be used as aversion therapy to discourage people from taking ethanol. Some other drugs, notably oral hypoglycaemic agents of the sulfonylurea class (e.g. chlorpropamide; see Ch. 25) and certain antibacterial drugs (e.g. nitrofurantoin; see Ch. 45) also occasionally produce similar reactions to ethanol. Interestingly, a Chinese herbal medicine, used traditionally to cure alcoholics, contains **daidzin**, a specific inhibitor of aldehyde dehydrogenase. In hamsters (which spontaneously consume alcohol in amounts that would defeat even the hardest two-legged drinker, while remaining, as far as one can tell in a hamster, completely sober), daidzin markedly inhibits alcohol consumption (see Keung & Vallee, 1993).

Genetic factors

In 50% of Asians, an inactive genetic variant of one of the aldehyde dehydrogenase isoforms (ALDH-1) is expressed; these individuals experience a disulfiram-like reaction after alcohol, and the incidence of alcoholism in this group is extremely low. Conversely, an isoform of alcohol dehydrogenase with reduced activity is also common in Asians, and this is associated with excessive drinking behaviour (Tanaka et al., 1997).

Metabolism of ethanol

- Ethanol is metabolised mainly by the liver, first by alcohol dehydrogenase to acetaldehyde, then by aldehyde dehydrogenase to acetate. About 25% of the acetaldehyde is metabolised extrahepatically.
- Small amounts of ethanol are excreted in urine and expired air.
- Hepatic metabolism shows saturation kinetics, mainly because of limited availability of NAD^+. Maximal rate of ethanol metabolism is about 10 ml/hour. Thus, plasma concentration falls linearly rather than exponentially.
- Acetaldehyde may produce toxic effects. Inhibition of aldehyde dehydrogenase by disulfiram accentuates nausea etc., caused by acetaldehyde, and can be used in aversion therapy.
- Methanol is similarly metabolised to formic acid, which is toxic, especially to retina.
- Asian races show a high rate of genetic polymorphism of alcohol and aldehyde dehydrogenase, associated with alcoholism and alcohol intolerance, respectively.

Metabolism and toxicity of methanol

▼ Methanol is metabolised in the same way as ethanol but produces formaldehyde instead of acetaldehyde from the first oxidation step. Formaldehyde is more reactive than acetaldehyde and reacts rapidly with proteins, causing the inactivation of enzymes involved in the tricarboxylic acid cycle. It is converted to another toxic metabolite, formic acid. This, unlike acetic acid, cannot be utilised in the tricarboxylic acid cycle and is liable to cause tissue damage. Conversion of alcohols to aldehydes occurs not only in the liver but also in the retina, catalysed by the dehydrogenase responsible for retinol–retinal conversion. Formation of formaldehyde in the retina accounts for one of the main toxic effects of methanol, namely blindness, which can occur after ingestion of as little as 10 g. Formic acid production, and derangement of the tricarboxylic acid cycle, also produce severe acidosis. Methanol is used as an industrial solvent and also to adulterate industrial ethanol in order to make it unfit to drink. Methanol poisoning is quite common, and it is treated by administration of large doses of ethanol, which acts to retard methanol metabolism by competition for alcohol dehydrogenase. This is often done in conjunction with haemodialysis to remove unchanged methanol, which has a small volume of distribution.

TOLERANCE AND DEPENDENCE

Tolerance to the effects of ethanol can be demonstrated in both humans and experimental animals, to the extent of a two- to threefold reduction in potency occurring over 1–3 weeks of continuing ethanol administration. A small component of this is the result of more rapid elimination of ethanol. The major component is tissue tolerance, which accounts for a roughly twofold decrease in potency and which can be observed in vitro (e.g. by measuring the inhibitory effect of ethanol on transmitter release from synaptosomes) as well as in vivo. The mechanism of this tolerance is not known for certain (see Little, 1991). Ethanol tolerance is associated with tolerance to many anaesthetic agents, and alcoholics are often difficult to anaesthetise with drugs such as halothane.

Chronic ethanol administration produces various changes in CNS neurons, which tend to oppose the acute cellular effects that it produces (see above). There is a small reduction in the density of $GABA_A$-receptors, and a proliferation of voltage-gated calcium channels and NMDA-receptors. The effect on calcium channels has received particular attention (see Charness et al., 1989). The acute effect of ethanol (see above) is to reduce Ca^{2+} entry through voltage-gated calcium channels, and thus to reduce transmitter release. During chronic exposure to ethanol, Ca^{2+} entry recovers owing to a proliferation of calcium channels, and when ethanol is withdrawn, depolarisation-evoked Ca^{2+} entry and transmitter release are increased above normal, which is possibly associated with the physical withdrawal symptoms. Consistent with this explanation, calcium-channel-blocking drugs of the dihydropyridine type (see Ch. 17) reduce the effects of ethanol withdrawal in experimental animals (see Little, 1991).

A well-defined physical abstinence syndrome develops in response to ethanol withdrawal. As with most other dependence-producing drugs, this is probably important as a short-term factor in sustaining the drug habit, but other (mainly psychological) factors are more important in the longer term. The physical abstinence syndrome usually subsides in a few days, but the craving for ethanol and the tendency to relapse last for very much longer.

The physical abstinence syndrome in humans, in severe form, develops after about 8 hours. In the first stage, the main symptoms are tremor, nausea, sweating, fever and, sometimes, hallucinations. These last for about 24 hours. This phase may be followed by epilepsy-like seizures. Over the next few days, the condition of 'delirium tremens' develops, in which the patient becomes confused, agitated and often aggressive, and may suffer much more severe hallucinations. A similar syndrome of central and autonomic hyperactivity can be produced in experimental animals by ethanol withdrawal.

Alcohol dependence ('alcoholism') is common (4–5% of the population) and, as with smoking, difficult to treat effectively. The main pharmacological approaches (see Zernig et al., 1997; Table 42.2) are as follows:

- To alleviate the acute abstinence syndrome during 'drying out': **benzodiazepines** (see Ch. 36) are effective; **clonidine** and **propranolol**, are also useful. Clonidine (α_2-adrenoceptor agonist) is believed to act by inhibiting the exaggerated transmitter release that occurs during withdrawal, while propranolol (β-adrenoceptor antagonist) blocks the effects of excessive sympathetic activity.
- To render alcohol consumption unpleasant: **disulfiram** (see above).
- To reduce alcohol-induced reward: **naltrexone** (opiate antagonist) is effective, for reasons that are poorly understood.
- To reduce craving: **acamprosate** is used. This recently introduced compound, a taurine analogue, is a weak antagonist at NMDA-receptors and may work by interfering in some way with synaptic plasicity. Several clinical trials have shown it to improve the success rate in achieving alcohol abstinence, with few unwanted effects.

CANNABIS

Extracts of the hemp plant, *Cannabis sativa*, which grows freely in temperate and tropical regions, contain the active substance Δ^9-tetrahydrocannabinol (THC; Fig. 42.8). Marijuana is the name given to the dried leaves and flower heads, prepared as a smoking mixture; hashish is the extracted resin. For centuries, these substances have been used for various medicinal purposes and as intoxicant preparations. Marijuana was brought to North America by immigrants, mainly in the 19th century, and began to be regarded as a social problem in the early years of this century; it was banned during the 1930s. Its use increased dramatically in the 1960s, and recent figures suggest that about 15% of the adult population in America and Western Europe have taken cannabis at some time, with a much higher proportion (close to 50%) among teenagers and young adults. A good scientific account is given by Iversen & Snyder (2000).

CHEMICAL ASPECTS

Cannabis extracts contain numerous related compounds, called cannabinoids, most of which are insoluble in water. The most abundant cannabinoids are THC, its precursor *cannabidiol*, and *cannabinol*, which is formed spontaneously from THC. THC is the most active pharmacologically, and also the most abundant, constituting about 1–10% by weight of marijuana and hashish preparations. A metabolite, 11-hydroxy-THC, is more active than

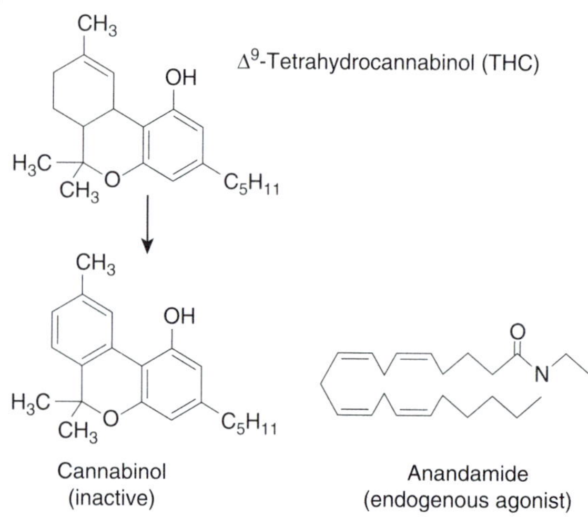

Fig. 42.8 Structure of cannabinoids. Anandamide is an arachidonic acid derivative that is present in the brain and believed to be an endogenous agonist for cannabinoid receptors.

THC itself and probably contributes to the pharmacological effect. Radioimmunoassays have been developed for cannabinoids, but they lack sufficient chemical specificity to be able to distinguish THC from numerous other cannabinoids found in crude extracts, and from the various metabolites that are formed in vivo. Therefore, the assay of pharmacologically active THC in biological fluids still presents a problem.

PHARMACOLOGICAL EFFECTS

THC acts mainly on the CNS, producing a mixture of psychotomimetic and depressant effects, together with various centrally mediated peripheral autonomic effects (see review by Dewey, 1986).

The main subjective effects in humans consist of:

- a feeling of relaxation and well-being, similar to the effect of ethanol, but without the accompanying aggression
- a feeling of sharpened sensory awareness, with sounds and sights seeming more intense and fantastic.

These effects are similar to, but usually less pronounced than, those produced by psychotomimetic drugs such as LSD (lysergic acid diethylamide; see Ch. 41). Subjects report that time passes extremely slowly. The alarming sensations and paranoid delusions that often occur with LSD are seldom experienced after cannabis.

Central effects that can be directly measured in human and animal studies include:

- impairment of short-term memory, and simple learning tasks—subjective feelings of confidence and heightened creativity are not reflected in actual performance
- impairment of motor coordination (e.g. driving performance)
- catalepsy—the retention of fixed unnatural postures
- analgesia
- antiemetic action
- increased appetite.

The main peripheral effects of cannabis are:

- tachycardia, which can be prevented by drugs that block sympathetic transmission
- vasodilatation, which is particularly marked on the scleral and conjunctival vessels, producing a bloodshot appearance characteristic of cannabis smokers
- reduction of intraocular pressure
- bronchodilatation.

RECEPTORS AND ENDOGENOUS LIGANDS

Cannabinoids, being highly lipid soluble, were originally thought to act in a similar way to general anaesthetic agents, but the identification of specific cannabinoid receptors in the brain and in the periphery dismissed this idea. Cannabinoid receptors (see Abood & Martin, 1996; Pertwee, 1997) are typical members of the family of G-protein-coupled receptors (see Ch. 3), linked to inhibition of adenylate cyclase. The receptors are also coupled to potassium channel activation and calcium channel inhibition, and thereby exert an inhibitory effect on transmitter release. These cellular effects closely resemble those of opioids. Brain cannabinoid receptors (CB_1 subtype) are abundant in the hippocampus (memory impairment), cerebellum and substantia nigra (motor disturbance), and mesolimbic dopamine pathways (reward), as well as in the cortex. The peripheral cannabinoid receptor (CB_2 subtype) shows only about 45% amino acid homology with CB_1 and is located mainly in the lymphoid system. This was an unexpected finding but may account for the inhibitory effects on immune function that have been reported with cannabis. The discovery of specific cannabinoid receptors in the brain naturally led to a search for an endogenous chemical mediator, and the discovery of *anandamide*, an amide derivative of arachidonic acid (see Fig. 42.8), which produces short-lasting cannabinoid-like effects when injected into the brain. The physiological role of this *endocannabinoid* system has attracted much recent interest (see Piomelli et al., 2000). The peripheral CB_2-receptor shows a different pharmacological specificity from the CB_1-receptor, but so far very little is known about its function. Agonists and antagonists specific for each type have been developed (see Pertwee, 1997). A potent CB_1-receptor antagonist, SR141716A, produces effects opposite to those of cannabinoid agonists, namely increased locomotor activity, improved short-term memory, as well as enhanced transmitter release in peripheral tissues, implying a degree of tonic activation of CB_1-receptors under physiological conditions.

The effects of cannabis on intraocular pressure, bronchial smooth muscle, pain perception and the vomiting reflex are of potential therapeutic value, and certain cannabinoid derivatives, e.g. **nabilone**, have been developed as therapeutic agents. The pronounced central effects produced by these compounds, including their possible addictive properties (see below), limit their usefulness. As there is little evidence for subtypes of the CB_1-receptor—which might offer the possibility of developing ligands with more selective central effects—therapeutic developments on this front are currently stalled.

TOLERANCE AND DEPENDENCE

Tolerance to cannabis, and physical dependence, occur only to a minor degree and mainly in heavy users. The abstinence symptoms are similar to those of ethanol or opiate withdrawal, namely nausea, agitation, irritability, confusion, tachycardia, sweating, etc. but are relatively mild and do not result in a compulsive urge to take the drug. Psychological dependence does not seem to occur with cannabis, and overall it cannot be classified as addictive (see review by Abood & Martin, 1992).

PHARMACOKINETIC ASPECTS

The effect of cannabis, taken by smoking or by intravenous injection, takes about 1 hour to develop fully and lasts for 2–3 hours. A small fraction is converted to 11-hydroxy-THC, which is more active than THC itself, but most is converted mainly to inactive metabolites. It is partly conjugated and undergoes

Cannabis

- Main active constituent is Δ^9-tetrahydro cannabinol (THC), though pharmacologically active metabolites may be important.
- Actions on CNS include both depressant and psychotomimetic effects.
- Subjectively, subjects experience euphoria and a feeling of relaxation, with sharpened sensory awareness.
- Objective tests show impairment of learning, memory and motor performance.
- THC also shows analgesic and antiemetic activity, as well as causing catalepsy and hypothermia in animal tests.
- Peripheral actions include vasodilatation, reduction of intraocular pressure and bronchodilatation.
- Cannabinoid receptors belong to the G-protein-coupled receptor family, linked to inhibition of adenylate cyclase and effects on calcium and potassium channel function, causing inhibition of synaptic transmission. The brain receptor (CB_1) differs from the peripheral receptor (CB_2), which is expressed mainly in cells of the immune system. Selective agonists and antagonists have been developed.
- Anandamide, an arachidonic acid derivative, is an endogenous ligand for the CNS cannabinoid receptor; its function has not yet been ascertained.
- Cannabinoids are less liable than opiates, nicotine or alcohol to cause dependence but may have long-term psychological effects.
- Nabilone, a THC analogue, has been developed for its antiemetic property.
- Though cannabinoids are not available for clinical use, trials are in progress for symptomatic treatment of multiple sclerosis and AIDS.

enterohepatic recirculation. Being highly lipophilic, THC and its metabolites are sequestered in body fat, and excretion continues for several days after a single dose.

ADVERSE EFFECTS

THC is relatively safe in overdose, producing drowsiness and confusion, but not respiratory or cardiovascular effects that threaten life. In this respect, it is safer than most abused substances, particularly opiates and ethanol. Even in low doses, THC and synthetic derivatives such as nabilone produce euphoria and drowsiness, sometimes accompanied by sensory distortion and hallucinations. These effects, together with the legal restrictions on the use of THC, preclude the widespread therapeutic use of cannabinoids.

THC produces teratogenic and mutagenic effects in rodents, and an increased incidence of chromosome breaks in circulating white cells has been reported in humans. Such breaks are, however, by no means unique to cannabis, and epidemiological studies have not shown any increased risk of fetal malformation or cancer among cannabis users.

Certain endocrine effects occur in humans, notably a decrease in plasma testosterone and a reduction of sperm count. One study showed a reduction of more than 50% in both plasma testosterone and sperm count in subjects smoking 10 or more marijuana cigarettes per week.

It is very difficult to assess the evidence that cannabis causes long-term psychological changes. It has been suggested that it can cause schizophrenia, and that it leads to a gradually developing state of apathy and underachievement, but it is very difficult to prove causation even where a positive association has been found.

The long-running argument over the legalisation of cannabis centres mainly on the seriousness of these adverse effects. Opponents of legalisation argue that it would be folly to change the law in favour of the use by the public at large of a substance which could turn out to have serious toxic effects. Proponents of a change argue that the present law is clearly ineffective and encourages crime, and that cannabis is undoubtedly safer than either ethanol or tobacco.

CLINICAL USE OF CANNABIS—A CONTROVERSIAL TOPIC

Anecdotal evidence suggests that smoking cannabis may be efficacious in a number of conditions, particularly the following: relief of pain and muscle spasms associated with multiple sclerosis; relief of other types of chronic neuropathic pain, including AIDS-related pain; improvement of appetite and prevention of wasting in AIDS; relief of chemotherapy-induced nausea (see British Medical Association, 1997). Currently, the use of cannabis is illegal in most countries, and cannabis products cannot be prescribed for medical use. Responding to public pressure, the Canadian government has relaxed these restrictions, allowing cannabis to be used for certain medical purposes. In UK, official clinical trials are in progress, though strict toxicological evaluation will be required before any product can be registered. In the USA, the federal government has so far resisted pressure to liberalise the use of cannabis.

REFERENCES AND FURTHER READING

Abood M E, Martin B R 1992 Neurobiology of marijuana abuse. Trends Pharmacol Sci 13: 201–206

Balfour D J K, Fagerstrom K O 1996 Pharmacology of nicotine and its therapeutic use in smoking cessation and neurodegenerative disorders. Pharmacol Ther 72: 51–81 (*Review of the pharmacology of nicotine and its usefulness as replacement therapy*)

Benowitz N L 1993 Nicotine replacement therapy. Drugs 45: 157–170

Benowitz N L 1996 Pharmacology of nicotine: addiction and therapeutics. Annu Rev Pharmacol 36: 597–613 (*General review article, including information on potential therapeutic uses of nicotine other than reduction of smoking*)

British Medical Association (Morgan D R, Ashton C (eds)) 1997 Therapeutic uses of cannabis. Harwood Medical, Amsterdam (*Report on potential clinical uses of cannabis, which led to formal trials being initiated*)

Charness M E, Simon R P, Greenberg D A 1989 Ethanol and the nervous system. N Engl J Med 321: 442–454

Dewey W L 1986 Cannabinoid pharmacology. Pharmacol Rev 38: 151–178

Friedman L, Fleming N F, Roberts D H, Hyman S E 1996 Source book of substance abuse and addiction. Williams & Wilkins, Baltimore, MD (*Useful source of factual information*)

Groenbaek M et al. 1994 Influence of sex, age, body mass index and smoking on alcohol intake and mortality. Br Med J 308: 302–306 (*Large-scale Danish study showing reduced coronary mortality at moderate levels of drinking with increase at high levels*)

Hyman S E, Malenka R C 2001 Addiction and the brain: the neurobiology of compulsion and its persistence. Nat Rev Neurosci 2: 695–705 (*Reviews long-term changes in brain associated with addiction, emphasising semi-permanent alterations in gene expression*)

Iversen LL, Snyder S H 2000 The science of marijuana. Oxford University Press, New York (*Short textbook presenting all aspects of cannabis*)

Jones S, Sudweeks S, Yakel J L 1999 Nicotinic receptors in the brain: correlating physiology with function. Trends Neurosci 22: 555–561

Keung W-M, Vallee B L 1993 Daidzin and daidzein suppress free-choice ethanol intake by Syrian golden hamsters. Proc Natl Acad Sci USA 90: 10008–10012

Koob g F 1996 Drug addiction: the yin and yang of hedonic homeostasis. Neuron 16: 893–896

Lieber C S 1995 Medical disorders of alcoholism. N Engl J Med 333: 1058–1065 (*Review focussing on ethanol-induced liver damage in relation to ethanol metabolism*)

Lister R G, Nutt D J 1987 Is Ro 15-4513 a specific alcohol antagonist? Trends Neurosci 6: 223–225

Little H J 1991 Mechanisms that may underlie the behavioural effects of ethanol. Prog Neurobiol 36: 171–194

Lovinger D M 1997 Alcohols and neurotransmitters-gated ion channels: past present and future. Naunyn-Schmiedeberg Arch Pharmacol 356: 267–282 (*Review article arguing that alcohol effects depend on interaction with synaptic ion channels*)

Maldonado R, Saiardi A, Valverde O, Samad T A, Roques B P, Borelli E 1997 Absence of opiate rewarding effects in mice lacking dopamine D_2 receptors. Nature 388: 586–589 (*Use of transgenic animals to demonstrate role of dopamine receptors in reward properties of opiates*)

Mottram D 1988 Drugs in sport. E & F N Spon, London

Nestler E J 2001a Molecular basis of long-term plasticity underlying addiction. Nat Rev Neurosci 2: 119–128 (*Good review article focussing on long-term changes in gene expression associated with drug dependence*)

Nestler E J 2001b Genes and addiction. Nat Genet 26: 277–281 (*Review of determined, and ongoing, efforts to identify the genes involved*)

O'Brien C P 1997 A range of research-based pharmacotherapies for addiction. Science 278: 66–70 (*Useful overview of pharmacological approaches to treatment*)

Pertwee R G 1997 Pharmacology of cannabinoid CB_1 and CB_2 receptors. Pharmacol Ther 74: 129–180 (*Comprehensive review of properties of cannabinoid receptors and their ligands*)

Peto R, Lopez A D, Boreham J, Thun M, Heath C, Doll R 1996 Mortality from smoking worldwide. Br Med Bull 52: 12–21.

Peto R, Chen Z-M, Boreham J 1999 Tobacco—the growing epidemic. Nat Med 3: 15–17

Picciotto M R, Zoli M, Rimondini R et al. 1998 Acetylcholine receptors containing the β_2 subunit are involved in the reinforcing properties of nicotine. Nature 391: 173–177 (*Shows that knocking out the β_2-subunit of the nicotinic acetylcholine receptor, which is expressed by mesolimbic neurons, abolishes the normal reward and self-administration properties of nicotine*)

Piomelli D, Giffrida A, Calignano F, de Foscea R 2000 The endocannabinoid system as a target for therapeutic drugs. Trends Pharmacol Sci 21: 218–224.

Royal College of Physicians Reports 1971, 1977 Smoking or health. Pitman Medical, Tunbridge Wells

Shuckit M A 1995 Drug and alcohol abuse. Plenum Medical, New York

Spanagel & Weiss 1999 The dopamine hyopthesis of reward: past and current research. Trends Neurosci 22: 521–527 (*Summarises evidence for activation of mesolimbic dopamine pathways as a factor in drug dependence*)

Tabakoff B, Hoffman P L 1996 Alcohol addiction: an enigma among us. Neuron 16: 909–912 (*Review of alcohol actions at the cellular and molecular level—ignore the silly title*)

Tanaka F, Shiratori Y, Yokusuka O, Imazeki F, Tsukada Y, Omata M 1997 Polymorphism of alcohol-metabolizing genes affects drinking behaviour and alcoholic liver disease in Japanese men. Alcohol Clin Exp Res 21: 596–601 (*Describes polymorphism of aldehyde and alcohol dehydrogenases, and their effect on drinking behaviour*)

Zernig G, Fabisch K, Fabisch H 1997 Pharmacotherapy of alcohol dependence. Trends Pharmacol Sci 18: 229–231 (*Short review of drug therapies used in alcoholism*)

43 Local anaesthetics

Overview 612

Local anaesthetics 612

Other drugs that affect sodium channels 616
— Tetrodotoxin and saxitoxin 616
— Agents that affect sodium channel gating 618

OVERVIEW

As described in Chapter 4, the property of electrical excitability is what enables the membranes of nerve and muscle cells to generate propagated action potentials, which are essential for communication in the nervous system and for the initiation of mechanical activity in cardiac and striated muscle. Electrical excitability depends mainly on voltage-gated sodium channels, which open transiently when the membrane is depolarised. Here we discuss local anaesthetics, which act mainly by blocking sodium channels, and mention briefly other drugs that affect sodium channel function

There are, broadly speaking, two ways in which channel function may be modified, namely block of the channels and modification of gating behaviour. Either mechanism can cause an increase or a decrease of electrical excitability. Thus, blocking sodium channels reduces excitability, whereas block of potassium channels tends to increase it. Similarly, an agent that affects sodium channel gating so as to increase channel opening will tend to increase excitability and vice versa.

LOCAL ANAESTHETICS

Though many drugs block voltage-sensitive sodium channels and inhibit the generation of the action potential, the only drugs in this category that are clinically useful are the local anaesthetics, various antiepileptic drugs (see Ch. 39) and class I antidysrhythmic drugs (see Ch. 17).

History

Coca leaves have been chewed for their psychotropic effects for thousands of years (see Ch. 41) by South American Indians, who knew about the numbing effect they produced on the mouth and tongue. Cocaine was isolated in 1860 and proposed as a local anaesthetic for surgical procedures. Sigmund Freud, who tried unsuccessfully to make use of its 'psychic energising' power, gave some cocaine to his ophthalmologist friend in Vienna, Carl Köller, who reported in 1884 that reversible corneal anaesthesia could be produced by dropping cocaine into the eye. The idea was rapidly taken up, and within a few years cocaine anaesthesia was introduced into dentistry and general surgery. A synthetic substitute, **procaine** was discovered in 1905, and many other useful compounds were later developed.

Chemical aspects

Local anaesthetic molecules consist of an aromatic part linked by an ester or amide bond to a basic side-chain (Fig. 43.1). They are weak bases, with pK_a values mainly in the range 8–9; consequently, they are mainly, but not completely, ionised at physiological pH. This is important in relation to their ability to penetrate the nerve sheath and axon membrane; quaternary derivatives, which are fully ionised irrespective of pH, are ineffective as local anaesthetics. **Benzocaine**, an atypical local anaesthetic, has no basic group.

The presence of the ester or amide bond in local anaesthetic molecules is important because of its susceptibility to metabolic hydrolysis. The ester-containing compounds are usually inactivated in the plasma and tissues (mainly liver) by non-specific esterases. Amides are more stable, and these anaesthetics generally have longer plasma half-lives.

Mechanism of action

Local anaesthetics block the initiation and propagation of action potentials by preventing the voltage-dependent increase in Na^+ conductance (see Fig. 4.5). Though they exert a variety of non-specific effects on membrane function, their main action is to block sodium channels, which they do by physically plugging the transmembrane pore, interacting with residues of the S6

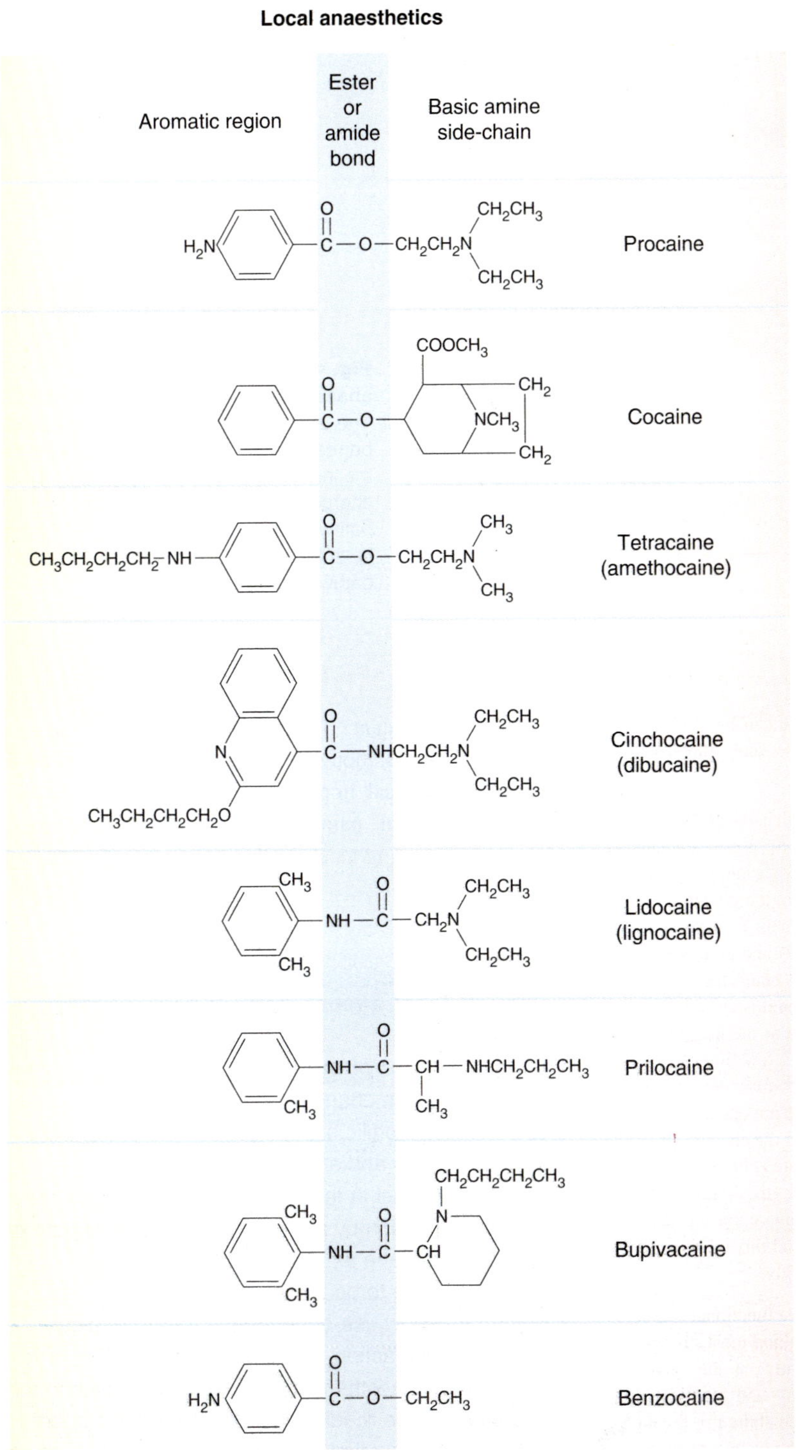

Fig. 43.1 Structures of local anaesthetics. The general structure of local anaesthetic molecules consists of aromatic group (left), ester or amide group (shaded) and amine group (right). Benzocaine is an exception, lacking a side-chain amino group.

transmembrane helical domain (see Strichartz & Ritchie, 1987; Hille, 1992; Ragsdale et al., 1994).

▼ Local anaesthetic activity is strongly pH dependent, being increased at alkaline pH (i.e. when the proportion of ionised molecules is low) and vice versa. This is because the compound needs to penetrate the nerve sheath and the axon membrane to reach the inner end of the sodium channel (where the local anaesthetic-binding site resides). Because the ionised form is not membrane permeant, penetration is very poor at acid pH. Once inside the axon, it is the ionised form of the local anaesthetic molecule that

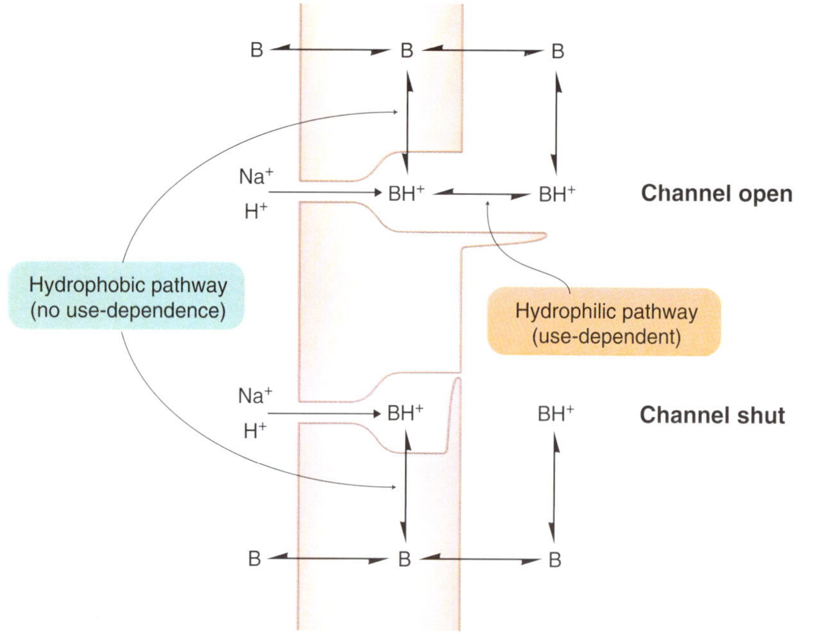

Fig. 43.2 Interaction of local anaesthetics with sodium channels. The blocking site within the channel can be reached via the open channel gate on the inner surface of the membrane by the charged species BH^+ (hydrophilic pathway), or directly from the membrane by the uncharged species B (hydrophilic pathway).

binds to the channel (Fig. 43.2). This pH-dependence can be clinically important, since inflamed tissues are often acidic and, therefore, somewhat resistant to local anaesthetic agents.

Further analysis of local anaesthesic action (see Strichartz & Ritchie, 1987) has shown that many drugs exhibit the property of 'use-dependent' block of sodium channels, as well as affecting, to some extent, the gating of the channels. Use-dependence means that the more the channels are opened, the greater the block becomes. It is a prominent feature of the action of many class I antidysrhythmic drugs (Ch. 17) and antiepileptic drugs (Ch. 39); it occurs because the blocking molecule enters the channel much more readily when the channel is open than when it is closed. With quaternary local anaesthetics working from the inside of the membrane, the channels must be cycled through their open state a few times before the blocking effect appears. With tertiary local anaesthetics, by comparison, block can develop even if the channels are not open, and it is likely that the blocking molecule (uncharged) can enter the channel either directly from the membrane phase or via the open gate (Fig. 43.2). The relative importance of these two blocking pathways—the hydrophobic pathway via the membrane, and the hydrophilic pathway via the inner mouth of the channel—varies according to the lipid solubility of the drug, and the degree of use-dependence varies correspondingly.

As discussed in Chapter 4, the channel can exist in three functional states: resting, open and inactivated. Many local anaesthetics bind most strongly to the inactivated state of the channel. Consequently, at any given membrane potential, the equilibrium between resting and inactivated channels will, in the presence of a local anaesthetic, be shifted in favour of the inactivated state, and this factor contributes to the overall blocking effect. The passage of a train of action potentials causes the channels to cycle through the open and inactivated states, both of which are more likely to bind local anaesthetic molecules than the resting state; thus, both mechanisms contribute to use-dependence.

In general, local anaesthetics block conduction in small-diameter nerve fibres more readily than in large fibres. Since nociceptive impulses are carried by Aδ- and C-fibres, pain sensation is blocked more readily than other sensory modalities (touch, proprioception, etc.). Motor axons, being large in diameter, are also relatively resistant. The differences in sensitivity among different nerve fibres, though easily measured experimentally, are not of much practical importance, and it is rarely possible to produce a block of pain sensation without affecting other modalities and causing local paralysis.

Action of local anaesthetics (LAs)

- LAs block action potential generation by blocking sodium channels.
- LAs are amphiphilic molecules, with a hydrophobic aromatic group and a basic amine group.
- LAs probably act in their cationic form but must reach their site of action by penetrating the nerve sheath and axonal membrane as unionised species; they, therefore, have to be weak bases.
- Many LAs show use-dependence (depth of block increases with action potential frequency). This arises:
  - —because anaesthetic molecules gain access to the channel more readily when the channel is open
  - —because anaesthetic molecules have higher affinity for inactivated than for resting channels.
- Use-dependence is mainly of importance in relation to antidysrhythmic and antiepileptic effects of sodium channel blockers.
- LAs block conduction in the following order: small myelinated axons, non-myelinated axons, large myelinated axons. Nociceptive and sympathetic transmission is thus blocked first.

Table 43.1 Properties of local anaesthetics

Drug	Onset	Duration	Tissue penetration	Plasma half-life (h)	Main unwanted effects	Notes
Cocaine	Medium	Medium	Good	~1	Cardiovascular and CNS effects owing to block of amine uptake	Rarely used, only as spray for upper respiratory tract
Procaine	Medium	Short	Poor	<1	CNS: restlessness, shivering, anxiety, occasionally convulsions followed by respiratory depression CVS: bradycardia and decreased caridac output, vasodilatation, which can cause cardiovascular collapse	The first synthetic agent No longer used
Lidocaine (lignocaine)	Rapid	Medium	Good	~2	As procaine, but less tendency to cause CNS effects	Widely used for local anaesthesia Also used intravenously for treating ventricular dysrythmias (Ch. 17) Mepivacaine is similar
Tetracaine (amethocaine)	Very slow	Long	Moderate	~1	As lidocaine	Used mainly for spinal and corneal anaesthesia
Bupivacaine	Slow	Long	Moderate	~2	As lidocaine, but greater cardiotoxicity	Widely used because of long duration of action Ropivacaine is similar, with less cardiotoxocity Levobupivacaine, recently introduced, causes less cardiotoxicity and CNS depression than the racemate
Prilocaine	Medium	Medium	Moderate	~2	No vasodilator activity Can cause methaemoglobinaemia	Widely used, not for obstetric analgesia because of risk of neonatal methaemoglobinaemia

Local anaesthetics, as their name implies, are mainly used to produce local nerve block. In concentrations too low to cause nerve block, however, they are able to suppress the spontaneous discharge in sensory neurons that is believed to be responsible for neuropathic pain (see Ch. 40). Drugs undergoing trial for oral use as analgesics in such pain states include two antidysrhythmic drugs, **tocainide** and **mexiletine** (see Ch. 17).

The properties of individual local anaesthetic drugs are summarised in Table 43.1.

Unwanted effects

The main unwanted effects of local anaesthetics involve the central nervous system (CNS) and cardiovascular system, and they constitute the main source of hazard when local anaesthetics are used clinically. Most local anaesthetics produce a mixture of stimulant and depressant effects on the CNS, often resulting in restlessness and tremor, with subjective effects ranging from confusion to extreme agitation. The tremor can progress to actual convulsions, and further increasing the dose produces CNS depression. The main threat to life comes from respiratory depression in this phase. The only local anaesthetic with markedly different CNS effects is **cocaine** (see Ch. 41), which produces euphoria at doses well below those that cause other CNS effects. This relates to its specific effect on monoamine uptake, an effect not shared by other local anaesthetics. **Procaine** is particularly liable to produce unwanted central effects and has been superseded in clinical use by agents such as **lidocaine** and **prilocaine**, the central effects of which are much less pronounced. Studies with **bupivacaine** (Table 43.1), a widely used long-acting local anaesthetic prepared as a racemic mixture of two optical isomers, suggested that its CNS and cardiac effects are mainly caused by the *S*(+)-isomer. The *R*(−)-isomer (**levobupivacaine**) proved to have a better margin of safety and has now been introduced.

The cardiovascular effects of local anaesthetics result mainly from myocardial depression and vasodilatation. Reduction of myocardial contractility probably results indirectly from an inhibition of the Na^+ current in cardiac muscle (see Ch. 17). The resulting decrease of $[Na^+]_i$, in turn, reduces intracellular Ca^{2+} stores (see Ch. 4), and this reduces the force of contraction. The antidysrhythmic effect of some local anaesthetics (especially lidocaine) is clinically useful.

Vasodilatation, mainly affecting arterioles, results partly from a direct effect on vascular smooth muscle and partly from inhibition of the sympathetic nervous system. The combined myocardial depression and vasodilatation leads to a fall in blood pressure, which may be sudden and life threatening. Cocaine is an exception in respect of its cardiovascular effects, because of its ability to inhibit noradrenaline reuptake (see Ch. 11). This produces an enhancement of sympathetic activity, leading to tachycardia, increased cardiac output, vasoconstriction and increased arterial pressure.

Though local anaesthetics are usually administered in such a way as to minimise their spread to other parts of the body, they are ultimately absorbed into the systemic circulation. They may also be injected into veins or arteries by accident. The most dangerous unwanted effects result from actions on the CNS and cardiovascular system discussed above, namely restlessness and convulsions followed by respiratory depression, and hypotension, or even cardiac arrest. Hypersensitivity reactions sometimes occur with local anaesthetics, usually in the form of allergic dermatitis, but rarely as an acute anaphylactic reaction. Other unwanted effects that are specific to particular drugs include mucosal irritation (cocaine) and methaemoglobinaemia (which occurs after large doses of **prilocaine**, because of the production of a toxic metabolite).

Pharmacokinetic aspects

Local anaesthetics vary a good deal in the rapidity with which they penetrate tissues, and this affects the rate at which they cause nerve block when injected into tissues and the rate of onset of, and recovery from, anaesthesia (Table 43.1). It also affects their usefulness as surface anaesthetics for application to mucous membranes.

Most of the ester-linked local anaesthetics (e.g. **tetracaine** (amethocaine)) are rapidly hydrolysed by plasma cholinesterase, and their plasma half-life is short. Procaine—no longer used—is hydrolysed to *p*-aminobenzoic acid, a folate precursor that interferes with the antibacterial effect of sulfonamides (see Ch. 51). The amide-linked drugs (e.g. lidocaine and prilocaine) are metabolised mainly in the liver, usually by N-dealkylation rather than cleavage of the amide bond, and the metabolites are often pharmacologically active.

Benzocaine is an unusual local anaesthetic of very low solubility that is used as a dry powder to dress painful skin ulcers. The drug is slowly released and produces long-lasting surface anaesthesia.

Unwanted effects and pharmacokinetics of local anaesthetics (LAs)

- LAs are either esters or amides. Esters are rapidly hydrolysed by plasma cholinesterase, and amides are metabolised in the liver. Plasma half-lives are generally short, about 1–2 hours.
- Unwanted effects result mainly from escape of LAs into systemic circulation.
- Main unwanted effects are:
  - —CNS effects, agitation, confusion, tremors progressing to convulsions and respiratory depression
  - —cardiovascular effects, namely myocardial depression and vasodilatation, leading to fall in blood pressure
  - —occasional hypersensitivity reactions.
- LAs vary in the rapidity with which they penetrate tissues, and in their duration of action. Lidocaine penetrates tissues readily and is suitable for surface application; bupivacaine has a particularly long duration of action.

The routes of administration, uses and main adverse effects of local anaesthetics are summarised in Table 43.2.

Future directions

Currently available local anaesthetic agents do not distinguish between the many sodium channel subtypes that are known to be expressed in different tissues (see Ch. 4). It is expected that, with the molecular characterisation of these channels and a better understanding of their role in pathophysiological situations, selective blocking agents can be developed for use in a wide variety of clinical situations, including epilepsy, neurodegenerative diseases, stroke, neuropathic pain, myopathies, etc., which are discussed elsewhere in this book. There is much activity in this area, so stay tuned.

OTHER DRUGS THAT AFFECT SODIUM CHANNELS

TETRODOTOXIN AND SAXITOXIN

▼ We should not be surprised that nature, rather than medicinal chemistry, has provided the most potent and selective agents that block sodium channels of excitable tissues. Tetrodotoxin (TTX) is produced by a marine bacterium and accumulates in the tissues of a poisonous Pacific fish, the puffer fish, so called because when alarmed it inflates itself to an almost spherical spiny ball. It is evidently a species highly preoccupied with defence, but the Japanese are not easily put off and the puffer fish is regarded by them as a special delicacy. To serve it in public restaurants, however, the chef must be registered as sufficiently skilled in removing

Table 43.2 Methods of administration, uses and adverse effects of local anesthetics (LAs)

Method	Uses	Drugs	Notes and adverse effects
Surface anaesthesia	Nose, mouth, bronchial tree (usually in spray form), cornea, urinary tract Not effective for skin[a]	Lidocaine, tetracaine, (amethocaine) dibucaine, benzocaine	Risk of systemic toxicity when high concentrations and large areas are involved
Infiltration anaesthesia	Direct injection into tissues to reach nerve branches and terminals Used in minor surgery	Most	**Epinephrine (adrenaline)** or **felypressin** often added as vasoconstrictors (not with fingers or toes, for fear of causing ischaemic tissue damage) Only suitable for small areas; otherwise, serious risk of systemic toxicity
Intravenous regional anaesthesia	LA injected intravenously distal to a pressure cuff to arrest blood flow; remains effective until the circulation is restored Used for limb surgery	Mainly lidocaine, prilocaine	Risk of systemic toxicity when cuff is released prematurely; risk is small if cuff remains inflated for at least 20 minutes
Nerve-block anaesthesia	LA is injected close to nerve trunks (e.g. brachial plexus, intercostal or dental nerves) to produce a loss of sensation peripherally Used for surgery, dentistry, analgesia	Most	Less LA needed than for infiltration anaesthesia Accurate placement of the needle is important Onset of anaesthesia may be slow Duration of anaesthesia may be increased by addition of vasoconstrictor
Spinal anaesthesia	LA injected into the subarachnoid space (containing CSF) to act on spinal roots and spinal cord Glucose sometimes added so that spread of LA can be limited by tilting patient Used for surgery to abdomen, pelvis or leg, mainly when general anesthesia cannot be used	Mainly lidocaine	Main risks are bradycardia and hypotension (owing to sympathetic block), respiratory depression (owing to effects on phrenic nerve or respiratory center); avoided by minimising cranial spread Postoperative urinary retention (block of pelvic autonomic outflow) is common
Epidural anaesthesia[b]	LA injected into epidural space, blocking spinal roots Uses as for spinal anesthesia; also for painless childbirth	Mainly lidocaine, bupivacaine	Unwanted effects similar to those of spinal anaesthesia but less probable, because longitudinal spread of LA is reduced Postoperative urinary retention common

[a]Surface anaesthesia does not work well on the skin, though a non-crystalline mixture of lidocaine and prilocaine (**eutectic mixture of local anesthetics** or **EMLA)** has been developed for application to the skin, producing complete anaesthesia in about 1 hour.
[b]Intrathecal or epidural administration of LA in combination with an opiate (see Ch. 40) produces more effective analgesia than can be achieved with the opiate alone. Only a small concentration of LA is needed, insufficient to produce appreciable loss of sensation or other side-effects. The mechanism of this synergism is unknown, but the procedure is proving useful in pain treatment.

the toxic organs (especially liver and ovaries) so as to make the flesh safe to eat. Accidental tetrodotoxin poisoning is quite common, nonetheless. Historical records of long sea-voyages often contained reference to attacks of severe weakness, progressing to complete paralysis and death, caused by eating puffer fish.

Saxitoxin (STX) is produced by a marine microorganism, which sometimes proliferates in very large numbers and even colours the sea, giving the 'red tide' phenomenon. At such times, marine shellfish can accumulate the toxin and become poisonous to humans.

These toxins, unlike conventional local anaesthetics, act exclusively from the outside of the membrane. Both are complex molecules, bearing a positively charged guanidinium moiety. The guanidinium ion is able to permeate voltage-sensitive sodium channels, and this part of the TTX or STX molecule lodges in the channel, while the rest of the molecule blocks its outer mouth. In contrast to the local anaesthetics, there is no interaction between the gating and blocking reactions with TTX or STX—their association and dissociation are independent of whether the channel is open or closed. Some voltage-sensitive sodium channels are insensitive to TTX, notably those of cardiac muscle and nociceptive peripheral sensory neurons, the latter being of interest as a possible target for novel analgesic agents (see Ch. 40).

TTX and STX are unsuitable for clinical use as local anaesthetics, being expensive to obtain from their exotic sources and poor at penetrating tissues because of their very low lipid solubility. They have, however, been important as experimental tools for the isolation and cloning of sodium channels (see Ch. 4).

AGENTS THAT AFFECT SODIUM CHANNEL GATING

▼ Various substances, mostly complex and ornate molecules, are known that modify sodium channel gating in such a way as to increase the probability of opening of the channels (see Hille, 1992). They include various toxins, mainly from frog skin (e.g. batrachotoxin), scorpion or sea anemone venoms, plant alkaloids such as veratridine, and insecticides such as DDT and the pyrethrins. They facilitate sodium channel activation, so that sodium channels open at the normal resting potential; they also inhibit inactivation, so the channels fail to close if the membrane remains depolarised. The membrane thus becomes hyperexcitable, and the action potential is prolonged. Spontaneous discharges occur at first, but the cells eventually become permanently depolarised and inexcitable. All of these substances affect the heart, producing extrasystoles and other dysrhythmias, culminating in fibrillation; they also cause spontaneous discharges in nerve and muscle, leading to twitching and convulsions. The very high lipid solubility of substances like DDT makes them effective as insecticides, for they are readily absorbed through the integument. Drugs in this class are useful as experimental tools for studying sodium channels but have no clinical uses.

REFERENCES AND FURTHER READING

Hille B 1992 Ionic channels of excitable membranes. Sinauer, Sunderland, MA (*Excellent clearly written textbook for those wanting more than the basic minimum*)

Ragsdale D R, McPhee J C, Scheuer T, Catterall W A 1994 Molecular determinants of state-dependent block of sodium channels by local anesthetics. Science 265: 1724–1728 (*Use of site-directed mutations of the sodium channel to show that local anaesthetics bind to residues in the S6 transmembrane domain*)

Strichartz G R, Ritchie J M 1987 The action of local anaesthetics on ion channels of excitable tissues. In: Strichartz G R (ed) Local anaesthetics. Handbook of experimental pharmacology. Springer-Verlag, Berlin, vol. 81, pp. 21–52 (*Excellent review of actions of local anaesthetics—other articles in the same volume cover more clinical aspects*)

SECTION 5

DRUGS USED IN THE TREATMENT OF INFECTIONS AND CANCER

44 Basic principles of chemotherapy

Overview 620

Background 620

The molecular basis of chemotherapy 620
Biochemical reactions as potential targets 621
The formed structures of the cell as potential targets 627

Resistance to antibacterial drugs 629
Genetic determinants of antibiotic resistance 629
Biochemical mechanisms of resistance to antibiotics 631
Current status of antibiotic resistance in bacteria 632

OVERVIEW

Agents that are selectively toxic to invading parasites are necessary to combat the many infectious conditions that humans are heir to: diseases caused by viruses, bacteria, protozoa, fungi and helminths. The use of drugs with selective toxicity against these invading parasites is termed *chemotherapy and the development of such agents during the past 80 years constitutes one of the most important therapeutic advances in the history of medicine. The feasibility of such selective toxicity depends on the existence of exploitable biochemical differences between the infecting organism and the host. The bulk of the chapters in this section of the book describe the drugs used against the organisms mentioned above. In this introductory chapter, we consider very broadly the overall exploitable biochemical differences between us and our invading parasites (as well as our internal 'invaders': cancer cells) and outline the molecular aspects of drug action against them.**

The success in developing drugs to attack the invaders has been paralleled by the success of the invaders in developing strategies against the drugs, resulting in the emergence of *drug resistance*. And at present the parasites—particularly some bacteria—may be close to getting the upper hand. So in this chapter we stress particularly the mechanisms of resistance and the means by which it is spread.

*Nowadays the term chemotherapy is often used restrictively, referring to the treatment of cancer rather than parasitic diseases. In this introductory chapter, we stick to the original meaning but extend the term to cover cancer chemotherapy, since similar mechanisms can be involved.

BACKGROUND

The term chemotherapy was coined by Ehrlich at the beginning of the century to describe the use of synthetic chemicals to destroy infective agents. In recent years, the definition of the term has been broadened to include antibiotics—substances produced by some microorganisms (or by pharmaceutical chemists) that kill or inhibit the growth of other microorganisms. Here, we broaden it still further to include cancer chemotherapy

THE MOLECULAR BASIS OF CHEMOTHERAPY

Chemotherapeutic agents are chemicals that are intended to be toxic for the pathogenic organism but innocuous for the host. Before discussing the molecular basis of such selective toxicity, we need to define what we mean by infectious organism. The word 'microbe' is generally used to describe bacteria, viruses and fungi, and the word 'parasite' to describe protozoa and helminths. In this book, we are only concerned with those organisms that cause disease. The immune response of the human host makes no distinction between the above categories when they cause disease, while the dictionary definition of parasite covers all of them. Accordingly, to simplify discussion, we shall be using the term parasite for any organism that can cause disease.** That leaves the mysterious prions (see Ch. 34), which cause disease but resist classification—the despair of taxonomists.

Living organisms are classified as either prokaryotes—consisting of cells without nuclei (the bacteria)—or eukaryotes—consisting of cells with nuclei (e.g. protozoa, fungi, helminths). In a separate category are the viruses, which are not, properly

**It is difficult to distinguish between 'commensals'—organisms that are parasitic without causing disease—and disease-causing organisms, since it is now clear that many so-called commensals can cause disease if the immune system of the host is compromised.

speaking, cells at all because they do not have their own biochemical machinery for generating energy or for any sort of synthesis. Viruses need to utilise the metabolic machinery of the host cell and they thus present a particular kind of problem for chemotherapeutic attack.

In yet another category are cancer cells—host cells that have become malignant, i.e. they have escaped from the regulating devices which control normal cells. Cancer cells can be considered to be, in a special sense, 'foreign' or 'parasitic', but are clearly more similar to normal host cells than are any of the organisms in the categories considered above, and this makes them an especially difficult problem for selective toxicity.

Let us now go on to discuss the biochemical differences between us and our disease-causing parasites and consider the extent to which these can be exploited for chemotherapy.

Virtually all living creatures, host and parasite alike, have the same basic blueprint: DNA (an exception being the RNA viruses) and some biochemical processes are common to many, even all, organisms. Finding agents that affect parasite but not human host necessitates finding either qualitative or quantitative biochemical differences between them.

Bacteria cause more infectious disease than any other parasites, so let us start with a bacterial cell and ask what such a cell has to do in order to grow and divide. Figure 44.1 shows in simplified diagrammatic form the main structures and functions of a 'generalised' bacterial cell. Surrounding the cell is the *cell wall*, which characteristically contains peptidoglycan in all forms of bacteria except mycoplasma. Peptidoglycan is unique to prokaryotic cells and has no counterpart in eukaryotes. Within the cell wall is the *plasma membrane*, which is similar to that of the eukaryotic cell, consisting of a phospholipid bilayer and proteins. However, in bacteria the plasma membrane does not contain any sterols and this may result in differential penetration of chemicals. It functions as a selectively permeable membrane with specific transport mechanisms for various types of nutrient. The function of the cell wall is to support this underlying plasma membrane, which is subject to an internal osmotic pressure of about 5 atmospheres in Gram-negative organisms, and about 20 atmospheres in Gram-positive organisms.* The plasma membrane and cell wall together comprise the envelope.

Within the plasma membrane is the *cytoplasm*. As in eukaryotic cells, this contains all the soluble proteins (most having enzymic functions), the ribosomes involved in protein synthesis, all the small molecule intermediates involved in metabolism and all the inorganic ions. However, the bacterial cell, unlike the eukaryotic cell, has no nucleus; instead, the genetic material, in the form of a single chromosome that holds all the genetic information of the cell, lies in the cytoplasm with no surrounding nuclear membrane. In further contrast to eukaryotic cells, there are no mitochondria—all the energy generation goes on in the plasma membrane.

These, then, are the essential structures of the generalised bacterial cell. Some bacteria have additional components such as

*The terms Gram positive and Gram negative refer to whether or not the cell stains with a particular combination of dyes. More detail of the differences between Gram-positive and Gram-negative organisms is given in Chapter 45.

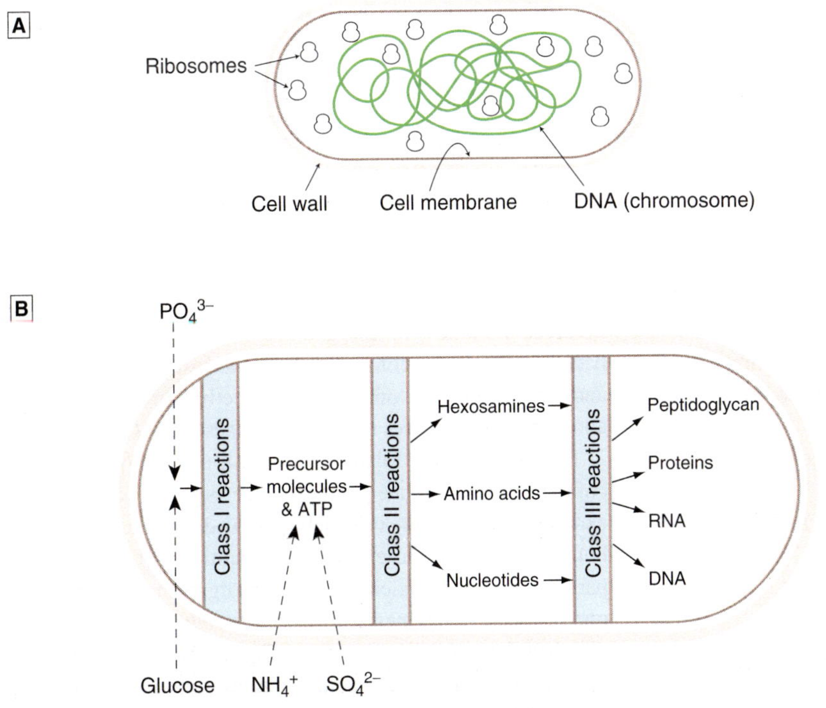

Fig. 44.1 Diagrams of structure and metabolism of a bacterial cell. [A] Schematic representation of a bacterial cell. [B] Flow diagram showing the synthesis of the main types of macromolecule of a bacterial cell. Class I reactions result in the synthesis of the precursor molecules necessary for class II reactions, which result in the synthesis of the constituent molecules; these are then assembled into macromolecules by class III reactions. (Modified from: Mandelstam J, McQuillen K, Dawes I (eds) 1982 Biochemistry of bacterial growth, Blackwell Scientific, Oxford.)

a capsule and/or one or more flagella, but the only additional structure with relevance for chemotherapy is the *outer membrane*, outside the cell wall, which is found in Gram-negative bacteria and which may prevent penetration of antibacterial agents (see Ch. 45, p. 637). It also prevents easy access of lysozyme (an enzyme that can break down cell wall structures and is found in white blood cells and tissue fluids such as tears) to the peptidoglycan of the cell wall.

Having outlined the essential structures of the bacterial cell, we need now to consider the biochemical reactions involved in their formation (Fig. 44.1). There are three general classes of reaction.

- *Class* I The utilisation of glucose or some alternative carbon source for the generation of energy (ATP) and simple carbon compounds (such as the intermediates of the tricarboxylic acid cycle), which are used as precursors in the next class of reactions.
- *Class* II The utilisation of the energy and precursors to make all the necessary small molecules: amino acids, nucleotides, phospholipids, amino sugars, carbohydrates and growth factors.
- *Class* III Assembly of the small molecules into macromolecules: proteins, RNA, DNA, polysaccharides and peptidoglycan.

These reactions are potential targets for attack by antibacterial drugs. Other potential targets are the formed structures, for example the cell membrane or, in higher organisms, the microtubules (targets in fungi and cancer cells). Specific types of cell may be targets in some higher organisms (e.g. muscle tissue in helminths).

In considering these targets, emphasis will be placed on bacteria, but reference will also be made to protozoa, helminths, fungi, cancer cells and, where possible, viruses. The classification that follows is clearly not a rigid one; a drug may affect reactions in more than one class or more than one subgroup of reactions within a class.

The molecular basis of chemotherapy

- To be effective, chemotherapeutic drugs should be toxic for invading organisms and innocuous for the host; such selective toxicity depends on there being exploitable biochemical differences between the parasite (e.g. a bacterium) and the host.
- Three general classes of biochemical reaction are potential targets for chemotherapy of bacteria. The characteristics of each class are:
  - —class I: glucose and other carbon sources are used to produce simple carbon compounds
  - —class II: energy and class I compounds are used to make small molecules, e.g. amino acids, nucleotides, etc.
  - —class III: small molecules are built into larger molecules, e.g. proteins, nucleic acids, peptidoglycan (in bacteria), etc.

BIOCHEMICAL REACTIONS AS POTENTIAL TARGETS

CLASS I REACTIONS

Class I reactions are not promising targets, for two reasons. First, there is no very marked difference between bacteria and humans cells in the mechanism for obtaining energy from glucose, since both use the Embden–Meyerhof pathway and the tricarboxylic acid cycle. Second, even if the glucose pathways were to be blocked, a large variety of other compounds (amino acids, lactate, etc.) could be used by bacteria as alternatives.

CLASS II REACTIONS

Class II reactions are better targets since some pathways involved in class II reactions exist in parasitic but not in humans cells. For instance, humans cells have in the course of evolution lost the ability, possessed by bacteria, to synthesise some amino acids—the so-called 'essential' amino acids—and also the growth factors (termed 'vitamins' in humans physiology). Any such difference represents a potential target. Another type of target occurs when a pathway is identical in both bacteria and humans but has differential sensitivity to drugs.

Folate

The synthesis of folate is an example of a metabolic pathway found in bacteria but not in humans. Folate is required for DNA synthesis in both bacteria and in humans (see Chs 21 and 45). Humans cannot synthesise it but obtain it from the diet and have evolved a transport mechanism for taking it up into the cells. By contrast, most species of bacteria, as well as the asexual forms of malarial protozoa, have not evolved the necessary transport mechanisms and they cannot make use of preformed folate. They must, of necessity, synthesise their own folate. This is a prime example of a difference that has proved to be useful for chemotherapy. **Sulfonamides** contain the sulfanilamide moiety—a structural analogue of *p*-aminobenzoic acid (PABA), which is essential in the synthesis of folate (see Figs 21.2 and 45.1). Sulfonamides compete with PABA for the enzyme involved in folate synthesis and thus inhibit the metabolism of the bacteria. They are consequently bacteriostatic not bactericidal and are, therefore, only really effective in the presence of adequate host defences (which are discussed in Ch. 15).

The utilisation of folate, in the form of tetrahydrofolate, as a cofactor in thymidylate synthesis (see Figs 21.3 and 50.9) is an example of a pathway in which there is differential sensitivity of humans and bacterial enzymes to chemicals (Table 44.1). This pathway is virtually identical in microorganisms and humans, but one of the key enzymes, *dihydrofolate reductase*, which reduces dihydrofolate to tetrahydrofolate (Fig. 21.2), is many times more sensitive to the folate antagonist **trimethoprim** in bacteria than in humans. In some malarial protozoa, this enzyme is somewhat less sensitive to trimethoprim than is the bacterial enzyme. The relative IC_{50} values (the concentration causing 50% inhibition) for bacterial, malarial, protozoal and mammalian enzymes are given in Table 44.1, as are those for **pyrimethamine**, primarily an antimalarial agent (Ch. 48). Another antimalarial drug that inhibits the protozoal enzyme specifically is **proguanil.** The humans enzyme, by comparison, is very sensitive to the effect of the folate analogue **methotrexate** (Table 44.1), and this compound is used in the chemotherapy of certain cancers (see Ch. 50). Methotrexate is inactive in bacteria because, being very similar in structure to folate, it requires active uptake by cells. Trimethoprim and pyrimethamine enter the cells by diffusion.

The use of sequential blockade with a combination of two drugs, which affect the same pathway in the parasite at different points, for example sulfonamides and the folate antagonists (Fig. 45.2), may be more successful than the use of either alone (e.g. in the treatment of *Pneumocystis carinii* pneumonia). Furthermore, lower concentrations of each drug are effective when the two are used together. Thus, pyrimethamine and a sulfonamide (**sulfadoxine**) are used to treat falciparum malaria (pp. 679–680). An antibacterial formulation that contains both a sulfonamide and trimethoprim is **co-trimoxazole** (p. 639); though this is less effective than when originally introduced because of the development of resistance to the sulfonamide.

Table 44.1 Specificity of inhibitors of dihydrofolate reductase

Inhibitor	IC_{50} (μmol/l) for dihydrofolate reductase		
	Human	Protozoal	Bacterial
Trimethoprim	260	0.07	0.005
Pyrimethamine	0.7	0.0005	2.5
Methotrexate	0.001	~0.1[a]	Inactive

[a]Tested on *Plasmodium berghei*, a rodent malaria.

Pyrimidine and purine analogues

The pyrimidine analogue **fluorouracil**, which is used in cancer chemotherapy (Ch. 50), is converted to a fraudulent nucleotide that interferes with thymidylate synthesis. Other cancer chemotherapy agents that give rise to fraudulent nucleotides are the purine analogues **mercaptopurine** and **tioguanine**. **Flucytosine**, an antifungal drug (Ch. 47), is deaminated to fluorouracil within the cell; selectivity for fungal cells results because this deamination occurs to a much lesser extent in the humans host.

CLASS III REACTIONS

Class III reactions are particularly good targets for selective toxicity because every cell has to make its own macromolecules—these cannot just be picked up from the environment—and there are very distinct differences between mammalian cells and parasitic cells in the pathways involved in class III reactions.

The synthesis of peptidoglycan

Peptidoglycan constitutes the cell wall of bacteria and does not occur in eukaryotes. It is the equivalent of a non-stretchable string bag enclosing the whole bacterium. For some bacteria (the Gram-negative organisms), the bag consists of a single thickness, but for others (Gram-positive organisms), it is up to 40 layers thick. Each layer consists of multiple backbones of amino sugars—alternating *N*-acetylglucosamine and *N*-acetylmuramic acid residues (Fig. 44.2)—the latter having short peptide side-chains that are cross-linked to form a latticework. The cross-links differ in different species. In staphylococci they consist of five glycine residues (Fig. 44.2). This cross-linking is responsible for the strength that allows the cell wall to resist the high internal osmotic pressure. The peptidoglycan is, in fact, one gigantic molecule with a molecular weight of many millions, constituting up to 10–15% of the dry weight of the cell.

In synthesising the peptidoglycan layer, the cell has the problem of using cytoplasmic components to build up this very large insoluble structure on the outside of the cell membrane. To do this, it is necessary to transport the components, which are synthesised within the cell and which are individually

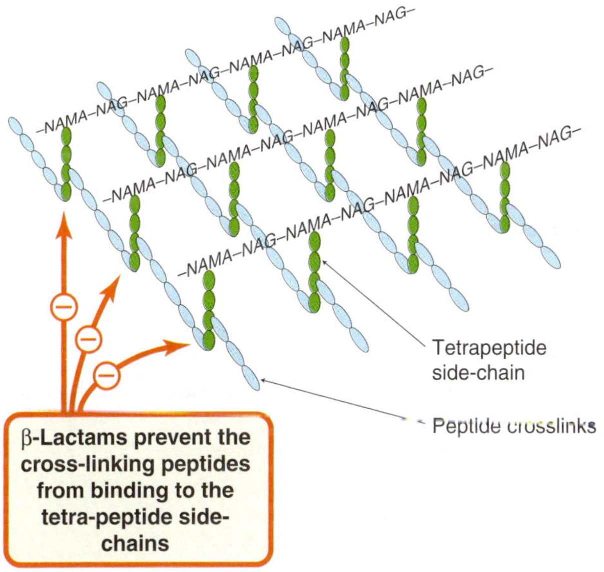

Fig. 44.2 Schematic diagram of a single layer of peptidoglycan from a bacterial cell (e.g. *Staphylococcus aureus*) showing the site of action of the β-lactam antibiotics (more detail in Fig. 44.3). In *Staphylococcus aureus* the peptide cross-links consist of five glycine residues. Gram-positive bacteria have several layers of peptidoglycan. (NAMA, *N*-acetylmuramic acid; NAG, *N*-acetylglucosamine.)

hydrophilic, piecemeal through the hydrophobic cell membrane. This is accomplished by linking them to a very large lipid carrier, containing 55 carbon atoms, which 'tows' them across the membrane. The process of peptidoglycan synthesis is outlined in Figure 44.3. First, *N*-acetylmuramic acid, which has attached to it both UDP and a pentapeptide, is transferred to the C_{55} lipid carrier in the membrane, with the release of UMP. This is followed by a reaction with UDP-*N*-acetylglucosamine, resulting in the formation of a disaccharide carrying the pentapeptide and attached to the carrier. This disaccharide with peptide attached is the basic building block of the peptidoglycan. In *Staphylococcus aureus*, the five glycine residues are attached to the peptide chain at this stage, as is shown in Figure 44.3. The 'building block' is now transported to the outside of the cell and added to the growing end of the peptidoglycan, the 'acceptor', with the release of the C_{55} lipid, which still has two phosphates attached. The lipid then loses one phosphate group and thus becomes available for another cycle. Cross-linking between the peptide side-chains of the sugar residues in the peptidoglycan layer then occurs, the hydrolytic removal of the terminal alanine supplying the requisite energy.

This synthesis of peptidoglycan can be blocked at several points by antibiotics (Fig. 44.3 and Ch. 45). **Cycloserine**, which is a structural analogue of D-alanine, prevents the addition of the two terminal alanines to the initial tripeptide side-chain on *N*-acetylmuramic acid, by competitive inhibition**. Vancomycin** inhibits the release of the building block unit from the carrier, thus preventing its addition to the growing end of the peptidoglycan. **Bacitracin** interferes with the regeneration of the lipid carrier by blocking its dephosphorylation. **Penicillins, cephalosporins** and other β-lactams inhibit the final transpeptidation that establishes the cross-links by forming covalent bonds with penicillin-binding proteins that have transpeptidase and carboxypeptidase activities.

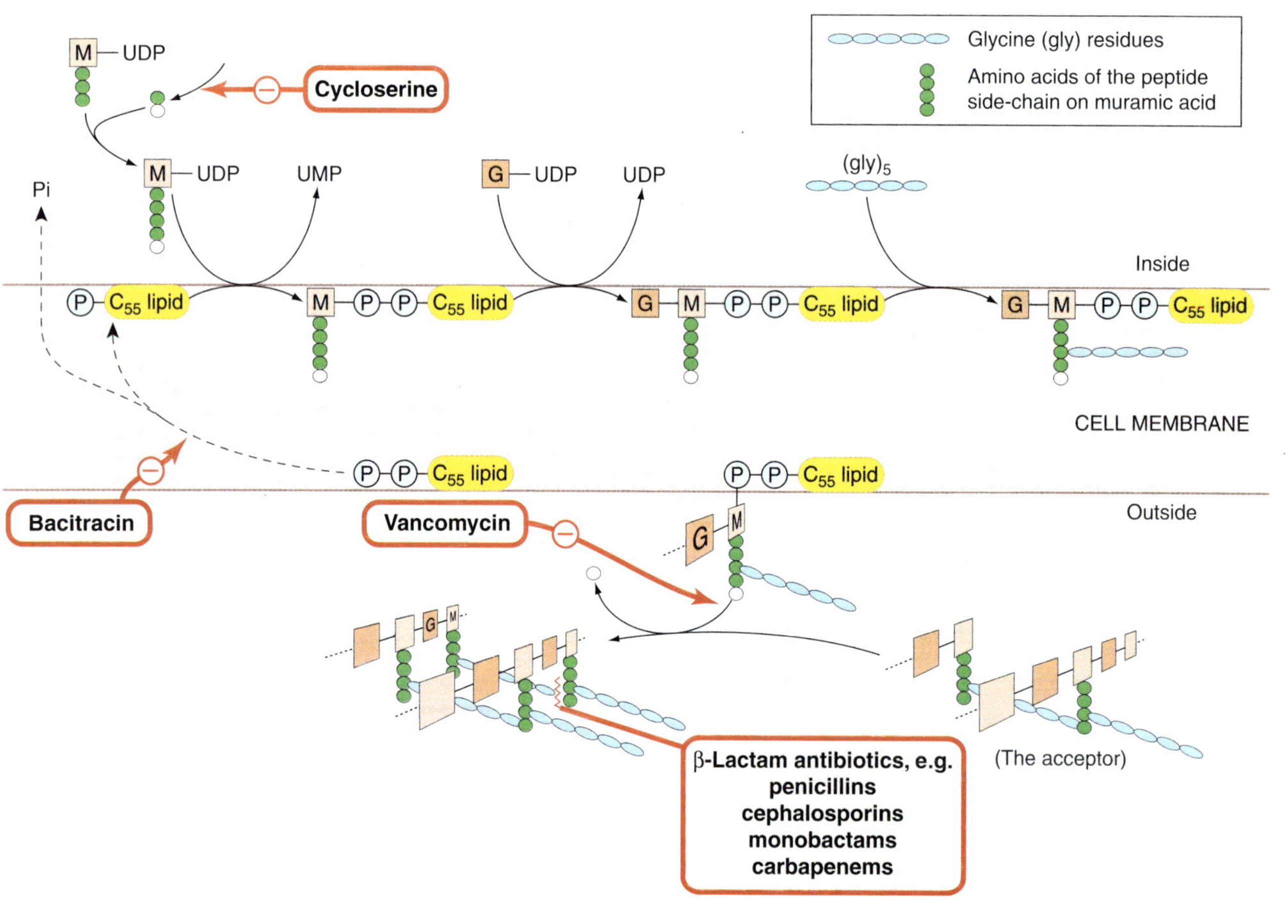

Fig. 44.3 Schematic diagram of the biosynthesis of peptidoglycan in a bacterial cell (e.g. *Staphylococcus aureus*) with the sites of action of various antibiotics. The hydrophilic disaccharide–pentapeptide is transferred across the lipid cell membrane attached to a large lipid (C_{55} lipid) by a pyrophosphate bridge (–P–P–). On the outside, it is enzymically attached to the 'acceptor' (the growing peptidoglycan layer). The final reaction is a transpeptidation, in which the loose end of the $(gly)_5$ chain is attached to a peptide side-chain of an M in the acceptor and during which the terminal amino acid (alanine) is lost. The lipid is regenerated by loss of a phosphate group (Pi) before functioning again as a carrier. (M, *N*-acetylmuramic acid; G, *N*-acetylglucosamine.)

Protein synthesis

Protein synthesis takes place in the ribosomes—cytoplasmic nucleoprotein structures. Ribosomes are different in eukaryotes and prokaryotes and this provides the basis for the selective antimicrobial action of some antibiotics. The bacterial ribosome consists of a 50S subunit and a 30S subunit (Fig. 44.4) whereas in the mammalian ribosome the subunits are 60S and 40S. The other elements involved in peptide synthesis are messenger RNA (mRNA), which forms the template for protein synthesis, and transfer RNA (tRNA), which brings the individual amino acids to the ribosome. The ribosome has three binding sites for tRNA, the A, P and E sites.

mRNA, which is transcribed from DNA (see below), becomes attached to the 30S subunit of the ribosome.

The 50S subunit then binds to the 30S subunit to form a 70S* subunit, which moves along the mRNA so that successive codons** of the messenger pass along the ribosome from the A position to the P position (Fig. 44.4).

A simplified version of protein synthesis in bacteria is shown in Figure 44.3. Antibiotics may affect protein synthesis at any one of these stages (Fig. 44.4 and Ch. 45).

Nucleic acid synthesis

The nucleic acids of the cell are DNA and RNA. There are three types of RNA: mRNA, tRNA and ribosomal RNA (rRNA). (The rRNA is an integral part of the ribosome, being necessary for its assembly, having a role in the binding of mRNA and having peptidyl transferase activity.) All are involved in protein synthesis (see above).

DNA is the template for the synthesis of both DNA and RNA. It exists in the cell as a double helix. Each chain or strand is a linear polymer of nucleotides. Each nucleotide consists of a base linked to a sugar (deoxyribose) and a phosphate. There are two purine bases, adenine (A) and guanine (G), and two pyrimidine bases, cytosine (C) and thymine (T). The chain is made up of alternating sugar and phosphate groups with the bases attached (Fig. 44.5). Specific hydrogen bonding between G and C and between A and T on each strand (i.e. complementary base-pairing) is the basis of the double-strand structure of DNA (Fig. 44.5). The DNA helix is itself coiled. In the test-tube, the coil has 10 base pairs per turn. In vivo, the coil is unwound by about 1 turn in 20 forming a *negative supercoil.*

Initiation of DNA synthesis requires first the activity of a protein that causes separation of the strands. The replication process inserts a positive supercoil. This is relaxed by DNA gyrase (also called topoisomerase II) (Fig. 44.6). During the synthesis of DNA, nucleotide units—each consisting of a base linked to a sugar and three phosphate groups—are added by base-pairing with the complementary residues in the template. Condensation occurs with the elimination of two of the phosphate groups, catalysed by DNA polymerase (Fig. 44.7).

RNA exists as a single, not a double, strand. The sugar moiety here is ribose, and the ribonucleotides contain the bases adenine, guanine, cytosine and uracil (U).

*You query whether 30S + 50S = 70S? Yes it does because we are talking about Svedberg units, which measure sedimentation rate not mass.

**A codon is a triplet consisting of three nucleotides that codes for a specific amino acid.

It is possible to interfere with nucleic acid synthesis in five different ways:

- by inhibiting the synthesis of the nucleotides
- by altering the base-pairing properties of the template
- by inhibiting either DNA or RNA polymerase
- by inhibiting DNA gyrase
- by direct effects on DNA itself.

Inhibition of the synthesis of the nucleotides

This can be accomplished by an effect on reactions earlier in the metabolic pathway. Examples of agents that have such an effect have been described under class II reactions.

Alteration of the base-pairing properties of the template

Agents that intercalate in the DNA have this effect. Examples are the acridines (proflavine, **acriflavine**), which are used topically as antiseptics. The acridines double the distance between adjacent base-pairs and cause a frameshift mutation (Fig. 44.8), whereas some purine and pyrimidine analogues cause mispairing.

Inhibition of either DNA or RNA polymerase

Dactinomycin (**actinomycin D**) binds to the guanine residues in DNA and blocks the movement of RNA polymerase, thus preventing transcription and consequently inhibiting protein

Biochemical reactions as potential targets for chemotherapy

- Class I reactions are poor targets.
- Class II reactions are better targets:
  - —folate synthesis in bacteria is inhibited by sulfonamides
  - —Folate utilisation is inhibited by folate antagonists, e.g. trimethoprim in bacteria, pyrimethamine in the malarial parasite, methotrexate (an anticancer drug) in humans
  - —pyrimidine analogues (e.g. fluorouracil) and purine analogues (e.g. mercaptopurine) give rise to fraudulent nucleotides; they are used to treat cancer.
- Class III reactions are important targets:
  - —peptidoglycan synthesis in bacteria can be selectively inhibited by β-lactam antibiotics, e.g. penicillin.
  - —protein synthesis can be selectively inhibited in bacteria by antibiotics that prevent binding of tRNA (e.g. tetracyclines), cause misreading of mRNA (e.g. aminoglycosides), inhibit transpeptidation (e.g. chloramphenicol), inhibit translocation of tRNA from A site to P site (e.g. erythromycin).
  - —nucleic acid synthesis can be inhibited by altering base-pairing of DNA template (e.g. vidarabine, an antiviral agent), inhibiting DNA polymerase (e.g. aciclovir and foscarnet, both antiviral agents) or inhibiting DNA gyrase (e.g. ciprofloxacin and antibacterial agent).

A The elements involved in protein synthesis are shown: a ribosome (with 3 binding sites for transfer RNA (tRNA): the P, A and E sites), messenger RNA (mRNA) and tRNA. The different mRNA codons (triplets of 3 nucleotides which code for specific amino acids) are represented by dots, dashes and straight or wavy lines and are shown in different colours. A tRNA with the growing peptide chain (consisting so far of Met–Leu–Trp: MLT) is in the P site, bound by codon:anticodon recognition (i.e. by complementary base-pairing). The incoming tRNA carries valine (V), covalently linked.

B The incoming tRNA binds to the A site by complementary base-pairing.

C Transpeptidation occurs, i.e. the peptide chain on the tRNA in the P site is transferred to the tRNA on the A site. The peptide chain attached to the tRNA in the A site now consists of Met–Leu–Trp–Val (MLTV). The tRNA in the P site has been 'discharged', i.e. has lost its peptide.

D The discharged tRNA is now transferred from the P site to the E site; the tRNA with the growing peptide chain is translocated from the A site to the P site and the ribosome moves on one codon, relative to the messenger.

E The tRNA from which the peptide chain has been removed is ejected. A new tRNA, with amino acid (M) attached and with the relevant anticodon, now moves into the A site, and the whole process is repeated.

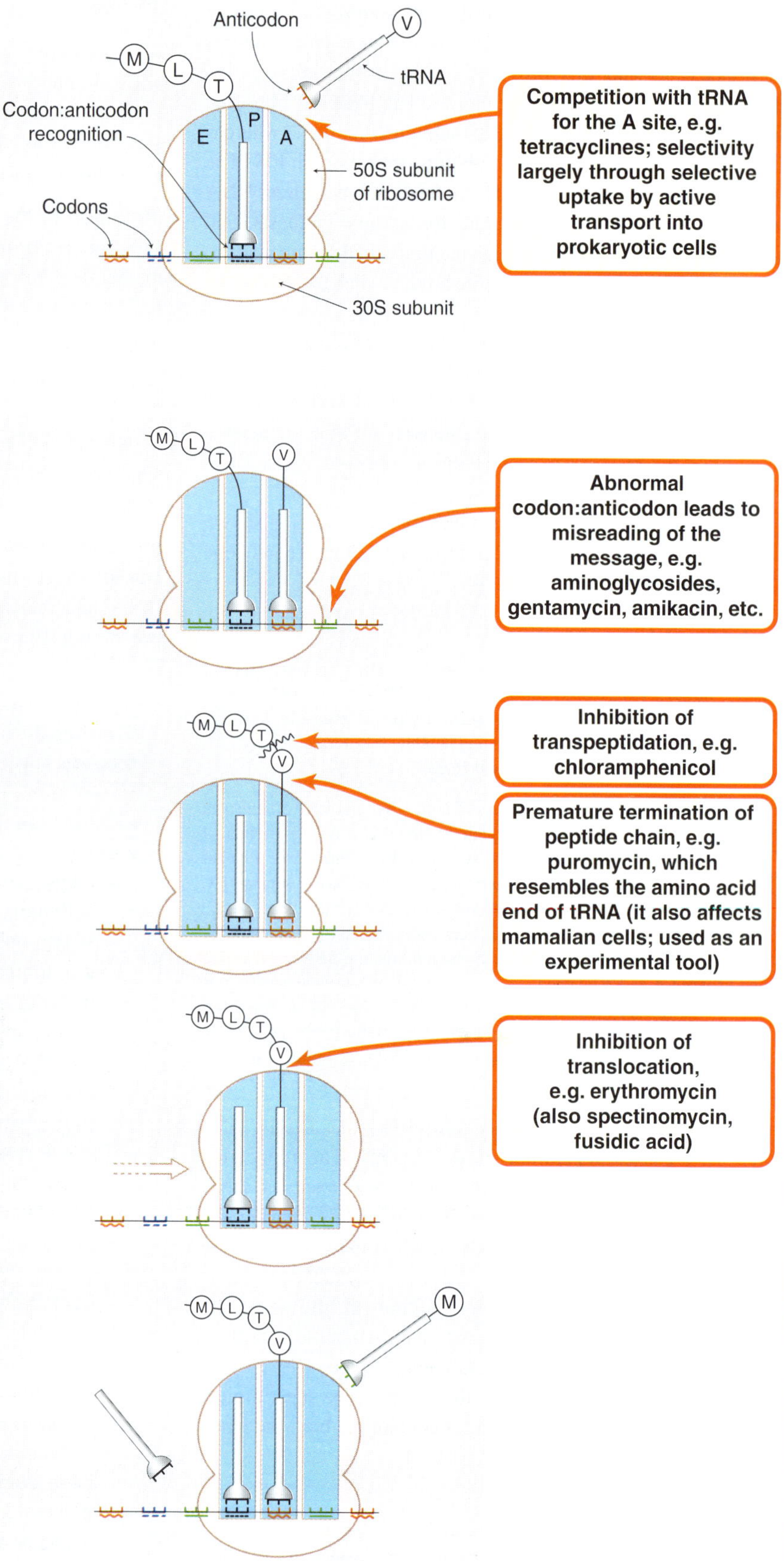

Fig. 44.4 Schematic diagram of bacterial protein synthesis indicating the points at which antibiotics inhibit the process.

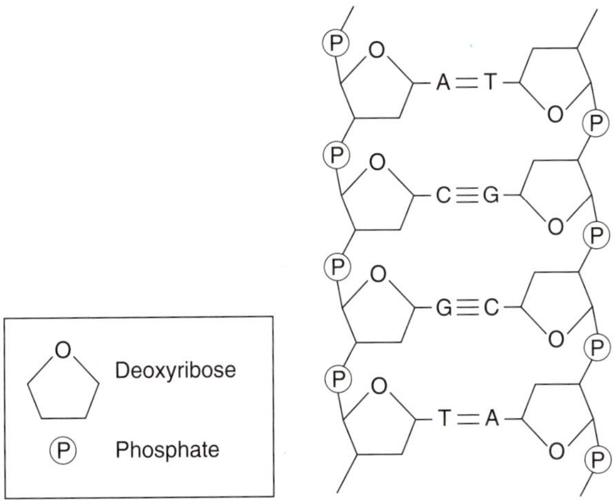

Fig. 44.5 Structure of DNA. Each strand of DNA consists of a sugar–phosphate backbone with purine or pyrimidine bases attached. The purines are adenine (A) or guanine (G) and the pyrimidines are cytosine (C) or thymine (T). The sugar is deoxyribose. Complementarity between the two strands of DNA is maintained by hydrogen bonds (either 2 or 3) between bases.

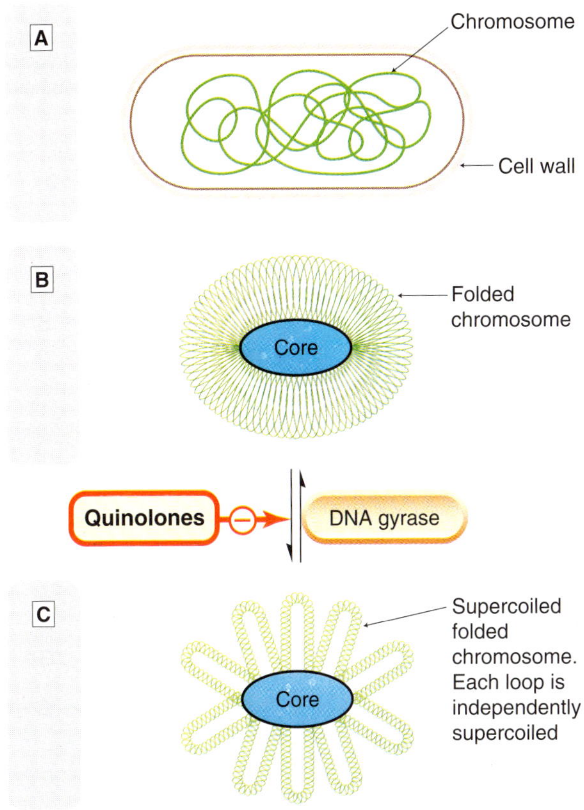

Fig. 44.6 Schematic diagram of the action of DNA gyrase: the site of action for quinolone antibacterials.
A Conventional diagram used to depict a bacterial cell and chromosome (e.g. *Escherichia coli*). Note that the *E. coli* chromosome is 1300 mm long and is contained in a cell envelope of 2 μm × 1 μm; this is approximately equivalent to a 50 m length of cotton folded into a matchbox. B Chromosome folded around RNA core, and then C supercoiled by DNA gyrase (topoisomerase II). Quinolone and antibacterials interfere with the action of this enzyme. (Modified from: Smith J T 1985 In: Greenwood D, O'Grady F (eds) Scientific basis of antimicrobial therapy. Cambridge University Press, p. 69.)

synthesis. It is used in cancer chemotherapy in humans (Ch. 50) and also as an experimental tool, but it is not useful as an antibacterial agent. Specific inhibitors of bacterial RNA polymerase that act by binding to this enzyme in prokaryotic but not in eukaryotic cells include **rifamycin** and **rifampicin**, which are active, in particular, against *Mycobacterium tuberculosis*, the tubercle bacillus (Ch. 45). **Aciclovir** (an analogue of guanine) is phosphorylated in cells infected with herpes virus, the initial phosphorylation being by a virus-specific kinase to give the aciclovir trisphosphate, which has an inhibitory action on the DNA polymerase of the herpes virus (Ch. 46).

RNA retroviruses have a *reverse transcriptase* (viral RNA-dependent DNA polymerase) that makes a DNA copy of the viral RNA, the viral DNA copy being integrated into the host cell DNA as a 'provirus'. Various agents (**zidovudine**, **didanosine**) are phosphorylated by cellular enzymes to the trisphosphate form, which competes with the equivalent host cell trisphosphates essential for the formation of proviral DNA by the viral reverse transcriptase.

Cytarabine (cytosine arabinoside) is used in cancer chemotherapy (Ch. 50). Its trisphosphate derivative is a potent inhibitor of DNA polymerase in mammalian cells. **Foscarnet** inhibits viral RNA polymerase by attaching to the pyrophosphate binding site.

Inhibition of DNA gyrase

Figure 44.6 is a simplified version of the action of DNA gyrase. The **fluoroquinolones** (**cinoxacin**, **ciprofloxacin**, **nalidixic acid** and **norfloxacin**) act by inhibiting DNA gyrase and these chemotherapeutic agents are used particularly in infections with Gram-negative organisms (Ch. 45, p. 647). These drugs are selective for the bacterial enzyme because it is structurally different from the mammalian enzyme. Some anticancer agents, for example **doxorubicin** (p. 703), act on the mammalian topoisomerase II.

Direct effects on DNA itself

Alkylating agents form covalent bonds with bases in the DNA and prevent replication. Compounds with this action are used only in cancer chemotherapy and include *nitrogen mustard derivatives* and *nitrosoureas* (Ch. 50). **Mitomycin** also binds covalently to DNA. No antibacterial agents work by these mechanisms.

THE FORMED STRUCTURES OF THE CELL AS POTENTIAL TARGETS

THE MEMBRANE

The plasma membrane of bacterial cells is fairly similar to that in mammalian cells in that it consists of a phospholipid bilayer in

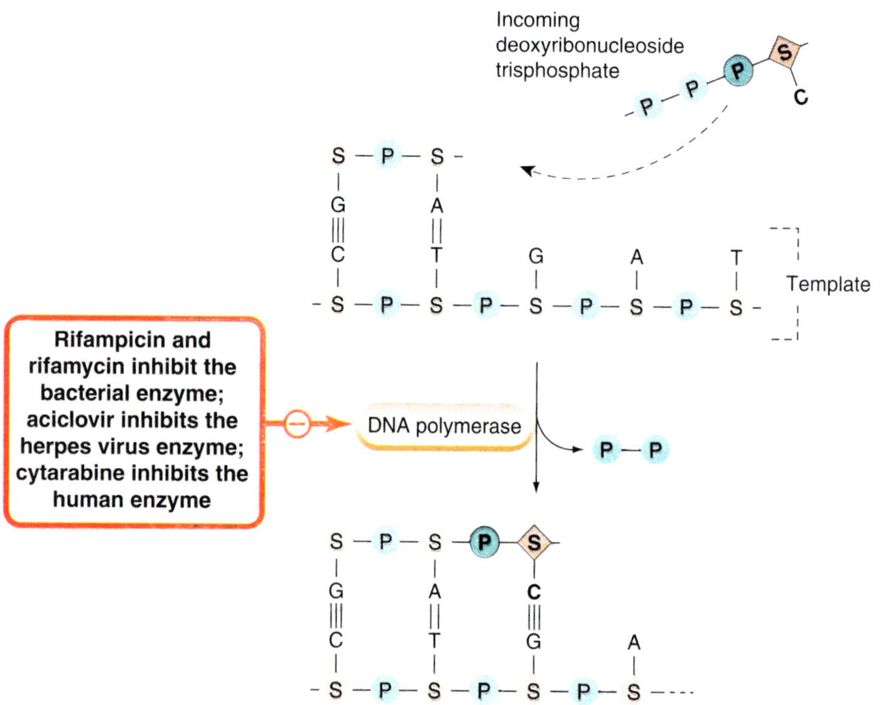

Fig. 44.7 Schematic diagram of DNA replication showing some antibiotics that inhibit it by action on DNA polymerase. Nucleotides are added, one at a time, by base-pairing to an exposed template strand and are then covalently joined together in a reaction catalysed by DNA polymerase. The units that pair with the complementary residues in the template consist of a base linked to a sugar and three phosphate groups. Condensation occurs with the elimination of two phosphates. The elements added to the template are shown in darker colours and bold type. (P, phosphate; S, sugar; A, adenine; T, thymine; G, guanine; C, cytosine.)

mRNA (normal)	UCU Ser	UUU Phe	CUU Leu	AUU Ile	GUU Val	UCU... Ser
mRNA (mutant)	UCU Ser	UUG Leu	UCU Ser	UAU Tyr	UGU Cys	UUC... Phe

Fig. 44.8 An example of the effect on RNA and protein synthesis of a frameshift mutation in the DNA. A frameshift mutation is one that involves a deletion of a base or an insertion of an extra base. In the above example an extra cytosine has been inserted in the DNA template with the result that when mRNA is formed, it has an additional guanine (G), as indicated in red. The effect is to alter that codon and all the succeeding ones (shown in blue), so that a completely different protein is synthesised, as indicated by the different amino acids (Leu instead of Phe, Ser instead of Leu, etc.). (G, guanine; C, cytosine; A, adenine; U, uracil.)

which proteins are embedded. Nevertheless, this structure can be more easily disrupted in certain bacteria and some fungi than in mammalian cells.

Polymixins are cationic detergent antibiotics that have a selective effect on bacterial cell membranes. They are peptides that contain both hydrophilic and lipophilic groups separated within the molecule. They interact with the phospholipids of the cell membrane and disrupt its structure; they are, therefore, bactericidal (Ch. 45).

Fungal cells, unlike mammalian and bacterial cells, have large amounts of ergosterol in the plasma membrane. The ergosterol facilitates the attachment of polyene antibiotics (e.g. **nystatin** and **amphotericin**; Ch. 47), which act as ionophores and cause leakage of cations.

Azoles, such as **itraconazole**, have antifungal action by inhibiting synthesis of ergosterol, altering membrane fluidity and thus the function of membrane-associated enzymes. The azoles also affect Gram-positive bacteria, their selectivity being associated with the presence of high levels of free fatty acids in the membrane of susceptible organisms (Ch. 47).

DNA

Bleomycin, an anticancer antibiotic, causes fragmentation of the DNA strands following free radical formation (Ch. 50).

INTRACELLULAR ORGANELLES

Microtubules and/or microfilaments

The *benzimidazoles* (e.g. **albendazole**) have anthelminthic action by binding selectively to parasite tubulin and preventing microtubule formation (Ch. 49).

The *vinca alkaloids* **vinblastine** and **vincristine** are anticancer agents that disrupt the functioning of microtubules during cell division (Ch. 50).

Food vacuoles

The erythrocytic form of the malaria plasmodium feeds on host haemoglobin, which is digested by proteases in the parasite food vacuole, the final product, haem, being detoxified by

Formed structures of the cell

- The plasma membrane is affected by:
  - —amphotericin, which acts as an ionophore in fungal cells
  - —azoles, which inhibit fungal membrane ergosterol synthesis.
- Microtubule function is disrupted by:
  - —vinca alkaloids (anticancer drugs)
  - —benzimidazoles (anthelminthics).
- Muscle fibres are affected by:
  - —avermectins (anthelminthics), which increase Cl^- permeability
  - —pyrantel (anthelminthic) stimulates nematode nicotinic receptors, eventually causing muscle paralysis.

polymerisation. **Chloroquine** has antimalarial action by inhibiting plasmodial haem polymerase (Ch. 48).

MUSCLE FIBRES

Some anthelminthic drugs have a selective action on muscle cells in helminths (Ch. 49).

Piperazine acts as an agonist on parasite-specific chloride channels gated by gamma-aminobutyric acid (GABA) in nematode muscle, hyperpolarising the muscle fibre membrane and paralysing the worm; **avermectins** increase chloride permeability in helminth muscle—possibly by a similar mechanism.

Pyrantel and **levamisole** act as agonists at nematode acetylcholine nicotinic receptors on muscle, causing contraction followed by paralysis (Ch. 49).

RESISTANCE TO ANTIBACTERIAL DRUGS

Since the 1940s, the development of effective and safe drugs to deal with bacterial infections has revolutionised medical treatment, and the morbidity and mortality from microbial disease have been dramatically reduced. Unfortunately, the development of effective antibacterial drugs has been accompanied by the emergence of drug-resistant organisms. This is not unexpected, it being an evolutionary principle that organisms adapt genetically to changes in their environment. Since the doubling time of bacteria can be as short as 20 minutes, there may be many generations in even a few hours, providing ample opportunity for evolutionary adaptation. The phenomenon of resistance imposes serious constraints on the options available for the medical treatment of many bacterial infections. Resistance to chemotherapeutic agents can also develop in protozoa, in multicellular parasites (see Foley and Tilley, 1997; Martin and Robertson, 2000; St Georgiev, 2000) and in populations of malignant cells (discussed in Ch. 50). However, in this chapter, discussion will be confined mainly to the mechanisms of resistance in bacteria.*

Antibiotic resistance in bacteria spreads at three levels:

- by transfer of bacteria between people
- by transfer of resistance genes between bacteria (usually on plasmids)
- by transfer of resistance genes between genetic elements within bacteria, on transposons. (Transposons are defined and explained below.)

Understanding the mechanisms involved in resistance to antibiotics is of importance both for the sensible use of these drugs in clinical practice and for the development of new antibacterial drugs to circumvent resistance. One result of the studies of resistance has been the development of new techniques using R plasmids and resistance genes for the cloning of foreign DNA. This cloning has been used rewardingly in many branches of biology and also in the production, by bacteria, of biologically active peptides such as mammalian hormones.

GENETIC DETERMINANTS OF ANTIBIOTIC RESISTANCE

CHROMOSOMAL DETERMINANTS: MUTATIONS

The spontaneous mutation rate in bacterial populations for any particular gene is very low—about 1 per 10^6–10^8 cells per cell division, i.e. the probability is that 1 cell in, say, 10 million will, on division, give rise to a daughter cell containing a mutation in a particular gene. However, since in an infection there are likely to be very many more cells than this, the probability of a mutation causing a change from drug sensitivity to drug resistance can be quite high with some species of bacteria and with some drugs. Fortunately, with most infective species and with most antibiotics, a few mutants are not sufficient to produce resistance. If an infecting bacterial population containing some mutants resistant to a particular antibiotic is exposed to that antibiotic, the mutants will have an enormous selective advantage. Luckily, in most cases the drastic reduction of the population by the antibiotic enables the host's natural defences (see Ch. 15) to deal effectively with the invading pathogens. However, this will not occur if the infection is caused by a population of microorganisms that are all resistant to the drug.

For most organisms, resistance resulting from chromosomal mutation is not of great clinical relevance, possibly because the mutants often have reduced pathogenicity; but it is important in methicillin-resistant staphylococcal infections (see below) and in infections caused by mycobacteria, particularly in tuberculosis.

EXTRACHROMOSOMAL DETERMINANTS: PLASMIDS

Many species of bacteria contain, in addition to the chromosome, extrachromosomal genetic elements called *plasmids* that exist

*Resistance to anticancer agents is considered in Chapter 50; resistance to antimalarial drugs is considered in Chapter 48.

free in the cytoplasm. These are genetic elements, other than the chromosome, that can replicate on their own They are closed loops of DNA that can consist of a single gene or many genes, up to 500 or more. With some plasmids, only a few copies may be present, with others there may be many copies, depending on the type; and there may be more than one type of plasmid in each bacterial cell. Plasmids that carry genes for resistance to antibiotics ('*r* genes') are referred to as R plasmids. Much of the drug resistance encountered in clinical medicine is plasmid determined. It is not known how these genes arose.

THE TRANSFER OF RESISTANCE GENES BETWEEN GENETIC ELEMENTS WITHIN THE BACTERIUM

Transposons

Some stretches of DNA can be fairly readily transferred (transposed) from one plasmid to another and also from plasmid to chromosome or vice versa. This is because integration of these segments of DNA, which are called transposons, into the acceptor DNA can occur independently of the normal mechanism of homologous genetic recombination. During the process of integration, the transposon can replicate (Fig. 44.9) and this results in a copy in both the donor and the acceptor DNA molecules. (Transposons, unlike plasmids, are not able to replicate on their own; moreover not all transposons replicate during transfer.) Transposons may carry one or more resistance genes (see below) and can 'hitch-hike' on a plasmid to a new species of bacterium; even if the plasmid is unable to replicate in the new host, the transposon may transfer to the new host's chromosome or to its indigenous plasmids. This probably accounts for the widespread distribution of certain of the resistance genes on different R plasmids and among unrelated bacteria.

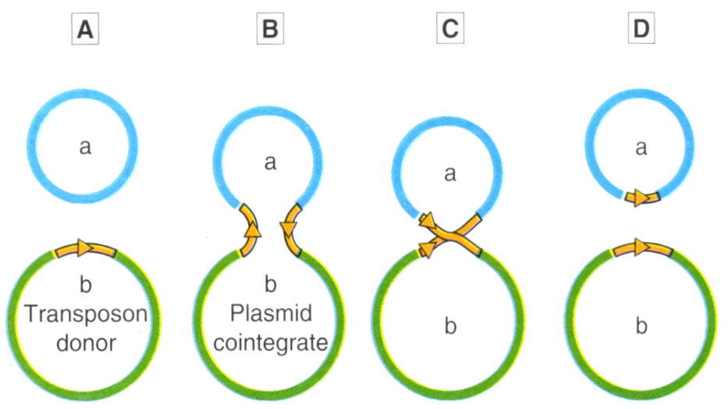

Fig. 44.9 An example of the transfer and replication of a transposon (which may carry genes coding for resistance to antibiotics). A Two plasmids, a and b, with plasmid b containing a transposon (shown in brown). B An enzyme encoded by the transposon cuts DNA of both donor plasmid and target plasmid a, to form a 'cointegrate'. During this process, the transposon replicates. C An enzyme encoded by the transposon 'resolves' the cointegrate. D Both plasmids now contain the transposon DNA.

Gene cassettes and integrons

Plasmids and transposons do not complete the tally of mechanisms that natural selection has provided to confound the hopes of the microbiologist/chemotherapist. Resistance—in fact, multidrug resistance—can also be spread by another mobile element: the *gene cassette* (an addition to the already arcane terminology of bacterial geneticists), which consists of a resistance gene attached to a small recognition site. Several cassettes may be packaged together in a multicassette array, which can, in turn, be integrated into a larger mobile DNA unit, termed an *integron*. The integron (which can be located on a transposon) contains a gene for the enzyme, an *integrase* (recombinase), that inserts the cassette(s) at unique sites on the integron.* This system—transposon/ integron/multiresistance cassette array—allows particularly rapid and efficient transfer of multidrug resistance between genetic elements within the bacterium (and between bacteria on plasmids, see below).

THE TRANSFER OF RESISTANCE GENES BETWEEN BACTERIA

The transfer of resistance genes between bacteria of the same species and of different species is of fundamental importance in the spread of resistance to antibiotics. There are three mechanisms for gene transfer: conjugation, transduction and transformation.

Conjugation

Conjugation involves cell-to-cell contact during which chromosomal or extrachromosomal DNA is transferred from one bacterium to another. It is the main mechanism for the spread of resistance. The ability to conjugate is encoded in conjugative plasmids; these are plasmids that contain transfer genes, which, in coliform bacteria, code for the production, by the host bacterium, of surface tubules of protein that connect the two cells—sex pili. The conjugative plasmid then passes across from one bacterium to the other, which is usually of the same species. Many Gram-negative and some Gram-positive bacteria can conjugate. Some plasmids cross the species barrier and, accepting one host as readily as another, are suggestively described as promiscuous plasmids. Many R plasmids are conjugative. Non-conjugative plasmids, if they coexist in a 'donor' cell with conjugative plasmids, can hitch-hike from one bacterium to the other with the conjugative plasmids. The transfer of resistance by conjugation is significant in populations of bacteria that are normally found at high densities, as in the gut.

Transduction

Transduction is a process by which plasmid DNA is enclosed in a bacterial virus (or phage) and transferred to another bacterium of the same species. It is a relatively ineffective means of transfer of genetic material, but there is evidence that it is clinically

*In addition there are cassette-like elements that determine pathogenicity.

important in the transmission of resistance genes between strains of staphylococci and between strains of streptococci.

Transformation

In a few species, a bacterium can, under natural conditions, undergo transformation by taking up naked DNA from its environment and incorporating it into its genome through the normal cross-over mechanism. This is possible only when the incoming DNA comes from a cell belonging to the same strain as the host bacterium or one that is very closely related. Transformation is probably not of importance in the clinical problem of drug resistance.

BIOCHEMICAL MECHANISMS OF RESISTANCE TO ANTIBIOTICS

THE PRODUCTION OF AN ENZYME THAT INACTIVATES THE DRUG

Inactivation of β-lactam antibiotics

The most important example of resistance caused by inactivation is that of the β-lactam antibiotics. The enzymes concerned are β-lactamases, which cleave the β-lactam ring of penicillins and cephalosporins (see Ch. 45). Cross-resistance between the two classes of antibiotic is not complete because some β-lactamases have a preference for penicillins and some for cephalosporins.

Resistance to antibiotics

- Resistance in bacterial populations can be spread from person to person by bacteria, from bacterium to bacterium by plasmids, from plasmid to plasmid (or chromosome) by transposons.
- Plasmids are extrachromosomal genetic elements that can replicate independently and can carry genes coding for resistance to antibiotics (*r* genes).
- The main method of transfer of *r* genes from one bacterium to another is by conjugative plasmids, which can cause the bacterium to make a connecting tube between bacteria, through which the plasmid itself (and other plasmids) can pass.
- A less-common method of transfer is by transduction, i.e. the transmission of an *r*-gene-carrying plasmid into a bacterium by a bacterial virus (phage).
- Transposons are stretches of DNA that can be transposed from one plasmid to another, and also from plasmid to chromosome and vice versa. For example an *r*-gene-carrying transposon in one plasmid codes for enzymes that cause integration of that plasmid into another plasmid, followed by their separation; during this the transposon replicates so that both plasmids will then contain the *r*-gene-carrying transposon.

Staphylococci are the principal bacteria producing β-lactamase, and the genes coding for the enzymes are on plasmids that can be transferred by transduction. In staphylococci, the enzyme is inducible (i.e. its synthesis is not expressed in the absence of the drug) but minute, sub-inhibitory, concentrations derepress the gene and result in a 50- to 80-fold increase in production. The enzyme is able to pass through the envelope and inactivate antibiotic molecules in the surrounding medium. The serious clinical problem posed by the staphylococci with resistance resulting from β-lactamase production was tackled by developing semisynthetic penicillins (such as **methicillin**) and new β-lactam antibiotics (**monobactams** and **carbapenems**), which were not susceptible, and cephalosporins (such as **cephamandole**), which were less susceptible to inactivation by these enzymes. (However, see below for 'methicillin-resistant' staphylococci.)

Gram-negative organisms can also produce β-lactamases, which are a significant factor in their resistance to the semisynthetic broad-spectrum β-lactam antibiotics. In these organisms, the enzymes may be determined by either chromosomal genes or by plasmid genes. In the former, the enzymes may be inducible. In the latter they are produced constitutively (i.e. they are synthesised even when the substrate is absent) and remain attached to sites in the cell wall, preventing access of the drug to the membrane-associated target site; they do not inactivate the drug in the surrounding medium. Many of these β-lactamases are encoded by transposons, some of which may also carry resistance determinants to several other antibiotics.

Inactivation of chloramphenicol

Chloramphenicol inactivation is brought about by chloramphenicol acetyltransferase produced by resistant strains of both Gram-positive and Gram-negative organisms, the resistance gene being plasmid-borne. In Gram-negative bacteria, the enzyme is produced constitutively, which results in levels of resistance fivefold higher than in Gram-positive bacteria, in which the enzyme is inducible.

Inactivation of aminoglycosides

Inactivation of *aminoglycosides* may be brought about by phosphorylation, adenylation or acetylation and the requisite enzymes have been found in both Gram-negative and Gram-positive organisms. The resistance genes are carried on plasmids and several are found on transposons.

ALTERATION OF DRUG-SENSITIVE SITE OR DRUG-BINDING SITE

The protein on the 30S subunit of the ribosome, which is the binding site for aminoglycosides, may be altered as the result of a chromosomal mutation. A plasmid-mediated alteration of the binding-site protein on the 50S subunit underlies resistance to **erythromycin**, and decreased binding of **fluoroquinolones** because of a point mutation in the DNA gyrase A protein has recently been described. An altered DNA-dependent RNA polymerase determined by a chromosomal mutation is the basis for resistance to **rifampicin**.

In addition to resistance to *β-lactams* through production of β-lactamase (as described above), some strains of *S. aureus* have become resistant even to some β-lactams that are not significantly inactivated by β-lactamase (e.g. methicillin), owing to expression of an additional β-lactam-binding protein coded for by a mutated chromosomal gene.

DECREASED DRUG ACCUMULATION IN THE BACTERIUM

An important example of decreased drug accumulation is the plasmid-mediated resistance to tetracyclines in both Gram-positive and Gram-negative bacteria. The resistance genes in the plasmid code for inducible proteins in the bacterial membrane, which promote energy-dependent efflux of the tetracyclines and hence resistance. This type of resistance is common and has reduced the value of the **tetracyclines** in humans and veterinary medicine. Resistance of *S. aureus* to **erythromycin** and the other macrolides and to **fluoroquinolones** can also be the result of energy-dependent efflux. In addition, there is also recent evidence of plasmid-determined inhibition of 'porin' synthesis, which could affect those hydrophilic antibiotics that enter the bacterium via these water-filled channels in the outer membrane.

Altered permeability as a result of chromosomal mutations involving the polysaccharide components of the outer membrane of Gram-negative organisms may confer enhanced resistance to **ampicillin**.

Mutations affecting envelope components have been reported to affect the accumulation of *aminoglycosides*, *β-lactams*, **chloramphenicol,** *peptide antibiotics* and **tetracycline**.

THE DEVELOPMENT OF A PATHWAY THAT BYPASSES THE REACTION INHIBITED BY THE ANTIBIOTIC

Resistance to **trimethoprim** is the result of plasmid-directed synthesis of a dihydrofolate reductase with low or zero affinity for trimethoprim. It is transferred by transduction and may be spread by transposons.

Sulfonamide resistance in many bacteria is plasmid mediated and results from the production of a form of dihydropteroate synthetase with a low affinity for sulfonamides but no change in affinity for *PABA*. Bacteria causing serious infections have been found to carry plasmids with resistance genes to both sulfonamides and trimethoprim.

CURRENT STATUS OF ANTIBIOTIC RESISTANCE IN BACTERIA

The most disturbing development of resistance has been in staphylococci, many strains of which are now resistant to almost all currently available antibiotics. In addition to resistance to some *β-lactams* owing to production of β-lactamase and the production of an additional β-lactam-binding protein, which renders them resistant to **methicillin** (see above), *S. aureus* may also manifest resistance to other antibiotics as follows:

- to **streptomycin** (owing to chromosomally determined alteration of target site)
- to *aminoglycosides* in general (owing to altered target site and plasmid-determined inactivating enzymes)
- to **chloramphenicol** and the *macrolides* (owing to plasmid-determined enzymes)
- to **trimethoprim** (owing to transposon-encoded drug-resistant dihydrofolate reductase)
- to **sulfonamides** (owing to chromosomally determined increased production of PABA)
- to **rifampicin** (thought to be caused by chromosomally determined and plasmid-determined increases in efflux of the drug)
- to **fusidic acid** (owing to chromosomally determined decreased affinity of the target site or a plasmid-encoded decreased permeability to the drug)
- to *quinolones*, for example **ciprofloxacin**, **norfloxacin** (owing to chromosomally determined reduced uptake).

Infections with these organisms, referred to as 'methicillin-resistant *Staphylococcus aureus*' (MRSA), have become a serious problem, particularly in hospitals, where they can spread rapidly among elderly and/or seriously ill patients, and patients with burns or wounds. In a number of hospitals, surgical wards have had to be closed because of the high rates of infection among patients. Until recently, the glycopeptide **vancomycin** was the antibiotic of last resort against MRSA, but, ominously, in 1997, strains of MRSA showing decreased susceptibility to this drug were isolated from hospitalised patients in the USA and Japan.* The vancomycin resistance seems to have developed

Biochemical mechanisms of resistance to antibiotics

- Production of enzymes that inactivate the drug, e.g. β-lactamases, which inactivate penicillin; acetyltransferases, which inactivate chloramphenicol; kinases and other enzymes, which inactivate aminoglycosides.
- Alteration of the drug-binding sites: this occurs with aminoglycosides, erythromycin, penicillin.
- Reduction of drug uptake by the bacterium, e.g. tetracyclines.
- Alteration of enzyme pathways, e.g. dihydrofolate reductase becomes insensitive to trimethoprim.

*Noble et al. have been able to transfer high-level vancomycin resistance from enterococci to staphylococci. If this occurred in a clinical environment it would be disastrous. Some microbiologists have suggested that Noble and his team should be autoclaved. (Noble W C 1992 FEMS Microbiol Lett 72: 195–198.)

Multidrug resistance

- Many pathogenic bacteria have developed resistance to the commonly used antibiotics; some examples are:
  - —some strains of staphylococci and enterococci are resistant to virtually all current antibiotics, resistance being transferred by transposons and/or plasmids; these organisms can cause serious and virtually untreatable nosocomial infections
  - —some strains of *Mycobacterium tuberculosis* have become resistant to most antituberculosis agents.

spontaneously. This could have major clinical consequences—and not only for nosocomial* infections with MRSA. It had been thought that antibiotic-resistant bacteria were dangerous only to seriously ill, hospitalised patients in that the genetic load of multiple resistance genes would lead to reduced virulence; however, there is now evidence that the spectrum and frequency of disease produced by methicillin-susceptible and methicillin-resistant staphylococci are similar.**

In the last few years, enterococci have been rapidly developing resistance to many chemotherapeutic agents and have emerged as the second most common nosocomial pathogen. Non-pathogenic enterococci are ubiquitously present in the intestine, have intrinsic resistance to many antibacterial drugs and can readily become resistant to other agents by taking up plasmids and transposons carrying the relevant resistance genes; this resistance is easily transferred to invading pathogenic enterococci.

Enterococci, already multiresistant, have recently developed resistance to vancomycin, thought to be achieved by replacement of the last two amino acids, D-Ala–D-Ala, with D-Ala–D-lactate in the five amino acid residue chain attached to *N*-acetylglucosamine–N-acetylmuramic acid (G-M) in the first steps of peptidoglycan synthesis (see Fig. 44.3 and Ch. 45). This is becoming a major problem in hospitalised patients. A particular concern is the possibility of transfer of vancomycin resistance from enterococci to staphylococci, since they can coexist in the same patient.

Furthermore, many other pathogens are developing or have developed resistance to commonly used drugs.*** The list includes, among others, *Pseudomonas aeruginosa*, *Streptococcus pyogenes*, *Streptococcus pneumoniae*, *Neisseria meningitidis*, *Neisseria gonorrhoeae*, *Haemophilius influenzae*, *Haemophilius ducreyi* as well as *Mycobacterium*, *Campylobacter* and *Bacteroides* species (see Jacobi & Archer, 1991). Some strains of *M. tuberculosis* are now able to evade every antibiotic in the clinician's armamentarium, and tuberculosis, once considered easily treatable, is now reported to be causing more deaths worldwide than malaria and AIDS together.

Extensive efforts are currently under way in many countries to find new antibiotics effective against the rapidly growing ranks of multiresistant bacteria, and several new potentially effective compounds are in the pipeline (see Bush & Macielag, 2000); however, nature has endowed microorganisms with fiendishly effective adaptive mechanisms for dealing with our pharmaceutical attack, and so far several have been effortlessly keeping pace with our attempts to deal with them.

*Nosocomial infections are those acquired in hospital.

**Reports from Iceland indicate that multidrug-resistant and non-resistant pneumococci can be equally virulent; and in South Africa, mortality from meningitis caused by penicillin-resistant pneumococci was reported to be higher than that from penicillin-susceptible pneumococci.

***It should be emphasised that one reason for our current inability to win the war against these microbe foes is that antibiotics are often used indiscriminately and to excess.

REFERENCES AND FURTHER READING

Amyes S G B 2001 Magic bullets, lost horizons: the rise and fall of antibiotics. Taylor and Francis, London (*Thought-provoking book by a bacteriologist with wide experience in bacterial resistance and genetics. He opines that unless the problem of antibiotic resistance is solved in the next 5 years, 'we are going to slip further into the abyss of uncontrollable infection'*)

Bush K, Macielag M 2000 New approaches in the treatment of bacterial infections. Curr Opin Chem Biol 4: 433–439 (*Concise discussion of new antibacterial agents in phase II or phase III trial or already approved*)

Courvalin P, Trieu-Cout 2001 Minimizing potential resistance: the molecular view. Clin Infect Dis 33: S138–S146 (*Reviews the potential contribution of molecular biology to preventing the spread of resistant bacieria*)

Croft S L 1997 The current status of antiparasite chemotherapy. Parasitology 114: S3–S15 (*Comprehensive coverage of current drugs for protozoal, coccidial and helminth infections with outline of approaches to possible future agents*)

Foley M, Tilley L 1997 Quinoline antimalarials: mechanisms of action and resistance. Int J Parasitol 27: 231–240 (*Good, short review; useful diagrams*)

Hawkey P M 1998 The origins and molecular basis of antibiotic resistance. Br Med J 7159: 657–659 (*Succinct overview of resistance: useful simple diagrams. This is one of 12 papers/articles on resistance in this issue of the journal*)

Jacobi G A, Archer G L 1991 Mechanisms of disease: new mechanisms of bacterial resistance to antimicrobial agents. N Engl J Med 324: 601–602

Jones M E, Peters E et al. 1997 Widespread occurrence of integrons causing multiple antibiotic resistance in bacteria. Lancet 349: 1742–1743

Knodler L A, Celli J, Finlay B B 2001 Pathogenic trickery: deception of host cell processes. Mol Cell Biol 2: 578–588 (*Discusses bacterial ploys to subvert or block normal host cellular processes: mimicking the ligands for host cell receptors or signalling pathways. Useful list of examples*)

Levy S B 1998a Antibacterial resistance: bacteria on the defence. Br Med J 7159: 612–613 (*Resistance seen from the point of view of the bacterium. This is one of seven editorial articles on the subject of resistance in this issue of the journal*)

Levy S B 1998b The challenge of antibiotic resistance. Sci Am March: 32–39 (*Simple, clear review by an expert in the field; excellent diagrams*)

Martin R J, Robertson A P 2000 Electrophysiological investigation of anthelmintic resistance. Parasitology 120(suppl): S87–S94 (*Uses patch-*

clamp technique to study ion channels in resistant and non-resistant nematode tissue)

Michel M, Gutman L 1997 Methicillin-resistant *Staphylococcus aureus* and vancomycin-resistant enterococci: therapeutic realities and possibilities. Lancet 349: 1901–1906 (*Good review article; useful diagram; suggests schemes for medical management of infections caused by resistant organisms*)

Recchia G D, Hall R M 1995 Gene cassettes: a new class of mobile element. Microbiology 141: 3015–3027 (*Detailed coverage*)

St Georgiev V 2000 Membrane transporters and antifungal drug resistance. Curr Drug Targets 1: 261–184 (*Discusses various aspects of multidrug resistance in disease-causing fungi in the context of targeted drug development*)

Tabaqchali S 1997 Vancomycin-resistant *Staphylococcus aureus*: apocalypse now? Lancet 350: 1644

Tan Y T, Tillett D J, McKay I A 2000 Molecular strategies for overcoming antibiotic resistance in bacteria. Mol Med Today 6: 309–314 (*Succinct article reviewing strategies to exploit advances in molecular biology to develop new antibiotics that overcome resistance. Useful glossary of relevant terms*)

van Belkum A 2000 Molecular epidemiology of methicilln-resistant *Staphylococcus aureus* strains: state of affairs and tomorrow's possibilities. Microb Drug Resist 6: 173–187

Walsh C 2000 Molecular mechanisms that confer antibacterial drug resistance. Nature 406: 775–781 (*Excellent review outlining the mechanisms of action of antibiotics and the resistance ploys of bacteria. Very good diagrams*)

Zasloff M 2002 Antimicrobial peptides of multicellular organisms. Nature 415: 389–395 (*Thought-provoking article about the potent, broad-spectrum antimicrobial peptides possessed by both animals and plants, which are used to fend off a wide range of microbes. It is suggested that exploiting these might be one answer to the problem of antibiotic resistance*)

Antibacterial drugs

45

Overview 635

Introduction 635

Antimicrobial agents that interfere with the synthesis or action of folate 637
- Sulfonamides 637
- Trimethoprim 639

Beta-lactam antibiotics 639
- Penicillin 639
- Cephalosporins and cephamycins 641
- Other β-lactam antibiotics 642

Antimicrobial agents affecting bacterial protein synthesis 643
- Tetracyclines 643
- Chloramphenicol 644
- Aminoglycosides 645
- Macrolides 646
- Streptogramins 646
- Lincosamides 646
- Oxalazidonones 647
- Fusidic acid 647

Antimicrobial agents affecting topoisomerase II 647
- Fluoroquinolones 647

Miscellaneous antibacterial agents 648

Antimycobacterial agents 649
- Drugs used to treat tuberculosis 649
- Drugs used to treat leprosy 651

Possible new antibacterial drugs 652

OVERVIEW

A detailed classification of the bacteria of medical importance is beyond the scope of this book. However, a short list of the commoner and/or more important microorganisms that cause disease is given in Table 45.1. Individual chemotherapeutic agents are dealt with briefly in this chapter and a general indication of their main antibacterial actions is given in Table 45.1. Some of the main diseases that may be caused by the organisms are included in the table but it should be understood that most of the organisms may, on occasion, produce other pathological conditions.

INTRODUCTION

In Table 45.1, many of the organisms are classified as either Gram-positive or Gram-negative. This classification is based on whether the organisms do or do not stain with Gram's stain, but it has a significance far beyond that of an empirical staining reaction. Gram-positive and Gram-negative organisms are different in several respects, not least in the structure of the cell wall, which has implications for the action of antibiotics.

The cell wall of Gram-positive organisms is a relatively simple structure, 15–50 nm thick. It consists of about 50% peptidoglycan (see p. 623 and Fig. 44.2), about 40–45% acidic polymer (which results in the cell surface being highly polar and carrying a negative charge) and about 5–10% proteins and polysaccharides. The strongly polar polymer layer influences the penetration of ionised molecules and favours the penetration of positively charged compounds, such as **streptomycin**, into the cell.

The cell wall of Gram-negative organisms is much more complex. From the plasma membrane outwards it consists of the following

- a periplasmic space containing enzymes and other components
- a peptidoglycan layer 2 nm in thickness and forming 5% of the cell wall mass; this is often linked to lipoprotein molecules which project outwards
- an outer membrane consisting of a lipid bilayer similar in some respects to the plasma membrane; it contains protein molecules and on its inner aspect has lipoprotein that is linked to the peptidoglycan
- complex polysaccharides forming important components of the outer surface; these are different in different strains of bacteria and are the main determinants of the antigenicity of the organism. The complex polysaccharides constitute the *endotoxins*, which, in vivo, trigger various aspects of the

Table 45.1 General choice of antibiotics against common or important microorganisms[a]

Microorganism[b]	First choice antibiotic(s)[c]	Second choice antibiotic(s)[c]
Gram-positive cocci		
Staphylococcus (boils, infection of wounds, etc.)		
Non β-lactamase-producing	Benzylpenicillin (penicillin G) or phenoxymethylpenicillin (penicillin V)	A cephalosporin or vancomycin
β-lactamase-producing	A β-lactamase-resistant penicillin (e.g. flucloxacillin)	A cephalosporin or vancomycin, or a macrolide, or a quinolone
Methicillin-resistant	Vancomycin ± gentamicin ± rifampicin	Co-trimoxazole, or ciprofloxacin, or a macrolide ± fusidic acid, or rifampicin
Methicillin/vancomycin resistant	Quinupristin/dalfopristin or linezolid	
Streptococcus, haemolytic types (septic infections e.g. bacteraemia, scarlet fever, toxic shock syndrome)	Benzylpenicillin or phenoxymethylpenicillin ± an aminoglycoside	A cephalosporin, or a macrolide, or vancomycin
Enterococcus (endocarditis)	Benzylpenicillin + gentamicin	Vancomycin
Pneumococcus (pneumonia)	Benzylpenicillin or phenoxymethylpenicillin or ampicillin, or a macrolide	A cephalosporin
Gram-negative cocci		
Morasella catarrhalis (sinusitis)	Amoxicillin + clavulanic acid	Ciproxafloxacin
Neisseria gonorrhoeae (gonorrhoea)	Amoxicillin + clavulanic acid, or ceftriaxone	Cefotaxime, or a quinolone
Neisseria meningitidis (meningitis)	Benzylpenicillin	Chloramphenicol, or cefotaxime, or minocycline
Gram-positive rods		
Corynebacterium (diphtheria)	A macrolide	Benzylpenicillin
Clostridium (tetanus, gangrene)	Benzylpenicillin	A tetracycline, or a cephalosporin
Listeria monocytogenes (rare cause of meningitis and generalised infection in neonates)	Amoxicillin ± an aminoglycoside	Erythromycin ± an aminoglycoside
Gram-negative rods		
Enterobacteriaceae (coliform organisms)		
Escherichia coli, Enterobacter, Klebsiella		
Infections of urinary tract	An oral cephalosporin, or a quinolone	Extended-spectrum penicillin
Septicaemia	An aminoglycoside (intravenous) or cefuroxime	Imipenem or a quinolone
Shigella (dysentery)	A quinolone	Ampicillin or trimethoprim
Salmonella (typhoid, paratyphoid)	A quinolone or ceftriaxone	Amoxicillin or chloramphenicol or trimethoprim
Haemophilus influenzae (infections of the respiratory tract, ear, sinuses; meningitis)	Ampicillin or cefuroxime	Cefuroxime (not for meningitis) or chloramphenicol
Bordetella pertussis (whooping cough)	A macrolide	Ampicillin
Pasteurella multocida (wound infections, abscess)	Amoxicillin + clavulanic acid	Ampicillin
Vibrio cholerae (cholera)	A tetracycline	A quinolone
Legionella pneumophila (pneumonia, Legionnaire's disease)	A macrolide ± rifampicin	
Helicobacter pylori (associated with peptic ulcer)	Metronidazole + amoxicillin + ranitidine[d] (2-week regimen)	Clarithromycin + metronidazole
Pseudomonas aeruginosa		
Urinary tract infection	A quinolone	Antipseudomonal penicillins

Table 45.1 *continued*

Other infections (of burns etc.)	Antipseudomonal penicillins + tobramycin[e]	Imipenem ± an aminoglycoside, or ceftazidime
Brucella (brucellosis)	Doxycycline + rifampicin	
Bacteroides fragilis		
Oropharyngeal infection	Benzylpenicillin	Metronidazole or clindamycin
Gastrointestinal infection	Metronidazole, clindamycin	Imipenem
Gram-negative anaerobic rods (other than *B. fragilis*)	Benzylpenicillin or metronidazole	A cephalosporin or clindamycin
Campylobacter (diarrhoea)	A macrolide or a quinolone	A tetracycline or gentamicin
Spirochaetes		
Treponema (syphilis, yaws)	Benzylpenicillin	A macrolide or ceftriaxone
Borrelia recurrentis (relapsing fever)	A tetracycline	Benzylpenicillin
Borrelia burgdorferi (Lyme disease)	A tetracycline	
Leptospira (Weil's disease)	Benzylpenicillin	A tetracycline
Rickettsiae (typhus, tick-bite fever, Q fever, etc.)	A tetracycline	A quinolone
Other organisms		
Mycoplasma pneumoniae	A tetracycline or a macrolide	Ciprofloxacin
Chlamydia (trachoma, psittacosis, urogenital infections)	A tetracycline	
Actinomyces (abscesses)	Benzylpenicillin	A tetracycline
Pneumocystis (pneumonia, especially in AIDS patients)	Co-trimoxazole (high dose)	Pentamidine or atovaquone or trimetrexate
Nocardia (lung disease, brain abscess)	Co-trimoxazole	

[a]This table is not meant to be a definitive guide for clinical treatment but a general indication of the main antimicrobial actions and thus of the overall usefulness of commonly used antibiotics. For a more comprehensive list, see Laurence et al. (1997).
[b]Only the main diseases caused by each organism are mentioned (in parentheses).
[c]± signifies that an agent is to be used with or without another agent; if agents are to be used concomitantly, a plus sign only is used.
[d]An antiulcer drug, not an antibiotic (see Ch. 24).
[e]Not in the same syringe.

inflammatory reaction, activating complement, causing fever, etc. (see Ch. 15). In addition, there are proteins in the outer membrane that form transmembrane water-filled channels, termed 'porins', through which hydrophilic antibiotics can move freely.

Difficulty in penetrating this complex outer layer is probably the reason why some antibiotics are less active against Gram-negative than Gram-positive bacteria. This is the basis of the extraordinary insusceptibility to most antibiotics of *Pseudomonas aeruginosa*, a pathogen which can cause life-threatening infections in neutropenic patients and patients with burns and wounds.

The lipopolysaccharide of the cell wall is also a major barrier to penetration.

Antibiotics for which penetration is a problem include **benzylpenicillin** (penicillin G), **methicillin**, the **macrolides**, **rifampicin**, **fusidic acid**, **vancomycin**, **bacitracin** and **novobiocin**.

ANTIMICROBIAL AGENTS THAT INTERFERE WITH THE SYNTHESIS OR ACTION OF FOLATE

SULFONAMIDES

In the 1930s, Domagk first demonstrated that a chemotherapeutic agent could influence the course of a bacterial infection. The drug was **prontosil**, a dye which proved to be a pro-drug, inactive in vitro and needing to be metabolised in vivo to give the active product—**sulfanilamide** (Fig. 45.1). Many sulfonamides have been developed since and they are still useful drugs.

Examples of sulfonamides in clinical use are **sulfadiazine** (Fig. 45.1), **sulfadimidine**, **sulfamethoxazole** (short-acting), **sulfametopyrazine** (long-acting), **sulfasalazine** (poorly absorbed in the gastrointestinal tract, see also Chs 16 and 24) and **sulfamethoxazole** (given with trimethoprim, the combination constitutes **co-trimoxazole**).

Mechanism of action

Sulfanilamide is a structural analogue of *p*-aminobenzoic acid (PABA; see Fig. 45.1), which is essential for the synthesis of folic acid in bacteria. As explained in Chapter 44, folate is required for the synthesis of the precursors of DNA and RNA both in bacteria and mammals, but mammals obtain their folic acid in their diet whereas bacteria need to synthesise it. Sulfonamides compete with PABA for the enzyme *dihydropteroate synthetase*, and the effect of the sulfonamide may be overcome by adding excess PABA. This is why some local anaesthetics, for example **procaine** (see Ch. 43), which are PABA esters, can antagonise the antibacterial effect of these agents.

The action of a sulfonamide is to inhibit growth of the bacteria, not to kill them, i.e. it is *bacteriostatic* rather than *bactericidal*. The action is negated by the presence of pus and the products of tissue breakdown since these contain thymidine and purines, which bacteria use to bypass the need for folic acid. Resistance, which is common, is plasmid mediated (see Ch. 44) and results from the synthesis of an enzyme insensitive to the drug.

Clinical uses of sulfonamides

- Combined with trimethoprim (co-trimoxazole) for *Pneumocystis carinii*.
- Combined with pyrimethamine for drug-resistant malaria (Table 48.1), and for toxoplasmosis.
- In inflammatory bowel disease and as an anti-inflammatory drug—sulfasalazine (sulfapyridine–aminosalicylate combination) is used.
- For infected burns (silver sulfadiazine given topically).
- For some sexually transmitted infections (e.g. trachoma, chlamydia, chancroid).
- For respiratory infections; use now confined to a few special problems (e.g. infection with *Nocardia*).
- For acute urinary tract infection (now seldom used).

Pharmacokinetic aspects

Most sulfonamides are readily absorbed in the gastrointestinal tract and reach maximum concentrations in the plasma in 4–6 hours.

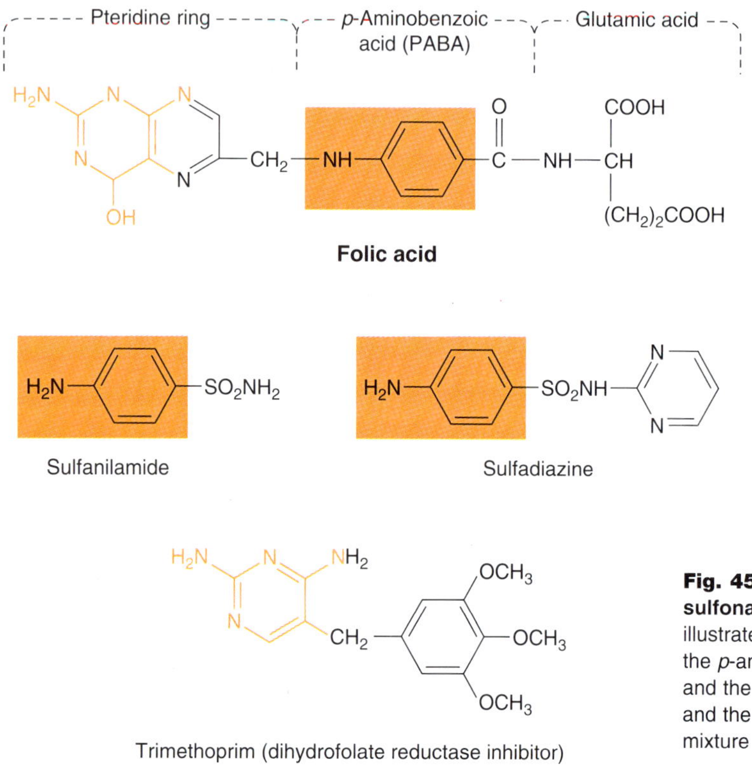

Fig. 45.1 Structures of two representative sulfonamides and trimethoprim. The structures illustrate the relationship between the sulfonamides and the *p*-aminobenzoic acid moiety in folic acid (orange box), and the possible relationship between the antifolate drugs and the pteridine moiety (orange). Co-trimoxazole is a mixture of sulfamethoxazole and trimethoprim.

They are usually not given topically, mainly because of the risk of sensitisation and allergic reactions. The drugs pass into inflammatory exudates and cross the placental and blood–brain barriers.

They are metabolised mainly in the liver, the major product being an acetylated derivative which lacks antibacterial action.

Unwanted effects

Mild-to-moderate side-effects are nausea and vomiting, headache and mental depression. Cyanosis caused by methaemoglobinaemia may occur and is a lot less alarming than it looks. Serious adverse effects that necessitate cessation of therapy include hepatitis, hypersensitivity reactions (rashes, fever, anaphylactoid reactions), bone marrow depression and crystalluria. This last results from the precipitation of acetylated metabolites in the urine.

TRIMETHOPRIM

In structure, trimethoprim (Fig. 45.1) resembles the pteridine moiety of folate. The similarity is close enough to confuse the relevant bacterial enzyme. Trimethoprim is chemically related to the antimalarial drug **pyrimethamine** (Fig. 48.4); both are *folate antagonists*. Bacterial dihydrofolate reductase is many times more sensitive to trimethoprim than is the equivalent enzyme in humans (Table 44.1).

Trimethoprim is active against most common bacterial pathogens, and it too is bacteriostatic. It is sometimes given as a mixture with sulfamethoxazole in a combination called **co-trimoxazole** (Fig. 45.1). Since sulfonamides affect an earlier stage in the same metabolic pathway in bacteria, i.e. folate synthesis, they can potentiate the action of trimethoprim. This is illustrated in Figure 45.2.

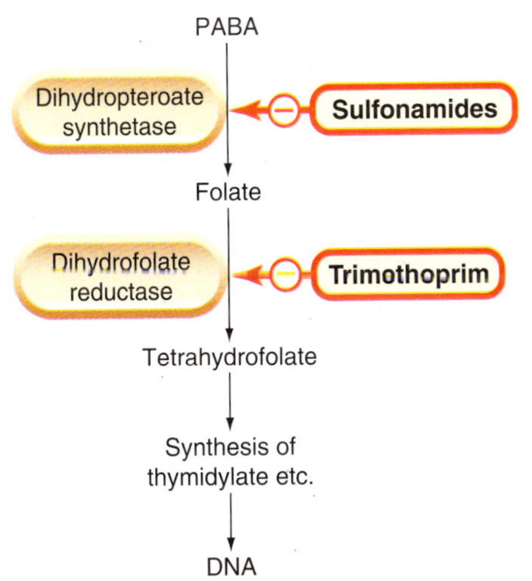

Fig. 45.2 The action of sulfonamides and trimethoprim on bacterial folate synthesis. See Figure 21.2 for more detail of tetrahydrofolate synthesis, and Table 44.1 for comparisons of antifolate drugs. (PABA, *p*-aminobenzoic acid.)

Clinical uses of trimethoprim/co-trimoxazole

- For urinary tract and respiratory infections; trimethoprim, used on its own, is usually preferred
- For infection with *Pneumocystis carinii*, which causes pneumonia in patients with AIDS; co-trimoxazole is used in high dose.

Antimicrobial agents that interfere with the synthesis or action of folate

- Sulfonamides are bacteriostatic; they act by interfering with folate synthesis and thus with nucleotide synthesis. Unwanted effects include crystalluria and hypersensitivities.
- Trimethoprim is bacteriostatic. It acts by folate antagonism.
- Co-trimoxazole is a mixture of trimethoprim with sulfamethoxazole, which affects bacterial nucleotide synthesis at two points.

Pharmacokinetic aspects

Trimethoprim is given orally, is fully absorbed in the gastrointestinal tract and widely distributed throughout the tissues and body fluids. It reaches high concentrations in the lungs and kidneys and fairly high concentrations in the cerebrospinal fluid (CSF). When given with sulfamethoxazole, about half of each is excreted within 24 hours. Since trimethoprim is a weak base, its elimination by the kidney increases with decreasing urinary pH.

The clinical use of trimethoprim is given in the box.

Unwanted effects

Unwanted effects of trimethoprim include nausea, vomiting, blood disorders and skin rashes. Folate deficiency, with resultant megaloblastic anaemia (see Ch. 21)—a toxic effect related to the pharmacological action of trimethoprim—can be prevented by giving folinic acid.

BETA-LACTAM ANTIBIOTICS

PENICILLIN

In 1928, Alexander Fleming, working at St Mary's Hospital in London, observed that a culture plate on which staphylococci were being grown had become contaminated with a mould of the genus *Penicillium*, and that bacterial growth in the vicinity of the mould had been inhibited. He isolated the mould in pure culture and demonstrated that it produced an antibacterial substance, which he called penicillin. This substance was subsequently extracted and its antibacterial effects analysed by Florey and Chain and their colleagues at Oxford in 1940. They showed that it had powerful chemotherapeutic properties in infected mice and that it was non-toxic. Its remarkable antibacterial effects in humans were clearly demonstrated in 1941. A small amount of penicillin, extracted laboriously from crude cultures in the laboratories of the Dunn School of Pathology in Oxford, was tested on a policeman who had staphylococcal and streptococcal septicaemia with multiple abscesses, and osteomyelitis with discharging sinuses. He was in great pain and was desperately ill. (Sulfonamides were available but would have had no effect in the presence of pus; see p. 638.) Intravenous injections of penicillin were given every 3 hours. All the patient's urine was collected and each day the excreted penicillin was extracted and used again. After 5 days, the patient's condition was vastly improved; his temperature was normal, he was eating well and there was obvious resolution of the abscesses. Furthermore, there seemed to be no toxic effects of the drug. Then the supply of penicillin ran out, his condition gradually deteriorated and he died a month later. This was the first evidence of the dramatic antibacterial effect of penicillin given *systemically* in humans. It is not generally known that *topical* penicillin had been used with success in five patients with eye infections 10 years previously by Paine—a graduate of St Mary's—who had obtained some penicillin mould from Fleming. The penicillins are extremely effective antibiotics and are very widely used. Penicillins may be destroyed by enzymes—amidases and β-lactamases (penicillinases) (see Fig. 45.3).

Mechanisms of action

All β-lactam antibiotics interfere with the synthesis of the bacterial cell wall peptidoglycan (see Ch. 44; Fig. 44.3). After attachment to binding sites on bacteria (termed *penicillin-binding proteins*, of which there may be seven or more types in different organisms), they inhibit the transpeptidation enzyme that cross-links the peptide chains attached to the backbone of the peptidoglycan.

The final bactericidal event is the inactivation of an inhibitor of the autolytic enzymes in the cell wall; this leads to lysis of the bacterium. Some organisms have defective autolytic enzymes and are inhibited but not lysed—they are referred to as 'tolerant'. Resistance to penicillin may result from a number of different causes and is discussed in detail in Ch. 44.

Types of penicillin and their antimicrobial activity

The first penicillin was the naturally occurring **benzylpenicillin** and its congeners such as **phenoxymethylpenicillin**. Benzylpenicillin is active against a wide range of organisms and is the drug of first choice for many infections (see Table 45.1 and the clinical box on p. 641). Its main drawbacks are poor absorption in the gastrointestinal tract (which means it must be

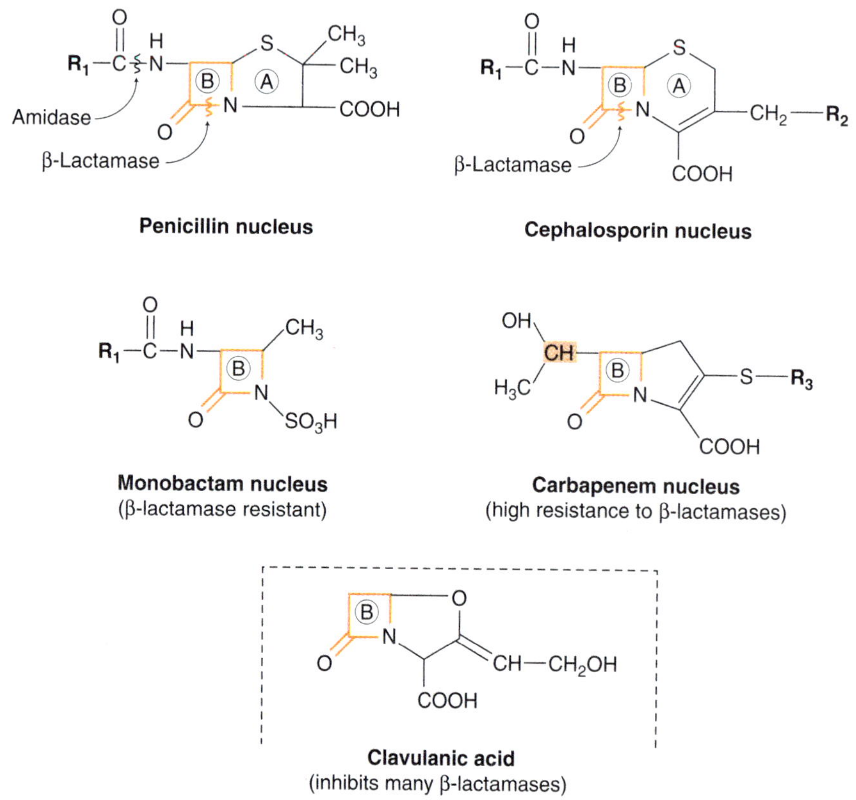

Fig. 45.3 Basic structures of four groups of β-lactam antibiotics and clavulanic acid. The structures illustrate the β-lactam ring (marked B), and the sites of action of bacterial enzymes that inactivate these antibiotics (A, thiazolidine ring). Various substituents are added at R_1, R_2, R_3, to produce agents with different properties. In carbapenems, the stereochemical configuration of the part of the β-lactam ring shown shaded in orange here is different from the corresponding part of the penicillin and cephalosporin molecules; this is probably the basis of the β-lactamase resistance of the carbapenems. The β-lactam ring of clavulanic acid is thought to bind strongly to β-lactamase, meanwhile protecting other β-lactams from the enzyme.

given by injection) and its susceptibility to bacterial β-lactamases.

Various semisynthetic penicillins have been prepared by adding different side-chains to the penicillin nucleus (at R_1 in Fig. 45.3). In this way *β-lactamase-resistant penicillins* (e.g. **flucloxacillin**) and *broad-spectrum penicillins* (e.g. **ampicillin, pivampicillin** and **amoxicillin**) have been produced. *Extended-spectrum penicillins* (e.g. **carbenacillin, ticarcilin** and **aziocillin**) with antipseudomonal activity have also been developed and have gone some way to overcoming the problem of serious infections caused by *P. aeruginosa*.

Pharmacokinetic aspects

When given orally, different penicillins are absorbed to differing degrees depending on their stability in acid and their adsorption to food. Penicillins can be given by intramuscular or intravenous injection. Intrathecal administration is inadvisable, particularly with **benzylpenicillin**, as it can cause convulsions. The drugs are widely distributed in the body fluids, passing into joints, into pleural and pericardial cavities, into the bile, the saliva and the milk and across the placenta. Being lipid insoluble they do not enter mammalian cells. They, therefore, do not cross the blood–brain barrier unless the meninges are inflamed, in which case they readily reach therapeutically effective concentrations in the CSF.

Elimination of most penicillins is mainly renal and occurs rapidly, 90% being by tubular secretion. The relatively short plasma half-life is a potential problem in the clinical use of **benzylpenicillin**, although since penicillin works by preventing cell wall synthesis in dividing organisms, intermittent rather than continuous exposure to the drug can be an advantage.

Clinical uses of the penicillins

- Penicillins are given by mouth or, in more severe infections, intravenously, and often in combination with other antibiotics.
- Uses include:
  —bacterial meningitis (e.g. caused by *Neisseria meningitidis, Streptococcus pneumoniae*): benzylpenicillin, high doses intravenously
  —bone and joint infections (e.g. with *Staphylococcus aureus*): flucloxacillin
  —skin and soft tissue infections (e.g. with *Streptococcus pyogenes* or *S. aureus*): benzylpenicillin, flucloxacillin; animal bites: co-amoxiclav
  —pharyngitis (from *S. pyogenes*): phenoxylmethylpenicillin
  —otitis media (organisms commonly include *S. pyogenes, Haemophilus influenzae*): amoxicillin
  —bronchitis (mixed infections common): amoxicillin
  —pneumonia: amoxicillin
  —urinary tract infections (e.g. with *Escherichia coli*): amoxicillin
  —gonorrhea: amoxicillin (plus probenecid)
  —syphilis: procaine benzylpenicillin
  —endocarditis (e.g. with *Streptococcus viridans* or *Enterococcus faecalis*)
  —serious infections with *Pseudomonas aeruginosa*: piperacillin.
- This list is not exhaustive. Treatment with penicillins is sometimes started empirically, if the likely causative organism is one thought to be susceptible to penicillin, while awaiting the results of laboratory tests to identify the organism and determine its antibiotic susceptibility.

Clinical use of the penicillins

Penicillins, often combined with other antibiotics, are crucially important in antibacterial chemotherapy. They are the drugs of choice for many infections. A list of clinical uses is given in the box. See also Table 45.1.

Unwanted effects

Penicillins are relatively free from direct toxic effects (other than their proconvulsant effect when given intrathecally). The main unwanted effects are *hypersensitivity reactions*, caused by the degradation products of penicillin, which combine with host protein and become antigenic. Skin rashes and fever are common; a delayed type of serum sickness occurs infrequently. Much more serious is *acute anaphylactic shock*, which may, in some cases, be fatal but is fortunately very rare.

Penicillins, particularly the broad-spectrum type given orally, alter the bacterial flora in the gut. This can be associated with gastrointestinal disturbances and, in some cases, with suprainfection by microorganisms not sensitive to penicillin.

CEPHALOSPORINS AND CEPHAMYCINS

Cephalosporins N and C, which are chemically related to penicillin, and cephalosporin P, a steroid antibiotic that resembles fusidic acid (see below) were first isolated from *Cephalosporium* fungus. The cephamycins are β-lactam antibiotics produced by *Streptomyces* organisms and they are closely related to the cephalosporins.

Semisynthetic *broad-spectrum cephalosporins* have been produced by addition, to the cephalosporin C nucleus, of different side-chains at R_1 and/or R_2 (see Fig. 45.3). These agents are water soluble and relatively acid stable. They vary in susceptibility to β-lactamases.

There are now a very large number of cephalosporins and cephamycins available for clinical use. Some of these drugs are described in Table 45.2.

Mechanism of action

The mechanism of action of these agents is the same as that of the penicillins—interference with bacterial peptidoglycan synthesis after binding to the β-lactam-binding proteins. This is described in detail in Chapter 44 and illustrated in Figure 44.3. Resistance

Table 45.2 Cephalosporins and cephamycins

Categories with examples	Important properties	Similar drugs
Oral drugs		
Cefalexin ($t_{1/2}$ 1 h)	An example of the first-generation compounds that have reasonable activity against Gram-positive organisms and modest activity against Gram-negative organisms	Cefachlor ($t_{1/2}$ 0.8 h) is a second-generation compound with greater potency against Gram- negative organisms, but it can cause unwanted cutaneous lesions
Parenteral drugs		
Cefuroxime ($t_{1/2}$1.5 h)	An example of the second-generation compounds that show only moderate activity against most Gram-positive organisms but reasonable potency against Gram-negative organisms	Cephamandole, cefoxitin ($t_{1/2}$ of both ~1 h), good activity against Gram-negative organisms, resistant to β-lactamase from Gram-negative rods, good potency against *Bacteroides fragilis*, bowel flora
Cefotaxime ($t_{1/2}$ 1 h)	An example of the third-generation compounds, which are less active against Gram-positive bacteria than those of the second generation but more active against Gram-negative bacteria. Has some activity against pseudomonads	Ceftizoxime ($t_{1/2}$1.5 h); ceftriaxone ($t_{1/2}$ 8.5 h), excreted largely in the bile; cefperazone ($t_{1/2}$ 2 h), excreted mainly in the bile, can cause decrease of vitamin K-dependent clotting factors

to this group of drugs has increased because of plasmid-encoded or chromosomal β-lactamase. Nearly all Gram-negative bacteria have a chromosomal gene coding for a β-lactamase that is more active in hydrolysing cephalosporins than penicillins; in several organisms a single-step mutation can result in high-level constitutive production of this enzyme. Resistance also occurs if there is decreased penetration of the drug as a result of alterations to outer membrane proteins or mutations of the binding-site proteins.

Pharmacokinetic aspects

Some cephalosporins may be given orally (see Table 45.2) but most are given parenterally, intramuscularly (which may be painful with some agents) or intravenously. After absorption they are widely distributed in the body. Some, such as **cefoperazone**, **cefotaxime**, **cefuroxime** and **ceftriaxone**, also cross the blood–brain barrier. Excretion is mostly via the kidney, largely by tubular secretion, but 40% of ceftriaxone and 75% of cefoperazone is eliminated in the bile.

Clinical uses of the cephalosporins

- Septicaemia (e.g. cefuroxime, cefotaxime)
- Pneumonia caused by susceptible organisms
- Meningitis (e.g. cefriaxone, cefotaxime)
- Biliary tract infection
- Urinary tract infection (especially in pregnancy, or in patients unresponsive to other drugs)
- Sinusitis (e.g. cefadroxil).

Clinical use

Some clinical uses of the cephalosporins are given in Table 45.2 and in the clinical box.

Unwanted effects

Hypersensitivity reactions, very similar to those that occur with penicillin, may be seen. Some cross-reactions occur; about 10% of penicillin-sensitive individuals will have allergic reactions to cephalosporins. Nephrotoxicity has been reported (especially with cefradine) as has intolerance to alcohol. Diarrhoea can occur with oral cephalosporins and cefoperazone

OTHER β-LACTAM ANTIBIOTICS

CARBAPENEMS AND MONOBACTAMS

Carbapenems and monobactams (see Fig. 45.3) were developed to deal with β-lactamase-producing Gram-negative organisms resistant to penicillins.

CARBAPENEMS

Imipenem, an example of a carbapenem, acts in the same way as the other β-lactams (see Fig. 45.3). It has a very broad spectrum of antimicrobial activity, being active against many aerobic and anaerobic Gram-positive and Gram-negative organisms. However, many of the 'methicillin-resistant' staphylococci (see p. 629) are less susceptible, and resistant strains of *P. aeruginosa* have emerged during therapy. Imipenem was originally resistant to all β-lactamases but some organisms now have chromosomal genes that code for imipenem-hydrolysing β-lactamases.

Unwanted effects are similar to those seen with other β-lactams, nausea and vomiting being the most frequently seen. Neurotoxicity can occur with high plasma concentrations.

Beta-lactam antibiotics

- Bactericidal by interference with peptidoglycan synthesis.

Penicillins

- The first choice for many infections.
- Benzylpenicillin
  - —given by injection, short half-life and is destroyed by β-lactamases
  - —spectrum: Gram-positive and Gram-negative cocci and some Gram-negative bacteria
  - —many staphylococci are now resistant.
- Beta-lactamase-resistant penicillins, e.g. flucloxacillin
  - —given orally
  - —spectrum: as for benzylpenicillin.
  - —many staphylococci are now resistant.
- Broad-spectrum penicillins, e.g. amoxicillin
  - —given orally; they are destroyed by β-lactamases
  - —spectrum: as for benzylpenicillin (though less potent); they are also active against Gram-negative bacteria.
- Extended-spectrum penicillins, e.g. ticarcillin
  - —given orally; they are susceptible to β-lactamases
  - —spectrum: as for broad-spectrum penicillins; they are also active against pseudomonads.
- Unwanted effects of penicillins: mainly hypersensitivities
- A combination of clavulanic acid plus amoxicillin or ticarcillin is effective against many β-lactamase-producing organisms.

Cephalosporins and cephamycins

- Second choice for many infections.
- Oral drugs, e.g. cefachlor, are used in urinary infections.
- Parenteral drugs, e.g. cefuroxime, which is active against *S. aureus, H. influenzae,* Enterobacteriaceae.
- Unwanted effects: mainly hypersensitivities.

Carbapenems

- Imipenem is used with cilastin, which blocks its breakdown in the kidney.
- Imipenem is a broad-spectrum antibiotic.

Monobactams

- Aztreonam. This is active only against Gram-negative aerobic bacteria and is resistant to most β-lactamases.

MONOBACTAMS

The main monobactam is **aztreonam**, a simple monocyclic β-lactam with a complex substituent at R_3 (see Fig. 45.3), which is resistant to most β-lactamases. This has an unusual spectrum—being active only against Gram-negative aerobic rods, including pseudomonads, *Neisseria meningitidis* and *Haemophilus influenzae*; it has no action against Gram-positive organisms or anaerobes.

It is given parenterally and has a plasma half-life of 2 hours.

Unwanted effects are, in general, similar to those of other β-lactam antibiotics, but this agent does not necessarily cross-react immunologically with penicillin and its products and so does not usually cause allergic reactions in penicillin-sensitive individuals.

ANTIMICROBIAL AGENTS AFFECTING BACTERIAL PROTEIN SYNTHESIS

TETRACYCLINES

Tetracyclines are broad-spectrum antibiotics. The group includes **tetracycline**, **oxytetracycline**, **doxycyclin**e and **minocycline**.

Mechanism of action

Tetracyclines act by inhibiting protein synthesis after uptake into susceptible organisms by active transport. This action is described in detail in Chapter 44 (p. 625 and Fig. 44.4). The tetracyclines are bacteriostatic, not bactericidal.

Antibacterial spectrum

The spectrum of antimicrobial activity of the tetracyclines is very wide and includes Gram-positive and Gram-negative bacteria, *Mycoplasma*, *Rickettsia*, *Chlamydia* spp., spirochaetes and some protozoa (e.g. amoebae). **Minocycline** is also effective against *N. meningitidis* and has been used to eradicate this organism from the nasopharynx of carriers. However, many strains of organisms have become resistant to these agents and this has decreased their usefulness (see p. 629). Resistance is transmitted mainly by

Clinical uses of tetracyclines

- Antibiotics of first choice for rickettsial, mycoplasma and chlamydial infections, brucellosis, cholera, plague and Lyme disease.
- Second choice for infections with several different organisms (see Table 45.1).
- They are useful in mixed infections of the respiratory tract and in acne.
- A use of **democloxyxline** distinct from its antimicrobial action is for chronic hyponatraemia caused by inappropriate secretion of antidiuretic hormone (for example by some malignant lung tumours); the drug inhibits the action of this hormone (Ch. 23).

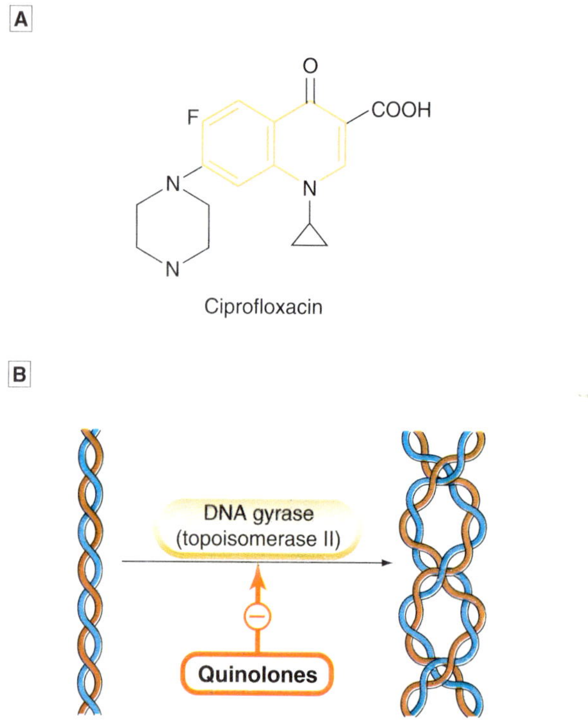

Fig. 45.4 A simplified diagram of the mechanism of action of the fluoroquinolones. A An example of a quinolone (the quinolone moiety is shown in orange). **B** Schematic diagram of (left) the double helix and (right) the double helix in supercoiled form. (See also Fig. 44.6.) In essence, the DNA gyrase unwinds the RNA-induced positive supercoil (not shown) and introduces a negative supercoil.

plasmids and, since the genes controlling resistance to tetracyclines are closely associated with genes for resistance to other antibiotics, organisms may become resistant to many drugs simultaneously.

Pharmacokinetic aspects

The tetracyclines are usually given orally but can be given parenterally. The absorption of most preparations from the gut is irregular and incomplete, and it is improved in the absence of food. Since tetracyclines chelate metal ions (calcium, magnesium, iron, aluminium), forming non-absorbable complexes, absorption is decreased in the presence of milk, certain antacids and iron preparations. **Minocycline** and **doxycycline** are virtually completely absorbed

The clinical use of the tetracyclines is given in the box on page 643.

Unwanted effects

The commonest unwanted effects are gastrointestinal disturbances caused initially by direct irritation and later to modification of the gut flora. Vitamin B complex deficiency can occur as can suprainfection.

Because they chelate Ca^{2+}, tetracyclines are deposited in growing bones and teeth, causing staining and sometimes dental hypoplasia and bone deformities. They should, therefore, not be given to children, pregnant women or nursing mothers. Another hazard in pregnant women is hepatotoxicity.

Phototoxicity (sensitisation to sunlight) has been seen, more particularly with **demeclocycline**. **Minocycline** can produce dose-related vestibular disturbances (dizziness and nausea). High doses of tetracyclines can decrease protein synthesis in host cells—an anti-anabolic effect—which could result in renal damage. Long-term therapy can cause disturbances of the bone marrow.

CHLORAMPHENICOL

Chloramphenicol was originally isolated from cultures of *Streptomyces*. The mechanism of action is by inhibition of protein synthesis as described in Chapter 44 (p. 625 and Fig. 44.4). Chloramphenicol binds to the 50S subunit of the bacterial ribosome at the same site as do **erythromycin** and **clindamycin**.

Antibacterial spectrum

Chloramphenicol has a wide spectrum of antimicrobial activity, including Gram-negative and Gram-positive organisms and rickettsiae. It is bacteriostatic for most organisms but bactericidal to *H. influenzae*. Resistance is caused by the production of chloramphenicol acetyltransferase (see p. 631) and is plasmid mediated.

Pharmacokinetic aspects

Given orally, chloramphenicol is rapidly and completely absorbed and reaches its maximum concentration in the plasma within 2 hours; it can also be given parenterally. It is widely distributed throughout the tissues and body fluids including the CSF, in which its concentration may be 60% of that in the blood. In the plasma it is 30–50% protein-bound and its half-life is approximately 2 hours. About 10% is excreted unchanged in the urine, and the remainder is inactivated in the liver.

The clinical use of chloramphenicol is given in the box.

Clinical uses of chloramphenicol

- Clinical use of chloramphenicol should be reserved for serious infections in which the benefit of the drug is greater than the risk of toxicity (see below), such as:
  - —infections caused by *Haemophilus influenzae* resistant to other drugs
  - —meningitis in patients in whom penicillin cannot be used.
- It is also safe and effective in bacterial conjunctivitis (given topically).
- It is effective in typhoid fever but ciprofloxacin or amoxicillin and co-trimoxazole are similarly effective and less toxic.
- Other possible uses are given in Table 45.1.

Unwanted effects

The most important unwanted effect of chloramphenicol is severe, idiosyncratic depression of the bone marrow resulting in pancytopenia (a decrease in all blood cell elements)—an effect which, though rare, can occur even with very low doses in some individuals.

Chloramphenicol should be used with great care in newborns because inadequate inactivation and excretion of the drug (see Ch. 51) can result in the 'grey baby syndrome'—vomiting, diarrhoea, flaccidity, low temperature and an ashen-grey colour—which carries a 40% mortality; if its use is essential, plasma concentrations should be determined and the dose adjusted accordingly. Hypersensitivity reactions can occur, as can gastrointestinal disturbances and other sequelae of alteration of the intestinal microbial flora.

AMINOGLYCOSIDES

The aminoglycosides are a group of antibiotics of complex chemical structure, resembling each other in antimicrobial activity, pharmacokinetic characteristics and toxicity. The main agents are **gentamicin**, **streptomycin**, **amikacin**, **tobramycin**, **netilmicin** and **neomycin**.

Mechanism of action

Aminoglycosides inhibit bacterial protein synthesis (see Ch. 44, p. 625).

Their penetration through the cell membrane of the bacterium depends partly on oxygen-dependent active transport by a polyamine carrier system and they have minimal action against anaerobic organisms. Chloramphenicol blocks this transport system. The effect of the aminoglycosides is bactericidal and is enhanced by agents that interfere with cell wall synthesis.

Resistance

Resistance to aminoglycosides is becoming a problem. It occurs by several different mechanisms (see pp. 631–632), the most important being inactivation by microbial enzymes of which there are nine or more. **Amikacin** was designed as a poor substrate for these enzymes; but some organisms have developed enzymes that inactivate this agent as well.

Resistance as a result of failure of penetration can be largely overcome by the concomitant use of **penicillin** and/or **vancomycin**.

Antibacterial spectrum

The aminoglycosides are effective against many aerobic Gram-negative and some Gram-positive organisms (see Table 45.1).

They are most widely used against Gram-negative enteric organisms and in sepsis. They may be given together with a penicillin in infections caused by streptococci, *Listeria* sp. and *P. aeruginosa* (see Table 45.1). **Gentamicin** is the aminoglycoside most commonly used, though **tobramycin** is the preferred member of this group for *P. aeruginosa* infections. **Amikacin** has the widest antimicrobial spectrum and along with **netilmicin** can be effective in infections with organisms resistant to gentamicin and tobramycin.

Pharmacokinetic aspects

The aminoglycosides are polycations and highly polar. They are not absorbed in the gastrointestinal tract and are usually given intramuscularly or intravenously. They do not cross the blood–brain barrier, penetrate the vitreous humour of the eye or reach high concentrations in secretions and body fluids, though high concentrations can be attained in joint and pleural fluids. They may, however, cross the placenta. The plasma half-life is 2–3 hours. Elimination is virtually entirely by glomerular filtration in the kidney, 50–60% of a dose being excreted unchanged within 24 hours. If renal function is impaired, accumulation occurs rapidly with a resultant increase in those toxic effects (such as ototoxicity and nephrotoxicity, see below) that are dose related.

Clinical use

Clinical uses of the aminoglycosides are given in Table 45.1.

Unwanted effects

Serious, dose-related toxic effects, which may increase as treatment proceeds, can occur with the aminoglycosides, the main hazards being ototoxicity and nephrotoxicity.

The *ototoxicity* involves progressive damage to, and destruction of, the sensory cells in the cochlea and vestibular organ of the ear. The result, usually irreversible, may be vertigo, ataxia and loss of balance in the case of vestibular damage, and auditory disturbances, including deafness, in the case of cochlear damage. Any aminoglycoside may produce both types of effect, but **streptomycin** and **gentamicin** are more likely to interfere with vestibular function whereas **neomycin** and **amikacin** affect mostly hearing. **Netilmicin** is less ototoxic than other aminoglycosides and is preferred when prolonged use is necessary. Ototoxicity is potentiated by the concomitant use of other ototoxic drugs (e.g. loop diuretics, p. 363).

The *nephrotoxicity* consists of damage to the kidney tubules and can be reversed if the use of the drugs is stopped. Nephrotoxicity is more likely to occur in patients with pre-existing renal disease or in conditions in which urine volume is reduced; concomitant use of other nephrotoxic agents (e.g. *cephalosporins*) increases the risk. Note that as the elimination of these drugs is almost entirely renal, their nephrotoxic action can impair their own excretion and a vicious cycle can be set up. Plasma concentrations should be monitored regularly. **Spectinomycin** is related to the aminoglycosides in structure. Its use is confined to the treatment of gonorrhoea in patients allergic to penicillin or those whose infections are caused by penicillin-resistant gonococci.

A rare but serious toxic reaction is paralysis caused by neuromuscular blockade, usually only seen if the agents are given concurrently with neuromuscular-blocking agents. It results from inhibition of the Ca^{2+} uptake necessary for the exocytotic release of acetylcholine (see Ch. 10).

MACROLIDES

For 40 years, **erythromycin** was the only macrolide antibiotic in general clinical use. (The term 'macrolide' relates to the structure—a many-membered lactone ring to which one or more deoxy sugars are attached.) Several additional macrolide and related antibiotics are now available, the two most important of which are **clarithromycin** and **azithromycin**.

Mechanism of action

The macrolides inhibit bacterial protein synthesis by an effect on translocation (Fig. 44.4). Their action may be bactericidal or bacteriostatic, the effect depending on the concentration and on the type of microorganism. The drugs bind to the 50S subunit of the bacterial ribosome; the binding site is the same as that of **chloramphenicol** and **clindamycin** and the three types of agent could compete, if given concurrently.

Antimicrobial spectrum

The antimicrobial spectrum of **erythromycin** is very similar to that of penicillin and it has proved to be a safe and effective alternative for penicillin-sensitive patients. Erythromycin is effective against Gram-positive bacteria and spirochaetes but not against most Gram-negative organisms, exceptions being *Neisseria gonorrhoeae* and, to a lesser extent, *H. influenzae*. *Mycoplasma pneumoniae*, *Legionella* sp. and some chlamydial organisms are also susceptible (see Table 45.1) Resistance can occur and results from a plasmid-controlled alteration of the binding site for erythromycin on the bacterial ribosome (Fig. 44.4).

Azithromycin is less active against Gram-positive bacteria than erythromycin, is considerably more effective against *H. influenzae* and may be more active against *Legionella*. It has excellent action against *Toxoplasma gondii* (p. 685), killing the cysts.

Clarithromycin is as active, and its metabolite is twice as active, against *H. influenzae* as erythromycin; it is also effective against *Mycobacterium avium-intercellulare* (which can infect immunologically compromised individuals and elderly patients with chronic lung disease) and it may be useful in leprosy and against *Helicobacter pylori* (see Ch. 24). Both these macrolides are effective in Lyme disease.

Pharmacokinetic aspects

The macrolides are administered orally, **azithromycin** and **clarithromycin** being more acid stable than **erythromycin**. Erythromycin can also be given parenterally, though intravenous injections can be followed by local thrombophlebitis. They all diffuse readily into most tissues but do not cross the blood–brain barrier and there is poor penetration into synovial fluid. The plasma half-life of erythromycin is about 90 minutes; that of clarithromycin is three times longer and that of azithromycin 8–16 times longer. Macrolides enter and are concentrated within phagocytes—azithromycin concentrations in phagocyte lysosomes can be 40 times higher than in the blood—and they can enhance phagocyte killing of bacteria.

Erythromycin is partly inactivated in the liver; azithromycin is more resistant to inactivation and clarithromycin is converted to an active metabolite. (Effects on the P450 cytochrome system can affect the bioavailability of other drugs; see Ch. 51.) The major route of elimination is in the bile.

Clinical use

The clinical use of the macrolides is given in Table 45.1.

Unwanted effects

Gastrointestinal disturbances are common and unpleasant but not serious. With erythromycin, the following have also been reported: hypersensitivity reactions such as skin rashes and fever, transient hearing disturbances, and, rarely, with treatment longer than 2 weeks, cholestatic jaundice.

Opportunistic infections of the gastrointestinal tract or vagina can occur.

STREPTOGRAMINS

Quinupristin and **dalfopristin** are members of the streptogramin family of compounds isolated from *Streptomyces pristinaespiralis*. These agents have a cyclic peptide structure. They act by inhibiting protein synthesis. Individually, quinupristin and dalfopristin exhibit only very modest bacteriostatic activity but combined together as an intravenous injection they are active against many Gram-positive bacteria..

Quinupristin/dalfopristin (3 parts to 7 parts weight for weight) is an effective approach to the treatment of serious infections usually where no other antibacterial is suitable. For example, the combination is effective against methicillin-sensitive *Staphylococcus aureus* and is also active against vancomycin-resistant *Enterococcal faecium*. The mechanism of action is to inhibit protein formation by binding to the 50S subunit of the bacterial ribosome. Dalfopristin changes the structure of the ribosome so as to promote the binding of quinupristin, which probably explains the improved effectiveness of the drugs when administered together.

Both quinupristin and dalfopristin are broken down in the liver and must, therefore, be given as an intravenous infusion. The half-life of each compound is 1–2 hours.

Unwanted effects

Unwanted effects include infusion site inflammation and pain, arthralgia, myalgia and nausea, vomiting and diarrhoea. To date, resistance to quinupristin and dalfopristine does not seem to be a major problem.

LINCOSAMIDES

Clindamycin is active against Gram-positive cocci, including many penicillin-resistant staphylococci, and many anaerobic bacteria such as *Bacteroides* species.

Its mechanism of action involves inhibition of protein synthesis similar to that of the macrolides and chloramphenicol (Fig. 44.4).

Clindamycin can be given orally or parenterally and is widely distributed in tissues (including bone) and body fluids but does not cross the blood–brain barrier. There is active uptake into leucocytes. Its half-life is 21 hours. Some is metabolised in the liver, and the metabolites, which are active, are excreted in the bile and the urine.

Unwanted effects

Unwanted effects consist mainly of gastrointestinal disturbances. A potentially lethal condition, *pseudomembranous colitis*, can occur; this is an acute inflammation of the colon caused by a necrotising toxin produced by a clindamycin-resistant organism, *Clostridium difficile*, which may be part of the normal faecal flora.* Vancomycin, given orally, and metronidazole (see below) are effective in the treatment of this condition.

Its *clinical use* is in infections caused by *Bacteroides* organisms and for staphylococcal infections of bones and joints. It is also used topically, as eye drops, for staphylococcal conjunctivitis.

Antimicrobial agents affecting bacterial protein synthesis

- *Tetracyclines,* e.g. **minocycline**. These are orally active, bacteriostatic, broad-spectrum antibiotics. Resistance is increasing. Gastrointestinal disorders are common. They chelate calcium and are deposited in growing bone. They are contraindicated in children and pregnant women.
- **Chloramphenicol**. This is an orally active, bacteriostatic, broad-spectrum antibiotic. Serious toxic effects are possible, including bone marrow depression, grey baby syndrome. It should be reserved for life-threatening infections.
- *Aminoglycosides,* e.g. **gentamicin**. These are given by injection. They are bactericidal, broad-spectrum antibiotics (but with low activity against anaerobes, streptococci and pneumococci). Resistance is increasing. The main unwanted effects are dose-related nephrotoxicity and ototoxicity. Serum levels should be monitored. (Streptomycin is an antituberculosis aminoglycoside.)
- *Macrolides,* e.g. **erythromycin**. Can be given orally and parenterally. They are bactericidal/bacteriostatic. The antibacterial spectrum is the same as for penicillin. Erythromycin can cause jaundice. Newer agents are clarithromycin and azithromycin.
- **Clindamycin**. Can be given orally and parenterally. It can cause pseudomembranous colitis.
- **Quinupristin/dalfopristin**. Given by intravenous infusion as a combination. Considerably less active when administered separately. Active against several strains of drug-resistant bacteria.
- **Fusidic acid**. This is a narrow-spectrum antibiotic that acts by inhibiting protein synthesis. It penetrates bone. Unwanted effects include gastrointestinal disorders.
- **Linezolid**. Given orally or by intravenous injection. Active against several strains of drug-resistant bacteria.

OXALIZIDONONES

Linezolid is the first oxalizidonone antibiotic drug to be introduced. It is active against a wide variety of Gram-positive bacteria and is particularly useful for the treatment of drug-resistant bacteria such as methicillin-resistant *S. aureus,* penicillin-resistant *Streptococcus pneumoniae* and vancomycin-resistant enterococci. The drug is also effective against some anaerobes such as *C. difficile*. Linezolid can be used to treat pneumonia, septicaemia and skin and soft tissue infections.

Its mechanism of action is to inhibit bacterial protein synthesis by binding to a site on the 50S ribosomal subunit.

Linezolid can be given orally or as an intravenous infusion in serious infection. After oral administration, peak plasma concentrations are achieved quickly with a half-life of 5–7 hours. Metabolism is by oxidation of the morpholine ring structure.

Unwanted effects

Unwanted effects include thrombocytopenia, diarrhoea, nausea and, rarely, rash and dizziness. Resistance is not yet a major problem but has been seen in patients with enterococcal infection. The drug is usually restricted to serious bacterial infections where other antibiotics have failed

FUSIDIC ACID

Fusidic acid is a narrow-spectrum steroid antibiotic active mainly against Gram-positive bacteria. It acts by inhibiting protein synthesis (Fig. 44.4).

Sodium fusidate is well absorbed from the gut and is distributed widely in the tissues. Some is excreted in the bile and some metabolised.

Unwanted effects

Unwanted effects such as gastrointestinal disturbances are fairly common. Skin eruptions and jaundice can occur. It is also used topically for staphylococcal conjunctivitis.

ANTIMICROBIAL AGENTS AFFECTING TOPOISOMERASE II

FLUOROQUINOLONES

The fluoroquinolones include the broad-spectrum agents **ciprofloxacin**, **levofloxacin,** **ofloxacin**, **norfloxacin**,

*This can also occur with some penicillins and cephalosporins.

acrosoxacin and **pefloxacin**, and the narrower-spectrum drugs used in urinary tract infections—**cinoxacin**, and **nalidixic acid**. (The last named was the first quinolone and is not fluorinated.) As explained on page 627, these agents inhibit topoisomerase II (a DNA gyrase), the enzyme that produces a negative supercoil in DNA and thus permits transcription or replication (see Fig. 45.4).

Antibacterial spectrum and clinical use

Ciprofloxacin is the most commonly used fluoroquinolone and will be described as the type agent. It is a broad-spectrum antibiotic, effective against both Gram-positive and Gram-negative organisms.. It has excellent activity against the Enterobacteriaceae (the enteric Gram-negative bacilli), including many organisms resistant to penicillins, cephalosporins and aminoglycosides, and it is also effective against *H. influenzae*, penicillinase-producing *N. gonorrhoeae*, *Campylobacter* sp. and pseudomonads. Of the Gram-positive organisms, streptococci and pneumococci are only weakly inhibited and there is a high incidence of staphylococcal resistance. Ciprofloxacin should be avoided in methicillin-resistant staphylococcal infections.

Clinically, the fluoroquinolones are best used for infections with facultative and aerobic Gram-negative rods and cocci.* Resistant strains of *S. aureus* and *P. aeruginosa* have emerged.

Pharmacokinetic aspects

Given orally, the fluoroquinolones are well absorbed. The half-life of ciprofloxacin and norfloxacin is 3 hours, that of ofloxacin is 5 hours and that of perfloxacin is 10 hours. The drugs concentrate in many tissues, particularly in the kidney, prostate and lung. All quinolones are concentrated in phagocytes. Most do not cross the blood–brain barrier except for pefloxacin and ofloxacin, which reach, in the CSF, 40% and 90%, respectively, of their serum concentrations. **Aluminium** and **magnesium antacids** interfere with the absorption of the quinolones. Elimination of ciprofloxacin, norfloxacin and enofloxacin is partly by hepatic metabolism by P450 enzymes (which they can inhibit, giving rise to interactions with other drugs; see below) and partly by renal excretion. Pefloxacin is metabolised to norfloxacin. Ofloxacin is excreted in the urine.

The clinical use of the fluoroquinolones is given in the box.

Unwanted effects

Unwanted effects are infrequent, usually mild and disappear if the agents are withdrawn. They consist mainly of gastrointestinal disorders and skin rashes. Arthropathy has been reported in young individuals. CNS symptoms—headache, dizziness—have occurred and, less frequently, convulsions, which have been associated with CNS pathology or concurrent use of theophylline or a non-steroidal anti-inflammatory drug.

*When ciprofloxacin was introduced, some clinical pharmacologists and microbiologists suggested, sensibly, that to prevent emergence of resistance, it should be reserved for organisms resistant to other drugs. However, it was estimated that, in 1989, it was prescribed for 1 in 44 of Americans; so it would seem that the horse has not only left the stable but has bolted.

Clinical uses of the fluoroquinolones

- Complicated urinary tract infections (norfloxacin, ofloxacin)
- *Pseudomonas aeruginosa* respiratory infections in patients with cystic fibrosis
- Invasive external otitis caused by *P. aeruginosa*
- Chronic Gram-negative bacillary osteomyelitis
- Eradication of *Salmonella typhi* in carriers
- Gonorrhoea (norfloxacin, ofloxacin)
- Bacterial prostatitis (norfloxacin)
- Cervicitis (ofloxacin)
- Anthrax.

Antimicrobial agents affecting DNA topoisomerase II

- These drugs—the fluoroquinolones, e.g. ciprofloxacin—interfere with the supercoiling of DNA.
- **Ciprofloxacin** has a wide antibacterial spectrum, being especially active against Gram-negative enteric coliform organisms including many organisms resistant to penicillins, cephalosporins and aminoglycosides; it is also effective against *Haemophilus influenzae*, penicillinase-producing *Neisseria gonorrhoeae*, *Campylobacter* sp. and pseudomonads. There is a high incidence of staphylococcal resistance. It is active orally with a half life of 4.5 hours.
- Unwanted effects include gastrointestinal tract upsets, hypersensitivity reactions and, rarely, CNS disturbances.

There is a clinically important interaction between **ciprofloxacin** and **theophylline** (through inhibition of P450 enzymes), which can lead to theophylline toxicity in asthmatics treated with the fluoroquinolones; theophylline toxicity is discussed in Chapter 22.

MISCELLANEOUS ANTIBACTERIAL AGENTS

The main glycopeptide antibiotic is **vancomycin. Teicoplanin** is similar but longer lasting. Vancomycin is bactericidal (except against streptococci) and acts by inhibiting cell wall synthesis (see Fig. 44.3). It is effective mainly against Gram-positive bacteria and has been used against methicillin-resistant staphylococci.

Vancomycin is not absorbed from the gut and is only given by the oral route for treatment of gastrointestinal infection with *C.*

difficile. For parenteral use it is given intravenously and has a plasma half-life of about 8 hours.

The *clinical use* of vancomycin is limited mainly to pseudomembranous colitis (see **clindamycin,** p. 647) and the treatment of some multiresistant staphylococcal infections. It is also valuable in severe staphylococcal infections in patients allergic both to *penicillins* and *cephalosporins*, and in some forms of endocarditis.

Unwanted effects include fever, rashes and local phlebitis at the site of injection. Ototoxicity and nephrotoxicity can occur and hypersensitivity reactions are seen occasionally.

Nitrofurantoin is a synthetic compound active against a range of Gram-positive and Gram-negative organisms. The development of resistance in susceptible organisms is rare and there is no cross-resistance. Its mechanism of action is not known. It is given orally and is rapidly and totally absorbed from the gastrointestinal tract and very rapidly excreted by the kidney.

The *clinical use* of nitrofurantoin is confined to the treatment of urinary tract infections.

Unwanted effects such as gastrointestinal disturbances are relatively common, and hypersensitivity reactions involving the skin and the bone marrow (e.g. leucopenia) can occur. Hepatotoxicity and peripheral neuropathy have been reported.

The polymixin antibiotics in use are **polymixin B** and **colistin** (polymixin E). They have cationic detergent properties and their mechanism of action involves interaction with the phospholipid of the cell membrane and disruption of its structure (Ch. 44, p. 628). They have a selective, rapidly bactericidal action on Gram-negative bacilli, especially pseudomonads and coliform organisms. They are not absorbed from the gastrointestinal tract.

Unwanted effects may be serious and include neurotoxicity and nephrotoxicity.

Clinical use of these drugs is limited by their toxicity and is confined largely to gut sterilisation and topical treatment of ear, eye or skin infections caused by susceptible organisms.

Metronidazole was introduced as an antiprotozoal agent (see p. 683) but it is also active against anaerobic bacteria such as *Bacteroides*, *Clostridia* sp. and some streptococci. It is effective in the therapy of pseudomembranous colitis, a clostridial infection sometimes associated with antibiotic therapy (see p. 647) and is important in the treatment of serious anaerobic infections (e.g. sepsis secondary to bowel disease).

> **Miscellaneous antibacterial agents**
>
> - *Glycopeptide* antibiotics, e.g. **vancomycin**. Vancomycin is bactericidal, acting by inhibiting cell wall synthesis. It is used intravenously for multiresistant staphylococcal infections and orally for pseudomembranous colitis. Unwanted effects include ototoxicity and nephrotoxicity.
> - *Polymixins*, e.g. **colistin**. They are bactericidal, acting by disrupting bacterial cell membranes. They are seriously neurotoxic and nephrotoxic and are only used topically.

ANTIMYCOBACTERIAL AGENTS

The main mycobacterial infections in humans are *tuberculosis* and *leprosy*—both typically chronic infections, caused, respectively, by *Mycobacterium tuberculosis* and *Mycobacterium leprae*. A particular problem with both these conditions is that after phagocytosis, the microorganism can survive inside macrophages, unless these are 'activated' by cytokines produced by T helper 1 lymphocytes (see Ch. 15).

DRUGS USED TO TREAT TUBERCULOSIS

Tuberculosis was for centuries a major killer disease; then 40 years or so ago, new drugs were developed and put to use and tuberculosis came to be seen as an easily curable condition. This is so no longer—the mycobacterium which causes it has come back to haunt us: multidrug-resistant strains are now common and strains with increased virulence have emerged (Bloom & Small, 1998). Tuberculosis is a major threat; killing about 2 million people each year. The World Health Organization estimates that 1 billion people will be newly infected in the period 2000–2020, resulting in 35 million more deaths. It has become clear that there is an ominous synergy between mycobacteria (e.g. *M. tuberculosis*, *M. avium-intercellulare*) and the human immunodeficiency virus (HIV). In Africa, about 15% of HIV-associated deaths are caused by tuberculosis. Tuberculosis is out of control in many parts of the world and it is now the world's leading cause of death from a single agent.

Against this increasingly worrisome background, the first-line drugs are **isoniazid**, **rifampicin**, **rifabutin, ethambutol** and **pyrazinamide**. Some second-line drugs available are **capreomycin**, **cycloserine**, **streptomycin** (rarely used now in the UK), **clarithromycin** and **ciprofloxacin**; these may be used for infections with tubercle bacilli likely to be resistant to first-line drugs or when the first-line agents have to be abandoned because of unwanted reactions.

To decrease the possibility of the emergence of resistant organisms, compound drug therapy is employed, involving the following:

- a first *initial* phase of about 2 months consisting of three drugs used concomitantly: isoniazid, rifampicin, pyrazinamide (plus ethambutol if the organism is suspected to be resistant)
- a second, *continuation* phase, of 4 months, consisting of two drugs: isoniazid and rifampicin; longer-term treatment is needed for patients with meningitis, bone/joint involvement or drug-resistant infection.

ISONIAZID

The antibacterial activity of isoniazid is limited to mycobacteria. It is bacteriostatic against resting organisms but can kill dividing bacteria. It passes freely into mammalian cells and is thus effective against intracellular organisms. The mechanism of its action is not clear. There is evidence that it inhibits the synthesis of mycolic acids, important constituents of the cell wall and peculiar to mycobacteria. It is also reported to combine with an enzyme that is uniquely found in isoniazid-sensitive strains of mycobacteria; this results in disorganisation of the metabolism of the cell. Resistance can occur and is caused by reduced penetration of the drug. Cross-resistance with other tuberculostatic drugs does not occur.

Pharmacokinetic aspects

Isoniazid is readily absorbed from the gastrointestinal tract and is widely distributed throughout the tissues and body fluids, including the CSF. An important point is that it penetrates well into 'caseous' tuberculous lesions (i.e. necrotic lesions, with a cheese-like consistency). Metabolism, which involves largely acetylation, depends on genetic factors that determine whether a person is a slow or rapid acetylator of the drug (see Chs 8 and 51), slow inactivators having a better therapeutic response. The half-life in slow inactivators is 3 hours and in rapid inactivators, 1 hour. Isoniazid is excreted in the urine partly as unchanged drug and partly in the acetylated or otherwise inactivated form.

Unwanted effects

Unwanted effects depend on the dosage and occur in about 5% of individuals, the commonest being allergic skin eruptions. A variety of other adverse reactions have been reported, including fever, hepatotoxicity, haematological changes, arthritic symptoms and vasculitis. Adverse effects involving the central or peripheral nervous systems are largely consequences of a deficiency of pyridoxine and are common in malnourished patients unless prevented by administration of this substance. Pyridoxal-hydrazone formation occurs mainly in slow acetylators. Isoniazid may cause haemolytic anaemia in individuals with glucose 6-phosphate dehydrogenase deficiency and it decreases the metabolism of the antiepileptic agents **phenytoin**, **ethosuximide** and **carbamazepine**, resulting in an increase in the plasma concentration and toxicity of these drugs.

RIFAMPICIN (RIFAMPIN)

Rifampicin acts by binding to, and inhibiting, DNA-dependent RNA polymerase in prokaryotic but not in eukaryotic cells (Ch. 44, p. 627). It is one of the most active antituberculosis agents known. It is also active against most Gram-positive bacteria as well as many Gram-negative species. It enters phagocytic cells and can kill intracellular microorganisms including the tubercle bacillus. Resistance can develop rapidly in a one-step process and is thought to be caused by chemical modification of microbial DNA-dependent RNA polymerase, resulting from a chromosomal mutation (see Ch. 44, p. 629).

Pharmacokinetic aspects

Rifampicin is given orally and is widely distributed in the tissues and body fluids, giving an orange tinge to saliva, sputum, tears and sweat. In the CSF, it reaches 10–40% of its serum concentration. It is excreted partly in the urine and partly in the bile, some of it undergoing enterohepatic cycling. The metabolite retains antibacterial activity but is less well absorbed from the gastrointestinal tract. The half-life is 1–5 hours, becoming shorter during treatment owing to induction of the hepatic microsomal enzymes.

Unwanted effects

Unwanted effects are relatively infrequent. The commonest are skin eruptions, fever and gastrointestinal disturbances. Liver damage with jaundice has been reported and has proved fatal in a very small proportion of patients. Liver function should be assessed before treatment is started. Rifampicin causes induction of hepatic metabolising enzymes, resulting in an increase in the degradation of warfarin, glucocorticoids, narcotic analgesics, oral antidiabetic drugs, dapsone and estrogens, the last leading to failure of oral contraceptives.

ETHAMBUTOL

Ethambutol has no effect on organisms other than mycobacteria. It is taken up by the bacteria and after a period of 24 hours it inhibits their growth. The mechanism of action is unknown. Resistance emerges rapidly if the drug is used on its own.

It is given orally and is well absorbed, reaching therapeutic plasma concentrations within 4 hours. In the blood it is taken up by erythrocytes and slowly released. It is partly metabolised and is excreted in the urine. The half-life is 3–4 hours. It can reach therapeutic concentrations in the CSF in tuberculous meningitis.

Unwanted effects

Unwanted effects are uncommon, the most important being optic neuritis, which is dose related and is more likely to occur if renal function is decreased. It results in visual disturbances: initially red/green colour blindness followed by a decrease in visual acuity. Colour vision should be monitored during prolonged treatment.

PYRAZINAMIDE

Pyrazinamide is inactive at neutral pH but tuberculostatic at acid pH. It is effective against the intracellular organisms in macrophages, since, after phagocytosis, the organisms are contained in phagolysosomes in which the pH is low. Resistance develops rather readily but cross-resistance with isoniazid does not occur.

The drug is well absorbed after oral administration and is widely distributed, penetrating well into the meninges. It is excreted through the kidney, mainly by glomerular filtration.

Unwanted effects

Unwanted effects include gout, which is associated with high concentrations of plasma urates. Gastrointestinal upsets, malaise and fever are reported. With the high doses previously used, serious hepatic damage was a possibility; this is now less likely with lower doses and shorter courses, but nevertheless, liver function should be assessed before treatment.

CAPREOMYCIN

Capreomycin is a peptide antibiotic given by intramuscular injection. There is some cross-reaction with the aminoglycoside **kanamycin**.

Unwanted effects are kidney damage and injury to the eighth nerve with deafness and ataxia. The drug should not be given at the same time as streptomycin or other drugs that may damage the eighth nerve.

Antituberculosis drugs

- To avoid emergence of resistant organisms, compound therapy is used, e.g. three drugs initially, then two drugs later.

First-line drugs

- **Isoniazid** kills actively growing mycobacteria within host cells; mechanism of action unknown. Given orally it penetrates necrotic lesions, also the cebrospinal fluid (CSF). 'Slow acetylators' (genetically determined) respond well. It has low toxicity. Pyridoxine deficiency increases risk of neurotoxicity. No cross-resistance with other agents.
- **Rifampicin** is a potent, orally active drug that inhibits mycobacterial RNA polymerase. It penetrates CSF. Unwanted effects are infrequent (but serious liver damage has occurred). It induces hepatic drug-metabolising enzymes. Resistance can develop rapidly.
- **Ethambutol** inhibits growth of mycobacteria by unknown mechanism. It is given orally and can penetrate CSF. Unwanted effects are uncommon; optic neuritis can occur. Resistance can emerge rapidly.
- **Pyrazinamide** is tuberculostatic against intracellular mycobacteria by an unknown mechanism. Given orally, it penetrates CSF. Resistance can develop rapidly. Unwanted effects: increased plasma urate, liver toxicity with high doses.

Second-line drugs

- **Capreomycin** is given intramuscularly. Unwanted effects include damage to kidney and to VIIIth nerve.
- **Cycloserine** is broad spectrum. It inhibits an early stage of peptidoglycan synthesis. Given orally it penetrates the CSF. Unwanted effects affect mostly CNS.
- **Streptomycin**, an aminoglycoside antibiotic, acts by inhibiting bacterial protein synthesis. It is given intramuscularly. Unwanted effects are ototoxicity (mainly vestibular) and nephrotoxicity. Infrequently used now.

CYCLOSERINE

Cycloserine is a broad-spectrum antibiotic inhibiting the growth of many bacteria including coliforms and mycobacteria. It is water soluble and destroyed at acid pH. It competitively inhibits cell wall synthesis by preventing the formation both of D-alanine and of the D-Ala– D-Ala dipeptide that is added to the initial tripeptide side-chain on *N*-acetylmuramic acid, i.e. it prevents completion of the major building block of peptidoglycan (see Fig. 44.3). After being given orally it is rapidly absorbed and reaches peak concentrations within 4 hours. It is distributed throughout the tissues and body fluids, concentrations in the CSF being equivalent to the concentration in the blood. Most of the drug is eliminated in active form in the urine, but some (approximately 35%) is metabolised.

Cycloserine has unwanted effects mainly on the CNS. A wide variety of disturbances may occur, ranging from headache and irritability to depression, convulsions and psychotic states. Its use is limited to tuberculosis that is resistant to other drugs.

DRUGS USED TO TREAT LEPROSY

There are approximately 11 million individuals with leprosy worldwide, most being in Africa, Asia and parts of South America. About 600 000–700 000 new cases are detected each year. Multidrug treatment regimens initiated by the World Health Organization in 1982 are improving the outlook for this disease. Paucibacillary leprosy—leprosy with few bacilli, which is mainly *tuberculoid** in type—is treated for 6 months with **dapsone**, and **rifampicin**. Multibacillary leprosy—leprosy with numerous bacilli, which is mainly *lepromatous** in type—is treated for at least 2 years with **rifampicin**, **dapsone** and **clofazimine**. The effect of therapy with minocycline or the fluoroquinolones is being investigated.

DAPSONE

Dapsone is chemically related to the **sulfonamides** and, since its action is antagonised by PABA, probably acts by inhibition of folate synthesis.

Resistance to dapsone is increasing and treatment with combinations of drugs is now recommended.

Dapsone is given orally and is well absorbed and widely distributed through the body water and all tissues. The plasma half-life is 24–48 hours but some dapsone remains in certain tissues (liver, kidney, and, to some extent, skin and muscle) for

*The basis of the difference appears to be that the T cells of patients with tuberculoid leprosy vigorously produce interferon γ, which enables macrophages to kill intracellular microbes, whereas in lepromatous leprosy, the immune response is dominated by interleukin-4, which blocks the action of interferon γ. See Chapter 15.

much longer periods. There is enterohepatic recycling of the drug but some is acetylated and excreted in the urine. Dapsone is also used to treat *dermatitis herpetiformis*, a chronic blistering skin condition associated with coeliac disease.

Unwanted effects

Unwanted effects occur fairly frequently and include haemolysis of red cells (usually not severe enough to lead to frank anaemia), methaemoglobinaemia, anorexia, nausea and vomiting, fever, allergic dermatitis and neuropathy. Lepra reactions (an exacerbation of lepromatous lesions) can occur and a syndrome resembling infectious mononucleosis, but which can be fatal, has occasionally been seen.

RIFAMPICIN

Rifampicin is discussed under 'Drugs used to treat tuberculosis'.

CLOFAZIMINE

Clofazimine is a dye of complex structure. It has anti-inflammatory activity and is also, therefore, useful in patients in whom dapsone causes inflammatory side-effects. Its mechanism of action against leprosy bacilli may involve an action on DNA.

It is given orally and tends to accumulate in the body, being sequestered in the mononuclear phagocyte system. The antileprotic effect is delayed and is usually not seen for 6–7 weeks. The plasma half-life may be as long as 8 weeks.

Unwanted effects

Unwanted effects may be related to the fact that clofazimine is a dye. Consequently, the skin and urine can develop a reddish colour and the lesions a blue-black discoloration. Dose-related nausea, giddiness, headache and gastrointestinal disturbances can also occur.

Antileprosy drugs

- For tuberculoid leprosy: dapsone and rifampicin.
- For lepromatous leprosy: dapsone, rifampicin and clofazimine.
- **Dapsone** is sulfonamide-like and may inhibit folate synthesis. It is given orally. Unwanted effects are fairly frequent, a few are serious. Resistance is increasing.
- **Clofazimine** is a dye which is given orally and can cumulate by sequestering in macrophages. Action is delayed for 6–7 weeks and its half-life is 8 weeks. Unwanted effects include red skin and urine, sometimes gastrointesinal disturbances.
- Rifampicin (see box on antituberculous drugs).

POSSIBLE NEW ANTIBACTERIAL DRUGS

The 1990s has seen a rise in drug-resistant bacteria ('superbugs') mainly as a consequence of the overuse of antibiotics. Vancomycin resistance has risen from 0.5% in 1989 to 18% in 1997 and similar rises in antibiotic resistance of *Staphylococcus* and *Enterococcus* spp. have been reported the world over (see Ch. 44). New antibiotic agents that act against such resistant organisms are, therefore, actively being sought (reviewed by Bax et al., 2000; Bryskier, 2000). These include:

- **everninomycin**, an oligosaccharide with activity against resistant *S. aureus*, currently in phase III trials
- new macrolide derivatives (e.g. **ketolides**, effective against multiresistant organisms, currently in phase III trials)
- new fluoroquinolone compounds such as **gemifloxanone, moxifloxacillin** and **gatifloxacin**, which are effective against multidrug resistant *S. pneumoniae* and will likely be targetted against serious respiratory tract infections
- clues to the identification of additional drugs with novel mechanisms may come from the genome sequences of drug-resistant bacterial strains several of which, including methicillin-resistant *S. aureus*, have been reported; numerous bacterial genes encoding for proteins which might be targets for antibiotic drugs have been identified.

REFERENCES AND FURTHER READING

Allington D R, Rivey M P 2001 Quinupristine/dalfopristin: a therapeutic review. Clin Ther 23: 24–44

Ball P 2001 Future of the quinolones. Sem Resp Infect 16: 215–224 (*Good overview of this class of drugs*)

Bax R, Mullan N, Verhoef J 2000 The millenium bugs—the need for and development of new antibacterials. Int J Antimicrob Agents 16: 51–59

Blondeau J M 1999 Expanded activity and utility of the new fluoroquinolones: a review. Clin Ther 21: 3–15 (*Good overview*)

Bloom B R, Small P M 1998 The evolving relation between humans and *Mycobacterium tuberculosis*. Lancet 338: 677–678 (*Editorial comment*)

Blumer J L 1997 Meropenem: evaluation of a new generation carbapenem. Int J Antimicrob Agents 8: 73–92

Bryskier A 2000 Ketolides–telithromycin, an example of a new class of antibacterial agents. Clin Microbiol Infect 6: 661–669

Cohn D L, Bustreo F, Raviglioni M C 1997 Drug-resistant tuberculosis: review of the worldwide situation and the WHO/IUATLD global surveillance project. Clin Infect Dis 24: S121–S130

Courvalin P 1996 Evasion of antibiotic action by bacteria. J Antimicrob Chemother 37: 855–869 (*Covers recent developments in the understanding of the genetics and biochemical mechanisms of resistance*)

Duran J M, Amsden G W 2000 Azithromycin: indications for the future? Exp Opin Pharmacother 1: 489–505

Finch R 1990 The penicillins today. Br Med J 300: 1289–1290

Fish D N, North D S 2001 Gatifloxacin, an advanced 8-methoxy fluoroquinolone. Pharmacotherapy 21: 35–59 (*Comprehensive evaluation of the effects of a novel fluoroquinolone*)

Gold H S, Moellering R C 1996 Antimicrobial drug resistance. N Engl J Med 335: 1445–1453 (*Excellent well-referenced review; covers mechanisms of resistance of important organisms to the main drugs; has useful table of therapeutic and preventive strategies, culled from the*

literature)
Greenwood D (ed) 1995 Antimicrobial chemotherapy, 3rd edn. Oxford University Press, Oxford
Heym B, Honoré N et al. 1994 Implications of multidrug resistance for the future of short-course chemotherapy of tuberculosis: a molecular study. Lancet 344: 293–298
Howie J 1986 Penicillin: 1929–1940. Br Med J 293: 158–159
Iseman M D 1993 Treatment of multidrug-resistant tuberculosis. N Engl J Med 329: 784–791
Jacoby G A, Archer G L 1991a Mechanisms of disease: new mechanisms of bacterial resistance to antimicrobial agents. N Engl J Med 324: 601–612
Jacoby G A, Medeiros A 1991b More extended-spectrum β-lactamases. Antimicrob Agents Chemother 35: 1697–1704
Laurence D R, Bennett P N, Brown M J 1997 Clinical pharmacology, 8th edn. Churchill Livingstone, Edinburgh
Livermore D M 2000 Antibiotic resistance in staphylococci. J Antimicrob Agents 16: S3–S10 (*Overview of problems of bacterial resistance*)
Loferer H 2000 Mining bacterial genomes for antimicrobial targets. Mol Med Today 6: 470–474 (*An interesting article focussing on the way in which a better understanding of the bacterial genome may lead to new drugs*)
Lowy F D 1998 *Staphylococcus aureus* infections. N Engl J Med 339: 520–541 (*Basis of* S. aureus *pathogenesis of infection, resistance; extensive references; impressive diagrams*)
Moellering R C 1985 Principles of anti-infective therapy. In: Mandell G L, Douglas R G, Bennett J E (eds) Principles and practice of infectious disease. John Wiley, New York
Michel M, Gutman L 1997 Methicillin-resistant *Staphylococcus aureus* and vancomycin-resistant enterococci: therapeutic realities and possibilities. Lancet 349: 1901–1906 (*Excellent review article; good diagrams*)
Nicas T I, Zeckel M L, Braun D K 1997 Beyond vancomycin: new therapies to meet the challenge of glycopeptide resistance. Trends Microbiol 5: 240–249
Perry C M, Jarvis B 2001 Linezolid: a review of its use in the management of serious gram-positive infections. Drugs 61: 525–551
Quagliarello V J, Scheld W M 1997 Treatment of bacterial meningitis. N Engl J Med 336: 708–716
Raoult D, Drancourt M 1994 Antimicrobial therapy of rickettsial diseases. Antimicrob Agents Chemother 35: 2457–2462
Sato K, Hoshino K, Mitsuhashi S 1992 Mode of action of the new quinolones: the inhibitory action on DNA gyrase. Prog Drug Res 38: 121–132
Shimada J, Hori S 1992 Adverse effects of fluoroquinolones. Prog Drug Res 38: 133–143
Stojiljkovic I, Evavold B D, Kumar V 2001 Antimicrobial properties of porphyrins. Expert Opin Invest Drugs 10: 309–320
Tillotson G S 1996 Quinolones: structure activity relationships and future predictions. J Med Microbiol 44: 320–324
Woodford N, Johnson A P et al. 1995 Current perspectives on glycopeptide resistance. Clin Microbiol Rev 8: 585–615 (*Comprehensive review*)

46

Antiviral drugs

Overview 654

Background information about viruses 654
- An outline of virus structure 654
- Examples of pathogenic viruses 654
- Virus function and life history 655

The host–virus interaction 655
- Host defences against viruses 655
- Viral ploys to invade host cells and circumvent host defences 656

HIV and AIDS 657

Antiviral drugs 659
- Anti-HIV drugs 659
- Other antiviral drugs 662
- Potential future developments in antiviral therapy 664

OVERVIEW

This chapter is about the drugs used to treat infections caused by viruses. We give first some necessary information about viruses: a simple outline of virus structure, a list of the main pathogenic viruses and a brief summary of the life history of an infectious virus. We go on to consider the host–virus interaction: the defences of the human host against viruses and the strategies that viruses employ to elude these. We then cover in some detail the pathogenesis of infection with the human immunodeficiency virus (HIV) and describe the various individual antiviral drugs, dealing first with anti-HIV drugs and then with other antiviral agents.

BACKGROUND INFORMATION ABOUT VIRUSES

AN OUTLINE OF VIRUS STRUCTURE

Viruses are small infective agents consisting essentially of nucleic acid (either RNA or DNA) enclosed in a protein coat or capsid (Fig. 46.1). The coat plus the nucleic acid core is termed the nucleocapsid. Some viruses have, in addition, a lipoprotein envelope, which may contain antigenic viral glycoproteins, as well as host phospholipids acquired when the virus nucleocapsid buds through the nuclear membrane or plasma membrane of the host cell. Certain viruses also contain enzymes that initiate their replication in the host cell. The whole infective particle is termed a virion. In different types of virus the genome may be double or single stranded.

For simple descriptions of viruses see Challand & Young (1997).

EXAMPLES OF PATHOGENIC VIRUSES

Some important examples of viruses and the diseases they cause are as follows:

- DNA viruses: poxviruses (smallpox), herpesviruses (chickenpox, shingles, cold sores, glandular fever), adenoviruses (sore throat, conjunctivitis) and papillomaviruses (warts)
- RNA viruses: orthomyxoviruses (influenza), paramyxoviruses (measles, mumps), rubella virus (German measles), rhabdoviruses (rabies), picornaviruses (colds, meningitis, poliomyelitis), retroviruses (acquired immunodeficiency syndrome (AIDS), T cell leukaemia), arenaviruses

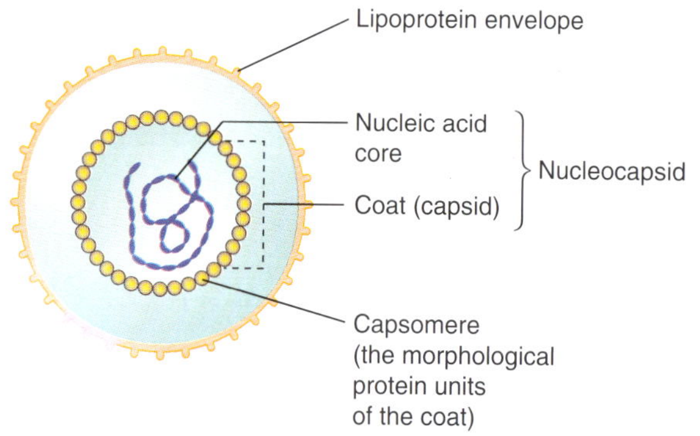

Fig. 46.1 Schematic diagram of the components of a virus particle or virion.

(meningitis, Lassa fever), hepadnaviruses (serum hepatitis) and arboviruses (arthropod-borne encephalitis and various fevers, e.g. yellow fever).

VIRUS FUNCTION AND LIFE HISTORY

Viruses are intracellular parasites with no metabolic machinery of their own. In order to replicate they have to attach to and enter a living host cell—animal, plant or bacterial—and use its metabolic processes. The binding sites on the virus are polypeptides on the envelope or capsid. The receptors on the host cell, to which the virus attaches, are normal membrane constituents—receptors for cytokines, neurotransmitters or hormones, ion channels, integral membrane glycoproteins, etc. Some examples of host cell receptors utilised by particular viruses are listed in Table 46.1. With many viruses, the receptor–virus complex enters the cell by receptor-mediated endocytosis during which the virus coat may be removed. Some bypass this route. Once in the host cell, the nucleic acid of the virus then uses the cell's machinery for synthesising nucleic acid and protein and the manufacture of new virus particles.

Table 46.1 Some host cell structures that can function as receptors for viruses

Host cell structure	Virus
CD4 glycoprotein on helper T lymphocytes	HIV (causing AIDS)
The receptor CCR5 for chemokines MCP-1 and RANTES	HIV (causing AIDS)
Chemokine receptor CXCR4 for cytokine SDF-1	HIV (causing AIDS)
Acetylcholine receptor on skeletal muscle	Rabies virus
Complement C3d receptor of B lymphocytes	Glandular fever virus
Interleukin-2 receptor on T lymphocytes	T cell leukaemia viruses
Beta-adrenoceptors	Infantile diarrhoea virus
MHC molecules	Adenovirus causing sore throat, conjunctivitis; T cell leukaemia viruses

HIV, human immodeficiency virus; AIDS, acquired immnodeficiency syndrome; MCP-1, monocyte chemoattractant protein-1; RANTES, regulated upon activation, normal T cell expressed and secreted; SDF-1, stromal cell-derived factor-1; MHC, major histocompatibility complex
Note: For more detail on complement, interleukin-2, the CD4 glycoprotein on helper T lymphocytes, MHC molecules, etc., see Chapter 15. For SDF-1, see Chapter 21.

Viral replication requires DNA or RNA synthesis, synthesis of viral proteins and glycosylation. A simplified account of viral replication is given here.

Replication in DNA viruses

There is generally entry of the viral DNA into the host cell nucleus, transcription of this viral DNA into mRNA by host cell RNA polymerase followed by translation of the mRNA into virus-specific proteins. Some of these proteins are enzymes that then synthesise more viral DNA as well as proteins of the coat and envelope. After assembly of coat proteins around the viral DNA, complete virions are released by budding or after cell lysis.

Replication in RNA viruses

Enzymes in the virion synthesise its mRNA or the viral RNA serves as its own mRNA. This is translated into various enzymes, including RNA polymerase (which directs the synthesis of more viral RNA), and also into structural proteins of the virion. Assembly and release of virions occurs as explained above. With these viruses the host cell nucleus is usually not involved in viral replication.*

Replication in retroviruses

The virion in retroviruses contains a reverse transcriptase (virus RNA-dependent DNA polymerase), which makes a DNA copy of the viral RNA. This DNA copy is integrated into the genome of the host cell and it is then termed a *provirus*. The provirus DNA is transcribed into both new genomic RNA and mRNA for translation into viral proteins. The completed viruses are released by budding and many can replicate without killing the host cell. Some RNA retroviruses can transform normal cells into malignant cells. HIV (see below) is an RNA retrovirus.

THE HOST–VIRUS INTERACTION

HOST DEFENCES AGAINST VIRUSES

The host reaction to virus infection involves the following devices.

- Deployment of the innate response and subsequently the adaptive response (Ch. 15, p. 218) occurs when the virus is detected in the tissues.
- Activation of cytotoxic $CD8^+$ T cells (cytotoxic lymphocytes, CTLs) follows virus entry to a host cell. The infected cell presents, on its surface, viral peptides complexed with major histocompatibility (MHC) class I molecules. This complex is recognised by CTLs,** which then kill the infected cell (Fig. 46.2). The killing mechanisms include:

*However, some RNA viruses, e.g. those causing influenza, replicate exclusively in the nucleus.

**MHC class I molecules are recognised by CTLs, MHC class II by $CD4^+$ T cells (see Ch. 15 for more detail).

—the release directly onto the infected cell of lytic proteins (perforins, granzymes) and/or
—triggering of the apoptotic pathway in the infected cell by activation of its Fas receptor (death receptor (p. 75) and/or
—release of cytokines (e.g. tumour necrosis factor (TNF)), which stimulate its Fas receptor (p. 75).

- Activation of natural killer (NK) cells (p. 222) occurs. If the virus escapes immune detection from CTLs by modifying the expression of the peptide–MHC complex by the infected cell (see below) it can still fall victim to NK cells. This NK reaction to the absence of normal MHC molecules might be called the 'mother turkey' strategy (kill everything that does not sound exactly like a baby turkey; see footnote on p. 222). But some viruses have a device for evading NK cells as well (see below).

VIRAL PLOYS TO INVADE HOST CELLS AND CIRCUMVENT HOST RESPONSES

Viruses have a variety of strategies to ensure successful infection, some entailing redirection of the host's response for the advantage of the virus (discussed by Tortorella et al., 2000).

Invasion of host cells

To invade the cells of the host, viruses use a stealth ploy: the expression of surface proteins that attach to host cell surface receptors enabling them to gain entry to the cell interior (Table 46.1).

Subversion of the immune response

Viruses can inhibit the action of the cytokines that orchestrate the innate and adaptive immune responses, such as interleukin-1, TNF-α and the antiviral interferons; (IFNs; see pp. 218, 241 and Fig. 15.3).

For example, some poxviruses, after infecting a cell, express proteins that match cytokine receptors—reducing the work of synthesising the proteins by expressing only the extracellular ligand-binding domains; these pseudoreceptors, when released, bind cytokines, preventing them from reaching their natural receptors on cells of the immune system and thus moderating the normal immune response to virus-infected cells.

Other viruses that can interfere with cytokine signalling include human cytomegalovirus, Epstein–Barr virus, herpesvirus and adenovirus.

Avoidance of immune detection and attack by killer cells

Once within host cells, viruses can escape immune detection and evade the killer attack by CTLs and NK cells in various ways:

- Interference with the surface proteins on the infected cells essential for killer cell attack. Some viruses can inhibit generation of the antigenic peptide and/or the presentation of MHC–peptide molecules. This turns off the signal that the cells are infected, enabling the viruses to remain undetected. Examples of viruses that can do this are adenovirus, herpes simplex virus, human cytomegalovirus, Epstein–Barr virus and influenza virus.
- Interference with the apoptotic pathway. Some viruses can subvert this pathway for their own purposes (e.g adenovirus, human cytomegalovirus, Epstein–Barr virus).

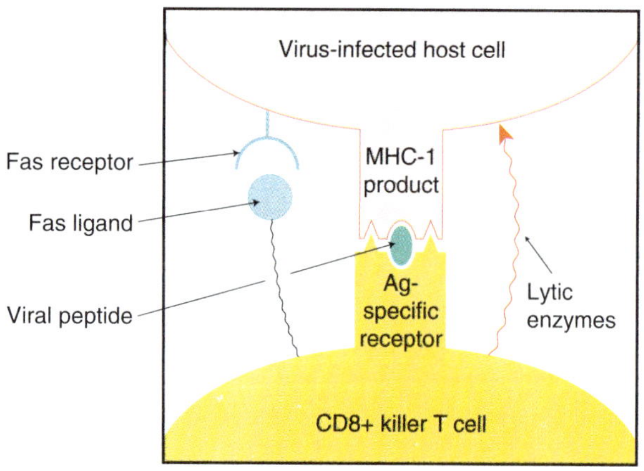

Fig. 46.2 The mechanisms whereby a CD8⁺ T cell kills a virus-infected host cell. The virus-infected host cell expresses a complex of virus peptide plus major histocompatibility complex class I (MCH-I) product on its surface; this is recognised by the CD8⁺ T cell, which then releases lytic enzymes into the virus-infected cell and also expresses a Fas ligand that triggers apoptosis in the infected cell by stimulating its Fas death receptor.

Viruses

- Viruses are small infective agents consisting essentially of nucleic acid (RNA or DNA) enclosed in a protein coat.
- They are not cells and, having no metabolic machinery of their own, are obligate intracellular parasites, i.e. they have to use the metabolic processes of the host cell, which they enter and infect.
- DNA viruses usually enter the host cell nucleus and direct the generation of new viruses.
- RNA viruses direct the generation of new viruses, usually without involving the host cell nucleus (the influenza virus is an exception in that it does involve the host cell nucleus).
- RNA retroviruses (e.g. HIV, T cell leukaemia virus) contain an enzyme, reverse transcriptase, which makes a DNA copy of the viral RNA. This DNA copy is integrated into the host cell genome and directs the generation of new virus particles.

- Some viruses, (e.g. cytomegalovirus) get round the 'mother turkey' approach of NK cells by adopting a 'baby turkey' ploy—they express a homologue of MHC class I (the equivalent of a baby turkey's noise) that is similar enough to the real thing to hoodwink NK cells.

It is evident that pathogenic viruses have many fiendish tactics for circumventing host defences; nevertheless, in most cases,* the host defences gain the upper hand and the majority of viral infections resolve spontaneously—except in the immunocompromised host.

Understanding the virus–host interaction is expected to lead to new types of antiviral therapy.

HIV AND AIDS

Infection with HIV** results in AIDS. In 2001, it was estimated that about 20 million people had died of AIDS; 30 million were HIV positive and there were 16 000 new infections daily. The epidemic is overwhelmingly centred on sub-Saharan Africa, where up to 35% of the adult population is infected with HIV (see Fig. 46.3).

For a review of the pathogenesis of AIDS, see Fauci (1996).

*HIV is an exception; and there are several other virus infections that have a high mortality: examples include Lassa fever and Ebola virus infection.

**In fact there are two viruses associated with AIDS—HIV-1 and HIV-2. HIV-1 causes most HIV infections worldwide; HIV-2 occurs in parts of Africa and India. In this chapter we are referring to both as HIV.

The interaction of HIV with the host's immune system is complex. The virus uses surface proteins of the immune system cells to gain entry to them. The cells of the immune system have the equivalent of 'name badges' that identify them. The surface protein CCR5 is a name badge on macrophages and dendritic cells and is the natural receptor for the β chemokines MCP-1 and RANTES.*** The surface glycoprotein CD4 is the name badge of a particular group of helper T lymphocytes (see Ch. 15; Fig. 15.3); it also occurs on macrophages and dendritic cells. A coreceptor (CXCR4) on the T cell is the normal receptor for a chemokine.

Virtually all HIV infections are initially caused by the transmission of virus that recognises the CCR5 and CD4 name badges and infects the cells displaying them. When, during the subsequent infection, immune surveillance breaks down, other strains of HIV arise that recognise both the CD4 and CXCR4 name badges. A surface glycoprotein, gp120, on the HIV envelope binds to CD4 and also to a chemokine coreceptor (CXCR4) on the T cell. Another viral glycoprotein, gp41, then causes fusion of the viral envelope with the plasma membrane of the T cell (Fig. 46.4).

Within the cell, HIV is integrated with the host DNA (the provirus form), undergoing transcription and generating new virions when the cell is activated (Fig. 46.4). In an untreated

***MCP in monocyte chemoattractant protein and RANTES is regulated upon activation normal T cell expressed and secreted. RANTES is being renamed CCL5 (see p. 221).

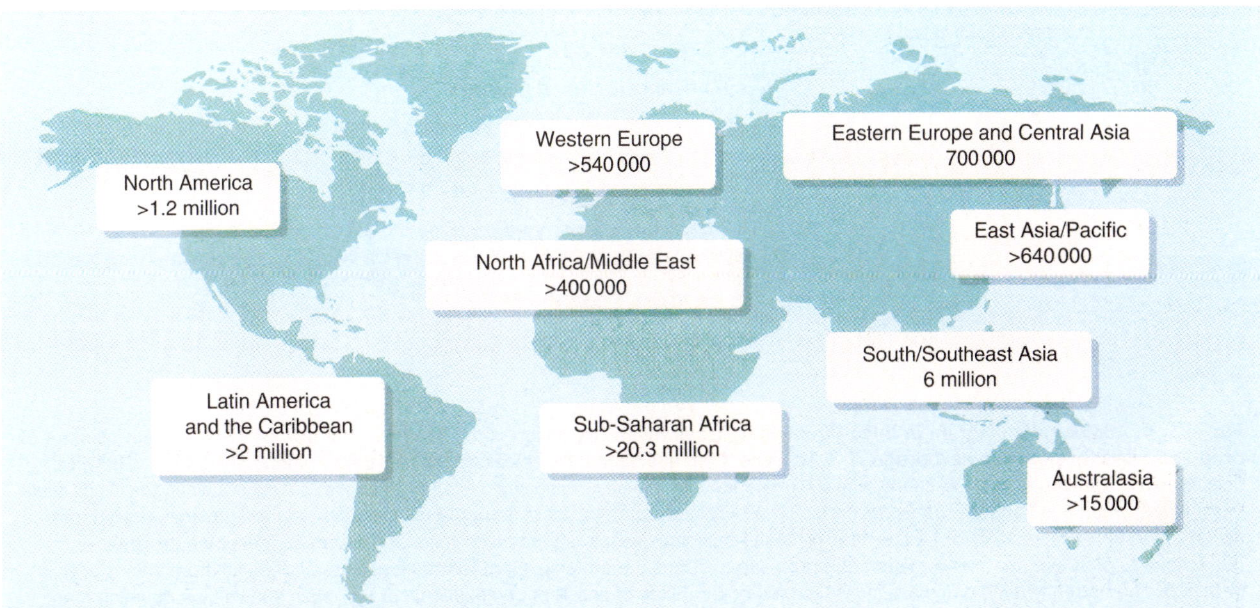

Fig. 46.3 Figures for the number of individuals with HIV/AIDS infection at the end of 2000. (Adapted from Grant A D, de Kock K M 2001 Br Med J 322:1475.)

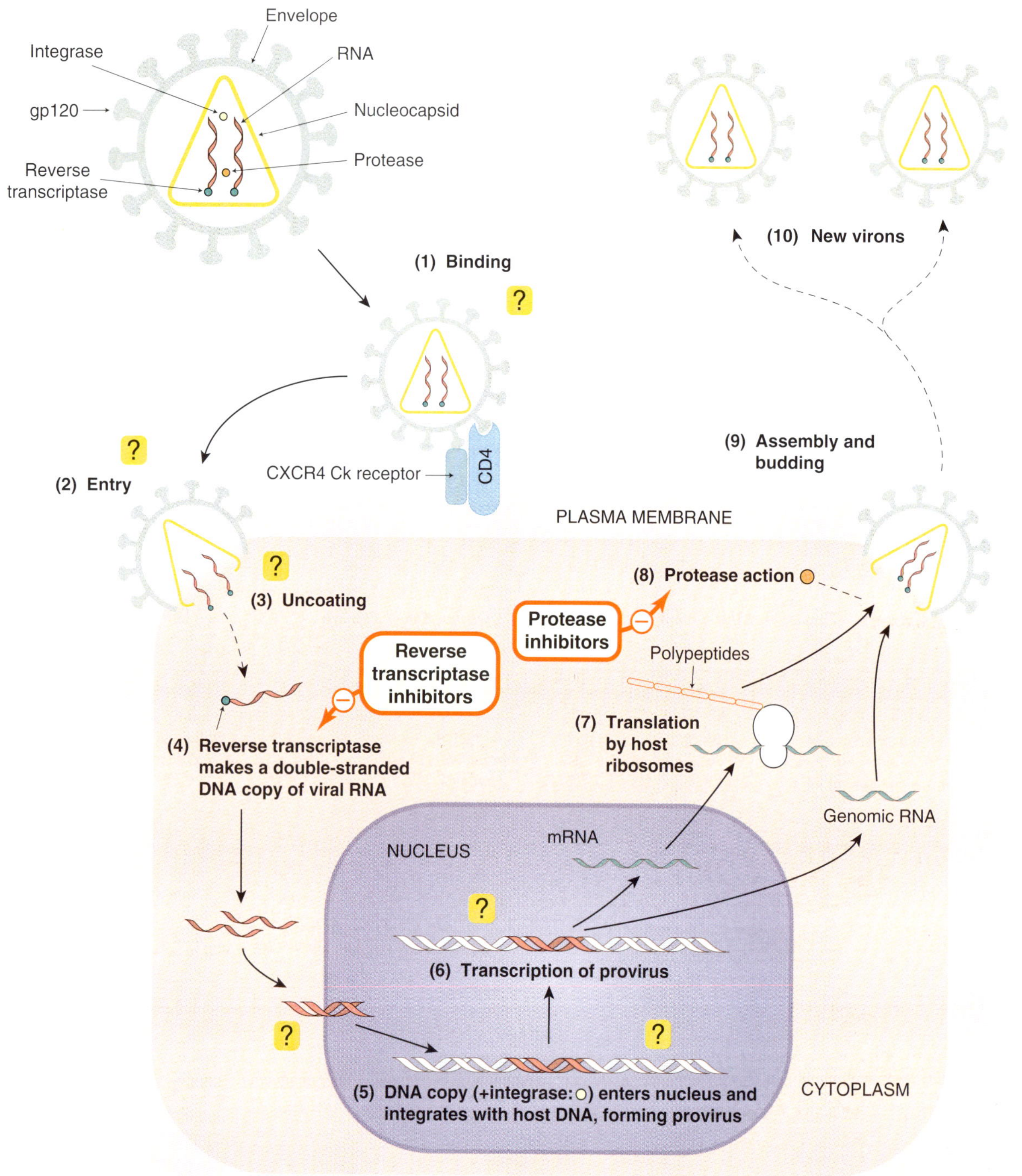

Fig. 46. 4 Schematic diagram of infection of $CD4^+$ T cell by an HIV virion with the sites of action of the two main classes of drug and sites for possible new drugs. The 10 steps, from attachment to the cell to release of new virions, are shown. The virus uses the CD4 coreceptor and the chemokine (Ck) receptor CXCR4 as binding sites. Step 6, transcription, occurs when the T cell itself is activated; when this happens, transcription factor NF-κB initiates transcription of both host cell DNA and the provirus. Step 8, the action of the viral protease, involves the cleaving of the polypeptides into structural proteins and enzymes (integrase, reverse transcriptase, protease) for the new virion (the protease and thus the protesase inhibitors actually act on the immature virions after budding). The currently used drugs are shown in pink boxes. Sites of action of potential new drugs, each shown by a question mark, include binding of the virion (by modification of the gp120–CD4 or gp120–CXCR4 interaction), entry of virion, uncoating of virion, translocation of viral complementary DNA into nucleus, integration of viral cDNA into host cell DNA, inhibition of the gene coding for the HIV core protein, inhibition of budding.

subject, some 10^{10} new virus particles may be produced each day. Much of intracellular HIV can remain silent for a long time before being stimulated into activity when that particular T cell clone meets its intended antigen partner and starts to proliferate.

Antibodies are produced to various HIV components but it is the action of CTLs* that initially prevents HIV spread, mainly by killing HIV-infected cells but also by releasing anti-HIV factors.

There is a progressive loss of CD4 helper T cells (see Fig. 46.5); this is the defining characteristic of HIV infection. The reason for this loss is not clear; it may be a result of killing by CTLs, direct virus-induced damage, etc.

Viral replication is error-prone and there are approximately 10^4–10^5 mutations per day at each site in the HIV genome, so HIV soon escapes the CTLs that recognise it initially. Although other CTLs recognise the mutated virus protein(s), further mutations, in turn, allow escape from these CTLs. It is suggested that wave after wave of CTLs act against new mutants as they arise, gradually diminishing the T cell repertoire, already being seriously diminished by loss of CD4 helper T cells, until eventually the immune response fails.

There is considerable variation in the progress of the disease but the usual clinical course of an untreated HIV infection is shown in Figure 45.5. There is usually an initial acute influenza-like illness associated with an increase in the number of virus particles in the blood, their widespread dissemination through the tissues and the seeding of lymphoid tissue with the virion particles. Within a few weeks, the viraemia is reduced by the action of CTLs as specified above.

The acute illness is followed by a symptom-free period during which there is reduction in the viraemia accompanied by silent virus replication in the lymph nodes, associated with damage to lymph node architecture and the loss of CD4 lymphocytes and dendritic cells. Clinical latency (median, 10 years) comes to an end when the immune response finally fails and the signs and symptoms of AIDS appear—opportunistic infections (e.g. with *Pneumocystis carinii* or the tubercle bacillus), neurological disease (e.g. confusion, paralysis, dementia), bone marrow depression and cancers. Chronic gastrointestinal infections contribute to the severe weight loss. Cardiovascular damage and kidney damage can also occur. In an untreated patient, death usually follows within 2 years. The advent of complex combination drug regimens has changed the prognosis—in countries that can employ it.

*CD4$^+$ helper T cells are important in the development of CD8$^+$ T cells (see Fig. 15.4).

ANTIVIRAL DRUGS

Because viruses share many of the metabolic processes of the host cell, it is difficult to find drugs that are selective for the pathogen. However, there are some enzymes that are virus specific and these are potential targets for drugs. Most currently available antiviral agents are only effective while the virus is replicating.

We deal first with anti-HIV drugs and then with other antiviral agents.

ANTI-HIV DRUGS

There are two main classes of anti-HIV drug: reverse transcriptase inhibitors and protease inhibitors. Each class has a different mechanism of action (Fig 46.4) and combinations are used in the therapy of HIV/AIDS. The reverse transcriptase inhibitors are subdivided into nucleoside reverse transcriptase inhibitors and non-nucleoside reverse transcriptase inhibitors.

As stated above, the use of combination treatment changed the prognosis of HIV/AIDS. The combination treatment is known as highly active antiretroviral therapy (HAART). A typical HAART combination would involve two nucleoside reverse transcriptase

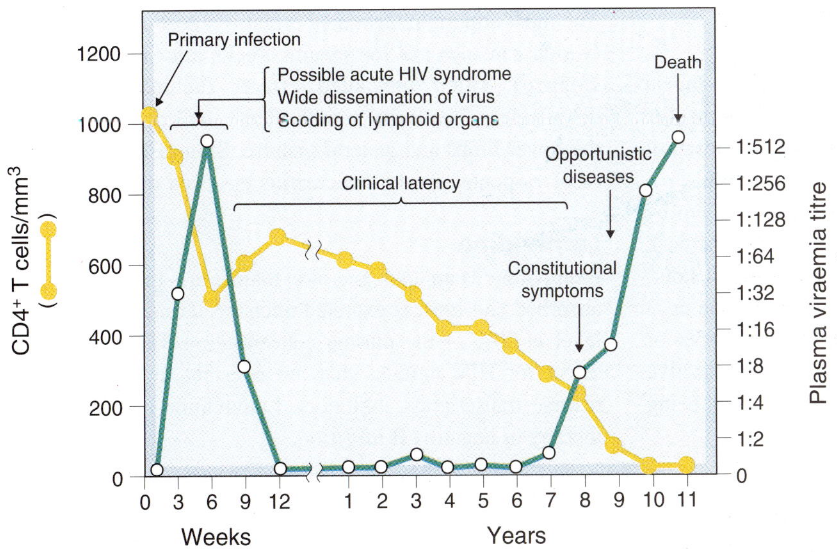

Fig. 46.5 Schematic outline of the course of HIV infection. (CD4$^+$ T cell titre is often given as cells/mm^3, which is equivalent to cells × 10^6 cells/l.) (Adapted from Pantaleo et al. 1993 N Engl J Med 328: 327–335.)

inhibitors with either a non-nucleoside reverse transcriptase inhibitor or one or two protease inhibitors.

With a HAART regimen, HIV replication is inhibited, the presence in the plasma of HIV RNA is reduced to undetectable levels and patient survival is prolonged. But the regimen is complex, has many unwanted effects, is difficult to adhere to and may well have to be lifelong because HIV will not have been eradicated. The virus will be lying latent in memory T cells, integrated into the host genome and forming a source for potential reactivation if the drugs are stopped.

At present, there is no cross-resistance between the three groups of drugs; but it needs to be borne in mind the virus has a high mutation rate—so resistance could be a problem in the future. The HIV virus has certainly not yet been outsmarted.

With all three groups, unwelcome drug interactions can occur and there may be interindividual variations in absorption. Some drugs penetrate poorly into the brain and this could lead to local proliferation of the virus.

NUCLEOSIDE REVERSE TRANSCRIPTASE INHIBITORS

This class includes **zidovudine** (AZT), **abacavir** (ABC), **lamivudine** (3TC), **didanosine** (ddI), **zalcitabine** (ddC) and **stavudine** (d4T). HAART regimens are often given only by a list of these abbreviations.

Mechanism of action

All are phosphorylated by host cell enzymes to give the 5'-trisphosphate. The 5′-trisphosphate moiety competes with the equivalent host cellular trisphosphates, which are essential substrates for the formation of proviral DNA by viral reverse transcriptase (viral RNA-dependent DNA polymerase); the incorporation of the 5′-trisphosphate moiety into the growing viral DNA chain results in chain termination.

Mammalian alpha DNA polymerase is relatively resistant to the effect. However, gamma DNA polymerase in the host cell mitochondria is fairly sensitive to the compound and this may be the basis of some unwanted effects.

Zidovudine

Zidovudine is an analogue of thymidine. It can prolong life in HIV-infected individuals and moderate HIV-associated dementia. Given to the parturient mother and then to the newborn infant it can reduce mother-to-baby transmission by more than 20%.

It is administered orally twice daily but can also be given by intravenous infusion. The bioavailability is 60–80% and the peak plasma concentration occurs at 30 minutes. Its half-life is 1 hour, and the intracellular half-life of the active trisphosphate is 3 hours. The concentration in cerebrospinal fluid (CSF) is 65% of the plasma level. Most of the drug is metabolised to the inactive glucuronide in the liver, only 20% of the active form being excreted in the urine.

Unwanted effects

Anaemia and neutropenia are common, particularly with long-term administration.* Other unwanted effects include gastrointestinal disturbances, paraesthesia, skin rash, insomnia, fever, headaches, abnormalities of liver function and, more particularly, myopathy. Confusion, anxiety, depression and a 'flu-like syndrome are also reported. The prophylactic short-term use of the drug in fit individuals, after specific exposure to the virus, is associated with only minor, reversible unwanted effects.

Resistance to the antiviral action of zidovudine

Because of rapid mutation, the virus is a constantly moving target, thus the therapeutic response wanes with long-term use, particularly in late-stage disease. Furthermore, resistant strains can be transferred between individuals. Other factors that underlie the loss of efficacy of the drug are decreased activation of zidovudine to the trisphosphate and increased virus load owing to reduction in immune mechanisms.

Didanosine

Didanosine is an analogue of deoxyadenosine. It is given orally, rapidly absorbed and is actively secreted by the kidney tubules. The level in the CSF reaches ~20% of the plasma concentration. The plasma half-life is 30 minutes but the intracellular half-life is more than 12 hours.

Unwanted effects

The main unwanted effect—occurring in >30% of patients—is dose-related pain and sensory loss in the feet. Dose-related pancreatitis occurs in 5–10% of patients and has been fatal in a few. Headache and gastrointestinal disturbance are also common and insomnia, skin rashes, bone marrow depression (less marked than with zidovudine) and alterations of liver function have been reported.

Zalcitabine

Zalcitabine is a homologue of cytosine. It is activated in the T cell by a different phosphorylation pathway from zidovudine. It is given orally. Its plasma half-life is 20 minutes and its intracellular half-life is nearly 3 hours; the CSF level is 20% of that in the plasma.

Unwanted effects

The most important unwanted effect is a dose-related neuropathy (which can increase for several weeks after the drug has been stopped). Other unwanted effects include gastrointestinal disturbances, headache, mouth ulcers, nail changes, oedema of the lower limbs and general malaise. Skin rashes occur but may resolve spontaneously. Pancreatitis has been reported.

Lamividine

Lamuvidine is an analogue of cytosine. It is given orally, is well absorbed and most is excreted unchanged in the urine. The CSF level is 20% of the plasma concentration. Used alone it could select for HIV mutants that are resistant to both it and other reverse transcriptase inhibitors. Lamuvidine is also used in the therapy of hepatitis B infection.

---

*Administration of **epoetin** (erythropoietin) and **molgramostim** (recombinant human granulocyte–macrophage colony-stimulating factor) (Ch. 21, p. 336) may alleviate these problems.

Unwanted effects

Unwanted effects are generally mild and include headache and gastrointestinal disorders.

Stavudine

Stavudine is a thymidine analogue. It is given orally, has a plasma half-life of 1 hour and most is eliminated via the kidney by active tubular secretion. The CSF level is 55% of that in the plasma. The main unwanted effect is dose-dependent peripheral neuropathy. Other adverse effects include joint pain and pancreatitis.

Abacavir

Abacavir is a guanosine analogue and has so far proved to be more effective than most other nucleoside reverse transcriptase inhibitors. It is well absorbed after oral administration and is metabolised in the liver to inactive compounds. The CSF level is 33% of that in the plasma.

Unwanted effects

Unwanted effects include a generalised hypersensitivity reaction (rare but potentially fatal), skin rashes and gastrointestinal disorders.

NON-NUCLEOSIDE REVERSE TRANSCRIPTASE INHIBITORS

Non-nucleoside reverse transcriptase inhibitors are chemically diverse compounds that bind to the reverse transcriptase near the catalytic site and denature it. Most non-nucleoside reverse transcriptase inhibitors are inducers, substrates or inhibitors to varying degrees of the liver cytochrome P450 enzymes. Currently available drugs are **efavirenz** (EFZ) and **nevirapine** (NVP).

Nevirapine

Nevirapine is given orally, its bioavailability is >90% and its CSF level is 45% of that in the plasma. It is metabolised in the liver and the metabolite is excreted in the urine. Nevirapine can prevent mother-to-baby transmission of HIV if given to the parturient mother and the neonate.

Unwanted effects

Rash occurs in about 17% of patients. If not carefully monitored, this may develop in some cases into life-threatening skin conditions: Stevens–Johnson syndrome or toxic epidermal necrolysis. Fulminant hepatitis has occasionally occurred. More common adverse effects are headache, fever and lethargy.

Efavirenz

Efavirenz is given orally, once daily because of its plasma half-life (~50 hours). It is 99% bound to plasma albumin and its CSF concentration is ~1% of that in the plasma. It is inactivated in the liver.

Unwanted effects

The unwanted effects are relatively mild and consist mainly of CNS symptoms (dizziness, confusion, dysphoria), which resolve as therapy is continued. Skin rashes occur in about 25% of patients and gastrointestinal disorders are experienced in 2%. Drug interactions could be a hazard and animal studies indicate that fetal abnormalities could occur.

PROTEASE INHIBITORS

In HIV, the mRNA transcribed from the provirus is translated into two biochemically inert polyproteins. A virus-specific protease then converts the polyproteins into various structural and functional proteins by cleavage at the appropriate positions (see Fig. 46.4). Since this protease does not occur in the host, it is a good target for chemotherapeutic intervention. HIV-specific protease inhibitors bind to the site where cleavage occurs, and their use, in combination with reverse transcriptase inhibitors, has transformed the therapy of AIDS. Examples of current protease inhibitors are **saquinavir** (SQV), **nelfinavir** (NFV), **indinavir** (IDV), **ritonavir** (RTV), and **amprenavir** (AMP).

They are all given orally, saquinavir being subject to extensive first-pass metabolism. CSF levels are negligible with saquinavir and highest with indinavir (76% of the plasma concentration). Nelfinavir and ritonavir are best taken with food and saquinavir within 2 hours of a meal.

Unwanted effects

All can cause gastrointestinal disorders and all may be associated with metabolic abnormalities such as insulin resistance, high blood sugar and hyperlipidaemia. Long-term use may lead to an unusual redistribution of cutaneous fat: less subcutaneous fat, increased abdominal fat, breast enlargement, 'buffalo humps'.

Raised concentrations of liver enzymes in the blood are reported with ritonavir and indinavir. Ritonavir and amprenavir can cause paraesthesias around the mouth, and in the hands and feet, and patients taking indinavir may develop kidney stones. A small percentage of patients on amprenavir have developed serious rashes, including Stevens–Johnson syndrome.

All inhibit the cytochrome P450 enzymes (indinavir and saquinavir to a lesser extent than ritonavir) and can interact with other drugs handled by this system. All can increase the plasma concentration of benzodiazepines.

Treatment of HIV/AIDS

A consensus on the use of retroviral therapy in AIDS has emerged based on the following principles.

- Monitor plasma viral load and $CD4^+$ cell count.
- Start treatment before immunodeficiency becomes evident.
- Aim to reduce plasma viral concentration as much as possible for as long as possible.
- Use combinations of at least three drugs, e.g. two reverse transcriptase inhibitors and one protease inhibitor.
- Change to a new regimen if plasma viral concentration increases.

Drugs for HIV infection

- Reverse transcriptase inhibitors (RTIs).
- Nucleoside RTIs (NRTIs) are phosphorylated by host cell enzymes to give the 5′-trisphosphate, which competes with the equivalent host cellular trisphosphates that are essential substrates for the formation of proviral DNA by viral reverse transcriptase. Examples are zidovudine and abacavir. They are used in combination with protease inhibitors. Unwanted effects with zidovudine (often serious) are blood dycrasias, gastrointestinal disturbances, myopathy, CNS disturbances. Unwanted effects with abacavir are generalised hypersensitivity reactions (rare but serious).
- Non-nucleoside RTIs (NNRTIs) are chemically diverse compounds that bind to the reverse transcriptase near the catalytic site and denature it. An example is nevirapine. This can prevent mother-to-newborn transmission. Main unwanted effect is rash; Stevens–Johnson syndrome may occur. Drug interactions can be a hazard.
- Protease inhibitors inhibit cleavage of the translated inert protein into functional and structural proteins. They are used in combination with reverse transcriptase inhibitors. An example is saquinavir. All inhibit the liver P450 enzymes. Main unwanted effects are metabolic disorders, altered distribution of fat (some fat wasting, some fat accumulation).
- Combination therapy is essential, e.g. two NRTIs with either a NNRTI or one or two protease inhibitors.

NEW TARGETS FOR ANTI-HIV DRUGS

The sites of potential attack by new drugs are shown in Figure 46.4.

OTHER ANTIVIRAL DRUGS

Drugs that affect viruses other than HIV act by inhibition of viral DNA polymerase or inhibition of attachment to the host cell.

DNA POLYMERASE INHIBITORS

Aciclovir (acyclovir)

The era of effective selective antiviral therapy began with aciclovir. This agent is a guanosine derivative with a high specificity for herpes simplex and varicella–zoster viruses. Herpes simplex can cause cold sores, conjunctivitis, mouth ulcers, genital infections* and, rarely but very seriously, encephalitis; in immunocompromised patients it is much more aggressive. Varicella–zoster viruses cause shingles and chickenpox. Herpes simplex is more susceptible to aciclovir than varicella–zoster. Epstein–Barr virus (a herpesvirus which causes glandular fever) is also slightly sensitive. Aciclovir has a small but reproducible effect against cytomegalovirus—a herpesvirus that can affect the fetus, with catastrophic consequences, and can cause a glandular-fever-like syndrome in adults and severe disease (e.g. retinitis, which can result in blindness) in individuals with decreased immune responses as a result of AIDS or the administration of immunosuppressants.

*Venereologists (now called 'sexually transmitted disease physicians', references to Venus presumably being no longer acceptable) with a taste for cynical humour ask 'What is the difference between true love and genital herpes?', their answer being that genital herpes is for ever. It may not be.

Mechanism of action

Aciclovir is converted to the monophosphate by thymidine kinase, and happily the virus-specific form of this enzyme is very much more effective in carrying out the phosphorylation than the enzyme of the host cell; it is, therefore, only adequately activated in infected cells. The host cell's kinases then convert the monophosphate to the trisphosphate. It is the aciclovir trisphosphate that inhibits viral DNA polymerase, terminating the nucleotide chain. It is 30 times more potent against the herpesvirus enzyme than the host enzyme. Aciclovir trisphosphate is fairly rapidly broken down within the host cells, presumably by cellular phosphatases. Resistance caused by changes in the viral genes coding for thymidine kinase or DNA polymerase has been reported and aciclovir-resistant herpes simplex virus has been the cause of pneumonia, encephalitis and mucocutaneous infections in immunocompromised patients.

Pharmacokinetic aspects

Aciclovir can be given orally, intravenously or topically. When it is given orally, only 20% of the dose is absorbed and peak plasma concentrations are reached in 1–2 hours. The drug is widely distributed, reaching concentrations in the CSF that are 50% of those in the plasma. It is excreted by the kidneys, partly by glomerular filtration and partly by tubular secretion.

Clinical use of aciclovir

- Treatment of varicella–zoster infections (shingles), orally in immunocompetent patients, intravenously in immunocompromised patients.
- Treatment of herpes simplex infections (genital herpes, mucocutaneous herpes and herpes encephalitis).
- Treatment of varicella (chickenpox) in immunocompromised patients.
- Prophylactically in patients who are to be treated with immunosuppressant drugs or radiotherapy and who are at risk of herpesvirus infection owing to reactivation of a latent virus.
- Prophylactically in individuals who suffer from frequent recurrences of genital infection with herpes simplex virus.

Unwanted effects

Unwanted effects are minimal. Local inflammation can occur during intravenous injection if there is extravasation of the solution. Renal dysfunction has been reported when aciclovir is given intravenously; slow infusion reduces the risk. Nausea and headache can occur and, rarely, encephalopathy.

Other drugs similar to aciclovir

Other drugs similar to aciclovir are **valaciclovir** and **famciclovir**.

Valaciclovir is a pro-drug of aciclovir. Famciclovir is metabolised to penciclovir, the active compound, in vivo. **Penciclovir** has a similar action to aciclovir.

Ganciclovir

Ganciclovir, an acyclic analogue of guanosine, is the drug of choice for cytomegalovirus infection, which occurs particularly in immunocompromised individuals. It is a frequent opportunistic infection in AIDS patients and has been a formidable obstacle to successful transplantation of organs and bone marrow (which necessitates immunosuppressive therapy).

Like aciclovir, ganciclovir has to be activated to the trisphosphate and in this form it competes with guanosine trisphosphate for incorporation into viral DNA. It suppresses viral DNA replication, but unlike aciclovir it does not act as a chain terminator nor is it rapidly broken down, being shown to persist in cells infected with cytomegalovirus for 18–20 hours.

Ganciclovir is given intravenously, excreted in the urine and has a half-life of 4 hours.

Unwanted effects

Ganciclovir has serious unwanted actions, including bone marrow depression and potential carcinogenicity; it is, therefore, used only for life- or sight-threatening cytomegalovirus infections in patients who are immunocompromised. Oral administration can be used for maintenance therapy in AIDS patients.

Tribavirin (ribavirin)

Tribavirin is a synthetic nucleoside, similar in structure to guanosine. It is thought to act either by altering virus nucleotide pools or by interfering with the synthesis of viral mRNA. It inhibits a wide range of DNA and RNA viruses including many that affect the lower airways. In aerosol form, it has been used to treat influenza and infections with respiratory syncytial virus (an RNA paramyxovirus).

It has been shown to be effective in Lassa fever, an extremely serious arenavirus infection; given intravenously within the first 6 days of onset, it has been shown to reduce to 9% a case-fatality rate previously 76%.

Foscarnet (phosphonoformate)

Foscarnet is a synthetic non-nucleoside analogue of pyrophosphate that inhibits viral DNA polymerase by binding directly to the pyrophosphate-binding site. It can cause serious nephrotoxicity. Given by intravenous infusion, it is a second-line drug in cytomegalovirus eye infection in immunocompromised patients.

INHIBITION OF ATTACHMENT TO OR PENETRATION OF HOST CELLS

Amantadine

Amantadine* is active against influenza A virus (an RNA virus) but has no action against influenza B virus. **Rimantadine** is similar in its effects.

Mechanism of action

At two stages of viral replication within the host cell, a viral membrane protein, M_2, functions as an ion channel. The stages are (i) the fusion of viral membrane and endosome membrane and (ii) the later stage of assembly and release of new virions at the host cell surface. Amantadine blocks this ion channel.

Pharmacokinetic aspects

Given orally, amantadine is well absorbed, reaches high levels in secretions (e.g. saliva) and most is excreted unchanged via the kidney. Aerosol administration is feasible.

Unwanted effects

Unwanted effects are relatively infrequent, occurring in 5–10% of patients, and are not serious. Dizziness, insomnia and slurred speech are the most common adverse effects.

Zanamivir

In influenza virus, the action of neuraminidase is involved in the budding of new virus from infected cells. The neuraminidase inhibitor **zanamivir**, active against both influenza A and B viruses, is licensed for use early in the infection. It is available as a powder for inhalation.

IMMUNOMODULATORS

Immunomodulators are drugs that act by moderating the immune response to viruses or use an immune mechanism to target a virus.

Immunoglobulin

Pooled immunoglobulin contains antibodies against various viruses present in the population. The antibodies are directed against the virus envelope and can 'neutralise' some viruses and prevent their attachment to host cells. If used before the onset of signs and symptoms, it may attenuate or prevent measles, infectious hepatitis, German measles, rabies or poliomyelitis. Hyperimmune globulin, specific against particular viruses, is used against hepatitis B, varicella–zoster and rabies.

Interferon

The IFNs are a family of inducible proteins synthesised by mammalian cells and now produced by recombinant DNA technology. There are at least three types, α, β, and γ, constituting a family of hormones involved in cell growth and regulation and modulation of immune reactions. IFNγ, termed 'immune

*Also used for its mildly beneficial effect in Parkinson's disease.

Antiviral drugs

- Antiviral drugs, other than anti-HIV drugs, act by the following mechanisms.
- Inhibition of penetration of host cell
  - —amantadine inhibits uncoating and is effective against influenza A virus
  - —gammaglobulin 'neutralises' viruses.
- Inhibition of transcription of the viral genome DNA polymerase inhibitors:
  - —aciclovir, a guanosine derivative, selectively inhibits viral DNA polymerase; effective against herpesviruses; minimal unwanted effects
  - —ganciclovir, also a guanosine derivative, is phosphorylated and then incorporated into viral DNA, suppressing its replication; used in cytomegalovirus infection, especially retinitis in AIDS patients; it can have serious unwanted effects
  - —tribavirin is similar to guanosine and is thought to interfere with synthesis of viral mRNA; it can inhibit many DNA and RNA viruses
  - —foscarnet inhibits viral DNA polymerase by attaching to the pyrophosphate binding site; it is fairly effective in cytomegalovirus infection.
- Immunomodulators
  - —interferons induce, in the host cells' ribosomes, enzymes which inhibit viral mRNA; they are used in hepatitis B infection and may be useful in AIDS
  - —immunoglobulins (IgGs), directed against virus envelope, can neutralise some viruses; general pooled IgG and specific hyperimmune IgGs are both available.

interferon' (see p. 225), is produced mainly by T lymphocytes as part of an immunological response to both viral and non-viral antigens, the latter including bacteria and their products, rickettsiae, protozoa, fungal polysaccharides and a range of polymeric chemicals and other cytokines. IFNα and IFNβ are produced by B and T lymphocytes, macrophages and fibroblasts in response to the presence of viruses and cytokines. The general actions of the IFNs are described briefly in Chapter 15.

Mechanism of antiviral action of interferons

The IFNs work by inducing, in the ribosomes of the host's cells, the production of enzymes that inhibit the translation of viral mRNA into viral proteins and thus stop the reproduction of the viruses. IFNs bind to specific receptors on cell membranes, which may be gangliosides. They inhibit the replication of most viruses in vitro.

Pharmacokinetic aspects

Given intravenously, IFNs have a half-life of 2–4 hours. With intramuscular injections, peak blood concentrations are reached in 5–8 hours. They do not cross the blood–brain barrier.

Clinical use

Interferon alfa-2a is used for treatment of hepatitis B infections and AIDS-related Kaposi sarcomas; **interferon alfa-2b** is used for hepatitis C. There are reports that IFNs can prevent re-activation of herpes simplex after trigeminal root section and can prevent spread of herpes zoster in cancer patients.

When used for antiviral chemotherapy, IFNs act partly by augmenting the host's immune response (see Ch. 15).

Unwanted effects

Unwanted effects are common and include fever, lassitude, headache and myalgia. Repeated injections cause chronic malaise. Bone marrow depression, rashes, alopecia and disturbances in cardiovascular, thyroid and hepatic function can also occur.

Palivisumab

Palivisumab is a monoclonal antibody (see Ch. 15) directed against a glycoprotein on the surface of respiratory syncytial virus and it is used (as an intramuscular injection) in infants to prevent infection by this organism.

POTENTIAL FUTURE DEVELOPMENTS IN ANTIVIRAL THERAPY

At the beginning of the 1990s, there were only five drugs available to treat viral infections; 10 years later there are more than 30. New strategies—based on the growing understanding of the biology of pathogenic viruses and their action on and in host cells—could well, if vigorously implemented, have the potential to target the viruses causing most viral diseases; see de Clercq (2002).

REFERENCES AND FURTHER READING

Balfour H H 1999 Antiviral drugs. N Engl J Med 340: 1255–1268 (*An excellent, comprehensive review of antiviral agents (other than those used for HIV) Describes their mechanisms of action, adverse effects and clinical use. Useful tables*)

Bartlett J G, Moore R D 1998 Improving HIV therapy. Sci Am July: 64–73 (*Simple crisp description of HIV–host interaction (with excellent 3D illustrations) and tabular outline of drugs used*)

Cairns J S, D'Souza M P 1998 Chemokines and HIV-1 second receptors: the therapeutic connection. Nat Med 4: 563–568 (*Excellent review of therapeutic strategies that target the chemokine receptors used by HIV-1 to invade host cells*)

Carr A, Cooper D A 2000 Adverse effects of antiretroviral therapy. Lancet 356: 1423–1430 (*A review which focuses on the pathogenesis, clinical features and management of the main unwanted actions of current antiretroviral drugs*)

Challand R, Young R J 1997 Antiviral chemotherapy. Biochemical and Medicinal Chemistry Series. Spectrum, USA (*Emphasis on medicinal chemistry*)

Cohn J A 1997 Recent advances: HIV-1 infection. Br Med J 314: 487–491 (*Short, clear coverage of clinical course of HIV infection, laboratory tests, and the newly licensed drugs: nucleoside and non-nucleoside reverse transcriptase inhibitors and protease inhibitors*)

de Clercq E 2002 Strategies in the design of antiviral drugs. Nat Rev Drug Discov 1:13–24 (*Outstanding article on the rationale behind current and future strategies for antiviral drug development*)
Fauci A S 1996 Host factors and the pathogenesis of HIV-induced disease. Nature 384: 529–534 (*Comprehensive coverage of immune mechanisms—particularly cytokines and chemokines and their receptors—in AIDS pathogenesis*)
Flexner C 1998 HIV-protease inhibitors. N Engl J Med 338: 1281–1292 (*Excellent, comprehensive review covering mechanisms of action, clinical and pharmacokinetic properties, potential drug resistance and possible treatment failure*)
Flexner C 2000 Dual protease inhibitor therapy in HIV-infected patients: Pharmacologic rationale and clinical benefits. Annu Rev Pharmacol Toxicol 40: 649–674 (*Review emphasising interactions between individual protease inhibitors and the potential benefits and disadvantages of dual therapy*)
Gallo R C, Lusso P 1997 Chemokines and HIV infection. Curr Opin Infect Dis 10: 12–17 (*Clear coverage of chemokine receptors as coreceptors for HIV, and the clinical relevance for HIV infection*)
Gubareva L, Kaiser L, Hayden F G 2000 Influenza virus neuraminidase inhibitors Lancet 355: 827–835 (*Admirable coverage of this topic. Lucid summary and clear diagrams of the influenza virus and its replication cycle. Description of the structure and the action of, and resistance, to zanamivir and oseltamivir and the relevant pharmacokinetic aspects and clinical efficacy*)
Guidotti L G, Chisari F V 2001 Noncytolytic control of viral infections by the innate and adaptive immune response. Annu Rev Immunol 19: 65–91 (*Detailed review emphasising the role of cytokines (e.g. IFNα/β) in the control of viral infections. Points out that antiviral cytokines IFNγ and TNF-α can purge viruses from infected cells and improve the immune response to viral infections*)
Hammer S M 2002 Increasing choices for HIV therapy. N Engl J Med 346: 2022–2023 (*Succinct article. See also Walmsley et al. N Engl J Med 346: 2039–2046*)
Hirsch M S 2002 HIV drug resistance—a chink in the armor. N Engl J Med 347: 438–439 (*Editorial on the challenge of drug-resistant HIV. See also Little S J et al. N Engl J Med 346: 385–394*)
Horuk R 2001 Chemokine receptors. Cytokine Growth Factor Rev 12: 313–335 (*Comprehensive review focussing on recent findings in chemokine receptor research and discussing the molecular, physiological and biochemical properties of each chemokine receptor*)
Kärre K, Welsh R M 1997 Viral decoy vetoes killer cell. Nature 386: 446–447 (*Covers invasion ploys of HIV and the response of megakaryocyte cells; very readable; useful diagram*)
Kitabwalla M, Ruprecht R M 2002 RNA interference—a new weapon against HIV and beyond. N Engl J Med 347: 1364–1368 (*An article in the series 'Clinical implications of basic research'*)
Lauer G M, Walker B D 2001 Hepatitis C virus infection. N Engl J Med 345: 41–52 (*Comprehensive review of pathogenesis, clinical characteristics, natural history and treatment of hepatitis C infection*)
Lee W M 1997 Hepatitis B virus infection N Engl J Med 337: 1733–1746 (*Detailed coverage of the epidemiology and pathogenesis of hepatitis B, the life cycle of the virus in the human host and the treatment of the disease. Clear diagram of the parasite–host interaction in the liver*)
Levy J A 1996 Infection by human immunodeficiency virus: CD4 is not enough. N Engl J Med 335: 1528–1530 (*Excellent explanatory diagram of interaction of virus with CD4 and coreceptors on human cell*)
Levy J A 2001 The importance of the innate immune system in controlling HIV infection and disease. Trends Immunol 22: 312–316 (*Stresses the role of innate immunity in the response to HIV. Neat tables of (i) components of the innate and adaptive immune systems and (ii) non-cytotoxic CD8$^+$ cell response to HIV*)
Mindel A, Tenant-Flowers M 2001 Natural history and management of early HIV infection. Br Med J 322: 1290–1293 (*A clinical review covering the current classification of HIV disease, clinical manifestations of primary HIV infection and general management of HIV patients*)
Moore J P, Stevenson M 2000 New targets for inhibitors of HIV-1 replication. Nat Rev Mol Cell Biol 1: 40–49 (*Excellent coverage of stages of the viral life cycle that might be susceptible to new drugs: attachment to host cell, membrane fusion, integration, accessory gene function, and assembly. Outlines various potentially promising chemical compounds*)
Morgan R A 1999 Genetic strategies to inhibit HIV. Mol Med Today 5: 454–458 (*Discusses recent progress in gene therapy strategies. Good diagram of potential targets for gene therapy*)
Murphy P M 2001 Viral exploitation and subversion of the immune system through chemokine mimicry. Nat Immunol 2: 116–122 (*Excellent description of virus–immune system interaction*)
Pantaleo G, Fauci A S 1996 Immunopathogenesis of HIV infection. Annu Rev Microbiol 50: 825–854 (*Detailed review of inter-relation of HIV infection and immune responses; discusses how this affects the progression of the disease in different individuals: rapid progressors, typical progressors, long-term non-progressors and long-term survivors*)
Patick A K, Potts K E 1998 Protease inhibitors as antiviral agents. Clin Microbiol Rev 11: 614–627 (*A useful review that summarises some of the general features of the viral proteases of the HIV virus, the human rhinovirus and the viruses causing herpes simplex and hepatitis C. The authors discuss the clinically useful inhibitors of HIV protease in some detail and outline the possible development of inhibitors of the proteases of the other viruses*)
Richman D D 2001 HIV chemotherapy. Nature 410: 995–1001 (*Outstanding article. Covers pathogenesis and natural history of HIV infection and the impact on viral dynamics and immune function of antiretroviral therapy. Discusses the main antiretroviral drugs, drug resistance of HIV and targets for new drugs. Excellent informative figures and full set of references*)
Tortorella D, Gewurz B E et al. 2000 Viral subversion of the immune system. Annu Rev Immunol 18: 861–926 (*A comprehensive clearly written review of the various mechanisms by which viruses elude detection and destruction by the host's immune system*)
Wain-Hobson S 1997 Down or out in blood and lymph. Nature 387: 123–124 (*Short 'News and Views' article on recent advances; very readable*)
Weiss R A 2001 Gulliver's travels in HIVland. Nature 410: 963–967 (*HIV and AIDS as if seen through the eyes of Lemuel Gulliver*)
Weller I V D, Williams I G 2001 Antiretroviral drugs. Br Med J 322: 1410–1412 (*Part of a BMJ series on the ABC of AIDS. Clear, succinct coverage. Gives antiretroviral regimens, recommendations for starting anti-HIV therapy and gives a helpful list of targets for new drug development*)
Werther G 1998 Not all is dead in the HIV-1 graveyard. Lancet 351: 308–309 (*Short article about reservoir of latent infection*)
Whitley R J, Roizman B 2001 Herpes simplex virus infections. Lancet 357: 1513–1518 (*A concise review of the viral replication cycle and the pathogenesis and treatment of herpes simplex virus infections*)

47 Antifungal drugs

Overview 666

Fungal infections 666

Drugs used for fungal infections 666
— Antifungal antibiotics 667
— Synthetic antifungal agents 668

Potential new antifungal therapies 670

OVERVIEW

Many of the fungi that can cause infections live in association with humans as commensals or are present in the environment; but until recently, serious superficial infections were relatively uncommon and systemic infections very uncommon indeed—at least in cool and temperate climatic zones. In these zones, a fungal infection usually meant athlete's foot or oral or vaginal thrush, which caused discomfort but were hardly life-threatening.

Since the 1970s, there has been a steady increase in the incidence of serious secondary systemic fungal infections. One of the factors aiding the spread of fungal disease has been the widespread use of broad-spectrum antibiotics, which eliminate or decrease the non-pathogenic bacterial populations that normally compete with fungi. Another has been the increased number of individuals with reduced immune responses caused by the acquired immunodeficiency syndrome (AIDS) or by the action of immunosuppressant drugs or cancer chemotherapy agents; this has led to an increased prevalence of opportunistic infections, i.e. infections with fungi that rarely cause disease in healthy individuals.

In other parts of the world a number of fungal infections occur as primary infection. These are now seen more often out of their normal geographical location because of the increase in international travel.

FUNGAL INFECTIONS

Fungal infections are termed mycoses and, in general, can be divided into superficial infections (affecting skin, nails, scalp or mucous membranes) and systemic infections (affecting deeper tissues and organs).

In the UK, the commonest systemic fungal disease is systemic candidiasis—an infection with a yeast-like organism. Other more serious conditions are cryptococcal meningitis or endocarditis, pulmonary aspergillosis, and rhinocerebral mucormycosis. Invasive pulmonary aspergillosis is now a leading cause of death in recipients of bone marrow transplants. Colonisation of the lungs of patients with asthma or cystic fibrosis by *Aspergillus* can lead to a similar condition, termed allergic bronchopulmonary aspergillosis. Whilst anyone can succumb to a fungal infection, some are more at risk than others. Older people, diabetics, pregnant women and burn wound victims are all more prone to fungal infections such as candidiasis.

In other parts of the world, the commonest systemic fungal infections are blastomycosis, histoplasmosis, coccidiomycosis and paracoccidiomycosis; these are often primary infections, i.e. they are not secondary to reduced immunological function or altered commensal microorganisms.

Superficial fungal infections can be classified into the *dermatomycoses* and *candidiasis*. Dermatomycoses are infections of the skin, hair and nails most commonly caused by *Trichophyton*, *Microsporum* and *Epidermophyton* spp., which cause various types of 'ringworm' or tinea. *Tinea capitis* affects the scalp, *Tinea cruris*, the groin, *Tinea pedis*, the feet (causing athlete's foot) and *Tinea corporis*, the body. In superficial candidiasis, the yeast-like organism infects the mucous membranes of the mouth (thrush), vagina or skin.

The drugs used in fungal infections are described briefly below and their clinical use is outlined in Table 47.1.

DRUGS USED FOR FUNGAL INFECTIONS

The mainstay of fungal drug therapy, **amphotericin**, was first used almost 50 years ago. Since then, many compounds have been discovered (Table 47.2), in contrast to antiprotozoal (Ch. 48) and anthelminthic (Ch. 49) drugs, where relatively few new agents have been introduced. For a detailed coverage of antifungal drugs, see Hoeprich (1995) and Groll et al. (1998).

Table 47.1 Outline of the uses of antifungal drugs

Disease	Drug used
Systemic infections	
Systemic candidiasis	Amphotericin ± flucytosine, [a]fluconazole
Cryptococcosis (meningitis)	Amphotericin ± flucytosine, [a]fluconazole, itraconazole
Systemic aspergillosis	Itraconazole, [a]amphotericin
Blastomycosis	Itraconazole, [a]amphotericin
Histoplasmosis	Amphotericin, itraconazole, fluconazole
Coccidiomycosis	Fluconazole, itraconazole, amphotericin
Paracoccidiomycosis	Fluconazole, itraconazole, amphotericin
Mucormycosis	Amphotericin ± flucytosine[a]
Disseminated sporotrichosis	Amphotericin, itraconazole
Superficial infections	
Dermatomycosis	
Tinea pedis (athlete's foot)	A topical azole, or oral itraconazole
Tinea corporis (skin ringworm)	A topical azole, oral terbinafine, oral itraconazole
Tinea cruris	A topical azole, oral terbinafine, oral itraconazole
Tinea capitis	Oral itraconazole
Tinea unguium (nail infection)	Oral or topical terbinafine, topical amorolfine
Candidiasis	
Skin	A topical azole, topical nystatin
Mouth (thrush)	A topical azole or nystatin, oral fluconazole
Vagina	A topical azole, oral fluconazole
Chronic mucocutaneous candidiasis	Fluconazole, ketoconazole[b]

[a]Drugs of choice.
[b]The potential benefits of treatment should be carefully weighed against the risk of liver damage.

ANTIFUNGAL ANTIBIOTICS

AMPHOTERICIN

Amphotericin is a macrolide antibiotic of complex structure, characterised by a many-membered ring of carbon atoms.

Mechanism of action

Amphotericin binds to cell membranes (like other polyene antibiotics; see Ch. 44) and interferes with permeability and with transport functions. It forms a pore in the membrane, the hydrophilic core of the molecule creating a transmembrane ion channel. One of the consequences of this is a loss of intracellular K^+. Amphotericin has a selective action, binding avidly to the membranes of fungi and some protozoa, less avidly to mammalian cells and not at all to bacteria. The relative specificity for fungi may be the result of the drug's greater avidity for ergosterol (the fungal membrane sterol) than for cholesterol, the main sterol in the plasma membrane of animal cells. It is active against most fungi and yeasts.

Amphotericin enhances the antifungal effect of **flucytosine** (see below).

Table 47.2 Discovery of antifungal drugs

Decade	Drug
1950s	Amphotericin
1960s	Griseofulvin
1970s	Flucytosine, clotrimazole, miconazole
1980s	Ketoconazole, fluconazole, itraconazole
1990s	Terbinafine, naftifine, different formulations[a] of amphotericin
2000s	Caspofungin
Under development	Voriconazole[b], posaconazol[b], ravuconazole[b], micafungin (FK463)[b], sordarins, pradimicin, nikkimycin

[a]Different formulations: liposomes, nanosomes, nanoparticles.
[b]Undergoing clinical trials.

Pharmacokinetic aspects

Given orally, amphotericin is poorly absorbed; it is, therefore, only given by this route for fungal infections of the gastrointestinal tract. It can also be given topically. For systemic infections it is complexed with sodium deoxycholate and given as a suspension by slow intravenous injection. The significant side-effects of this compound (see below) have triggered a search for additional formulations and/or delivery systems with reduced toxicity (for a review of this approach see Walsh et al., 2000). Other preparations available for intravenous infusion include amphotericin complexed with lipids or with β-cyclodextrin or encapsulated in liposomes or nanospheres. Long-circulating or so-called 'stealth' liposomes containing amphotericin have been used to good effect.

Amphotericin is very highly protein bound and is found in fairly high concentrations in inflammatory exudates. It normally crosses the blood–brain barrier poorly, but penetration may be improved when the meninges are inflamed since intravenous amphotericin, used with flucytosine, is effective in *cryptococcal meningitis*. It is excreted very slowly via the kidney, traces being found in the urine for 2 months or more after administration has ceased.

Unwanted effects

The commonest and most serious unwanted effect of amphotericin is renal toxicity. Some degree of reduction of renal function occurs in more than 80% of patients receiving the drug; although this generally recovers after treatment is stopped, some impairment of glomerular filtration may remain. Hypokalaemia occurs in 25% of patients, requiring potassium chloride supplementation. Hypomagnesaemia also occurs and anaemia can be a further problem. Other unwanted effects include impaired hepatic function, thrombocytopenia, and anaphylactic reactions. Injection frequently results initially in chills, fever, tinnitus and headache, and about one in five patients vomit. The drug is irritant to the endothelium of the veins, and local thrombophlebitis is sometimes seen after intravenous injection. Intrathecal injections can cause neurotoxicity, and topical applications cause a skin rash. The liposome-encapsulated and lipid-complexed preparations cause fewer adverse reactions but are considerably more expensive.

NYSTATIN

Nystatin is a polyene macrolide antibiotic similar in structure to amphotericin and with the same mechanism of action. There is virtually no absorption from the mucous membranes of the body or from skin and its use is limited to fungal infections of the skin and the gastrointestinal tract.

GRISEOFULVIN

Griseofulvin is a narrow-spectrum antifungal agent isolated from cultures of *Penicillium griseofulvum*. It is fungistatic and it acts by interacting with microtubules and interfering with mitosis. It can be used to treat dermatophyte infections of skin or nails, but treatment needs to be very prolonged.

Pharmacokinetic aspects

Griseofulvin is given orally. It is poorly soluble in water and absorption varies with the type of preparation, in particular with particle size. Peak plasma concentrations are reached in about 5 hours. It is taken up selectively by newly formed skin and concentrated in the keratin.

The plasma half-life is 24 hours, but it is retained in the skin for much longer. It potently induces cytochrome P450 enzymes and causes several clinically important drug interactions.

Unwanted effects

Unwanted effects with griseofulvin use are infrequent but the drug can cause gastrointestinal upsets, headache and photosensitivity. Allergic reactions (rashes, fever) may also occur.

SYNTHETIC ANTIFUNGAL AGENTS

AZOLES

The azoles are a group of synthetic fungistatic agents with a broad spectrum of activity. The main drugs available are **fluconazole**, **itraconazole**, **ketoconazole**, **miconazole** and **econazole**. For reviews, see Como & Dismukes (1994), Hoeprich (1995) and Neely & Ghannoun (2000).

Mechanism of action of the azoles

The azoles inhibit the fungal cytochrome P450 3A (CYP3A) enzyme, lanosine 14α-demethylase, which is responsible for converting lanosterol to ergosterol, the main sterol in the fungal cell membrane. The resulting depletion of ergosterol alters the fluidity of the membrane and this interferes with the action of membrane-associated enzymes. The net effect is an inhibition of replication. Azoles also inhibit the transformation of candidal yeast cells into hyphae—the invasive and pathogenic form of the parasite. The depletion of membrane ergosterol reduces the binding sites for amphotericin.

Ketoconazole

Ketoconazole was the first azole that could be given orally to treat systemic fungal infections. It is effective against several different types of fungus (see Table 47.1). It is, however, toxic (see below) and relapse is common after apparently successful treatment. It is well absorbed from the gastrointestinal tract. It is distributed widely throughout the tissues and tissue fluids but does not reach therapeutic concentrations in the central nervous system (CNS) unless high doses are given. It is inactivated in the liver and excreted in bile and in urine. Its half-life in the plasma is 8 hours.

Unwanted effects

The main hazard of ketoconazole is liver toxicity, which is rare but can prove fatal. It may occur without overt clinical evidence and may progress even after stopping the drug. Other side-effects that occur are gastrointestinal disturbances and pruritus. Inhibition of adrenocortical steroid and testosterone synthesis has been recorded with high doses, the latter resulting in gynaecomastia in some male patients. There may be adverse interactions with other drugs. Ciclosporin, terfenadine and astemizole all interfere with the metabolising enzymes, causing increased plasma concentrations of ketoconazole or the interacting drug or both. Rifampicin, histamine H_2-receptor antagonists and antacids decrease the absorption of ketoconazole.

Fluconazole

Fluconazole can be given orally or intravenously. It reaches high concentrations in the cerebrospinal fluid (CSF) and ocular fluids and may become the drug of first choice for most types of fungal meningitis. Fungicidal concentrations are also achieved in vaginal tissue, saliva, skin and nails. It has a half-life of ~25 hours; 90% is excreted unchanged in the urine and 10% in the faeces.

Unwanted effects

Unwanted effects, which are generally mild, include nausea, headache and abdominal pain. However, exfoliative skin lesions (including, on occasion, Stevens–Johnson syndrome*) have been seen in some individuals—primarily in AIDS patients who are being treated with multiple drugs.

Hepatitis has been reported, though this is rare, and fluconazole, in the doses usually used, does not produce the inhibition of hepatic drug metabolism and of steroidogenesis that occurs with ketoconazole.

Itraconazole

Itraconazole is given orally and, after absorption (which is variable), undergoes extensive hepatic metabolism. It is highly lipid soluble (and water insoluble) and a formulation in which the drug is retained within pockets of β-cyclodextrin is available. In this form, itraconazole can be administered intravenously, thereby overcoming the problem of variable absorption from the gastrointestinal tract. Adminstered orally, its half-life is about 36 hours and it is excreted in the urine. It does not penetrate the CSF.

Unwanted effects

Gastrointestinal disturbances, headache and dizziness can occur. Rare unwanted effects are hepatitis, hypokalaemia and impotence. Allergic skin reactions have been reported (including Stevens–Johnson syndrome; see above). Inhibition of steroidogenesis has not been reported. Drug interactions as a result of inhibition of cytochrome P450 enzymes occur (similar to those described above for ketoconazole).

Miconazole

Miconazole is given orally for infections of the gastrointestinal tract. It has a short plasma half-life and needs to be given every 8 hours. It reaches therapeutic concentrations in bone, joints and lung tissue but not in the CNS, and it is inactivated in the liver. It can also be given topically.

*This is a severe and usually fatal condition involving blistering of the skin, mouth, eyes and genitalia, often accompanied by fever, polyarthritis and kidney failure.

Unwanted effects

Unwanted effects are relatively infrequent, those most commonly seen being gastrointestinal disturbances, but pruritus, blood dyscrasias and hyponatraemia are also reported. There can be problems during the process of injection—the occurrence of anaphylactic reactions, dysrhythmias and fevers. The drug can have an irritant action on the venous endothelium. Because of the possibility of adverse interactions, concomitant administration with the histamine H_1-receptor antagonists terfenadine and astemizole should be avoided.

Other azoles

Clotrimazole, **econazole**, **tioconazole** and **sulconazole** are azole antifungal agents used only for topical application. Clotrimazole interferes with amino acid transport into the fungus by an action on the cell membrane. It is active against a wide range of fungi, including candidal organisms.

FLUCYTOSINE

Flucytosine is a synthetic antifungal agent that, given orally, is active against a limited range of systemic fungal infections, being effective mainly in those caused by yeast. If given alone, drug resistance commonly arises during treatment so it is usually combined with amphotericin for severe infections such as cryptococcal meningitis.

Mechanism of action

Flucytosine is converted to the antimetabolite 5-fluorouracil (5-FU) in fungal but not human cells. 5-FU inhibits thymidylate synthetase and thus DNA synthesis (see Chs 44 and 50). Resistant mutants may emerge rapidly so this drug should not be used alone.

Pharmacokinetic aspects

Flucytosine is usually given by intravenous infusion but can also be given orally. It is widely distributed throughout the body fluids including the CSF. About 90% is excreted unchanged via the kidneys, and the plasma half-life is 3–5 hours. The dosage should be reduced if renal function is impaired.

Unwanted effects

Unwanted effects are infrequent. Gastrointestinal disturbances, anaemia, neutropenia, thrombocytopenia and alopecia have occurred, but these are usually mild and are reversed when therapy ceases. Uracil is reported to decrease the toxic effects on the bone marrow without impairing the antimycotic action. Hepatitis has been reported but is rare.

TERBINAFINE

Terbinafine is a highly lipophilic, keratinophilic fungicidal compound active against a wide range of skin pathogens. It acts by selectively inhibiting the enzyme *squalene epoxidase,* which is involved in the synthesis of ergosterol from squalene in the fungal cell wall. The accumulation of squalene within the cell is toxic to the organism.

It is used to treat fungal infections of the nails. Given orally, it is rapidly absorbed and is taken up by skin, nails and adipose tissue. Given topically, it penetrates skin and mucous membranes. It is metabolised in the liver by the cytochrome P450 system and the metabolites are excreted in the urine. Given topically, it penetrates skin and mucous membranes. **Naftifine** is similar in action to terbinafine.

Unwanted effects

Unwanted effects occur in about 10% of individuals and are usually mild and self-limiting. They include gastrointestinal disturbances, rashes, pruritus, headache and dizziness. Joint and muscle pains have been reported and, more rarely, hepatitis.

ECHINOCANDINS

The echinocandins inhibit the synthesis of 1,3-β-glucan, a glucose polymer that is necessary for maintaining the structure of fungal cell walls. In the absence of this polymer, fungal cells lose integrity and lysis follows quickly.

Echinocandins comprise a ring of six amino acids linked to a lipophilic side-chain. All drugs in this group are based on the structure of echinocandin B, which is found naturally in *Aspergillus nidulans*.

Caspofungin (available in the USA, not available in the UK) is active in vitro against a wide variety of fungi and has proved effective in the treatment of candidiasis and forms of invasive aspergillosis that are refractory to amphotericin. Oral absorption is poor and caspofungin is extensively protein bound in the bloodstream. After intravenous administration, it exhibits a half-life in humans of 9–10 hours and once daily therapy is, therefore, feasible.

Micafungin (FK463) is currently undergoing clinical trials. It is very effective against *Aspergillus* and *Candida* spp. even in patients who are immunocompromised with AIDS.

Amorolfine is a morpholine derivative that interferes with fungal sterol synthesis. It is given locally as a lacquer and is reported to be effective against fungal infections of the nails.

POTENTIAL NEW ANTIFUNGAL THERAPIES

Increasing numbers of fungal strains are becoming resistant to the currently used antifungal drugs. Fortunately, drug resistance is not transferable in fungi—though this is small comfort to a patient infected with a resistant strain. An additional problem is that new strains of commensal-turned-pathogenic fungi have emerged.

Fungal infections are on the rise and new and better antifungal agents are being sought. Encouragingly, new compounds are in development some with novel mechanisms of action (for review, see Neely & Ghannoun, 2000).

Several 'new generation' azoles are currently undergoing phase III clinical trials. None of these has yet been approved for clinical use but **voriconazole** is probably the most advanced. It has a promisingly broad spectrum of antifungal activity and has the advantage of being active against fluconazole-resistant strains of *Candida* and *Cryptococcus*. In clinical trials, it has proved as, or more, effective as amphotericin. It can be admistered orally or intravenously and has few side-effects other than transient visual disturbances. Further azoles under development include **posaconazole** and **ravuconazole**.

Drugs that reduce fungal cell wall viability are also a major focus for study. **Pradimicin** and like agents exhibit antifungal activity by virtue of binding mannosides, which are important components of the cell wall. **Nikkomycins** have a similar effect by preventing the formation of chitin, another cell wall component. The pharmacology of drugs that target the fungal cell wall has been reviewed by Georgopapadakou (2001).

Fungal protein synthesis could be yet another target for antifungal drug development since such synthesis requires an elongation factor that is missing from human cells. The **sordarins** are effective against yeast fungi since they inhibit fungal elongation factor 2, which is an important step in fungal protein production.

An entirely different approach, also being tested, is to enhance the host's ability to confront the fungal pathogen. Recombinant forms of human granulocyte colony-stimulating factor (see Ch. 21), for example **lenograstim** and **molgramostim**, can increase the neutrophil count in neutropenic patients with fungal infections. Animal studies also suggest an antifungal-enhancing effect of cytokines such as interleukins 1, 12 and 15. Small-scale clinical studies of granulocyte colony-stimulating factor either with or without amphotericin have proved equivocal, and more clinical work is needed to determine whether combination antifungal agent/cytokine treatment is likely be effective.

The possibility of developing an antifungal vaccine was first put forward in the 1960s. Fungi are several orders of magnitude more complex than bacteria or even viruses, for which vaccines are available, and despite some limited success in animals there are as yet no antifungal vaccines available for clinical use.

REFERENCES AND FURTHER READING

Bonn D 1997 New antifungals make mayhem for mycoses. Lancet 350: 870 *(Succinct summary article)*

Como J A, Dismukes W E 1994 Oral azoles as systemic antifungal chemotherapy. N Engl J Med 330: 263–272 *(Comprehensive review)*

Georgopapadakou N 2001 Update on antifungals targeted to the cell wall: focus on beta-1,3-glucan synthase inhibitors. Expert Opin Investig Drugs 10:269–280

Groll A M, Piscitelli S C, Walsh T J 1998 Clinical pharmacology of systemic antifungal events. Adv Pharmacol vol. 44 (*A comprehensive review of agents in clinical use, current investigational compounds and putative targets for antifungal drug developments*)

Hartsel S, Bolard J 1996 Amphotericin B: new life for an old drug. Trends Pharmacol Sci 17: 445–449

Hoeprich P D 1995 Antifungal chemotherapy. Prog Drug Res 44: 88–127 *(Detailed coverage of main classes of drug: chemical formulae, mode of action, pharmacokinetics, adverse effects)*

Kauffman C A 2001 Fungal infections in older adults. Clin Infect Dis 33: 550–555 *(Interesting account of fungal infections and their treatment)*
Lambert H P, O'Grady F W 1992 Antifungal agents. In: Lambert H P, O'Grady F W (eds) Antibiotic and chemotherapy. Churchill Livingstone, Edinburgh
Neely M N, Ghannoun M A 2000 The exciting future of antifungal therapy. Eur J. Clin Microbiol Infect Dis 19: 897–914 *(Good overview of antifungal drugs)*
Polak A, Hartman P G 1991 Antifungal chemotherapy—are we winning? Prog Drug Res 37: 181–265
Ryley J F (ed) 1990 Chemotherapy of fungal diseases. Springer-Verlag, Berlin
Walsh T J 1992 Invasive fungal infections: problems and challenges for developing new antifungal compounds. In: Sutcliffe J A, Georgopapadakou N H (eds) Emerging targets in antibacterial and antifungal therapy. Chapman & Hall, New York, ch. 13
Walsh T J, Viviani M A, Arathoon E et al. 2000 New targets and delivery systems for antifungal therapy. Med Mycol 38(suppl. 1): 335–347
Yamaguchi H, Kobayashi G S, Takahashi H 1992 (eds) Recent progress in antifungal chemotherapy. Marcel Dekker, New York

48 Antiprotozoal drugs

Overview 672

Host–parasite interactions 672

Malaria 673
- The life cycle of the malaria parasite 673
- Antimalarial drugs 676
- Potential new antimalarial drugs 682

Pneumocystis pneumonia and its treatment 682

Amoebiasis and amoebicidal drugs 682

Leishmaniasis and leishmanicidal drugs 683

Trypanosomiasis and trypanosomicidal drugs 684

Trichomoniasis and trichomonicidal drugs 684

Toxoplasmosis and toxoplasmocidal drugs 684

New approaches to antiprotozoal therapy 685

OVERVIEW

The main protozoa that produce disease in humans are those causing malaria, amoebiasis, leishmaniasis, trypanosomiasis and trichomoniasis. In this chapter, we explore the underlying causes of each of these diseases and discuss the principal drugs used in their treatment.

HOST–PARASITE INTERACTIONS

Mammals have developed very efficient mechanisms for dealing with invading parasites, and some of these parasites have, in turn, evolved clever tactics to evade the defensive responses of the host. One parasite ploy is to take refuge within the cells of the host where antibodies cannot reach them. Most protozoa do this, some (plasmodia species) taking up residence in red cells, some (leishmania species) infecting macrophages exclusively and some (various trypanosome species) invading many cell types. The host has, in turn, evolved strategies to deal with these intracellular parasites, namely cell-mediated immune responses involving primarily the T helper (Th) 1 pathway cytokines, such as interleukin (IL)-2, tumour necrosis factor (TNF)-β and interferon (IFN) γ, that activate macrophages and cytotoxic CD8+ T cells (Ch. 15). Activated macrophages kill intracellular parasites, and cytotoxic T cells collaborate with macrophages by producing macrophage-activating cytokines.

The Th1 pathway responses can be downregulated by Th2 pathway cytokines such as TGF-β, IL-4 and IL-10 (p. 224). Some intracellular parasites have evolved mechanisms for manipulating the Th1/Th2 balance to their own advantage by stimulating production of the Th2 cytokines that downregulate cell-mediated immune reactions. For example, the invasion of macrophages by *Leishmania* species is associated with induction of TGF-β; the invasion of T cells, B cells and macrophages by trypanosomes is associated with induction of IL-10. Similar mechanisms occur during worm infestations (see Ch. 49).

Toxoplasma gondii, has evolved a different ploy—upregulation of some host responses. The main, definitive host of this protozoon is the cat, but humans can inadvertently become intermediate hosts, harbouring the asexual form of the parasite. In most individuals, the disease is asymptomatic, though it can severely damage the developing fetus and can cause fatal generalised infection in patients with the acquired immnodeficiency syndrome (AIDS) or other cause of immunosuppression. In humans, *T. gondii* infects numerous cell types and has a highly virulent replicative stage; it is, therefore, important to the parasite that its proliferative capacity is regulated so as to ensure the survival of its host. To do this, it stimulates production of IFNγ, thus modulating the host's cell-mediated responses, which then promote encystment of the parasite in the tissues.*

Improved understanding of host–protozoon relationships has opened up new vistas for the development of antiprotozoal agents. The possibility of using cytokine analogues and/or antagonists to treat disease caused by protozoa is already being investigated (for review, see Odeh, 2001).

*The encysted parasite is waiting patiently for its intermediate host to be eaten by its main host, a cat—a somewhat flawed stratagem when the intermediate host is a human.

MALARIA

Malaria is mosquito-borne and is one of the major killer diseases of the world. The statistics involved are staggering. According to the World Health Organization (WHO), malaria is a significant public health problem in more than 90 countries inhabited by some 2400 million people (about 40% of the world's population) (see Fig. 48.1). There are an estimated 300–500 million clinical cases each year with more than 90% of these occurring in sub-Saharan Africa. Malaria causes up to 2.7 million deaths per year with the vast majority of these among young children in Africa, especially in remote rural areas with limited or no access to medical care. In fact, in some parts of Africa, malaria kills 3000 children under 5 years of age each day. Such a death toll is very much greater than that associated with, for example, AIDS. Other high-risk groups include women during pregnancy, refugees and labourers entering endemic regions. Malaria also imposes a huge economic burden on countries where the disease is rife.*

The symptoms of malaria include fever, shivering, pain in the joints, headache, repeated vomiting, generalised convulsions and coma. Symptoms only become apparent 7–9 days after being bitten by an infected mosquito. By far the most dangerous of the parasites is *Plasmodium falciparum*.

About 50 years ago, the WHO attempted to eradicate malaria using the powerful 'residual' insecticides and the highly effective antimalarial drugs that had become available. By the end of the 1950s, the incidence of malaria had dropped dramatically. However, during the 1970s it became clear that the attempt at eradication had failed—largely owing to the increasing resistance of the mosquito to the insecticides and of the parasite to the drugs. Sadly, it is now the case that malaria has re-emerged in several countries where it was previously under control or indeed eradicated. Sporadic cases—the result of air travel—are quite common in Western Europe and the USA, where the risk of transmission is negligible.**

THE LIFE CYCLE OF THE MALARIA PARASITE

The life cycle consists of a *sexual cycle*, which takes place in the female anopheline mosquito, and an *asexual cycle*, which occurs in humans (Fig. 48.2). With the bite of an infected female mosquito, *sporozoites*—usually few in number—are injected and reach the bloodstream. Within 30 minutes, they disappear from the blood and enter the parenchymal cells of the liver, where, during the next 10–14 days, they undergo a *pre-erythrocytic stage* of development and multiplication. At the end of this stage, the parasitised liver cells rupture and a host of *merozoites* are released. These bind to and enter the red cells of the blood and form motile intracellular parasites termed *trophozoites*. The development and multiplication of the plasmodia within these cells constitutes the *erythrocytic stage*. During maturation within the red cell, the parasite remodels the host cell, inserting parasite proteins and phospholipids into the red cell membrane. The host's haemoglobin is digested and transported to the parasite's food vacuole, where it provides a source of amino acids. Free haem, which would be toxic to the plasmodium, is rendered harmless by polymerisation to *haemozoin*. Some antimalarial drugs act by inhibiting the haem polymerase (see below).

Following mitotic replication of its nucleus, the parasite in the red cell is called a *schizont*, and its rapid growth and division, *schizogony*, another phase of multiplication, results in the production of further merozoites, which are released when the red cell ruptures. These merozoites then bind to and enter fresh red cells and the erythrocytic cycle starts all over again.

In certain forms of malaria, some sporozoites on entering the liver cells form *hypnozoites*, or 'sleeping' forms of the parasite, which can be reactivated to continue an *exoerythrocytic cycle* of multiplication. The dormancy can last for months or years.

Malaria parasites can multiply in the body at a phenomenal rate—a single parasite of *Plasmodium vivax* being capable of giving rise to 250 million merozoites in 14 days. To appreciate the action required of an antimalarial drug, note that destruction of 94% of the parasites every 48 hours will only *maintain* equilibrium and will not reduce their number or their propensity

Malaria

- Malaria is caused by various species of plasmodia. The female anopheline mosquito injects sporozoites (the asexual form of the parasite), which can develop in the liver into:
  —schizonts (the pre-erythrocytic stage), which liberate merozoites: these infect red blood cells, forming motile trophozoites, which, after development, release another batch of erythrocyte-infecting merozoites causing fever; this constitutes the erythrocytic cycle
  —dormant hypnozoites, which may liberate merozoites later (the exoerythrocytic stage).
- The main malarial parasites causing 'tertian' malaria (by definition fever 'every third day', though various patterns are seen) are:
  —*P. vivax*, which causes benign tertian malaria
  —*P. falciparum*, which causes malignant tertian malaria; unlike *P. vivax*, this plasmodium has no exoerythrocytic stage.
- Some merozoites develop into gametocytes, the sexual forms of the parasite; these, when ingested by the mosquito, give rise to further stages of the parasite's life cycle within the insect.

*Taking into account factors such as initial poverty, economic policy etc. it has been calculated that countries with intensive malaria grow 1.3% less per person per year than malaria-free zones and that a 1.1% reduction in malaria is associated with a 0.3% higher rate of economic growth.

**As an example of such 'airport malaria', the UK registered 2364 cases of malaria in 1997. All of them imported by travellers. 'Weekend malaria', which occurs when city dwellers in Africa spend weekends in the countryside, is also becoming more of a problem.

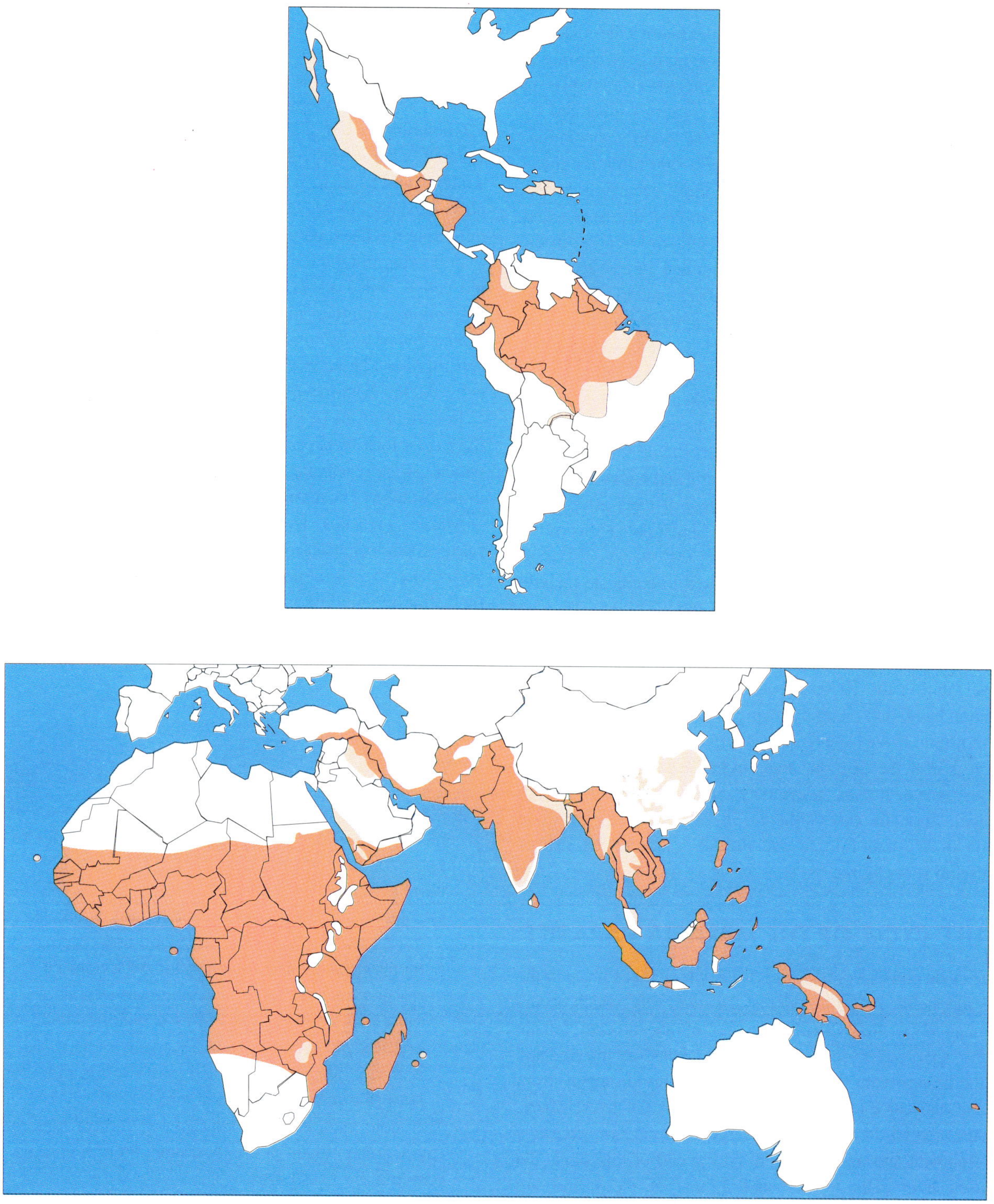

Fig. 48.1 Geographic distribution of malaria. Dark shade indicates, areas where malaria transmission occurs; light shade indicates areas with limited risk; unshaded areas are those in which malaria has disappeared, been eradicated or never existed. (Map from US Department of Health and Human Services, National Center for Infectious Diseases, 2000.)

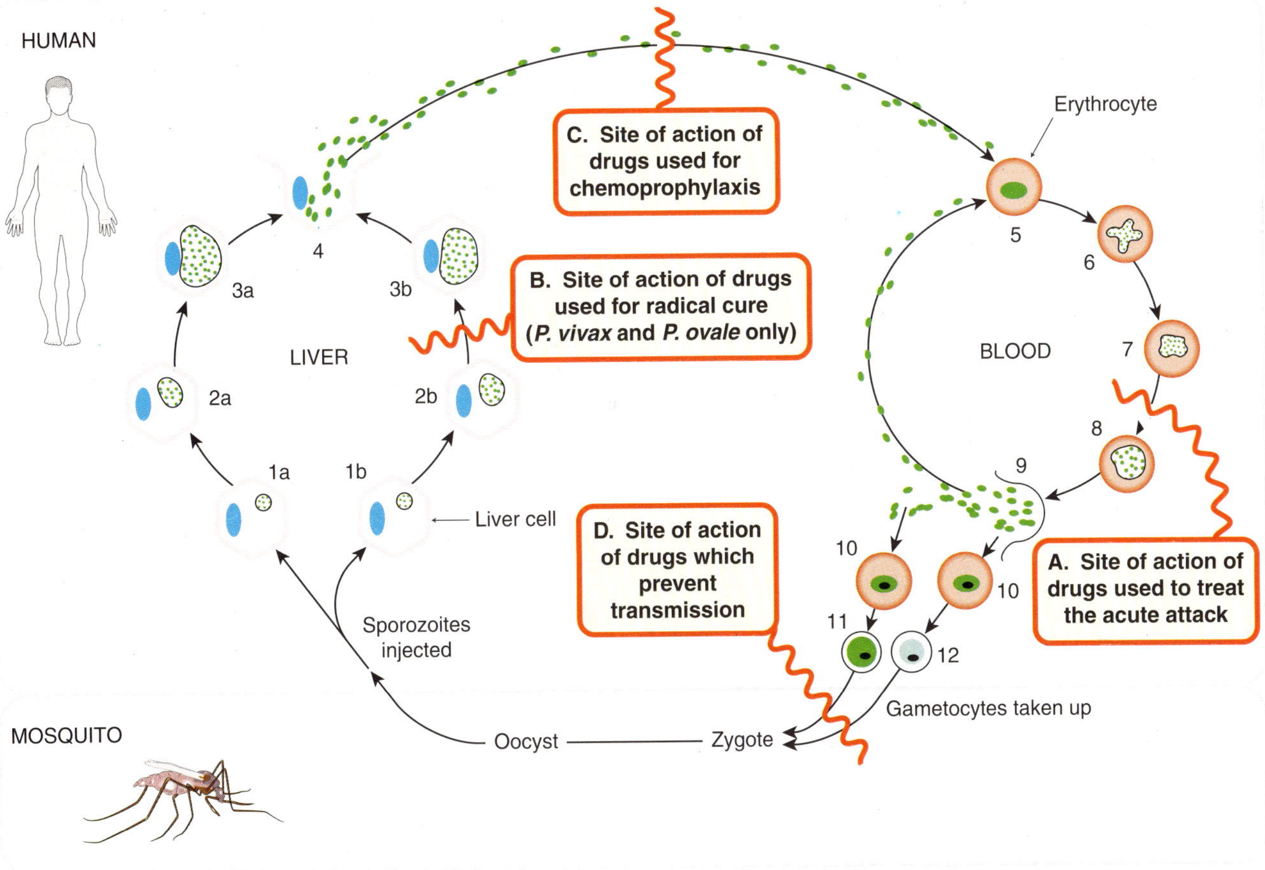

Fig. 48.2 The life cycle of the malarial parasite and the site of action of antimalarial drugs. The pre- or exoerythrocytic cycle in the liver and the erythrocytic cycle in the blood are shown: 1a. Entry of sporozoite into liver cell (the parasite is shown as a small circle containing dots and the liver cell nucleus as a white oval). 2a and 3a. Development of the schizont in liver cell. 4. Rupture of liver cell with release of merozoites (some may enter liver cells to give resting forms of the parasite, hypnozoites). 5. Entry of a merozoite into a red cell 6. Trophozoite in red cell. 7 and 8. Development of schizont in red cell. 9. Rupture of red cell with release of merozoites, most of which parasitise other red cells. 10–12. Entry of some merozoites into red cells and development of male and female gametocytes. 1b. Resting form of parasite in liver (hypnozoite). 2b and 3b. Growth and multiplication of hypnozoites. Sites of drug action: A. Drugs used to treat the acute attack (also called 'blood schizonticidal agents' or 'drugs for suppressive or clinical cure'). B. Drugs that affect the exoerythrocytic hypnozoites and result in radical cure of *P. vivax* and *P. ovale*. C. Drugs that block the link between the exoerythrocytic stage and the erythrocytic stage; they are used for chemoprophylaxis (also termed 'causal prophylactics') and prevent the development of malarial attacks. D. Drugs that prevent transmission and thus prevent increase of the human reservoir of the disease.

for proliferation. Some merozoites, on entering red cells, differentiate into male and female forms of the parasite, called *gametocytes*. These can only complete their cycle when taken up by the mosquito, when it sucks the blood of an infected host. The cycle in the mosquito involves fertilisation of the female gametocyte by the male gametocyte with the formation of a zygote, which develops into an oocyst (sporocyst). A further stage of division and multiplication takes place, leading to rupture of the sporocyst with release of sporozoites, which then migrate to the mosquito's salivary glands and enter another human host with the mosquito's bite.

The periodic episodes of fever that characterise malaria result from the synchronised rupture of red cells with release of merozoites and cell debris. The rise in temperature is associated with a rise in the concentration of TNF-α in the plasma.

Relapses of malaria are likely to occur with those forms of malaria that have an exoerythrocytic cycle, because the dormant hypnozoite form in the liver can emerge after an interval of weeks or months to start the infection again.

The chief species of human malaria parasites are as follows:

- *P. falciparum*, which has an erythrocytic cycle of 48 hours in humans, produces *malignant tertian malaria*—'tertian' because the fever was believed to recur every third day, 'malignant' because it is the most severe form of malaria and can be fatal. The plasmodium induces, on the infected red

Antimalarial therapy and the parasite life cycle

- Drugs used to treat the acute attack of malaria (i.e. for suppressive or clinical cure) act on the parasites in the blood; they can cure infections with parasites (e.g. *P. falciparum*) that have no exoerythrocytic stage.
- Drugs used for chemoprophylaxis (causal prophylactics) (i.e. to prevent malarial attacks when in a malarious area) act on merozoites emerging from liver cells.
- Drugs used for radical cure are active against parasites in the liver.
- Some drugs act on gametocytes and prevent transmission by the mosquito.

cell's membrane, receptors for the adhesion molecules on vascular endothelial cells (see p. 221). These parasitised red cells then stick to uninfected red cells forming clusters (rosettes). They also adhere to and pack the vessels of the microcirculation, interfering with tissue blood flow and causing organ dysfunction, for example renal failure and encephalopathy (cerebral malaria). *P. falciparum* does not have an exoerythrocytic stage, so if the erythrocytic stage is eradicated, relapses do not occur (Fig. 48.2).

- *P. vivax* produces benign tertian malaria—'benign' because it is less severe than falciparum malaria and rarely fatal. Exoerythrocytic forms may persist for years and cause relapses (Fig. 48.2).
- *P. ovale*, which has a 48-hour cycle and an exoerythrocytic stage, is the cause of a rare form of malaria (see Fig. 48.2).
- *P. malariae* has a 72-hour cycle, causes *quartan malaria* and has no exoerythrocytic cycle (Fig. 48.2).

Immunity to malaria occurs and can protect many individuals living in malarious areas. It involves mostly cell-mediated reactions (Ch. 15) the details of which are now gradually being elucidated. The immunity is lost if the individual is absent from the area for more than 6 months.

ANTIMALARIAL DRUGS

The best way to treat malaria is to avoid the disease in the first place by preventing mosquito bites. Travellers to infected areas should always take simple precautions such as wearing clothes that cover much of the skin and using insect repellents in living, and especially in sleeping, areas since mosquitoes tend to bite between dusk and dawn. Bed nets sprayed with insecticides such as **permethrin** can also be very effective. Some drugs can be used prophylactically to prevent malaria while others are directed towards treating acute attacks. In general, antimalarial drugs are classified in terms of the action against the different stages of the life cycle of the parasite (Fig. 48.2).

Drugs used to treat the acute attack

Blood schizonticidal agents (Fig. 48.2, site A) are used to treat the acute attack—they are also known as drugs for suppressive or clinical cure. They act on the erythrocytic forms of the plasmodium. In infections with *P. falciparum* or *P. malariae*, which have no exoerythrocytic stage, these drugs effect a cure; with *P. vivax* or *P. ovale*, the drugs suppress the actual attack but exoerythrocytic forms can cause later relapses.

This group of drugs includes *quinoline–methanols* (e.g. **quinine** and **mefloquine**), various *4-aminoquinolines* (e.g. **chloroquine**), the phenanthrene **halofantrine**, and agents that interfere either with the synthesis of folate (e.g. **sulfones**) or with its action (e.g. **pyrimethamine** and **proguanil**) as well as the hydroxynaphthoquinone compound **atovaquone**. Combinations of these agents are frequently used. Some antibiotics, such as **tetracycline** and **doxycycline** (see Ch. 45), have proved useful when combined with the above agents. Compounds derived from qinghaosu, for example **artemether, arteflene** and **artesunate**, have also proved effective.

For a brief summary of currently recommended treatment regimens, see Table 48.1. A more detailed coverage of the treatment of malaria is given by Newton & White (1999).

Drugs that effect radical cure

Tissue schizonticidal agents effect a radical cure by acting on the parasites in the liver (Fig. 48.2, site B). Only the 8-aminoquinolines (e.g. **primaquine** and **tafenoquine**) have this action. These drugs also destroy gametocytes and thus reduce the spread of infection.

Drugs used for chemoprophylaxis

Drugs used for chemoprophylaxis (also known as *causal prophylactic* drugs) block the link between the exoerythrocytic stage and the erythrocytic stage and thus prevent the development of malarial attacks. True causal prophylaxis—the prevention of infection by the killing of the sporozoites on entry into the host—is not feasible with the drugs at present in use, though it may be achieved in the future with vaccines. Prevention of the development of clinical attacks can, however, be effected by chemoprophylactic drugs that kill the parasites when they emerge from the liver after the pre-erythrocytic stage (Fig. 48.2, site C). The drugs used for this purpose are mainly those listed above: **chloroquine**, **mefloquine**, **proguanil**, **pyrimethamine**, **dapsone** and **doxycycline**. They are often used in combinations.

Chemoprophylactic agents are given to individuals who intend travelling to an area where malaria is endemic. Administration should start 1 week before entering the area and should be continued throughout the stay and for at least a month afterwards. No chemoprophylactic regimen is 100% effective and the choice of drug is difficult. In addition to the normal criteria used in selecting a drug, the unwanted effects of some antimalarial agents need to be borne in mind and weighed against the risk of a serious, possibly fatal, parasitaemia. A further problem is the

Table 48.1 Summary of drugs used for treatment and chemoprophylaxis of malaria[a]

Infections	Drugs for the treatment of the clinical attack[b]	Drugs for chemoprophylaxis[c]
All plasmodial infections except chloroquine-resistant *P. falciparum*[d]	Oral chloroquine[e] or sulfadoxine–pyrimethamine	Oral chloroquine or proguanil
Infection with chloroquine-resistant *P. falciparum*[d]	Oral quinine[f] plus: (i) tetracycline or (ii) doxycycline[g] or oral halofantrine[h] or oral mefloquine[i]	Oral chloroquine plus: (i) proguanil or (ii) doxycycline[g] or (iii) pyrimethamine–dapsone or oral mefloquine[j]

[a]The specific combinations of drugs used may vary in different malarious areas.
[b]Severe malaria can be treated by intravenous infusion of chloroquine (up to 24 hours) but oral dosing should be used as soon as the patient can take tablets by mouth. See White (1996) for more detail.
[c]See Bradley & Warhurst (1995) for more detail.
[d]Chloroquine-resistant *P. falciparum* is now very widespread, and in some areas *P. vivax* has also became resistant. If there is any doubt about drug sensitivity then the infection should be assumed to be resistant.
[e]Hydroxychloroquine can be substituted.
[f]If oral administration is not feasible, quinine is given by slow intravenous infusion.
[g]Contraindicated in children under 12, pregnant women and nursing mothers.
[h]Can cause cardiac problems. Should not be taken with fatty foods.
[i]Has a fairly high incidence of adverse effects.
[j]Should not be used for chemoprophylaxis unless there is a high risk of chloroquine-resistant malaria.

complexity of the regimens, which require different drugs to be taken at different times, and the fact that different agents may be required for different travel destinations.

For a brief summary of currently recommended regimens of chemoprophylaxis, see Table 48.1. More detailed coverage is given by Bradley & Warhurst (1995) and Rosenblatt (1999).

Drugs used to prevent transmission

Some drugs (e.g. **primaquine, proguanil** and **pyrimethamine**) have the additional action of destroying the gametocytes (Fig. 48.2, site D), preventing transmission by the mosquito and thus preventing the increase of the human reservoir of the disease—but they are rarely used for this action alone.

4-AMINOQUINOLINES

The main 4-aminoquinoline used clinically is **chloroquine** (Fig. 48.3). **Amodiaquine** has very similar action to chloroquine. It was withdrawn several years ago because it caused agranulocytosis but has now been re-introduced in several areas of the world where chloroquine resistance is endemic.

Chloroquine

Chloroquine is a very potent blood schizonticidal drug (Fig. 48.2, site A), effective against the erythrocytic forms of all four plasmodial species (if sensitive to the drug), but it does not have any effect on sporozoites, hypnozoites or gametocytes. It has a complex mechanism of action that is not fully understood. It is uncharged at neutral pH and can, therefore, diffuse freely into the parasite lysosome. At the acid pH of the lysosome, it is converted to a protonated, membrane-impermeable form and is 'trapped' inside the parasite. At high concentrations, chloroquine inhibits protein, RNA and DNA synthesis but these effects are unlikely to be involved in its antimalarial activity. Chloroquine acts mainly on haem disposal by preventing digestion of haemoglobin by the parasite and thus reducing the supply of amino acids necessary for parasite viability. It also inhibits haem polymerase—the enzyme that polymerises toxic free haem to haemozoin—rendering it harmless.

Resistance

P. falciparum is now resistant to chloroquine in most parts of the world. Resistance appears to result from enhanced efflux of the drug from parasitic vesicles as a result of increased expression of the human multidrug resistance transporter *P-glycoprotein* (see Chs 7 and 50). Resistance of *P. vivax* to chloroquine is also a growing problem in many parts of the world.

Pharmacological actions

Chloroquine is a disease-modifying antirheumatoid drug (p. 256) and also has some quinidine-like actions on the heart.

The *clinical use* of chloroquine is given in Table 48.1.

Administration and pharmacokinetic aspects

Chloroquine is given orally, is completely absorbed, is extensively distributed throughout the tissues and is concentrated in parasitised red cells. In severe falciparum malaria it may be given by frequent intramuscular or subcutaneous injection of small doses or by slow continuous intravenous infusion.

As explained above, chloroquine concentrates particularly in parasitised red cells. It is released slowly from the tissues and metabolised in the liver. It is excreted in the urine, 70% as unchanged drug and 30% as metabolites. Elimination is slow, the major phase having a half-life of 50 hours, and a residue persists for weeks or months.

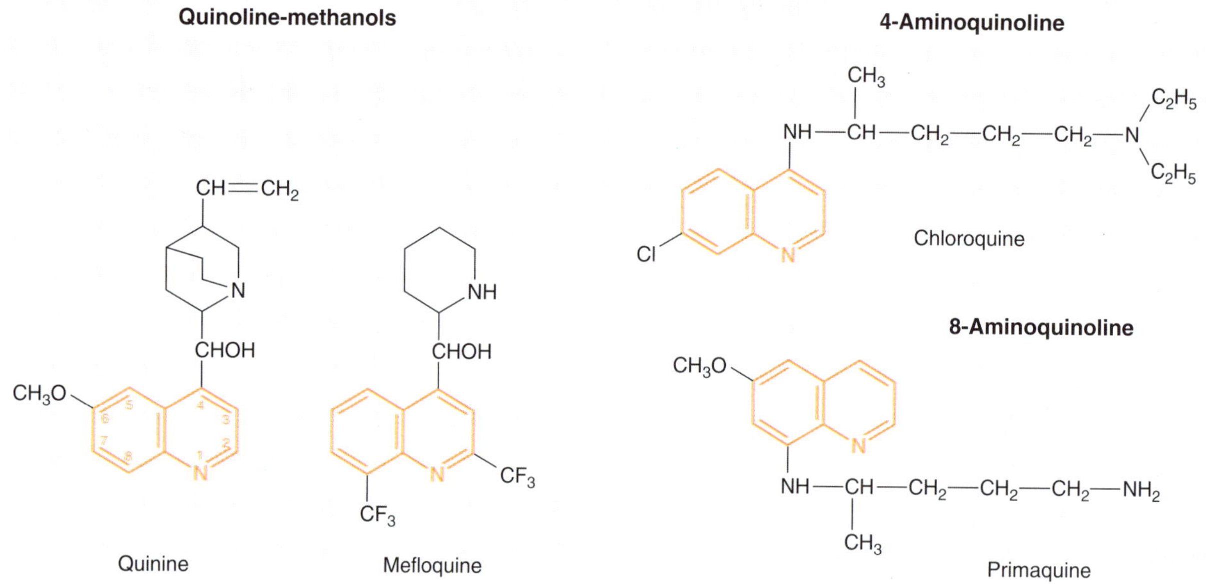

Fig. 48.3 **Structures of some quinoline antimalarial drugs.** The quinoline moiety is shown in orange.

Unwanted effects

Chloroquine has few adverse effects when given for chemoprophylaxis. With the larger doses used to treat the clinical attack of malaria, unwanted effects can occasionally occur, including nausea and vomiting, dizziness and blurring of vision, headache, and urticarial symptoms. Large doses have sometimes resulted in retinopathies. Bolus intravenous injections of chloroquine can cause hypotension and, if high doses are used, fatal dysrhythmias.

Chloroquine is considered to be safe for use by pregnant women.

QUINOLINE–METHANOLS

The two most widely used quinoline–methanols are **quinine** and **mefloquine** (Fig. 48.3).

Quinine

Quinine is an alkaloid derived from cinchona bark. It is a blood schizonticidal drug effective against the erythrocytic forms of all four species of plasmodium (Fig. 48.2, site A), but it has no effect on exoerythrocytic forms or on the gametocytes of *P. falciparum*. Its mechanism of action is, like that of chloroquine, associated with inhibition of the parasite's haem polymerase; but quinine is not so extensively concentrated in the plasmodium as chloroquine so other mechanisms could also be involved.

With the emergence and spread of chloroquine resistance, quinine is now the main chemotherapeutic agent for *P. falciparum*.

Pharmacological actions

Pharmacological actions on host tissue include a depressant action on the heart, a mild oxytocic effect on the uterus in pregnancy, a slight blocking action on the neuromuscular junction and a weak antipyretic effect.

The *clinical use* of quinine is given in Table 48.1.

Pharmacokinetic aspects

Quinine is usually given orally in a 7-day course, but it can be given by slow intravenous infusion for severe *P. falciparum* infections and in patients who are vomiting. A loading dose may be required, but bolus intravenous administration is contraindicated because of the risk of cardiac dysrhythmias. It is well absorbed from the gastrointestinal tract and is metabolised in the liver, the metabolites being excreted in the urine within about 24 hours. The half life is 10 hours.

Unwanted effects

Given orally, quinine is bitter, so compliance is poor. It is irritant to the gastric mucosa and can cause nausea and vomiting. If the concentration in the plasma exceeds 30–60 μmol/l, 'cinchonism' is likely to occur—nausea, dizziness, tinnitus, headache and blurring of vision. Excessive plasma levels of quinine can result in hypotension, cardiac dysrhythmias and severe central nervous system (CNS) disturbances such as delirium and coma.

Other rarer unwanted reactions that have been reported are hypoglycaemia, blood dyscrasias (especially thrombocytopenia) and hypersensitivity reactions.

Quinine can stimulate insulin release. Patients with marked falciparum parasitaemia can have low blood sugar for this reason and also because of glucose consumption by the parasite. This can cause diagnostic confusion between coma caused by cerebral malaria and hypoglycaemic coma—which responds to glucose.

Blackwater fever, a severe and often fatal condition in which acute haemolytic anaemia is associated with renal failure, is a rare result of treating malaria with quinine or of erratic and inappropriate use of quinine for a 'fever'.

Resistance

Some degree of resistance is developing. Like chloroquine, resistance is conferred by increased expression of P-glycoprotein, which effectively pumps the drug out of the parasite.

Mefloquine

Mefloquine (Fig. 48.3) is a blood schizonticidal quinoline–methanol compound, active against *P. falciparum* and *P. vivax* (Fig. 48.2, site A); however, it has no effect on hepatic forms of the parasites, so treatment of *P. vivax* infections should be followed by a course of primaquine (see below) to eradicate the hypnozoites. Mefloquine is frequently combined with pyrimethamine.

The antiparasite action is associated with inhibition of the haem polymerase; however, since mefloquine, like quinine, is not as extensively concentrated in the parasite as chloroquine, other mechanisms might also be involved.

Resistance has occurred in *P. falciparum* in some areas—particularly in southeast Asia—and is thought to be caused, as with quinine, by increased expression in the parasite of the P-glycoprotein (see Chs 5, 7 and 50).

The *clinical use* of mefloquine is given in Table 48.1.

Pharmacokinetic aspects

Mefloquine is given orally and is rapidly absorbed. It has a slow onset of action and a very long plasma half-life (up to 30 days), which may be the result of enterohepatic cycling or tissue storage.

Unwanted effects

When mefloquine is used for treatment of the acute attack, about 50% of subjects complain of gastrointestinal disturbances. Transient CNS toxicity—giddiness, confusion, dysphoria and insomnia—can occur and there have been a few reports of aberrant atrioventricular conduction and serious, but rare, skin diseases. Mefloquine may rarely provoke severe neuropsychiatric reactions. Mefloquine is contraindicated in pregnant women and in women liable to become pregnant within 3 months of stopping the drug, because of its long half-life and uncertainty about its possible teratogenicity.

When used for chemoprophylaxis the unwanted actions are usually milder, but the drug should not be used in this way unless there is a high risk of acquiring chloroquine-resistant malaria.

PHENANTHRENE–METHANOLS

Halofantrine

Halofantrine is a blood schizonticidal drug. It is one of a group of compounds that were studied during the Second World War and found to have antimalarial activity but were not developed when chloroquine was found to be successful. However, as chloroquine resistance developed, halofantrine came in from the cold. It is active against strains of *P. falciparum* that are resistant to **chloroquine, pyrimethamine** and **quinine**. It is effective against the erythrocytic form of *P. vivax* (Fig. 48.2, site A) but not the hypnozoites. However, it is not usually used for vivax malaria since this is generally susceptible to chloroquine. Cross-resistance between halofantrine and mefloquine in falciparum infections has been reported. Its mechanism of action is not known.

The *clinical use* of halofantrine is given in Table 48.1.

Pharmacokinetic aspects

Halofantrine is given orally. It is slowly and rather irregularly absorbed, with a peak plasma concentration approximately 4–6 hours after ingestion and a half-life of 1–2 days, though its main metabolite, which has equal potency, has a half-life of 3–5 days. Absorption is substantially increased by a fatty meal and elimination is in the faeces.

Unwanted effects

Abdominal pain, gastrointestinal disturbances, headache, a transient rise in hepatic enzymes and cough occur. Pruritus is reported but is less marked than with chloroquine. Halofantrine can produce changes in cardiac rhythm (most notably a lengthening of the Q–T interval) particularly if given with other dysrhythmia-inducing drugs, and it should be used with caution in patients with a history of dysrhythmia. It has caused sudden cardiac death. Rarer reactions are haemolytic anaemia and convulsions. Because of such unwanted actions, halofantrine is no longer used for 'standby' treatment of malaria and it is now reserved for infections caused by resistant organisms. However, even in this case, decreasing sensitivity and resistance of *P. falciparum* have been reported.

DRUGS AFFECTING THE SYNTHESIS OR UTILISATION OF FOLATE

Antifolate drugs are classified into type 1 and type 2 compounds. The type 1 antifolates are the sulfonamides and the sulfones, which inhibit the synthesis of folate by competing with *p*-aminobenzoic acid (see Chs 44 and 45). The type 2 antifolates are drugs such as **pyrimethamine** and **proguanil**, which prevent the utilisation of folate by inhibiting the conversion of dihydrofolate to tetrahydrofolate by *dihydrofolate reductase*. Combinations of folate antagonists (type 2) with drugs inhibiting folate synthesis (type 1) cause sequential blockade, affecting the same pathway at different points; these combinations thus have synergistic action (see Fig. 45.2).

Pyrimethamine is a 2,4,diaminopyrimidine (see Fig. 48.4) and is similar in structure to trimethoprim (see Fig. 45.1). The structure of **proguanil** is different but it can assume a configuration similar to that of pyrimethamine (see Fig. 48.4). These compounds inhibit the formation of tetrahydrofolate with the consequences for DNA synthesis outlined in Chapter 50 (p. 701). As explained in Chapters 44 and 45, some agents (pyrimethamine, proguanil) have a greater affinity for the plasmodial enzyme than for the human enzyme. They have a slow action against the erythrocytic forms of the parasite (Fig. 48.2, site A) and proguanil is believed to have an additional effect on the initial hepatic stage (1a to 3a in Fig. 48.2) but not on the hypnozoites of *P. vivax* (Fig. 48.2, Site B). Pyrimethamine is only used in combination with either dapsone or a sulfonamide.

The main sulfonamide used in malaria treatment is **sulfadoxine** and the only sulfone used is **dapsone** (see Fig. 48.4). Details of these drugs are given in Chapter 45. The sulfonamides and sulfones are active against the erythrocytic forms of *P. falciparum* but are less active against those of *P. vivax*; they have no activity against the sporozoite or hypnozoite forms of the plasmodia. Pyrimethamine–sulfadoxine has been extensively used for chloroquine-resistant malaria but resistance to this combination has developed in many areas.

The *clinical use* of these drugs is given in Table 48.1.

Pharmacokinetic aspects

Both pyrimethamine and proguanil are given orally and are well absorbed, though the process is slow. Pyrimethamine has a plasma half-life of 4 days and effective 'suppressive' plasma concentrations may last for 14 days; it is taken once a week. The half-life of proguanil is 16 hours. It is a pro-drug, metabolised in the liver to its active form, cycloguanil, which is excreted mainly in the urine. It must be taken daily. Details of the pharmacokinetics of dapsone are given in Chapter 45 (p. 651).

Unwanted effects

These drugs have few untoward effects if used carefully in therapeutic doses. Larger doses of the pyrimethamine–dapsone combination can cause serious reactions such as haemolytic anaemia, agranulocytosis and eosinophilic alveolitis. The pyrimethamine–sulfadoxine combination can cause serious skin reactions, blood dyscrasias and allergic alveolitis; it is no longer recommended for chemoprophylaxis. In high doses, pyrimethamine may inhibit mammalian dihydrofolate reductase and cause a megaloblastic anaemia (see Ch. 21); folic acid supplements should be given if this drug is used during pregnancy. Resistance to antifolate drugs arises from single point mutations in the genes encoding parasite dihydrofolate reductase.

8-AMINOQUINOLINES

The only 8-aminoquinoline licensed for current use is **primaquine** (see Fig. 48.3). **Etaquine** and **tafenoquine** are more active and slowly metabolised analogues of primaquine and are currently undergoing clinical evaluation. The mechanism of action of these compounds is not known.

The antimalarial action of these drugs is exerted against the liver hypnozoites and they can effect a radical cure of those forms of malaria in which the parasites have a dormant stage in the liver—*P. vivax* and *P. ovale*. Primaquine does not affect sporozoites and has little if any action against the erythrocytic stage of the parasite. However, it has a gametocidal action and is the most effective antimalarial drug for *preventing transmission* of the disease in all four species of plasmodia. It is almost invariably used in combination with another drug, usually **chloroquine**. Resistance to primaquine is rare, though evidence

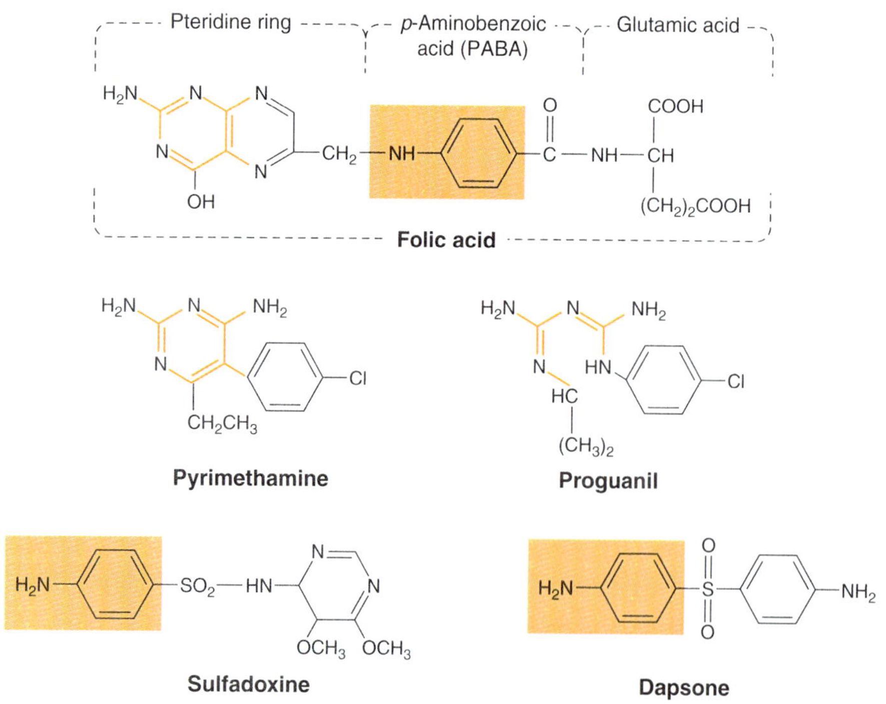

Fig. 48.4 Structures of some antimalarial drugs which act on the folic acid pathway of the plasmodia. Folate antagonists (pyrimethamine, proguanil) inhibit dihydrofolate reductase; the relationship between these drugs and the pteridine moiety is shown in orange. Sulfones (e.g. dapsone) and sulfonamides (e.g. sulfadoxine) compete with *p*-aminobenzoic acid for dihydropteroate synthetase (relationship shown in orange box). (See also Fig. 45.1.)

of a decreased sensitivity of some *P. vivax* strains has been reported. The pharmacology of primaquine and like drugs has been reviewed by Shanks et al. (2001).

Pharmacokinetic aspects

Primaquine is given orally and is well absorbed. Its metabolism is rapid and very little drug is present in the body after 10–12 hours. The half-life is 3–6 hours. Tafenoquine is broken down much more slowly and, therefore, has the advantage that it can be given on a weekly basis.

Unwanted effects

Primaquine has few unwanted effects in most patients when used in normal therapeutic dosage. Dose-related gastrointestinal symptoms can occur and large doses may cause methaemoglobinaemia with cyanosis. This antimalarial drug can, however, cause haemolysis in individuals with an X-chromosome-linked genetic metabolic condition—a deficiency of glucose 6-phosphate dehydrogenase in the red cells. When this deficiency is present, the red cells are not able to regenerate NADPH, its concentration being reduced by the oxidant metabolic derivatives of primaquine. As a consequence, the metabolic functions of the red cells are impaired and haemolysis occurs. Primaquine metabolites have greater haemolytic activity than the parent compound. The deficiency of the enzyme occurs in up to 15% of Black males and is also fairly common in some other ethnic groups. Glucose 6-phosphate dehydrogenase activity should be estimated before giving primaquine.

ANTIBIOTICS USED IN MALARIA

Some antibiotics, for example **doxycycline** and **tetracycline**, have a place in the treatment of the acute attack of malaria and in chemoprophylaxis; see page 676 above and Table 48.1. Details of these antibiotics are given in Chapter 45 (p. 643).

QINGHAOSU (ARTEMISININ) AND RELATED COMPOUNDS

The qinghaosu-based compounds are derived from the herb qing hao, a traditional Chinese remedy for malaria. The scientific name, conferred on the herb by Linnaeus, is *Artemisia*.* **Artemisinin**, a chemical extract from *Artemisia*, is poorly soluble in water and a fast-acting blood schizonticide effective in treating the acute attack of malaria (including chloroquine-resistant and cerebral malaria). **Artesunate**, a water-soluble derivative, and the synthetic analogues **artemether** and **artether** have higher activity and are better absorbed. The compounds are concentrated in parasitised red cells. The mechanism of action is not known; it may involve damage to the parasite membrane by carbon-centred free radicals (generated by the breakdown of ferrous protoporphyrin IX) or covalent alkylation of proteins. These compounds do not have any effect on liver hypnozoites and are not useful for chemoprophylaxis. Artemisinin can be given orally, intramuscularly or by suppository, artemether orally or intramuscularly, artesunate intramuscularly or intravenously. They are rapidly absorbed and widely distributed, and are converted in the liver to the active metabolite dihydroartemisinin. The half-life of artemisinin is about 4 hours, of artesunate 45 minutes and of artemether 4–11 hours.

Unwanted effects

There have been few unwanted effects reported to date. Transient heart block, decrease in blood neutrophil count and brief episodes of fever have been reported. In animal studies, artemisinin causes an unusual injury to some brainstem nuclei, particularly those involved in auditory function. However, there have been no reported incidences of neurotoxicity in humans. So far, there have also been no reported cases of resistance.

In rodent studies, artemisinin potentiated the effects of mefloquine, primaquine, and tetracycline, was additive with chloroquine and antagonised the sulfonamides and the folate antagonists. For this reason, artemisinin derivatives are frequently used in combination with other antimalarial drugs.

In randomised trials, the qinghaosu compounds have cured attacks of malaria, including cerebral malaria, more rapidly and with fewer unwanted effects than other antimalarial agents. Artemisinin and derivatives are effective against multidrug-resistant *P. falciparum* in sub-Saharan Africa and, combined with mefloquine, against multidrug-resistant *P. falciparum* in southeast Asia. However, the preclinical and clinical data are at present insufficient to satisfy the drug regulatory requirements in many countries. For reviews of this topic, see Hien & White (1993) and Olliaro et al. (2001).

HYDROXYNAPHTHOQUINONE DRUGS

Atavaquone is used for the treatment of malaria and has some ability to prevent its development. It acts primarily to inhibit the parasite's mitochondrial electron transport chain, possibly by mimicking the natural substrate *ubiquinone*.

Atavaquone and the antifolate drug **proguanil** are usually used in combination since they act together to cause a synergistic antimalarial effect. The mechanism underlying this effect is not known but synergy is specific for this particular pair of drugs since other antifolate drugs or electron transport inhibitors have no such effect. When combined with proguanil, atavaquone is highly effective and well tolerated.

Few side-effects of such combination treatment have been reported, but abdominal pain, nausea and vomiting can occur. Pregnant or breastfeeding women should not take atavaquone.

Resistance to atavaquone is rapid and results from a single point mutation in the gene for cytochrome *b*. Resistance to combined treatment with atavaquone and proguanil is less common.

*The herbs are noted for their extreme bitterness and their name derives from Artemisia, wife and sister of the fourth century king of Halicarnassus; her sorrow on his death led her to mix his ashes with whatever she drank to make it bitter.

Antimalarial drugs

- Chloroquine is a blood schizonticide acting by inhibiting haem polymerase—the enzyme that renders harmless the otherwise toxic free haem (derived from haemoglobin digestion). It is usually given orally (half-life 50 hours) and it is concentrated in the parasite. Unwanted effects include gastrointestinal disturbances, dizziness, urticaria; bolus intravenous injections can cause dysrhythmias.
- Quinine is a blood schizonticide. It is given orally (half-life 10 hours) but can be given by intravenous infusion if necessary. Unwanted effects include gastrointestinal tract upsets, tinnitus, blurred vision and, with large doses, dysrhythmias and CNS disturbances. 'Blackwater fever' is very occasionally associated with its administration. It is usually given in combination therapy with:
  - —pyrimethamine, a folate antagonist that acts as a slow blood schizonticide and is given orally (half-life 4 days), and either
  - —dapsone, a sulfone, given orally (half-life 24–48 hours), or
  - —sulfadoxine, a long-acting sulfonamide (half-life 7–9 days).
- Proguanil, a folate antagonist, is a slow blood schizonticide with some action on the primary liver forms of *P. vivax*. It is given orally (half-life 16 hours).
- Mefloquine is a blood schizonticidal agent active against *P. falciparum* and *P. vivax*. It is given orally and acts by inhibiting the parasite's haem polymerase. The onset of action is slow and the half-life is 30 days. The main unwanted effects are gastrointestinal disturbances, neurotoxicity (e.g. convulsions), psychiatric problems.
- Halofantrine is a blood schizonticidal agent active against all species of malarial parasite, including multiresistant *P. falciparum*. It is given orally but is irregularly absorbed. The half-life of the parent drug is 1–2 days and that of the active metabolite is 3–5 days. Common unwanted effects (abdominal pain, gastrointestinal disturbances, headache) are fewer than with mefloquine, but serious cardiac problems sometimes occur.
- Pimaquine is effective against the liver hypnozoites and is also active against gametocytes. Given orally, its half-life is 36 hours. Unwanted effects are mainly gastrointestinal tract disturbances and, with large doses, methaemoglobinaemia. Haemolysis is produced in individuals with genetic deficiency of erythrocyte glucose 6-phosphate dehydrogenase.
- Artemisinin derivatives are widely used in Asia and Africa but are not licensed in Europe or the USA. They are fast-acting blood schizonticidal agents that are effective against both *P. falciparum* and *P. vivax*. Artesunate is water soluble and can be given orally or by intravenous, intramuscular or rectal administration. Side-effects are rare.
- Atavaquone (in combination with proguanil) is used for the treatment of acute, uncomplicated *P. falciparum* malaria. The drug combination is effective orally. It is given at regular intervals over 3-4 days. Side-effects include diarrhoea, nausea and vomiting. Resistance to atavaquone develops rapidly if it is given alone.

POTENTIAL NEW ANTIMALARIAL DRUGS

Several new drugs are currently under test for antimalarial activity with positive results in animals and in preliminary trials in humans. One of these, **pyonaridine,** has been used in China for almost 10 years. It is active against *P. falciparum* and *P. vivax* and is also active in chloroquine-resistant *P. falciparum*. It is effective orally and has low toxicity. The mechanism of action is unknown.

Lumefantrine is structurally related to quinine and is effective against *P. falciparum* particularly when combined with either mefloquine or artemisinin derivatives.

PNEUMOCYSTIS PNEUMONIA AND ITS TREATMENT

First recognised in 1909, *Pneumocystis carinii* was presumed to belong to the protozoa, but recent studies have shown that it shares structural features with both protozoa and fungi, leaving its precise classification uncertain. Previously considered to be an innocuous microorganism widely distributed in the animal kingdom without causing disease, it now causes opportunistic infection in patients with AIDS. *P. carinii* pneumonia (PCP) is often the presenting symptom in an AIDS patient and it is a leading cause of death.

Many drugs have been used to treat PCP. High-dose **co-trimoxazole** (Ch. 45) is the drug of choice, with parenteral **pentamidine** (see above) as an alternative. Other treatment regimens include **trimethoprim–dapsone**, or **atovaquone** or **clindamycin– primaquine**.

AMOEBIASIS AND AMOEBICIDAL DRUGS

Amoebiasis is an infection with *Entamoeba histolytica* produced by the ingestion of cysts of this organism. In the intestine, the cysts develop into trophozoites that adhere to colonic epithelial cells by means of a lectin on the parasite membrane, which has similarity to host adherence proteins (Ch. 15). The trophozoite then lyses the host cell (hence histolytica) and invades the submucosa, where it may secrete a factor that inhibits IFNγ-activated macrophages, which would otherwise kill it. These processes may result in dysentery, though in many subjects a chronic intestinal infection can be present in the absence of dysentery. The parasite may invade the liver, leading to the development of liver abscesses, and in some subjects an amoebic granuloma (an *amoeboma*) develops in the intestinal wall. Some individuals are 'carriers'—they harbour the parasite without developing overt disease, but the cysts are present in their faeces and they can infect other individuals. The cysts can survive outside the body for at least a week in a moist and cool environment.

The use of drugs in treating this condition depends largely on the site and type of infection, and different drugs may be effective in acute amoebic dysentery, in chronic intestinal amoebiasis, in extra-intestinal infection and in the carrier state.

The main drugs currently used are **metronidazole, tinidazole** and **diloxanide**. These agents may be used in combination.

The drugs of choice for the various forms of amoebiasis are as follows:

- for acute invasive intestinal amoebiasis resulting in acute severe amoebic dysentery: metronidazole (or tinidazole) followed by diloxanide
- for chronic intestinal amoebiasis: diloxanide
- for hepatic amoebiasis: metronidazole followed by diloxanide
- for the carrier state: diloxanide.

Metronidazole

Metronidazole kills the trophozoites of *E. histolytica* but has no effect on the cysts. It is the most effective drug available for invasive amoebiasis involving the intestine or the liver, but it is less effective against organisms in the lumen of the gut.

The action of metronidazole is thought to be through damage to the DNA of the trophozoite by toxic oxygen products generated from the drug by the parasite.

Pharmacokinetic aspects

Metronidazole is usually given orally and is rapidly and completely absorbed, giving peak plasma concentration in 1–3 hours, with a half-life of about 7 hours. Rectal and intravenous preparations are also available. It is distributed rapidly throughout the tissues, reaching high concentrations in the body fluids, including the cerebrospinal fluid. Some is metabolised but most is excreted in urine.

Unwanted effects

There are few unwanted effects with therapeutic doses. It has a metallic, bitter taste in the mouth. Minor gastrointestinal disturbances have been reported as have CNS symptoms (dizziness, headache, sensory neuropathies). The drug interferes with alcohol metabolism and alcohol should be strictly avoided. Metronidazole should not be used in pregnancy.

Tinidazole and **nimorazole** are similar to metronidazole. Tinidazole is eliminated more slowly than metronidazole, having a half-life of 12–14 hours.

Unwanted effects are similar to those seen with metronidazole.

Diloxanide

Both diloxanide itself and, more particularly, an insoluble ester, **diloxanide furoate**, are effective against the non-invasive intestinal parasite. The drugs have a direct amoebicidal action, affecting the amoebae before encystment. Diloxanide furoate is given orally, the unabsorbed moiety being the amoebicidal agent. It has no serious adverse effects.

LEISHMANIASIS AND LEISHMANICIDAL DRUGS

There are a variety of *Leishmania* organisms that cause disease, mainly in tropical and subtropical regions. The WHO estimates that there are about 1 million cases worldwide, with 400 000 new cases each year. With increasing international travel, leishmaniasis is being imported into areas where it was not previously seen and opportunistic infections are now being reported (particularly in AIDS patients).

The parasite exists in two forms—a flagellated form, found in a sandfly (the insect vector) that feeds on warm-blooded animals, and a non-flagellated form, which occurs in the bitten mammalian host. In the latter, the parasite is taken up by the mononuclear phagocyte system where it remains alive and viable.

There are several clinical types of leishmaniasis:

- a simple skin infection that may heal spontaneously
- a mucocutaneous form in which there may be large ulcers of the mucous membranes
- a visceral form (kala azar) where the parasite spreads through the bloodstream and causes hepatomegaly and splenomegaly, anaemia and intermittent fever.

The main drugs used in visceral leishmaniasis are **pentavalent antimony compounds**, **sodium stibogluconate** and **meglumine antimoniate**, but resistance to these agents is increasing.

Sodium stibogluconate is given intramuscularly or by slow intravenous injection in a 10-day course. It is rapidly eliminated in the urine—70% being excreted within 6 hours. More than one course may be required. Unwanted effects are anorexia, vomiting, bradycardia and hypotension. Treatment may also be associated with increased incidence of herpes zoster. Coughing and substernal pain may occur during intravenous infusion. The mechanism of action of sodium stibogluconate is not clear but the drug may increase production of oxygen free radicals, which are toxic to the parasite.

Miltefosine is also effective in the treatment of both cutaneous and visceral leishmaniasis. The drug may be given orally and is well tolerated. Side-effects are mild and include nausea and vomiting. In vitro, miltefosine activates macrophages and T cells to synthesise cytokines, although it is unlikely that this action accounts for its clinical effectiveness.

Pentamidine isethionate (see below) can be used in antimony-resistant leishmaniasis.

Drugs used in amoebiasis

- Amoebiasis is caused by infection with *Entamoeba histolytica*, which causes dysentery associated with invasion of the intestinal wall and, rarely, of the liver. The organism may be present in motile invasive form or as a cyst.
- Metronidazole (half-life 7 hours) is given orally and is active against the invasive form in gut and liver but not the cysts. Unwanted effects, which are rare, include gastrointestinal disturbances and CNS symptoms.
- Diloxanide is given orally with no serious unwanted effects; it is active, while unabsorbed, against the non-invasive form in the gastrointestinal tract.

Other drugs used in leishmaniasis are liposomally incorporated **amphotericin** (also used as an antifungal agent; p. 667) and **metronidazole** (see above), which is effective against cutaneous lesions.

Current drug usage and possible future approaches to the treatment of leishmaniasis are discussed by Murrey (2000).

TRYPANOSOMIASIS AND TRYPANOSOMICIDAL DRUGS

There are three main species of trypanosome that cause disease in humans—*Trypanosoma gambiense* and *T. rhodesiense*, which cause sleeping sickness in Africa, and *T. cruzi*, which causes Chagas' disease in South America. About 25 000 new cases of sleeping sickness are reported each year and 50 million people are classed as at risk of contracting the disease. In both types of disease there is an initial local lesion at the site of entry, followed by bouts of parasitaemia and fever. Damage to organs is caused by the toxins released, involving the CNS (in sleeping sickness), and the heart and sometimes liver, spleen, bone and the intestine (in Chagas' disease).

The main drugs used for African sleeping sickness are **suramin**, with **pentamidine** as an alternative, in the haemolymphatic stage of the disease and the arsenical **melarsoprol** for the late stage with CNS involvement (see Wang, 1995; Denise & Barrett, 2001). **Megazol** has good activity against *T. gambiense* in vitro and in a mouse model in vivo. The mechanism of action may involve generation of free radicals that are toxic to trypanosomes. Unfortunately, there are few (if any) new drugs in the clinical pipe-line and if resistance should develop to these agents, the number of deaths from this condition is set to rise (Keiser et al., 2001).

Drugs used in Chagas' disease include **primaquine** (see above), **puromycin** (see Ch. 45), **nifurtimox** and **benznidazole** (the latter two used in the acute disease only and not available in the UK); however, there is, in essence, no really effective treatment for this condition.

Suramin

Suramin was introduced into the therapy of trypanosomiasis in 1920. It does not kill the parasites immediately but induces biochemical changes that result in the organisms being cleared from the circulation after an interval of 24 hours.

The drug binds firmly to host plasma proteins and the complex enters the trypanosome by endocytosis; it is then liberated by lysosomal proteases. It has a selective action on trypanosomal enzymes.

It is given by slow intravenous injection. The blood concentration drops rapidly during the first few hours and then more slowly over the succeeding days. A low concentration remains for 3–4 months. It tends to accumulate in the mononuclear phagocyte system of the host and is also found in the cells of the proximal tubule in the kidney.

Unwanted effects

Suramin is relatively toxic, particularly in a malnourished patient, the main toxic effect being in the kidney. Other slowly developing adverse effects reported include optic atrophy, adrenal insufficiency, skin rashes, haemolytic anaemia and agranulocytosis. A small proportion of individuals have an immediate idiosyncratic reaction to suramin injection—nausea, vomiting, shock, seizures, and loss of consciousness.

Pentamidine isethionate

Pentamidine has a direct trypanocidal action in vitro. It is rapidly taken up in the parasites by a high-affinity energy-dependent carrier and is thought to interact with the DNA. Pentamidine is given intravenously or by deep intramuscular injection, usually daily for 10–15 days; after absorption from the injection site, it soon leaves the circulation. It is eliminated slowly—only 50% of a dose being excreted over 5 days. Fairly high concentrations of the drug persist in the kidney, the liver and the spleen for several months. Its usefulness is limited by its unwanted effects—an immediate decrease in blood pressure, with tachycardia, breathlessness and vomiting, and later serious toxicity, such as kidney damage, hepatic impairment, blood dyscrasias and hypoglycaemia.

TRICHOMONIASIS AND TRICHOMONICIDAL DRUGS

The principal *Trichomonas* organism that produces disease in humans is *T. vaginalis*. Virulent strains cause inflammation of the vagina in females and sometimes of the urethra in males.

The main drug used in therapy is **metronidazole** (p. 683) although resistance to metronidazole is on the increase. High doses of **tinidazole** are also effective with few side effects.

TOXOPLASMOSIS AND TOXOPLASMOCIDAL DRUGS

T. gondii is a protozoan that infects cats and other animals. Oocysts in the infected animal's faeces can infect humans, giving rise to sporozoites, then to trophozoites and finally to cysts in the tissues. In many individuals, toxoplasmosis is self-limiting or even asymptomatic, but infection with the protozoan during pregnancy can cause serious disease in the fetus. Immunocompromised individuals (e.g. AIDS patients) are also very susceptible.

The treatment of choice is **pyrimethamine–sulfadiazine** (to be avoided in pregnant patients); **trimethoprim–sulfamethoxazole** or parenteral **pentamidine** is also used and, more recently, **azithromycin** has shown promise.

NEW APPROACHES TO ANTIPROTOZOAL THERAPY

ENZYME INHIBITORS

Protozoan enzymes for which inhibitors are being sought include:

- *T. cruzi* protease (cruzain), which is essential for parasite replication
- *T. cruzi* trans-sialidase, which promotes attachment to host cells
- proteosomes in plasmodia.
- cysteine/aspartate proteinase
- DNA topoisomerases.

Proteosomes are large complexes containing the enzymes responsible for ubiquitin-dependent proteolysis, which is thought to be involved in the remodelling that the plasmodium undergoes in its life cycle in the host. Proteosome inhibitors such as **lactacystin** (specific irreversible inhibitor of the 20S proteosome) inhibit development of the erythrocytic stage of *P. falciparum* and are active in parasitised rats. Lactacystin also reduces replication of *Trypanosoma* and *Entamoeba* spp.

Parasitic enzymes that degrade haemoglobin (cysteine/asparate proteinases) are also potential targets for antimalarial drugs. Two proteinase enzymes (*plasmepsins I* and *II*), which split haemoglobin to yield free haem, have been identified. Blocking these enzymes prevents haemoglobin degradation, causing death of the parasite. Although similar enzymes do occur in the host's cells, the degree of homology with their parasitic counterparts is low enough to raise hopes that selective inhibitors may be useful. Several peptides that block these enzymes have been found but as yet, no 'lead compounds' suitable for clinical exploration.

DNA topoisomerases are enzymes that enable DNA to untwist prior to replication (see Ch. 44) and their inhibition would prevent parasite growth. Some **fluoroquinolone** derivatives (Ch. 45) and **anilinoacridine**-based inhibitors of this enzyme have been show to have activity against *P. falciparum*.

VACCINES

Clinical trials of vaccines directed either at destroying sporozoites and infected hepatocytes or at attacking parasites within blood cells and thereby limiting replication are under way. Some evidence of protection by these vaccines has been obtained but there are many problems and a safe and effective vaccine is probably still many years away.

CYTOKINE-BASED THERAPIES

The relationship between host and parasite is determined largely by host cytokines and chemokines and, as more understanding of the role of cytokines is gained, the possibility of utilising this approach for therapy is being studied. Agents under consideration include peptide antagonists at cytokine receptors, anti-cytokine antibodies and mutant cytokines. IL-2 has been shown to protect monkeys against malaria (for reviews, see Brenier-Pinchart, 2001; Odeh, 2001).

REFERENCES AND FURTHER READING

Berent A R, Craig A G 1997 *Plasmodium falciparum*—sticky jams and PECAM pie. Nat Med 3: 1315–1316 (*Deals with malaria parasites and host adhesion molecules*)

Brenier-Pinchart M-P, Pelloux H, Derouich-Guergour D et al. 2001 Chemokines in host–parasite interactions. Trends in Parasitol: 17: 292-296 (*Good review of role of immune system*)

Bradley D J, Warhurst D 1995 Malaria prophylaxis: guidelines for travellers. Br Med J 310: 709–714 (*Excellent review of chemoprophylaxis regimens*)

Bryson H M, Goa K L 1992 Halofantrine. A review of its antimalarial activity, pharmacokinetic properties and therapeutic potential. Drugs 43: 236–258

Cox F E G 1992 Malaria: getting into the liver. Nature 359: 361–362

Croft S L 1997 The current status of antiparasite chemotherapy. Parasitology 114: S3–S15 (*Comprehensive coverage of current drugs and outline of approaches to possible future agents*)

Denise H, Barrett M P 2001 Uptake and mode of action of drugs used against sleeping sickness. Biochem Pharmacol 61: 1–5 (*Good coverage of drug therapy*)

Foley M, Tilley L 1997 Quinoline antimalarials: mechanisms of action and resistance. Int J Parasitol 27: 231–240 (*Good, short review; useful diagrams*)

Haldar K 1996 Sphingolipid synthesis and membrane formation by *Plasmodium*. (*Biochemical insights into effects of parasite growth within red cell; potential targets for new drugs*)

Hien T T, White N J 1993 Qinghaosu. Lancet 341: 603–608 (*Good background article on qinghaosu*)

Holt R A, Subramanian G M et al. 2002 The genome sequence of the malaria mosquito *Anopheles gambiae*. Science 298: 129–149

Hudson A T 1993 Atovaquone—a novel broad-spectrum anti-infective drug. Parasitol Today 9: 66–68

Hughes W, Leoung G et al. 1993 Comparison of atovaquone (556C80) with trimethoprim–sulfamethoxazole to treat *Pneumocystis carinii* pneumonia in patients with AIDS. N Engl J Med 328: 1521–1527

Kalinna B H 1997 DNA vaccines for parasitic infections. Immunobiol Cell Biol 75: 370–375

Keiser J, Stich A, Burri C 2001 New drugs for the treatment of human African trypanosomiasis: research and development. Trends Parasitol 17: 42-49 (*Excellent review on an increasingly threatening disease*)

Krishna S 1997 Malaria. Br Med J 315: 730–732 (*Good, short review in series 'Science, medicine and the future'; useful diagram*)

Lell B, Luckner D et al. 1998 Randomised placebo-controlled study of

atovaquone plus proguanil for malaria prophylaxis in children. Lancet 351: 709–713 (*States that this is highly effective and well tolerated*)
Martinez-Palomo A, Espinosa-Cantellano M 1998 Amoebiasis: new understandings and new goals. Parasitol Today 14: 1–3
Masur H 1992 Prevention and treatment of *Pneumocystis* pneumonia. N Engl J Med 327: 1853–1860
Mishra M, Biswas U K et al. 1992 Amphotericin versus pentamidine in antimony-unresponsive kala-azar. Lancet 340: 1256–1257
Murphy G S, Basri H et al. 1993 Vivax malaria resistant to treatment and prophylaxis with chloroquine. Lancet 341: 96–100
Murrey H W (2000) Treatment of visceral leishmaniasis (kala-azar): a decade of progress and future approaches. Int J Infect Dis 4: 158-177 (*Clear account of present clinical therapy and potential new drugs*)
Newton P, White N 1999 Malaria: new developments in treatment and prevention. Annu Rev Med 50: 179-192 (*Excellent review of drug treatment and management of malaria*)
Nosten F, Ter Kuile F O et al. 1993 Cardiac effects of antimalarial treatment with halofantrine. Lancet 341: 1054–1056
O'Brien C 1997 Beating the malaria parasite at its own game. Lancet 350: 192 (*Clear, succinct coverage of mechanisms of action and resistance of current antimalarials and potential new drugs; useful diagram*)
Odeh M (2001) The role of tumour necrosis factor-alpha in the pathogenesis of complicated falciparum malaria. Cytokine 14: 11–18
Olliaro P L, Haynes R K, Meunier B et al. 2001 Possible modes of action of artemisin-type compounds. Trends Parasitol 17: 266–268
Petri W A, Clark C G 1993 International seminar on amebiasis. Parasitol Today 9: 73–76
Radloff P D, Phillips J et al. 1996 Atovaquone and proguanil for *Plasmodium falciparum* malaria. Lancet 347: 1511–1514
Reed S G 1995 Cytokine control of the macrophage parasites *Leishmania* and *Trypanosoma cruzi*. In: Boothroyd J C, Komuniecki R (eds) Molecular approaches to parasitology. Wiley-Liss, New York, pp. 443–453 (*Thought-provoking coverage of interaction between parasites and host cytokines*)
Riley E 1997 Malaria vaccines: current status and future prospects. J Pharm Pharmacol 49(suppl 2): 21–27
Rosenblatt J E 1999 Antiparasitic agents. Mayo Clin Proc 74: 1161-1175 (*Broad review article, wide coverage*)
Shanks G D, Kain K C, Keystone J S 2001 Malaria chemoprophylaxis in the age of drug resistance. II Drugs that may be available in the future. Clin Infect Dis 33: 381–385 (*A useful look ahead to new drugs*)
Sher A 1995 Regulation of cell-mediated immunity by parasites: the ups and downs of an important host adaptation. In: Boothroyd J C, Komuniecki R (eds) Molecular approaches to parasitology. Wiley-Liss, New York, pp. 431–442 (*Thought-provoking coverage of host–parasite interactions*)
Targett G A 1998 Malaria—variety is the price of life. Nat Med 4: 267–268 (*The biological roles of the surface proteins of malaria-infected red cells*)
Ter Kuile F O, Dolan G et al. 1993 Halofantrine versus mefloquine in treatment of multidrug-resistant falciparum malaria. Lancet 341: 1044–1049
Wang C C 1995 Molecular mechanisms and therapeutic approaches to the treatment of African trypanosomiasis. Annu Rev Pharmacol Toxicol 35: 93–127 (*Detailed review*)
Warren E, George S et al. 1997 Advances in the treatment and prophylaxis of *Pneumocystis carinii* pneumonia. Pharmacotherapy 17: 900–916
Winstanley P 1996 Pyronaridine: a promising drug for Africa? Lancet 347: 2–3
Wirth D F 1995 Drug resistance and transfection in *Plasmodium*. In: Boothroyd J C, Komuniecki R (eds) Molecular approaches to parasitology. Wiley-Liss, New York, pp. 227–241

Anthelminthic drugs

49

Overview 687

Helminth infections 687

Anthelminthic drugs 688

Resistance to anthelminthic drugs 691

New approaches to anthelminthic therapy 691

OVERVIEW

Many humans harbour helminths (worms) of one species or another. In some cases these infections result mainly in discomfort and do not cause substantial ill health, an example being threadworms in children. Other worm infections, such as schistosomiasis (bilharzia) and hookworm disease, can produce very serious morbidity. In many countries, particularly those in tropical and subtropical regions, almost all the indigenous population is infected with hookworms and/or other helminths and the problem of the treatment of helminthiasis is, therefore, one of very great practical importance. In addition, worm infections are also a major cause for concern in veterinary medicine, affecting both domestic pets and farm animals.

HELMINTH INFECTIONS

Humans are the primary (definitive) hosts for most, but not all, helminth infections; in other words, most worms reproduce sexually in the human host, producing eggs or larvae that pass out of the body and infect the secondary (intermediate) host.

There are two clinically important types of worm infections—those in which the worm lives in the host's alimentary canal and those in which the worm lives in other tissues of the host's body.

The main examples of worms that live in the host's alimentary canal are:

- **Tapeworms (cestodes)**: *Taenia saginata, Taenia solium, Hymenolepis nana, Diphyllobothrium latum*. In Asia, Africa and parts of America, about 85 million people harbour one or other of these tapeworm species. Only the first two are likely to be seen in the UK. The usual intermediate hosts of the two most common tapeworms (*T. saginata* and *T. solium*) are cattle and pigs, respectively. Humans become infected by eating raw or undercooked meat containing the larvae, which have encysted in the animals' muscle tissue. (In some circumstances, the larval stage of *T. solium* can develop in humans, resulting in *cysticercosis*, a condition characterised by encysted larvae in the muscles and the viscera or, more seriously, in the eye or the brain.) *H. nana* can have both the adult stage (the intestinal worm) and the larval stage in the same host, which may be human or rodent, though some insects (fleas, grain beetles) can also serve as intermediate hosts. The infection is usually asymptomatic. *D. latum* has two sequential intermediate hosts—a freshwater crustacean and a freshwater fish. Humans become infected by eating raw or incompletely cooked fish containing the larvae. Vitamin B_{12} deficiency sometimes occurs (see Ch. 21).
- **Intestinal roundworms (nematodes)**: *Ascaris lumbricoides* (common roundworm), *Enterobius vermicularis* (threadworm, called pinworm in the USA), *Trichuris trichiura* (whipworm), *Strongyloides stercoralis* (threadworm in USA), *Necator americanus, Ankylostoma duodenale* (hookworms).

The main examples of worms that live in the tissues of the host are:

- **Trematodes or flukes**: *Schistosoma haematobium, Schistosoma mansoni, Schistosoma japonicum*. These cause schistosomiasis (bilharzia). The adult worms of both sexes live and mate in the veins or venules of the gut wall or the bladder. The female lays eggs that pass into the bladder or gut and produce inflammation of these organs, resulting in haematuria in the former case and, occasionally, loss of blood in the faeces in the latter. The eggs hatch in water after discharge from the body and give rise to *miracidia*, which enter the secondary host—a particular species of snail. After a period of development in this host, free-swimming *cercariae* emerge. These are capable of infecting humans by penetration of the skin. About 200 million people are infected with one or other of the schistosomes.
- **Tissue roundworms**: *Trichinella spiralis, Dracunculus medinensis* (guinea-worm) and the filariae, which include *Wuchereria bancrofti, Loa loa, Onchocerca volvulus* and *Brugia malayi*. The adult filariae live in the lymphatics,

connective tissues or mesentery of the host and produce live embryos or microfilariae, which find their way into the bloodstream. They may be ingested by mosquitoes or similar biting insects when they feed. After a period of development within this secondary host, the larvae pass to the mouthparts of the insect and are re-injected into humans. Major filarial diseases are caused by *Wuchereria* or *Brugia*, which cause obstruction of lymphatic vessels producing elephantiasis; other related diseases are onchocerciasis (in which the presence of microfilariae in the eye causes 'river-blindness') and loiasis (in which the microfilariae cause inflammation in the skin and other tissues). In guinea-worm infection, larvae released from crustaceans in wells and water-holes are ingested and migrate from the intestinal tract to mature and mate in the tissues; the gravid female then migrates to the subcutaneous tissues of the leg or the foot where she may protrude through an ulcer in the skin. The worm may be up to a metre in length and has to be removed surgically or by slow mechanical winding of the worm on to a stick over a period of days.* *T. spiralis* causes trichinosis; the larvae from the viviparous female worms in the intestine migrate to skeletal muscle, where they become encysted.
- **Hydatid tapeworm**: *Echinococcus* species. These are cestodes for which canines are the primary (definitive) hosts, and sheep the intermediate hosts. The primary, intestinal stage does not occur in humans, but under certain circumstances humans can function as the intermediate host, in which case the larvae develop into hydatid cysts within the tissues.

Some nematodes that usually live in the gastrointestinal tract of animals may infect humans and penetrate tissues. A skin infestation, termed creeping eruption or cutaneous larva migrans, is caused by the larvae of dog and cat hookworms. Toxocariasis or visceral larva migrans is caused by larvae of cat and dog roundworms of the *Toxocara* genus.

One of the consequences of nematode infection is activation of the host's immune system. The processes involved are similar to those which take place during protozoal infections (see Ch. 48). Typically, enhanced T helper (Th) 1 responses occur accompanied by eosinophilia and IgE production. Nitric oxide (synthesised by inducible nitric oxide synthase) and peroxynitrite are most probably used by the host to kill the parasitic worms (Ch. 14). Some nematodes have evolved mechanisms for overcoming attack by the host's immune system. The larvae of *S. mansoni*, for example, activate lung endothelial cells to produce interleukin-6 in an attempt to downregulate Th1 pathways and thus escape the inflammatory reaction that develops in the infected host. The interaction of nematodes with the host's immune system is reviewed by Loukas & Prociv (2001).

*In 1980 there were 2 million cases of guinea-worm infection worldwide. In 1986 the World Health Organization initiated a programme to eradicate this worm. The target date, set in 1990, was 1995. At that date the total number of cases had fallen by about 95%, mainly because of public health measures. However, 160 000 cases were still reported that year. The number of cases has fallen again subsequently and many parts of the world are now more or less completely free of the condition.

ANTHELMINTHIC DRUGS

To be an effective anthelminthic, a drug must be able to penetrate the cuticle of the worm or gain access to its alimentary tract. This in itself presents difficulties for the design of good anthelminthic drugs since some worms are exclusively haemophagous (blood eating) while others are best described as 'tissue grazers'. The route and dose of anthelminthic is, therefore, important and must be chosen carefully since parasitic worms cannot be relied upon to consume sufficient amounts of the drug to be effective (for a review of this and other problems associated with anthelminthic drug use, see Geary et al. (1999)).

An anthelminthic drug can act by causing paralysis of the worm, or by damaging its cuticle, leading to partial digestion or to rejection by immune mechanisms. Anthelminthic drugs can also interfere with the metabolism of the worm, and since the metabolic requirements of these parasites vary greatly from one species to another, drugs that are highly effective against one type of worm can be ineffective against others. Individual drugs are described briefly below; indications for their use are given in Table 49.1. For a comprehensive coverage of antiparasitic drugs and their use in humans and animals, see Liu & Weller (1996) and Martin et al. (1997).

BENZIMIDAZOLES

The benzimidazole anthelminthics include **mebendazole, thiabendazole** and **albendazole.** These compounds are broad-spectrum agents and constitute one of the main groups of anthelminthics used clinically. They bind to free β-tubulin, inhibiting its polymerisation and thus interfering with microtubule-dependent glucose uptake by the worm. They have a selective inhibitory action on helminth microtubular function, being 250–400 times more potent in helminth than in mammalian tissue. The effect takes time to develop and the worms may not be expelled for several days.

Only 10% of mebendazole is absorbed after oral administration; a fatty meal increases absorption. It is rapidly metabolised, the products being excreted in the urine and the bile within 24–48 hours. It is given as a single dose for threadworm and twice daily for 3 days for hookworm and roundworm infestations. Thiabendazole is rapidly absorbed from the gastrointestinal tract, very rapidly metabolised and excreted in the urine in conjugated form. It is given twice daily for 3 days for guinea-worm and strongyloides infestations, and for up to 5 days for hookworm and roundworm infestations.

Unwanted effects are few with mebendazole though gastrointestinal disturbances can occasionally occur. Unwanted effects with thiabendazole are more frequent but usually transient, the commonest being gastrointestinal disturbances,

Table 49.1 Drugs used in helminth infections

Helminth	Drugs used
Threadworm (pinworm)[a] (*Enterobius vermicularis*)	Mebendazole,[b] albendazole,[b] (piperazine, pyrantel)
Strongyloides stercoralis (called threadworm in the USA)	Albendazole,[b] thiabendazole, ivermectin[c]
Common roundworm (*Ascaris lumbricoides*)	Mebendazole,[b] pyrantel (piperazine), levamisole[c]
Other roundworm (filariae)	
Wuchereria bancrofti, Loa loa	Diethylcarbamazine, ivermectin
Onchocerca volvulus	Ivermectin
Guinea-worm (*Dracunculus medinensis*)	Praziquantel,[b] (mebendazole, metronidazole)[d]
Trichiniasis (*Trichinella spiralis*)	Thiabendazole,[b] mebendazole,[b] (pyrantel)
Cysticercosis (infection with larval *Taenia solium*)	Praziquantel,[b] albendazole
Tapeworm (*Taenia saginata, T. solium*)	Praziquantel,[b] niclosamide
Hydatid disease[e] (*Echinococcus granulosus*)	Albendazole,[b] praziquantel
Hookworm (*Ankylostoma duodenale, Necator americanus*)	Mebendazole,[b] albendazole,[b] pyrantel
Whipworm (*Trichuris trichiura*)	Mebendazole,[b] albendazole,[b] diethylcarbamazine
Blood flukes (*Schistosoma* species)	
S. haematobium	Praziquantel[b]
S. mansoni	Praziquantel,[b] oxamniquine
S. japonicum	Praziquantel[b]
Cutaneous larva migrans (*Ankylostoma caninum*)	Albendazole,[b] thiabendazole (diethylcarbamazine)
Visceral larva migrans (*Toxacara canis*)	Albendazole,[b] thiabendazole (diethylcarbamazine)

Based largely on Liu & Weller (1996), Croft (1997) and Geary et al. (1999)
[a]Combination of hygienic measures with anthelminthics essential.
[b]Indicates drug of first choice. Drugs less commonly used are given in parentheses.
[c]Available in the UK on a 'named patient' basis.
[d]See Chapter 48.
[e]Surgery may be needed for cysts.

though headache, dizziness and drowsiness have been reported and allergic reactions (fever, rashes) can occur.

Albendazole is a broad-spectrum anthelminthic. Given orally it is rapidly absorbed and metabolised to the sulfoxide and sulfone, which may be responsible for its anthelminthic actions. The plasma concentration of its active metabolite is 100 times greater than that of mebendazole.

Unwanted effects—mainly gastrointestinal disturbances—are not common and usually do not require discontinuation of the drug.

PRAZIQUANTEL

Praziquantel is a broad-spectrum anthelminthic drug. It is the drug of choice for all species of schistosomes and is effective in cysticercosis, for which there was previously no effective therapy.

It acts by increasing the permeability of the nematode to Ca^{2+} thereby causing contraction of the musculature and eventual paralysis and death of the worm. Praziquantel also modifies the parasite so that it becomes susceptible to the host's normal immune responses (see Sher, 1995).

The drug affects not only the adult schistosomes but also the immature forms and the cercariae—the form of the parasite that infects humans by penetrating the skin.

Praziquantel has no pharmacological effects in humans in therapeutic dosage. Given orally it is quickly absorbed; much of the drug is rapidly metabolised to inactive metabolites on first passage through the liver and the metabolites are excreted in the urine. The plasma half-life of the parent compound is 60–90 minutes.

Mild *unwanted effects* occur but are usually transitory and rarely of clinical importance. They include gastrointestinal disturbance, dizziness, aching in muscles and joints, skin eruptions and low-grade fever. Some effects are more marked in patients with a heavy worm load and may be caused by products released from the dead worms.

PIPERAZINE

Piperazine can be used to treat infections with the common roundworm (*A. lumbricoides*) and the threadworm (*E. vermicularis*). It reversibly inhibits neuromuscular transmission in the worm, probably by acting like gamma-aminobutyric acid (GABA), the inhibitory neurotransmitter on GABA-gated chloride channels in nematode muscle. The paralysed worms are expelled alive.

Piperazine is given orally and some but not all is absorbed. It is partly metabolised and the remainder is eliminated, unchanged, via the kidney. The drug has singularly little pharmacological action in the host.

Unwanted effects are uncommon but gastrointestinal disturbances, urticaria and bronchospasm occur occasionally and some patients experience dizziness, paraesthesias, vertigo, incoordination.

Used to treat roundworm, piperazine is effective in a single dose. For threadworm, a longer course (7 days) at lower dosage is necessary. This drug has been largely superseded by the benzimidazoles.

PYRANTEL

Pyrantel is a derivative of tetrahydropyrimidine that is thought to act by depolarising the helminth neuromuscular junction, causing spasm and paralysis. It also has some anticholinesterase activity. There is poor absorption from the gastrointestinal tract after oral dosing—more than 50% of the drug being eliminated in the faeces.

It is generally regarded as a safe drug. *Unwanted effects* are mild and transitory and involve mostly gastrointestinal upsets. Dizziness and fever have been reported, but no serious effects on blood, kidney or liver. It is not widely used and has been largely superseded by the benzimidazoles.

NICLOSAMIDE

Niclosamide was the drug of choice for tapeworm infections but has now largely been superseded by praziquantel. The scolex (the head of the worm with the parts that attach to the host intestinal cells) and a proximal segment are irreversibly damaged by the drug; the worm separates from the intestinal wall and is expelled. For *T. solium*, the drug is given in a single dose after a light meal, followed by a purgative 2 hours later. A purgative is necessary because the damaged tapeworm segments may release ova, which are not affected by the drug, so there is a theoretical possibility that cysticercosis may develop. For other tapeworm infections, it is not necessary to give a purgative after administration of niclosamide. There is negligible absorption of the drug from the gastrointestinal tract.

Unwanted effects are few, infrequent and transient. Nausea and vomiting can occur.

OXAMNIQUINE

Oxamniquine is active against *S. mansoni*, affecting both mature and immature forms, although its use has now been largely superseded by praziquantel. The mechanism of action may involve intercalation in the DNA and its selective action may be related to the ability of the parasite to concentrate the drug. Resistance has occurred in some geographical areas. It is given orally, is well absorbed, and is metabolised in the gut wall and in the liver to inactive metabolites that are excreted in the urine. It has a short half-life of 1–2 hours and is eliminated from the plasma by 10–12 hours.

Unwanted effects of transient dizziness and headache are reported in 30–95% of patients in various studies, and gastrointestinal disturbances in 10–20% of patients. Symptoms caused by central nervous system stimulation may occur and include hallucinations and convulsions. Allergic manifestations and other symptoms, which appear several days after treatment has stopped, may be related to the release of products from the dead fluke.

DIETHYLCARBAMAZINE

Diethylcarbamazine is a piperazine derivative that is active in filarial infections caused by *W. bancrofti* and *L. loa*. Diethylcarbamazine rapidly removes the microfilariae from the blood circulation and has a limited effect on the adult worms in the lymphatics, but it has little action on microfilariae in vitro. It has been suggested that it modifies the parasite so that it becomes susceptible to the host's normal immune responses. It may also interfere with the parasite's arachidonate metabolism.

The drug is given orally, is absorbed and is distributed throughout the cells and tissues of the body, excepting adipose tissue. It is partly metabolised and both the parent drug and its metabolites are excreted in the urine, being cleared from the body within about 48 hours.

Unwanted effects are common but transient, subsiding within a day or so even if the drug is continued. Side-effects from the drug itself are gastrointestinal disturbances, arthralgias, headache and a general feeling of weakness. Allergic side-effects referable to the products of the filariae are common and vary with the species of worm. In general these start during the first day's treatment and last 3–7 days; they include skin reactions, enlargement of lymph glands, dizziness, tachycardia and gastrointestinal and respiratory disturbances. When these symptoms disappear, larger doses of the drug can be given without further problem. The drug is not used in patients with onchocerciasis, in whom it can have serious unwanted effects.

LEVAMISOLE

Levamisole (available in the UK on a 'named patient' basis*) is effective in infections with the common roundworm (*A.*

lumbricoides). It has a nicotine-like action, stimulating and subsequently blocking the neuromuscular junctions. The paralysed worms are then passed in the faeces. Ova are not killed. The drug is given orally, is rapidly absorbed and is widely distributed. It crosses the blood–brain barrier. It is metabolised in the liver to inactive metabolites, which are excreted via the kidney. Its plasma half-life is 4 hours.

When single-dose therapy is used, *unwanted effects* are few and soon subside. They include gastrointestinal disturbances, dizziness and skin eruptions. High concentrations can have nicotinic actions on autonomic ganglia in the mammalian host.

IVERMECTIN

Ivermectin (available in the UK on a 'named patient' basis*) is a semisynthetic agent derived from a group of natural substances, the avermectins, obtained from an actinomycete. It has potent anthelminthic activity against filaria in humans, being the drug of choice for onchocerciasis, which causes river blindness; it has also given good results against *W. bancrofti,* which causes elephantiasis. A single dose kills the immature microfilariae of *O. volvulus* but not the adult worms. Ivermectin reduces the incidence of onchocercal blindness by up to 80%. The drug also has activity against infections with some roundworms: common round worms, whipworms, threadworms—both the UK variety (*E. vermicularis*) and the US variety (*S. stercoralis*)—but not hookworms.

It is given orally and has a half-life of 11 hours.

Ivermectin is thought to kill the worm either by opening glutamate-gated chloride channels (found only in invertebrates) and increasing Cl^- conductance or by binding to a novel allosteric site on the acetylcholine nicotinic receptor to cause an increase in transmission leading to motor paralysis (Martin et al., 1998).

Unwanted effects include skin rashes, fever, giddiness, headaches and pains in muscles, joints and lymph glands. In general, the drug is well tolerated.

*A relatively rare situation in which the physician seeks approval from a pharmaceutical company to use one of their drugs in a named individual. The drug is either a 'newcomer' which has shown particular promise in clinical trials but has not yet been licensed or, as in these instances, an established drug that has not been licensed because the company has not applied for a product licence (possibly for commercial reasons).

RESISTANCE TO ANTHELMINTHIC DRUGS

Resistance to anthelminthic drugs is a widespread and growing problem not only in humans but also most particularly in the animal health market.

During the 1990s, sheep (and to a lesser extent cattle) helminth infections have developed varying degrees of resistance to a number of different anthelminthic drugs. Nematodes that develop such resistance pass this ability on to their offspring, leading in quick succession to treatment failure and the persistence of the worm infection.

Little is known of the molecular mechanisms involved in nematode resistance. However, benzimidazole resistance has been attributed to an impairment of high-affinity binding to parasite β-tubulin whilst levamisole and pyrantel resistance is associated with changes in the structure of the target acetylcholine nicotinic receptor (Robertson et al., 2000).

The complete nucleotide sequence of the genome of the free-living nematode *Caenorhabditis elegans* has been reported. This may make it possible to create transgenic *C. elegans* that expresses mutations found in resistant parasitic worms and this may provide a better understanding of the mechanisms underlying resistance (see Prichard & Tait, 2001).

NEW APPROACHES TO ANTHELMINTHIC THERAPY

Despite the enormity of the clinical problem, few new anthelminthic drugs have been introduced in the last few years or indeed can be expected in the next few.

Nitazoxanide kills both protozoa and helminths in humans whereas **paraherquamide** has excellent activity against nematode parasites in sheep and cattle and is still effective against worms resistant to other anthelminthics. In each of these cases, the mechanism of action at the molecular level is not known.

An alternative approach to eradication of worms is the development of antiparasite vaccines. Several of these have been produced for animal use including, for example, a cathepsin L vaccine against *F. hepatica.* Several other parasitic worms are being targeted with vaccines and it is hoped that this work will lead to the development of new and more broad-spectrum worm vaccines for human as well as for animal use (see Dalton & Mulcahy, 2001).

REFERENCES AND FURTHER READING

Burnham G M 1997 Ivermectin where *Loa loa* is endemic. Br Med J 350: 2–3
Burnham G M 1998 Onchocerciasis. Lancet 351: 1341–1346
Cairncross S 1995 Victory over guineaworm disease: partial or pyrrhic? Lancet 346: 1440
Cook G C 1992 Use of protozoan and anthelmintic drugs during pregnancy: side-effects and contraindications. J Infect 25: 1–9
Croft S L 1997 The current status of antiparasite chemotherapy. Parasitology 114: S3–S15 (*Comprehensive coverage of current drugs and outline of approaches to possible future agents*)
Dalton J P, Mulcahy G 2001 Parasite vaccines—a reality? Vet Parasit 98: 149–167 (*Interesting discussion of the promise and pitfalls of vaccines*)
Day T A, Bennett J L, Pax R A 1992 Praziquantel: the enigmatic antiparasitic. Parasitol Today 8: 342–344
Fisher M H, Mrozik H 1992 The chemistry and pharmacology of the avermectins. Annu Rev Pharmacol Toxicol 32: 537–553

Geary T G, Sangster N C, Thompson D P 1999 Frontiers in anthelmintic pharmacology. Vet Parasitol 84: 275–295 (*Thoughtful account of the difficulties associated with drug treatment*)
Klein R D, Geary T G 1996 Prospects for rational approaches to anthelmintic discovery. Parasitology 113: S217–S234
Liu L X, Weller P F 1996 Antiparasitic drugs. N Engl J Med 334: 1178–1184 (*Excellent coverage of antiparasitic drugs and their clinical use*)
Loukas A, Prociv P 2001 Immune responses in hookworm infections. Clin Microbiol Rev 14: 689–703 (*An interesting account of the response of the immune system to worm infections*)
Martin R J, Robertson A P, Bjorn H 1997 Target sites of anthelminthics. Parasitology 114(suppl): S111–S124
Martin R J, Murray I, Robertson A P et al. 1998 Anthelmintics and ion-channels: after a puncture, use a patch. Int J Parasitol 28: 849–862
Moodley M, Moosa A 1989 Treatment of neurocysticercosis: is praziquantel the new hope? Lancet i: 262–263
Pearce E J, MacDonald A S 2002 The immunobiology of schistosomiasis. Nat Rev Immunol 2: 499–512
Prichard R, Tait A 2001 The role of molecular biology in veterinary parasitology. Vet Parasitol 98: 169–194 (*Excellent review of the application of molecular biology to understanding the problem of drug resistance and to the development of new anthelminthic agents*)
Robertson A P, Bjorn H E, Martin R J 2000 Pyrantel resistance alters nematode nicotinic acetylcholine receptor single channel properties. Eur J Pharmacol 394: 1–8
Sher A 1995 Regulation of cell-mediated immunity by parasites: the ups and downs of an important host adaptation. In: Boothroyd J C, Komuniecki R (eds) Molecular approaches to parasitology. Wiley-Liss, New York, pp. 431–442 (*Thought-provoking coverage of host–parasite interaction*)
Thompson D P, Klein R D, Geary T G 1996 Prospects for rational approaches to anthelmintic discovery. Parasitology 113: S217–S234
Whitworth J 1992 Treatment of onchocerciasis with ivermectin in Sierra Leone. Parasitol Today 8: 138–140
World Health Organization 1995 WHO model prescribing information: drugs used in parasitic diseases, 2nd edn. WHO, Geneva

50 Cancer chemotherapy

Overview 693

Background 693

The pathogenesis of cancer 693
- The genesis of a cancer cell 694
- The special characteristics of cancer cells 694

General principles of action of cytotoxic anticancer drugs 696

Drugs used in cancer chemotherapy 698
- Alkylating agents and related compounds 698
- Antimetabolites 701
- Cytotoxic antibiotics 703
- Plant derivatives 704
- Hormones 704
- Radioactive isotopes 705
- Miscellaneous agents 705

Resistance to anticancer drugs 706

Treatment schedules 707

Techniques for dealing with emesis and myelosuppression 707

Possible future strategies for cancer chemotherapy 707

OVERVIEW

In this chapter we deal with cancer and anticancer therapy, emphasising first the pathogenesis of cancer before proceeding to describe the drugs used therapeutically. Finally we consider the extent to which new knowledge of cancer biology is leading to new treatments.

BACKGROUND

Cancer is a disease in which there is uncontrolled multiplication and spread within the body of abnormal forms of the body's own cells. It is one of the major causes of death in the developed nations—at least one in five of the population of Europe and North America can expect to die of cancer. Figures for the last 100 years or so give the impression that the disease is increasing in these countries, but cancer is largely a disease of the later age groups, and with the advances in public health and medical science many more people live to the age where they are liable to get cancer.

The terms cancer, malignant neoplasm* and malignant tumour are synonymous; they are distinguished from benign tumours by the properties of dedifferentiation, invasiveness and the ability to metastasise (spread to other parts of the body). (Both benign and malignant tumours manifest uncontrolled proliferation.) In this chapter, we shall be concerned only with the therapy of malignant neoplasia or cancer. The appearance of these abnormal characteristics reflects altered patterns of gene expression in the cancer cells, resulting from genetic mutations.

There are three main approaches to treating established cancer—surgical excision, irradiation and chemotherapy—and the role of each of these depends on the type of tumour and the stage of its development. Chemotherapy can be used on its own or as an adjunct to other forms of therapy.

Other approaches to cancer treatment, for example, approaches based on knowledge of the pathobiology of cancer, are being investigated (see below) and are beginning to produce results.

Chemotherapy of cancer, as compared with that of bacterial disease, presents a difficult problem. In biochemical terms, microorganisms are both quantitatively and qualitatively different from human cells (see Ch. 44); however cancer cells and normal cells are so similar in many respects that it is more difficult to find general, exploitable, biochemical differences between them.

THE PATHOGENESIS OF CANCER

In the decade leading up to this edition (2003), there have been numerous advances in the understanding of the pathogenesis of cancer and, as a result, significant progress has been made and is still being made in the development of novel anticancer drugs. To understand the action and drawbacks of current anticancer drugs and how drugs now in the pipeline and future agents will act, it is important to consider in more detail the pathobiology of this disease.

*Neoplasm means 'new growth'.

Cancer cells manifest, to varying degrees, four characteristics that distinguish them from normal cells:

- uncontrolled proliferation
- dedifferentiation and loss of function
- invasiveness
- metastasis.

THE GENESIS OF A CANCER CELL

A normal cell turns into a cancer cell because of one or more mutations in its DNA, which can be inherited* or acquired. The development of cancer is a complex multistage process, involving not only more than one genetic change but usually also other, epigenetic factors (hormonal action, co-carcinogen and tumour promoter effects, etc.) that are not in themselves cancer producing but which increase the likelihood that the genetic mutation(s) will result in cancer. Here, in considering the biology of cancer, we concentrate on genetic changes.

There are two main categories of genetic change that lead to cancer:

- the activation of proto-oncogenes to oncogenes
- the inactivation of tumour suppressor genes.

These changes are a result of point mutations, gene amplification or chromosomal translocation, often due to the action of certain viruses or chemical carcinogens.

Activation of proto-oncogenes to oncogenes

Proto-oncogenes are genes that normally control cell division, apoptosis and differentiation but which can be converted to oncogenes by viral or carcinogen action.

Inactivation of tumour suppressor genes

Normal cells contain genes that have the ability to suppress malignant change—termed tumour suppressor genes (anti-oncogenes)—and there is now good evidence that mutations of these genes are involved in many different cancers.The loss of function of tumour suppressor genes can be the critical event in carcinogenesis.

About 30 tumour suppressor genes and 100 dominant oncogenes have been identified.

THE SPECIAL CHARACTERISTICS OF CANCER CELLS

UNCONTROLLED PROLIFERATION

The proliferation of cancer cells is not controlled by the processes that normally regulate cell division and tissue growth. It is this, rather than their *rate* of proliferation, that distinguishes them from normal cells. Some normal cells (such as neurons) have little or no capacity to divide and proliferate, but others, for example in the bone marrow and the epithelium of the gastrointestinal tract, have the property of continuous rapid division. Some cancer cells multiply slowly (e.g. those in plasma cell tumours) and some fast (e.g. the cells of Burkitt's lymphoma). It is, therefore, not generally true that cancer cells proliferate faster than normal cells. The significant point about cancer cells is not that they proliferate faster than normal cells but that their proliferation is not subject to normal regulatory processes.

What are the changes that leads to the uncontrolled proliferation of tumour cells? Inactivation of tumour suppressor genes or transformation of proto-oncogenes into oncogenes can confer autonomy of growth on a cell and thus result in uncontrolled proliferation by producing changes in:

- growth factors and their receptors** (Fig. 50.1)
- the growth factor pathways**—the cytosolic and nuclear transducers (Fig. 50.1)
- the cell cycle transducers*—e.g. cyclins, cyclin-dependent kinases (cdks) or the cdk inhibitors (Fig. 50.1)
- the apoptotic mechanisms* that normally dispose of abnormal cells
- telomerase expression
- local blood vessels, resulting from tumour-directed angiogenesis.

Potentially all the genes coding for the above components could be regarded as oncogenes or tumour suppressor genes (see Fig. 50.1) though not all are equally prone to malignant transformation. And it should be understood that malignant transformation of several components is needed for the development of cancer.

Apoptosis and the genesis of a cancer cell

Apoptosis is programmed cell death (Ch. 5) and anti-apoptotic genetic lesions are necessary for cancer to develop. In fact development of resistance to apoptosis is a hallmark of cancer. Decreased apoptosis can be brought about by inactivation of pro-apototic factors or by activation of anti-apoptotic factors.

Telomerase expression

Telomeres are specialised structures that cap the ends of chromosomes — like the small metal tubes on the end of shoe-laces — protecting them from degradation, rearrangement and fusion with other chromosomes. Put simply, DNA polymerase cannot easily duplicate the last few nucleotides at the ends of DNA and telomeres prevent loss of the 'end' genes. With each round of cell division, a portion of the telomere is eroded, so that eventually it becomes non-functional. At this point, DNA replication ceases and the cell becomes senescent.

Germline cells, stem cells and the proliferating cells of the gastrointestinal tract, bone marrow, etc. express *telomerase*—an

*It is not the cancer itself that is inherited but a gene that has mutated and now predisposes to cancer. Examples are the tumour suppressor genes *BRCA1* and *BRCA2*; women who inherit a single defective copy of either of these genes have a significantly increased risk of developing breast cancer.

*These are dealt with in detail in Chapter 5.

**These are dealt with in Chapters 3 and 5.

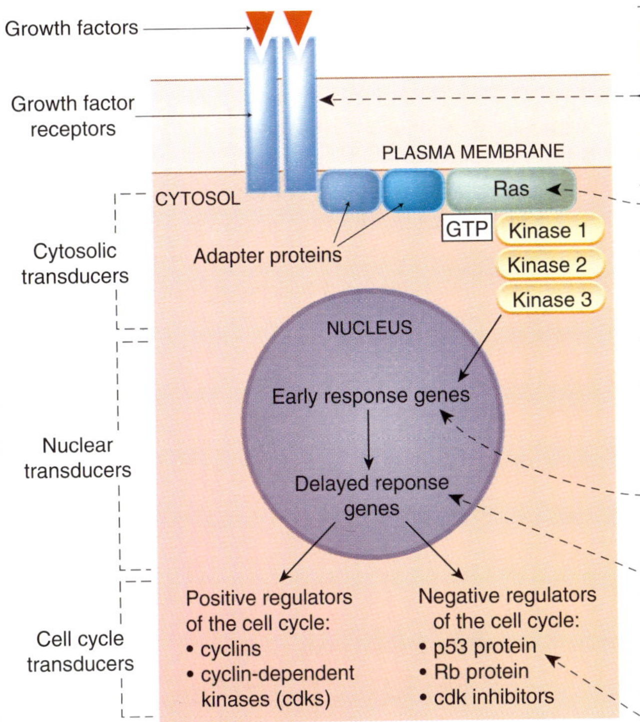

Proto-oncogene	Proto-oncogene products	Cancer	Anticancer drugs
Genes for growth factors e.g. for IGF	Growth factors e.g. IGF	Prostate, breast colorectal, etc.	Research in progress. WTS
Gene for EGF receptors (e.g. c-*erbB*)	Her2*, (a receptor tyrosine kinase)	Breast	Inhibited by **trastuzumab**
Gene for PDGF (c-*sis*)	PDGF (a receptor tyrosine kinase)	Chronic myeloid leukaemia	Inhibited by **imatinib** (aka Gleevec)
c-ras	Ras proteins	30% of all tumours	Ras inhibitors in clinical trial
abl	Abl tyrosine kinase (cytoplasmic)	Chronic myeloid leukaemia	Inhibited by **imatinib** (aka Gleevec)
c-src	Cytoplasmic tyrosine kinase	Breast, pancreas, bone	Research in progress. WTS
Genes for JAK, Lck		Leukemias	
c-jun/c-fos	Transcription factors (Jun, Fos, Myc)	Colorectal	
c-myc		Lung, neural tissue	

Fig. 50.1 The signal transduction pathway initiated by growth factors leading to the production of the cell cycle regulators, and its relationship to cancer development. A few examples of proto-oncogenes and the products they code for are given in the table, with examples of the cancers that are associated with their conversion to oncogenes. Drugs (some available, others in the pipeline) are also shown. Many growth factor receptors are receptor tyrosine kinases, the cytosolic transducers including adapter proteins that bind to phosphorylated tyrosine residues in the receptors. Ras proteins are guanine nucleotide-binding proteins and have GTPase action; decreased GTPase action means Ras remains activated. (EGF, epidermal growth factor; IGF, insulin-like growth factor; PDGF, platelet-derived growth factor; WTS, Watch this space.) *Her2 is also termed her2/neu.

enzyme that maintains and stabilises telomeres. Most fully differentiated somatic cells do not express telomerase, but about 95% of late-stage malignant tumours do express it and it is suggested that this enzyme can confer 'immortality' on a cancer cell.

The control of tumour-related blood vessels

The factors described above lead to the uncontrolled proliferation of individual cancer cells. We need also to consider factors that influence the total tumour mass. The actual growth of a solid tumour depends on the development of its own blood supply. Tumours 1–2 mm in diameter can receive nutrients by diffusion, but any further expansion requires the development of new blood vessels—*angiogenesis* (see p. 221). Angiogenesis occurs in response to growth factors produced by the growing tumour (see Griffioen & Molema, 2000; Carmeliet & Jain, 2000).

DEDIFFERENTIATION AND LOSS OF FUNCTION

The multiplication of normal cells involves division of the stem cells in a particular tissue to give rise to daughter cells. These daughter cells eventually differentiate to become the mature cells of the relevant tissue and carry out their programmed functions. For example, fibroblasts become capable of secreting and organising extracellular matrix, muscle cells become capable of contraction, and so on. One of the main characteristics of cancer cells is that they dedifferentiate—to a varying degree in different tumours. In general, poorly differentiated cancers multiply faster and have a poorer prognosis than well-differentiated cancers.

INVASIVENESS

Normal cells are not found outside their 'designated' tissue of origin; for example, liver cells are not found in the bladder, and pancreatic cells are not found in the testis. This is because during differentiation and during the growth of tissues and organs, normal cells develop certain spatial relationships with respect to each other. These relationships are maintained by various tissue-specific survival factors—anti-apoptotic factors (see Ch. 5). Any cells that escape accidentally lose these survival signals and undergo apoptosis.

Consequently, although the cells of the normal mucosal epithelium of the rectum proliferate continuously as the lining is shed, they remain as a lining epithelium. A cancer of the rectal mucosa, by comparison, invades the tissues in the other layers of the rectum and may invade the tissues of other pelvic organs. Cancer cells have not only lost, through mutation, the restraints that act on normal cells, they are also particularly adept at secreting enzymes (e.g. metalloproteinases; see Ch. 5) that break down the extracellular matrix, enabling the cancer cells to slip through.

METASTASES

Metastases are secondary tumours formed by cells that have been released from the initial or primary tumour and have reached other sites through blood vessels or lymphatics, or as a result of being shed into body cavities. Metastases are the principal cause of mortality and morbidity in most cancers and constitute a major problem for cancer therapy.

As discussed above, it has become clear that dislodgment or aberrant migration of normal cells would lead to their programmed cell death as a result of withdrawal of the necessary anti-apoptotic factors. Cancer cells that have the ability to metastasise have undergone a series of genetic changes which alter their responses to the regulatory factors that control the tissue siting of normal cells, thus enabling them to establish themselves 'extraterritorially'. Tumour-induced growth of new blood vessels locally (see above) makes metastasis easier and more likely.

Secondary tumours occur more frequently in some tissues than others. For example, the metastases of mammary cancers are often found in lung, bone and brain. The basis of this selective metastasis is now known. Breast cancer cells express chemokine receptors such as CXR4 on their surfaces. Chemokines that recognise these receptors are expressed at high level in some tissues (lung, bone, brain) and circulating cancer cells are attracted to these tissues but not others (e.g. kidney) in which high levels of these chemokines do not occur.

GENERAL PRINCIPLES OF ACTION OF CYTOTOXIC ANTICANCER DRUGS

In experiments with rapidly growing transplantable leukaemias in mice, it has been found that a given therapeutic dose of a cytotoxic drug destroys a constant fraction of the malignant cells. Thus a dose which kills 99.99% of cells, if used to treat a tumour with 10^{11} cells, will still leave 10 million (10^7) viable malignant cells. As the same principle holds for similar fast-growing tumours in humans, schedules for chemotherapy of these tumours are necessarily aimed at producing as near a total cell kill as possible because, in contrast to the situation with microorganisms, little reliance can be placed on the host's immunological defence mechanisms against the remaining cancer cells.

One of the major difficulties in the use of cancer chemotherapy is that a tumour is usually far advanced before it is diagnosed. Let us suppose that a tumour arises from a single cell and that the growth is exponential—as it may well be in the initial stages. Doubling times vary with different tumours, for example being, very roughly, 24 hours with Burkitt's lymphoma, 2 weeks with some leukaemias, and 3 months with mammary cancers. Approximately 30 doublings would be required to produce a cell mass with a diameter of 2 cm, containing 10^9 cells. A tumour that size is within the limits of diagnostic procedures, though it might be unnoticed in many organs, such as the liver. Another 10 doublings would produce 10^{12} cells—a tumour mass that is likely to be lethal, and which would measure about 20 cm in diameter if it were all in one clump. The neoplasm would, therefore, be silent for the first three quarters or more of its existence, and the

Cancer pathogenesis and cancer chemotherapy: general principles

- The term cancer refers to a malignant neoplasm (new growth).
- Cancer arises as a result of a series of genetic and epigenetic changes, the main genetic lesions being:
  - —inactivation of tumour suppressor genes, e.g. *p53*
  - —the activation of oncogenes (mutation of the normal genes controlling cell division and other processes).
- Cancer cells have four characteristics that distinguish them from normal cells:
  - —uncontrolled proliferation
  - —loss of function because of lack of capacity to differentiate
  - —invasiveness
  - —the ability to metastasise.
- Cancer cells have uncontrolled proliferation owing to changes in:
  - —growth factors and/or their receptors
  - —intracellular signalling pathways, particularly those controlling the cell cycle and apoptosis
  - —telomerase expression
  - —tumour-related angiogenesis.
- Most anticancer drugs are antiproliferative—most damage DNA and thereby initiate apoptosis. They also affect rapidly dividing normal cells and are thus likely to depress bone marrow, impair healing, depress growth, cause sterility and hair loss, and be teratogenic. Most cause nausea and vomiting.

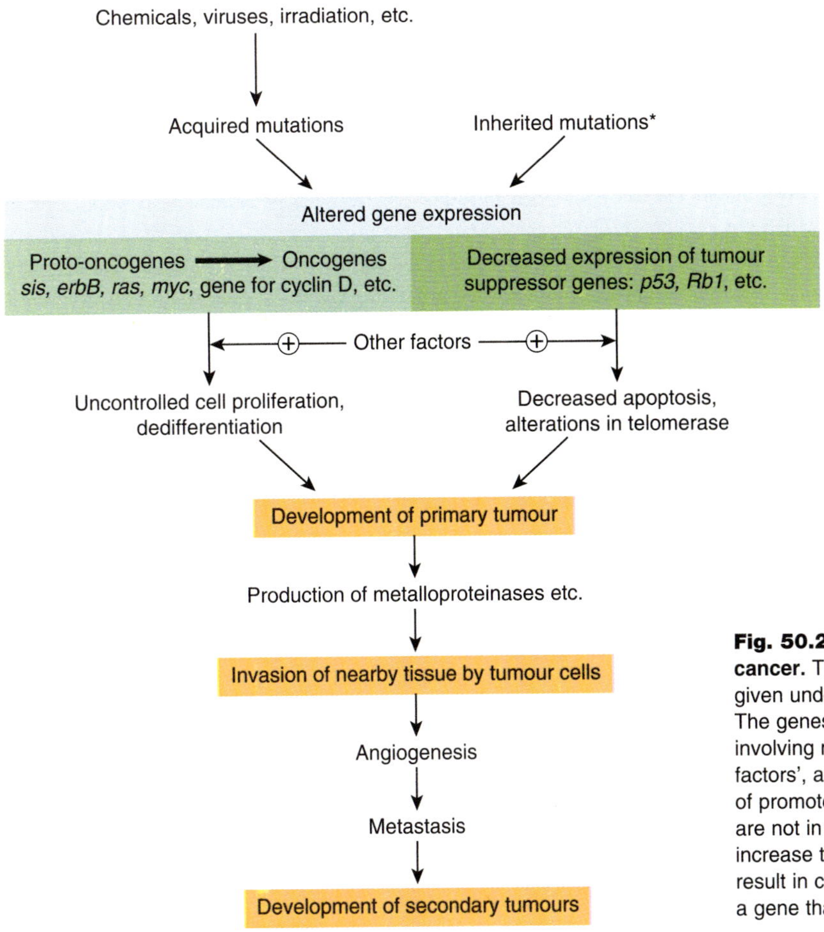

Fig. 50.2 Simplified outline of the genesis of cancer. The diagram summarises the information given under the pathobiology of cancer in the text. The genesis of cancer is usually multifactorial, involving more than one genetic change. 'Other factors', as specified above, may involve the actions of promoters, co-carcinogens, hormones, etc. that are not in themselves carcinogenic but which increase the likelihood that genetic mutation(s) will result in cancer. *It is not cancer that is inherited but a gene that has mutated and predisposes to cancer.

problem of stopping its development after diagnosis, when there are very large numbers of malignant cells, is considerable.

However, continuous exponential growth of this sort does not usually occur. With most solid tumours (for example of lung, stomach, uterus and so on), as opposed to leukaemias (the tumours of white blood cells), the growth rate falls as the neoplasm gets larger. This is partly because the tumour tends to outgrow its ability to maintain its blood supply, with resultant necrosis of some of its bulk, and partly because not all the cells proliferate continuously. The cells of a solid tumour can be considered as belonging to three compartments:

- compartment A consists of dividing cells, possibly being continuously in cell cycle (pp. 69–72)
- compartment B consists of resting cells (in G_0 phase): cells which, though not dividing, are potentially able to do so
- compartment C consists of cells that are no longer able to divide but which contribute to the tumour volume.

Essentially only cells in compartment A, which may form as little as 5% of some solid tumours, are susceptible to the main currently available cytotoxic drugs, as is explained below. The cells in compartment C do not constitute a problem—it is the existence of cells in compartment B that makes cancer chemotherapy difficult, because these cells are not very sensitive to cytotoxic drugs but are liable to re-enter compartment A following a course of chemotherapy.

Most currently used anticancer drugs, in particular those which are 'cytotoxic', affect only the first of the characteristics of cancer cells outlined previously—the process of cell division, i.e. they are antiproliferative; they have no specific inhibitory effect on invasiveness, the loss of differentiation or the tendency to metastasise. For many, their antiproliferative action results mainly from an action during S phase of the cell cycle, and the resultant damage to DNA initiates apoptosis (see above and pp. 72–73). Furthermore, because their main effect is on cell division, they will affect all rapidly dividing normal tissues and thus they are likely to produce, to a greater or lesser extent, the following general toxic effects:

- bone marrow toxicity (myelosuppression) with decreased leucocyte production and thus decreased resistance to infection

- impaired wound healing
- loss of hair (alopecia)
- damage to gastrointestinal epithelium
- depression of growth in children
- sterility
- teratogenicity.

They can also, in certain circumstances, be *carcinogenic* (i.e. they may themselves cause cancer). In addition, if there is rapid cell destruction with extensive purine catabolism, urates may precipitate in the renal tubules and cause *kidney damage*. Finally, virtually all cytotoxic drugs produce severe *nausea* and *vomiting*, which has been called 'the inbuilt deterrent' to patient compliance in completing a course of treatment with these agents (see p. 373). Some compounds have particular toxic effects that are specific for them. These will be dealt with under the individual drugs.

DRUGS USED IN CANCER CHEMOTHERAPY

The main anticancer drugs can be divided into the following general categories.

- Cytotoxic drugs:* the mechanism of action of these drugs is discussed more fully below and summarised in Figure 50.3; they include
  —alkylating agents and related compounds, which act by forming covalent bonds with DNA and thus impeding DNA replication
  —antimetabolites, which block or subvert one or more of the metabolic pathways involved in DNA synthesis
  —cytotoxic antibiotics, i.e. substances of microbial origin that prevent mammalian cell division
  —plant derivatives (vinca alkaloids, taxanes, campothecins): most of these specifically affect microtubule function and hence the formation of the mitotic spindle.
- Hormones—of which the most important are steroids, namely glucocorticoids, estrogens and androgens—and drugs that suppress hormone secretion or antagonise hormone action.
- Miscellaneous agents that do not fit into the above categories. This group includes a number of recently developed drugs designed to affect specific tumour-related targets.

For detailed coverage of the pharmacology of anticancer drugs see Chabner & Longo (1996).

The clinical use of anticancer drugs is the province of the specialist oncologist and is not covered in detail here. In the following sections, we concentrate on mechanisms of action and outline the main unwanted effects of commonly used anticancer agents.

*The term 'cytotoxic drug' applies to any drug that can damage or kill cells. In practice, it is used more restrictively to mean drugs that inhibit cell division and are potentially useful in cancer chemotherapy.

ALKYLATING AGENTS AND RELATED COMPOUNDS

Alkylating agents and related compounds contain chemical groups that can form covalent bonds with particular nucleophilic substances in the cell. With alkylating agents themselves, the main step is the formation of a carbonium ion—a carbon atom with only six electrons in its outer shell. Such ions are highly reactive and react instantaneously with an electron donor such as amine, hydroxyl or sulfhydryl groups. Most of the cytotoxic anticancer alkylating agents are bifunctional, i.e. they have two alkylating groups (Fig. 50.4).

The nitrogen at position 7 (N7) of guanine, being strongly nucleophilic, is probably the main molecular target for alkylation in DNA (Fig. 50.5), although N1 and N3 of adenine and N3 of cytosine may also be affected. A bifunctional agent, being able to react with two groups, can cause intra- or interchain cross-linking (Fig. 50.4). This can interfere not only with transcription but also with replication, which is probably the critical effect of anticancer alkylating agents. Other effects of alkylation at guanine N7 are excision of the guanine base with main chain scission, or pairing of the alkylated guanine with thymine instead of cytosine and eventual substitution of the GC pair by an AT pair.

Anticancer drugs: alkylating agents and related compounds

- Alkylating agents have alkyl groups that can form covalent bonds with cell substituents; a carbonium ion is the reactive intermediate. Most have two alkylating groups and can cross-link two nucleophilic sites such as the N7 of guanine in DNA. Cross-linking can cause defective replication through pairing of alkylguanine and thymine, leading to substitution of AT for GC, or it can cause excision of guanine and chain breakage.
- Their principal effect occurs during DNA synthesis; the resulting DNA damage triggers apoptosis.
- Unwanted effects include myelosuppression, sterility and risk of non-lymphocytic leukaemia.
- The main alkylating agents are:
  —nitrogen mustards, e.g. cyclophosphamide, which is activated to give aldophosphamide, which is then converted to phosphoramide mustard (the cytotoxic molecule) and acrolein (which causes bladder damage that can be ameliorated by masna); cyclophosphamide myelosuppression affects particularly the lymphocytes
  —nitrosoureas, e.g. lomustine, may act on non-dividing cells, can cross the blood–brain barrier, and cause delayed, cumulative myelotoxicity.
- Cisplatin causes intrastrand linking in DNA; it has low myelotoxicity but causes sever nausea and vomiting and can be nephrotoxic. It has revolutionised the treatment of germ cell tumours.

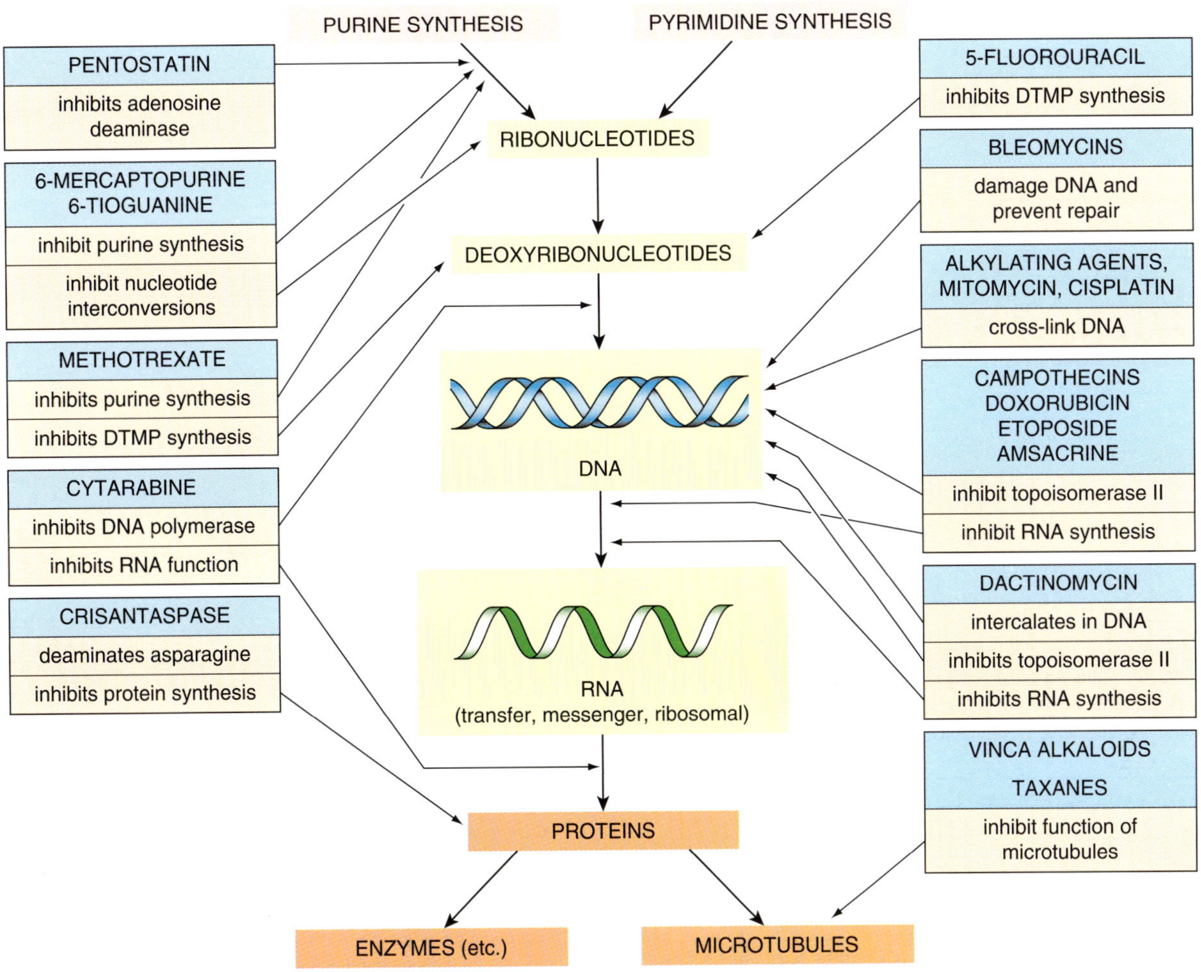

Fig. 50.3 Summary of the main sites of action of cytotoxic agents that act on dividing cells. For some groups of drugs, only one or two examples are given. (DTMP, 2′-deoxythymidylate.) (Adapted from: Calabresi P, Parks R E 1980. In: Gilman A G, Goodman L S, Gilman A (eds) The pharmacological basis of therapeutics, 6th edn. Macmillan, New York.)

The main action occurs during replication, when some parts of the DNA are unpaired and more susceptible to alkylation; i.e. the effects are made manifest during S phase, resulting in a block at G_2 (see Fig. 5.4) and subsequent apoptotic cell death.

All alkylating agents depress bone marrow function and cause gastrointestinal disturbances. With prolonged use, two further unwanted effects occur: depression of gametogenesis (particularly in men), leading to sterility, and an increased risk of acute non-lymphocytic leukaemia and other malignancies.

A large number of alkylating agents are available for use in cancer chemotherapy. Only a few commonly used ones will be dealt with here.

Nitrogen mustards

Nitrogen mustards are related to sulfur mustard, the 'mustard gas' used during the First World War, and their basic formula is R-*N*-bis-(2-chloroethyl); see Figure 50.5. In the body, each 2-chloroethyl side-chain undergoes an intramolecular cyclisation with the release of a Cl^-. The highly reactive ethylene immonium derivative so formed can interact with DNA (see Figs 50.4 and 50.5) and other molecules.

Cyclophosphamide is probably the most commonly used alkylating agent. It is inactive until metabolised in the liver by the P450 mixed function oxidases (see Fig. 50.6 and Ch. 8). It has a pronounced effect on lymphocytes and can be used as an immunosuppressant (see Ch. 16). It is usually given orally or by intravenous injection but may also be given intramuscularly. Important toxic effects are nausea and vomiting, bone marrow depression and haemorrhagic cystitis. This last effect (which also occurs with the related drug **ifosfamide**) is caused by the metabolite acrolein and can be ameliorated by increasing fluid intake and administering compounds that are sulfhydryl donors, such as *N*-acetylcysteine or mesna (sodium-2-mercaptoethane sulfonate). These agents interact specifically with acrolein, forming a non-toxic compound. See also Chapters 8 and 52.

Estramustine is a combination of mustine (see above) with an estrogen. It has both cytotoxic and hormonal action.

Other nitrogen mustards used are **melphalan** and **chlorambucil**.

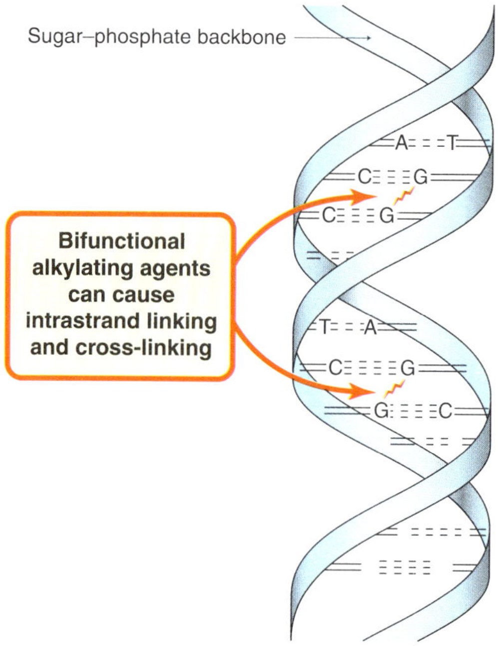

Fig. 50.4 The possible effects of bifunctional alkylating agents on DNA: cross-linking two guanines. (G, guanine; C, cytosine; A, adenine; T, thymine.)

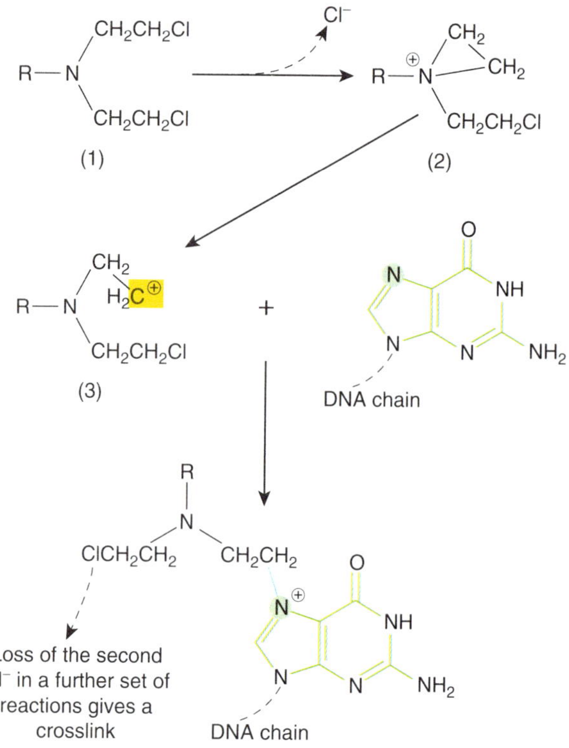

Fig. 50.5 An example of alkylation and cross-linking of DNA by a nitrogen mustard. A bis(chloroethyl)amine (1) undergoes intramolecular cyclisation forming an unstable ethylene immonium cation (2) and releasing Cl^-, the tertiary amine being transformed to a quaternary ammonium compound. The strained ring of the ethylene immonium intermediate opens to form a reactive carbonium ion (in yellow box) (3), which reacts immediately with N7 of guanine (in green circle) to give 7-alkylguanine (bond shown in blue), the N7 being converted to a quaternary ammonium nitrogen. These reactions can then be repeated with the other $-CH_2CH_2Cl$ to give a cross-link.

Nitrosoureas

Examples of the nitrosoureas are the chloroethylnitrosoureas **lomustine** and **carmustine**, which, because they are lipid soluble and can, therefore, cross the blood–brain barrier, may be used against tumours of the brain and meninges. However, most nitrosoureas have a severe cumulative depressive effect on the bone marrow that starts 3–6 weeks after initiation of treatment.

Busulphan

Busulphan has a selective effect on the bone marrow, depressing the formation of granulocytes and platelets in low dosage and red cells in higher dosage. It has little or no effect on lymphoid tissue or the gastrointestinal tract. It is used in chronic granulocytic leukaemia.

Other alkylating agents

Other alkylating agents are **thiotepa** and **treosulphan**.

Cisplatin

Cisplatin is a water-soluble planar coordination complex containing a central platinum atom surrounded by two chlorine atoms and two ammonia groups. Its action is analogous to that of the alkylating agents. When it enters the cell, Cl^- dissociates leaving a reactive complex that reacts with water and then interacts with DNA. It causes intrastrand cross-linking—probably between N7 and O6 of adjacent guanine molecules—which results in local denaturation of the DNA chain.

Cisplatin is given by slow intravenous injection or infusion. It is seriously nephrotoxic unless regimens of hydration and diuresis are instituted. It has low myelotoxicity but causes very severe nausea and vomiting. The 5-HT_3-receptor antagonists (e.g. **ondansetron**; see Chs 12 and 24) are very effective in preventing this and have transformed cancer chemotherapy with cisplatin. Tinnitus and hearing loss in the high frequency range may occur, as may peripheral neuropathies, hyperuricaemia and anaphylactic reactions.

It has revolutionised the treatment of solid tumours of the testes and ovary.

Carboplatin is a derivative of cisplatin. It causes less nephrotoxicity, neurotoxicity and ototoxicity, and less severe nausea and vomiting than cisplatin, but is more myelotoxic.

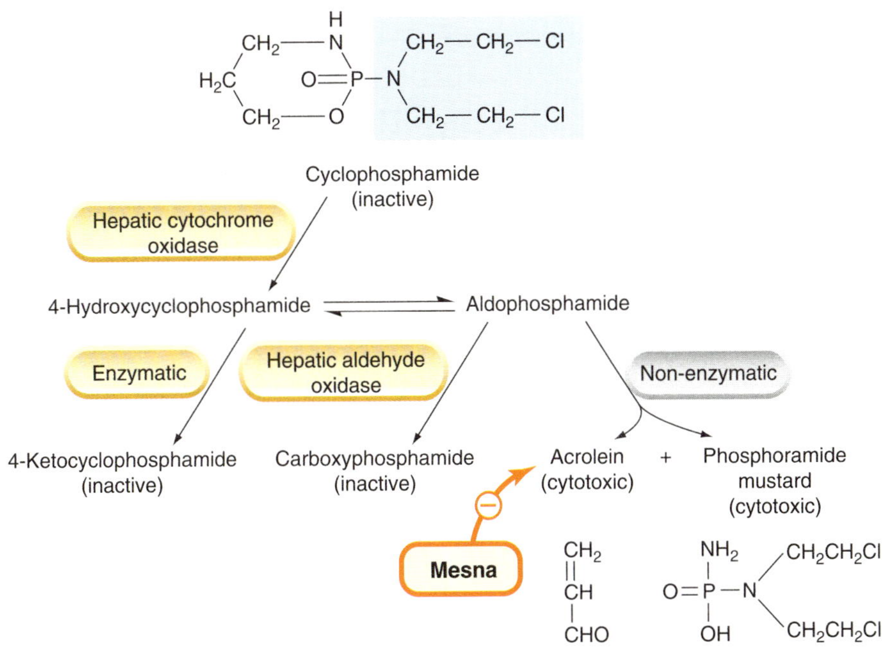

Fig. 50.6 The metabolism of cyclophosphamide. Cyclophosphamide is inactive until metabolised in the liver by P450 mixed function oxidases to 4-hydroxycyclophosphamide, which forms aldophosphamide reversibly. Aldophosphamide is conveyed to other tissues where it is converted to phosphoramide mustard, the actual cytotoxic molecule, and acrolein, which is responsible for unwanted effects. The part of the cyclophosphamide molecule that gives rise to the active metabolites is shown in the blue box. Mesna (sodium 2-mercaptoethane sulfonate) interacts with acrolein, forming a non-toxic compound.

Dacarbazine

Dacarbazine, a pro-drug, is activated in the liver, and the resulting compound is subsequently cleaved in the target cell to release an alkylating derivative. Unwanted effects include myelotoxicity and severe nausea and vomiting.

ANTIMETABOLITES

Folate antagonists

The main folate antagonist is **methotrexate**: it is one of the most widely used antimetabolites in cancer chemotherapy.

Folates are essential for the synthesis of purine nucleotides and thymidylate, which in turn are essential for DNA synthesis and cell division. (This topic is also dealt with in Chs 21, 44 and 48.) The main action of the folate antagonists is to interfere with thymidylate synthesis.

In structure, folates consist of three elements: a pteridine ring, *p*-aminobenzoic acid (PABA) and glutamic acid (Fig. 50.7). Folates are actively taken up into cells where they are converted to polyglutamates. In order to act as coenzymes, folates must be reduced to tetrahydrofolate (FH_4). This reaction is catalysed by *dihydrofolate reductase* and occurs in two steps, first to dihydrofolate (FH_2), then to FH_4 (Fig. 50.8). FH_4 functions as a cofactor in the transfer of one-carbon units, a process which is essential both for the methylation of uracil in 2-deoxyuridylate (DUMP) to form thymidylate (DTMP), and thus for the synthesis of DNA, and also for the de novo synthesis of purines.

During the formation of DTMP from DUMP, FH_4 is converted back to FH_2. **Methotrexate** has a higher affinity for dihydrofolate reductase than has FH_2; it thus inhibits the enzyme (Fig. 50.8) and depletes intracellular FH_4. The binding of methotrexate to dihydrofolate reductase involves an additional hydrogen bond or ionic bond not present when FH_2 binds. The reaction most sensitive to FH_4 depletion is DTMP formation.

Methotrexate is usually given orally but can also be given intramuscularly, intravenously or intrathecally.

The drug has low lipid solubility and thus does not readily cross the blood–brain barrier. It is actively taken up into cells by the transport system used by folate and is metabolised to polyglutamate derivatives, which are retained in the cell for weeks (months in some tissues) in the absence of extracellular drug.

Resistance to methotrexate may develop in tumour cells, a variety of mechanisms being involved (see below, pp. 706–707).

Unwanted effects are depression of the bone marrow and damage to the epithelium of the gastrointestinal tract. Pneumonitis can occur. In addition, when high-dose regimens are used, there may be nephrotoxicity, caused by precipitation of the drug or a metabolite in the renal tubules. High-dose regimens (doses 10 times greater than the standard doses), sometimes used in patients with methotrexate resistance, must be followed by 'rescue' with folinic acid (a form of FH_4).

Pyrimidine analogues

Fluorouracil—an analogue of uracil—interferes with DTMP synthesis (Fig. 50.8). It is converted into a 'fraudulent' nucleotide: fluorodeoxyuridine monophosphate (FDUMP). This interacts with thymidylate synthetase but cannot be converted

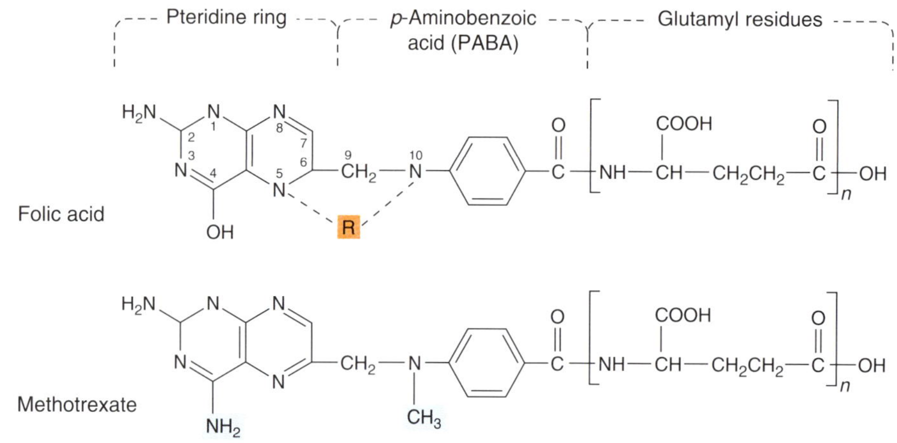

Fig. 50.7 Structure of folic acid and methotrexate. Both compounds are shown as polyglutamates. In tetrahydrofolate, one-carbon groups (R, in orange box) are transported on N5 or N10 or both (shown dotted). (See Figs 21.2 and 21.3.) The points at which methotrexate differs from endogenous folic acid are shown in the blue boxes.

into DTMP. The result is inhibition of DNA synthesis but not RNA or protein synthesis.

Fluorouracil is usually given parenterally. The main unwanted effects are gastrointestinal epithelial damage and myelotoxicity. Cerebellar disturbances can occur.

Cytarabine (cytosine arabinoside) is an analogue of the naturally occurring nucleoside 2′-deoxycytidine. Cytarabine enters the target cell and undergoes the same phosphorylation reactions as the physiological nucleoside to give the cytosine arabinoside trisphosphate; this inhibits DNA polymerase (see Fig. 50.9). The main unwanted effects are on the bone marrow and the gastrointestinal tract. It causes nausea and vomiting.

Gemcitabine, a promising new analogue of cytarabine, has fewer unwanted actions—an influenza-like syndrome and mild myelotoxicity.

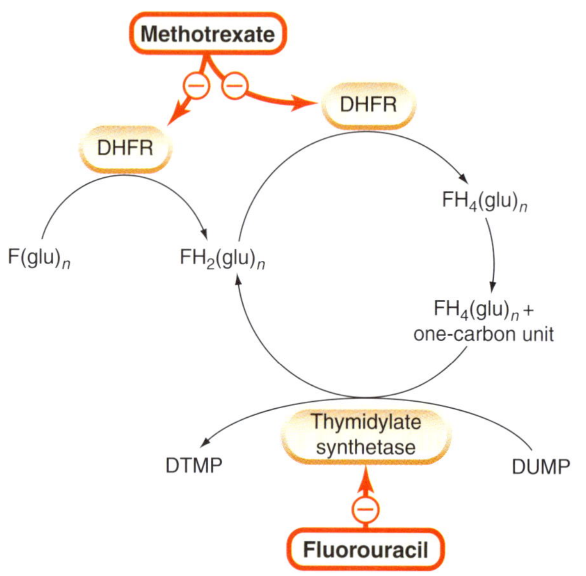

Fig. 50.8 Simplified diagram of action of methotrexate and fluorouracil on thymidylate synthesis. Tetrahydrofolate polyglutamate $FH_4\,(glu)_n$ functions as a carrier of a one-carbon unit, providing the methyl group necessary for the conversion of 2′-deoxyuridylate (DUMP) to 2′-deoxythymidylate (DTMP) by thymidylate synthetase. This one-carbon transfer results in the oxidation of $FH_4\,(glu)_n$ to $FH_2\,(glu)_n$. Fluorouracil is converted to FDUMP, which inhibits thymidylate synthetase. (DHFR, dihydrofolate reductase.)

Purine analogues

The main anticancer purine analogues include **fludarabine, pentostatin, cladribine, mercaptopurine** and **tioguanine**.

Anticancer drugs: antimetabolites

- Antimetabolites block or subvert pathways in DNA synthesis.
- Folate antagonists. Methotrexate inhibits dihydrofolate reductase, preventing generation of tetrahydrofolate; the main result is interference with thymidylate synthesis. Methotrexate is taken up into cells by the folate carrier and, like folate, is converted to the polyglutamate form. Normal cells affected by high doses can be 'rescued' by folinic acid. Unwanted effects are myelosuppression and possible nephroxtoxicity.
- Pyrimidine analogues. Fluorouracil is converted to a fraudulent nucleotide and inhibits thymidylate synthesis. Cytarabine in its trisphosphate form inhibits DNA polymerase; they are potent myelosuppressives.
- Purine analogues. Mercaptopurine is converted into fraudulent nucleotide. Fludarabine in its trisphosphate form inhibits DNA polymerase; it is myelosuppressive. Pentostatin inhibits adenosine deaminase—a critical pathway in purine metabolism.

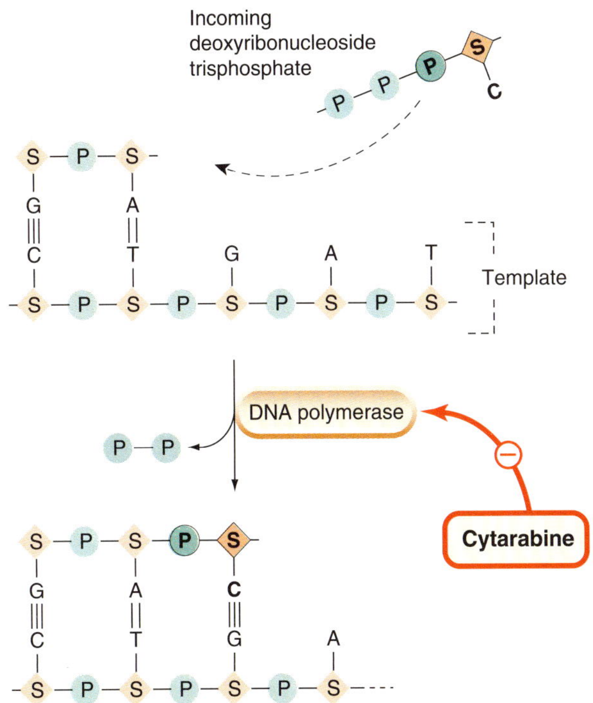

Fig. 50.9 The mechanism of action of cytarabine (cytosine arabinoside). For details of DNA polymerase action see Figure 44.7. Cytarabine is an analogue of cytosine.

Fludarabine is metabolised to the trisphosphate and inhibits DNA synthesis by actions similar to cytarabine. It is myelosuppressive.

Pentostatin has a different mechanism of action. It inhibits adenosine deaminase, the enzyme that catalyses deamination of adenosine to inosine. This action can interfere with critical pathways in purine metabolism and can have significant effects on cell proliferation.

CYTOTOXIC ANTIBIOTICS

Antitumour antibiotics produce their effects mainly by direct action on DNA.

The anthracyclines

The main anticancer anthracycline antibiotic is **doxorubicin**. Others are **idarubicin, epirubicin, aclarubicin**, and mitoxantrone (**mitozantrone**).

Doxorubicin has several cytotoxic actions. It binds to DNA and inhibits both DNA and RNA synthesis, but its main cytotoxic action appears to be mediated through an effect on topoisomerase II (a DNA gyrase; see Ch. 44, p. 627), the activity of which is markedly increased in proliferating cells. The significance of the enzyme lies in the fact that, during replication of the DNA helix, reversible swivelling needs to take place around the replication fork in order to prevent the daughter DNA molecule becoming inextricably entangled during mitotic segregation. The swivel is produced by topoisomerase II, which nicks both DNA strands and subsequently reseals the breaks. Doxorubicin intercalates in the DNA and its effect is, in essence, to stabilise the DNA–topoisomerase II complex after the strands have been nicked, thus causing the process to seize up at this point.

It is given by intravenous infusion. Extravasation at the injection site can cause local necrosis.

In addition to the general unwanted effects (pp. 697–698), doxorubicin can cause cumulative, dose-related cardiac damage, leading to dysrhythmias and heart failure. This action may be the result of generation of free radicals. Marked hair loss frequently occurs.

Epirubicin and mitozantrone are structurally related to doxorubicin. Mitozantrone has dose-related cardiotoxicity and causes bone marrow suppression. Epirubicin is less cardiotoxic than doxorubicin.

Dactinomycin

Dactinomycin intercalates in the minor groove of DNA between adjacent guanosine–cytosine pairs, interfering with the movement of RNA polymerase along the gene and thus preventing transcription. There is also evidence that it has a similar action to the anthracyclines on topoisomerase II. It can have all the toxic effects outlined above (pp. 697–698).

Bleomycins

The bleomycins are a group of metal-chelating glycopeptide antibiotics that degrade preformed DNA, causing chain fragmentation and release of free bases. Their action on DNA is thought to involve chelation of ferrous iron and interaction with oxygen, resulting in the oxidation of the iron and generation of superoxide and/or hydroxyl radicals. Bleomycin is most effective in the G_2 phase of the cell cycle and mitosis, but it is also active against non-dividing cells (i.e. cells in the G_0 phase; Fig. 5.4). In contrast to most anticancer drugs, bleomycin causes little myelosuppression. Its most serious toxic effect is pulmonary fibrosis, which occurs in 10% of patients treated and is reported to be fatal in 1%. Allergic reactions can occur. About half the patients manifest mucocutaneous reactions (the palms are frequently affected) and many develop hyperpyrexia.

Mitomycin

Mitomycin, after enzymic activation in the cells, functions as a bifunctional alkylating agent, alkylating preferentially at O6 of guanine. It cross-links DNA and may also degrade DNA through the generation of free radicals. It causes marked myelosuppression and can also cause kidney damage and fibrosis of lung tissue.

Procarbazine

Procarbazine inhibits DNA and RNA synthesis and interferes with mitosis at interphase. Its effects may be mediated by the production of active metabolites. It is given orally and its main use is in Hodgkin's disease.

Anticancer drugs: cytotoxic antibiotics

- Doxorubicin inhibits DNA and RNA synthesis; the DNA effect is mainly through interference with topoisomerase II action. Unwanted effects include nausea and vomiting, myelosuppression and hair loss; it is cardiotoxic in high doses.
- Bleomycin causes fragmentation of DNA chains. It can act on non-dividing cells. Unwanted effects include fever, allergies, mucocutaneous reactions and pulmonary fibrosis. There is virtually no myelosuppression.
- Dactinomycin intercalates in DNA, interfering with RNA polymerase and inhibiting transcription. It also interferes with the action of topoisomerase II. Unwanted effects include nausea, vomiting and myelosuppression.
- Mitomycin is activated to give an alkylating metabolite.

It interacts with some agents: it causes disulfiram-like actions with alcohol (see Ch. 51), exacerbates the effects of central nervous system (CNS) depressants and, because it is a weak monoamine oxidase inhibitor, can produce hypertension if given with certain sympathomimetic agents. It causes the usual unwanted effects (pp. 697–698): thus it can be leukaemogenic, carcinogenic and teratogenic. Allergic skin reactions may necessitate cessation of treatment.

Hydroxycarbamide

Hydroxycarbamide (hydroxyurea) is a urea analogue that inhibits ribonucleotide reductase, thus interfering with the conversion of ribonucleotides to deoxyribonucleotides. It has the usual unwanted effects (pp. 697–698), bone marrow depression being significant.

PLANT DERIVATIVES

Vinca alkaloids

The main vinca alkaloids are **vincristine, vinblastine** and **vindesine**. They act by binding to tubulin and inhibiting its polymerisation into microtubules, which prevents spindle formation in mitosing cells and causes arrest at metaphase. Their effects only become manifest during mitosis. They also inhibit other cellular activities that involve the microtubules, such as leucocyte phagocytosis and chemotaxis as well as axonal transport in neurons.

The vinca alkaloids are relatively non-toxic. Vincristine has very mild myelosuppressive activity but causes paraesthesias (sensory changes) and muscle weakness fairly frequently. Vinblastine is less neurotoxic but causes leucopenia, while vindesine has both moderate myelotoxicity and neurotoxicity.

A new vinca alkaloid is **vinorelbine**.

Taxanes

The taxanes **paclitaxel** and **docelatel** act on microtubules, stabilising them (in effect 'freezing' them) in the polymerised state. This has repercussions similar to those described above for the vinca alkaloids. Paclitaxel is given by intravenous infusion and docelatel by mouth. Both have a place in the treatment of breast cancers; paclitaxel, given with carboplatin, is the treatment of choice for ovarian cancer.

Unwanted effects, which can be serious, include bone marrow suppression and cumulative neurotoxicity. Resistant fluid retention (particularly oedema of the legs) can occur with docelatel. Hypersensitivity to both compounds is liable to occur and requires pretreatment with corticosteroids and antihistamines.

Etoposide

Etoposide is derived from mandrake root. Its mode of action is not clearly known but it may act by inhibiting mitochondrial function and nucleoside transport, as well as having an effect on topoisomerase II similar to that seen with doxorubicin (see above).

Unwanted effects include nausea and vomiting, myelosuppression and hair loss.

Campothecins

The campothecins **irinotecan** and **topotecan** bind to and inhibit topoisomerase I, high levels of which occur throughout the cell cycle. Diarrhoea and reversible bone marrow depression occur but, in general, these drugs have fewer unwanted effects than most other anticancer agents.

HORMONES

Tumours derived from hormone-sensitive tissues may be hormone dependent. Their growth can be inhibited by hormones with opposing actions, by hormone antagonists or by agents that inhibit the synthesis of the relevant hormones. Hormones or hormone analogues that themselves have inhibitory actions on particular tissues can be used in treatment of tumours of those tissues.

Anticancer drugs: plant derivatives

- Vincristine inhibits mitosis at metaphase by binding to tubulin. It is relatively non-toxic but can cause unwanted neuromuscular effects.
- Etoposide inhibits DNA synthesis by an action on topoisomerse II and also inhibits mitochondrial function. Common unwanted effects include vomiting, myelosuppression and alopecia.
- Paclitaxel stabilises microtubules, inhibiting mitosis; it is relatively toxic and hypersensitvity reactions occur.
- Irinotecan binds to and inhibits topoisomerase 1; it has relatively few toxic effects.

Glucocorticoids

Glucocorticoids have inhibitory effects on lymphocyte proliferation (see Ch. 12) and are used in leukaemias and lymphomas. They are also used in a supportive role in other cancers on the basis of their effect on raised intracranial pressure.

Estrogens

Estrogens, such as **fosfestrol** (a pro-drug, activated by acid phosphatase in prostatic tissue to yield stilbestrol), block the effect of androgens in androgen-dependent prostatic tumours, though this is a minor use; these tumours are best treated with gonadotrophin-releasing hormone analogues (see below).

Estrogens can be used to recruit resting mammary cancer cells (i.e. cells in compartment B; see above) into the proliferating pool of cells (i.e. into compartment A), thus allowing a greater killing efficacy of the cytotoxic drugs that are then given.

Progestogens

Progestogens such as **megestrol** and **medroxyprogesterone** have been useful in endometrial neoplasms and in renal tumours.

The hormone dependency of tumours treated with steroids is related to the presence of steroid receptors in the malignant cells.

Gonadotrophin-releasing hormone analogues

As explained in Chapter 29 (p. 437), analogues of the gonadotrophin-releasing hormones, such as **goserelin**, can, under certain circumstances, inhibit gonadotrophin release. This agent can be used to treat advanced breast cancer in premenopausal women and prostate cancer. The surge of testosterone secretion that can occur in patients with prostate cancer treated in this way can be prevented by an antiandrogen such as **cyproterone** (p. 437).

An analogue of somatostatin, **octreotide** (see p. 406), is used to treat various hormone-secreting tumours of the gastrointestinal tract such as VIPomas, glucagonomas, carcinoid syndrome and gastrinomas. These tumours express somatostatin receptors, activation of which inhibits cell proliferation as well as hormone secretion.

Hormone antagonists

Hormone antagonists can be effective in several hormone-sensitive tumours.

Anti-estrogens

An anti-estrogen, **tamoxifen** (p. 433), is remarkably effective in some cases of hormone-dependent breast cancer and may have a role in preventing these cancers. In breast tissue, tamoxifen competes with endogenous oestrogens for the oestrogen receptors and inhibits the transcription of oestrogen-responsive genes. Tamoxifen is also reported to have cardioprotective effects, partly by virtue of its ability to protect low density lipoproteins against oxidative damage.

Anti-androgens

Androgen antagonists, **flutamide** and **cyproterone**, are used in prostate tumours.

Anticancer agents: hormones and radioactive isotopes

- Hormones or their antagonists are used in hormone-sensitive tumours:
  - —glucocorticoids for leukaemias and lymphomas
  - —tamoxifen for breast tumours
  - —gonadotrophin-releasing hormone analogues for prostate and breast tumours
  - —anti-androgens for prostate cancer
  - —inhibitors of sex hormone synthesis for postmenopausal breast cancer.
- Radioactive iostopes can be targeted at specific tissues, e.g. ^{131}I for thyroid tumours.

Adrenal hormone synthesis inhibitors

Several agents that inhibit synthesis of adrenal hormones have effects in postmenopausal breast cancer. The drugs used are **formestane**, which acts at a late stage of sex hormone synthesis to inhibite the enzyme aromatase, which metabolises androgens to oestrogens (see Fig. 29.3), and **trilostane** and **aminoglutethimide** (see Fig. 27.4) which inhibit sex hormone synthesis at an early stage. Replacement of corticosteroids is necessary with these latter two agents.

RADIOACTIVE ISOTOPES

Radioactive isotopes have a place in the therapy of certain tumours; for example, **radioactive iodine** ($^{131}1$) is used in treating thyroid tumours (discussed in Ch. 28).

MISCELLANEOUS AGENTS

Crisantaspase

Crisantaspase is a preparation of the enzyme asparaginase, given intramuscularly or intravenously. It breaks down asparagine to aspartic acid and ammonia. It is active against tumour cells that, having lost the capacity to synthesise asparagine, now require an exogenous source of it, e.g. acute lymphoblastic leukaemia cells. Most normal body cells are able to synthesise asparagine, and the drug thus has a fairly selective action on certain tumours. It has very little suppressive effect on the bone marrow, the mucosa of the gastrointestinal tract or hair follicles. It causes nausea and vomiting and it can cause CNS depression, anaphylactic reactions and liver damage.

Mitotane

Mitotane interferes with the synthesis of adrenocortical steroids (Ch. 27) having eventually a cytotoxic action on cells in the adrenal cortex. It is used solely for tumours of these cells.

Anticancer drugs: miscellaneous agents

- Procarbazine inhibits DNA and RNA synthesis and interferes with mitosis.
- Crisantaspase is active against acute lymphoblastic leukaemia cells, which cannot synthesise asparagine.
- Hydroxycarbamide (hydroxyurea) inhibits ribonucleotide reductase.
- Amsacrine acts on topoisomerase II.
- Mitoxantrone (mitozantrone) causes DNA chain breakage.
- Mitotane stops synthesis of adrenocortical steroids
- Monoclonal antibodies: riruximab targets a B cell surface protein and is used for B cell lymphomas; trastuzumab targets epidermal growth factor receptor and is used for breast cancer.
- Imatinib inhibits gene signalling pathways and is used for chronic myeloid leukaemia.

Amsacrine

Amsacrine has a mechanism of action similar to that of doxorubicin (p. 703). Bone marrow depression and cardiac toxicity have been reported.

Monoclonal antibodies

Monoclonal antibodies are immunoglobulins produced by cell culture selected to react with antigen specifically expressed on cancer cells (pp. 241–242). Some are 'humanised', which means they are hybrids or chimerae of human antibodies with a murine or primate backbone. They attach to the specific antigen with the Fab portions of the molecule, leaving the Fc portion jutting out. This activates the host's immune mechanisms and the cancer cell is killed by complement-mediated lysis (see p. 220) or attack by killer cells (see p. 222). Some monoclonal antibodies attach to and inactivate growth factor receptors on cancer cells, thus inhibiting the survival pathway and promoting apoptosis (Figs 5.4 and 50.1).

Two monoclonal antibodies are already in clinical use: rituximab and trastuzumab.

Rituximab

Rituximab is a monoclonal antibody that attaches to CD20 protein* on B cells and kills by complement-mediated lysis or by inducing apoptosis. It sensitises resistant cells (see below) to chemotherapeutic drugs.

It is given by infusion and its plasma half-life is approximately 3 days when first given, increasing with each administration to about 8 days by the fourth administration.

*Polymers of CD20 proteins are thought to form a calcium channel implicated in cell activation.

It is used for B-cell lymphomas, being effective in 40-50% of cases when combined with standard chemotherapy.

Unwanted effects include hypotension, chills and fever during the initial infusions and subsequent hypersensitivity reactions. A 'cytokine-release' reaction can occur and has been fatal. The drug may make cardiovascular disorders worse.

Trastuzumab

Trastuzumab is a humanised murine monoclonal antibody that binds to a protein termed Her2/neu (was called HER2), which is a member of the epidermal growth factor receptor family—receptors with integral tyrosine kinase activity (Fig. 50.1). There is some evidence that, in addition to inducing host immune responses, trastuzumab induces cell cycle inhibitors p21 and p27 (Fig. 50.2).

In about 25% of breast cancer patients, the tumour cells overexpress this receptor and the cancer proliferates rapidly. Early results show that trastuzumab given with standard chemotherapy has resulted in a 79% 1-year survival rate in treatment-naive patients with this aggressive form of breast cancer.

Unwanted effects are similar to those with rituximab.

Imatinib mesylate

Imatinib mesylate (aka Gleevec, Glivec) is a small molecule inhibitor of signalling pathway kinases. It inhibits not only platelet-derived growth factor (a receptor tyrosine kinase; Fig. 50.1) but also other aspects of signal transduction, specifically a cytoplasmic kinase (Bcr/Abl kinase, see Fig. 50.1) considered to be a unique factor in the pathogenesis of chronic myeloid leukaemia. It has recently been licensed for the treatment of this tumour.

Biological response modifiers

Agents that enhance the host's response are referred to as biological response modifiers. Some, for example, **interferon γ**, **aldesleukin** (a preparation of interleukin-2) and **tretinoin**, are in use for selected tumours. Tretinoin is a powerful inducer of differentiation in leukaemic cells and is used as an adjunct to chemotherapy.

RESISTANCE TO ANTICANCER DRUGS

The resistance that neoplastic cells manifest to cytotoxic drugs can be primary (present when the drug is first given) or acquired (developing during treatment with the drug). Acquired resistance may result from either adaptation of the tumour cells or mutation, with the emergence of cells that are less affected or unaffected by the drug and that consequently have a selective advantage over the sensitive cells. The following are examples of various mechanisms of resistance.

- Decreased accumulation of cytotoxic drugs in cells as a result of the increased expression of cell surface, energy-dependent drug transport proteins. These are responsible for multidrug resistance to many structurally dissimilar anticancer drugs (doxorubicin, vinblastine, dactinomycin, etc; see Gottesman et al. (2002)). An important member of this group is P-glycoprotein (PGP/MDR1). The physiological role of P-glycoprotein is thought to be the protection of cells against environmental toxins. It functions as a hydrophobic 'vacuum cleaner', picking up drugs as they enter the cell membrane and expelling them. Non-cytotoxic agents that reverse multidrug resistance are being investigated.

- A decrease in the amount of drug taken up by the cell (methotrexate).
- Insufficient activation of the drug (mercaptopurine, fluorouracil, cytarabine). By this it is meant that there may be decreased metabolism of these agents so that they do not enter the pathways where they would normally exert their effects. For example, fluorouracil may not be converted to FDUMP, cytarabine may not undergo phosphorylation; mercaptopurine may not be converted into a 'fraudulent' nucleotide.
- Increase in inactivation (cytarabine, mercaptopurine).
- Increased concentration of target enzyme (methotrexate).
- Decreased requirement for substrate (crisantaspase).
- Increased utilisation of alternative metabolic pathways (antimetabolites).
- Rapid repair of drug-induced lesions (alkylating agents).
- Altered activity of target, for example modified topoisomerase II (doxorubicin).
- Mutations in the *p53* gene and overexpression of the *bcl-2* gene family (several cytotoxic drugs).

TREATMENT SCHEDULES

Treatment with combinations of several anticancer agents increases the cytotoxicity against cancer cells without necessarily increasing the general toxicity. For example, **methotrexate**, with mainly myelosuppressive toxicity, may be used in a regimen with **vincristine**, which has mainly neurotoxicity. The few drugs with low myelotoxicity, such as **cisplatin** and **bleomycin**, are good candidates for combination regimens. Treatment with combinations of drugs also decreases the possibility of the development of resistance to individual agents. Drugs are often given in large doses intermittently in several courses, with intervals of 2–3 weeks between courses, rather than in small doses continuously, because this permits the bone marrow to regenerate during the intervals. Furthermore, it has been shown that the same total dose of an agent is more effective when given in one or two large doses than in multiple small doses.

The possible clinical applications of drug action during the cell cycle

Cells that are constantly replicating constitute the 'growth fraction' of the tumour. Anticancer drugs can be classified in terms of their actions at particular phases on the cell cycle as shown below and it has been proposed that this information could be of value in selecting agents for clinical use. However, not all authorities agree that treatment schedules based on these principles are better than purely empirical schedules.

- Phase-specific agents, i.e. acting at a specific phase of the cell cycle. The vinca alkaloids act in mitosis. Cytarabine, hydroxycarbamide, fluorouracil, methotrexate and mercaptopurine act in S phase. Some of these compounds have some action during G_1 phase and thus may slow the entry of a cell into S phase, where it would be more susceptible to the drug.
- Cycle-specific agents, i.e. acting at all stages of the cell cycle and not having much effect on cells out of cycle: alkylating agents, dactinomycin, doxorubicin and cisplatin.
- Cycle non-specific agents, i.e. acting on cells whether in cycle or not: bleomycins and nitrosoureas.

TECHNIQUES FOR DEALING WITH EMESIS AND MYELOSUPPRESSION

EMESIS

The nausea and vomiting induced by many cancer chemotherapy agents constitutes an 'inbuilt deterrent' to patient compliance (see also Ch. 24, p. 373). It is a particular problem with **cisplatin** but also complicates therapy with many other compounds, such as the alkylating agents. 5-HT_3-receptor antagonists such as **ondansetron** or **granisetron** (see Chs 12 and 24) are effective against cytotoxic-drug-induced vomiting. Of the other antiemetic agents available (see pp. 373–375), **metoclopramide** in high dose, given intravenously, has proved useful, and it is often combined with **dexamethasone** (Ch. 27) or **lorazepam** (Ch. 36) therapy. As metoclopramide commonly causes extrapyramidal side-effects in children and young adults, **diphenhydramine** (Ch. 16) can be used instead.

MYELOSUPPRESSION

Myelosuppression limits the use of many anticancer agents. Regimens to overcome the problem have included removing some of the patient's bone marrow prior to giving cytotoxic agents, purging it of cancer cells (e.g. with specific monoclonal antibodies; see below) and replacing it afterwards. Administering **molgramostim**, then harvesting stem cells from the blood and multiplying them up in vitro with the relevant haemopoietic growth factors (Ch. 23), is now frequently used. The use of haemopoietic growth factors after replacement of the marrow has been successful in some cases. A further possibility is the introduction, into the extracted bone marrow, of the mutated gene that confers multidrug resistance, so that when replaced, the marrow cells (but not the cancer cells) will be resistant to the cytotoxic action of the anticancer drugs.

POSSIBLE FUTURE STRATEGIES FOR CANCER CHEMOTHERAPY

Some of the main drawbacks of the current chemotherapy of cancer are:

General approaches to cancer therapy

- Kill or remove malignant cells:
  —cytotoxic drugs*
  —surgery*
  —irradiation*
  —targeted cytotoxic agents (e.g. antibody-linked toxins or radioactive agents).**
- Inactivate components of oncogene signalling pathway:
  —inhibitors of growth factor receptors, e.g. receptor tyrosine kinases*
  —inhibitors of adapter proteins (e.g. Ras), cytoplasmic kinases, cyclins, cyclin-dependent kinases, etc.***
  —antisense oligonucleotides**
  —inhibitors of anti-apoptotic factors or stimulators of pro-apoptotic factors***
- Restore function of tumour suppressor genes:
  —gene therapy.**
- Employ tissue-specific proliferation inhibitors:
  —estrogens, antiestrogens, androgens, anti-androgens, glucocorticoids, gonadotrophin-releasing hormone analogues.
- Inhibit tumour growth, invasion, metastasis:
  —inhibitors of angiogenesis**
  —matrix metalloproteinase inhibitors.**
- Enhance host immune response
  —cytokine-based therapies**
  —gene therapy-based approaches**
  —cell-based approaches (e.g. antitumour T cells).***
- Reverse drug resistance
  —inhibitors of multidrug resistance transport.**

*Therapies in general use.
**Therapies in development.
***Potential approaches.

- virtually all anticancer drugs target cell proliferation not the more lethal properties of invasiveness and metastasis
- current anticancer drugs are, in the main, non-specific cell killers rather than being aimed at the particular changes which make a cell malignant (see pp. 694–696)
- the development of resistance (particularly multidrug resistance) to anticancer drugs (see above)
- total elimination of malignant cells is not possible with many tumours using therapeutic doses (see p. 696), and the host's immune response is often not adequate to deal with the remaining cells.

Attempts are being made to overcome these problems—the first two by developing new approaches based on the advances in knowledge of the pathobiology of the cancer cell and by using selective targeting of anticancer compounds, the third by developing agents that reverse multidrug resistance and the fourth by boosting or augmenting the host's immune responses to the tumour.

APPROACHES BASED ON THE PATHOBIOLOGY OF THE CANCER CELL

In the decade preceeding this 5th edition, there have been significant advances in our knowledge of the biology of the cancer cell—as discussed above. In Figures 50.1 and 50.2, some of the major factors in the production of malignancy are outlined. Figure 50.1 shows some recently introduced anticancer drugs and targets for development of further drugs. Further possibilities are given below.

Labelled monoclonal antibodies

Monoclonal antibodies that target the extracellular domains of receptors are under investigation. Some already in clinical use are discussed above (p. 706); see also White et al. (2001). Monoclonal antibodies conjugated with radioisotopes (e.g. yttrium) are in clinical trial and are also being used to purge bone marrow (see p. 242).

The Ras protein

Ras proteins (Fig. 50.1) regulate signalling pathways by acting as on/off switches. Farnesyl protein transferases are important in the localisation of Ras to the plasma membrane. Farnesyl protein transferase inhibitors are in clinical trial.

Tyrosine kinases of tumour cells

Small molecule inhibitors of the internal enzymic domains of receptor tyrosine kinases are proving efficacious. **Imatinib** is already in use (p. 706). Two others are in clinical trial: **iressa**, which interferes with epidermal-growth factor receptor signalling, and **tarceva**, which directly inhibits this receptor signalling.

Inhibitors of the kinase cascade shown in Figure 50.1 are also potential targets and an inhibitor of Raf-1, the first kinase in the cascade, is in clinical trial.

Cyclins and cyclin-dependent kinases

Small molecule inhibitors of cdks are being vigorously investigated (see Ch. 5). **Flavopiridol** is in clinical trial.

Telomerase inhibitors

Agents that inhibit telomerase (see p. 695) could prove to be wide-spectrum anticancer agents, since many tumours express telomerase. This possibility is being explored.

Angiogenesis and metalloproteinase inhibitors

Tumour cells produce metalloproteinases and angiogenic factors that facilitate tumour growth, invasion of normal tissue and metastases (see pp. 78, 221 and 695). Targetting the mechanisms involved has the potential to be successful. Several angiogenesis inhibitors (see Griffioen, 2000; Rosen, 2000; Claesson & Welsh, 2001) and several agents that inhibit metalloproteinases are in clinical trial.

Cyclooxygenase inhibitors

There is epidemiological evidence that long-continued use of non-steroidal anti-inflammatory drugs, which inhibit cyclooxygenase (COX), protects against cancer of the gastrointestinal tract. Furthermore there is good evidence that COX-2 is overexpressed in about 85% of cancers. The COX-2 inhibitor **celecoxib** (Ch. 15) reduces mammary tumour incidence in animal models and cause regression of existing tumours. COX-2 is now considered to be a potentially important target for anticancer drug development (see Dempke et al., 2001; Gupta & Dubois, 2001).

p53 as anticancer target

More than 50% of human tumours carry a mutation of the *p53* gene (see pp. 72–73 and Fig. 50.1) and there have been many attempts to capitalise on this. Virally mediated introduction of the wild-type (normal) *p53* gene has not been very successful; but therapy with oncolytic virus ONYX-015, given into the tumour in conjunction with standard chemotherapy, has given good preliminary results. ONYX-015 replicates in and lyses tumour cells but not cells expressing normal p53 protein.

Antisense oligonucleotides

Antisense oligonucleotides are synthetic sequences of single-stranded DNA complementary to specific coding regions of mRNA, which can inhibit gene expression in some tumour cells. An antisense drug, **augmerosen**, downregulates Bcl-2. In an early clinical trial, it sensitised malignant melanoma to standard anticancer drugs.

REVERSAL OF MULTIDRUG RESISTANCE

Several non-cytotoxic drugs (e.g. calcium channel blockers) can reverse multidrug resistance. Development of related compounds could make it feasible to overcome this type of resistance. In addition, the use of antibodies, immunotoxins, antisense oligonucleotides (see above) or liposome-encapsulated agents could be useful in the elimination of cells with multidrug resistance (reviewed by Gottesman & Pastan, 1993).

ENHANCEMENT OF THE HOST'S RESPONSE TO CANCER

Drugs that enhance the host's response to cancer are classified as biological response modifiers. Some biological response modifiers are already in use: e.g. interferon α is used in some lymphomas, aldesleukin (recombinant interleukin-2) is used in selected renal tumours. Further investigation of the efficacy of immunotherapy for tumours may be fruitful (e.g. the use of antitumour T cells) and cancer experts have been exhorted to get to grips with 'immunobabble'.

A combination of the various novel approaches to anticancer treatment cited above may be of even more potential value than their use alone. One way or another, it is likely that significant advances in the treatment of cancer will occur in the not too distant future.

REFERENCES AND FURTHER READING

Adjei A A 2001 Blocking oncogenic Ras signaling for cancer therapy. J Natl Cancer Institute. 93: 1062–1074 (*Gives details of Ras processing, activation, mutations, cytoplamsic targets and physiological role, and outlines therapeutic implications*)

Anderson W F 2000 Gene therapy scores against cancer. Nat Med 6: 862–863 (*Short crisp article*)

Armstrong A C, Eaton D, Ewing J C 2001 Cellular immunotherapy for cancer. Br Med J 323: 1289–1293 (*Brief discussion of rationale and possible future exploitation of tumour cell and dendritic cell vaccines and T cell therapy*)

Blume-Jensen P, Hunter T 2001 Oncogenic kinase signalling. Nature 411: 355–365 (*Excellent article. Emphasises oncogenic receptor-tyrosine kinases and cytoplasmic-tyrosine kinases. Useful figures and tables. Note that there are eight other relevant articles in the same issue of Nature*)

Buys C H C M 2000 Telomeres, telomerase and cancer. N Engl J Med 342: 1282–1283 (*Clear concise coverage*)

Carmeliet P, Jain R K 2000 Angiogenesis in cancer and other diseases. Nature 407: 249–257 (*Gives details of mechanisms involved in angiogenesis, lists biological activators and inhibitors, and agents in clinical trials. Excellent figures*)

Carter P 2001 Improving the efficacy of antibody-based cancer therapies. Nat Rev Cancer 1: 118–128 (*Review considering the possible future use of monoclonal antibodies to treat cancer. Lists antibodies in advanced clinical trials*)

Chabner B A, Longo D L 1996 Cancer chemotherapy and biotherapy, 2nd edn. Lippincott-Raven, Philadelphia, PA (*Textbook with comprehensive coverage of the anticancer drugs used then, most still used*)

Chambers A F, Groom A C, MacDonald I C 2002 Dissemination and growth of cancer cells in metastatic sites. Nat Rev Cancer 2: 563–57 (*Review. Stresses that metastases rather than primary tumours are responsible for most cancer deaths; discusses the mechanisms involved in metastasis and raises the possibility of targetting these in anticancer drug development*)

Dempke W, Rie C et al. 2001 Cyclooxygenase-2: a novel target for cancer chemotherapy. J Cancer Res Clin Oncol 127: 411–417 (*Discusses role of COX-2 in apoptosis, angiogenesis and invasiveness*)

English J M, Cobb M H 2002 Pharmacological inhibitors of MAPK pathways. Trends in Pharmacol Sci 23: 40–45 (*Lists mitogen activated protein kinases (MAPKs) and discusses small molecule inhibitors under investigation*)

Favoni R E, de Cupis A 2000 The role of polypeptide growth factors in human carcinomas: new targets for a novel pharmacological approach. Pharmacol Rev 52: 179–206 (*Thorough coverage. Outlines growth factor signalling; describes 14 growth factor families and their possible role in cancer; discusses possible drug action on signalling pathways*)

Gottesman M M, Fojo T, Bates S E 2002 Multidrug resistance in cancer: role of ATP-dependent transporters. Nat Rev Cancer 2: 48–56 (*Outlines cellular mechanisms of resistance; describes ATP-dependent transporters, emphasising those in human cancer. Considers resistance reversal strategies*)

Gottesman M M, Pastan I 1993 Biochemistry of multidrug resistance mediated by the multidrug transporter. Annu Rev Biochem 62: 385–427 (*Clear review*)

Greider C W, Blackburn E H 1996 Telomeres, telomerase and cancer. Sci Am Feb: 80–85 (*Simple, clear overview with high-quality figures*)

Griffioen A, Molema G 2000 Angiogenesis: potentials for pharmacologic intervention in the treatment of cancer, cardiovascular diseases and chronic inflammation. Pharmacol Rev 52: 237–268 (*Comprehensive review covering virtually all aspects of angiogenesis and the potential methods of modifying it*)

Gupta R A, Dubois R N 2001 Colorectal cancer prevention and treatment by inhibition of cyclooxygenase-2. Nat Rev Cancer 1: 11–21 (*Reviews evidence from human, animal and cell culture studies that COX-2 may be implicated in the development of colorectal cancer and points out that inhibition of COX-2 would be a viable target for cancer prevention and/or therapy*)

Haber D A, Fearon E R 1998 The promise of cancer genetics. Lancet 351(SII): 1–8 (*Excellent coverage; detailed tables of mutations in proto-oncogenes and tumour-suppressor genes in human cancers*)

Houghton A N, Scheinberg D 2000 Monoclonal antibody therapies — a 'constant' threat to cancer. Nat Med 6: 373–374 (*Lucid article: very useful diagram*)

Norman K L, Farassati F, Lee P W K 2001 Oncolytic viruses and cancer therapy. Cytokine Growth Factor Rev 12: 271–282 (*Describes mechanisms of action and efficacy of three oncolytic viruses in clinical trial*)

Overall C M, López-Otin C 2002 Strategies for MMO inhibition in cancer: innovations for the post-trial era. Nat Rev Cancer 2: 6577–7672 (*Review. Points out that it is now well known that matrix metaloproteinases (MMPs) are required for tumour metastasis and discusses various approaches that could be used to target MMPs for new anticancer drugs*)

Reed J C 2002 Apoptosis-based therapies. Nat Rev Drug Discov 1: 111–121 (*Excellent coverage, useful tables, good diagrams*)

Rosen L 2000 Antiangiogenic strategies and agents in clinical trial. Oncologist 5: 20–27 (*Succinct coverage; useful summary tables*)

Rosenberg S A 2001 Progress in human tumour immunology and immunotherapy. Nature 411: 380–384 (*Commendable coverage of current status*)

Savage D G, Antman K H 2002 Imatinib mesylate—a new oral targeted therapy. N Engl J Med 346: 683–693 (*Review with detailed coverage of the new biological agent for chronic myelogenous leukaemia. Very good diagrams*)

Senderowicz A M, Sausville E A 2000 Preclinical and clinical development of cyclin-dependent kinase modulators. J Natl Cancer Inst 92: 376–387 (*Outlines cell cycle control and targets for intervention and discusses preclinical pharmacology of agents in clinical trial*)

Sikic B I 1999 New approaches in cancer treatment. Ann Oncol 10: S149–S153 (*Pithy coverage of monoclonal antibodies, angiogenic inhibitors, agents for supportive care. Very useful tables*)

Smith I E 2002 New drugs for breast cancer Lancet 360: 790–792 (*Succinct coverage*)

Streiter R M 2001 Chemokines: not just leucocyte attractants in the promotion of cancer. Nat Immunol 2: 285–286 (*Elegant, crisp article on the role of chemokines in tumour growth, invasion and metastasis. Good diagram*)

Talapatra S, Thompson C B 2001 Growth factor signaling in cell survival: implications for cancer treatment. J Pharmacol Exp Ther 298: 873–878 (*Succinct overview of death-receptor-induced apoptosis, the role of growth factors in preventing it, and potential drugs*)

Wagner R W, Flanagan W M 1997 Antisense technology and prospects for therapy of viral infections and cancer. Mol Med Today Jan: 31–38

Weinberg R A 1996 How cancer arises. Sci Am Sept: 42–48 (*Simple, clear overview, listing main oncogenes, tumour suppressor genes and the cell cycle; excellent diagrams*)

White C A, Weaver R L, Grillo-Löpez 2001 Antibody-targeted immunotherapy for treatment of malignancy. Annu Rev Med 52: 125–145 (*Clear, comprehensive review; has tables of monoclonals and radiolabelled monoclonals in clinical trial*)

Workman P, Kaye S B (eds) 2002 Cancer therapeutics. A Trends Guide with eleven reviews on various new potential approaches to the development of anticancer drugs. S Trends Mol Med Suppl 8: S1–S73 (*A series of short reviews covering the main approaches to developing novel anticancer drugs*)

Yarden Y, Sliwkowski M X 2001 Untangling the ErbB signalling network. Nat Mol Cell Biol 2: 127–137 (*Describes ErbBs epidermal growth factor receptors, their ligands and their signalling pathways, their involvement in cancer and their potential as targets for anticancer drugs*)

Zörnig M, Hueber A-O et al. 2001 Apoptosis regulators and their role in tumorigenesis. Biochim Biophys Acta 1551: F1–F37 (*Extensive review describing the genes and mechanisms involved in apoptosis and summarising the evidence that impaired apoptosis is a prerequisite for cancer development*)

Zwick E, Baaange J, Ullrich A 2002 Receptor tyrosine kinases as targets for anticancer drugs. Trends Mol Med 8: 17–23 (*Review. Points out that receptor tryosine kinases (RTKs) are the main mediators of extracellular signals for cell proliferation and discusses strategies for targetting RTKs for anticancer therapy. Lists RTK-based anticancer drugs in clinical trial*)

SECTION 6

SPECIAL TOPICS

51 Individual variation and drug interaction

Overview 712

Effects of ethnicity 712

Effects of age 713

Effects of pregnancy 714

Genetic factors 714

Idiosyncratic reactions 716

Effects of disease 717

Drug interactions 718

Individual variation

- Variability is a serious problem; if not taken into account it can result in:
  - —lack of efficacy
  - —unexpected side-effects.
- Types of variability may be classified as:
  - —pharmacokinetic
  - —pharmacodynamic
  - —idiosyncratic.
- The main causes of variability are:
  - —age
  - —genetic factors
  - —immunological factors (Ch. 52)
  - —pathological states (e.g. kidney or liver disease)
  - —drug interactions.

OVERVIEW

Therapeutics would be a great deal easier if responses to the same dose of drug were always the same. In reality, inter- and even intraindividual variation is often substantial. Physicians need to be aware of the sources of such variation to prescribe drugs safely and effectively. Variation can be caused by different concentrations at sites of drug action or by different responses to the same drug concentration. The first kind is called pharmacokinetic variation and can occur because of differences in absorption, distribution, metabolism or excretion (Chs 7 and 8). The second kind is called pharmacodynamic variation.

Variation is usually quantitative in the sense that the drug produces a larger or smaller effect, or acts for a longer or shorter time, while still exerting qualitatively the same effect. In other cases, the action is qualitatively different. These are known as idiosyncratic reactions (the OED defines an idiosyncrasy as 'the physical constitution peculiar to an individual or class') and are often caused by genetic or immunological differences between individuals.

Effects on drug absorption and elimination of bioavailability, food intake and gastric and urinary pH were discussed in Chapters 7 and 8. In this chapter we describe other important factors responsible for variation in drug response, namely:

- ethnicity
- age
- pregnancy
- genetic factors
- idiosyncratic reactions
- disease
- drug interactions.

EFFECTS OF ETHNICITY

Ethnic differences in drug responsiveness can be important. For example, Chinese subjects differ from Caucasians in the way that they metabolise ethanol, producing a higher plasma concentration of acetaldehyde, which can cause flushing and palpitations (Ch. 52). Chinese subjects are considerably more sensitive to the cardiovascular effects of propranolol (Ch. 11) than Caucasians, whereas Afro-Caribbean individuals are less sensitive. Despite their increased sensitivity to β-adrenoceptor antagonists, Chinese subjects metabolise propranolol faster than Caucasians, implying that the difference relates to pharmacodynamic differences in sensitivity at or beyond the β-adrenoceptors. It is probable that many such ethnic differences are genetic in origin (genetic factors are discussed later in this chapter), but environmental factors, for example relating to diet, may also contribute.

EFFECTS OF AGE

The main reason that age affects drug action is that drug elimination is less efficient in newborn babies and in old people, so that drugs commonly produce greater and more prolonged effects at the extremes of life. Other age-related factors, such as variations in pharmacodynamic sensitivity, are also important with some drugs. Physiological factors (e.g. altered cardiovascular reflexes) and pathological factors (e.g. hypothermia), which are common in elderly people, also influence drug effects. Body composition changes with age, fat contributing a greater proportion to body mass in the elderly, with consequent changes in distribution volume of drugs. Elderly people consume more drugs than do younger adults, so the potential for drug interactions is also increased.

EFFECT OF AGE ON RENAL EXCRETION OF DRUGS

Glomerular filtration rate (GFR) in the newborn, normalised to body surface area, is only about 20% of the adult value, and tubular function is also reduced. Accordingly, plasma elimination half-lives of renally eliminated drugs are longer in neonates than in adults (Table 51.1). In babies born at term, renal function increases to values similar to those in young adults in less than a week, and indeed continues to increase to a maximum of approximately twice the adult value at 6 months of age. The increase in renal function occurs more slowly in premature infants. Renal immaturity in premature infants can have a very large effect on drug elimination. For example, in premature newborn babies the antibiotic gentamicin has a plasma half-life of 18 hours or greater, compared with 1–4 hours for adults and approximately 10 hours for babies born at term. It is, therefore, necessary to reduce and/or space out doses to avoid toxicity in premature babies.

GFR declines slowly from about 20 years of age, falling by about 25% at 50 years and by 50% at 75 years. Figure 51.1 shows that the renal clearance of digoxin in young and old subjects is

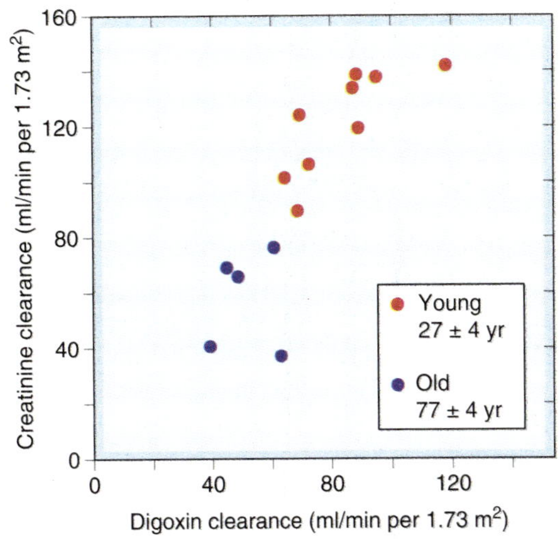

Fig. 51.1 Relationship between renal function (measured as creatinine clearance) and digoxin clearance in young and old subjects. (From: Ewy G A et al. 1969 Circulation 34: 452.)

Table 51.1 Effect of age on plasma elimination half-lives of various drugs

Drug	Mean or range of half-life (h)		
	Term neonate[a]	Adult	Elderly
Drugs that are mainly excreted unchanged in the urine			
Gentamicin	10	2	4
Lithium	120	24	48
Digoxin	200	40	80
Drugs that are mainly metabolised			
Diazepam	25–100	15–25	50–150
Phenytoin	10–30	10–30	10–30
Sulfamethoxypyridazine	140	60	100

[a]Even greater differences from mean adult values occur in premature babies.
Data from: Reidenberg 1971 Renal function and drug action. Saunders, Philadelphia, PA; and Dollery 1991 Therapeutic drugs. Churchill Livingstone, Edinburgh

closely correlated with creatinine clearance, a measure of GFR. Consequently, chronic administration over the years of the same daily dose of digoxin to an individual as he or she ages leads to a progressive increase in plasma concentration, and this is a common cause of glycoside toxicity in elderly people (see Ch. 17).

▼ The age-related decline in GFR is not reflected by an increase in plasma creatinine concentration, as distinct from creatinine clearance. Plasma creatinine typically remains within the normal adult range in elderly persons despite substantially diminished GFR. This is because creatinine synthesis is reduced in elderly persons because of their reduced muscle mass. Consequently a 'normal' plasma creatinine in an elderly person does not indicate that they have a normal GFR. Failure to recognise this and reduce the dose of drugs that are eliminated by renal excretion can lead to drug toxicity.

EFFECT OF AGE ON DRUG METABOLISM

Several enzymes that are important for drug metabolism, for example hepatic microsomal oxidase, glucuronyltransferase, acetyltransferase and plasma esterases, have low activity in neonates, especially if they have been born prematurely. These enzymes take 8 weeks or longer to reach the adult level of activity. The relative lack of conjugating activity in the newborn can have serious consequences, as in kernicterus caused by drug displacement of bilirubin from its binding sites on albumin (see below) and in the 'grey baby' syndrome caused by the antibiotic **chloramphenicol** (see Ch. 45). This sometimes-fatal condition, at first thought to be a specific biochemical sensitivity to the drug in young babies, actually results simply from accumulation of very high tissue concentrations of chloramphenicol because of slow hepatic conjugation. Chloramphenicol is no more toxic to babies than to adults provided the dose is reduced to make allowance for this. Slow conjugation is also one reason why morphine (which is excreted mainly as the glucuronide) is not used as an analgesic in labour, since drug transferred via the placenta has a long half-life in the newborn baby and can cause prolonged respiratory depression.

The activity of hepatic microsomal enzymes declines slowly (and very variably) with age, and the distribution volume of lipid-soluble drugs increases, because the proportion of the body that is fat increases with advancing age. The increasing half-life of the anxiolytic drug **diazepam** with advancing age (Fig. 51.2) is one consequence of this. Some other benzodiazepines and their active metabolites show even greater age-related increases in half-life. Since half-life determines the time course of drug accumulation during repeated dosing (Ch. 8) insidious effects, developing over days or weeks, can occur in elderly people and may be misattributed to age-related memory impairment rather than to drug accumulation. The effect of age is less marked for many other drugs, but even though the mean half-life may not change much, there is often a striking increase in the variability of half-life between individuals with increasing age. This is important, because a population of old people will contain some individuals with grossly reduced rates of drug metabolism whereas such extremes do not occur so commonly in young adult populations. Drug regulatory authorities, therefore, usually require studies in elderly patients as part of drug evaluation.

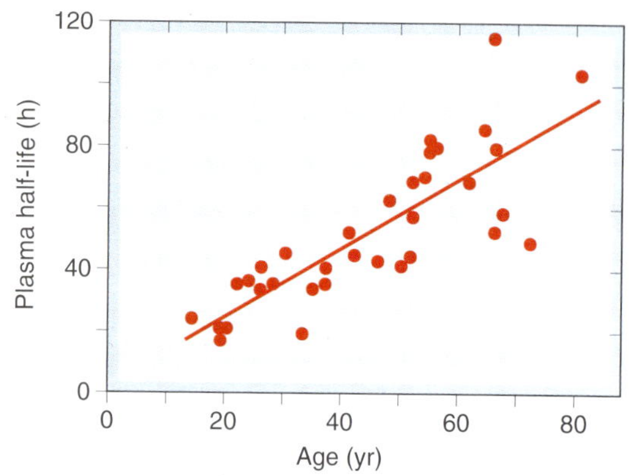

Fig. 51.2 Increasing plasma half-life for diazepam with age in 33 normal subjects. Note the increased variability as well as increased half-life with ageing.(From: Klotz U et al. 1975 J Clin Invest 55: 347.)

AGE-RELATED VARIATION IN SENSITIVITY TO DRUGS

The same plasma concentration of a drug can cause different effects in young and old subjects. Benzodiazepines (Ch. 36) exemplify this, producing more confusion and less sedation in elderly than in young subjects; similarly, hypotensive drugs (Ch. 18) cause postural hypotension more commonly in elderly than in younger adult patients.

EFFECTS OF PREGNANCY

Pregnancy causes several physiological changes that can influence drug disposition in mother and fetus. Maternal plasma albumin concentration is reduced, influencing drug protein binding (Ch. 7). Cardiac output is increased, leading to increased renal blood flow and glomerular filtration and increased renal elimination of drugs (Ch. 8). Lipophilic molecules rapidly traverse the placental barrier, whereas transfer of hypdrophobic drugs is slow, limiting fetal drug exposure following a single maternal dose. The placental barrier excludes some drugs (e.g. low-molecular-weight heparins; Ch. 20) so effectively that they can be administered chronically to the mother without causing effects in the fetus. However, drugs that *are* transferred to the fetus are *slowly* eliminated. The activity of most drug-metabolising enzymes in fetal liver is much less than in the adult. Furthermore, the fetal kidney is not an efficient route of elimination because excreted drug enters the amniotic fluid, which is swallowed by the fetus.

GENETIC FACTORS

Studies on identical and non-identical twins have shown that much individual variability is genetically determined. Thus half-life values for antipyrene, a probe of hepatic drug oxidation (Ch. 8), and for coumarin, an oral anticoagulant (Ch. 20), are 6–22 times less variable in identical than in fraternal twins. Genes influence pharmacokinetics, pharmacodynamics and the susceptibility to idiosyncratic reactions. To understand this better, it is necessary to recall some elementary genetics.

Mutations change the base sequence of DNA. This may, or may not,* result in a change in the amino acid sequence of the protein for which the gene codes. Most changes in protein structure are deleterious and so the altered gene dies out in future generations as a result of natural selection. Some changes may confer advantages, however, at least under some environmental circumstances. An example is the X-linked gene for glucose 6-phosphate dehydrogenase (G6PD); deficiency of this enzyme may confer partial resistance to malaria (a considerable selective advantage in parts of the world where this disease is common) at the expense of susceptibility to haemolysis in response to oxidative stress in the form of exposure to various dietary constituents, including drugs (see below and Ch. 52). This ambiguity gives rise to the abnormal gene being preserved in future generations, at a frequency that depends on the balance of selective pressures in the environment. Therefore, the frequency of G6PD deficiency follows the geographic distribution of malaria (see Fig. 48.1). The situation where several functionally distinct genes are common in a population is called a 'balanced polymorphism'. Now that genes can be sequenced readily, it has become apparent that such balanced polymorphisms are very common, although it is seldom known what is the selective advantage conferred by the mutant gene.

Polymorphisms can affect individual susceptibility to both dose-dependent and dose-independent adverse drug reactions. Determinants of susceptibility include kinetic factors (e.g. polymorphisms in the genes encoding cytochrome P450 enzymes) and dynamic factors (e.g. polymorphisms in drug targets (such as receptors and enzymes). More than one gene may be involved. There is, therefore, great excitement over the potential of the approach of profiling the whole genome for *single nucleotide polymorphisms* (SNPs) as a means of predicting individual susceptibility to adverse effects. If this proves successful, it could ultimately replace the current empirical approach to drug selection in diseases such as hypertension: instead of using one of a range of different drugs (such as **bendroflumethiazide** (**bendrofluazide**), **atenolol**, **nifedipine**, **trandolapril**) on a trial and error basis, and changing if there is lack of efficacy or poor tolerability, one would profile DNA from the individual and select a drug accordingly. During drug development, blood samples are now often stored in the hope of testing this approach, but it has yet to prove itself. Meanwhile, there are several clear-cut examples of single gene variations that do cause variations in drug responsiveness and these are considered below.

*The genetic code is 'redundant', i.e. more than one set of nucleotide base triplets codes for any one amino acid. If a mutation results in a base change that leads to a triplet that codes for the same amino acid as the original there is no change in the protein and consequently no change in function. Such mutations are neither advantageous nor disadvantageous so they will neither be eliminated by natural selection nor accumulate in the population at the expense of the wild-type gene.

GENETIC INFLUENCES ON DRUG METABOLISM

Figure 51.3 contrasts the approximately Gaussian distribution of plasma concentrations achieved 3 hours after administration of a dose of salicylate with the bimodal distribution of plasma concentrations after a dose of isoniazid. The isoniazid concentration was <20 µmol/l in about half the population, and in this group the mode was approximately 9 µmol/l. In the other half of the population (plasma concentration >20 µmol/l) the mode was approximately 30 µmol/l. The elimination of isoniazid depends mainly on acetylation, involving acetyl-CoA and an acetyltransferase enzyme (Ch. 44). White populations contain roughly equal numbers of 'fast acetylators' and 'slow acetylators' (i.e. a 'balanced polymorphism' as described above). The characteristic of fast or slow acetylation is controlled by a single recessive gene associated with low hepatic acetyltransferase activity. Other ethnic groups have different proportions of fast and slow acetylators. Isoniazid causes two distinct forms of toxicity. One is peripheral neuropathy, which is produced by isoniazid itself and is commoner in slow acetylators. The other is hepatotoxicity, which has been related to conversion of the acetylated metabolite to acetylhydrazine and is commoner in fast acetylators, at least in some populations. This type of genetic variation thus produces a qualitative change in the pattern of toxicity caused by the drug in different populations. Acetyltransferase is also important in the metabolism of other drugs, including hydralazine (Ch. 18), procainamide (Ch. 17) and various sulfonamides (Ch. 44).

Drugs for which such polymorphic variation is important include **phenytoin**, an anticonvulsant (Ch. 39); **debrisoquine**, a hypotensive drug that is obsolete therapeutically but useful because it is a convenient indicator for several other drugs metabolised by the same form of cytochrome P450 (Ch. 8); and **mercaptopurine**, an antitumour drug (Ch. 50).

Genetic factors

- Genetic variation is an important source of pharmacokinetic variability.
- There are several clear examples where genetic variation influences drug response, including:
  - —fast/slow acetylators (hydralazine, procainamide, isoniazid)
  - —plasma cholinesterase variants (suxamethonium)
  - —hydroxylase polymorphism (debrisoquine).
- In future, profiling an individual's DNA for single nucleotide polymorphisms (SNPs) could provide a way to anticipate drug responsiveness.

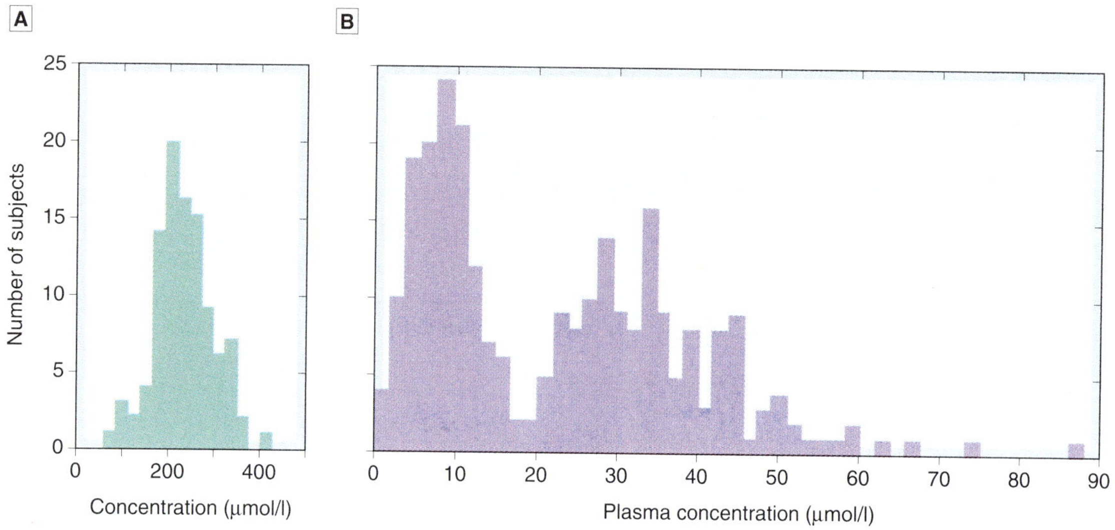

Fig. 51.3 Distribution of individual plasma concentrations for two drugs in humans. A Plasma salicylate concentration 3 hours after oral dosage with sodium salicylate at 0.19 mmol/kg. B Plasma isoniazid concentration 6 hours after oral dosage. Note the normally distributed values for salicylate, compared with the bimodal distribution of isoniazid. (From: (A) Evans & Clarke 1961 Br Med Bull 17: 234–280; (B) Price-Evans D A 1963 Am J Med 3: 639.)

Suxamethonium provides a well-studied example of genetic variation in the rate of drug metabolism as a result of a Mendelian autosomal recessive trait. This short-acting neuromuscular-blocking drug is widely used in anaesthesia and is normally rapidly hydrolysed by plasma cholinesterase (Ch. 10). About 1 in 3000 individuals fail to inactivate suxamethonium rapidly and experience prolonged neuromuscular block if treated with it; this is because a recessive gene gives rise to an abnormal type of plasma cholinesterase. The abnormal enzyme has a modified pattern of substrate and inhibitor specificity. It is detected by measuring the effect of the inhibitor dibucaine, which inhibits the abnormal enzyme less than the normal enzyme. Heterozygotes hydrolyse suxamethonium at a more or less normal rate, but their plasma cholinesterase has reduced sensitivity to dibucaine, intermediate between normals and homozygotes (Fig. 51.4). There are other, non-genetic, reasons why suxamethonium hydrolysis may be impaired in an individual patient (see p. 155), so it is important to discover whether this genetic abnormality is present in patients who experience prolonged paralysis following treatment with this drug, and to test family members who may be affected.

IDIOSYNCRATIC REACTIONS

An idiosyncratic reaction is a qualitatively abnormal, and usually harmful, drug effect that occurs in a small proportion of individuals. For example, chloramphenicol causes aplastic anaemia in approximately 1 in 50 000 patients (p. 645). In many cases, genetic anomalies are responsible, though the mechanisms are often poorly understood. G6PD deficiency (see above) is the basis for the most common known form of genetically determined adverse reaction to drugs, a discovery that stemmed from investigation of the antimalarial drug **primaquine** (Ch. 48), which, while well tolerated in most individuals, causes haemolysis leading to severe anaemia in 5–10% of Afro-Caribbean men. This reaction, in sensitive individuals, also occurs with other drugs, including **dapsone**, **doxorubicin** and some sulfonamide drugs, and after eating the bean Vicia fava or inhaling its pollen. This underlies the condition known as favism characterised in severely affected individuals by life-threatening haemolysis. This was described in antiquity in Mediterranean countries and in China. G6PD is necessary to maintain the content of reduced glutathione (GSH) in red cells, GSH being necessary to prevent haemolysis. Primaquine and related substances reduce red cell GSH harmlessly in normal cells but enough to cause haemolysis in G6PD-deficient cells. As explained above, heterozygote females, who show no tendency to haemolysis, have an increased resistance to malaria, providing a selective advantage that accounts for the persistence of the gene in regions where malaria is endemic.

The hepatic *porphyrias* are prototypic pharmacogenetic disorders. Although individually rare, they are clinically important. The well-intentioned use of sedative, antipsychotic or analgesic drugs in patients with undiagnosed hepatic porphyria can be lethal, whereas with appropriate supportive management most patients recover completely.* These disorders are

*Life expectancy, obtained from parish records, of patients with porphyria dignosed retrospectively within large kindreds in Scandinavia was normal until the advent and widespread use of barbiturates and opioids in the 19th century, when it plummeted.

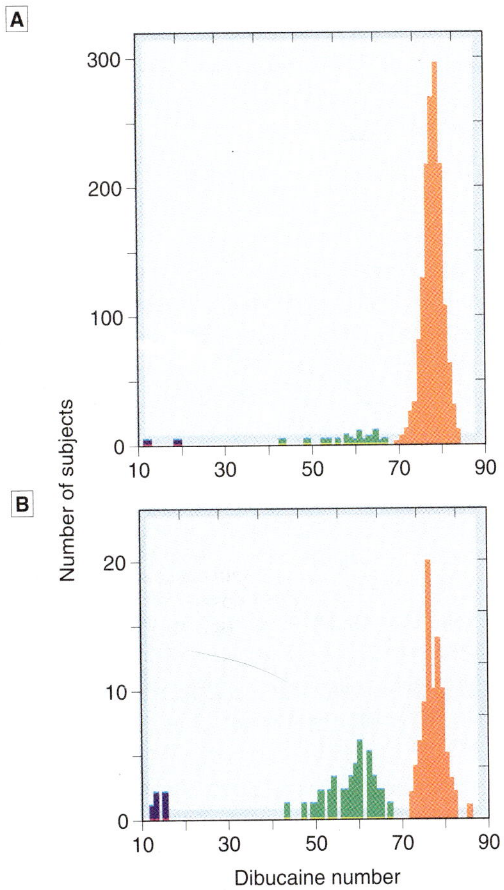

Fig. 51.4 Distribution of plasma cholinesterase phenotypes in humans. Dibucaine number is a measure of the percentage inhibition of plasma cholinesterase by 10^{-5} mol/l dibucaine. The abnormal enzyme has, in addition to low enzymic activity, a low dibucaine number. A Normal population. B Families of subjects with low or intermediate dibucaine numbers. (From: Kalow 1962 Pharmacogenetics. W. B. Saunders, Philadelphia, PA.)

characterised by absence of one of the enzymes required for haem synthesis, with the result that various porphyrin-containing haem precursors accumulate, giving rise to acute attacks of gastrointestinal, neurological and behavioural disturbances. Many drugs, especially but not exclusively those that induce hepatic mixed function P450 oxidase enzymes (e.g. barbiturates, **griseofulvin**, **carbamazepine**, estrogens), can precipitate acute attacks in susceptible individuals. Porphyrins are synthesised from δ-amino laevulinic acid (ALA), formed by ALA synthase in the liver. This enzyme is induced, like various other hepatic enzymes, by drugs such as barbiturates, resulting in increased ALA production and, hence, increased porphyrin accumulation.

Various other diseases cause genetically determined idiosyncratic reactions. These include *malignant hyperthermia*, a metabolic reaction to drugs including **suxamethonium** and various inhalational anaesthetic and antipsychotic drugs. It is caused by an inherited abnormality in the Ca^{2+} release channel of the sarcoplasmic reticulum in striated muscle, which is known as the ryanodine receptor (Ch. 4).

Immunological mechanisms underlie many idiosyncratic reactions. They are considered further in Chapter 52.

Idiosyncratic reactions

- Harmful, sometimes fatal, reactions that occur in a small minority of individuals.
- Reactions may occur with low doses.
- Genetic factors may be responsible (e.g. primaquine sensitivity, malignant hyperthermia), though often the cause is poorly understood (e.g. bone marrow depression with chloramphenicol).
- Immunological factors are also important (see Ch. 52).

EFFECTS OF DISEASE

Detailed consideration of the many diseases that are important as a cause of individual variation is beyond the scope of this book. Disease can cause pharmacokinetic or pharmacodynamic variation. Common disorders such as impaired renal or hepatic function predispose to toxicity by causing unexpectedly intense or prolonged drug effects. Drug absorption is slowed in conditions causing gastric stasis (e.g. *migraine*, *diabetic neuropathy*) and may be incomplete in patients with malabsorption owing to ileal or pancreatic disease or to oedema of the ileal mucosa caused by heart failure or nephrotic syndrome. *Nephrotic syndrome* (characterised by heavy proteinuria, oedema and a reduced concentration of albumin in plasma) alters drug absorption because of oedema of intestinal mucosa, alters drug disposition through changes in binding to plasma albumin and causes insensitivity to diuretics such as **furosemide** (frusemide) that act on ion transport mechanisms on the luminal surface of tubular epithelium (Ch. 23), through binding to albumin in tubular fluid. Hypothyroidism is associated with increased sensitivity to several widely used drugs (e.g. **pethidine**), for reasons that are poorly understood. *Hypothermia* (to which elderly persons, in particular, are predisposed) markedly reduces the clearance of many drugs.

Other disorders, although unusual, are important because they illustrate mechanisms that may prove to be of more general applicability. Examples include:

- diseases that influence receptors:
  —*myasthenia gravis*, an autoallergic disease characterised by antibodies to nicotinic acetylcholine receptors (Ch. 10)
  —*X-linked nephrogenic diabetes insipidus*, characterised by abnormal antidiuretic hormone (vasopressin) receptors
  —*familial hypercholesterolaemia*, an inherited disease of low density lipoprotein receptors (Ch. 19).

Variation due to disease

Pharmacokinetic alterations in:

- Absorption:
  - —gastric stasis (e.g. migraine)
  - —malabsorption (e.g. steatorrhoea from pancreatic insufficiency)
  - —oedema of ileal mucosa (e.g. heart failure, nephrotic syndrome).
- Distribution:
  - —altered plasma protein binding (e.g. of phenytoin in chronic renal failure)
  - —impaired blood–brain barrier (e.g. to penicillin in meningitis).
- Metabolism:
  - —chronic liver disease
  - —hypothermia.
- Excretion:
  - —acute and/or chronic renal failure.

Pharmacodynamic alterations in:

- Receptors (e.g. myasthenia gravis, nephrogenic diabetes insipidus, familial hypercholesterolaemia).
- Signal transduction (e.g. pseudohypoparathyroidism, familial precocious puberty).
- Unknown mechanisms (e.g. increased sensitivity to pethidine in hypothyroidism).

- diseases that influence signal transduction mechanisms:
  - —*pseudohypoparathyroidism*, which stems from impaired coupling of receptors with adenylate cyclase
  - —*familial precocious puberty*, and *hyperthyroidism caused by functioning thyroid adenomas*, which are each caused by mutations in G-protein-coupled receptors that result in the receptors remaining 'turned on' even in the absence of the hormones that are their natural agonists.

DRUG INTERACTIONS

Many patients, especially the elderly, are treated continuously with one or more drugs for chronic diseases such as hypertension, heart failure, osteoarthritis and so on. Acute events (e.g. infections, myocardial infarction) are treated with additional drugs. The potential for drug interactions is, therefore, substantial and 'polypharmacy' is an important factor to consider when prescribing in this group. Drugs can also interact with other dietary constituents (e.g. grapefruit juice, which downregulates expression of a specific isoform of P450, CYP3A4, in the gut wall) and herbal remedies (such as St John's wort), the latter becoming more widely used despite flimsy or absent evidence of safety or efficacy. The administration of one drug (A) can alter the action of another (B) by one of two general mechanisms:*

- modification of the pharmacological effect of B without altering its concentration in the tissue fluid (pharmacodynamic interaction)
- alteration of the concentration of B that reaches its site of action (pharmacokinetic interaction).

For such interactions to be important clinically, it is necessary that the therapeutic range of drug B is narrow (i.e. that a small reduction in effect will lead to loss of efficacy and/or a small increase in effect will lead to toxicity). For pharmacokinetic interactions to be clinically important it is also necessary that the concentration–response curve of drug B is steep (so that a small change in plasma concentration leads to a substantial change in effect). For many drugs, these conditions are not met: even quite large changes in plasma concentrations of relatively non-toxic drugs like **penicillin** are unlikely to give rise to clinical problems because there is usually a comfortable safety margin between plasma concentrations produced by usual doses and those resulting in either loss of efficacy or toxicity. Several drugs do have steep concentration–response relationships and a narrow therapeutic margin and, for these, drug interactions can cause major problems, for example with antithrombotic, antidysrhythmic and antiepileptic drugs, lithium and several antineoplastic and immunosuppressant drugs.

PHARMACODYNAMIC INTERACTION

Pharmacodynamic interaction can occur in many different ways (including those discussed under 'Drug antagonism' in Ch. 2). There are many mechanisms, and some examples of practical importance are probably more useful than attempts at classification.

- Beta-adrenoceptor antagonists diminish the effectiveness of β-adrenoceptor agonists, such as **salbutamol** or **terbutaline** (Ch. 11).
- Many diuretics lower plasma K^+ concentration (see Ch. 23), and thereby enhance some actions of cardiac glycosides and predispose to glycoside toxicity and to toxicity with type III antidysrhythmic drugs that prolong the cardiac action potential (Ch. 17).
- **Sildenafil** inhibits the isoform of phosphodiesterase (PDE type 5) that inactivates cGMP (Chs 14 and 29); consequently, it potentiates organic nitrates, which work by activating guanylate cyclase, and can cause severe hypotension in patients taking these drugs.
- Monoamine oxidase inhibitors increase the amount of noradrenaline stored in noradrenergic nerve terminals and

*A third category of pharmaceutical interactions should be mentioned, in which drugs interact in vitro so that one or both are inactivated. No pharmacological principles are involved, just chemistry. An example is the formation of a complex between **thiopental** and **suxamethonium**, which must not be mixed in the same syringe. **Heparin** is highly charged and interacts in this way with many basic drugs; it is sometimes used to keep intravenous lines or cannulae open and can inactivate basic drugs if they are injected without first clearing the line with saline.

thereby interact dangerously with drugs, such as **ephedrine** or **tyramine**, that work by releasing stored noradrenaline. This can also occur with tyramine-rich foods—particularly fermented cheeses such as Camembert (see Ch. 38).

- **Warfarin** competes with vitamin K, preventing hepatic synthesis of various coagulation factors (see Ch. 20). If vitamin K production in the intestine is inhibited (e.g. by antibiotics), the anticoagulant action of warfarin is increased.
- The risk of bleeding, especially from the stomach, caused by warfarin is increased by drugs that cause bleeding by different mechanisms (e.g. **aspirin**, which inhibits platelet thromboxane A_2 biosynthesis and which can damage the stomach; Ch. 16).
- Sulfonamides prevent the synthesis of folic acid by bacteria and other microorganisms; **trimethoprim** inhibits its reduction to tetrahydrofolate. Given together, the drugs have a synergistic action of value in treating *Pneumocystis carinii* (Ch. 45).
- Non-steroidal anti-inflammatory drugs (NSAIDs; Ch. 16), such as **ibuprofen** or **indometacin**, inhibit biosynthesis of prostaglandins, including renal vasodilator/natriuretic prostaglandins (PGE_2, PGI_2). If administered to patients receiving treatment for hypertension, they cause a variable but sometimes marked increase in blood pressure. If given to patients being treated with diuretics for chronic heart failure, they can cause salt and water retention and hence cardiac decompensation.*
- Histamine H_1-receptor antagonists, such as **mepyramine**, commonly cause drowsiness as an unwanted effect. This is more troublesome if such drugs are taken with alcohol, and it may lead to accidents at work or on the road.

PHARMACOKINETIC INTERACTION

All of the four major processes that determine pharmacokinetic behaviour—absorption, distribution, metabolism and excretion—can be affected by drugs. Pharmacokinetic interactions have received a great deal of attention, and examples have sprouted in the literature like mushrooms. Some of the more important mechanisms are given here, with examples.

Absorption

Gastrointestinal absorption is slowed by drugs that inhibit gastric emptying, such as **atropine** or opiates, or accelerated by drugs that hasten gastric emptying (e.g. **metoclopramide**; see Ch. 24). Alternatively, drug A may interact with drug B in the gut in such a way as to inhibit absorption of B (cf. pharmaceutical interactions; see footnote, p. 718). For example, Ca^{2+} (and also iron) forms an insoluble complex with tetracycline and retards its absorption; **colestyramine**, a bile acid-binding resin used to treat hypercholesterolaemia (Ch. 19), binds several drugs (e.g. **warfarin**, **digoxin**), preventing their absorption if administered simultaneously. Another example is the addition of **adrenaline** (epinephrine) to local anaesthetic injections: the resulting vasoconstriction slows the absorption of the anaesthetic, thus prolonging its local effect (Ch. 42).

Drug distribution

One drug may alter the distribution of another, but such interactions are seldom clinically important. Displacement of a drug from binding sites in plasma or tissues transiently increases the concentration of free (unbound) drug, but this is followed by increased elimination so a new steady state results, in which total drug concentration in plasma is reduced but the free drug concentration is similar to that before introduction of the second 'displacing' drug. There are several direct consequences of potential clinical importance:

- toxicity from the transient increase in concentration of free drug before the new steady state is reached.
- if dose is being adjusted according to measurements of total plasma concentration, it must be appreciated that the target therapeutic concentration range will be altered by coadministration of a displacing drug
- when the displacing drug additionally reduces elimination of the first, so the free concentration is increased not only acutely but also chronically at the new steady state, severe toxicity may ensue.

Though many drugs have appreciable affinity for plasma albumin and, therefore, might potentially be expected to interact in these ways, there are rather few instances of clinically important interactions of this type. Protein-bound drugs that are given in large enough dosage to act as 'displacing agents' include various **sulfonamides** and **chloral hydrate**; trichloracetic acid, a metabolite of chloral hydrate, binds very strongly to plasma albumin. Displacement of *bilirubin* from albumin by such drugs in jaundiced premature neonates could have clinically disastrous consequences: bilirubin metabolism is undeveloped in the premature liver and unbound bilirubin can cross the immature blood–brain barrier and cause *kernicterus* (staining of the basal ganglia by bilirubin). This causes a distressing and permanent disturbance of movement known as choreoathetosis, characterised by involuntary writhing and twisting movements in the child.

Phenytoin dose is adjusted according to measurement of its concentration in plasma, and such measurements do not routinely distinguish bound from free phenytoin (that is, they reflect the total concentration of drug). Introduction of a displacing drug in an epileptic patient stabilised on phenytoin (Ch. 39) reduces the total plasma phenytoin concentration owing to increased elimination of free drug, but there is no loss of efficacy because the concentration of unbound (active) phenytoin at the new steady state is unaltered. If it is not appreciated that the therapeutic range of plasma concentrations has been reduced in this way, an increased dose may be prescribed, resulting in toxicity.

*The interaction with diuretics may involve a pharmacokinetic interaction in addition to the pharmacodynamic effect described here, because NSAIDs can compete with weak acids, including diuretics, for renal tubular secretion, see below.

There are several instances where drugs that alter protein binding additionally reduce elimination of the displaced drug, causing clinically important interactions. **Phenylbutazone** displaces **warfarin** from binding sites on albumin and more importantly selectively inhibits metabolism of the pharmacologically active (*S*)-isomer (see below), prolonging prothrombin time and resulting in increased bleeding (Ch. 20). **Salicylates** displace **methotrexate** from binding sites on albumin and reduce its secretion into the nephron by competition with the anion secretory carrier (Ch. 8). **Quinidine** and several other antidysrhythmic drugs including **verapamil** and **amiodarone** (Ch. 17) displace **digoxin** from tissue-binding sites while simultaneously reducing its renal excretion; they, consequently, can cause severe dysrhythmias through digoxin toxicity.

Drug metabolism

Drugs can both inhibit (Table 51.2) and induce (Table 51.3) the drug-metabolising enzymes, giving rise to both hazard and advantage.

Enzyme induction

Enzyme induction (e.g. by barbiturates, ethanol or **rifampicin**; see Ch. 8) is also an important cause of drug interaction. Over 200 drugs cause enzyme induction and thereby decrease the pharmacological activity of a range of other drugs. Some examples are given in Table 51.3. Since the inducing agent is normally itself a substrate for the induced enzymes, the process can result in slowly developing tolerance. This pharmacokinetic kind of tolerance is generally less marked than pharmacodynamic tolerance to opioids (Ch. 40), but it is clinically important in starting treatment with **carbamazepine**. This is initiated at a low dose to avoid toxicity (since liver enzymes are not induced initially) and gradually increased over a period of a few weeks during which it induces its own metabolism.

Figure 51.5 shows how the antibiotic **rifampicin**, given for 3 days, reduces the effectiveness of **warfarin** as an anticoagulant. Conversely, enzyme induction can increase toxicity of a second drug if its toxic effects are mediated via a metabolite. **Paracetamol** toxicity is a case in point (see Fig. 52.1): it is caused by *N*-acetyl-*p*-benzoquinone imine, which is formed by cytochrome P450. Consequently, the risk of serious hepatic injury following paracetamol overdose is increased in patients whose cytochrome P450 system has been induced, for example by chronic use of alcohol. It is likely that part of the variability in rates of drug metabolism between individuals results from varying exposure to environmental contaminants, some of which are strong enzyme inducers.

Enzyme induction is exploited therapeutically, by administering **phenobarbital** to premature babies to induce glucuronyltransferase, thereby increasing bilirubin conjugation and reducing the risk of kernicterus (see above).

Enzyme inhibition

Enzyme inhibition, particularly of the P450 system, slows the metabolism and hence increases the action, of other drugs metabolised by the enzyme. Such effects can be clinically important and are major considerations in the treatment of patients with human immunodeficiency virus (HIV) infection with triple and quadruple therapy, since some protease inhibitors are potent inhibitors of P450 enzymes (Ch. 46). Another example is the interaction between the non-sedating antihistamine **terfenadine** and imidazole antifungal drugs such as **ketoconazole** and other drugs that inhibit the CYP3A subfamily of P450 enzymes (Ch. 8). This can result in prolongation of the **Q–T interval*** on the electrocardiogram and a form of ventricular tachycardia in susceptible individuals. *Grapefruit juice* reduces the metabolism of terfenadine and other drugs, including **ciclosporin** and several calcium channel antagonists.

Table 51.2 Examples of drugs that inhibit drug-metabolising enzymes

Drugs inhibiting enzyme action	Drugs with metabolism affected
Allopurinol	Mercaptopurine, azathioprine
Chloramphenicol	Phenytoin
Cimetidine	Amiodarone, phenytoin, pethidine
Ciprofloxacin	Theophylline
Corticosteroids	Tricyclic antidepressants, cyclophosphamide
Ciprofloxacin	Theophylline
Disulfiram	Warfarin
Erythromycin	Ciclosporin, theophylline
Monoamine oxidase inhibitors	Pethidine
Ritonavir	Saquinavir

Table 51.3 Examples of drugs that induce drug-metabolising enzymes

Drugs inducing enzyme action	Drugs with metabolism affected
Phenobarbital Rifampicin Griseofulvin Phenytoin Ethanol Carbamazepine	Warfarin Oral contraceptives Corticosteroids Ciclosporin Drugs listed in left-hand column will also be affected

*The Q–T interval (see Fig. 14.1) normally varies physiologically with the heart rate; this is corrected for by calculating a corrected Q–T interval (Q–Tc) by dividing by the square root of the R–R interval.

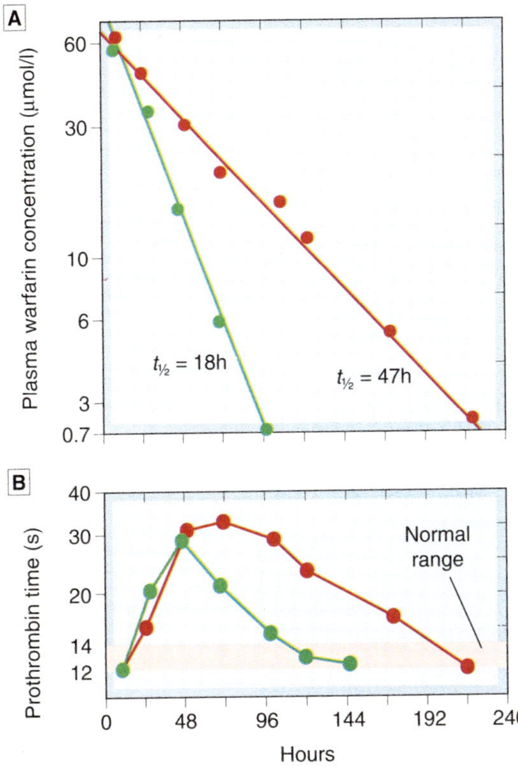

Fig. 51.5 Effect of rifampicin on the metabolism and anticoagulant action of warfarin. A Plasma concentration of warfarin (log scale) as a function of time following a single oral dose of 5 μmol/kg body weight. After the subject was given rifampicin (600 mg daily for a few days), the plasma half-life of warfarin decreased from 47 hours (red curve) to 18 hours (green curve). B The effect of a single dose of warfarin on prothrombin time under normal conditions (red curve) and after rifampicin administration (green curve). (Redrawn from: O'Reilly 1974 Ann Intern Med 81: 337.)

To make life even more difficult, several inhibitors of drug metabolism influence the metabolism of different stereoisomers selectively. Examples of drugs that inhibit the metabolism of the active (*S*)- and less active (*R*)-isomers of warfarin in this way are shown in Table 51.4.

The therapeutic effects of some drugs are a direct consequence of enzyme inhibition (e.g. the xanthine oxidase inhibitor allopurinol, used to prevent gout; Ch. 16). Xanthine oxidase metabolises several cytotoxic and immunosuppressant drugs, including **mercaptopurine** (the active metabolite of azathioprine), the action of which is thus potentiated and prolonged by allopurinol. **Disulfiram**, an inhibitor of aldehyde dehydrogenase used to produce an aversive reaction to ethanol (see Ch. 52), also inhibits metabolism of other drugs, including **warfarin**, which it potentiates. **Metronidazole**, an antimicrobial used to treat anaerobic bacterial infections and several protozoal diseases (Chs 45 and 48), also inhibits this enzyme, and patients prescribed it are advised to avoid alcohol for this reason.

Table 51.4 Stereoselective and non-stereoselective inhibition of warfarin metabolism

Inhibition of metabolism	Drug
Stereoselective for (S)-isomer	Phenylbutazone
	Metronidazole
	Sulfinpyrazone
	Trimethoprim–sulfamethoxazole
	Disulfiram
Stereoselective for (R)-isomer	Cimetidine[a]
	Omeprazole[a]
Non-stereoselective effect on both isomers	Amiodarone

[a]Minor effect only on prothrombin time.
From: Hirsh 1991 N Engl J Med 324: 1865–1875.

In other instances, inhibition of drug metabolism is less expected since enzyme inhibition is not the main mechanism of action of the offending agents. Thus **steroids** and **cimetidine** enhance the actions of a range of drugs including some antidepressant and cytotoxic drugs. The only rule for prescribers is: if in doubt about the existence of a possible interaction, look it up (e.g. in the British National Formulary, which has an invaluable appendix on drug interactions indicating which are of known clinical importance).

Haemodynamic effects

Variations in hepatic blood flow influence the rate of inactivation of drugs that are subject to extensive presystemic hepatic metabolism (e.g. **lidocaine** or **propranolol**). A reduced cardiac output reduces hepatic blood flow, so negative inotropes (e.g. propranolol) reduce the rate of metabolism of lidocaine by this mechanism.

Drug excretion

The main mechanisms by which one drug can affect the rate of renal excretion of another are:

- by altering protein binding, and hence filtration
- by inhibiting tubular secretion
- by altering urine flow and/or urine pH.

Inhibition of tubular secretion

Probenecid (Ch. 23) was developed expressly to inhibit **penicillin** secretion and thus prolong its action. It also inhibits the excretion of other drugs, including **zidovudine** (see Ch. 46). Other drugs have an incidental probenecid-like effect and can

Drug interactions

- These are many and varied; the rule is: if in doubt, look it up.
- Interactions may be pharmacodynamic or pharmacokinetic .
- Pharmacodynamic interactions are often predictable from the actions of the interacting drugs.
- Pharmacokinetic interactions can involve effects on:
  —absorption
  —distribution (e.g. competition for protein binding)
  —hepatic metabolism (induction or inhibition)
  —renal excretion.

Table 51.5 Examples of drugs that inhibit renal tubular secretion

Drugs causing inhibition	Drugs affected
Probenecid Sulfinpyrazone Phenylbutazone Sulfonamides Aspirin Thiazide diuretics Indometacin	Penicillin Azidothymidine Indometacin
Verapamil Amiodarone Quinidine	Digoxin
Indometacin	Furosemide (frusemide)
Aspirin Non-steroidal anti-inflammatory drugs	Methotrexate

enhance the actions of substances that rely on tubular secretion for their elimination. Table 51.5 gives some examples. Since diuretics act from within the tubular lumen, drugs that inhibit their secretion into the tubular fluid, such as NSAIDs, reduce their effect.

Alteration of urine flow and pH

Diuretics tend to increase the urinary excretion of other drugs, but this is seldom clinically important. Conversely, loop and thiazide diuretics indirectly increase the proximal tubular reabsorption of **lithium** (which is handled in a similar way as Na^+) and this can cause lithium toxicity in patients treated with lithium carbonate for mood disorders (Ch. 38). The effect of urinary pH on the excretion of weak acids and bases is put to use in the treatment of poisoning (see Ch. 8), but it is not a cause of accidental interactions.

REFERENCES AND FURTHER READING

Bailey D G, Malcolm J, Arnold O, Spence J D 1998 Grapefruit juice—drug interactions. Br J Clin Pharmacol 46: 101–110 (*Review*)

Barry M, Mulcahy F, Merry C, Gibbons S, Back D 1999 Pharmacokinetics and potential interactions amongst antiretroviral agents used to treat patients with HIV infection. Clin Pharmacokinet 36: 289–304 (*Multidrug combinations have transformed the outlook for patients with HIV infection. Drug interactions are one of the main problems associated with these*)

Carmichael D J S 1998 Handling of drugs in kidney disease. In: Davison A M, Grünfeld J-P, Kerr D, Ritz E Oxford textbook of clinical nephrology, 2nd edn. Oxford University Press, Oxford, pp. 2659–2678 (*Discusses the influence on pharmacokinetics of renal failure and nephrotic syndrome and outlines a practical approach to prescribing in such patients*)

Fugh-Berman A, Ernst E 2001 Herb–drug interactions: review and assessment of report reliability. Br J Clin Pharmacol 52: 587–595 (*Warfarin the most common drug, St John's wort the most common herb. More data needed! See also Fugh-Berman A 2000 Lancet 355: 134–138*)

Hanratty C G, McGlinchey P, Johnston G D, Passmore A P 2000 Differential pharmacokinetics of digoxin in elderly patients. Drugs Aging 17: 353–362 (*Reviews pharmacokinetics of digoxin in relation to age, concomitant disease and interacting drugs*)

Ito K, Iwatsubo T, Kanamitsu S, Ueda K, Suzuki H, Sugiyama Y 1998 Prediction of pharmacokinetic alterations caused by drug—drug interactions: metabolic interactions in the liver. Pharmacol Rev 50: 387–411 (*Can one predict pharmacokinetic changes from findings in isolated human hepatocytes? Reviews influences of plasma protein binding, hepatic upake, transport systems etc.*)

Lin J H, Liu A Y H 2001 Interindividual variability in inhibition and induction of cytochrome P450 enzymes. Annu Rev Pharmacol Toxicol 41: 535–567 (*Examines sources of interindividual variability in inhibition and induction of P450 enzymes*)

Morgan D J 1997 Drug disposition in mother and fetus. Clin Exp Pharmacol Physiol 24: 869–873 (*Review*)

Pirmohamed M, Park B K 2001 Genetic susceptibility to adverse drug reactions. Trends in Pharmacological Sciences 22: 298–304 (*Up-to-date review, with sensibly sceptical approach to possibility that genotyping will prove useful in preventing adverse drug reactions which 'needs to be proven by use of prospective controlled clinical trials'*)

Price-Evans D A 1993 Genetic factors in drug therapy, clinical and molecular pharmacogenetics. Cambridge University Press, Cambridge (*Scholarly tour de force. Also a surprisingly good read!*)

Rane A 1985 Drug metabolism and disposition in neonates and infancy. In: Wilkinson G R, Rawlins D M (eds) Drug metabolism and disposition. MTP Press, Lancaster, UK.

Ritter J M, Lewis L D, Mant T G K 1999 A textbook of clinical pharmacology, 4th edn. Edward Arnold, London (*Chapters on drugs at extremes of age, pregnancy and drug interactions provide an introduction*)

Roden D M, George A L 2002 The genetic basis of variability in drug responses. Nat Rev Drug Discov 1: 37–44 (*Discusses the concept that genetic variants determine much of the variability in response to drugs*)

Rowland M, Tozer T N 1995 Clinical pharmacokinetics, concepts and applications. Williams & Wilkins, Baltimore, MD, pp. 203–312 (*See section IV: 'Individualization'*)

Sproule B A, Hardy B G, Shulman K I 2000 Differential pharmacokinetics in elderly pateients. Drugs Aging 16: 165–177 (*Reviews age-related changes in pharmacodynamics as well as pharmacokinetics and drug*

interactions, all of which are clinically important)
Westphal J F 2000 Macrolide-induced clinically relevant drug interactions with cytochrome P450A (CYP) 3A4: an update focused on clarithromycin, azithromycin and dirithromycin. Br J Clin Pharmacol 50: 285–295 (*Review: theophylline, ciclosporine, warfarin, involvement of P-glycoprotein as well as metabolism*)
Wood A J J 2001 Racial differences in response to drugs—pointers to genetic differences. N Engl J Med 344: 1393–1396
Xie H-G, Kim R B, Wood A J J, Stein C M 2001 Molecular basis of ethnic differences in drug disposition and response. Annu Rev Pharmacol Toxicol 41: 815–850 (*Recent developments in understanding genetic variations that may underlie ethnic differences in drug-metabolising enzymes, transporters, receptors and second messenger systems*)
Zevin S, Benowitz N L 1999 Drug interactions with tobacco smoking—an update. Clin Pharmacokinet 36: 425–438 (*Polycyclic aromatic hydrocarbons in tobacco smoke induce various P450 enzymes. 'Cigarette smoking should be specifically studied in clinical trials of new drugs'*)

52 Harmful effects of drugs

Overview 724

Types of adverse drug reaction 724

Drug toxicity 725
- Toxicity testing 725
- General mechanisms of toxin-induced cell damage and cell death 725
- Mutagenesis and carcinogenicity 729
- Teratogenesis and drug-induced fetal damage 731
- Allergic reactions to drugs 735

OVERVIEW

Clinically important adverse drug reactions are diverse. Any organ system can be the principal target, or several systems can be involved simultaneously. The time course of an adverse drug effect sometimes closely shadows drug administration and discontinuation, but in other cases adverse effects are delayed, first appearing months or years after chronic treatment is started. Such events represent a huge challenge in terms of their initial recognition, and even when they have been well described, such reactions can be difficult to diagnose in individual patients. Some adverse effects occur typically at the end of treatment, when drug administration is stopped. Consequently, anticipating, avoiding, recognising and responding to adverse drug reactions are among the most challenging and important parts of clinical practice. In this chapter we discuss:

- **types of adverse drug reaction**
- **toxicity testing in animals**
- **general mechanisms of toxin-induced cell damage and cell death**
- **mutagenesis and carcinogenesis**
- **teratogenesis**
- **allergic reactions to drugs.**

TYPES OF ADVERSE DRUG REACTION

All drugs can produce harmful as well as beneficial effects. These are either related or unrelated to the principal pharmacological action of the drug. Adverse effects are of great concern to drug regulatory authorities, which are charged with establishing the safety as well as the efficacy of drugs before these are licensed for marketing. This concern is especially great for adverse effects that are unpredictable.

Adverse effects related to the main pharmacological action of the drug

Many adverse effects related to the main pharmacological action of the drug are predictable, at least if this action is well understood. They are sometimes referred to as type A ('augmented') adverse reactions (Rawlins & Thompson, 1985). Many such reactions have been described in previous chapters. For example, postural hypotension occurs with α_1-adrenoceptor antagonists, bleeding with anticoagulants, cardiac dysrhythmias with glycosides, sedation with anxiolytics and so on. In many instances, this type of unwanted effect is reversible, and the problem can often be dealt with by reducing the dose. Such effects are sometimes serious (e.g. intracerebral bleeding caused by anticoagulants, hypoglycaemic coma from insulin) and occasionally they are not easily reversible, for example drug dependence produced by opiate analgesics (see Ch. 42).

Adverse effects unrelated to the main pharmacological action of the drug

Adverse effects unrelated to the main pharmacological effect may be predictable when a drug is taken in *excessive dose* (e.g. **paracetamol** hepatotoxicity, **aspirin**-induced tinnitus, aminoglycoside ototoxicity), during *pregnancy* (e.g. **thalidomide** teratogenicity), or by patients with a *predisposing disorder* (e.g. **primaquine**–induced haemolysis in patients with glucose 6-phospate dehydrogenase (G6PD) deficiency, as described in Ch. 51).

Sometimes a predictable subsidiary pharmacological effect can have serious implications for rare susceptible individuals: there is concern over effects of drugs on the electrocardiographic Q–T interval for this reason (see Chs 8, 17 and 51).

Rare unpredictable adverse effects have also been mentioned in earlier chapters, including aplastic anaemia from

chloramphenicol, anaphylaxis in response to **penicillin** and oculomucocutaneous syndrome with **practolol**, a β_1-selective antagonist that had to be withdrawn because of this problem. These idiosyncratic reactions are termed type B ('bizarre') in the Rawlins & Thompson (1985) classification. They are usually severe—otherwise they would go unrecognised—and their existence is important in establishing the safety of medicines.

▼ If the incidence of an adverse reaction is 1 in 6000 patients exposed, approximately 18 000 patients would have to be exposed to the drug for three events to occur and approximately double that number for three events to be detected and their possible relationship to the drug recognised and reported, even if there were no background incidence of the event in question. Consequently, such reactions cannot be excluded by early-phase clinical trials (which might typically expose only 1–2000 individuals to the drug), and the association may only come to light after years of use. A recent example is an association between pulmonary hypertension or valvular heart disease with **fenfluramine**, an appetite suppressant that had been used for several years, and with **dexfenfluramine** its pharmacologically active isomer. Such experiences are not unique and call for prudence in prescribing newly introduced drugs. They also illustrate the need for continued monitoring by regulatory authorities after drugs have been licensed and marketed. Different countries have responded to this need in different ways, and harmonising the procedures of the different agencies involved is a major international challenge, currently being addressed through a body known as the International Conference on Harmonisation (ICH).

Idiosyncratic reactions are often initiated by a chemically reactive metabolite rather than the parent drug. Such indirect toxicity may be direct or immunological in nature. Examples include liver or kidney damage, bone marrow suppression, carcinogenesis and disordered fetal development. Such effects (which are by no means confined to drugs, being liable to occur with any kind of chemical) fall conventionally into the area of toxicology rather than pharmacology.

DRUG TOXICITY

TOXICITY TESTING

Toxicity testing in animals is carried out on new drugs to identify potential hazards before administering them to humans. It involves the use of a wide range of tests in different species, with long-term administration of the drug, regular monitoring for physiological or biochemical abnormalities, and a detailed postmortem examination at the end of the trial to detect any gross or histological abnormalities. Such studies are performed with doses well above the expected therapeutic range, and they determine which tissues or organs are likely 'targets' of toxic effects of the drug. Recovery studies are performed to assess whether toxic effects are reversible, and particular attention is paid to irreversible changes such as carcinogenesis or neurodegeneration. The basic premise is that toxic effects caused by a drug are similar in humans and other animals. This is inherently reasonable in view of the similarities between higher organisms at the cellular and molecular levels. There are, nevertheless, wide interspecies variations, especially in metabolising enzymes; consequently, a toxic metabolite formed in one species may not be formed in another and so toxicity testing in animals is not always a reliable guide. Toxic effects can range from negligible to so severe as to preclude further development of the compound. Intermediate levels of toxicity are more acceptable in drugs intended for the more severe illnesses (for example the acquired immunodeficiency syndrome (AIDS) or cancers) and decisions on whether or not to continue development are often difficult. If development does proceed, safety monitoring can be concentrated on the system 'flagged' as a potential target of toxicity by the animal studies.* *Safety* of a drug (as opposed to toxicity) can only be established during use in humans.

Types of drug toxicity

- Toxic effects of drugs can be:
  - —related to the principal pharmacological action, e.g. bleeding with anticoagulants
  - —unrelated to the principal pharmacological action, e.g. liver damage with paracetamol.
- Some adverse reactions that occur with ordinary therapeutic dosage are unpredictable, serious and uncommon (e.g. agranulocytosis with carbimazole). Such idiosyncratic reactions are almost inevitably only detected after widespread use of a new drug.
- Adverse effects unrelated to the main action of a drug are often caused by reactive metabolites and/or immunological reactions.

GENERAL MECHANISMS OF TOXIN-INDUCED CELL DAMAGE AND CELL DEATH

Toxic concentrations of drugs or drug metabolites can cause *necrosis;* however, programmed cell death (*apoptosis*; see Ch. 5) is increasingly recognised to be of paramount importance, especially in chronic toxicity.

Chemically reactive drug metabolites can form covalent bonds with target molecules or alter the target molecule by non-covalent interactions. Some metabolites do both. The liver is of great importance in drug metabolism (Ch. 8), and hepatocytes are exposed to high concentrations of nascent metabolites as these are formed by cytochrome P450-dependent drug oxidation. Drugs and their polar metabolites are concentrated in renal tubular fluid as water is reabsorbed, so renal tubules are exposed

*The value of toxicity testing is illustrated by experience with **triparanol**, a cholesterol-lowering drug marketed in the USA in 1959. Three years later a team from the Food and Drug Administration (FDA), acting on a tip-off, paid the manufacturer a surprise visit that revealed falsification of toxicology data demonstrating cataracts in rats and dogs. The drug was withdrawn, but some patients who had been taking it for a year or more also developed cataracts. Regulatory authorities now require that toxicity testing is performed under a tightly defined code of practice (Good Laboratory Practice), which incorporates many safeguards to minimise the risk of error or fraud.

to higher concentrations than are other tissues. Furthermore, renal vascular mechanisms are critical to the maintenance of glomerular filtration and are vulnerable to drugs that interfere with the control of afferent and efferent arteriolar contractility. It is, therefore, not surprising that hepatic or renal damage are common reasons for abandoning development of drugs during toxicity testing.

NON-COVALENT INTERACTIONS

Reactive metabolites of drugs can be involved in several related, potentially cytotoxic, non-covalent interactions including:

- lipid peroxidation
- generation of toxic oxygen radicals
- reactions causing depletion of glutathione (GSH)
- modification of sulfhydryl groups.

Some of these effects are also produced by covalent reactions.

Lipid peroxidation

Lipid peroxidation of polyunsaturated lipids can be initiated either by reactive metabolites or by reactive oxygen species generated by such metabolites (see below). Lipid peroxyradicals ($ROO^{\bullet}$) can produce lipid hydroperoxides (ROOH), which produce further lipid peroxyradicals. This chain reaction—a peroxidative cascade—may eventually affect much of the membrane lipid. Cell damage and eventually cell death can result from alteration of membrane permeability or from reactions of the products of lipid peroxidation with proteins. Defence mechanisms, for example glutathione peroxidase and vitamin E, protect against this, so lipid peroxidation may not, in itself, be sufficient to cause cell death.

Generation of toxic oxygen radicals

Generation of toxic oxygen radicals by reactive metabolites involves reduction of molecular oxygen to superoxide anion (O_2) followed by enzymic conversion to hydrogen peroxide (H_2O_2) or to reactive species such as the hydroperoxy ($HOO^{\bullet}$) and hydroxyl ($OH^{\bullet}$) radicals or singlet oxygen. These reactive oxygen species are cytotoxic, both directly and through lipid peroxidation (see above).

Depletion of glutathione

Reactions causing depletion of GSH result in oxidative stress, which is a disturbance in the pro-oxidant/antioxidant balance in cells in favour of the pro-oxidant state. It can be caused by accumulation of the normal oxidative products of cell metabolism, or by the action of toxic chemicals. The GSH redox cycle is a protective system that minimises cell damage from oxidative stress. GSH is normally maintained in a redox couple with its disulfide, GSSG. Oxidising species convert GSH to GSSG, GSH being regenerated by NADPH-dependent GSSG-reductase. When cellular GSH falls to about 20–30% of normal, cellular defence against toxic compounds is impaired and cell death can result.

Modification of sulfhydryl groups

Modification of sulfhydryl groups can be produced either by oxidising species that alter sulfhydryl groups reversibly or by covalent interaction. Free sulfhydryl groups have a critical role in the catalytic activity of many enzymes, and modification of such sulfhydryl groups results in inactivation. Important targets for sulfhydryl modification by reactive metabolites include the cytoskeletal protein actin, glutathione reductase (see above) and Ca^{2+}-transporting ATPases in the plasma membrane and endoplasmic reticulum. These maintain cytoplasmic Ca^{2+} concentration at approximately 0.1 μmol/l, in the face of an external Ca^{2+} concentration of more than 1 mmol/l. A sustained rise in cell Ca^{2+} occurs with inactivation of these enzymes (or with increased membrane permeability; see above), and this compromises cell viability. Lethal processes leading to cell death after acute Ca^{2+} overload include activation of degradative enzymes (neutral proteases, phospholipases, endonucleases) and protein kinases, mitochondrial damage and cytoskeletal alterations (e.g. modification of association between actin and actin-binding proteins).

COVALENT INTERACTIONS

Targets for covalent interactions include DNA, proteins/peptides, lipids and carbohydrates. Covalent bonding to DNA is a basic mechanism of action of mutagenic chemicals; this is dealt with below. Several non-mutagenic chemicals also form covalent

General mechanisms of cell damage and cell death

- Drug-induced cell damage/death is usually caused by reactive metabolites of the drug, involving non-covalent and/or covalent interactions with target molecules. Cell death is often 'self-inflicted', via triggering of apoptosis rather than caused by acute necrosis.
- Non-covalent interactions include:
  —lipid peroxidation; peroxyradicals produce hydroperoxides that produce further peroxyradicals and so on
  —generation of cytotoxic oxygen radicals
  —reactions causing depletion of glutathione, resulting in 'oxidative stress'
  —modification of sulfhydryl groups on key enzymes (e.g. Ca^{2+}-ATPases, glutathione disulfide reductase) and structural proteins.
- Covalent interactions, e.g. adduct formation between the metabolite of paracetamol (NAPBQI: *N*-acetyl-*p*-benzoquinone imine) and cellular macromolecules (Fig. 52.1). Covalent binding to protein can produce an immunogen; binding to DNA can cause carcinogenesis and teratogenesis.

bonds with macromolecules, but the relationship between this and cell damage is not clear. For example, the cholinesterase inhibitor **paraoxon** binds acetylcholinesterase at the neuromuscular junction and causes necrosis of skeletal muscle. One toxin from an exceptionally poisonous toadstool, *Amanita phalloides*, binds actin and another binds to RNA polymerase, interfering with actin depolymerisation and protein synthesis, respectively.

HEPATOTOXICITY

Many therapeutic drugs cause liver damage, manifested clinically as hepatitis or (in less severe cases) only as laboratory abnormalities (e.g. increased plasma aspartate transaminase activity). **Paracetamol**, **isoniazid**, **iproniazid** and **halothane** cause hepatotoxicity by the mechanisms of cell damage outlined above. Genetic differences in drug metabolism (see Ch. 51) have been implicated in some instances (e.g. **isoniazid**, **phenytoin**). Mild drug-induced abnormalities of liver function are not uncommon but the mechanism of liver injury is often uncertain (e.g. statins; Ch. 19). It is not always necessary to discontinue a drug when such mild laboratory abnormalities occur, but the occurrence of irreversible liver disease (cirrhosis) as a result of long-term low-dose **methotrexate** treatment (Ch. 16) for psoriasis (a chronic skin disease of unknown cause that is usually mild, if tiresome, but can rarely be very severe*) argues for caution. Hepatotoxicity of a different kind, namely reversible obstructive jaundice, occurs with **chlorpromazine** (Ch. 37) and **androgens** (Ch. 29).

Hepatotoxicity caused by toxic doses of **paracetamol** is clinically important (paracetamol was the fourth most common cause of death following self-poisoning in the UK in 1989). An outline of the initial reactions in which this drug is involved is given in Chapter 16 (p. 252). Because the body's handling of this drug exemplifies many of the general mechanisms of cell damage outlined above, the story is taken up again here. With toxic doses of paracetamol, the enzymes catalysing the normal conjugation reactions are saturated (see Ch. 16), and mixed-function oxidases convert the drug to the reactive metabolite *N*-acetyl-*p*-benzoquinone imine (NAPBQI). As explained in Chapters 8 and 51, paracetamol toxicity is increased in patients in whom P450 enzymes have been induced, for instance by chronic excessive consumption of alcohol. NAPBQI initiates several of the covalent and non-covalent interactions described above and illustrated in Figure 52.1. Oxidative stress from GSH depletion is important in

*Afficionados of Dennis Potter will recall the protagonist in the television drama 'The Singing Detective'; Potter was himself afflicted by the most severe form of the disease.

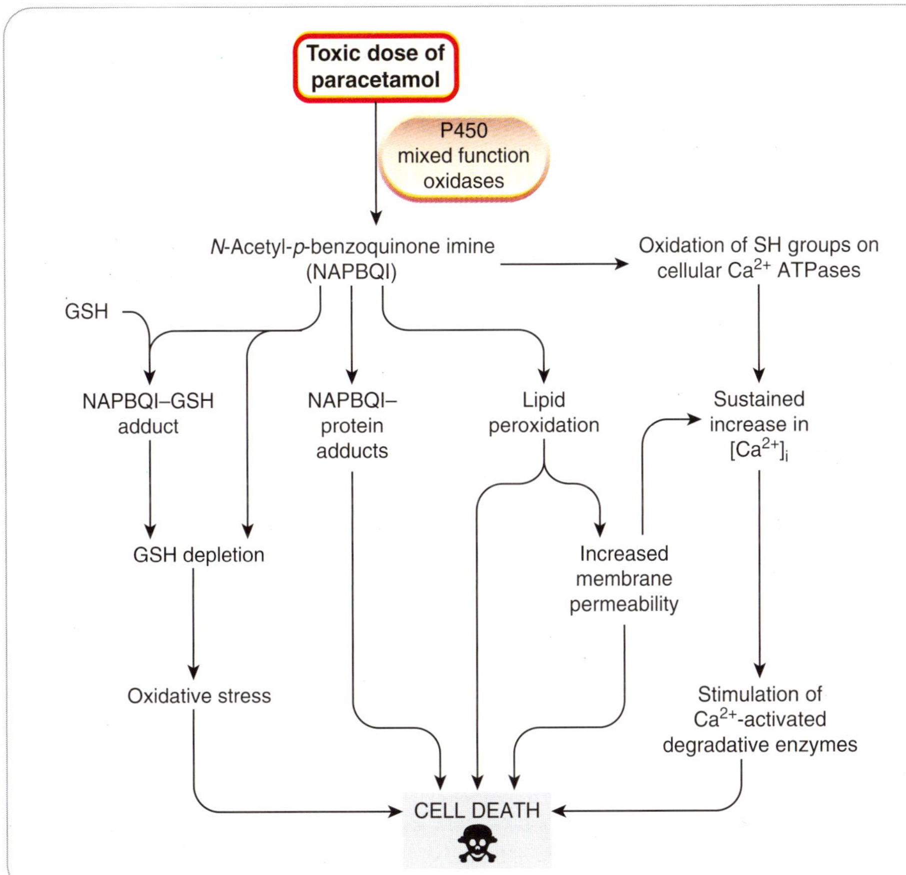

Fig. 52.1 Potential mechanisms of liver cell death resulting from the metabolism of paracetamol to *N*-acetyl-*p*-benzoquinone imine (NAPBQI). (GSH, glutathione.) (Based on data from: Boobis A R et al. 1989, and Nelson S D, Pearson P G 1990 Annu Rev Pharmacol Toxicol 30: 169.)

Hepatotoxicity

- Hepatocytes are exposed to reactive metabolites of drugs as these are formed by P450 enzymes.
- Liver damage can be produced by general mechanisms of cell injury; paracetamol exemplifies many of these (see Fig. 52.1).
- Some drugs (e.g. chlorpromazine) can cause reversible cholestatic jaundice.
- Immunological mechanisms are sometimes implicated (e.g. halothane).

leading to cell death, although the precise mechanism is not yet clear. Synthesis of new GSH depends on the availability of cysteine, the intracellular availability of which can be limiting. Acetylcysteine or methionine increase GSH availability and reduce mortality in patients with severe paracetamol poisoning.

Liver damage can also be produced by immunological mechanisms (see below), which have been particularly implicated in halothane hepatitis (see Ch. 35).

NEPHROTOXICITY

Drug-induced nephrotoxicity is a common clinical problem. Indeed, non-steroidal anti-inflammatory drugs (NSAIDs; Table 52.1) and angiotensin-converting enzyme inhibitors (ACEI) are currently among the commonest causes of acute renal failure. This is usually caused by the principal pharmacological actions of these drugs, which, although well tolerated in healthy people, cause renal failure in patients with diseases that jeopardise glomerular filtration. In patients with heart or liver disease, glomerular filtration rate (GFR) depends critically on vasodilator prostaglandin biosynthesis. This is inhibited by NSAIDs (Ch. 15) and hence these drugs reduce renal perfusion in such patients. Similarly, in patients with bilateral renal artery stenosis, GFR depends on angiotensin-II-mediated efferent arteriolar vasoconstriction (which is inhibited by ACEI; Ch. 18); acute renal impairment occurs on starting an ACEI drug and is reversible if the drug is discontinued promptly. Additionally, NSAIDs indirectly depress renin and aldosterone secretion by inhibiting renal prostaglandin I_2 biosynthesis, and ACEI depress angiotensin II-stimulated aldosterone secretion. Reduced aldosterone can cause hyperkalaemia, especially if GFR is also reduced.

In addition to these effects related to their main pharmacological action, NSAIDs can also cause an allergic interstitial nephritis. This is rare but severe and usually occurs several months to 1 year after starting treatment. It manifests clinically as acute renal failure, often accompanied by eosinophil leucocytes in the urine and proteinuria, or as nephrotic syndrome (heavy proteinuria, hypoalbuminuria and oedema). **Fenoprofen** is particularly liable to cause this type of renal damage, possibly because its metabolites bind irreversibly to albumin. Penicillins (Ch. 44), especially **meticillin**, also cause interstitial nephritis.

Analgesic nephropathy is a third kind of renal damage in which NSAIDs are implicated. This consists of renal papillary necrosis* and chronic *interstitial nephritis*. The clinical course is typically insidious but leads ultimately to end-stage chronic renal failure. It is associated with prolonged and massive overuse of analgesics. **Phenacetin** has particularly been incriminated, but **paracetamol** and NSAIDs have not been exonerated. The role of **caffeine**

*It is worth noting that the renal papilla is the part of the kidney exposed to the highest concentration of solutes, including drug metabolites; it also has a lower blood flow than other parts as a result of counter-current exchange in the vasa recta.

Table 52.1 Adverse effects of non-steroidal anti-inflammatory drugs on the kidney

Cause	Adverse effect
Principal pharmacological action (i.e. inhibition of prostaglandin biosynthesis)	Acute ischaemic renal failure Sodium retention (leading to or exacerbating hypertension and/or heart failure) Water retention Hyporeninaemic hypoaldosteronism (leading to hyperkalaemia)
Unrelated to principal pharmacological action (allergic-type interstitial nephritis)	Renal failure Proteinuria
Unknown whether or not related to principal pharmacological action (analgesic nephropathy)	Papillary necrosis Chronic renal failure

Adapted from: Murray & Brater 1993

Nephrotoxicity

- The kidney is exposed to high concentrations of drugs and drug metabolites as the urine is concentrated.
- Renal damage can be produced by general mechanisms of cell injury, which can cause papillary and/or tubular necrosis.
- Reduction in compensatory vasodilator prostaglandins can result in increased renal vascular resistance and decreased renal function.

(often included with analgesics and NSAIDs in combined preparations) is uncertain but could be important. It is possible that such analgesic-associated nephropathy is causally related to inhibition of renal prostaglandin synthesis, but its pathogenesis is not understood.

Captopril, in higher doses than are currently recommended, can cause heavy proteinuria (Ch. 18). This is the result of glomerular injury, which is also caused by some other drugs that, like captopril, contain a sulfhydryl group (e.g. **penicillamine**). It is, therefore, believed that it is this chemical feature rather than ACE inhibition per se that is responsible for this adverse effect.

Ciclosporin, used to prevent transplant rejection (Ch. 16), causes renal damage via renal vasoconstriction, which reduces GFR and causes hypertension. It alters renal prostaglandin biosynthesis.

Many drugs that cause hepatotoxicity (e.g. **paracetamol**) can also cause toxic damage to the kidney, most commonly by producing necrosis of renal tubular cells. The mechanisms involved are described above (p. 727).

MUTAGENESIS AND CARCINOGENICITY

Mutation is a change in the genotype of a cell that is passed on when the cell divides. Chemical agents cause mutation by covalent modification of DNA. Certain kinds of mutation result in carcinogenesis, because the affected DNA sequence codes for a protein that is involved in growth regulation. It usually requires more than one mutation in a cell to initiate the changes that result in malignancy, mutations in proto-oncogenes (which regulate cell growth) and tumour suppressor genes (which code for products that inhibit the transcription of oncogenes) being particularly implicated (see Ch. 5). Some oncogenes code for modified growth factors or growth factor receptors, or for elements of the intracellular transduction mechanism by which growth factors regulate cell proliferation (see p. 694). Growth factors are polypeptide mediators that stimulate cell division; examples are *epidermal growth factor* and *platelet-derived growth factor*. The receptors for these growth factors regulate a number of cellular processes through tyrosine phosphorylation (see Fig. 3.15). Though there are many details to be filled in, the complex connection between exposure to a mutagenic chemical and the development of a cancer is beginning to be understood.

Mutagenesis and carcinogenicity

- Mutagenesis involves alteration of the genotype of a cell by modification of DNA.
- Carcinogenesis involves alteration of proto-oncogenes or tumour suppressor genes by mutation; more than one mutation is usually required.
- Drugs are relatively uncommon (but not unimportant) causes of birth defects and cancers.

BIOCHEMICAL MECHANISMS OF MUTAGENESIS

▼ Most chemical carcinogens act by modifying bases in DNA, particularly guanine, the O6 and N7 positions of which readily combine covalently with reactive metabolites of chemical carcinogens. Substitution at the O6 position is the more likely to produce a permanent mutagenic effect, since N7 substitutions are usually quickly repaired.

The accessibility of bases in DNA to chemical attack is greatest when DNA is in the process of replication (i.e. during cell division). The likelihood of genetic damage by many mutagens is, therefore, related to the frequency of cell division. The developing fetus is particularly susceptible, and mutagens are also potentially teratogenic (see below). This is also important in relation to mutagenesis of germ cells, particularly in the female, because in humans the production of primary oocytes occurs by a rapid succession of mitotic divisions very early in embryogenesis. Each of these primary oocytes then undergoes only two further divisions much later in life at the time of ovulation. It is, consequently, during early pregnancy that germ cells of the developing female embryo are most likely to undergo mutagenesis, the mutations being transmitted to progeny conceived many years after exposure to the mutagen. In the male, germ cell divisions occur throughout life, and sensitivity to mutagens is continuously present.

The importance of drugs, in comparison with other chemicals such as pollutants and food additives, as a causative factor in mutagenesis has not been established, and such epidemiological evidence as exists suggests that they are uncommon (but not unimportant) causes of fetal malformations and cancers.

CARCINOGENESIS

Alteration of DNA is the first step in the complex, multistage process of carcinogenesis (see Ch. 5). Carcinogens are chemical substances that cause cancer, and can interact directly with DNA or act at a later stage to increase the likelihood that mutation will result in the production of a tumour (Fig. 52.2). Carcinogens are divided into two groups.

- *Genotoxic carcinogens* (i.e. mutagens, as discussed above). These are also termed 'initiators' and can be further divided into:
  —primary carcinogens, which act on DNA directly
  —secondary carcinogens, which must be converted to a reactive metabolite before they affect DNA Most important carcinogens fall into this category.

- *Epigenetic carcinogens* (i.e. agents that do not themselves cause genetic damage, but increase the likelihood that such damage will cause cancer). There are several different types of epigenetic carcinogen, the most important being:
  —promoters: these are not carcinogenic by themselves, but increase the likelihood of tumour development from genetically damaged cells; they can thus produce cancers when given after a genotoxic agent; examples include *phorbol esters*, bile acids, saccharin (in large doses) and *cigarette smoke* (which not only contains carcinogenic aromatic hydrocarbons but also has promoter activity)
  —co-carcinogens: these substances are not carcinogenic by themselves but enhance the effect of genotoxic agents when given simultaneously; examples include phorbol esters and various aromatic and aliphatic hydrocarbons; some chemicals have both genotoxic and promoter/co-carcinogenic activity
  —hormones: some tumours are hormone dependent (see Ch. 50), important examples being oestrogen-dependent breast cancers and androgen-dependent prostatic cancers. Endometrial hyperplasia induced by prolonged estrogen treatment increases the risk of uterine carcinoma unless countered by cyclical progestogen administration. This is probably the result of expression of a pre-existing change in the DNA during cellular proliferation. Hormone replacement therapy with estrogen for postmenopausal women with an intact uterus is, therefore, accompanied by cyclical treatment with a progestogen (Ch. 29).

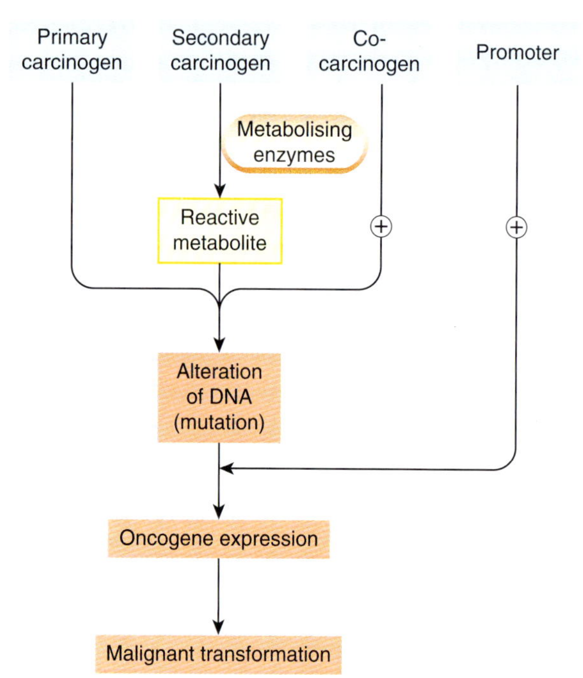

Fig. 52.2 Sequence of events in mutagenesis and carcinogenesis.

MEASUREMENT OF MUTAGENICITY AND CARCINOGENICITY

Much effort has gone into developing tests for detecting mutagenicity and carcinogenicity. These can be broadly divided into:

- *In vitro tests for mutagenicity*. These rapid tests are suitable for screening large numbers of compounds, but they can give positive results on compounds that are not subsequently shown to be carcinogenic in tests on whole animals, and they can miss known carcinogens.
- *Whole animal tests for carcinogenicity*. Such tests are expensive and time consuming, but they are usually required by drug regulatory authorities before a new drug is licensed for use in humans. The main limitation of this kind of study is that there are important species differences, mainly to do with the metabolism of the foreign compound and the formation of reactive products.
- *Whole animal tests for teratogenesis (reproductive-toxicity testing)*. Tests on pregnant animals are required for drugs that are to be used by women of reproductive potential, especially (obviously) if they are to be used during pregnancy. Similar limitations of such tests apply as with carcinogenicity testing.

In vitro tests for genotoxic carcinogens

Bacteria have great advantages as a test system for measuring mutagenicity because of their high replication rate. The most widely used assays are variations on the *Ames test*, which measures the rate of back-mutation (i.e. reversion from mutant to wild-type form) in a culture of *Salmonella typhimurium*.

▼ The normal, wild-type strain can grow in a medium containing no added amino acids, because it can synthesise all the amino acids it needs from simple carbon and nitrogen sources. The test makes use of the fact that a mutant form of the organism cannot make histidine in this way and, therefore, only grows on a medium containing this amino acid. The test involves growing the mutant form on a medium containing a small amount of histidine, the drug to be tested being added to the culture. After several divisions, the histidine becomes depleted, and the only cells that continue dividing are those that have back-mutated to the wild type. A count of colonies following subculture on plates deficient in histidine gives a measure of the mutation rate.

Primary carcinogens cause mutation by a direct action on bacterial DNA but most carcinogens have to be converted to an active metabolite (see above). Therefore, it is necessary to include, in the culture, enzymes that catalyse the necessary conversion. An extract of liver from a rat treated with phenobarbital to induce liver enzymes is usually employed. There are many variations based on the same principle.

Other short-term in vitro tests for genotoxic chemicals include measurements of mutagenesis in mouse lymphoma cells, and assays for chromosome aberrations and sister chromatid exchanges in Chinese hamster ovary (CHO) cells. However, all the in vitro tests give some false positives and some false negatives.

In vivo tests for carcinogenicity

In vivo tests for carcinogenicity entail detection of tumours in groups of test animals. Carcinogenicity tests are inevitably slow, since there is usually a latency of months or years before tumours

Carcinogens

- Carcinogens can be:
  - *genotoxic*, i.e. causing mutations directly (primary carcinogens) or after conversion to reactive metabolites (secondary carcinogens)
  - *epigenetic*, i.e. increasing the possibility that a mutagen will cause cancer, though not themselves mutagenic.
- Epigenetic carcinogens include 'promoters', which increase cancer rate if given after the mutagen, and 'co-carcinogens', which increase the rate if given with it. Phorbol esters have both actions.
- New drugs are tested for mutagenicity and carcinogenicity.
- The main test for mutagenicity measures back-mutation, in histidine-free medium, of a mutant *Salmonella typhimurium* (which, unlike the wild type, cannot grow without histidine) in the presence of:
  - the chemical to be tested
  - a liver microsomal enzyme preparation for generating reactive metabolites.

  Colony growth indicates that mutagenesis has occurred. The test is rapid and inexpensive, but some false positives and false negatives occur.
- Carcinogenicity testing:
  - involves chronic dosing of groups of animals
  - is expensive and time-consuming
  - there is no really suitable test for epigenetic carcinogens.

develop. Furthermore, tumours can develop spontaneously in control animals, and the results often provide only equivocal evidence of carcinogenicity of the test drug, making it difficult for industry and regulatory authorities to decide on further development and possible licensing of a product. None of the tests so far described can reliably detect epigenetic carcinogens. To do this, it is necessary to measure the effect of the test substance on tumour production with a threshold dose of a genotoxic agent. Such tests are being evaluated.

Few therapeutic drugs are known to increase the risk of cancer, the most important groups being drugs that act on DNA, i.e. cytotoxic and immunosuppressant drugs, and sex hormones (e.g. **estrogens**, which increase the occurrence of endometrial cancer and possibly also cancer of other sex hormone-responsive organs). **Pyrimethamine** (Ch. 47) is mutagenic in high concentrations, and carcinogenicity testing in strain A mice (but not other strains or species) was positive for a threefold increase in lung tumours. **Methoxsalen** (a psoralen used together with ultraviolet light (PUVA) in special skin disease centres for treatment of psoriasis) is both mutagenic and carcinogenic in animal models, and it may increase the incidence of skin cancer in humans.

TERATOGENESIS AND DRUG-INDUCED FETAL DAMAGE

The term teratogenesis is used to signify the production of gross structural malformations during fetal development, to distinguish it from other kinds of drug-induced fetal damage such as growth retardation, dysplasia (e.g. iodide-associated goitre) or the asymmetric limb reduction resulting from vasoconstriction caused by **cocaine** (see Ch. 42) in an otherwise normally developing limb. Examples of drugs that affect fetal development adversely are given in Table 52.2.

It has been known since about 1920 that external agents can affect fetal development, when it was discovered that X-irradiation during pregnancy could cause fetal malformation or death. Nearly 20 years later, the importance of rubella infection was recognised, but it was not until 1960 that drugs were implicated as causative agents in teratogenesis: the shocking experience with **thalidomide** led to a widespread reappraisal of many other drugs in clinical use, and to the setting up of drug regulatory bodies in many countries. Most birth defects (about 70%) occur with no recognisable causative factor. Drug or chemical exposure during pregnancy are believed to account for only about 1% of all fetal malformations. While this percentage may appear small, the total numbers affected are substantial.

MECHANISM OF TERATOGENESIS

The timing of the teratogenic insult in relation to the stage of fetal development is critical in determining the type and extent of damage produced. Mammalian fetal development passes through three phases (Table 52.3):

- blastocyst formation
- organogenesis
- histogenesis and maturation of function.

Cell division is the main process occurring during blastocyst formation. During this phase, drugs can cause death of the embryo by inhibiting cell division, but provided the embryo survives, its subsequent development does not generally seem to be compromised, although ethanol may affect development at this very early stage (Ch. 42).

It is during organogenesis, which occurs during days 17–60, that drugs can cause gross malformations. The structural organisation of the embryo occurs in a well-defined sequence: eye and brain, skeleton and limbs, heart and major vessels, palate, genitourinary system. The type of malformation produced thus depends on the time of exposure to the teratogen.

The cellular mechanisms by which teratogenic substances produce their effects are not at all well understood. There is a considerable overlap between mutagenicity and teratogenicity. In one large survey, among 78 compounds, 34 were both teratogenic and mutagenic, 19 were negative in both tests and 25 (among them thalidomide) were positive in one but not the other. It, therefore, seems that damage to DNA is important, but, as with carcinogenesis, it is certainly not the only factor. The control of morphogenesis is poorly understood; *vitamin A derivatives*

Table 52.2 Drugs reported to have adverse effects on human fetal development

Agent	Effect	Teratogenicity	See Chapter
Thalidomide	Phocomelia, heart defects, gut atresia, etc.	K	52
Penicillamine	Loose skin etc.	K	16
Warfarin	Saddle nose, retarded growth, defects of limbs, eyes, CNS	K	20
Corticosteroids	Cleft palate and congenital cataract—rare		27
Androgens	Masculinisation in female		29
Estrogens	Testicular atrophy in male		29
Stilbestrol	Vaginal adenosis in female fetus, also vaginal or cervical cancer	20+ years later	29
Anticonvulsants			
Phenytoin	Cleft lip/palate, microcephaly, mental retardation	K	39
Valproate	Neural tube defects, e.g. spina bifida	K	39
Carbamazepine	Retardation of fetal head growth	S	39
Cytotoxic drugs (especially folate antagonists)	Hydrocephalus, cleft palate, neural tube defects, etc.	K	49
Aminoglycosides	Deafness		44
Tetracycline	Staining of bones and teeth, thin tooth enamel, impaired bone growth	S	44
Ethanol	Fetal alcohol syndrome	K	52
Retinoids	Hydrocephalus etc.	K	51
Angiotensin-converting enzyme inhibitors	Oligohydramnios, renal failure	K	18

K, known teratogen (in experimental animals and/or humans); S, suspected teratogen (in experimental animals and/or humans).
Adapted from: Juchau 1989 Annu Rev Pharmacol Toxicol 29: 165.

Table 52.3 The nature of drug effects on fetal development

Stage	Gestation period in humans	Main cellular processes	Affected by
Blastocyst formation	0–16 days	Cell division	Cytotoxic drugs, ?alcohol
Organogenesis	17–60 days approximately	Division	Teratogens
		Migration	Teratogens
		Differentiation	Teratogens
		Death	Teratogens
Histogenesis and functional maturation	60 days to term	As above	Miscellaneous drugs, e.g. alcohol, nicotine, antithyroid drugs, steroids

(retinoids) are involved and are potent teratogens (see below). Known teratogens also include several drugs (e.g. **methotrexate** and **phenytoin**) that do not react directly with DNA but which inhibit its synthesis by their effects on *folate metabolism*. Administration of **folate** during pregnancy reduces the frequency of both spontaneous and drug-induced malformations, especially *neural tube defects*.

In the final stage of histogenesis and functional maturation, the fetus is dependent on an adequate supply of nutrients, and development is regulated by a variety of hormones. Gross structural malformations do not arise from exposure to mutagens at this stage, but drugs that interfere with the supply of nutrients or with the hormonal milieu may have deleterious effects on growth and development. Exposure of a female fetus to androgens at this stage can cause masculinisation. **Stilbestrol** was commonly given to pregnant women with a history of recurrent miscarriage during the 1950s (for unsound reasons) and causes dysplasia of the vagina of the infant and an increased incidence of carcinoma of the vagina in the teens and twenties. Angiotensin is believed to play an important part in the later stages of fetal development and in renal function in the fetus, and ACEI and angiotensin receptor antagonists ('sartans') cause oligohydramnios and renal failure if administered during later stages of pregnancy. They have also been associated with skull defects in experimental animals.

TESTING FOR TERATOGENICITY

The **thalidomide** disaster dramatically brought home the need for routine teratogenicity studies on new therapeutic drugs. Assessment of teratogenicity in humans is a particularly difficult problem, for various reasons. One is that the 'spontaneous' malformation rate is high (3–10% depending on the definition of a significant malformation) and highly variable between different regions, age groups and social classes. Large-scale studies are required, which take many years and much money to perform, and they usually give suggestive, rather than conclusive, results.

In vitro methods, based on the culture of cells, organs or whole embryos, have not so far been developed to a level where they satisfactorily predict teratogenesis in vivo, and most regulatory authorities require teratogenicity testing in one rodent (usually rat or mouse) and one non-rodent (usually rabbit) species. Pregnant females are dosed at various levels during the critical period of organogenesis, and the fetuses are examined for structural abnormalities. However, poor cross-species correlation means that tests of this kind are not reliably predictive in humans, and it is usually recommended that new drugs are not used in pregnancy unless it is essential.

SOME DEFINITE AND PROBABLE HUMAN TERATOGENS

Though many drugs have been found to be teratogenic in varying degrees in experimental animals, relatively few are known to be teratogenic in humans (see Table 52.2). Some of the more important are discussed below.

Thalidomide

Thalidomide is virtually unique in producing, at therapeutic dosage, virtually 100% malformed infants when taken in the first 3–6 weeks of gestation. It was introduced in 1957 as a hypnotic and sedative with the special feature that it was extremely safe in overdosage, and it was even recommended specifically for use in pregnancy (with the advertising slogan 'the safe hypnotic'). As was then normal, it had been subjected only to acute toxicity testing, and not to chronic toxicity* or teratogenicity testing. Thalidomide was marketed energetically and successfully, and the first suspicion of its teratogenicity arose early in 1961 with reports of a sudden increase in the incidence of phocomelia. This abnormality ('seal limbs') consists of an absence of development of the long bones of the arms and legs and had hitherto been virtually unknown. At this time approximately 1 000 000 tablets were being sold daily in West Germany. Reports of phocomelia came simultaneously from Hamburg and Sydney, and the connection with thalidomide was made. The drug was withdrawn late in 1961, by which time an estimated 10 000 malformed babies had been born (Fig. 52.3). In spite of intensive study, its mechanism of action remains poorly understood, although epidemiological investigation showed very clearly the correlation between the time of exposure and the type of malfunction produced (Table 52.4).

Cytotoxic drugs

Many alkylating agents (e.g. **chlorambucil** and **cyclophosphamide**) and antimetabolites (e.g. **azathioprine** and **mercaptopurine**) cause malformations when used in early pregnancy but more often lead to abortion (see Ch. 49). Folate antagonists (e.g. **methotrexate**) produce a much higher incidence

*A severe peripheral neuropathy, leading to irreversible paralysis and sensory loss, was reported within a year of the drug's introduction and subsequently confirmed in many reports. The drug company responsible was less than punctilious in acting on these reports (see Sjostrom H, Nilsson R 1972 Thalidomide and the power of the drug companies. Penguin Books, London), which were soon eclipsed by the discovery of teratogenic effects, but the neurotoxic effect was severe enough in its own right to have necessitated withdrawal of the drug from general use. Today, use of thalidomide has had a small resurgence related to several highly specialised applications. It is prescribed by specialists (in dermatology, and in HIV infection among others) under tightly controlled and restricted conditions.

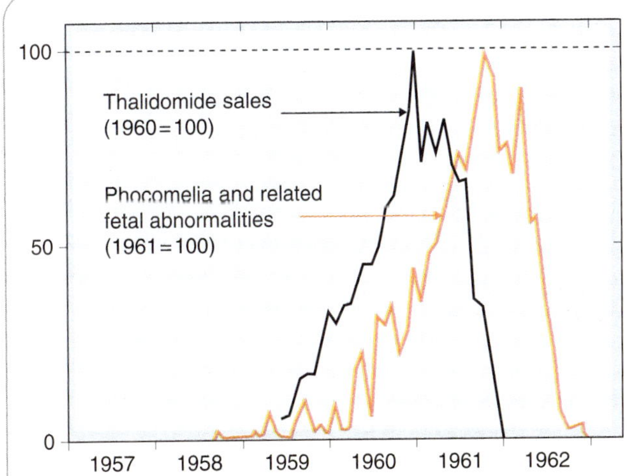

Fig. 52.3 Incidence of major fetal abnormalities in Western Europe following the introduction and withdrawal of thalidomide.

Table 52.4 Thalidomide teratogenesis

Day of gestation	Type of deformity
21–22	Malformation of ears Cranial nerve defects
24–27	Phocomelia of arms
28–29	Phocomelia of arms and legs
30–36	Malformation of hands Anorectal stenosis

of major malformations, evident in both live-born and still-born fetuses.

Retinoids

Etretinate, a retinoid (i.e. vitamin A derivative) with marked effects on epidermal differentiation, is a known teratogen and causes a high proportion of serious abnormalities (notably skeletal deformities) in exposed fetuses. Dermatologists use retinoids to treat skin diseases including several, such as acne and psoriasis, which are common in young women. Etretinate accumulates in subcutaneous fat and is eliminated extremely slowly, detectable amounts persisting for many months after chronic dosing is discontinued. Because of this, women should avoid pregnancy for at least 2 years after treatment. **Acitretin** is an active metabolite of etretinate. It is equally teratogenic, but tissue accumulation is less pronounced and elimination may, therefore, be more rapid.

Heavy metals

Lead, *cadmium* and *mercury* all cause fetal malformations in humans. The main evidence comes from *Minamata disease*, named after the locality in Japan where an epidemic occurred when the local population ate fish contaminated with methylmercury that had been used as an agricultural fungicide. This impaired brain development in exposed fetuses, resulting in cerebral palsy and mental retardation, often with microcephaly. Mercury, like other heavy metals, inactivates many enzymes by forming covalent bonds with sulfhydryl and other groups, and this is believed to be responsible for these developmental abnormalities.

Antiepileptic drugs

Congenital malformations are increased two- to threefold in babies of epileptic mothers. Interestingly, all existing antiepileptic drugs have been implicated including **phenytoin** (particularly cleft lip/palate), **valproate** (neural tube defects) and **carbamazepine** (spina bifida and hypospadias—a malformation of the male urethra) as well as newer agents (Ch. 39).

Teratogenesis and drug-induced fetal damage

- Teratogenesis means production of gross structural malformations of the fetus, e.g. the absence of limbs after thalidomide. Less-comprehensive damage can be produced by many other drugs (see Table 52.2). Less than 1% of congenital fetal defects are attributed to drugs given to the mother.
- Gross malformations are produced only if teratogens act during organogenesis. This occurs during the first 3 months of pregnancy but after blastocyst formation. Drug-induced fetal damage is rare during blastocyst formation (exception: fetal alcohol syndrome) and after the first 3 months (exception: angiotensin-converting enzyme inhibitors and sartans).
- The mechanisms of action of teratogens are not clearly understood, though DNA damage is a factor in many cases.
- New drugs are usually tested in pregnant females of at least one rodent and one non-rodent (e.g. rabbit) species.

Warfarin

Administration of warfarin (Ch. 20) in the first trimester is associated with nasal hypoplasia and various central nervous system (CNS) abnormalities, affecting roughly 25% of exposed babies. In the last trimester it must not be used because of the risk of intracranial haemorrhage in the baby during delivery.

Antiemetics

Antiemetics have been widely used to treat morning sickness in early pregnancy, and some are teratogenic in animals. Results of surveys in humans are inconclusive, providing no clear evidence of teratogenicity. Nevertheless, it is prudent to avoid the use of these drugs in pregnant patients if possible.

ASSESSMENT OF GENOTOXIC POTENTIAL

Registration of pharmaceuticals requires a comprehensive assessment of their genotoxic potential. Since no single test is adequate, the usual approach recommended by the International Conference on Harmonisation (ESRA Rapporteur 1997 4: 5–7) is to carry out a battery of in vitro and in vivo tests for genotoxicity. The following battery is often used:

- a test for gene mutation in bacteria
- an in vitro test with cytogenetic evaluation of chromosomal damage
- an in vivo test for chromosomal damage using rodent haemopoietic cells
- reproductive toxicity testing
- carcinogenicity testing.

ALLERGIC REACTIONS TO DRUGS

Allergic reactions of various kinds are a common form of adverse response to drugs. Most drugs, being low-molecular-weight substances, are not immunogenic in themselves. A drug or its metabolites can, however, act as a *hapten* by interacting with protein to form a stable conjugate that is immunogenic (Ch. 15). The immunological basis of some allergic drug reactions has been well worked out, but often it is inferred from the clinical characteristics of the reaction, and direct evidence of an immunological mechanism is lacking. The main criteria that are suggestive of an immune response are:

- the reaction has a time course different from that of the pharmacodynamic effect: it is either delayed in onset, occurring a few days after administration of the drug, or occurs only with repeated exposure to the drug
- sensitisation and/or the subsequent allergic reaction may occur with doses that are too small to elicit pharmacodynamic effects
- the reaction conforms to one of the clinical syndromes associated with allergy—types I, II, III and IV of the Gell & Coombs classification (below and Ch. 15)—and is unrelated to the pharmacodynamic effect of the drug.

The overall incidence of allergic drug reactions is variously reported as being between 2 and 25%. The great majority are relatively harmless skin eruptions. Serious reactions (e.g. anaphylaxis, haemolysis and bone marrow depression), which can be fatal, are rare. **Penicillins**, which are the commonest cause of drug-induced anaphylaxis, produce this response in an estimated 1 in 50 000 patients exposed. Skin eruptions can be severe, and fatalities occur with Stevens–Johnson syndrome (provoked, for example, by sulfonamides) and with toxic epidermal necrolysis (which can be caused by **allopurinol**).

Immunological mechanisms

The formation of an immunogenic conjugate between a small molecule and an endogenous protein requires covalent bonding. In most cases, reactive metabolites, rather than the drug itself, are responsible. Such reactive metabolites can be produced during drug oxidation or by photo-activation in the skin. They may also be produced by the action of toxic oxygen metabolites generated by activated leucocytes. Rarely (e.g. in drug-induced lupus erythematosus) the reactive moiety interacts to form an immunogen with nuclear components (DNA, histone) rather than proteins (see below). Conjugation with a macromolecule is usually essential, although penicillin is an exception because it can form sufficiently large polymers in solution to elicit an anaphylactic reaction in a sensitised individual even without conjugation to protein. Conjugates of penicillin and its metabolites with protein are also formed and can also act as immunogens.

Clinical types of allergic response to drugs

In the Gell & Coombs classification of hypersensitivity reactions (Ch. 15), types I, II and III are antibody-mediated reactions and type IV is cell mediated. Unwanted reactions to drugs involve both antibody- and cell-mediated reactions. The more important clinical manifestations of hypersensitivity include anaphylactic shock, haematological reactions, allergic liver damage and other hypersensitivity reactions.

Anaphylactic shock

Anaphylactic shock—a type I hypersensitivity response— is a sudden and life-threatening reaction that results from the release of histamine, leukotrienes and other mediators (Ch. 15). The main features include urticarial rash, swelling of soft tissues, bronchoconstriction and hypotension.

Penicillins are the drugs most likely to cause anaphylactic reactions, and they account for about 75% of anaphylactic deaths, reflecting the frequency with which they are used in clinical practice. Other drugs that can cause anaphylaxis include various enzymes, for example **streptokinase** (Ch. 20), **asparaginase** (Ch. 50); hormones, for example **corticotropin** (adrenocorticotrophic hormone; Ch. 27); **heparin** (Ch. 20); *dextrans*; *radiological contrast agents*; *vaccines*; and other *serological products*. Anaphylaxis with local anaesthetics (Ch. 43), the surface antiseptic chlorhexidine and with many other drugs has been reported but is uncommon. Anaphylaxis is treated by injection of **adrenaline** (**epinephrine**) which is life-saving in this circumstance, *corticosteroids* and *antihistamines*.

It is sometimes feasible to carry out a skin test for the presence of anaphylactic hypersensitivity, which involves injecting a minute dose intradermally. This is sometimes done if a patient reports that he or she is allergic to a particular drug. However, the test is not completely reliable. Furthermore, the test dose itself may elicit a severe reaction. The use of penicilloylpolylysine as a skin test reagent for penicillin allergy is an improvement over the use of penicillin itself, because it bypasses the need for conjugation of the test substance, thereby reducing the likelihood of a false negative. Other specialised tests are available to detect the presence of specific IgE in the plasma, or to measure histamine release from the patient's basophils, but these are not used routinely.

Other drug-induced type I hypersensitivity reactions include bronchospasm (Ch. 22) and urticaria.

Haematological reactions

Drug-induced haematological reactions can be produced by type II, III or IV hypersensitivity. Type II reactions can affect any or all of the formed elements of the blood, which may be destroyed by effects either on the circulating blood cells themselves or on their progenitors in the bone marrow. They involve antibody binding to a drug–macromolecule complex on the cell surface membrane. The antigen–antibody reaction activates complement leading to lysis (Fig. 15.1) or provokes attack by killer lymphocytes or phagocytic leucocytes. *Haemolytic anaemia* has been most commonly reported with sulfonamides and related drugs (Ch. 45) and with an antihypertensive drug, **methyldopa** (Ch. 11), which is still widely used to treat hypertension during pregnancy. With methyldopa, significant haemolysis occurs in less than 1% of patients, but the appearance of antibodies directed against the surface of red cells is detectable in 15% by the Coombs' test. The antibodies are directed against Rh antigens, but it is not known how methyldopa produces this effect.

Drug-induced agranulocytosis (complete absence of circulating neutrophils) is usually delayed 2–12 weeks after beginning drug treatment but may then be sudden in onset. It often presents with mouth ulcers, a severe sore throat or other infection. Serum from the patient lyses leucocytes from other individuals, and circulating antileucocyte antibodies can usually be detected immunologically. Drugs associated with agranulocytosis include NSAIDs (especially **phenylbutazone**; Ch. 16), **carbimazole** (Ch. 28) and **clozapine** (Ch. 37)). Sulfonamides and related drugs (e.g. thiazides and sulfonylureas) are uncommon but well-documented causes of agranulocytosis. This is a rare, but life-threatening condition, because the marked reduction of blood granulocytes makes the patient extremely vulnerable to bacterial infections. Recovery when the drug is stopped is often slow or absent. This type of antibody-mediated leucocyte destruction must be distinguished from the direct effect of cytotoxic drugs (see Ch. 50), most of which cause granulocytopenia. With these latter drugs, however, the effect is rapid in onset, predictably related to dose and reversible.

Thrombocytopenia (reduction in platelet numbers) can be caused by type II reactions to **quinine** (Ch. 48), **heparin** (Ch. 20) and thiazide diuretics (Ch. 23).

Some drugs (notably **chloramphenicol**) can suppress all three haemopoietic cell lineages giving rise to *aplastic anaemia* (anaemia with associated agranulocytosis and thrombocytopenia).

The distinction between type III and type IV hypersensitivity reactions in the causation of haematological reactions is not clear-cut, and it is likely that either or both mechanisms are often involved.

Allergic liver damage

Most drug-induced liver damage results from the direct toxic effects of drugs or their metabolites as described above. However, hypersensitivity reactions are sometimes involved, a particular example being **halothane**-induced hepatic necrosis (see Ch. 35). Trifluoracetylchloride, a reactive metabolite of halothane, couples to a macromolecule to form an immunogen. Most patients with halothane-induced liver damage have antibodies that react with halothane–carrier conjugates. There is evidence from rabbit experiments that the halothane–protein antigens can be expressed on the surface of hepatocytes. Destruction of the cells occurs by type II hypersensitivity reactions involving killer T cells. If antigen–antibody complexes are released by damaged cells, type III reactions can contribute.

Enflurane may also cause antibody-mediated liver damage, and apparent cross-sensitisation with halothane is reported.

Other hypersensitivity reactions

The clinical manifestations of type IV hypersensitivity reactions are diverse, ranging from minor skin rashes to generalised autoimmune disease. Fever may accompany these reactions. Skin rashes can be antibody mediated, but are usually cell mediated. They range from mild eruptions to fatal exfoliation. In some cases, the lesions are photosensitive, probably because of degradation of the drug to reactive substances in the presence of ultraviolet light.

Some drugs (notably **hydralazine** and **procainamide**) can produce an autoimmune syndrome resembling systemic lupus erythematosus. This is a multisystem disorder in which there is immunological damage to many organs and tissues (including joints, skin, lung, central nervous system and kidney) caused particularly, but not exclusively, by type III hypersensitivity reactions. The prodigious array of antibodies directed against 'self' components has been termed 'an autoimmune thunderstorm'. The antibodies react with determinants shared by many molecules, for example the phosphodiester backbone of DNA, RNA and phospholipids. In drug-induced systemic lupus erythematosus, the immunogen may result from the reactive drug moiety interacting with nuclear material, and in the effector phase, joint and pulmonary damage is common. The condition usually resolves when treatment with the offending drug is stopped.

Allergic reactions to drugs

- Drugs or their reactive metabolites can bind covalently to proteins to form immunogens. Penicillin (which can also be immunogenic by forming polymers) is an important example.
- Drug-induced allergic (hypersensitivity) reactions may be antibody mediated (types I, II, III) or cell mediated (type IV). Important clinical manifestations include:
  —anaphylactic shock (type I): this is life-threatening, by obstructing respiration; many drugs can cause the condition and most deaths are caused by penicillin
  —haematological reactions (type II, III or IV): these, along with examples of causative drugs, are haemolytic anaemia (sulfonamides and methyldopa), agranulocytosis, which can be irreversible (sulfonamides, chloramphenicol and carbimazole), and thrombocytopenia (quinine, heparin and thiazide diuretics)
  —allergic liver damage (type II, III): for example, the reactive metabolite of halothane couples to liver proteins to form an immunogen
  —skin rashes (type I, IV): these occur with many drugs, are usually type IV and usually mild, though some can be life threatening
  —drug-induced systemic lupus erythematosus (mainly type II): this involves antibodies to nuclear material.

REFERENCES AND FURTHER READING

Alison M R, Sarraf C E 1995 Apoptosis: regulation and relevance to toxicology. Hum Exp Toxicol 14: 234–247 (*Review*)

Anonymous 1997 Drug-induced agranulocytosis. Drug Ther Bull 35: 49–52 (*Considers which drugs are most commonly involved, how to minimise risk and how to manage*)

Boobis A R, Fawthrop D J, Davies D S 1989 Mechanisms of cell death. Trends Pharmacol Sci 10: 275–280 (*Oxidising species convert GSH to GSSG. GSH is usually regenerated by NADPH-dependent GSSG-reductase; but when the rate of GSH oxidation to GSSG exceeds the capacity of this enzyme, GSSG is removed from the cell by active transport*)

Briggs G G, Freeman R K, Sumner J Y 1994 Drugs in pregnancy and lactation, 4th edn. Williams & Wilkins, Baltimore, MD (*Invaluable reference guide to fetal and neonatal risk for clinicians caring for pregnant women*)

Brimblecombe R W, Dayan A D 1993 Preclinical toxicity testing. In: Burley D M, Clarke J M, Lasagna L (eds) Pharmaceutical medicine, 2nd edn. Edward Arnold, London. pp. 12–32 (*Scholarly review*)

Collins M D, Mayo G E 1999 Teratology of retinoids. Annu Rev Pharmacol Toxicol 39: 399-430 (*Overviews principles of teratology as they apply to the retinoids, describes signal transduction of retinoids and toxikinetics*)

De Weck A L 1983 Immunopathological mechanisms and clinical aspects of allergic reactions to drugs. In: De Weck A L, Bundgaard H (eds) Allergic responses to drugs. Handbook of experimental pharmacology. Springer-Verlag, Berlin, vol. 63, pp. 75–135

Farrar H C, Blumer J L 1991 Fetal effects of maternal drug exposure. Annu Rev Pharmacol 31: 525–547 (*Reviews teratology, fetal drug effects, teratogenesis and fetal pharmacology*)

Glassman A H, Bigger J T 2001 Antipsychotic drugs: prolonged QTc interval, torsade de pointes, and sudden death. Am J Psychiat 158: 1774-1782 (*Reviews mechanisms and risks of torsade and sudden death with antipsychotic drugs. The greatest risk is with thioridazine*)

Hanson J W, Streissguth A P, Smith D W 1978 The effects of moderate alcohol consumption during pregnancy on fetal growth and morphogenesis. J Paediatr 92: 457–460

Hay A 1988 How to identify a carcinogen. Nature 332: 782–783

Hinson J A, Roberts D W 1992 Role of covalent and noncovalent interactions in cell toxicity: effects on proteins. Annu Rev Pharmacol Toxicol 32: 471–510

Huff J, Haseman J, Rall D 1991 Scientific concepts, value, and significance of chemical carcinogenesis studies. Annu Rev Pharmacol Toxicol 31: 621–652

Jones J K, Idänpään-Heikkilä J E 1993 Adverse reactions, postmarketing surveillance and pharmacoepidemiology. In: Burley D M, Clarke J M, Lasagna L (eds) Pharmaceutical medicine, 2nd edn. Edward Arnold, London, pp. 145–180

Kenna J G, Knight T L, van Pelt F N A M 1993 Immunity of halothane metabolite-modified proteins in halothane hepatitis. Ann NY Acad Sci 685: 646–661

Lutz W K, Maier P 1988 Genotoxic and epigenetic chemical carcinogens: one process, different mechanisms. Trends Pharmacol Sci 9: 322–326

Moss A J 1993 Measurement of the QT interval and the risk of QTc prolongation: a review. Am J Cardiol 72: 23B–25B

Murray M D, Brater D C 1993 Renal toxicity of the nonsteroidal anti-inflammatory drugs. Annu Rev Pharmacol Toxicol 33: 435–465

Nicotera P, Bellomo G, Orrenius S 1992 Calcium-mediated mechanisms in chemically-induced cell death. Annu Rev Pharmacol Toxicol 32: 449–470 (*Discusses the role of Ca^{2+} in the early development of cell damage*)

Pirmohamed M, Breckenridge A M, Kitteringham N R et al. 1998 Adverse drug reactions. Br Med J 316: 1295-1298 (*Adverse drug reactions are estimated to account for 5% of all UK hospital admissions and to occur in an additional 10–20% of inpatients during the course of their admission*)

Pohl L R, Satoh H, Christ D D, Kenna J G 1988 The immunologic and metabolic basis of drug hypersensitivities. Annu Rev Pharmacol 28: 367–387

Pumford N R, Halmes N C 1997 Protein targets of xenobiotic reactive intermediates. Annu Rev Pharmacol Toxicol 37: 91–117 (*Intrinsic versus idiosyncratic toxicity*)

Raffray M, Cohen G M 1997 Apoptosis and necrosis in toxicology: a continuum or distinct modes of cell death? Pharmacol Ther 75: 153–177 (*Essentially distinct processes with only limited molecular overlap*)

Rawlins M D, Thomson J W 1985 Mechanisms of adverse drug reactions. In: Davies D M (ed) Textbook of adverse drug reactions, 3rd edn. Oxford University Press, Oxford, pp. 12–38 (*Type A/type B classification*)

Scales M D C 1993 Toxicity testing. In: Griffin J P, O'Grady J, Wells F O (eds) The textbook of pharmaceutical medicine. Queen's University Press, Belfast, pp. 53–79 (*Thoughtful review*)

Svensson C K, Cowen E W, Gaspari A A 2001 Cutaneous drug reactions. Pharmacol Rev 53: 357-380 (*Covers epidemiology, clinical morphology and mechanisms. Assesses current knowledge of four types of cutaneous drug reaction: immediate-type immune-mediated, delayed-type immune-mediated, photosensitivity and autoimmune. Also reviews the role of viral infection as predisposing factor*)

Timbrell J A 1982 Principles of biochemical toxicology. Taylor & Francis, London

Uetrecht J 1989 Mechanism of hypersensitivity reactions: proposed involvement of reactive metabolites generated by activated leucocytes. Trends Pharmacol Sci 10: 463–467

Venitt S 1981 Microbial tests in carcinogenesis studies. In: Gorrod J W 1981 Testing for toxicity. Taylor & Francis, London (*Describes some of the many variants of the Ames test*)

Weinberg R A 1984 Cellular oncogenes. Trends Biochem Sci 9: 131–133

Weisburge J H, Williams G M 1984 New, efficient approaches to test for carcinogenicity of chemicals based on their mechanisms of action. In: Zbinden G et al. (eds) Current problems in drug toxicology Libbey, Paris (*Scheme of classification of carcinogens*)

53 Gene therapy

Overview 738

Introduction 738

Technical aspects 739
- Gene delivery 739
- Controlling gene expression 741

Safety 743

Therapeutic aspects 743
- Single gene defects 743
- Gene therapy for cancer 743
- Gene therapy and infectious disease 744
- Gene therapy and cardiovascular disease 744
- Other gene-based approaches 744

OVERVIEW

Gene therapy is the genetic modification of cells to prevent, alleviate or cure disease. It has not yet led to licensed products but holds great promise. In this chapter we introduce the central concepts, discuss technical problems and approaches to dealing with these, describe safety issues and, finally, consider progress that has been made in specific therapeutic areas. We are confident that:

- **nucleic acid-based therapies will be developed that are safe and effective**
- **this will radically change medicine**
- **the full impact will not, however, be realised for many years.**

INTRODUCTION

The history of therapeutics has been punctuated by monumental innovations (e.g. surgery, immunisation, antibiotics) that are conceptually simple but have changed the world. Gene therapy has certainly not done that—yet. The concept of introducing nucleic acid into cells of the body in order to treat or prevent disease is, however, so appealing that vast resources (both public and private) have been committed to its development. There are several reasons for this appeal. First, the approach offers the potential for radical cure of single gene diseases such as cystic fibrosis and the haemoglobinopathies, which are collectively responsible for much misery throughout the world. Second, many much commoner conditions, including malignant, neurodegenerative and infectious diseases, have a large genetic component. Conventional treatment of such disorders is, as readers of this book will appreciate, woefully inadequate, so a completely new approach has enormous attraction. Finally, an ability to control gene expression could revolutionise the management of diseases in which there is no genetic component at all.* The gene for vascular endothelial growth factor is being used to stimulate the growth of new blood vessels around blockages in atherosclerotic arteries, and preliminary results have been encouraging. More mundanely, if a deficient protein (such as factor VIII, insulin or erythropoietin) could be synthesised in vivo in response to a single therapeutic intervention, this would have great practical advantages over recurrent injections of purified or synthetic protein in diseases such as haemophilia (Ch. 20), diabetes (Ch. 25) or chronic renal failure (Ch. 23).

Using modern techniques, it is possible to identify and clone genes, alter DNA or RNA in the laboratory and produce large amounts of this modified, recombinant, nucleic acid. Such recombinant nucleic acid, coding for a gene that it is hoped will have therapeutic effect, can be introduced into host chromosomes via plasmids and transposons (see Ch. 5). The gurus are emphatic that 'the conceptual part of the gene therapy revolution has indeed occurred…'—so where are the therapies? The devil, of course, is in the detail: in this case the details of

- pharmacokinetics: gene delivery to appropriate target cells
- pharmacodynamics controlled expression of the gene in question
- safety
- clinical efficacy and long-term practicability.

These problems are formidable: an analogy is to put oneself in the shoes of a barber-surgeon cutting for stone on Samuel Pepys. Such a practitioner would surely have imagined the concept of abdominal surgery (to relieve obstruction from a strangulated

*A lamb can be grown from the nucleus of a cell from the udder of an adult sheep: it does not take an H G Wells to contemplate applications (e.g. for amputees), although it must be admitted that this still appears far-fetched.

Definition and potential uses

- Gene therapy is the genetic modification of cells to prevent, alleviate or cure disease; current efforts are directed to somatic and not to germ cells.
- Potential applications:
  —radical cure of single gene diseases (e.g. cystic fibrosis, haemoglobinopathies)
  —amelioration of diseases with or without a genetic component, including many malignant, neurodegenerative and infectious diseases.

hernia or tumour for instance), but realisation of the dream would needs await discoveries in the fields of anaesthesia and aseptic technique in the 19th and 20th centuries.

In the case of gene therapy, perhaps the most fundamental hurdle is the delivery problem; here modern virology offers more than a whiff of the possibilities of gene delivery for therapeutic use, and other techniques are also available that can introduce functional nucleic acids into mammalian cells (see below). It is this sense of the possible in the setting, on the one hand, of a concept so simple that any broadsheet reader can apprehend it and, on the other, great prizes (humanitarian, scientific and commercial) that has led inevitably to great expectations and, perhaps equally inevitably, to frustration at the lack of practical progress.

There has been a consensus* that attempts at gene therapy should focus on somatic cells and a moratorium has been agreed on therapies intended to alter the DNA of germ cells and hence influence the next generation.

TECHNICAL ASPECTS

GENE DELIVERY

The transfer of recombinant nucleic acid into target cells—the 'drug distribution' problem—is critical to the success of gene therapy. Nucleic acid must pass from the extracellular space across the plasma and nuclear membranes, and it must then be incorporated into the chromosomes. Since DNA is highly negatively charged and single genes have molecular weights around 10^4 times greater than conventional drugs, the problem is of a different order from the equivalent stage of routine drug development. Various approaches have been developed, most of which involve inserting the therapeutic gene into a drug delivery system called a vector, often in the form of a suitably modified virus (see below).

There are two main strategies for delivering genes into patients: in vivo and ex vivo. The in vivo strategy is to inject a suspension of a vector containing the therapeutic gene directly into the patient, either intravenously—in which case some form of targeting of the vector to the organ or tissue on which it is intended to act is required—or into a tissue on which it is hoped that it will act (e.g. directly into a malignant tumour). The ex vivo strategy is to remove cells from the patient (e.g. stem cells from marrow or circulating blood, or myoblasts from a biopsy of striated muscle) treat them with the vector and inject the genetically altered cells back into the patient.

An ideal vector would be safe, highly efficient (i.e. insert the therapeutic gene into a large fraction of target cells) and selective in that it would lead to expression of the therapeutic protein in the target cells but not to the expression of viral proteins. It would cause persistent expression, avoiding the need for repeated treatment provided the cell into which it is inserted is itself long-lived. This is a problem with a therapeutic target such as the airway epithelium. This malfunctions in the autosomal recessive disorder *cystic fibrosis* owing to deficiency of a membrane Cl^- transporter known as the cystic fibrosis transport regulator (CFTR). Epithelial cells in the airways are continuously dying off and being replaced, so even if the *CFTR* gene were stably transfected into the epithelium, there would still be a need for periodic retreatment unless the gene can be inserted into the progenitor (stem) cells. Similar problems are anticipated in other cells that turn over continuously such as gastrointestinal epithelium and skin. (Repeat administration of therapeutic drugs is, of course, usually needed, but in the case of macromolecules and viruses this repetition causes problems associated with immune responses.)

Viral vectors

Viruses take over the metabolic machinery of the cells they invade, and some are expert at fusing with the cell's nucleic acid. Most strategies for gene delivery utilise these properties. While producing a tantalising glimpse of the possible,** there remain substantial practical problems with this approach, partly at least because as viruses have evolved the means to invade human cells, so humans have evolved enzymes and immune responses that thwart them. This is not all bad news, however, at least from the point of view of safety. For example, one therapeutic trial was halted by the US Food and Drug Administration (FDA) because of the appearance of the gene-bearing virus in seminal fluid of one recipient, raising fears that this could lead to transmission to an unborn child. Further investigation, however, revealed that the virus was not present in sperm, possibly because of mechanisms evolved to protect the genetic information in gametes from viral assault.

Retroviruses

Retroviral vectors have the attraction that, if introduced into stem cells, their effects are persistent because they become

*For some thoughtful dissenting views see: Stack G, Campbell J (eds) 'Engineering the human germline: an exploration of the science and ethics of altering the genes we pass to our children'. Oxford University Press, New York.

**Rather like a would-be abdominal surgeon in the 17th century contemplating the use of general anaesthesia when his only experience of it was intoxication with alcoholic beverages.

incorporated into and replicate with host DNA and so are passed down to each daughter during cell division. Against this, since they are inserted randomly into the chromosome, they may cause damage (see below). Furthermore, since they are relatively promiscuous as regards the cells they infect, they could produce undesired effects, including effects on germ cells, if administered in vivo. They are, therefore, currently used for ex vivo attempts at therapy. The life cycle of naturally occurring retroviruses is exploited to create vectors for use in gene therapy (see Fig. 53.1). For the future, it is hoped that it will be possible to alter the retroviral envelope to increase specificity, so that the vector could be administered systemically but would home in only on the desired target cell population. An example of this approach is the substitution of the envelope protein of a non-pathogenic vector (e.g. mouse leukaemia virus, which is not pathogenic for humans and has been evaluated as a potential retrovirus vector for use in humans) with the envelope protein of human vesicular stomatitis virus, in order specifically to target epithelial cells. Most retrovirus vectors are unable to penetrate the nuclear envelope and, therefore, only infect dividing cells since the nuclear membrane dissolves during cell division. Consequently, they do not infect non-dividing cells such as adult neurons.

Adrenovirus

Adenovirus vectors are popular because of the high transgene expression that can be achieved. They transfer genes to the nucleus of the host cell, but (unlike retroviruses) these are not inserted into the host genome and so do not produce effects that outlast subsequent cell divisions. Adenovirus vectors have been used to attempt in vivo gene therapy. The lack of insertion into host chromosomes obviates the risk of disturbing the function of vital cellular genes and the theoretical risk of carcinogenicity that this imparts (see below), but at the cost of producing only a temporary effect. Adenovirus vectors are genetically modified by making deletions in the viral genome, thereby making the virus unable to replicate and cause widespread infection in the host while at the same time creating space in the viral genome for the therapeutic transgene to be inserted. One of the first adenoviral vectors lacked part of a growth-controlling region called E_1. This defective virus is grown in a cell line that substitutes for the

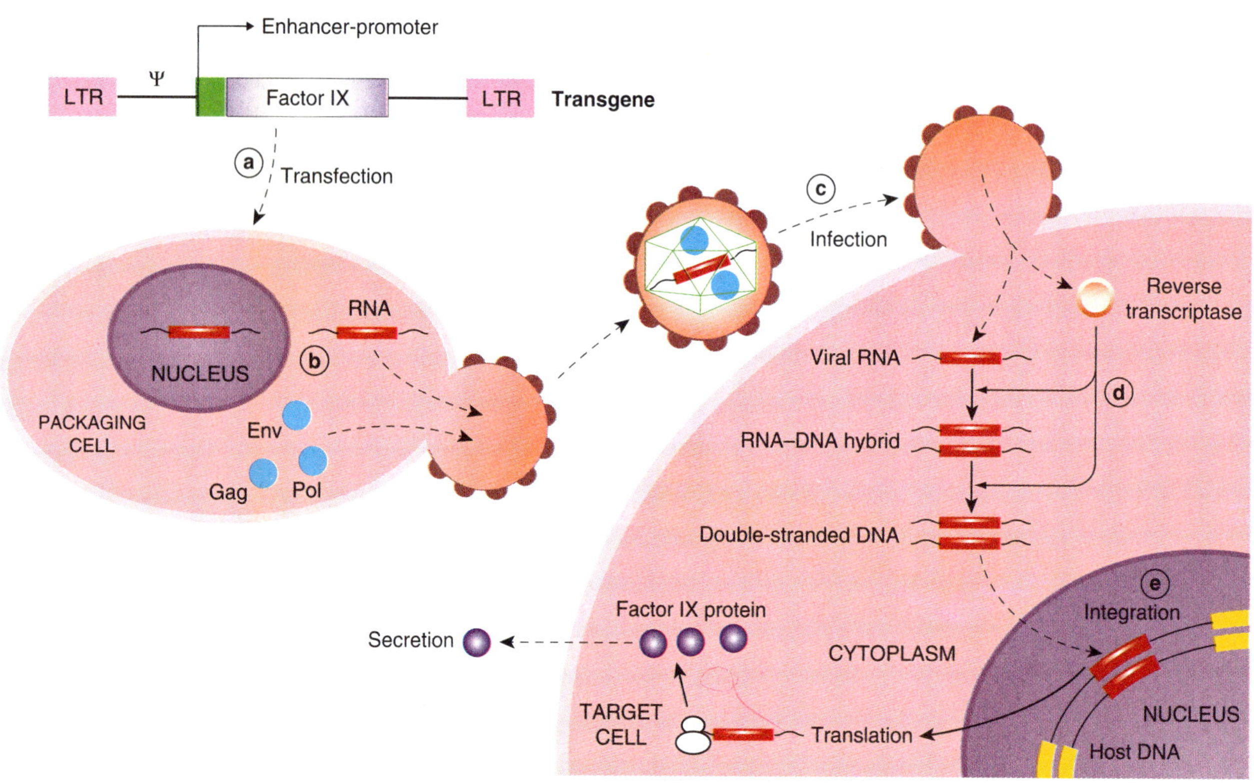

Fig. 53.1 Strategy for making retroviral vectors. The transgene (the example shows the gene for factor IX) in a vector backbone is introduced (a) into a packaging cell, where it is integrated into a chromosome in the nucleus, and (b) transcribed to make vector mRNA, which is packaged into the retroviral vector and shed from the packaging cell. It then infects the target cell (c). Virally encoded reverse transcriptase (d) converts vector RNA into an RNA–DNA hybrid, and then into double-stranded DNA, which is integrated (e) into the genome of the target cell. It can then be transcribed and translated to make factor IX protein. (Redrawn from: Verma I M, Somia N 1997 Nature 389: 239–242.)

missing E_1 function. Recombinant virus is produced by infecting complementing cells with a plasmid generated from the cloned DNA of therapeutic interest plus an expression cassette and portions of adenoviral DNA. Recombination between this and the 'backbone' of the E_1-deficient adenoviral genome results in a virus encoding the desired transgene. This approach led to seemingly spectacular results, demonstrating gene transfer to cell lines and animal models of disease, but it has been disappointing (especially for cystic fibrosis) in humans. The main problem has been that low doses (administered by aerosol to patients with this disease) have produced only very low efficiency transfer, whereas higher doses have resulted in inflammation and a host immune response, and short-lived expression of the gene. Furthermore, treatment cannot be repeated because of neutralising antibodies. This has led to manipulations of adenoviral vectors in attempts to reduce their immunogenicity, by mutating or removing the genes that are most strongly immunogenic, an approach that is currently very active.

Other viral vectors

Other potential viral vectors under investigation include adeno-associated virus, herpes virus, and disabled versions of human immunodeficiency virus (HIV). Adeno-associated virus associates with host DNA; it may be less immunogenic than other vectors but is hard to mass produce and has a small capacity; consequently, it cannot be used to carry large transgenes. Herpesvirus does not associate with host DNA but is very long lived in nervous tissue and could, therefore, have specific applications in treating neurological disease. HIV, unlike most other retroviruses (see above), can infect non-dividing cells such as neurons. It is possible to remove the genes from HIV that permit its replication and substitute marker genes that are expressed following injection into rat brain, and it is hoped that therapeutic genes could be inserted similarly. Alternatively, it may prove possible to transfer those genes that permit HIV to penetrate the nuclear envelope to other non-pathogenic retroviruses.

Non-viral vectors

Liposomes

Non-viral vectors include a variant of liposomes (Ch. 7). Plasmids (diameter up to approximately 2 μm) are too big to package in regular liposomes (diameter 0.025–0.1 μm), but larger particles can be made using positively charged lipids ('lipoplexes'), which interact with negative charges on cell membranes and negatively charged DNA, improving delivery into the cell nucleus and incorporation into the chromosome. Such particles have been used to deliver the genes for HLA-B7, interleukin-2 and CFTR. They are much less efficient than viruses and attempts are currently under way to improve this by incorporating various viral signal proteins (membrane fusion proteins, for example) in their outer coat. Meanwhile, direct injection into solid tumours (e.g. melanoma, breast, kidney and colon cancers) can achieve high local concentrations within the tumour.

Microspheres

Biologically erodable microspheres made from polyanhydride copolymers of fumaric and sebacic acids (see Ch. 7) can be loaded with plasmid DNA. A plasmid with bacterial β-galactosidase activity formulated in this way and given by mouth to rats can result in systemic absorption and expression of the bacterial enzyme in the rat liver, raising the possibility of oral gene therapy!

Plasmid DNA

Surprisingly, it has emerged that plasmid DNA itself ('naked DNA') can access the nucleus and be expressed, albeit much less efficiently than when it is packaged in a vector.* Such DNA carries no risk of viral replication and is not necessarily itself immunogenic,** but it cannot be targeted to a cell of interest. There is considerable interest in the possibility of using naked DNA for vaccines, since even very small amounts of foreign protein can stimulate an immune response. Such a vaccine for influenza is in clinical development, and more ambitious long-term targets include malaria, tuberculosis, chlamydia, helicobacter and hepatitis.

CONTROLLING GENE EXPRESSION

To realise the full potential of gene therapy, it will not, of course, be enough to transfer the gene selectively to the desired target cells and keep it there still expressing its product—difficult though these goals are. For many uses it will also be essential for the activity of the gene to be controlled. Historically, it was the realisation of how difficult this was going to be that diverted attention from the haemoglobinopathies (which were the first projected targets of gene therapy). Correction of these disorders demands an appropriate balance of α and β-globin chain synthesis in addition to synthesis of wild type rather than mutant polypeptide. For this and for many other potential applications, more or less precisely controlled gene expression will be essential. It has not yet proved possible to control transgenes in human recipients, but there are potential ways of achieving this. One hinges on the use of a tetracycline-inducible expression system. This was first applied in cultured cells, and subsequently to the mouse in vivo. Myoblasts were engineered for doxycycline-inducible and skeletal-muscle-specific expression of erythropoietin by using two retroviral vectors. After intramuscular injection of these cells, the transgene became detectable in skeletal muscle of the recipient, and it proved possible to switch erythropoietin production (and consequently the haematocrit) in the mouse on or off by treatment with **doxycycline** over a period of several months (Fig. 53.2). To carry

*The discovery came from its use—injected into striated muscle—as a 'negative' control that turned out positive.

**This is a theoretical concern, since antibodies directed against DNA are characteristic of several autoimmune diseases including systemic lupus erythematosus.

Gene delivery and expression

- Gene delivery is one of the main hurdles to making gene therapy practicable.
- Recombinant genes are transferred via a plasmid to a vector, often a suitably modified virus.
- There are two main strategies for delivering genes into patients:
  —in vivo injection of the vector containing the therapeutic gene directly into the patient (e.g. into a malignant tumour)
  —ex vivo treatment of cells from the patient (e.g. stem cells from marrow or circulating blood, or myoblasts from a biopsy of striated muscle) followed by reinjection into the patient.
- An ideal vector would be safe, efficient (i.e. insert the gene into a large fraction of target cells), selective (i.e. lead to expression of the therapeutic protein but not of viral proteins) and would cause persistent expression of the therapeutic gene.
- Viral vectors include retroviruses, adenoviruses, adeno-associated virus, herpesvirus and disabled human immnodeficiency virus (HIV).
- Retroviruses infect many different types of dividing cells and become incorporated randomly into host DNA.
- Adenoviruses are genetically modified by deletions in the genome that make them unable to replicate and that creates space for the therapeutic transgene. They transfer genes to the nucleus but not to the genome of the host cell. Problems with current adenovirus vectors include a strong immune response, inflammation and short-lived expression. Treatment cannot be repeated because of neutralising antibodies.
- Adeno-associated virus associates with host DNA and is non-immunogenic. However, it is hard to mass produce and has a small capacity.
- Herpesvirus does not associate with host DNA but is very long lived in nervous tissue and could, therefore, have specific applications in treating neurological disease.
- Disabled versions of HIV differ from most other retroviruses in that they infect non-dividing cells, including neurons.
- Non-viral vectors include:
  —a variant of liposomes (Ch. 7), made using positively charged lipids and called 'lipoplexes'
  —biologically erodable microspheres (see Ch. 7), which hold out a possibility of orally active gene therapy
  —plasmid DNA itself ('naked DNA'), which can access the nucleus and be expressed, albeit much less efficiently than when it is packaged in a vector; it is being used to develop new vaccines.
- Once a gene has been transferred, it will be essential, for many uses, for the activity of the therapeutic gene to be *controlled*. One promising approach to this is to use a tetracycline-inducible expression system.

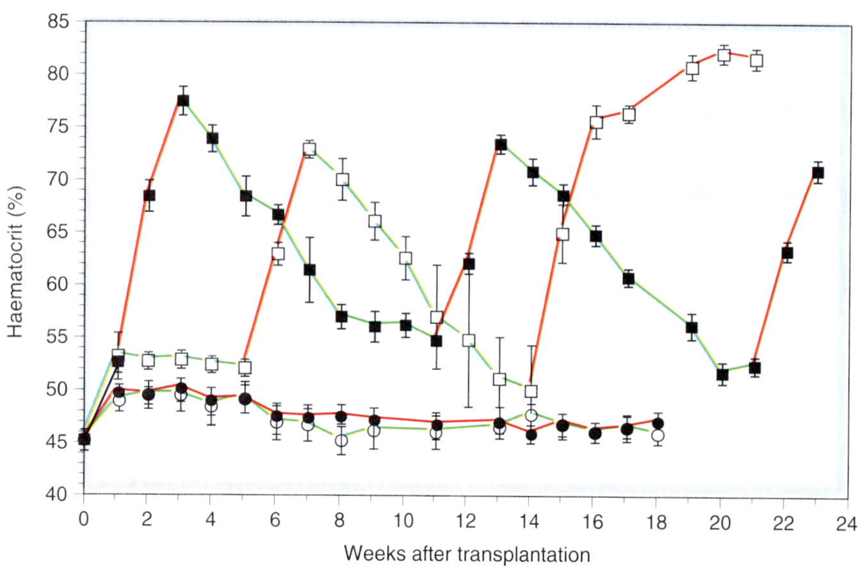

Fig. 53.2 Control of erythropoietin secretion by doxycycline in mice transplanted with myoblasts containing an erythropoietin transgene with (squares) or without (circles) a second transgene that confers doxycycline inducibility. Intermittent administration of doxycycline via drinking water (indicated in red) turned on the secretion of erythropoietin in the animals that had received the doxycycline-inducibility gene, and hence increased haematocrit, over a 5-month period. (From: Bohl D, Naffakh N, Heard J M 1997 Nat Med 3: 299–305.)

this strategy further, it will be necessary to discover ways whereby physiological stimuli can control expression of the therapeutic gene. This will clearly be a great deal more difficult for situations where very rapid responses (e.g. to changing blood glucose in a diabetic) are needed.

SAFETY

In addition to safety concerns specific to any particular therapy (e.g. polycythaemia, thrombosis and hypertension from overexpression of erythropoietin; see above and Fig. 53.2), a number of concerns relate generally to the use of viral vectors. These are selected to be non-pathogenic for humans, or modified to render them non-pathogenic, but there is a concern that such agents could acquire virulence during use. Viral proteins may be expressed that are immunogenic and can elicit an inflammatory response, which is harmful in some situations (e.g. in the airways in patients with cystic fibrosis). Viruses such as retroviruses, which insert randomly into host DNA, could damage the genome and interfere with the protective mechanisms that normally regulate the cell cycle (see Ch. 5). Consequently, if they happen to disrupt an essential function this could increase the risk of malignancy. That this risk is more than a theoretical possibility has recently become evident in a child treated for severe combined immunodeficiency (SCID; see below), who has developed a leukaemia-like illness. The retroviral vector was shown to have inserted itself into a gene called LMO-2. Mutations of LMO-2 are associated with childhood cancers.

Initial clinical experience was reassuring, but the tragic death of Jesse Gelsinger (an 18-year-old volunteer in a gene therapy trial for the non-fatal disease ornithine decarboxylase deficiency, which is controllable by diet and drugs) led to the appreciation that safety concerns related to immune-mediated responses to vectors are very real. Protocol violations became apparent and subsequently six further previously unreported deaths emerged in two other programmes. The possible influence of commercial interests on reporting of such events was much discussed.* The issue of the appropriate level of public scrutiny of such studies is under debate.

Safety

- There are safety concerns specific to any particular therapy (e.g. polycythaemia from overexpression of erythropoietin), and additional general concerns relating, for example, to vectors.
- Viral vectors:
  - —might acquire virulence during use
  - —contain viral proteins, which may be immunogenic
  - —can elicit an inflammatory response
  - —could damage the host genome and interfere with the cell cycle; this could cause malignancy.
- The limited clinical experience to date has not so far provided evidence of insurmountable problems.

THERAPEUTIC ASPECTS

SINGLE GENE DEFECTS

Single gene disorders are individually relatively uncommon. As mentioned above, the haemoglobinopathies were the first projected targets of gene therapy (in the 1980s), but early attempts were put on 'hold' because of the problem posed by the need to control precisely the expression of the genes encoding the different polypeptide chains of the haemoglobin molecule. Patients with thalassaemia** of identical genotype have diverse disease expression, because even in monogenic disorders other genes are also involved and environment influences the clinical manifestations (see Weatherall, 2000). The focus shifted to a rare genetic disorder called *adenine deaminase deficiency*, which results in SCID. This led to the first therapeutic gene transfer protocol to be approved by the US National Institutes of Health. Subsequently, a French team have treated 11 children with another form of SCID and have provided the first proof that gene therapy can cure a life-threatening disease but also evidence that retroviral vectors can cause malignancy (see above). Tight regulation of therapeutic protein biosynthesis may not be essential in some other disorders (e.g. cystic fibrosis and the haemophilias). Attempts at gene therapy for these and for other single gene disorders continue: protocols that have been approved for clinical trials by the recombinant DNA advisory committee include ones for α_1-antitrypsin deficiency (which causes chronic lung disease), chronic granulomatous disease (an X-linked disease in which neutrophils malfunction), familial hypercholesterolaemia (see Ch. 19), Duchenne muscular dystrophy (another X-linked disease, in which affected boys become progressively disabled) and various lysosomal storage disorders including Gaucher's disease and Hunter's syndrome (in which abnormal lipids or mucopolysaccharides accumulate in various organs).

GENE THERAPY FOR CANCER

Approximately half of all current clinical gene therapy research is on cancer. The first gene transfer experiment to be approved by the National Institutes of Health was a non-therapeutic protocol in the late 1980s designed to introduce a marker gene (conferring resistance to an analogue of **neomycin**) into a class of

*See for example 'Gene therapy under a cloud' and 'The balance of risk and benefit in gene-therapy trials' in the Lancet 2000, 355: 329 and 384, and 'The increasing opacity of gene therapy' in Nature 1999, 402: 107.

**The thalassaemias are the commonest group of monogenic diseases. They are characterised by unbalanced synthesis of the α- and β-chains of haemoglobin, and show enormous phenotypic variability. They occur throughout the world, and are common around the Mediterranean (*thalassa* is Greek for 'sea').

lymphocytes that infiltrate various tumours ('tumour infiltrating lymphocytes'). Gene transfer was performed ex vivo, and the cells reinjected into the patient in order to track their subsequent redistribution. This strategy has been useful in tracking other cells and hence identifying the cause of relapse following bone marrow transplantation for various leukaemias. Various therapeutic approaches are under investigation: there is excellent evidence from animal models for the potential usefulness of several of these, but experience with conventional antineoplastic drugs (Ch. 50) cautions against extrapolation to the clinical situation. Promising approaches include:

- restoring protective mechanisms such as p53 (see Ch. 5)
- inactivating oncogene expression (e.g. by a retroviral vector bearing a construct that produces an antisense transcript RNA to the k-*ras* oncogene; see below)
- delivering a gene to malignant cells, thus rendering them sensitive to drugs (e.g. that encoding thymidylate kinase, which activates **ganciclovir**)
- delivery of proteins to healthy host cells in order to protect them (e.g. addition of the multidrug resistance channel—see Ch. 50—to bone marrow cells ex vivo thereby rendering them resistant to drugs used in chemotherapy and protecting the patient from the neutropenia and thrombocytopenia that is otherwise predictably caused by such treatment)
- tagging cancer cells with genes that when expressed render malignant cells more visible to the immune system of the host and trigger a vigorous defensive response (e.g. for antigens such as HLA-B7 or cytokines such as granulocyte–macrophage colony-stimulating factor and interleukin-2).

Gap junctions between malignant cells may help to propagate the desired effect from cells that have taken up the therapeutic gene to neighbouring cells. Among studies using these approaches are ongoing clinical trials in head and neck cancer involving injection into the tumour of recombinant adenoviral vectors containing the human *p53* gene, and trials in glioblastoma (a brain tumour that affects 4000–5000 people in the UK each year) involving herpesvirus vectors carrying a gene to activate a pro-drug. The most clinically advanced programme for glioblastoma currently is a phase III trial using a retroviral vector encoding the herpes simplex virus gene for thymidylate kinase, which is administered into the tumour at the time of surgery and may render the tumour susceptible to drugs such as **ganciclovir**—see above.

Gene therapy for cancer

- Promising approaches include:
  —restoring protective mechanisms such as p53
  —inactivating oncogene expression
  —delivering a gene to malignant cells, thus rendering them sensitive to drugs
  —delivering a gene to healthy host cells to protect them from chemotherapy
  —tagging cancer cells with genes that make them immunogenic.

GENE THERAPY AND INFECTIOUS DISEASE

In addition to the approaches to vaccine development using naked DNA mentioned above, there is considerable interest in the potential of gene therapy for HIV infection. Currently, approximately 10% of all clinical gene therapy research is focussed on this area. The objectives are to stop HIV replicating in infected cells and to prevent it from spreading to uninfected cells, ideally by rendering stem cells (which differentiate into immune cells) resistant to HIV before they mature. Various strategies are under investigation including the use of genes that code for variants of HIV-directed proteins that serve as blocking agents (so-called 'dominant-negative' mutations, e.g. *rev*, which began clinical testing in 1995), RNA decoys and soluble forms of CD4 (the cellular receptor whereby HIV gains access to lymphocytes; Ch. 46) that will bind, and hopefully inactivate, HIV extracellularly.

GENE THERAPY AND CARDIOVASCULAR DISEASE

Vascular gene transfer is attractive, not least because cardiologists and vascular surgeons routinely perform invasive studies that offer the opportunity to administer gene therapy ex vivo (e.g. to a blood vessel that has been temporarily removed with the intention of reimplanting it as a graft) or locally in vivo (e.g. by injection though a catheter directly into a diseased coronary or femoral artery). Vascular gene transfer offers potential new treatments for several cardiovascular diseases (see Ylä-Herttuala and Martin, 2000). The nature of many vascular disorders such as restenosis following *angioplasty* (stretching up a narrowed artery using a balloon that can be inflated via a catheter) is such that transient gene expression might be all that is needed therapeutically. There is no shortage of attractive candidates for therapeutic overexpression in blood vessels, including nitric oxide or prostaglandin I_2 (prostacyclin) synthase, thymidylate kinase, cyclin, growth arrest homeobox and many others. Some of these have been studied in animal models of restenosis. Overexpression of vascular endothelial growth factor and fibroblast growth factor has been studied in this way and has increased blood flow and collateral vessel growth in ischaemic leg muscle and myocardium. This is a promising area.

OTHER GENE-BASED APPROACHES

So far, we have largely been considering the addition of whole genes, but there are other, related nucleic acid-based therapeutic strategies. One is to attempt to correct a gene that has been altered by mutation; this has the enormous theoretical advantage that the corrected gene would remain under physiological control, avoiding the problems discussed above on controlling gene expression. This approach is in its infancy and is beyond the range of this book.

Other therapeutic approaches that are, in effect, gene therapies are conventionally excluded from this terminology. These include organ transplantation to correct a gene deficiency (e.g. liver transplantation to correct low density lipoprotein receptor deficiency in homozygous familial hypercholesterolaemia; Ch. 19) or the use of conventional drugs to alter gene expression, for example the use of **hydroxycarbamide** (**hydroxyurea**) to increase the expression of γ-chain globin and hence increase fetal haemoglobin and ameliorate the severity of sickle cell anaemia.

Another method, known as the 'antisense oligonucleotide' approach—which we describe briefly here—has enormous theoretical appeal. This consists of the use of short (15–25) sequences of nucleotide bases (oligonucleotides) that are complementary to part of a gene or gene product that it is desired to inhibit. These snippets of genetic material can be designed to influence the expression of a gene either by forming a triplex (three-stranded helix) with a regulatory component of chromosomal DNA or by complexing a region of messenger RNA (mRNA). Oligonucleotides can cross plasma and nuclear membranes by endocytosis as well as by direct diffusion, despite their molecular size and charge. However, there are abundant enzymes that cleave foreign DNA in plasma and in cell cytoplasm so methylphosphorate analogues have been synthesised in which a methyl group substitutes for an oxygen atom in the nucleotide backbone. Another approach is the use of phosphothiorate analogues in which a negatively charged sulfur atom substitutes for an oxygen (so called 'S-oligomers'). This increases water solubility as well as conferring resistance to enzymic degradation. The oligomer needs to be at least 15 bases long to confer specificity and tight binding. Following parenteral administration, such oligomers distribute widely (although not to the central nervous system) and work in part by interfering with the transcription of mRNA and in part by stimulating its breakdown by ribonuclease H, which cleaves the bound mRNA. This approach is being investigated in clinical studies in patients with viral disease (including HIV infection) and malignancy (including the use of *bcl-2* antisense therapy administered subcutaneously in patients with non-Hodgkin lymphoma).

Other gene-based approaches

- Correction of a gene that has been altered by mutation would be ideal. This is in its infancy.
- 'Antisense oligonucleotides' are short (15–25) sequences of nucleotide bases (oligonucleotides) that are complementary to part of a gene or gene product that it is desired to inhibit. They influence the expression of a gene either by forming a triplex (three-stranded helix) with a regulatory component of chromosomal DNA or by complexing a region of mRNA.
- Oligonucleotides can cross plasma and nuclear membranes, but there are abundant enzymes that cleave foreign DNA so water-soluble methylphosphorate or phosphothiorate analogues, which are resistant to enzymic degradation, are used.
- This approach is being used in clinical trials in HIV infection and malignancy.

REFERENCES AND FURTHER READING

Scientific American published an issue devoted to gene therapy in June 1997, which is an excellent introduction, including articles by T Friedmann (*on 'overcoming the obstacles to gene therapy'*), P L Felgner (*on non-viral strategies for gene therapy*), R M Blaese (*on gene therapy for cancer*) and by D Y Ho and R M Sapolsky (*on gene therapy for the nervous system*)

Askari F K, McDonnell W M 1996 Antisense-oligonucleotide therapy. N Engl J Med 334: 316–318

Blau H M, Springer M L 1995a Gene therapy—a novel form of drug delivery. N Engl J Med 333: 1204–1207 (*Succinct molecular pharmacological view*)

Blau H M, Springer M L 1995b Muscle-mediated gene therapy. N Engl J Med 333: 1554–1556

Brenner M K 1996 Gene transfer to hematopoietic cells. N Engl J Med 335: 337–339 (*Pluripotent stem cells could provide stable populations of genetically altered cells within each haematopoietic lineage*)

Channon K M, George S E 1997 Improved adenoviral vectors: cautious optimism for gene therapy. Q J Med 90: 105–109 (*'Second generation' adenoviral vectors with the potential for long-term transgene expression with little or no chronic inflammatory response*)

Check E 2002 A tragic setback. Nature 420: 116–118 (*News feature describing efforts to explain the mechanism underlying a leukaemia-like illness in a child previously cured of severe combined immunodeficiency by gene therapy*)

Collins F S 1999 Shattuck lecture: medical and societal consequences of the human genome project. N Engl J Med 341:28-37 (*Thoughtful overview*)

Docherty K 1997 Gene therapy for diabetes mellitus. Clin Sci 92: 321–330 (*Reviews experimental approaches to engineering glucose-responsive B cell and non-B cell lines, and in vivo transfer of the insulin gene in animals*)

Friedmann T 1996 Human gene therapy—an immature genie, but certainly out of the bottle. Nat Med 2: 144–147 (*Commentary on the mood swings of the gene therapy community by a founding father*)

Guttmacher A E, Collins F S 2002 Genomic medicine—a primer. N Engl J Med 347: 1512–1520 (*First in a series on genomic medicine*)

Leiden J M 1995 Gene therapy—promise, pitfalls and prognosis. N Engl J Med 333: 871–872 (*Editorial discussing two negative trials in the same issue, one on adenoviral vector-mediated gene transfer in cystic fibrosis (pp. 823–831) and the other on myoblast transfer in the treatment of Duchenne muscular dystrophy (pp. 832–838)*)

Matteucci M D, Wagner R W 1996 In pursuit of antisense. Nature 384(suppl): 20–22 (*First-generation antisense oligodeoxynucleotides (ODNs) are undergoing clinical trial in HIV and cytomegalovirus infections, various malignancies and to prevent restenosis after balloon angioplasty; also discusses second- and third-generation phosphothiorate and other modifications of ODNs*)

Verma I M, Somia N 1997 Gene therapy—promises, problems and prospects. Nature 389: 239–242 (*The authors, from the Salk Institute,*

describe the principle of putting corrective genetic material into cells to alleviate disease, the practical obstacles to this, and the hopes that better delivery systems will overcome these)
Weatherall D J 2000 Single gene disorders or complex traits: lessons from the thalassaemias and other monogenic diseases. Br Med J 321: 1117–1120 (*Argues that relating genotype to phenotype is the challenge for genetic medicine over the next century*)
Weichselbaum R R, Kufe D 1997 Gene therapy of cancer. Lancet 349(suppl II): 10–12 (*Discusses vectors, selective transgene expression and transduction, therapeutic genes, immunogene therapy, gene replacement, transfer of resistance to cytotoxic therapy and clinical trials*)
Wilson J M 1996 Adenoviruses as gene-delivery vehicles. N Engl J Med 334: 1185–1187 (*Briefly reviews the development of adenovirus as vector for the* CFTR *gene, which is defective in patients with cystic fibrosis, and the problems that result from immune responses to such vectors*)
Ylä-Herttuala S, Martin JF 2000 Cardiovascular gene therapy. Lancet 355: 213–222 (*Reviews rationale, vectors, delivery, therapeutic targets, human trials, ethics and future directions*)

Drug discovery and development

54

Overview 747

The preclinical stages 747

Clinical development 749

Commercial aspects 750

A final note 751

OVERVIEW

With the development of the pharmaceutical industry towards the end of the 19th century, drug discovery became a highly focussed and managed process. Discovering new drugs moved from the domain of inventive doctors to that of scientists hired for the purpose. Today, the bulk of modern therapeutics, and of modern pharmacology, is based on drugs that came from the laboratories of pharmaceutical companies, without which neither the practise of therapeutics nor the science of pharmacology would be more than a pale fragment of what they have become.

In this final chapter, we give a brief overview of the modern approach to drug discovery, touching on the scientific principles involved in inventing a new drug, and also the various clinical, technical, commercial and regulatory criteria that it must satisfy. Our account is necessarily brief and superficial, and more detail can be found elsewhere (Smith, 1992; Drews, 1998).

THE PRECLINICAL STAGES

Figure 54.1 shows in an idealised way the stages of a 'typical' project, aimed at producing a marketable drug that meets a particular medical need (e.g. to retard the progression of Parkinson's disease or cardiac failure, or to prevent migraine attacks).

Broadly the process can be divided into three main components, namely:

- *drug discovery*, during which candidate molecules are chosen on the basis of their pharmacological properties
- *preclinical development*, during which a wide range of non-human studies (e.g. toxicity testing, pharmacokinetic analysis, formulation, etc.) are performed
- *clinical development*, during which the selected compound is tested for efficacy, side-effects and potential dangers in volunteers and patients.

These phases do not necessarily follow in strict succession as indicated in Figure 54.1 but generally overlap.

THE DRUG DISCOVERY PHASE

Given the task of planning a project to discover a new drug to treat, say Parkinson's disease, where does one start? Assuming that we are not simply trying to develop a slightly improved me-too version of a drug already in use,* we first need to choose a new target.

TARGET SELECTION

As discussed in Chapter 2, drug targets are, with few exception, functional proteins (e.g. receptors, enzymes, transport proteins). Though in the past, drug discovery programmes were often based—successfully—on measuring a complex resonse in vivo, such as prevention of experimentally induced seizures, lowering of blood sugar or suppression of an inflammatory response, without the need for prior identification of a drug target, nowadays it will be rare to start without a defined protein target, so the first step is *target identification*. This most often comes from biological intelligence. It was known, for example, that inhibiting angiotensin-converting enzyme lowers blood pressure by suppressing angiotensin II formation, so it made sense to look

*Many commercially successful drugs have in the past emerged from exactly such me-too projects, examples being the dozen or so β-adrenoceptor-blocking drugs developed in the wake of propranolol, or the recent gush of 'triptans' used to treat migraine. Quite small improvements (e.g. in pharmacokinetics or side-effects) coupled with aggressive marketing have often proved enough for clinical and commercial success, but the barriers are getting higher, so the emphasis has now shifted towards novel drug targets.

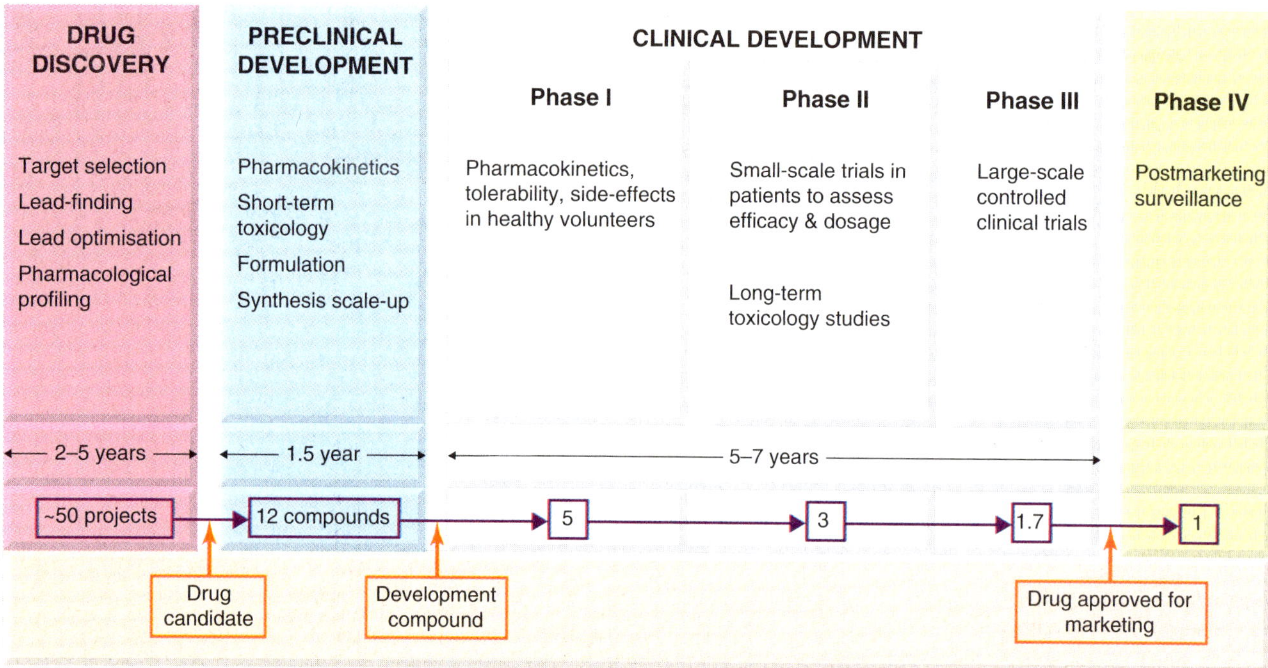

Fig. 54.1 The stages of development of a 'typical' new drug, i.e. a synthetic compound being developed for systemic use. Only the main activites undertaken at each stage are shown, and the details vary greatly according to the kind of drug being developed. Overall cost per marketed compound is £250–500 million and the typical time scale is 8–12 years. Only about 1 in 12 compounds entering development succeeds in reaching the market.

for antagonists for the vascular angiotensin II receptor—hence the successful 'sartan' series of antihyptensive drugs. Similarly, substance P was thought to play a role in pain management, so targeting its receptor (the NK-1 receptor) in a quest for new analgesic drugs was also rational (though in this case unsuccessful). Current therapeutic drugs address about 400 distinct targets, but there are still many proteins that are thought to play a role in disease for which we still have no cognate drug; many of these represent potential starting points for drug discovery.

Conventional biological wisdom, drawing on a rich fund of knowledge of disease mechanisms and chemical signalling pathways, remains the basis on which novel targets are most often chosen. However, looking ahead, there is no doubt that genomics will play an increasing role, by revealing new proteins involved in chemical signalling and new genes involved in disease. Space precludes discussion here of this burgeoning area: interested readers are referred to recent reviews (Drews, 1998; Dyer et al., 1999; Lenz et al., 2000).

LEAD-FINDING

When the biochemical target has been decided—usually after much discussion—and the feasibility of the project has been assessed, the next step is to find *lead compounds*. The usual approach involves cloning of the target protein—normally the human form, since the sequence variation among species is often associated with pharmacological differences, and it is essential to optimise for activity in humans. An assay system must then be developed, allowing the functional activity of the target protein to be measured. This could be a cell-free enzyme assay, a membrane-based binding assay or a cellular response assay. It must be engineered to run automatically, if possible with an optical readout (e.g. fluorescence or optical absorbance), and in a miniaturised multiwell plate format for reasons of speed and economy. Robotically controlled assay facilities capable of testing tens of thousands of compounds per day in several parallel assays are now commonplace in the pharmaceutical industry, and these have become the standard starting point for most drug discovery projects. For an update on how the technology is developing, see Sundberg (2000).

To keep such hungry monsters running requires very large compound libraries. Large companies will typically maintain a growing collection of a million or more synthetic compounds, which will be routinely screened whenever a new assay is set up. Whereas in the past, compounds were generally synthesised and purified one by one, often taking a week or more for each, the present tendency is to use *combinatorial chemistry*, which allows families of several hundreds or thousands of related compounds to be made simultaneously. By coupling such high-speed chemistry to high-throughput assay systems, the time taken over the initial lead-finding stage of projects has been reduced to a few months in most cases, having previously often taken several years. Despite the apparent mindlessness of the high-throughput random screening approach, it usually gives results in the form of lead compounds that have the appropriate pharmacological activity and are amenable to further chemical medification. Building and maintaining huge compound libraries is, however, a costly business, and it has to be realised that even the largest practicable compound collection represents only a minute fraction of the number of 'drug-like' molecules that exists in theory—estimated at about 10^{60}.

Natural products as lead compounds

Historically, natural products, derived mainly from fungal and plant sources, have proved to be a fruitful source of new therapeutic agents, particularly in the field of anti-infective, anti-cancer and immunosuppressant drugs. Familiar examples include penicillin, streptomycin and many other antibiotics, vinca alkaloids, taxol, ciclosporin and rapamycin. These substances presumably serve a specific protective function, having evolved so as to recognise with great precision vulnerable target molecules in their enemies or competitors. The surface of this resource has been barely scratched, and many companies are actively engaged in generating and testing natural product libraries for lead-finding purposes. Fungi and other microorganisms are particularly suitable for this, since they are ubiquitous, highly diverse and easy to collect and grow in the laboratory. The main disadvantage of natural products as lead compounds is that they are often complex molecules that are difficult to synthesise or modify by conventional synthetic chemistry; consequently lead optimisation may be difficult, and commercial production very expensive.

LEAD OPTIMISATION

Lead compounds found by random screening are the basis for the next stage, *lead optimisation*, where the aim (usually) is to increase the potency of the compound on its target, and to optimise it with respect to other properties, such as selectivity, metabolic stability, etc. In this phase, the tests applied include a broader range of assays on different test systems, including studies to measure the activity and time course of the compounds in vivo (where possible in animal models mimicking aspects of the clinical condition), checking for obvious side-effects, and usually for oral absorption. The objective of the lead optimisation phase is to identify one or more *drug candidates* suitable for further development.

As shown in Figure 54.1, only about one project in four succeeds in generating a drug candidate, and it can take up to 5 years. The most common problem is that 'lead optimisation' proves to be impossible: despite much ingenious and back-breaking chemistry, the lead compounds, like antisocial teenagers, refuse to give up their bad habits. In other cases, the compounds, though they produce the desired effects on the target molecule and have no other obvious defects, fail to produce the expected effects in animal models of the disease, implying that the target is probably not a good one. The virtuous minority proceed to the next phase, *preclinical development*.

PRECLINICAL DEVELOPMENT

The aim of preclinical development is to satisfy all the requirements that have to be met before a new compound is deemed ready to be tested for the first time in humans.

The work falls into four categories.

- *Pharmacological testing*, to check that the drug does not produce any potentially hazardous or serious unwanted effects, such as bronchoconstriction, cardiac dysrhythmias, blood pressure changes, ataxia, etc.
- *Preliminary toxicological testing*, to eliminate genotoxicity and to determine the maximum non-toxic dose of the drug (usually when given daily for 28 days, and tested in two species). The animals so treated are examined minutely postmortem at the end of the experiment to look for histological and biochemical evidence of tissue damage.
- *Pharmacokinetic testing*, including studies on the absorption, metabolism, distribution and elimination (ADME studies) in laboratory animals.
- *Chemical and pharmaceutical development*, to assess the feasibility of large-scale synthesis and purification, the stability of the compound under various conditions, and to develop a formulation suitable for clinical studies.

Much of the work of preclinical development, especially that relating to safety issues, is done under a formal code, known as *Good Laboratory Practice* (GLP), which covers such aspects as record-keeping procedures, data analysis, instrument calibration, staff trammg, etc. The aim of GLP is to eliminate human error as far as possible, and to ensure the reliability of the data submitted to the regulatory authority. Laboratories are regularly monitored for compliance to GLP standards. The strict discipline involved in working to this code is generally ill-suited to the creative approaches needed in the earlier stages of drug discovery, so GLP standards are not usually adopted until projects get beyond the discovery phase.

Roughly half of the compounds fail during the preclinical development phase; for the rest, a detailed dossier is prepared for submission to the regulatory authority (e.g. the Medicines Control Agency in the UK or the Food and Drug Administration in the USA), whose permission is required to proceed with studies in humans. This is not lightly given, and the regulatory authority may refuse permission or require further work to be done before giving approval.

CLINICAL DEVELOPMENT

Non-clinical development work continues throughout the clinical trials period, when much more data, particularly in relation to long-term toxicity in animals, has to be generated. If a drug is intended for long-term use in the clinic, the animal toxicology studies may have to be extended for up to 2 years and may include time-consuming studies for possible effects on fertility and fetal development. Failure of a compound at this stage is very costly, and considerable efforts are made to eliminate potentially toxic compounds much earlier in the drug discovery process by the use of in vitro, or even 'in silico', methods.

Clinical development proceeds through four distinct phases (for details see Friedman et al., 1996).

Phase I

Phase I trials are performed on a small group (normally 20–80) of normal healthy volunteers, and their aim is to check for several factors.

- *Safety*—Does the drug produce any potentially dangerous effects, e.g. on cardiovascular, respiratory, hepatic or renal function?
- *Tolerability*—Does the drug produce any unpleasant symptons, e.g. headache, nausea, drowsiness?
- *Pharmacokinetic properties*—Is the drug well absorbed? What is the time course of the plasma concentration? Is there evidence of accumulation or non-linear kinetics?
- *Pharmacodynamic effects* may also be tested—Does a novel analgesic compound block experimentally induced pain in humans? How does the effect vary with dose?

Phase II

Phase II studies are performed on groups of patients (normally 100–300) and are designed to test for efficacy in the clinical situation, as well as extending the phase I studies to include patients as well as healthy volunteers. Often such studies will cover several distinct clinical groups (e.g. depression, anxiety states, phobias, etc.) to give an indication of the possible therapeutic indication for the new compound, and the dose required. When new drug targets are being studied, it is not until these phase II trials are completed that the team finds out whether or not the initial hypothesis was correct, and lack of the expected efficacy is a common reason for failure.

Phase III

Phase III studies are the definitive double-blind randomised trials, commonly performed as multicentre trials on 1000–3000 patients, aimed at comparing the new drug with commonly used alternatives. These trials are extremely costly, difficult to organise and often take years to complete, particularly if the treatment is designed to retard the progression of a chronic disease. It is not uncommon for a drug that seemed highly effective in the limited patient groups tested in phase II to look much less impressive under the more rigorous conditions of phase III trials, particularly when the requirement of the regulatory authorities is that the drug should show distinct advantages over currently available therapies.

Increasingly, phase III trials are being required to include a pharmacoeconomic analysis (see Ch. 1), such that not only clinical but also economic benefits of the new treatment are assessed. The whole process has to comply with an elaborate code known as *Good Clinical Practice*, covering every detail of the patient group, data collection methods, recording of information, statistical analysis and documentation.

At the end of phase III, the drug will be submitted to the relevant regulatory authority for licensing. The dossier required for this is a massive detailed compilation of all of the preclinical and clinical data obtained. Evaluation by the regulatory authority normally takes a year or more, and further delays often arise when aspects of the submission have to be clarified or more data are required. Eventually, about two thirds of submissions gain marketing approval.

Phase IV

Phase IV studies comprise the obligatory postmarketing surveillance designed to detect any rare or long-term adverse effects resulting from the use of the drug in a clinical setting in many thousands of patients. Such events may necessitate limiting the use of the drug to particular patient groups, or even withdrawal of the drug (as recently happened when a cholesterol-lowering drug, cerivastatin, was withdrawn after a few cases of severe muscle degeneration were linked to its use).

BIOPHARMACEUTICALS

Biopharmaceuticals is the term used to describe therapeutic agents produced by biotechnology, rather than conventional synthetic chemistry. Such agents include many hormones, such as insulin, growth hormone, erythropoietin, as well as various therapeutic antibodies and vaccines (see Ch. 13), and cytokines, such as interferon (Ch. 15). Gene-based therapeutics (see Ch. 53), as well as cell-based transplantation procedures (see Ch. 38) are further examples of biopharmaceutical approaches, still in their infancy. The biotechnology industry, much of it directed towards therapeutics, has undergone explosive growth since its origins in the early 1980s, and the number of biopharmaceutical products registered for clinical use—currently about 25% of new products registered each year—is expected to rise. The underlying principles of biopharmaceuticals, and the process of developing them for clinical use, are rooted more in molecular and cell biology than in conventional pharmacology, and lie beyond the scope of this chapter. For more information, see Brooks (1999).

COMMERCIAL ASPECTS

Figure 54.1 shows the approximate time taken for such a project, the attrition rate (importantly) at each stage and the overall process based on averaged data for several large pharaceutical companies in recent years. The key messages are (i) that it is a high-risk business, with only about 1 project in 50 reaching its goal of putting a new drug on the market; (ii) that it takes a long time, about 12 years on average; and (iii) that it costs a lot of money to develop one drug (£250–500 million and rising rapidly, according to recent estimates*). For any one project, the costs escalate rapidly as development proceeds, phase II trials and

*The total R&D spend of the pharmaceutical industry, $20 billion in 2000, has doubled every 5 years since 1970.

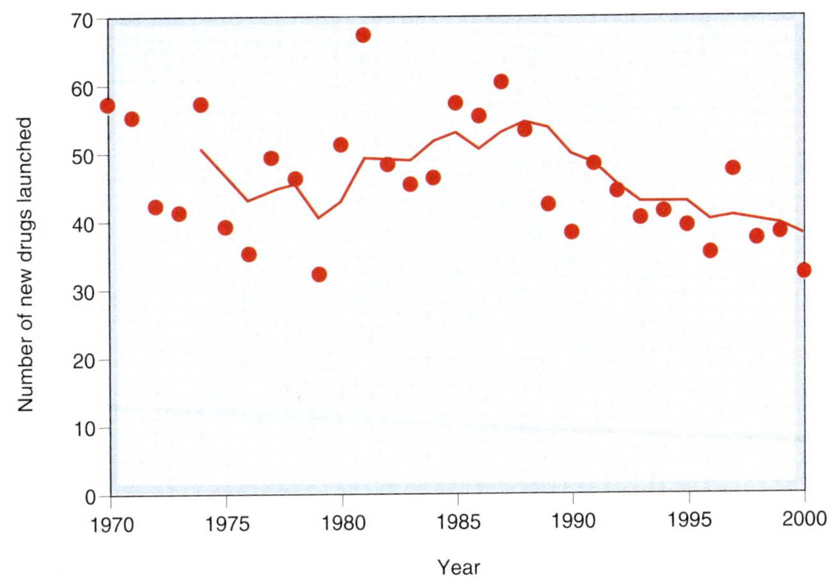

Fig. 54.2 The rate of introduction of new drugs into the major worldwide markets, showing the steady decline in the 1990s. The line shows the 5-year rolling average. (Figure taken with permission from Centre for Medicines Research R&D compendium, 2000.)

long-term toxicology studies being particularly expensive. The time factor is crucial, since the new drug has to be patented, usually at the end of the discovery phase, and the period of exclusivity (about 20 years) during which the company is free from competition in the market starts on that date. After 20 years, the patent expires, and other companies, which have not supported development costs, are free to make and sell the drug much more cheaply, so the revenues for the original company decrease rapidly thereafter. Reducing the development time after patenting is a major concern for all companies, but so far it has remained stubbornly fixed at around 10 years, partly because the regulatory authorities are demanding more clinical data before they will grant a licence. In practice, only about one drug in eight that goes on the market brings in enough revenue to cover its development costs. Success for the company relies on this one drug being a 'block buster' that pays for the rest.

Figure 54.2 illustrates the steady decline in the number of new drugs launched in the major markets worldwide, despite escalating costs and improved technology. There has been much speculation as to the causes, the optimistic view (see below) being that fewer but better drugs are being introduced, and that the recent technological jump has yet to make its impact.

A FINAL NOTE

Since the 1990s, the drug discovery process has been in the throes of a substantial methodological revolution, following the rapid ascendancy of molecular biology, genomics and informatics, amid high expectations that this would bring remarkable dividends in terms of speed, cost and success rate. High-throughput screening has undoubtedly emerged as a powerful lead-finding technology, but overall, the benefits are not yet clear: costs have risen steadily, the success rate has drifted downwards (the number of launches in 2000 being the lowest since 1979; Fig. 54.2) and development times have not decreased. None of this matters, of course, if the new drugs that are being developed improve the quality of medical care, and here there is room for optimism. In recent years, drugs aimed at new targets (e.g. selective serotinin reuptake inhibitors, statins, the kinase inhibitor imatinib, etc.) have made major contributions to patient care. These are 'pre-revolutionary' drugs. It is too soon for the new technologies to have made an impact on new drug registrations, but we can reasonably expect that their ability to make new targets available to the drug discovery machine will have a real effect on patient care.

REFERENCES AND FURTHER READING

Brooks G 1999 Biotechnology in healthcare: an introduction to biopharmaceuticals. Pharmaceutical Press, London

Drews J 1998 In quest of tomorrow's medicines. Springer, New York (*Thoughtful and non-technical account of the history, principles and future directions of drug discovery*)

Dyer M R, Cohen D, Herrling P L 1999 Functional genomics: from genes to new therapies. Drug Discovery Today 4: 109–114 (*General account of the impact of genomics on the drug dricovery process*)

Friedman L M, Furberg C D, de Mets D L 1996 Fundamentals of clinical trials, 3rd edn. Mosby, St Louis, MO (*Standard textbook*)

Lenz G R, Nash H M, Jindal S 2000 Chemical ligands, genomics and drug discovery. Drug Discovery Today 5: 145–155 (*Futuristic review, pointing to new approaches for finding lead compounds*)

Smith C G 1992 The process of new drug discovery and development. CRC Press, Boca Raton, FL (*Detailed account, useful but now somewhat out-of date in certain aspects*)

Sundberg S A 2000 High-throughput and ultra-high-throughput screening: solution and cell-based approaches. Curr Opin Biotechnol 11: 14–53

Appendix

Some important pharmacological agents

Students may feel overwhelmed by the number of drugs described in pharmacology textbooks. We would emphasise that it is more important to understand general pharmacological principles and to appreciate the pharmacology of the main classes of drug than to attempt to memorise details of individual agents. Specific drugs are best learned about when they are encountered in the setting of particular topics (e.g. noradrenergic transmission), during practical classes or (for therapeutic drugs) near a patient's bedside. The following list gives examples of some of the more important pharmacological agents. It is not intended as a starting point to learning pharmacology, and we would caution against attempting to memorise lists of names and properties. The examples we provide here are divided into agents of primary and secondary importance. In some geographic areas, one or another class of drug will have more or less importance (e.g. anthelminthics are very important in regions where schistosomiasis is common, less so in the UK), so these categories are meant only as a broad guide. The list includes not only drugs used therapeutically but also endogenous mediators/transmitters and certain important drugs used as experimental tools; these are shown in italics. A working knowledge of drugs in the 'primary importance' category, including effects and mode of action, and (for those used therapeutically) pharmacokinetic properties, side-effects, toxicity and main uses should be built up gradually as they are encountered during training. For drugs in the second category, it is usually sufficient to have awareness of the mechanism of action supplemented, where appropriate, by understanding how they differ from those in the primary category.

The choice of drugs in clinical use is inevitably somewhat arbitrary. Hospital formulary committees grapple with choosing which individual drugs of a therapeutic class to stock in the pharmacy. There is a play-off between stocking several individual drugs of one category, for each of which there is good evidence of efficacy for distinct indications, and stocking a more restricted choice based on assuming that efficacy is likely to be a common feature of different members of a class of drugs. Local variations will be encountered (e.g. as to which angiotensin-converting enzyme inhibitor (ACEI) or non-steroidal inflammatory drug (NSAID) is stocked in the hospital pharmacy). If the student or doctor comes to these (e.g. when changing to a job in a new hospital) with a sound appreciation of the general principles of pharmacology and of the specifics of the various classes of agent involved, he or she will be able to look up and understand the details of a specific agent favoured locally and use it sensibly. (Learning how to cope with change is one of the main educational objectives defined in the General Medical Council's recommendations on undergraduate medical training in 'Tomorrow's doctors' and this is one example of its importance.)

The drugs are grouped broadly as in the chapters of the text, and may appear more than once in the lists.

Primary	Secondary
1. Pharmacological agents and cholinergic transmission	
Agonists	
acetylcholine	carbachol
suxamethonium	nicotine
	pilocarpine
Antagonists	
atropine	tropicamide
	pirenzepine
tubocurarine	atracurium
	α-bungarotoxin
	vecuronium
hexamethonium	trimethaphan
Anticholinesterases and related drugs	
neostigmine	edrophonium
	dyflos
	(pralidoxime—cholinesterase reactivator)

2. Pharmacological agents and noradrenergic transmission

Primary	Secondary
Agonists	
adrenaline (epinephrine)	clonidine
noradrenaline (norepinephrine)	phenylephrine
isoprenaline (isoproterenol)	
salbutamol	
Antagonists	
propranolol	atenolol
prazosin	metoprolol
Drugs affecting noradrenergic neurons	
guanethidine	*tyramine*
	amphetamine
methyldopa	*cocaine*
	reserpine
	α-methyltyrosine
	imipramine
	phenelzine

3. Other peripheral mediators (5-hydroxytryptamine (5-HT), purines, peptides and nitric oxide) and agents related to them

Primary	Secondary
Drugs acting on 5-HT receptors	
5-hydroxytryptamine (5-HT, serotonin)	ergonovine
ondansetron	
methysergide	
sumatriptan	
Drugs acting on purinoceptors	
adenosine	theophylline
ATP	
ADP	
Renin–angiotensin system	
angiotensin	
captopril	
losartan	
Various peptides	
bradykinin	*atrial natriuretic peptide (ANP)*
endothelin	calcitonin
oxytocin	*calcitonin gene-related peptide (CGRP)*
vasopressin	*cholecystokinin*
	neuropeptide Y (NPY)
	octreotide
	substance P
	vasoactive intestinal polypeptide (VIP)
Nitric oxide	
nitric oxide (NO)	
L-N^{G}-monomethyl arginine (L-NMMA)	

4. Local hormones, inflammation and allergy (including anti-inflammatory and immunosuppressant drugs)

Primary	Secondary
Eicosanoids	**Leukotriene antagonists and 5-lipoxygenase inhibitors**
prostaglandins	montelukast
thromboxanes	zileutin
prostaglandin (prostacyclin)	
leukotrienes	
Cyclooxygenase inhibitors NSAIDs	
aspirin	
ibuprofen	
indometacin	
Histamine and antihistamines	
histamine	
mepyramine	terfenadine
	fexofenadine
ranitidine	cimetidine
Drugs used in gout	
allopurinol	colchicine
	probenecid
	sulfinpyrazone
Immunosuppressant drugs	
azathioprine	tacrolimus
ciclosporin	
methotrexate	
prednisolone	
Other disease modifying antirheumatic drugs	
	auranofin
	hydroxychloroquine
	penicillamine
	sulfasalazine
Other mediators	
cytokines (e.g. interleukins)	
platelet-activating factor (PAF)	
interferon beta	

5. Drugs affecting the cardiovascular system

Primary	Secondary
Antidysrhythmic drugs (Vaughan–Williams classification)	
Class I: lidocaine	flecainide
Class II: atenolol	metoprolol
Class III: amiodarone	sotalol
Class IV: verapamil	
Unclassified: adenosine	
digoxin	
Antianginal drugs	
Nitrates:	
glyceryl trinitrate	
isosorbide mononitrate	
β-Blockers: atenolol	metoprolol
Calcium antagonists:	
amlodipine	
nifedipine	diltiazem
Antihypertensive drugs	
Thiazide diuretics:	
bendroflumethiazide (bendrofluazide)	hydrochlorothiazide
β-Adrenoceptor antagonists:	
atenolol	
Angiotensin-converting enzyme inhibitors (ACEI) and angiotensin II (AT1 receptor) antagonists:	
captopril	lisinopril
enalapril	trandolapril
losartan	irbesartan
Calcium antagonists:	
amlodipine	
nifedipine	
α_1-Adrenoceptor antagonists:	
doxazosin	prazosin
	terazocin
Other vasodilators	
lisinopril	hydralazine
	minoxidil
	nitroprusside
Centrally acting drugs	
	methyldopa
	moxonidine
Drugs used in heart failure and shock	
Diuretics:	
furosemide (frusemide)	bendroflumethiazide (bendrofluazide)
amiloride	
ACEI:	
captopril	
enalapril	
Cardiac glycosides:	
digoxin	
Drugs acting on catecholamine receptors:	
	dobutamine
	dopamine
Drugs used to prevent atherosclerosis	
Statins: simvastatin	pravastatin
Fibrates: bezafibrate	gemfibrozil
Resins: colestyramine	colestipol

6. Drugs used in hemostasis and thrombosis

Primary	Secondary
Oral anticoagulants and antagonists	
warfarin	
vitamin K	
Heparin and ( ) antagonists	
heparin	(protamine)
low-molecular-weight heparins (e.g. tizaprin)	
Antiplatelet drugs	
aspirin	dipyridamole
	prostacyclin
	ticlopidine
Fibrinolytic drugs and ( ) inhibitors of fibrinolysis	
streptokinase	(tranexamic acid)
tissue plasminogen activator	

7. Drugs affecting the respiratory system

Primary	Secondary
β_2-Adrenoceptor agonists	
salbuterol	salmeterol
	terbutaline
Inhaled glucocorticoids:	
beclometasone propionate	
Inhaled muscarinic antagonists:	
ipratropium	
Xanthine alkaloids:	
theophylline	
Other inhaled drugs used for asthma prophylaxis:	cromoglycate
Leukotriene antagonists and 5-lipoxygenase inhibitors:	montelukast
	zileutin
Antitussive drugs	
	codeine

8. Drugs affecting the kidney

Primary	Secondary
Thiazide diuretics:	
bendroflumethiazide (bendrofluazide)	hydrochlorothiazide
chlorothiazide	
Loop diuretics:	
Furosemide (frusemide)	bumetanide
K⁺-sparing diuretics:	
spironolactone	triamterene
amiloride	
Osmotic diuretics:	mannitol
Carbonic anhydrase inhibitors:	acetazolamide
Antidiuretic hormone (vasopressin) (V2) agonist:	desmopressin

9. Drugs affecting the gastrointestinal system

Primary	Secondary
Ulcer-healing drugs	
H_2 receptor antagonists:	
ranitidine	cimetidine
Proton pump inhibitors:	
omeprazole	lansoprazole
Antibiotics for *Helicobacter pylori*:	
See Section 30	
Prostaglandin analogues:	misoprostol
Aluminium complexes:	sucralfate
Laxatives	
lactulose	
senna	
Anti-emetics	
domperidone	
metoclopramide	
ondansetron	
Emetics	
	ipecacuanha
Antidiarrheal drugs	
codeine	loperamide
Drugs for inflammatory bowel disease	
sulfasalazine	
Antispasmodics	
	hyoscine
	cyclizine

10. Drugs affecting the endocrine pancreas

Primary	Secondary
Hormones:	
insulin	*amylin*
glucagon	*somatostatin*
Sulfonylureas:	
tolbutamide	glibenclamide
	gliburide
Biguanides:	
metformin	
α-Glucosidase inhibitors	acarbose
Thiazolidinediones:	troglitazone

11. Thyroid hormones and antithyroid drugs

Primary	Secondary
Hormones and precursors	
thyroxine	liothyronine
	iodine/iodide
Antithyroid drugs	
carbimazole	propylthiouracil
	radioiodine (^{131}I)

12. Obesity

Primary	Secondary
	leptin
	neuropeptide Y

13. Anterior pituitary and adrenal glands

Primary	Secondary
Glucocorticoids:	
prednisolone	
hydrocortisone	
dexamethasone	
Mineralocorticoids:	
fludrocortisone	
Pituitary hormones:	corticotropin (ACTH)
	growth hormone
	somatostatin
	octreotide

Primary	Secondary
14. Sex hormones and related drugs	
Estrogens:	
estradiol	
Anti-estrogens:	
tamoxifen	clomiphene
Progestins:	
progesterone	norethindrone
Antiprogestogens:	
mifepristone	
Androgens:	
testosterone	
Anti-androgens:	
cyproterone	finasteride
Gonadotrophin-releasing hormone analogues:	buserelin

Primary	Secondary
15. Drugs acting on the uterus	
ergonovine	
oxytocin	
dinoprostone (PGE_2)	

Primary	Secondary
16. Drugs and bone	
parathyroid hormone (PTH)	calcitonin
vitamin D	calcium salts
estrogen	
etidronate	

Primary	Secondary
17. Hemopoietic system	
Hematinic drugs:	
ferrous sulfate	
folic acid	
vitamin B_{12}	
Hormones and growth factors:	epoetin (erythropoietin)
	filgrastim, lenograstim (granulocyte colony-stimulating factor)
	molgrastin (granulocyte–macrophage colony-stimulating factor)
	thrombopoietin

Primary	Secondary
18. Chemical mediators in the central nervous system	
Neurotransmitters and ( ) related drugs (see also lists 1–3)	
glutamate	
***NMDA*:**	(ketamine—NMDA channel blocker)
	(dizocilpine—NMDA channel blocker)
***kainic acid*:**	
glycine	(strychnine—glycine antagonist)
GABA	(baclofen—$GABA_B$-receptor agonist)
	(bicuculline—$GABA_A$-receptor antagonist)
Amines:	
noradrenaline (norepinephrine)	
dopamine	
5-HT	
acetylcholine	
histamine	melatonin

Primary	Secondary
19. Neurodegenerative diseases	
Parkinson's disease	
levodopa	selegiline
carbidopa	benztropine
bromocriptine	amantadine
	apomorphine
	MPTP
Amyotrophic lateral sclerosis	
	riluzole
Alzheimer's disease	
	donepezil

Primary	Secondary
20. General anesthetics	
Inhalational	
halothane	ether
enflurane	
isoflurane	
nitrous oxide	
Intravenous	
propofol	etomidate
	ketamine
	thiopental

21. Anxiolytic, hypnotic and related drugs

Primary	Secondary
Benzodiazepines and ( ) antagonists	
temazepam	nitrazepam
diazepam	lorazepam
	(flumazenil)
Barbiturates:	phenobarbital
Other:	buspirone ($5\text{-}HT_{1A}$ receptor agonist)

22. Antipsychotic drugs

Primary	Secondary
Classical	
chlorpromazine	fluphenazine
haloperidol	thioridazine
Atypical:	
clozapine	risperidone
olanzapine	sulpiride

23. Drugs used in affective disorders

Primary	Secondary
Tricyclic antidepressants:	
amitriptyline	imipramine
	mianserin
Selective serotonin (5-HT) reuptake inhibitors (SSRIs):	
fluoxetine	fluvoxamine
sertraline	
Monoamine oxidase inhibitors (MAOIs):	
moclobemide	phenelzine
	tranylcypromine
Atypical antidepressants	mianserin
	maprotiline
Antimanic drugs ('mood stabilisers')	
lithium	carbamazepine

24. Anti-epileptic drugs and centrally acting muscle relaxants

Primary	Secondary
phenytoin	phenobarbital
carbamazepine	diazepam
valproate	clonazepam
	ethosuximide
	vigabatrin
	gabapentin
	baclofen

25. Analgesics and related substances

Primary	Secondary
Opioids and ( ) antagonists	
morphine	fentanyl
codeine	methadone
pentazocine	diamorphine
(naloxone)	pethidine
Mild analgesics (see also under list 4):	
aspirin	
paracetamol	
Other analgesic drugs:	tramadol
	carbamazepine
	amitriptyline
Other compounds involved in nociception:	
enkephalins and *endorphins*	*dynorphin*
	substance P
	capsaicin

26. Central nervous system stimulants and psychotomimetics

Primary	Secondary
amphetamine	methylphenidate
cocaine	*MDMA* ('ecstasy')
caffeine	*LSD* (lysergic acid diethylamide)
	phencyclidine
	strychnine
	bicuculline
	pentylenetetrazol

27. Drug dependence and drug abuse

Primary	Secondary
opiates (morphine, heroin)	Δ^9-tetrahydrocannabinol (THC)
nicotine	*anandamide*
ethanol	solvents
cocaine	benzodiazepines
	amphetamine

28. Local anesthetics and other drugs that affect sodium or potassium channels

Primary	Secondary
Local anesthetics	
lidocaine	tetracaine (amethocaine)
Selective sodium channel antagonists	*tetrodotoxin (TTX)*
Potassium channel antagonists	tetraethylammonium (TEA) *4-aminopyridine* sulfonylureas (see list 10)
Potassium channel activators	cromakalim

29. Cancer chemotherapy

Primary	Secondary
Alkylating agents and related compounds:	
cyclophosphamide cisplatin	lomustine
Antimetabolites:	
cytarabine methotrexate	fluorouracil mercaptopurine
Cytotoxic antibiotics:	
doxorubicin	
Plant derivatives:	
vincristine paclitaxel	etoposide
Hormones and related drugs:	
prednisolone tamoxifen	

30. Antibacterial agents

Primary	Secondary
Bacterial cell wall inhibitors:	
benzylpenicillin fluloxacillin amoxicillin vancomycin	piperacillin cefadroxil cefotaxime ceftriaxone
Topoisomerase inhibitors:	
ciprofloxacin	
Folate inhibitors:	
trimethoprim	sulfonamides
Bacterial protein synthesis inhibitors:	
gentamicin tetracycline chloramphenicol erythromycin	amikacin clarithromycin
Anti-anerobe drugs:	
metronidazole	
Antimycobacterial agents:	
isoniazid rifampin pyrazinamide	ethambutol streptomycin dapsone

31. Antiviral agents

Primary	Secondary
DNA polymerase inhibitors:	
aciclovir	foscarnet ganciclovir tribavirin (ribavirin)
Reverse transcriptase inhibitors	
zidovudine (AZT)	didanosine zalcitabine
Protease inhibitors	
saquinavir	
Immunomodulators:	interferons

32. Antifungal drugs

Primary	Secondary
Polyene antibiotics:	
amphotericin B	nystatin
Azoles:	
fluconazole	miconazole
Antimetabolites:	flucytosine
Others:	terbinafine

Primary	Secondary
33. Antiprotozoal drugs	
Antimalarials:	
chloroquine	pyrimethamine plus sulfadoxine
quinine	artemesenin
primaquine	
For *Pneumocystis pneumoniae*:	
co-trimoxazole (high dose)	
Amebicidal drugs:	
metronidazole	
Leishmanicidal drugs:	antimonials (e.g. stibogluconate) pentamidine
Trypanosomicidal drugs:	suramin pentamidine
Toxoplasmicidal drugs:	pyrimethamine–sulfadiazine

Primary	Secondary
34. Anthelminthic drugs	
Broad spectrum:	mebendazole
Round worm, threadworm:	piperazine
Schistosomes:	praziquantel
River blindness:	ivermectin

This appendix is adapted from that in Dale M M, Dickenson A H, Haylett D G 1996 Companion to pharmacology, 2nd edn. Churchill Livingstone, Edinburgh, with permission.

Index

A

A cells (glucagon-secreting), 380
A_1/A_2 receptors, *see* Adenosine receptors
Abacavir, 661
ABC (abacavir), 661
Abciximab, 241, 325
Abortion, therapeutic, 235, 434, 443
Absence seizures (petit mal), 551–2
therapy, 556
Absorption, 98–101
of calcium in intestine, 449
of drugs, 98–101
delaying methods, 101
disease affecting, 717, 718
drugs affecting, 719
effects of variations in rate of, 115–16
warfarin interactions with drugs reducing, 322
of iron, 332
of potassium in kidney, 361
of sodium and chloride in kidney, 355
of water in kidney, 358
see also Reabsorption
Abstinence syndrome, *see* Withdrawal
Abuse, *see* Drug abuse
Acamprosate, 608
Acarbose, 391, 392
ACE, *see* Angiotensin-converting enzyme
Acetaldehyde, 606
Acetaminophen, *see* Paracetamol
Acetazolamide, 93, 146, 365
in glaucoma, 100, 146
renal actions/effects, 355
Acetylation reactions, 109
isoniazid and, 715
N-Acetyl-*p*-benzoquinone imine, 720, 727
Acetylcholine (ACh), 124, 126, 144, 483–5
action/effects, 136–7
airways, 340
CNS, 483–4
drugs affecting, 143–7
gastric, 369
historical observations, 123, 136
NO release, 137, 288
synaptic (incl. motor endplate/neuromuscular junction), 31, 140, 141, 148, 149–54
in CNS, 483–5
desensitisation with, 20
release, 139–41
adrenaline affects (at presynaptic terminal), 128
drugs affecting, 147, 154–5
Parkinson's disease and, 497
synthesis, 139–41
inhibitors, 154
Acetylcholine receptors, 137–9
ACh concentration reaching, 11
antagonists
muscarinic, *see* Muscarinic ACh receptor antagonists
non-depolarising blocking agents as, 150
in Parkinson's disease, 148, 499, 500
CNS, 483
locations, 138
muscarinic, *see* Muscarinic ACh receptors
nicotinic, *see* Nicotinic ACh receptors
structure, 29–30
Acetylcholinesterase (AChE), 140, 155, 159, 484–5
distribution and function, 155–6
CNS, 484–5
inhibitors, *see* Anticholinesterases
learning deficit with overexpression, 484
see also Cholinesterase
Acetylcysteine, 252, 728
Acetylsalicylic acid, *see* Aspirin
Aciclovir, 662–3
clinical use, 662
herpes viruses, 627, 662
mechanism of action, 627, 662
pharmacokinetics, 662
pro-drug of, 104, 663
unwanted effects, 663
Acid(s)
gastric, *see* Gastric acid
organic, secretion into renal tubule, 355
Acid–base balance, 360
kidney and, 360
salicylates affecting, 251
see also pH
Acidic drugs
pK_a values, 94
weakly
ionisation, 92, 93, 94, 112
renal excretion, 112
Acidification, urinary
drugs causing, 365
effects, 93
see also Acid–base balance; pH
Acidosis
metabolic, with salicylates, 251
respiratory, with salicylates, 251
Acipimox, 312
Acitretin, teratogenicity, 734
Aclarubicin, 703
Acridines, 625
Acromegaly, 385, 407
Acrosoxacin, 648
ACTH, *see* Adrenocorticotrophic hormone
Actin, 62
myocardial, 269
Actinomycin D (dactinomycin), action, 625–7, 703
Action (of drugs), 7–50
general principles, 7–21
molecular aspects, 22–47
targets for, *see* Targets
see also Interactions
Action potential, 55, 56, 57
cardiac (myocyte), 62, 265, 266
inhibition by class I antidysrhythmics, 274
myocardial damage affecting, 268
prolongation by class III antidysrhythmics, 275
seizures and, 553
site of action of drugs and toxins affecting channels involved in, 59
skeletal muscle, 62
smooth muscle, 62
Activated partial thromboplastin time, 320
Activator protein-1 (AP-1), 413
Active transport, 94
nephron, 355
Active zone, synaptic transmission, 66
Acyclovir, *see* Aciclovir
Adaptation, physiological, drug effect diminution due to, 21
Addiction, *see* Dependence
Addison's disease, 411, 418
Aδ-fibres, 563
Adenine deaminase deficiency, 743
Adeno-associated viruses as gene vectors, 741, 742
Adenohypophysis (anterior pituitary), 404–6, 407–11
glucocorticoid feedback effects, 416
testosterone feedback effects, 435
Adenosine, 128, 192, 194, 195, 277–8
actions/effects, 194, 195
in CNS, 485
in coronary flow regulation, 270
in haemostasis and thrombosis, 317
in myocardial ischaemic preconditioning, 269
in nociception, 195, 572
analogues, as analgesics, 583
therapeutic use, 269, 277–8
supraventricular tachycardia, 196, 278
see also ADP; ADP-ribose; AMP; ATP
Adenosine kinase inhibitors, 583
Adenosine receptors ($A_1/A_2/A_3$; formerly P_1), 194, 195, 485
agonists, 485
antagonists, 196
xanthines as, 196, 278, 346, 485, 590
Adenoviruses as gene vectors, 740, 742
Adenylate cyclase, 36, 41
drugs affecting, 294
opioid receptors and, 576
ADH, *see* Antidiuretic hormone
Adhesive proteins/molecules, cell surface and extracellular matrix, 73
vascular endothelium, 221
Adipose tissue, *see* Fat
ADL 8-2698, 103
Administration, routes of, 98–101
insulin, 387
local anaesthetics, 617
see also specific routes and specific drugs
ADP, 192
platelets and, 194
receptors, *see* P_{2x} receptors
ADP-ribose (cADPR), 54
Adrenal cortex, 411–19
insufficiency
diagnosis, 409
glucocorticoid-induced, 417
primary (Addison's disease), 411, 418
see also Hypothalamic–pituitary–adrenal axis
Adrenal steroids (corticosteroids – commonly called or implying glucocorticoids), 411–19
actions, 182, 348–9, 412, 413–17
anti-inflammatory, *see subheading below*
on blood glucose, 386
on bone, 416, 417, 450
on corticotrophin-releasing factor, 406
immunosuppressive, 258, 416–17, 418
on macrophages, 221
mechanisms/sites, 232, 348, 413–15
unwanted, *see subheading below*
anti-inflammatory actions, 231, 412, 416–17, 418
in inflammatory bowel disease, 377
clinical uses, 418
as antiemetic, 375

Adrenal steroids, *continued*
asthma, 348, 350
autoimmune disease, 228
chronic obstructive pulmonary disease, 350
hyperthyroidism, 427
inflammatory bowel disease, 377
neoplastic disease, 418, 705
shock, 303
inhaled, 100
pharmacokinetics, 417–18
receptors, *see* Steroid, receptors
sudden withdrawal, 417
synthesis/release, 411–13, 414
ACTH effects on, 409
anticancer agents inhibiting, 705
deficient, *see* Adrenal cortex, insufficiency
drugs (other than steroids) affecting, 413, 705
glucocorticoid therapy suppressing, 417
unwanted effects, 349, 417, 418
inhaled forms, 349
see also Androgens; Mineralocorticoids; Sex steroids
Adrenaline (epinephrine), 179
actions/effects, 8, 11, 179
on ACh release at presynaptic terminals, 128
on blood glucose, 386
historical perspectives, 122, 161, 162
unwanted/adverse, 179
clinical uses, 172, 179
in anaphylaxis and anaphylactic shock, 172, 303, 735
in local anaesthetic solutions, 101, 617, 719
pharmacokinetics, 179
Adrenergic transmission/neurons, *see* Noradrenergic neurons; Noradrenergic transmission
Adrenoceptor(s), 161–4
autonomic nervous system effects related to types of, 127
classification, 161–4
distribution, 163
drugs (in general) acting on, 168–76
structure–activity relationships, 168–72
Adrenoceptor agonists (in general; sympathomimetic amines), 169–72
actions/effects, 169–72, 179
pharmacokinetics, 179
unwanted effects, 179
clinical uses, 172
appetite suppressant, 402
partial, 164
Adrenoceptor antagonists/blockers (in general), 172–6, 180–1
actions/effects, 172–6
unwanted, 180
clinical use, 175, 180–1
mixed, 173, 179, 181
pharmacokinetics, 180–1
α-Adrenoceptor agonists, 162, 163, 171, 179
airway effects, 341
partial, ergot alkaloids as, 189
smooth muscle effects, 170
α-Adrenoceptor antagonists, 163, 172–3, 180
actions/effects, 172–3
ergot alkaloids as, 172, 189
unwanted, 173, 180
antipsychotics as, 529, 532
β-adrenoceptor antagonists and, compounds with activity of both, 173, 179, 181
clinical uses, 173, 175
α_1-Adrenoceptor(s), 162, 163
activation (and effects), 162, 163
agonists (selective), 163, 171, 179
antagonists (selective), 163, 172, 173, 180
adverse effects, 180
clinical uses (other than hypertension), 173, 175, 437
H_1-receptor antagonists as, 253
in hypertension, 173, 300, 301
distribution, 163
in smooth muscle, 170
α_{1A}-Adrenoceptor antagonists, 173, 175
α_2-Adrenoceptor(s), 162, 163
activation (and effects), 162, 163
agonists (selective), 163, 171, 179
alcoholism, 608
glaucoma, 146
migraine, 192
nicotine withdrawal, 603
antagonists (selective), 163, 172, 173, 180
in erectile dysfunction, 444
in migraine, 192
antidepressants downregulating, 539
distribution, 163
noradrenaline release and, 166
in smooth muscle, 170
β-Adrenoceptor(s), 34, 162, 163
airway, 341
antidepressants downregulating, 539
cardiac, *see* Heart
desensitisation, 20
methylxanthine effects, 590
smooth muscle, 170
β-Adrenoceptor agonists, 163, 179
actions/effects, 170–2, 179
ethnicity and, 712–13
clinical use, 172, 179
in heart failure, 279
in preterm labour, 443
interactions, 718
pharmacokinetics, 179
unwanted effects, 179
β-Adrenoceptor blockers/antagonists, 163, 173–6, 180
actions/effects, 174–5
α-adrenoceptor antagonists and, compounds with activity of both, 173, 179, 181
clinical uses
alcohol withdrawal, 608
angina prophylaxis, 282
anxiety, 175, 516, 517
dysrhythmias, 174, 274, 275, 276–7
glaucoma, 100, 146, 175
heart failure, 279, 302
hypertension, 174, 300, 301
hyperthyroidism, 427
migraine, 192, 193
myocardial infarction, 88, 271
phaeochromocytoma, 173
interactions, 718
unwanted effects, 175–6, 180, 276
asthmatics, 175, 346
β_1-Adrenoceptor(s), 162, 163
activation (and effects), 162, 163
agonists (selective), 163, 171
in heart failure, 279
antagonists (selective), 163, 180
actions/effects, 180
distribution, 163
β_2-Adrenoceptor(s), 162, 163, 345–6
activation (and effects), 162, 163
agonists (selective), 163, 171
in asthma, 172, 345–6, 348
in chronic obstructive pulmonary disease, 346
in pregnancy (as myometrial relaxants), 443
antagonists, 163, 181
bronchial smooth muscle, 170
distribution, 163
polymorphisms/mutations, 48
unwanted effects, 346
β_3-Adrenoceptor, 163
activation (and effects), 162, 163
agonists (selective), 170, 173
in obesity, 170, 173, 392, 402
distribution, 163
in obesity pathophysiology, 399, 400
Adrenocorticotrophic hormone (ACTH; corticotrophin), 405, 408–9
actions/effects, 405, 408–9
biosynthesis, 203, 408, 411–12
glucocorticoid feedback effects, 416
clinical use, 409
Adrenomedulin, 286
Adsorbent agents, 377
Adult respiratory distress syndrome, NO therapy, 213
Advanced glycation end-products, 386
Adverse/unwanted reactions (toxicity/side-effects), 724–37
in gene therapy, 743
idiosyncratic, *see* Idiosyncratic reactions
testing/measuring, 725
in preclinical development, 749
types, 724–5
see also Carcinogenesis; Excitotoxicity; Hypersensitivity reactions; Mutagenesis; Risk; Teratogens; Toxic metabolites *and specific drugs*
Affective (mood) disorders, 535–48
drugs used in, *see* Antidepressants; Mood-stabilising drugs
see also specific disorders
Afferent nerves/neurons/fibres, 123
airway, 340, 341
effector functions, 123
nociceptive, 562–3, 568
Affinity for receptors, 9, 10, 16
see also Binding
African sleeping sickness, 684
After-depolarisation in cardiac tissue, delayed, 267
After-load, 285
reduction, 302
Agar, 375
Age, effects of, 713–14
benzodiazepines and, 521
Aggression
antipsychotics reducing, 531
anxiolytics reducing, 516
benzodiazepines, 518–19
SSRIs increasing, reports, 545
Agonists, 8, 9, 18
binding curves with, 11
concentration–effect (dose–response) curves, *see* Dose–response (concentration–effect) curves
definition, 9
examples, 24
full, 9, 12, 13, 18
inverse, 14–15, 18, 23
occupancy of receptors by, *see* Occupancy
partial, 9, 12–13
trafficking, 38
see also specific agonists
Agouti-signalling protein and agouti-related peptide, 410
Agranulocytosis and granulocytopenia, drugs causing, 736
antipsychotic, 533
AIDS, *see* HIV disease
AIF (apoptotic initiating factor), 75
Airway
glands, regulation, 340
resistance, 340
beta-blocker effects, 175
measurement, 340
smooth muscle
adrenoceptors, 170
leukotriene actions, 236
regulation, 340
vasculature, regulation, 340
see also Lungs; Respiratory system
β-Alanine, 473
Albendazole, 628, 688, 689
unwanted effects, 689
Albumin, binding to, 96, 719
glucocorticoid, 417–18
thiopental, 513
warfarin, drugs displacing, 322
Alcohol, *see* Ethanol; Methanol
Alcohol dehydrogenase, 109, 606
Aldehyde dehydrogenase, 606
in catecholamine degradation, 167
inactive genetic variant of one isoform, 607
inhibitors, 606–7
interactions, 721
Aldesleukin, 706
Aldosterone, 67
action/effects, 67, 358, 412, 418–19
mechanisms, 418–19
antagonists, *see* Eplerenone; Spironolactone
secretion/release, 292, 358, 418–19
deficient, 418
deficient, heparin-induced, 321
excess, *see* Hyperaldosteronism
see also Renin–angiotensin(–aldosterone) system
Alemtuzumab, 241
Alendronate, 451

Alfacalcidol, 452
Alginates, 371
Alimentary tract, *see* Gastrointestinal tract
Alizapride, 374
Alkalinisation, urinary
drugs causing, 365
effects, 93
see also Acid–base balance; pH
Alkaloids, *see* Ergot alkaloids; Vinca alkaloids
Alkalosis, metabolic, with loop diuretics, 363
Alkylating agents (and related drugs), 698, 698–701
All-or-nothing responses, 83
Allergic asthma, development, 243–5
Allergic interstitial nephritis, 728
Allergy
to drugs, 735–6
to insulin, 388
to iodine, 427
H_1-receptor antagonists in, 253
see also Hypersensitivity reactions
Allodynia, 563, 563–4
Allograft rejection, *see* Transplant
Allopurinol, 254
actions/effects, 254
unwanted, 254, 735
interactions, 254, 721
pharmacokinetics, 254
α-adrenoceptors/receptors and blockers, see Adrenoceptors
α-phase of elimination, 117
α-toxins, 26
Alphaxolone, 471
Alprazolam, 517, 518
Alprenolol, 174
Alprostadil, erectile dysfunction, 444
Alteplase, 328
Alternative medicine, 3–4
Aluminium, Alzheimer's disease and, 371
Aluminium antacids (incl. hydroxide gel), 371
interactions with quinolones, 648
Alveolar concentration, minimal (MAC), anaesthetics, 504, 507
Alveolar ventilation, inhalation anaesthetics, 508
Alzheimer's disease, 494–7
aluminium and, 371
pathogenesis, 494–5
prevention of
aspirin in, 250
oestrogens in, 435
smoking and, 602
therapy, 496–7
Amantadine, 500, 663
in influenza, 663
in Parkinson's disease, 500, 663
pharmacokinetics, 663
unwanted effects, 663
American Lipid Research Clinics' trial, 312
Ames test, 730
Amethocaine, *see* Tetracaine
Amikacin, 645
Amiloride, 364
actions/effects, 67, 358, 361, 364
on potassium balance, 361
unwanted, 364
pharmacokinetics, 364
Amine(s) (as transmitters)
sympathomimetic, *see* Sympathomimetic amines
synthesis/release, 134
uptake/storage, 134
see also Catecholamines; Monoamines
Amino acid(s), in brain/CNS, 462–73
excitatory, *see* Excitatory amino acids; Excitotoxicity
inhibitory, 462, 470–3
metabolism/release, 462–3
Amino-acid decarboxylase, 185, 480
p-Aminobenzoic acid, sulfonamides competing with, 638
γ-Aminobutyric acid, *see* GABA
Aminoglutethamide, 413, 705
Aminoglycosides, 645, 647
clinical use, 645
mechanism of action, 645
pharmacokinetics, 93, 645
blood–brain barrier, 102
membrane permeation, 93
resistance, 645
mechanisms, 631, 632
S. aureus, 632
spectrum of activity, 645
unwanted effects, 645
δ-Amino-3–hydroxy-5–methyl-isoxazole receptors, see AMPA receptors
α-Aminolaevulinic acid synthase, 717
Aminophylline, 346
Aminopyridine(s)
cholinergic transmission enhanced by, 160
K^+ channels blocked by, 61
4-Aminoquinolines, 677
malaria, 676
rheumatoid disease, 256
8-Aminoquinolines
in malaria, 676
in rheumatoid disease, 256
4-Aminosalicylic acid, 378
5-Aminosalicylic acid
alone (=mesalazine), 99, 378
pro-drug (olsalazine), 99, 378
sulfapyridine combined with, *see* Sulfasalazine
Amiodarone, 277
adverse effects, 277, 313, 424
antidysrhythmic action, 274, 275, 277
interactions, 313, 720
pharmacokinetics, partitioning into tissues, 97
Amiphenazole, 585, 586, 587
Amitriptyline, 540
analgesic effects, 583
chemical aspects/structure, 542
unwanted effects, 540
Amlodipine, 283
Ammonium chloride and urinary pH, 365
Amnesia
with anaesthetics, 505
with benzodiazepines, 520
Amodiaquine, 677
Amoebiasis, 682–3
Amorolfine, 670
Amoxicillin, *H. pylori* eradication, 371
AMP, receptors, *see* P_{2X} receptors
cAMP (cyclic AMP), 36, 41
β-adrenoceptors and, 170
drugs increasing concentration, 294–5
glucocorticoids and, 415
habituation and, 596–7
lithium affecting hormone-induced production of, 548
Na^+ and Cl^- transport and, 68
see also CREB
AMPA receptors, 463, 465, 491
agonists, 465
antagonists, 465
synaptic transmission and, 468
functional role, 466–7
Amphetamines (amphetamine and related drugs), 177, 178, 180, 586
actions/effects, 180, 478, 526
behavioural, 478–80, 587–8
mode of action, 177, 586, 667
schizophrenia-like episodes, 526
unwanted/adverse, 180, 586, 589
clinical use, 589
appetite suppressants, 588, 589
dependence, 588–9
pharmacokinetics, 180, 589
structure, 587
tests of antidepressant potentiation of central actions, 538
tolerance, 588–9
Amphotericin, 666, 667–8
in fungal infections, 668
in leishmaniasis, 683
liposomal formulation, 105
mechanisms of action, 628
pharmacokinetics, 668
unwanted effects, 668
Ampicillin, 641
resistance mechanisms, 632
Amprenavir, 661
Amrinone, 279
Amsacrine, 706
Amygdaloid complex, dopaminergic pathways, 476
Amyl nitrite, 279
Amylin (islet amyloid polypeptide), 380, 385
agonists, 385
Amyloid-β and Alzheimer's disease, 494–5
Amyloid polypeptide, islet, *see* Amylin
Amyloid precursor protein, 494–5
Amyotrophic lateral sclerosis, 493
Anabolic agents, fluoride and statins as, 453
Anabolic effects of testosterone, 435
Anabolic steroids, 437
Anaemia, 330–1
aplastic, drugs causing, 736
haemolytic, *see* Haemolysis
iron-deficiency, iron administration, 332
megaloblastic, *see* Megaloblastic haemopoiesis and anaemia
pernicious, *see* Pernicious anaemia
Anaesthesia
epidural, 617
general, 503–14
premedication, 148
stages, 505–6
infiltration, 617
intravenous regional, 617
spinal, 617
surface, 617
surgical, 505
Anaesthetics, general, 460, 503–14
definition, 460
induction, *see* Induction, of anaesthesia
inhalational, 100, 504–5, 506–11
adverse effects/toxicity, 111, 507, 509, 717
mechanisms of actions, 504–5
metabolism, 508–9
obsolete/historical interest, 503–4, 510
pharmacokinetics, 506–7, 509
recovery with, 508–9
injected (intravenous etc.), 511–13
induction with, 511–12
recovery with, 512
unwanted effects/toxicity, 513
nervous system effects, 505–6
theories, 504–5
Anaesthetics, local, 612–18
actions/effects, 612–16
adrenaline (epinephrine) prolonging, 101, 617, 719
mechanisms, 612–15
unwanted, 615, 615–16, 617
administration, methods of, 617
chemical aspects, 612
future directions, 616
history, 612
pharmacokinetics, 616
structures, 613
uses, 615, 617
neuropathic pain, 583, 615
Analeptics, *see* Respiratory stimulants; Seizures, drugs inducing
Analgesia, 572–84
in general anaesthesia, 505, 506
morphine-induced, 576–7
see also Neuroleptanalgesia
Analgesic(s), 460, 572–84
bioassays, 84
definition, 460
in migraine, 192
narcotic, *see* Morphine-like drugs
nicotinic ACh receptor agonist as, 484, 599
NSAIDs as, 246, 250
prospective, 583–4
Analgesic nephropathy, 728–9
Anandamide, 486, 488, 568, 609
Anaphase, 72
Anaphylactic reactions (type I hypersensitivity incl. anaphylactic shock), 228
adrenaline in, 172, 303, 735
to drugs, 735
penicillin, 641, 735
Anaphylatoxin, 220
Anaphylaxis, slow reacting substance of, 235–6

Anaritide, 295
Androgens, 436–7
actions, 436
mechanism, 436
unwanted, 437, 727
clinical uses, 437
pharmacokinetics, 436–7
preparations, 436
synthesis, 432, 436
adrenal, 411, 414
males, 435
sites of drug action, 432
Angina/anginal pain, 174, 270–2, 279–84
stable, 270
therapy, 272, 279–84
unstable, 270–1
variant, 271
Angiogenesis, 69, 74
in cancer, 695
agents inhibiting, 708
in chronic inflammation, 229
endothelium in, 221, 288
inhibitors, 77, 708
stimulators, 78
Angioplasty, 744
coronary artery, 326
Angiotensin, 65
in brain, 200
see also Renin–angiotensin system
Angiotensin I, 290, 358
Angiotensin II, 286–7, 293
actions, 292, 293, 358
formation, 290, 291, 358
Angiotensin II receptor subtype I (AT_1), 292
antagonists, 204, 297–8
clinical uses, 298, 302, 386
development, 747
bradykinin receptor and, 40
Angiotensin II receptor subtype II, 292
Angiotensin III, 290
Angiotensin IV, 291, 317
Angiotensin-converting enzyme (ACE), 286, 291–2
Angiotensin-converting enzyme inhibitors, 296–7
clinical uses, 297
cardiac failure, 301–2
diabetics, 386
hypertension, 300
myocardial infarction, 271–2
peripheral vascular disease, 303
pharmacological effects, 296
unwanted effects, 297, 728, 729
Angiotensinogen, 290
Aniloacridine, 685
Animal(s)
as disease models, *see* Models
toxicity tests, 725
carcinogenicity, 730
teratogenicity, 730
Anion(s), organic, excretion, 361
Anion-bind resins, 312
Aniracetam, 470, 496
Ankylostoma spp.
caninum (cutaneous larva migrans), 688
therapy, 689
duodenale, 687
therapy, 689
Annexin-1, 415
Anorectic drugs, *see* Appetite suppressants
Antacids, 371, 453
clinical use, 372
Antagonism, 11–12, 18–19
chemical, 18
competitive, 11–12, 17
irreversible/non-equilibrium, 18, 19
reversible, 12, 18
non-competitive, 18
'misuse' of term, 18
pharmacokinetic, 18
physiological, 19
receptor-block, 18
surmountable vs non-surmountable, 11–12
Antagonists, 8, 18
binding curves with, 11
competitive
interaction with normal/inverse agonists, 14
irreversible, 16
reversible, 16
definition, 9
examples, 24
Anthelminthic drugs, 688–91
mechanism of action, 628, 629
new/in development, 691
resistance, 691
Anthracyclines, 703
Antiandrogens, 437
in prostate cancer, 437, 705
Antiarrhythmic drugs, *see* Antidysrhythmic drugs
Antibacterial drugs (commonly referred to as antibiotics), 635–53
antimalarial activity, 676, 681
biochemical reactions as targets for, 622–9
blood–brain barrier, 101, 102
choice, 635–6
combinations, 623
in diarrhoeal illness, 376
H. pylori eradication, 371
new, 633, 652
P. carinii pneumonia, 682
resistance to, 629–33, 652
biochemical mechanisms, 631–2
current status, 632
genetic determinants, 629–31
spread/transfer, 629, 629–31
in shock, 303
structural targets, 627–9
see also specific (types of) drugs
Antibiotics
biochemical reactions as targets for, 622–9
cytotoxic (anticancer), 703–4
definition of term, 620
for infections, *see* Antibacterial drugs; Antifungal drugs *etc.*
resistance to, *see* Resistance
Antibody (antibodies), 225–6
classes, 226
conjugation of drugs/toxins etc. with, 206, 708
in cancer therapy, 104, 708
cytotoxicity and, *see* Cytotoxic hypersensitivity; Cytotoxicity
in immune response (=humoral response), 224, 225–6
azathioprine effects, 258
in effector phase, 225–6
in induction phase, 225
monoclonal, *see* Monoclonal antibodies
see also Autoantibodies; Autoimmune disease; Immunoglobulins
Antibody-dependent cytotoxic hypersensitivity (type III hypersensitivity), 228, 735, 736
Anticholinergics, *see* Muscarinic ACh receptor antagonists
Anticholinesterases (cholinesterase inhibition), 23, 153, 153–4, 156–8
actions/effects, 157, 158
unwanted/toxic, 153, 158, 727
clinical uses, 156, 160–1
Alzheimer's disease, 496
myasthenia gravis, 159–60
tricyclic antidepressant CNS toxicity control, 544
irreversible, 157–8
medium-duration, 157
short-acting, 156–7
Anticoagulants, 319–23
clinical uses, 319
injectable
heparin, *see* Heparin
other than heparin, 319
mechanisms/sites of action, 316
oral (coumarins etc.), *see* Oral anticoagulants
Antidepressants (thymoleptics), 460, 538–47
actions/effects, 539
analgesic, 583
measurement, 538–9
mechanism, 539, 542, 546
antipsychotics acting as, 533
clinical effectiveness, 548
definition, 460
types, 538–47
see also specific types
Antidiarrhoeal agents, 376–7
Antidiuretic hormone (ADH; vasopressin; arginine vasopressin), 293, 358–9, 410–11
actions/effects, 200, 410
drugs affecting, 410
inhibitors, 359
renal, 358, 410
unwanted, 410
clinical use, 303
pharmacokinetics, 410–11
preparations (including analogues), 205, 411
receptors, 293, 358–9, 410
secretion/release, 410
defective, 410
regulation, 410
in shock, deficiency, 302
Antidysrhythmic drugs, 274–9
adenosine as, 196
class I (sodium channel blockers), 274
Ia, 274, 275
Ib, 274, 275
Ic, 274, 275
class II (beta-blockers), 174, 274, 275, 276–7
class III, 274, 275–6, 277
class IV (calcium antagonists), 274, 276, 277, 283
clinical uses, 274, 276, 277
interactions, 720
Antiemetic drugs, 373–5
antipsychotics as, 373–4, 531
in cancer chemotherapy, 707
H_1-receptors antagonists as, 253, 373, 375
metoclopramide, 374, 480
ondansetron, 373, 481
in Parkinson's disease therapy, 102, 500
with postcoital contraceptive, 441
site of action, 374
teratogenicity, 734
Antiepileptic (anticonvulsant) drugs, 553–60
actions/effects, 553–6
mechanisms, 553–6, 558, 559, 560
benzodiazepines as, 519–20, 554, 555, 558
clinical use (other than epilepsy)
as analgesics, 583
as mood stabilisers, 548
isoniazid interactions, 650
in status epilepticus, 100, 520, 555, 558
types, 555, 556–60
newer, 559–60
unwanted effects, 555
on fetal development, 732, 734
Antifibrinolytic drugs, 328–9
Antifolates (incl. folate antagonists), 334, 622–3
antibacterial, 622, 637–9
anticancer, 701
teratogenicity, 733–4
antimalarial, 622–3, 676, 679–80
structures, 680
mechanism of action, 622–3, 638
unwanted effects, 639
Antifungal drugs, 666–71
discovery
historical, 667
new agents (under development), 667, 670
mechanisms of action, 628
purine analogues, 623
Antigen(s)
MHC association with (=peptide–antigen complex), 226
presentation, 224
Antigen-presenting cells, 224
Antihelminthic drugs, *see* Anthelminthic drugs
Antihistamines (conventional term), *see* Histamine H_1 receptor
Antihypertensives, 299–300
ACE inhibitors, 300
adverse effects, 301
α-blockers, 173, 300, 301
β-blockers, 174, 300, 301
calcium antagonists, 293–4, 300, 301
diabetics, 386
diuretics, 300, 301, 363
hydralazine, 295
sites of action, 299

Anti-inflammatory drugs, 244–57
in asthma, 348–9
glucocorticoids as, *see* Adrenal steroids
non-steroidal, *see* Non-steroidal anti-inflammatory drugs
sites of action, 232
Anti-inflammatory modulator role
cytokines, 240
NO, 239
prostaglandins, 235
Antimalarial agents, 676–82
chemoprophylaxis, 676–8
chemotherapy, 676
in acute attacks, 676
for radical cure, 676
resistance, 677, 679, 681–2, 681–2
mechanism/site of action, 622–3, 629, 676–82
potential new, 682, 685
preventing transmission, 677, 680
site of action, 675
Antimetabolites (affecting metabolic pathways involved in DNA synthesis), 627, 698, 701–3
Antimigraine drugs, *see* Migraine
Antimonials, leishmaniasis, 683
Antimotility agents, 376–7
morphine-like drugs as, 376, 377, 577
Antimuscarinics, *see* Muscarinic ACh receptor antagonists
Antimycobacterial drugs, 649–52
Anti-oestrogens, 433–4
in cancer therapy, 703
uses, 433
Anti-oxidants, 493
Antiplatelet drugs, 323–7
aspirin as, 250
clinical uses, 326
peripheral vascular disease, 303
monoclonal antibodies as, 241, 325
warfarin interactions, 322
Antiprogestogens, 434
Antiprotozoal agents, 676–86
Antipsychotic drugs (antischizophrenic/neuroleptic drugs; major tranquilisers), 460, 528–34
actions/effects, 528–34
at 5-HT receptors, 482, 529, 532
mechanisms, 528–30
classification (typical/classical vs atypical), 528
clinical efficacy in schizophrenia, 533–4
clinical uses (other than schizophrenia), 533
antiemetic, 373–4, 531
definition, 460
as dopamine antagonists, 477, 478, 526–7, 528–30
general properties, 528
pharmacokinetics, 533
unwanted effects, 531–3
motor disturbances, 477, 478, 529, 531–2
Antipyretic agents, NSAIDs as, 235, 246, 250
Antiretroviral agents, 627
in HIV disease, 659–62
highly active (HAART), 659–60
new targets, 662
sites of action, 658
Antirheumatoid agents, 255–7
monoclonal antibodies as, 241, 242, 256–7
Antischizophrenic drugs, *see* Antipsychotic drugs
Antisense strategies (oligonucleotides), 745
cancer, 709, 745
Antispasmodics, 148, 377
Antithrombin III
action, 316
heparin binding to, 320
Antithrombin III-independent anticoagulants, 321
Antithrombotic agents, *see* Anticoagulants; Antiplatelet drugs; Fibrinolysis, drugs increasing
Antithyroid drugs, 425–7
Antituberculosis drugs, 649–51
1st-line, 649, 651
2nd-line, 649, 651
resistance, 633
measures preventing, 649
Antitussives (cough suppressants), 350
morphine-like drugs/opioids, 350, 577
Antiviral agents, 659–64
future developments, 664
mechanisms of action, 627
see also specific agents
Anturane Reinfarction Trial Research Group, 88–9
Anxiety, 515–24
animal models, 516
classification of anxiety disorders, 515
drugs treating, *see* Anxiolytic agents
nature, 515–16
Anxiolytic agents (hypnotics; sedatives; minor tranquilizers), 460, 515–24
animal tests, 516
β-blockers as, 175, 516, 517
buspirone as, 482, 517, 523
classification, 516–17
see also specific classes
definition, 460
human tests, 516
ondansetron as, 482, 523
AP-1, 413
Apaf-1, 76
Apathy with antipsychotics, 531
Aplastic anaemia, drug-induced, 736
Apoferritin, 332
Apomorphine, 478
in erectile dysfunction, 444
in Parkinson's disease, 102, 500
schizophrenia-like behaviour with, 526
Apoptosis, 74–8, 77–8, 491–3
in cancer, 77
resistance to, 694
defective, 77
inhibitors, 77
morphological changes, 75
myocardial infarction and, 271
neuronal, 490, 491–3
over-exuberant, 77
pathophysiological implications, 77
pathways to, 75
toxic reactions causing, 725
in viral infection, 656
interference with, 657
Appetite-stimulating factors, *see* Orexigenic factors
Appetite suppressants (anorectic/food intake-reducing agents), 401–2
amphetamines, 588, 589
smoking, 599
withdrawn, 401
Aprotinin, 329
APV (NMDA receptor antagonists), 468
Aquaporins, 359
Aqueous humour and intraocular pressure, 145
Aqueous pores, diffusion through, 92
Arachidonic acid, 231
insulin release and, 381
metabolism (and arachidonic acid cascade), 231, 232, 233
see also Eicosanoids *and specific enzymes involved*
Arachioline, 486
Area postrema (chemoreceptor trigger zone) in vomiting, 188, 372–3
Area under the curve (AUC), 116
Arecoline, 484
Argatroban, 321
L-Arginine, NO metabolism and, 210
Arginine vasopressin, *see* Antidiuretic hormone
Aromatase inhibitors, 705
Aromatic hydrocarbon receptor, 110
Arousal
cholinergic pathways and, 483–4
noradrenaline and, 475
Arrestins, 39
Arrhythmias, cardiac, *see* Dysrhythmias
Arsenical in trypanosomiasis, 684
Arteflene, 676
Artemesinin, 676, 681, 682
Artemether, 676, 681
Arteries
compliance, *see* Compliance
thrombus, 314–15
Arteriolar dilatation with Ca^{2+} antagonists, 301
Artesunate, 676, 681
Artether, 681
Arthritis
gouty, 254, 366
rheumatoid, *see* Antirheumatoid agents; Rheumatoid disease
Arthus reaction, 228
Ascaris lumbricoides (common roundworm), 687
therapy, 689, 690, 691
Ascorbic acid (vitamin C)
as anti-oxidant, 493
iron absorption, 331
Asparaginase, 705
Aspartate, 462
Aspirin (acetylsalicylic acid), 104, 245, 250–1, 323–4, 326
actions/effects, 23, 323–4
mechanisms, 247
unwanted, 250–1
clinical uses, 324
coronary artery disease (with aspirin), 325
myocardial infarction prevention, 271
myocardial infarction treatment, 324
nicotinic acid/acipimox-induced flushing, 312
peripheral vascular disease, 303
historical aspects, 104
interactions, 251
with warfarin, 251, 322
overdose, treatment, 112
partition in aqueous compartments, 94
Assays, *see* Bioassay; Measurement *and specific methods*
Asthma, 341–50
acute severe (status asthmaticus), 342, 349
hydrocortisone, 349
allergic, development, 342–5
β-blocker (e.g. propranolol) dangers, 175, 347
characteristics, 342
definition, 341, 343
drug treatment, 145, 148, 172, 237, 345–9
sites of action, 344
exercise-induced, 344
immediate phase, 342–4
late phase, 344–5
leukotriene role, 236
Astrocytes
glutamate and glutamine transport, 464
signalling role, 458
Atenolol, 174
antidysrhythmic action, 174, 276
phaeochromocytoma, 173
Atherogenesis (atheroma formation), 306–7
coronary, 270
prevention, 307
risk factors, 306
Atherosclerosis, 315
coronary, *see* Coronary artery disease
ethanol effects, 604–5
Atopic disease, immunotherapy, 242
Atorvastatin, 310
in familial homozygous hypercholesterolaemia, 311
Atosiban, 443
Atovaquone
malaria, 676, 681, 682
P. carinii pneumonia, 682
ATP, 165, 192–4
in CNS, 485
neurotransmission involving, 132, 165, 192–4
in co-transmission (with noradrenaline), 131
nociception and, 485, 570
receptors, *see* P_{2x} receptors; P_{2y} receptors
in shock, 302
ATP-sensitive K^+ channels, 46, 60, 294
islet B-cells, 380–1
sulfonylureas as blockers of, 389
ATPase, Na^+/K^+-, *see* Sodium pump
Atracurium, 149, 150, 151
pharmacokinetics, 151, 152
side-effects, 151
Atrial fibrillation, glycosides in, 278
Atrial natriuretic peptide (atriopeptin), 200, 272
in brain, 200
role/actions, 272
in kidney, 272, 359
synthetic form, 295
Atriopeptin, *see* Atrial natriuretic peptide

Atrioventricular conduction, depression/slowing/block
antidysrhythmics causing, 275, 276
glycosides causing, 278
Atropine, 100, 145, 147
actions/effects, 136
cardiac, 123
CNS, 146–7, 484
historical observations, 122, 123
antidepressant side-effects similar to
MAO inhibitor, 546
tricyclic, 543, 544
clinical uses, 147
biliary spasm, 378
poisoning, 146–7
Atropine methonitrate, 145, 147
Attapulgite, activated, 377
Attention, selective, defect in schizophrenia, 525–6
Attention deficit/hyperactivity disorder, 589
AUC (area under the curve), 116
Auerbach's plexus, 367
Augmerosen, 709
Auranofin, 255, 256
Aurothiomalate, sodium, 255, 256
Autoantibodies to nicotinic ACh receptor, 48, 159, 717
see also Autoimmune disease
Autocrine effects of NO, 212
Autocrine system, cytokines and, 224
Autoimmune disease, 228
drug-induced, 736
thyroid, 424
treatment, 228
see also Autoantibodies *and specific diseases*
Auto-inhibitory feedback, 128
noradrenaline release, 128, 165
Autonomic ganglia, *see* Ganglion
Autonomic nervous system, 122–83
anatomy, 123–6
chemical mediators/transmission in, 122–35
divisions, 123
see also Enteric nervous system; Parasympathetic nervous system; Sympathetic nervous system
physiology, 123–6, 127
airway, 340–1
cardiac, 272–4
gastrointestinal, 127, 367
historical aspects, 122–3
main effects, 127
Autoradiography, receptor distribution, 10
Autoreceptors
muscarinic M_2 as, 341
presynaptic, 128
Avermectins, 629
see also Ivermectin
Aversive therapies, 598
Axon reflex, 230
Azathioprine, 258
interactions, 254
metabolism to mercaptopurine, 111, 258
unwanted effects, 258
Azidothymidine, *see* Zidovudine
Azithromycin, 646
toxoplasmosis, 685
Azlocillin, 641
Azoles (incl. imidazoles), 668–9
amoebiasis, 683
bacterial infections, 649
fungal infections, 628
new agents, 670
mechanism of action, 668
trichomoniasis, 684
see also Benzimidazoles; Nitroindazole
AZT, *see* Zidovudine
Aztreonam, 643

B

B-cell (lymphocyte), 223
in effector phase of immune response, 224, 226
Th2-release cytokines stimulating, 225
B-cell (pancreatic; β-cell), 386
destruction in diabetes, 386
insulin secretion by, 380
drugs stimulating, 389
B-cell lymphoma, therapy, 242, 706, 745
Bacilli (rods), antibiotics choice, 636
Bacitracin, mechanism of action, 624
Baclofen, 472
in Huntington's disease, 501
intrathecal, 101
as muscle relaxant, 561
Bacteria
drugs acting against, *see* Antibacterial drugs
pathogen-associated molecular patterns on, 218
phagocytosis, 226
structures, 621–2, 635–7
formation, biochemical reactions involved in (as targets), 622–7, 637–52
formed, as targets, 627, 635–7
toxins, G-proteins and, 35
Bacteriophages, 630–1
Bacteriostatic agents, sulfonamides as, 622, 638
Bambuterol, 346
Barbiturates, 523
as antiepileptics, 555, 558
mechanism of action, 554
as anxiolytics, 517, 523
$GABA_A$ receptors and, 471
pharmacokinetics, 558
unwanted effects, 523, 558
Baroreceptor reflexes, adrenoceptor agonist effects, 170
Bartter's syndrome, 62
Basal ganglia
dopamine in, 478
in Parkinson's disease, 497
Basal nucleus of Meynert, cholinergic pathways, 483
Base(s) (alkali), organic, secretion into renal tubule, 355
see also Acid–base balance
Base(s) (nucleic acid), 625
pairing, nucleotide, agents affecting, 625
Basic drugs
pK_a values, 94
weakly
ionisation and distribution, 93, 94, 112
renal excretion, 112
Basiliximab, 241, 259–60
Basophils, 220, 221
antibodies and, 221
histamine, 229
Batrachotoxin, 60
Bax, 491
Bay K 8644, 282, 294
BAY41-2272, 294
Bcl-2
antisense therapy, 709, 745
apoptosis and, 76, 78, 491
Beclometasone dipropionate, 100, 412
in asthma, 348
Behaviour
drugs affecting
amphetamines, 478–80, 587–8
antipsychotics, 530–1
anxiolytics, measurement, 516
dopaminergic pathways and, 478–80
ethanol, 603
sex hormones, 431
see also Psychotropic drugs
in schizophrenia, 525
Bendroflu(methi)azide, 282
Benefit, determining, 89–90
Benserazide, 499
Benzatropine, 500
Benzimidazoles, 628, 688–9
Benznidazole, 684
Benzocaine, 612
pharmacokinetics, 616
Benzodiazepine(s), 130, 470, 517–22, 558
actions/effects, 23
clinical, *see subheading below*
mechanisms, 518, 554
structure related to, 517–18
unwanted, 521–2
antagonists, 471, 520, 522, 523
chemistry, 517–18
dependence, 522
GABA and, 471
inverse agonists, 520–1
pharmacokinetics/metabolism, 517
receptors and binding sites
endogenous ligand/modulator, 471, 520
GABA receptors, 23, 471, 518, 520
peripheral, 518
therapeutic use, 518–20
anaesthesia, 512, 514
anticonvulsant, 519–20, 554, 555, 558
anxiolytic, 516, 518–19
sedation/sleep induction, 519
tolerance, 522
withdrawal syndrome, 522, 558
Benzodiazepine-like mediator, endogenous, 471, 520
Benzomorphan series, 574
Benzoquimanide, 374
Benzothiazepines, 282
Benzpyrene metabolism, 109
Benztropine (benzatropine), 500
Benzylpenicillin (penicillin G), 640–1, 642
pharmacokinetics, 641
β-amyloid/Aβ and Alzheimer's disease, 494–5
β-cells, *see* B-cells (pancreatic)
β-lactam antibiotics, 639–43
mechanism of action, 624
resistance mechanisms, 631, 632
structures, 640
β-lactam-binding protein, 632
β-lactamases, 631, 632, 636
penicillins resistant to, 641, 643
Betamethasone, 412
Betanidine, 178
β-phase of elimination, 117
Bethanecol, 143, 144
clinical use, 145
Bezafibrate, 311
Bias in trials, avoidance, 87, 89
Bicarbonate, sodium, 371
clinical use
as antacid, 371
urinary alkalinisation, 365
gastric secretion, 368, 369
plasma pH increase with, 93
Bicarbonate ion
carbonic anhydrase inhibitor effects, 365
renal handling, 353, 355, 360, 361
Bicuculline, 471, 586, 587
Bigeminy, 278
Biguanides, 388, 391
Bile acid-binding resins, 312
Bilharzia, *see* Schistosomiasis
Biliary system, 378
drugs affecting, 378
excretion, 113–14
spasm, 378
stones, *see* Gallstones
Bilirubin metabolism, premature neonates, 719
Binding (of drugs), 7–19
of antibiotics to target site, resistance due to altered binding site, 631–2
to cells, 7–19
to proteins, 8
drug interactions concerning, 719–20
in plasma, 96
to receptors, 10–11
direct measurement, 10
quantitative aspects, 15–17
specificity, *see* Specificity
see also Affinity
Bioassays, 80–4
definition, 80
design, 82–3
general principles, 82–3
graded responses, 83
humans, 83–4
quantal responses, 83
standards and unknown preparations in, 82–3
uses, 8
Bioavailability, 99
definition, 99
'Biological clock', 485
Biological response modifiers in cancer, 706, 709
see also Immunomodulators
Biological variation, *see* Variation
Biopharmaceuticals, 750
Biotechnology, 4, 5

Bipolar affective disorder, 535, 548–9
  mood-stabilising drugs, 548–9, 556
Bisacodyl, 376
Bismuth chelate, 372
  clinical use, 371, 372
Bismuth subsalicylate, 377
Bisoprolol, 302
Bisphosphonates, 451
Blackwater fever, 679
Blastocyst, drugs affecting formation, 731, 732
Bleeding, *see* Haemorrhage
Bleomycin(s), 703
  in combination regimes, 707
  mechanism of action, 628, 703
  toxicity, 703
Blinding in trials, 87
β-blockers, *see* β-Adrenoceptor blockers
Blood
  coagulation, *see* Coagulation; Haemostasis
  5-HT in, 184
  lipoprotein transport, 307–9
  see also entries under Haem-
Blood–brain barrier, 101, 102–3, 460
Blood cell differentiation, *see* Haemopoiesis
Blood clot, definition, 314
Blood flow
  cerebral, in migraine, 190–1
  coronary, 270–2
  hepatic, drug interactions and, 721
Blood:gas partition coefficient of anaesthetics, 507
Blood pressure
  ACh effects, 136, 137
  low, *see* Hypotension
  raised/high, *see* Hypertension
  regulatory mechanisms, 298–9
    NO role, 213
    noradrenaline, 475–6
Blood vessels, *see* Vascular system
Blood volume
  drugs affecting, 286
  replacement therapy, 303
  see also Hypovolaemia
BMS 182874, 289
Body
  compartments, *see* Compartments
  distribution of drugs in, *see* Distribution
  fat, *see* Fat
  weight, *see* Weight
Body mass index, 394
  excessively large, 394, 399
Bone, 446–54
  disorders, and drug therapy, 451–2
  formation, drugs stimulating, 452–3
  glucocorticoid effects, 416, 417, 450
  metabolism
    disorders, 451–2
    hormones involved, 449–50
  oestrogen effects, 450
  remodelling, 446–50
    hormones involved, 446, 447, 449–50
    site of drug action on, 447
  structure/composition, 446
    disorders, 451
  turnover (of mineral), 448–9
Bone marrow
  depression, *see* Myelosuppression
  purging and replacement, 707
Bosentan, 204, 295
Botulinum toxin, 66, 561, 585
  ACh release inhibited by, 155
  use, 561
Bovine spongiform encephalopathy, 501
Bowel, *see* Intestine
Bowman's capsule, 354
Boyle, Robert, 2
BQ-123, 289
Bradycardia, 265
  drugs inducing, 153, 165, 578
  drugs treating, 148
Bradykinin, 237–9, 569
  inactivation, 238
  in inflammation, 238–9
  in nociception, 569
  receptors, 239, 569
  angiotensin (AT_1) receptor and, 40
  antagonists, 238, 239, 569
  source and formation, 237–8
Brain
  anaesthetic effects, 505
  degenerative disease, *see* Neurodegeneration
  fetal development, cocaine effects, 590
  5-HT_{1A} receptors, 186
  ischaemia, *see* Ischaemia
  migraine pathophysiology and, 191
  peptides in, 200
  tumours, gene therapy, 744
  see also Blood–brain barrier; Central nervous system; Cerebrum *and specific parts of brain*
Brain-derived neurotrophic factors and epilepsy, 553
Brainstem, vomiting centre (area postrema; chemoreceptor trigger zone), 188, 372–3
Bran, 375
Breast (mammary gland)
  antipsychotic effects, 532
  cancer
    hormone replacement therapy and, 435
    hormone therapy in, 705
    monoclonal antibody therapy, 706
    oral contraceptives and, 440
  see also Lactation
Bretylium, 177
Bromocriptine, 189
  unwanted reactions, 189
    schizophrenia-like behaviour, 526
  uses, 407
    acromegaly, 407
    Parkinson's disease, 500
    prolactin suppression, 407, 408, 480
Bronchi
  hyper-reactivity/hyper-responsiveness in asthma, 342
  secretions
    muscarinic agonist effects, 144
    muscarinic antagonist effects, 146
  smooth muscle, *see* Airway
  see also Airway
Bronchial asthma, *see* Asthma
Bronchitis, chronic, 349
  smoking and, 601
Bronchoconstriction/bronchospasm
  adrenoceptor antagonists inducing, 175
  in asthma, 342
  mediators causing
    adenosine, 195
    leukotrienes, 236
    PAF, 237
Bronchodilators, 345–8
  in asthma, 345–8
  inhalational administration, 100
Brown fat cells, 396–7
Brugia malayi, 688
Budesonide, 412
  in asthma, 348
Bulk flow transfer, 91
Bulk laxatives, 375
Bumetanide, 362
Bungarotoxin
  α-bungarotoxin, 26, 155
  β-bungarotoxin, 155
Bupivacaine, 615
Buprenorphine, 574, 580, 582
  biliary spasm, 378
Bupropion, 402, 541, 602–3
Buserelin, 437
Buspirone, 523
  anxiolytic effects, 482, 517, 523
  side-effects, 523
Busulphan, 700
Butoxamine, 181
Butyrophenones, antipsychotic, 528
  antiemetic effects, 374
Butyrylcholinesterase, 155–6, 159

C

C-fibres
  capsaicin destroying, 568
  pain sensation and, 563
C-natriuretic peptide, 286
C-peptide (insulin), 380
C3, 220
  activation/splitting, 220
C3a, 220
C3b (opsonin), 220, 221
C5–C9, 220
Cadmium, fetal toxicity, 734
Caffeine, 346
  actions/effects, 196, 485, 590
    central stimulant, 590, 591
  Ca^{2+} sensitivity of ryanodine receptors and, 54
  clinical use, 591
CAG repeat, 501
Calcifediol (25-hydroxy-vitamin D_3), 450
Calcitonin, 421, 450, 452
  actions/effects, 448, 450
    unwanted, 452
  synthesis, and gene splicing, 203
  use/administration, 452
    as analgesic, 583
    in osteoporosis, 452
Calcitonin gene-related peptide (CGRP), 132
  amylin and, structural homology, 385
  capsaicin causing release, 568
  inflammation and, 564
  synthesis, and gene splicing, 203
Calcitonin receptor-like receptor, 40
Calcitriol (1,25-dihydroxycholecalciferol), 450
Calcium (bone mineral), 446
  metabolism, 448–9
    parathormone and, 449–50
    vitamin D and, 450
Calcium (ions), 37–8, 51–5
  balance/homeostasis/metabolism/transport
    bone, *see* Calcium (bone mineral)
    capsaicin and, 568
    cardiac, 264, 265, 267
    entry mechanisms, 52–4
    excitotoxicity and, 491
    extrusion mechanisms, 54
    glucocorticoids and, 416
    glutamate/NMDA receptors and, 466, 468
    inositol phosphates and, 37–8
    insulin release and, 381
    loop diuretics and, 362
    vascular smooth muscle tone and, 286
  chemical mediator release and role of, 65
  ion channels activated by, 47
    K^+ channels, 46, 60, 61
  muscle contraction and, 62–3
  NO synthase and, 210
  see also Hypercalcaemia; Hypocalcaemia
Calcium antagonists, *see* Calcium channel blockers
Calcium channel(s), 46, 52–5, 282
  ethanol effects, 608
  ligand-gated, 52–3
  store-operated, 46, 53, 54
  types, 52
    L, *see* L-type Ca^{2+} channels
    T, *see* T-type Ca^{2+} channels
  voltage-gated, 46, 52, 53
    cardiac function and, 264–5
Calcium channel blockers/antagonists, 282–4
  adverse effects, 283–4
  cardiovascular effects (in general), 272, 283, 293–4
  clinical uses, 282–4
    angina, 282–4
    dysrhythmias, 274, 276, 277, 283
    epilepsy, 554, 555
    hypertension, 293–4, 300, 301
    migraine, 192
    myocardial infarction, 272
    as vasodilators, 283, 293–4, 298
  by dihydropyridines, 23
  pharmacokinetics, 283
Calcium release channels, 46
Calcium salts, 452
  clinical uses, 453
  unwanted effects, 452
Calcium-sensing receptors, 32
Calculi, biliary, *see* Gallstones
Calmodulin, 55
  NO synthase and, 210

Campothecins, 704
Canal of Schlemm, muscarinic agonist actions, 145
Cancer (malignant tumours/neoplasms), 693–710
apoptosis and, *see* Apoptosis
breast, *see* Breast
colorectal, aspirin prophylaxis, 250
endometrial, *see* Endometrium
glucocorticoid use, 418, 705
growth factors and their receptors and, 48, 694, 695
liver, oral contraceptives and, 440
lung, 601
ovarian, oral contraceptives and, 440
pathogenesis, *see* Carcinogenesis
prostate, 437, 438
smoking and, 601
spread, 696
therapy, 693–710
drug, *see* Chemotherapy, cancer
hormonal, *see* Hormone therapy
novel approaches, 104, 708–9, 743–4, 745
other approaches, 693
vaginal, stilboestrol and, 433
see also specific types
Cancer cells, 621
apoptosis, *see* Apoptosis
dedifferentiation/loss of function, 695
genesis, 694
invasiveness, 695–6
new treatment approaches based on pathobiology, 708–9
proliferation, uncontrolled, 77, 694–5
Candoxatril, 295
Cannabinoid(s), 375
actions/effects, 609
antiemetic, 374
in cannabis, 608
tolerance and dependence, 609–10
Cannabinoid receptors, 486, 488, 609
agonists/activators, 583–4
analgesic affects, 583–4
endogenous, 486, 488, 568, 609
antagonists, 377, 609
Cannabis (marijuana; hashish), 608–10
adverse effects, 610
clinical uses, 610
multiple sclerosis, 561
effects, 609
legislation, 610
pharmacokinetics, 609–10
Capreomycin, 651
Capsaicin, 567, 568
uses, 568
Capsofungin, 670
Captopril, 296
pharmacological effects, 296–7
unwanted effects, 297
Carbachol, 138, 143, 144
Carbamazepine, 555, 556, 559, 560
actions/effects
as analgesic, 583
as antiepileptic, 560
as mood stabiliser, 548
unwanted, 557, 560, 734
interactions, 720
isoniazid, 650
pharmacokinetics, 555, 557
Carbapenems, 631, 642–3
structure, 640
unwanted effects, 643
Carbenicillin, 641
Carbenoxolone, 372
Carbidopa, 176, 178, 181
in Parkinson's disease, 499
Carbimazole, 425, 427
pharmacokinetics, 425–6
Carbohydrate metabolism, insulin effects, 382
Carbon monoxide
as CNS mediator, 487
from tobacco smoke, harmful effects, 602
Carbonic anhydrase, 355, 360
gastric acid secretion and, 368
inhibitors, 365
in glaucoma, 100
mechanism of action, 355, 361
Carboplatin, 700
Carboprost, 442, 443
Carboxyhaemoglobin, 602
γ-Carboxylation of glutamate residues, *see* Glutamate residues
Carboxypeptidase, kinin inactivation, 239
Carcinogen(s), 729–30
cytotoxic drugs as, 698
epigenetic, 730
genotoxic, *see* Genotoxic carcinogens
tests for, 730–1
Carcinogenesis, 693–6, 697, 729–31
apoptosis and, 77
Carcinoid syndrome, 185
Cardiac actions/function *etc*, *see* Heart
Cardiomyocytes, *see* Myocytes
Cardiotonic steroids, *see* Glycosides, cardiac
Cardiovascular system, *see* Heart; Vascular system
'CARE' trial, 310
Carrier molecules, 24
drugs transported by, 24, 92, 94–5
in kidney, 112
inhibitors and false substrates, 25
see also Transport
Carteolol, 146
Carvedilol, 173, 181
in heart failure, 302
Cascade superfusion technique, 82
Caspases, 75–6, 76, 491
Huntington's disease and, 501
inhibitors, 78
Catabolism, *see* Degradative metabolism
Catalase, 493
Catalepsy with antipsychotics, 530–1
Catecholamines, 166–7
airway regulation and, 341
cardiac effects, 170, 273
degradation, 167–8
dysrhythmias and, 268
metabolic effects, 170–1
structure–activity relationships, 169
structures, 161
synthesis, 164
uptake, 166–7
see also specific catecholamines
Catechol-*O*-methyl transferase (COMT), 167, 168, 476
inhibitors, 499, 500
Cathartics (purgatives), 375–6
Cations, organic, excretion, 361
Caveolae and caveolin and endothelial NOS, 209–10
C-C chemokines, 240, 241
CCK, *see* Cholecystokinin
CCNU (lomustine), 700
CCR5 co-receptor on T cells (and HIV), 657
antagonist, 242
CD4, 224
HIV recognition of/binding to, *see* HIV
$CD4^+$ helper lymphocytes
HIV and, *see* HIV; HIV disease
in immune response, 224
glucocorticoid effects, 416
uncommitted, *see* Th1 and Th2 cells
CD8, 224
$CD8^+$ (cytotoxic) T cells, 224, 225, 226
viral infection and, 655, 656
HIV and, 659
CD20, monoclonal antibody to (rituximab), 242, 706
Cefachlor, 642
Cefalexin, 642
Cefotaxime, 642
Cefoxitin, 642
Cefperazone, 642
Ceftizoxime, 642
Ceftriaxone, 642
Cefuroxime, 642
Celecoxib, 245, 252, 370
anticancer properties, 709
Cell(s)
barriers/membranes, *see* Membranes; Wall
binding of drugs to, 7–19
cancer, *see* Cancer cells
damage/death, mechanisms
drug toxicity and, 725–9
in myocardial infarction, 271
neuronal, 490–3
see also Apoptosis; Necrosis
function, mechanisms of regulation, 51–79
hypersensitivity reactions (type III) mediated by, 228, 735, 736
in immune response, *see* Immune response
in inflammation, 220–2
mediators derived from, 222
proliferation, *see* Proliferation
removal (dead cells), 76–7
structures, *see specific structures*
see also specific cell types
Cell cycle, 69–73
cancer cells, 694, 695
drug effects on, 707
regulators, 70–3
cloning and therapeutic use, 78
negative, 72–3
positive, 70–2
Central nervous system, 456–618
ADH effects, 410
alcohol toxicity, 604
amino acid transmitters, *see* Amino acids
anaesthetic effects, 505
anticholinesterase effects, 158
autonomic nervous system conveying output from, 123, 125
blood–brain barrier, 101, 102–3, 460
cannabis effects, 609
cycloserine toxicity, 651
depressants (abused), 595
ethanol, 603–4
ethanol enhancing effects or other depressants, 604
dopamine in, *see* Dopamine
drug action in (general aspects), 459–60
targets, 458–9
fluoroquinolone effects, 648
histamine actions, 231
histamine H_1 antagonist effects, 253
5-HT in, *see* 5-Hydroxytryptamine
5-HT receptors (and agonist/antagonist actions) in, 186, 188, 481
inflammation, 227
lithium adverse effects, 549
local anaesthetic effects, unwanted, 615–16
MAO inhibitor toxicity, 546
morphine/opioid effects, 576–7
MPTP toxicity, 497–8
muscarinic agonist effects, 145
muscarinic antagonist effects/uses, 146–7
muscle relaxants acting on, 560–1
nicotine effects, 599
NO role, 212
noradrenaline in, *see* Noradrenaline
pain in disorders of, 566
in respiratory regulation, 340
salicylate toxicity, 251
stimulants, *see* Psychomotor stimulants; Respiratory stimulants; Seizures, drugs inducing
tricyclic antidepressant toxicity, 544
vitamin B_{12} deficiency effects, 333
xanthine effects, 346
unwanted, 346, 347
see also Neurotoxicity
Central nervous system-type muscarinic ACh receptors, 137, 138
Cephaeline, 373
Cephalosporins, 641–2, 643
broad-spectrum, 641
clinical use, 642
mechanism of action, 624, 641–2
pharmacokinetics, 642
resistance, 642
structure, 640
unwanted effects, 642
Cephamandole, 631, 642
Cephamycins, 641–2, 643
Cerebral vasospasm following subarachnoid haemorrhage, reducing, 283
Cerebrovascular accident, *see* Stroke
Cerebrum
blood flow, migraine and, 190–1
ischaemia, *see* Ischaemia

oedema, osmotic diuretics, 365
see also Brain
Cerivastatin, withdrawn, 311, 750
Cestodes, *see* Tapeworms
Cetirizine, 253
CGP35348, 473
CGRP, *see* Calcitonin gene-related peptide
Chagas' disease (*T. cruzi*), 684, 685
Chalk, 377
Channels, *see* Ion channels *and specific ion channels*
Charcoal, 377
Cheese (tyramine) reaction with MAO inhibitors, 546, 546–7, 719
Chemical antagonism, 18
Chemical mediators/factors, *see* Mediators
Chemical sympathectomy, 176
Chemokines, 219, 240–1
as drug targets, 242
metastases and, 696
Chemoreceptor trigger zone (area postrema) in vomiting, 188, 372–3
Chemotaxin(s), 221
in asthma, 344
leukotrienes as, 236
PAF as, 237
Chemotherapy, 620–710
definition, 620
molecular basis, 620–9
resistance to, *see* Resistance
Chemotherapy, cancer, 696–709
agents used in, 698–706
cytotoxic, *see* Cytotoxic agents
see also specific drugs
combination schedules, 707
future strategies, 707–8
resistance, *see* Multidrug resistance; Resistance
toxicity, 697–8
fetal, 733–4
management, 707
Chenodeoxycholic acid, 378
Chest pain, cardiac, *see* Angina
Chickenpox, 662
Chief cells, 368
Children
absence seizures, 551–2
attention deficit and hyperactivity disorder, 589
development, *see* Development
growth, *see* Growth
see also Neonates
Chloral hydrate, 322, 517
Chlorambucil, 699
Chloramphenicol
clinical use, 644
mechanisms of action, 644, 646
pharmacokinetics, 644
resistance
mechanisms, 631, 632
S. aureus, 632
spectrum of activity, 644
unwanted effects, 645, 716
neonates, 645, 714
Chlordiazepoxide, 517, 518
Chloride (ions) transport, 67–8
gastric, 368
renal, 256, 353, 355
thiazide effects, 363
Chloride channels, GABA receptors/benzodiazepines and, 23, 471
Chloroform, 504, 509, 511
7-Chloro-kynurenic acid, 469
p-Chlorophenylalanine (PCPA), 480, 482
Chloroquine, 256, 677, 682
actions/effects, 677
mechanisms, 629, 677
unwanted, 678
in malaria, 677, 682
primaquine with, 680
resistance, 677
pharmacokinetics, 677
partitioning into tissues, 97
in rheumatoid disease, 256
Chlorothiazide–bile acid resin interactions, 312
Chlorpheniramine, 253
Chlorpromazine, 528
as antiemetic, 374
in Huntington's disease, 501
pharmacokinetics, 96, 533
side-effects/toxicity, 529, 727
Chlorpropamide, 389
Cholecalciferol, 453
Cholecystokinin (CCK)
antagonists
as anxiolytics, 524
as appetite suppressants, 402
biosynthesis, 203
food intake and, 397
Cholelithiasis, *see* Gallstones
Cholera toxin, 35
Cholesterol
abnormally high levels, *see* Hypercholesterolaemia
drugs inhibiting synthesis, *see* HMG-CoA reductase inhibitors
metabolism, 307, 308
in glucocorticoid synthesis, 413
in sex hormone synthesis, 432
in vitamin D synthesis, 453
transport, 307, 308
Cholesterol and Recurrent Events trial, 310
Cholesterol gallstones, *see* Gallstones
Choline, 139
Choline acetyltransferase, 139
Alzheimer's disease and, 496
Cholinergic transmission, 136–60
CNS, 483
Alzheimer's disease and, 495–6
function, 483–4
Parkinson's disease and, 497
effects of drugs, 143–60
electrical events, 141–3
physiology, 128, 139–43
Cholinesterase, 140, 155–60
distribution, 155–6
function, 155–6
genetic variants, 153
inhibition, *see* Anticholinesterases
reactivation, 158, 159
types, *see also* Acetylcholinesterase; Butyrylcholinesterase
Choreiform movements in Huntington's disease, 501
Chorionic gonadotrophin, human, 431, 438
Christmas disease, 318
Chromaffinomas (phaeochromocytomas), 173
Chromogranin A, 165
Chromosomes, *see* DNA; Genes; Mutations
Chronic obstructive pulmonary disease, 349–50
β_2-agonists, 346
Churg–Strauss syndrome, 347
Chylomicrons, 307, 309
Chymase, 297
Ciclosporin, 206, 257–8
actions/effects, 23
mechanisms, 225, 257–8
unwanted, 258, 729
pharmacokinetics, 258
Cigaglitazone, 390, 391
Cigarettes, *see* Nicotine; Smoking
Ciliary muscle, muscarinic agonist actions, 144
Cilostazol, 295
peripheral vascular disease, 303–4
Cimetidine, 230, 369, 370
actions, 369
interactions, 370, 721
pharmacokinetics, 370
unwanted effects, 370
Cinnarizine, 253, 373
Cinoxacin, 627, 648
CIP family, 72
Ciprofibrate, 311
Ciprofloxacin, 627, 647, 648
diarrhoeal illness, 376
pharmacokinetics, 648
S. aureus resistance, 632
spectrum of activity, 648
Circadian rhythms, 485
Circulation, *see* Enterohepatic circulation; Heart; Vascular system
Circus movement, 268
Cisapride, 376
Cisplatin, 700–1
in combination regimes, 707
Citalopram, 540, 544
Citrates, sodium and potassium, 365
Cladribine, 702
Clarithromycin, 646
H. pylori eradication, 371
Clavulanic acid, 642
Clearance
in hypothermia, 717
renal, drug elimination expressed as, 113
in single-compartment pharmacokinetic model, 114–15
see also Elimination
Clenbuterol, 171, 179
Clindamycin, 646–7
clinical use, 647
P. carinii pneumonia, with primaquine, 682
mechanism of action, 646
unwanted effects, 647
Clinical development/testing, 747, 749–50
phases, 749–50
Clinical outcome, measures, 87–8
Clinical trials (phase III studies), 81, 86–9, 730
bias, avoidance, 86–7, 88
diabetes, 387
hybrid design, 87
lipid-lowering drugs
bile acid-binding resins, 312
probucol, 312
statins, 310
myocardial infarction, 88, 88–9
organisation, 86, 88–9
principles, 86
sample size, 87
sequential, 87, 88
stroke prevention, 325
Clioquinol, Alzheimer's disease, 497
Clobazam, 555, 558
Clofazimine, 652
Clofibrate, 311
adverse effects, 311
Clomiphene, 433, 437
clinical use, 434
Clomipramine, 540
chemical aspects/structure, 542
Clonazepam, 517, 518
as anticonvulsant, 520, 555, 558
Clonidine, 146, 172, 179, 475
in alcohol withdrawal, 608
in glaucoma, 146
in migraine, 192
in nicotine dependence, 603
Cloning
neuropeptides, 199–200
receptors, 26
Clopenthixol, 529
Clopidogrel, 325, 326
clinical uses
coronary artery disease, 325
peripheral vascular disease, 303
Clostridium botulinum toxin, *see* Botulinum toxin
Clostridium difficile pseudomembranous colitis, *see* Pseudomembranous colitis
Clostridium tetani toxin, 473, 585
Clot, blood, definition, 314
Clotrimazole, 669
Clotting, *see* Coagulation
Clozapine, 529, 530, 532
CNQX and synaptic transmission, 468
Coagulation (clotting), 315–23
defects, 318–19
acquired, 318–19
inherited, 318
disseminated intravascular, 317
inflammation and, 220
oestrogens increasing, 432
pathway/cascade, 315–17
drugs acting on, 317–23
unwanted, *see* Thrombosis
see also Anticoagulants; Clot *and specific clotting factors*
Coated implantable devices, 105
Cobalamins, *see* Vitamin B_{12}

Cocaine, 178, 181, 586, 589–90, 615
actions/effects, 178, 181, 589
adverse, 181, 590, 615, 616
mechanism, 586
historical aspects, 589, 612
pharmacokinetics, 181, 589–90
Co-carcinogens, 730
Cocci, antibiotic choice, 636
Codeine (3-methylmorphine), 575, 580, 581
antimotility effects, 377
assay of analgesic action, 84
cough suppression, 350, 577
pharmacokinetics, 579, 580
Cognition/intellect
enhancers, 496
amphetamines as, 588
ethanol impairing, 603
Colchicine, 254–5
actions/effects, 22, 254–5
on ADH, 410
in gout, 254–5
unwanted, 255, 359
pharmacokinetics, 255
Cold extremities with β-blockers, 176
Colestipol, 312
Colestyramine, 312
interactions, 99, 312, 719
Colistin, 649
Colitis
pseudomembranous, *see* Pseudomembranous colitis
ulcerative, 377–8
Collagens, extracellular matrix, 73
Collateral vessels in angina, dilatation, 280
Collecting tubules and ducts, 359–60
active potassium absorption, 361
drugs acting on, 359
hormones acting on, 358, 359
Colony-stimulating factors (CSFs), 336, 337–8
actions/effects, 337–8
unwanted, 338
clinical uses, 338
cancer chemotherapy, 338, 707
fungal infections, 670
pharmacokinetics, 338
Colorectal cancer, aspirin prophylaxis, 250
Combinatorial chemistry, 748
Compartments (in body)
fluid, 101–4
pharmacokinetic models and, 114–17
well-stirred, 91, 114
see also specific compartments and Partitioning
Competitive antagonism, *see* Antagonism
Competitive inhibition
of enzymes, 23
of transport, 94
Complement system (in inflammation), 220, 226
activation, 220, 226
alternative pathway, 220
classical pathway, 220, 226
Complementary (alternative) medicine, 3–4
Compliance, arterial/aortic, 286
drugs affecting, 286
Concentration (of drug)
drug–receptor interactions and, 15–16
pharmacokinetic models and, 115–16
Concentration–effect, *see* Dose–response curves
Conditional mutagenesis, 86
Conditioning, 596
Conduction, block
cardiac, *see* Heart, conduction slowing/block
by local anaesthetics, 614
Conflict tests
animals, 516
humans, 516
Congenital abnormalities, drug-induced, *see* Fetal development; Teratogens
Conjugates
drug-antibody, *see* Antibody
drug-toxin, 206
reactions forming, 109
Conjugation, bacterial, 630
Conn's syndrome, 411, 418
Consciousness, loss in anaesthesia, 506
Consent, informed, 86
Constipation, 375–6
morphine-like drug-induced, 577
treatment, 375–6
Contraceptives, hormonal, 439–41
female, 434, 439–41
male, 441
oral, *see* Oral contraceptives
Contraction, muscle, 62–4, 65
cardiac (myocardium), 268–9
drugs increasing contractility, 278–9, 302, 616
smooth muscle, 62–3
excitation and, coupling, 63
uterine, *see* Uterus
smooth muscle, vascular, 286
mediators causing, 286, 287
see also Vasoconstriction
Controls in trials, 86
Convoluted tubules, 354–5
distal, *see* Distal tubules
proximal, 354–5
Convulsions and convulsants, *see* Seizures
Coronary artery
angioplasty, 326
atherosclerosis, *see* Coronary artery disease
blood flow, 270–2
spasm, 271, 280
vasodilation, *see* Vasodilation
Coronary artery disease (ischaemic heart disease incl. atherosclerosis), 270–2
clopidrogel + aspirin, 325
dysrhythmias in, 265
ethanol reducing mortality, 604–5
oestrogen replacement reducing incidence, 435
smoking and, 601
see also Angina; Myocardial infarction
Corpus luteum (in menstrual cycle and pregnancy), 431
Corpus striatum
cholinergic neurons of, Parkinson's disease and, 497
dopaminergic pathways, 476
Cortical spreading depression, 191
Corticosteroid(s), *see* Adrenal steroids; Mineralocorticoids; Steroids
Corticosteroid-binding globulin, 417
Corticosterone, 411, 412
Corticotrophin, *see* Adrenocorticotrophic hormone
Corticotrophin-releasing factor, 405, 406, 412–13
depression and, 537
glucocorticoid feedback effects on secretion, 416
Cortisol, *see* Hydrocortisone
Cortisone, 412
Costs, 5
Cotransmission, 130–1, 132, 133
noradrenaline/ATP, 131
peptides as, 200
Co-transport (symport) systems, 354, 355, 356
Co-trimoxazole (sulfamethoxazole–trimethoprim), 623, 638
P. carinii pneumonia, 682
toxoplasmosis, 685
Cough, 350
suppressants (antitussives), morphine-like drugs, 350, 577
Coumarins, *see* Oral anticoagulants
Counter-current mechanism (exchange and multiplier), 352, 356, 359–60
Covalent interactions, targets for, 726–7
Cranial outflow of parasympathetic nervous system, 125
Craving, *see* Psychological dependence
CREB (cAMP response element-binding protein) and habituation, 597
Cretinism, 424
Creutzfeldt–Jakob disease, 501
growth hormone preparations and, 407
Crisantapase, 705
Crohn's disease, 377–8
Cromakalim, K^+ channels and, 62
Cromoglicate, 349, 350
Cromokalim, 294
Cross-over design, 86
CSFs, *see* Colony-stimulating factors
Curare, 150
Cushing's syndrome, 411
diagnosis, 418
glucocorticoid-induced, 416, 417
Cutaneous administration/reactions etc., *see* Skin
Cutaneous larva migrans, *see Ankylostoma* spp.
C-X-C chemokines, 240, 241
Cyclazocine, 574
Cyclic nucleotides, drugs increasing concentration, 294
see also AMP; GMP
Cyclin(s), 70–2
Cyclin-dependent kinases (cdks), 70–2
inhibitors, 708
Cyclizine, 253, 373
Cyclo-oxygenase (COX), 231
forms, 234, 244–5
inhibitors, *see* Non-steroidal anti-inflammatory drugs
roles, 244–5, 247
Cyclopentolate, 145, 147
Cyclophilin, 258
Cyclophosphamide, 699–700
interactions, 254
metabolism, 699, 700
unwanted effects, 111, 699
Cycloplegia, 146
Cycloserine, 651
mechanism of action, 624, 651
unwanted effects, 651
Cyclosporin, *see* Ciclosporin
Cyclothiazide, 470
Cyproheptadine, 188, 193, 253
carcinoid syndrome, 192
migraine, 192, 193
Cyproterone, 437
prostate cancer, 705
Cysteinyl leukotrienes, 235, 236
actions, 236
in inflammation, 236–7
receptors and receptor antagonists, *see* Leukotrienes
Cystic fibrosis, gene therapy, 739
Cystic fibrosis transmembrane conductance regulator, 67–8, 739
Cysticercosis (*T. solium*), 687
therapy, 689, 690
Cytarabine, 627, 702, 703
Cytochrome *c* and apoptosis, 76
Cytochrome P450 system, *see* P450 mono-oxygenase system
Cytokines
in asthma, 342, 344, 345
in bone remodelling, 446–8
classifications, 239–40
definition, 218, 239
glucocorticoid effects on, 348, 416
in inflammatory/immune response, 218–19, 239–41
T cell-released, 224, 225
receptors, 42
therapeutic targeting, 241, 260
malaria, 685
rheumatoid disease, 256–7
in viral infection
inhibition of action, 656
release, 656
see also Growth factors *and specific cytokines*
Cytomegalovirus
avoiding immune response, 657
drug therapy, 662
Cytoplasm, bacterial, 621
Cytoprotective agents
Ca^{2+} antagonists as, in ischaemic tissue, 283
gastric mucosal, 372
see also Neuroprotection
Cytosine arabinoside, 627, 702, 703
Cytotoxic agents, 698–706
in cancer therapy, 698–706
antibody–drug conjugates, 104, 708
categories, 698
combination schedules, 707
general principles of action, 696–8
mechanisms of action, 623, 627, 628, 698, 699, 701, 702, 703, 708
resistance to, *see* Resistance
definition, 698
toxicity, 697–8
fetal, 733–4
management, 707
see also specific agents

Cytotoxic hypersensitivity, antibody-dependent (type III hypersensitivity), 228, 735, 736
Cytotoxic T cells, *see* CD8+ T cells
Cytotoxicity, cellular, antibodies and, 226

D

D cells (somatostatin-secreting), 380, 385
D4T (stavudine), 661
Dacarbazine, 701
Daclizumab, 241, 259–60
Dactinomycin (actinomycin D), action, 625–7, 703
Daidzin, 607
Dale, Sir Henry Hallett
  adrenoceptor classification, 161, 162
  muscarinic vs. nicotinic activity of ACh, classification, 136–7
  neurotransmitter principles, 126
Dalfopristin, 646, 647
Danazol, 437, 438
Dantrolene
  in malignant hyperthermia, 54, 154
  ryanodine receptors and, 54
Dapsone, 651–2
  dermatitis herpetiformis, 652
  leprosy, 651–2
  malaria, 676, 680
    pyrimethamine with, unwanted effects, 680
  P. carinii pneumonia, with trimethoprim, 682
  structure, 680
  unwanted reactions, 680
Dazoxiben, 327
ddC (zalcitabine), 660
ddI, *see* Didanosine
Death, cell, *see* Apoptosis; Cell; Necrosis
Debrisoquine, 109, 715
Decamethonium, 149, 152
Decongestion, nasal, 172
Dedifferentiation, cancer cells, 695
Defence, host
  cancer, enhancement, 709
  immune system in, *see* Immune response
  NO in, 212, 213
  viral infections, 655–6
    evasion by virus, 656–7
Deferiprone, 333
Degradative metabolism (catabolism)
  catecholamines, 167–8
  5-HT, 185
  increased, tolerance, 21
  NO, 210–12
  pro-drugs, 23
  prostanoids, 234
Delayed (type IV) hypersensitivity, 228, 735, 736
Delirium tremens, 608
Delivery systems, 104–5
  gene, 739–41
  see also Formulation
δ-opioid receptors, 574
  opioid drug and peptide selectivity for, 575
  role, 574, 575
Delusions in schizophrenia, 525
Demeclocycline, 643
  ADH affected by, 410
  unwanted effects, 359, 644
Dementia, Alzheimer's type, *see* Alzheimer's disease
Denervation, supersensitivity to neurotransmitters with, 126–8
Deoxyadenosylcobalamin (ado-B_{12}), 335, 336
Deoxycortone, 412
Deoxythymidylate synthesis, *see* Thymidylate
Deoxyuridylate, deoxythymidylate synthesis from, *see* Thymidylate
Dependence (addiction), 594–611
  alcohol, *see* Ethanol
  amphetamines, 588–9
  benzodiazepine, 522
  cannabis, 609–10
  cocaine, 589
  morphine-like drugs, 578–9, 597
  nature, 595–6
  nicotine, *see* Nicotine
  pharmacological approaches (in general), 598
  physical, *see* Physical dependence
  psychological, *see* Psychological dependence
  see also Habituation
Depolarisation, 55
  in cardiac tissue, 265
    Ca^{2+} channel responses to, 282
    partial, 268
  in cholinergic transmission, 141
    block, 142–3
    neuromuscular blockers causing, *see* Depolarising blocking agents
  seizure-related, 553
  see also After-depolarisation; Paroxysmal depolarising shift
Depolarising blocking agents, 148, 152–4
  non-depolarising drugs compared with, 153
  unwanted/dangerous effects, 153–4
Depot preparations, *see* Intramuscular injection; Subcutaneous implants
Depression (mood), 535–48
  animal models, 538
  bipolar, *see* Bipolar affective disorder
  drug therapy, *see* Antidepressants
  electroconvulsive therapy, 538, 547–8
  endogenous, 535
  monoamine theory, 536–8
  nature, 535
  reactive, 535
  reserpine inducing, 176
  unipolar, 535
Depression (synaptic transmission), long-term, *see* Long-term depression
Dermatitis herpetiformis, 652
Dermatomycosis, 666, 667
Descending inhibitory pathway and pain, 565–6
Desensitisation (tachyphylaxis), 19–21
  G-protein-coupled receptors, 38–9, 41
  nicotinic receptors, 143
Desferrioxamine, 333
Desflurane, 507, 510, 511
  adverse effects, 507
Desipramine, 178, 540
  chemical aspects/structure, 542
  unwanted effects, 540, 543
Desmopressin, 411
Desogestrol, 434
  in combined pill, 439
Development (drug), 747–51
  antibiotics
    antibacterials, 633, 652
    antifungals, 667, 671
    antiprotozoals, 682, 685
  bioassay, 81
  new targets in, 77–8
    selection, 747–8
Development (human)
  fetal, *see* Fetal development
  retinoic acid in, 44–5
  thyroid hormones in, 423–4
  see also Growth
Dexamethasone, actions/effects, 412
  antiemetic, 375
    in cancer chemotherapy, 707
Dexamethasone suppression test, 418
  in depression, 537
Dexfenfluramine
  adverse effects, 725
  as anorectic, 588
Dextroamphetamine, 587
Dextromethorphan, antitussive actions, 350
Dextropropoxyphene, 574, 575, 580, 581
Dezocine, 582
D4T (stavudine), 661
Diabetes Control and Complications Trial, 387
Diabetes insipidus, 410
  thiazide diuretic effects in, 363
  X-linked nephrogenic, 717
Diabetes mellitus, 385–92
  β-blockers and, 175, 176–7
  drug therapy, 387–92
    new agents, 392
  erectile dysfunction in, 215, 216
  type 1, *see* Insulin-dependent diabetes
  type 2, *see* Non-insulin-dependent diabetes mellitus
  types other than type 1/2, 387
Diacetylmorphine, *see* Diamorphine
Diacylglycerol, 37, 38
Diamorphine (diacetylmorphine; heroin), 580, 581
  euphoric effects, 577
Diarrhoea, 376–7
Diazepam, 471, 517
  in anaesthesia, 512
  as anticonvulsant, 520, 555, 558
  pharmacokinetics, 517, 520, 521
    age-related differences, 714
    elimination, 111, 117
  rectal, 100
Diazepam-binding inhibitor, 471, 520
Diazoxide, 363
  K^+ channels and, 62
Dichloroisoprenaline, 173
Diclofenac, 245
Dicycloverine (dicyclomine), 148, 377
Didanosine (ddI; dideoxyinosine), 627, 660
  pharmacokinetics, 660
  unwanted effects, 660
Dideoxycytosine (zalcitabine), 660
Dideoxyinosine, *see* Didanosine
Diet
  in diabetes (type 2), 387
  folate in, 334
  iron in, 331
  mechanism explaining difficulty in maintaining weight loss by, 400
  see also Appetite; Food; Malnutrition; Nutrient deficiency
Diethyl ether, *see* Ether
Diethylcarbamazine, 690
Diethylstilboestrol, *see* Stilboestrol
Differentiation defects in cancer, 695
Diffusion (of drugs), 91
  in aqueous pores, 92
  coefficient of, 91
  facilitated, 94
  in lipid, 92, 92–4
  in renal tubule, 112–13
Diflunisal, 245
Digoxin, 278–9
  actions, 278
  adverse effects, 278
  calcium extrusion and, 54
  interactions, with bile acid-binding resins, 312
  pharmacokinetics, 279
    age affecting, 713–14
    formulation affecting intestinal absorption, 98
  uses, 279
    heart failure, 279, 302
Dihydrocodeine, 581
Dihydroergotamine, 188, 189
  Alzheimer's disease, 496
Dihydrofolate, metabolism
  bacterial, 622
  human, 334
Dihydrofolate reductase, 334, 701
  inhibition, 334, 622–3, 679
    by methotrexate, 623, 701
    by trimethoprim, 622–3, 639
Dihydropteroate reductase and sulfonamides, 638
Dihydropyridines, 23
  in angina, 282
  Ca^{2+} channels and, 23, 52
  in myocardial infarction, 272
  receptor, skeletal muscle, 62
  vasodilatory effects, 293
Dihydrotestosterone, 436
1,25-Dihydroxycholecalciferol, 450
Dihydroxymandellic acid synthesis, 167
Dihydroxyphenylacetic acid production, 476
Dihydroxyphenylalanine, *see* DOPA
Dihydroxyvitamin D_3, 450
Diloxanide/diloxanide furoate, 683
Diltiazem
  actions
    anti-anginal, 282
    dysrhythmic and antidysrhythmic, 277, 283
    vasodilatory, 293
Dimaprit, 230

Dimenhydrinate, 253, 373
Dimethylphenylpiperazinium, 147
1,3-Dimethylxanthine, *see* Theophylline
Dinoprostone, 442
  clinical use, 443
Diphenhydramine, 253
  as antiemetic, 253, 373
    cancer chemotherapy, 707
  as hypnotic, 517
Diphenoxylate, 377
Diphyllobothrium latum, 687
Dipyridamole, 278, 280, 325, 326
  stroke prevention, 325
Discovery, 747–51
Disease (in general)
  individual variation due to, 717–18
  models, *see* Models
  oral anticoagulant action affected in, 322
  receptors and, 48, 717–18
Disease-modifying antirheumatoid drugs (DMARDs), 255–6
Disopyramide, 274, 275, 276
Disposition, drug, 97
  see also Absorption; Distribution; Elimination; Metabolism
Disseminated intravascular coagulation, 317
Distal tubules, 356
  diuretic acting on, *see* Thiazide diuretics
Distribution (of drugs), 101–4
  disease affecting, 718
  drugs affecting, 719–20
  volume of, *see* Volume of distribution
Disulfiram, 165, 607, 608
  in alcohol aversion therapy, 607, 608
  interactions, 721
Disulfiram-like effect of chlorpropamide, 389
Diuresis, ethanol-induced, 604
Diuretics, 362–5
  in cardiac failure, 300
  in hypertension, 300, 301, 363
  interactions, 718, 722
  loop, *see* Loop diuretics
  in nephrotic syndrome, insensitivity to, 717
  osmotic, 364–5
  potassium-sparing, *see* Potassium-sparing diuretics
  thiazide, *see* Thiazide diuretics
Dizocilpine (MK801), 469
  as NMDA receptor channel blocker, 466, 469, 527
DNA
  alkylation, 698, 698–701
  cloned, receptors, 26
  damage
    anticancer drugs acting by, 628, 703
    apoptosis with, 76
  insulin and, 384
  platinum drug interactions, 700
  structure, 625, 627
  synthesis/replication, 625–7
    antibacterial agents interfering with, 627
    anticancer agents (antimetabolites) interfering with, 627, 698, 701–3
    antiviral agents interfering with, 627, 660–1, 662–3
    in DNA viruses, 655
    folate in, 334
  transcription, *see* Transcription
  vaccination with, 741, 742
  see also Genes; Mutagenesis; Mutations; Nucleic acid synthesis
DNA-binding domain of receptors, 44, 45
  glucocorticoid receptors, 413, 415
DNA gyrase inhibitors, *see* Topoisomerase inhibitors
DNA polymerase inhibition, 625–6, 628
  cancer cells, 702
  viruses, 622, 662–3
    herpes, 627
DNA technology, 5
  see also Cloning; Molecular techniques
DNA topoisomerase inhibitors, *see* Topoisomerase inhibitors
DNA viruses, 654
  diseases caused, 654
  replication, 655
Dobutamine, 179
  clinical use, 179
    heart failure, 279, 302
    shock, 303
Docelatel, 704
Docosahexaenoic acid, 313
Docusate sodium, 375
Dolasetron, 373
Domoic acid, 491
Domperidone, 102
  antiemetic effects, 374
    in Parkinson's disease therapy, 102, 500
    in postcoital contraception, 441
Donepezil, 496
DOPA (dihydroxyphenylalanine)
  dopamine synthesis from, 164
  synthesis, 164
DOPA decarboxylase, inhibition, 176, 178, 181
  in Parkinson's disease therapy, 499
L-Dopa, *see* Levodopa
Dopamine, 128, 130, 162, 476–80
  in CNS/brain, 476–80
    distribution/synthesis/release, 476, 477
    functions, 478–80
    Parkinson's disease and, *see* Parkinson's disease
    schizophrenia and, 526–7
  in neurotransmission, 128, 130
  noradrenaline synthesis from, 165
  pituitary and, 406
  release
    amphetamine effects, 588
    antiparkinsonian drugs increasing, 499, 500
  reuptake inhibitor, 541
    as appetite suppressant, 402
  synthesis, 164
  vasodilatory effects, 132, 294
Dopamine-β-hydroxylase, 165
Dopamine receptor(s), 477–8
  CNS, 477–8
  D_1 type/family (D_1/D_5), 477, 479
  D_2 type/family (= D_2/D_3/D_4), 477, 479
  D_3, 477
  D_4, 477
    genetic polymorphism, 527
  peripheral, 478
  in schizophrenia, 526
    antipsychotics effects, 528–30
Dopamine receptor agonists, 479
  actions, 407
    schizophrenia-like episodes, 526
  clinical uses
    in acromegaly, 407
    in erectile dysfunction, 444
    Parkinson's disease, 500
    prolactin suppression, 407
  D1, 479
  D2, 479
Dopamine receptor antagonists, 479
  D1, 479
    in hypertension, 300
  D2, 479
    antiemetic actions, 374, 375
    antipsychotics as, 478, 526–7, 528–30
    prokinetic actions, 376
  in Huntington's disease, 501
  prolactin release stimulated by, 407
Dopaminergic pathways in CNS, 476–7
  antipsychotic effects, 528–30
  function, 478–80
  Huntington's disease and, 501
  limbic/mesolimbic system, 476, 596, 600
  opioid dependence and, 579
  reward and, 596, 600
Dorsal horn
  morphine action, 576
  nociceptive pathways, 564–5
Dorzolamide, 100, 146
Dose (amount/quantity)
  loading, 115
  repeated, pharmacokinetic effects, 115
Dose ratio, antagonism and, 12, 17
Dose–response (concentration–effect) curves, 11
  in bioassays, 83
  irreversible antagonist effects on, 19
Double-blinding, 87
Double compartment (two-compartment) model of pharmacokinetics, 116–17
Downregulation, receptor, 20
Doxapram, 585, 586, 587
Doxazosin, 173
  in hypertension, 300
Doxepin, chemical aspects/structure, 542
Doxorubicin, 703
  mechanisms of action, 627, 703
Doxycycline, 643
  in malaria, 676, 681
  pharmacokinetics, 644
DP (PGD_2) receptors, 234
Dracunculus medinensis, *see* Guinea worm
Driving and alcohol, 603–4
Dronabinol, 375
Droperidol
  as antiemetic, 374
  in neuroleptoanalgesia, 512
Drug abuse, 594–611
  definition, 595
  see also Dependence *and specific drugs*
Ductus arteriosus
  delayed closure, COX inhibitors as cause of, 443
  patency, prostanoids and, 235
Duodenal ulcers, *see* Peptic ulcers
Duteplase, 328
Dwarfism, pituitary, 407
Dyflos, 156, 157, 158
Dyhydrogesterone, 434
Dynorphin, 572
Dyskinesia
  with levodopa, 49–500
  tardive, with antipsychotics, 531–2
Dyslipidaemia (implying hyperlipidaemia/hyperlipoproteinaemia), 309–13
  classification, 309
  drug treatment, *see* Lipid-lowering drugs
Dysmenorrhea, 442
Dysrhythmias, cardiac, 265–8
  classification, 265
  drugs causing
    adrenoceptor agonists, 170
    adrenoceptor antagonists, 175
    depolarising drugs, 153
    general anaesthetics, 506
    glycosides, 278
    morphine-like drugs, 578
    tricyclic antidepressants, 543, 544
  drugs treating, *see* Antidysrhythmic drugs
Dysrhythmias, cardiac post-myocardial infarction/damage, 265, 267
Dystonias with antipsychotics, 531

E

Ear, aminoglycoside toxicity, 645
Echinocandins, 670
Echinococcus spp., *see* Hydatid disease
Econazole, 669
Economic issues, *see* Pharmacoeconomics
Ecothiopate, 146, 156, 157, 158, 160
'Ecstasy', *see* Methylenedioxymethamphetamine
Ectopic beats (incl. ectopic pacemaker activity), 267
  antidysrhythmic drugs, 276
  glycosides causing, 278
ED_{50}, 89
Edrophonium, 156, 160
EEG, *see* Electroencephalography
Efavirenz, 661
Effect
  dose and, *see* Dose–response curves
  measuring, *see* Measurement
Effective dose, 50[percent] (ED_{50}), 89
Effector(s)
  afferent nerves as, 123
  receptors and
    G-protein-coupled receptors, 41
    types of linkage, 27
  for various types of drug targets, 24–5
Effector phase of immune response, 223–4

Efferent pathways
airway, 340, 340–1
somatic, 123
Efficacy
agonists and, 9, 13, 14
therapeutic (therapeutic effectiveness), in clinical trials, 84, 86
Effort, *see* Exercise
Ehrlich, Paul, 7, 102
Eicosanoids (arachidonic acid metabolites), 66, 231–7, 361–2
actions
in CNS, 486, 487
in inflammatory/immune response, 222, 225
on insulin secretion, 381
renal, 361–2
biosynthesis, 231–4
nomenclature, 234
structure, 231
see also Prostanoids *and specific eicosanoids*
Eicosapentaenoic acid, 313
Electrical events, cholinergic transmission, 141–3
Electrically excitation of cell membranes, *see* Excitation
Electroconvulsive therapy, 538, 547–8
Electroencephalography (EEG)
arousal monitoring, 483–4
in epilepsy, 550
Electrolyte balance
in diarrhoeal illness, maintenance, 376
salicylates affecting, 251
see also Ions
Eledoisin, 570
Elimination (incl. excretion), 106, 111–14
drugs promoting, *see* Diuretics
of drugs/metabolites, 106, 111–14
age affecting, 713–14
drugs affecting, 362–5, 721–2
renal, *see* Kidney
see also Clearance
Elimination rate constant, 115
Eliprodil, 466
Elliott, TR, 122
Embolus and embolism, 315
see also Thromboembolism
Emesis, *see* Vomiting
Emetine, 373
Emetogenicity, *see* Vomiting
EMLA, 617
Emodin, 376
Emotions in depression, 535
Emphysema, 349–50
Enalakiren, 296
Enalapril, 111, 296
Encainide, 275, 276
Encephalopathy
salicylate-induced, 251
spongiform, 501
End-diastolic volume, 269
Endocrine system, 380–428
actions/effects (of drugs) on
antipsychotics, 532
cannabis, 610
ethanol, 604
gastrointestinal tract regulation by, 367
in reproduction, 429–39
see also Neuroendocrine system
Endocrine therapy (cancer), *see* Hormone therapy
Endometrial cancer, oestrogens and risk of, 730
HRT, 435, 730
oral contraceptives and, 440
Endoplasmic reticulum, Ca^{2+} channels, 54
Endorphins, 203, 572
Endothelial NOS, 209–10
Endothelin, 200, 287, 288–90, 293
action/function, 289, 290, 293
biosynthesis, 288–9
in brain, 200
discovery, 288
distribution, 288–9
receptors, 288, 289–90
agonists, 290
antagonists, 204, 289, 290, 295
secretion, 288–9
Endothelium (and endothelial cells), vascular, 286–90, 317
in diabetes, dysfunction, 215, 216
mediators derived from, *see* Mediators, vascular
movement of drug across, 91–2
role, 221–2
in angiogenesis, 221, 288
in atherogenesis/atherosclerosis, 306–7
in haemostasis and thrombosis, 317
in inflammation, 221–2
Endothelium-derived hyperpolarising factor, 287
Endothelium-derived relaxing factor, 208, 209, 286
see also Nitric oxide
Endotoxin, *see* Lipopolysaccharide
Endplate(s), motor, *see* Neuromuscular junction
Endplate potential at cholinergic synapses, 141
Energy balance (metabolism/stores/expenditure), 394–7
agents increasing expenditure, 402
catecholamine and adrenoceptor agonist effects, 170
regulation, 396–7, 398
cAMP in, 36, 37
homeostatic mechanisms in, 394, 394–6
obesity as disorder of, 399–401
Enflurane, 507, 510–11
adverse effects, 507, 511, 736
metabolism, 509
Enkephalin(s), 203, 572
Enkephalinase inhibitors, 583
Enprofylline, 346
Enrofloxacin, 648
Entacapone, 499, 500
Entamoeba histolytica (amoebiasis), 682–3
Enteric nervous system, 123, 125, 367
Enterobacteriaceae, antibiotic choice, 636
Enterobius vermicularis (threadworm in UK/pinworm in USA), 687
therapy, 689, 690, 691
Enterochromaffin cells, 184
Enterococci, antibiotic resistance, 633
Enterohepatic circulation, 113–14
Enterostatin, 402
Enzyme(s), 23
age-related differences, 714
as drug target, 23
false substrates, 23
examples, 24–5
inactivation, antibiotic resistance via, 631
induction, 109–10, 720
inhibitors, 720–1
as antiprotozoals, 685
competitive, 23
examples, 24–5
polymorphic/genetic variation, 715
see also specific (types of) enzymes
Eosinophils, 220
in inflammation, 220, 221, 237
PAF and, 237
EP (PGE_2) receptors, 234
Ephedrine, 177, 178, 180
Epibatidine, 149, 484, 583, 599
Epidural anaesthesia, 617
Epigenetic carcinogens, 730
Epilepsy, 550–60
drugs in, *see* Antiepileptic drugs
mechanisms and animal models, 552–3
types, 550–1
see also Seizures
Epinephrine, *see* Adrenaline
Epirubicin, 703
Epithelium
as barrier to drug, 91
ion transport, 66–8
as route of administration, 100
Eplerenone, 419
Epoietin, *see* Erythropoietin
Epoprostenol (synthetic prostacyclin), 325–7
in shock, 303
Epstein–Barr virus, therapy, 662
Eptifibatide, 325
Equilibrium constant, 15–16
Erection (penile), 443–4
dysfunction (impotence), 443–4
causes, 443–4
in diabetes, 215, 216
treatment, 215, 295
physiology, 443
Ergocalciferol, 450
Ergometrine, 189, 442
actions/effects, 190, 442
mechanism, 190, 442
unwanted, 442
clinical uses, 442
in migraine, 190
obstetric, 443
Ergonovine, 189
Ergot alkaloids, 188–90
actions/effects, 172, 189
unwanted, 189, 190
clinical uses, 189, 190
Ergotamine, 188, 189, 193
in migraine, 190, 192, 193
unwanted effects, 193
Errors in trials, 87, 89
Erythrocytes (red cells), 330
destruction, excessive, *see* Haemolysis
function, 330
Plasmodium life cycle in, 673, 674, 675
drugs acting at, 677, 680
Erythromycin, 646, 647
diarrhoeal illness, 376
interactions, 646
mechanism of action, 644, 646
pharmacokinetics, 646
resistance, 646
mechanisms, 631, 632
spectrum of activity, 646
unwanted effects, 646
Erythropoietin, 336–7, 338
recombinant forms (epoietin), 336
clinical use, 337
pharmacokinetics, 337
unwanted effects, 337
transgenic, 741, 742
Eserine, *see* Physostigmine
Esterified steroid hormones, 101
Estramustine, 699
ET receptors, *see* Endothelin
Etacrynic acid, 362
Etanercept, 241, 256, 257
Etaquine, 680
Ethacrynic acid, *see* Etacrynic acid
Ethambutol, 650
Ethanol (alcohol), 603–8
actions/effects, 603–5
vasodilatory, 295
dependence (alcoholism), 607–8
treatment, 608
interactions
metronidazole, 721
tricyclic antidepressants, 544
pharmacokinetics, 605–7
elimination, 117
ethnic differences, 712
metabolism, 109, 605–7
tolerance, 607–8
Ether, diethyl, 503, 507, 511
toxicity, 507
Ethics, trials, 86
Ethinyloestradiol in combined pill, 439
Ethnicity, variations in response due to, 712–13
Ethosuximide, 555, 557, 560
isoniazid interactions, 650
mechanism of action, 554
Ethynodiol, 434
in combined pill, 439
Etodalac, 245
Etomidate, 512, 513
Etoposide, 704
Etorphine, 574, 581
Etretinate, teratogenicity, 734
Euphoria
amphetamine-induced, 588
cocaine-induced, 615
morphine/opioid-induced, 577
European stroke prevention trial (ESPS-2), 325
Eutectic mixture of local anaesthetics (EMLA), 617
Evernimomycin, 652
Evidence-based medicine, 86

Excitation/excitability, electrical (of membranes), 55–62
ion channels and, 55–62
muscle contraction and, coupling, 63
Excitatory amino acids, 462–70
metabolism and release, 462–3
neurotoxicity, *see* Excitotoxicity
Excitatory postsynaptic potentials in cholinergic transmission
fast, 141
slow, 142
Excitement stage (anaesthesia), 505
Excitotoxicity, 53, 491
epilepsy and, 553
glutamate, *see* Glutamate
mechanisms, 491, 492
Excretion, *see* Elimination
Exercise/effort
asthma induced by, 344
obesity and, 400–1
Exocrine glands (and their secretions), 127
airway, 340
muscarinic receptors, 127, 138
agonist effects, 144
antagonist effects, 146
Exocytosis, 65, 65–6
Exoerythrocytic (pre-erythrocytic) stage, malaria parasite, 673, 675
Exons, 203
Experimental models of disease, *see* Models
Extracellular fluid compartment, 101, 102
drugs distributed in, 104
Extracellular matrix, growth factors and cell interactions with, 73–4
Extrapyramidal motor system
antipsychotic side-effects, 529, 531–2
dopamine and, 476
Huntington's disease and, 498
Parkinson's disease and, 498
Extrinsic factor, *see* Vitamin B_{12}
Exudate in inflammation, 220
Eye
adrenoceptors, 127
autonomic effects on, 127
muscarinic receptors, 127
agonist actions, 144
antagonist actions/uses, 146
pressure, *see* Glaucoma
sildenafil adverse effects, 444
Eye drops, 100

F

Facilitated diffusion, 94
Factors, clotting
factor II/IIa, *see* Prothrombin; Prothrombin time; Thrombin
factor V Leiden, 317
factor VII, 317
factor VIII deficiency, 318
factor IX deficiency, 318
factor Xa, 316
heparin–antithrombin III complex and, 320
prothrombin interactions, 318
factor XII, *see* Hageman factor
Faecal softeners, 376
Famciclovir, 104, 663
Famotidine, 370
Farnesyl transferase inhibitors, 708
Fas receptor and viral infection, 656
Fasciculations with suxamethonium, 153
Fasciola hepatica, 691
Fast excitatory postsynaptic potentials in cholinergic transmission, 141
Fast phase of elimination, 117
Fat, body (fat cells and adipose tissue), 395, 396–7
energy stores in, sensors, 395
insulin and, 382, 395
partitioning into, *see* Partitioning
in thermogenesis, 396–7
see also Lipid; Oil
Fat:water partition coefficient, 96
Fatigue
amphetamines reducing, 588
with β-blockers, 176
Favism, 716
Feeding, *see* Appetite
Felbamate, 558, 559
Felypressin, 411
in infiltration anaesthesia, 617
Females, reproductive system
hormonal contraceptives, 434, 439–41
neurohormonal control, 429–31
Feminisation, alcoholics, 604
Fenbufen, 245
Fenfluramine, 587
adverse effects, 725
as anorectic, 588
Fenofibrate, 311
Fenoldopam, 300
Fenoprofen, nephrotoxicity, 728
Fenoterol, 346
Fentanyl, 573, 580, 581
neuroleptoanalgesia induced by, 512
Ferritin, 331, 332
Ferrous iron salts, 332–3
Fertility, reduced, treatment, 437
Fetal development (drugs adversely affecting), 731–2
cannabis/THC, 610
cocaine, 590
ethanol, 605
mechanisms of damage, 731–4
see also Teratogens
Fever/pyrexia
NSAIDs, 235, 246, 250
oral anticoagulants affected in, 322
PGE involvement, 235
see also Hyperpyrexia
Fexofenadine, 111
Fibrates (fibric acid derivatives), 311–12
adverse effects, 311
clinical use, 311
mechanism of action, 311
Fibric acid derivatives, *see* Fibrates
Fibrillation
atrial, glycosides in, 278
ventricular, post-myocardial infarction, 265
Fibrin formation, 220, 315–17
extrinsic pathway, 315–16
intrinsic pathway, 316
Fibrinolysis (thrombolysis), 327–9
drugs increasing, 328
clinical use, 328
unwanted effects/contraindications, 328
drugs inhibiting, 328–9
in inflammation, 220
Fibroblasts
in chronic inflammation, 229
glucocorticoid effects, 416
Filarial infections, 687
therapy, 689, 691
Filgrastim, 336, 338
fungal infections, 670
Filtration, glomerular, *see* Glomerulus
Finasteride, 437
clinical uses, 432
sites of action, 432
First-order kinetics, 115
First-pass (presystemic) metabolism, 110
Fish oils, 313
FK-binding protein, 258
FK463 (micafungin), 670
FK506 (tacrolismus), 258
FLAP (5-lipoxygenase-activating protein), 235
Flare (with axon reflex), 230
Flavoperidol, 708
Flecainide, 274, 275, 276
with probucol, avoidance, 313
Fluconazole, 668, 669
Flucytosine, 623, 669
amphotericin interactions, 667
mechanism of action, 669
pharmacokinetics, 669
unwanted effects, 669
Fludarabine, 702, 703
Fludrocortisone, 419
actions, 412
use, 419
Fluid
compartments, 101–4
renal transport/balance, 353, 356
see also Water
Fluid exudate in inflammation, 220
Fluid replacement (and volume replacement)
diarrhoea, 376
shock, 303
Flukes (trematodes), 687
therapy, 689
Flumazenil, 471, 520, 522, 523
ethanol depressant effects reversed by, 603
Flunitrazepam, 505
Fluoride
anabolic actions, 453
generated from anaesthetics, 509
Fluoroquinolones, *see* Quinolones
Fluorouracil, 623, 701–2
flucytosine converted to, 669
intestinal absorption, 98
mechanism of action, 623, 702–3
unwanted effects, 702
Fluoxetine, 482, 540, 544
in anxiety, 524
Flupenthixol, 529
Fluphenazine, 529
Flurazepam, 517
Flutamide, 437, 438
Fluticasone propionate, 348
Fluvoxamine, 540, 544
Focal (partial) seizures, 551, 556
Folate, *see* Folic acid
Folate polyglutamates, 334, 335, 701
Folic acid/folate (pteroylglutamic acid) in humans, 333–5, 336
actions, 334
antagonists in cancer therapy, *see* Antifolates
clinical use, 335
deficiency, 333, 335
trimethoprim-induced, 639
pharmacokinetics/metabolism, 334, 335–6
unwanted effects, 334–5
Folic acid/folate (pteroylglutamic acid) in parasites/microbes, synthesis and utilisation, 622–3
drugs affecting, *see* Antifolates
Folinic acid, 334
Follicle
Graafian, 430, 431
thyroid, 421
iodide uptake by, 421, 422
Follicle-stimulating hormone, 405, 438
in females
inhibition of release by combined pill, 439
release/actions, 430
GnRH in regulation of release, 437
in males, release/actions, 435, 435–6
recombinant, 438
Follicular phase of menstrual cycle, 430–1
Follitrophin, 438
Food
drugs hastening transit, 375–6
intake
drugs reducing, *see* Appetite suppressants
obesity and, 400
regulation, 395, 397
MAO inhibitor reactions with, 546–7, 719
see also Diet; Malnutrition; Nutrient deficiency; Orexigenic factors
Food vacuole, plasmodial, 628–9
Formaldehyde from methanol, 607
Formestane, 705
Formic acid from methanol, 607
Formoterol, 346
Formulation and intestinal absorption, 98
see also Delivery systems
Foscarnet (phosphonoformate), 627, 663
Fosfestrol, 705
4S trial (Scandinavian Simvastatin Survival Study), 310
FP ($PGF_{2\alpha}$) receptors, 234
Frame-shift mutations, agents inducing, 625, 628
Frank–Starling law, 269

Frederickson/WHO classification of hyperlipoproteinaemia, 309
Free radicals (reactive oxygen species)
generation of
atherogenesis and, 307
drug-induced, 726
neurodegeneration and, 493
NO reacting with, 487
NSAIDs as scavengers of, 247
Fructose, 606
Frusemide, *see* Furosemide
Fungal infections, 666–71
drugs inhibiting, *see* Antifungal drugs
superficial, 666, 667
systemic, 666, 667
Furosemide (frusemide), 362
dose–response curves, 357
in nephrotic syndrome, insensitivity, 717
Fusidic acid, 647
S. aureus resistance, 632

G

G_0 phase of cell cycle, 69
regulators in, 70–1
G_1 phase of cell cycle, 69
activation into, 70
regulators in, 71–2
G_2 phase of cell cycle, 69
regulators in, 72
G-CSF, *see* Granulocyte-CSF
G-protein(s), 32–44
classes, 35
mutations, 48
role, 33–4, 38–9
targets, 36–41
G-protein-coupled receptor(s) (metabotropic/7-transmembrane receptors), 27, 28–9, 32–44
activation, 33
constitutive, 33
agonists, specificity, 38
desensitisation, 38–9, 41
dimerisation, 40
glutamate, *see* Glutamate receptors
opioid receptors as, 576
presynaptic, 128
signal transduction by, 33–5, 36–8
structure, 27, 28, 32–3, 34
variations, 34–5
typical, adrenoceptors as, 162
G-protein-coupled receptor kinases (GRKs), 39
GABA (γ-aminobutyric acid), 128, 130, 462, 470–2
epilepsy and, 553
antiepileptic drugs and, 554, 558, 559
function, 470–1
in neurotransmission, 132, 470
in nociception, 572
interactions
benzodiazepines, 518
pentobarbital, 523
synthesis/storage, 470
GABA receptors, 471
agonists, 464
in Huntington's disease, 501
as muscle relaxants, 561
benzodiazepines and, 23, 471, 518, 520
structure, 471
$GABA_A$ receptors, 471
chloride channels and, 23, 471
drugs acting on, 471, 472
antiepileptics, 554, 555
benzodiazepines, 471, 518, 520
ethanol, 603
endogenous modulators, 471, 520
$GABA_B$ receptors, 471
drugs acting on, 471–3
muscle relaxants, 561
GABA-transaminase, 462, 470
vigabatrin and, 470, 559
Gabapentin, 558–9
as analgesic, 583
as antiepileptic, 559, 560
mechanisms of action, 553
as mood stabiliser, 548
pharmacokinetics, 560
pro-drug, 560
unwanted effects, 560
Galantamine, 130, 496
Gallamine, 138, 150, 151
unwanted effects, 150, 151
Gallstones/choleliths (incl. cholesterol stones), 378
clofibrate-induced, 311
Galvanic skin response and anxiety, 516
Gametocytes, plasmodial, 675
drugs acting against, 677, 680
Gamma-aminobutyric acid, *see* GABA
Ganciclovir, 663
Ganglion/ganglia, autonomic (ganglionic synapse), 123–5
blockers, 147–9, 150
clinical uses, 149
effects, 148–9
cholinergic transmission at, 141, 142
stimulants, 147, 150
see also Postganglionic neurons; Preganglionic neurons
Ganglionic-type nicotinic ACh receptors, 137, 138
Gastric acid secretion, 368–72
drugs inhibiting/neutralising, 369–71
clinical use, 372
sites of action, 369
regulation, 368–9
histamine in, 230, 368, 368–9
Gastric inhibitory polypeptide, 381
Gastric secretion
of acid, *see* Gastric acid secretion
of bicarbonate, 368, 369
ethanol stimulating, 604
Gastric ulcers, *see* Peptic ulcers
Gastrin, 367, 368, 368–9
receptors, 368, 369
antagonists, 368
Gastritis, ethanol-induced, 604, 605
Gastrointestinal tract, 367–89
actions on (of drugs/metabolites), 369–78
β-agonists, 170
colchicine, unwanted, 255
5-HT, 185–6
morphine-like drugs, 577
muscarinic receptor antagonists, 146, 148
NSAIDs, unwanted, 248–9, 370
prostanoids, 235
autonomic nervous system, 127, 367
drug absorption from, 98–9
functions relevant to pharmacology, 367–8
hormones, *see* Hormones
innervation, 367
motility, *see* Motility
movement, 375–7
drugs decreasing, 376–7
drugs increasing, 375–6
Gate control theory of pain, 564–5
Gatifloxacin, 652
Gating (of ion channels), 45, 46
Ca$_{2+}$ channels, 53
of ligand-gated ion channels, 30–1, 46, 47
of voltage-gated ion channels, 46, 47
GDP and G-proteins, 33, 34
Gemcitabine, 702
Gemeprost, 442
clinical use, 443
Gemfibrozil, 311
Gemifloxanone, 652
Gemtuzumab, 241
Gene(s)
delivery, in gene therapy, 739–41
expression, gene therapy requiring control of, 741–3
mutations/defects, *see* Mutagenesis; Mutations
splicing, *see* mRNA
transcription, *see* Transcription
Gene cassettes and antibacterial resistance, 630
Gene therapy, 4, 738–46
cancer, 743–4
infections, 744
safety, 743
technical aspects, 739–41
General anaesthesia, *see* Anaesthesia; Anaesthetics, general
Generalised anxiety disorder, 515
Generalised seizures, 551–2
Genetic disorders of coagulation, 318
Genetic factors
diabetes, 386
drug abuse/dependence, 597
alcohol, 607
in individual variations in response, 714–16
drug metabolism, 715–16
idiosyncratic reactions, 716–17
see also Pharmacogenetics; Pharmacogenomics
obesity, 400
schizophrenia, 526
Genetic mechanisms, antibacterial drug resistance, 629–31
Genetic models of disease, 85–6
Genetic variants, cholinesterase, 153
Genotoxic carcinogens, 729
tests for, 734
Gentamicin, 645, 647
Gepirone, 523
Gestodene, 434
in combined pill, 439
Gigantism, 407
Gla proteins, *see* Glutamate residues, γ-carboxylation
Gland(s), *see* Exocrine glands *and specific glands*
Glaucoma (raised intraocular pressure), 100, 145
drugs causing
muscarinic antagonists, 146
suxamethonium, 153
drugs used, 146
anticholinesterases, 153
β-blockers (incl. timolol), 100, 146, 175
carbonic anhydrase inhibitor (acetazolamide), 100, 146
muscarinic agonists, 145
osmotic diuretics, 365
prostaglandin analogue, 235
Glial cells, signalling role, 458
see also Astrocytes
Glibenclamide, 389, 390
Glioblastoma, gene therapy, 744
Glipizide, 389
Glitazones, *see* Thiazolidinediones
Globin and NO, 211
Glomerulus, 352
filtration, 111–12, 354
age and, 713–14
drugs modifying content of filtrate, 364–5
Glucagon, 279, 384–5
actions, 385, 386
myocardial contractility, 279
clinical uses, 385
synthesis/secretion, 384–5
see also Secretin/glucagon receptor family
Glucagon-like peptide, 381
Glucocorticoids, *see* Adrenal steroids
Glucokinase, 380
Gluconeogenesis
glucagon effects, 385
insulin effects, 382
Glucose
blood levels
abnormal, *see* Hyperglycaemia; Hypoglycaemia
regulation, 380, 384, 385, 386
glutamate synthesis from, 462
oxidation, glucagon effects, 385
synthesis, *see* Gluconeogenesis
tolerance, oral contraceptives and, 440
Glucose-6-phosphate dehydrogenase deficiency, 715, 716
primaquine and, 681
α-Glucosidase inhibitor, 391, 392
Glucuronide formation, 109
morphine, 579
Glucuronyl transferase induction, 720
Glutamate (in CNS), 462–70
action (in general), 463
epilepsy and, 553

Glutamate, *continued*
ethanol effects on excitatory effects of, 603
excitotoxicity, 491
ischaemic brain damage and, 493–4
nociception and, 572
schizophrenia and, 527
storage/release (from synaptic vesicles), 463
synthesis, 462–3
transport, 463, 464
Glutamate receptors, 463–70
agonists and positive modulators, 464, 465, 470
antagonists, 465, 468, 468–70
as analgesics, 583
nociceptive transmission and, 565
functional role, 466
metabotropic, 33, 463, 465, 491
antagonists, 468
role, 467
subtypes, 463–6
metabotropic, *see subheading above*
NMDA-type, *see* NMDA receptors
therapeutic use, 469–70
Glutamate residues, γ-carboxylation (Gla proteins), 318
oral anticoagulants interfering with, 319
Glutamic acid decarboxylase, 470
Glutamine, 462
Glutathione
as anti-oxidant, 493
drug-induced depletion, 716, 726, 727–8
Glycation end-products, advanced, 386
Glyceryl trinitrate (nitroglycerine), 213, 281
in angina, 279, 281
in cardiac failure, 302
sublingual, 99–100
Glycine, 462, 472
NMDA/glutamate receptors and, 466
receptor, 472
agonists, 464
antagonists, 472, 472
Glycogen
breakdown (glycogenolysis)
glucagon effects, 385
insulin effects, 382
metabolism, cAMP regulation, 36, 37
synthesis
glucagon effects, 385
insulin effects, 384
Glycolysis, insulin increasing, 382
Glycopeptide antibiotics, 648–9
Glycoprotein IIb/IIIa receptor antagonists, 241, 325, 326
clinical uses, 325
myocardial infarction prophylaxis, 271
Glycosides, cardiac, 278–9
actions, 278–9
adverse, 278
mechanisms, 278–9
chemistry, 278
clinical uses, 279
see also Digoxin
Glycosuria in diabetes, 385
GM-CSF, *see* Granulocyte–macrophage–CSF
GMP, cyclic (cGMP)
drugs increasing concentration, 294–5
NO effects on production, 212, 487
urine measurement, 214
Goitre
diffuse toxic, 424
simple non-toxic, 425
toxic nodular, 424
Gold compounds, 255–6
Gonadorelin, 406
Gonadotrophin(s), 438–9
actions
menstrual cycle, 430
pregnancy, 431
clinical use, 438–9
human chorionic, 431, 438
pharmacokinetics, 438–9
preparations, 438
release, 438
danazol inhibiting, 438
men, 435
women, 430, 431
see also Follicle-stimulating hormone; Luteinising hormone
Gonadotrophin-releasing hormone, 20, 405, 406, 437
menstrual cycle and, 430
synthetic forms, 438
Gonadotrophin-releasing hormone analogues (agonists/antagonists), 437–8
as anticancer agents, 438, 705
Goserelin, 437
in cancer, 705
Gout, 254–5, 366
GPIIa/IIIb receptor antagonists, *see* Glycoprotein IIb/IIIa receptor antagonists
GR32191, 326
GR205171 (vofopitant), 375
Graafian follicle, 430, 431
Graded responses in bioassays, 83
Gram-negative organisms, 635–7
antibiotic choice, 636
Gram-positive organisms, 635
antibiotic choice, 636
Grand mal, *see* Tonic–clonic seizures
Granisetron, 373
in cancer chemotherapy, 707
Granulocyte (polymorphonuclear cells)
absence/deficiency, *see* Agranulocytosis and granulocytopenia
in inflammation, 220–1
see also Basophils; Eosinophils; Neutrophils
Granulocyte-CSF, 337
actions, 337
recombinant, *see* Filgrastim
Granulocyte-macrophage-CSF, 337
actions, 338
recombinant, *see* Molgramostim
Grapefruit juice, 720
Graves' disease, 424
'Grey baby syndrome', 645, 714
Griseofulvin, 668
Growth
cell, and proliferation, *see* Proliferation
humans (children)
glucocorticoid-related disorders, 417
growth hormone-related disorders, 407
thyroid hormones affecting, 423
Growth factors
asthma and, 345
in cancer (and growth factor receptors), 48, 694, 695
cell and extracellular matrix interactions with, 73–4
cell cycle and, 70, 71
haemopoietic, 336–8
clinical use, 337, 338, 707
in inflammation, 240
as neural mediators, 199
in signal transduction, 70, 78
see also specific factors
Growth hormone (somatotrophin), 405, 407
actions/effects, 407
on blood glucose, 386
clinical use, 407
production/secretion, 407
disorders, 407
regulation, 407
Growth hormone-release inhibiting factor, *see* Somatostatin
Growth hormone-releasing factor (GHRF), 405, 406, 407
GTP and G-proteins, 34
Guam, dementia–paralysis–parkinsonism of, 491
Guanethidine, 177, 178
in hypertension, 300
in hyperthyroidism, 427
Guanine nucleotides, G-proteins and, 34
see also GDP; GMP; GTP
Guanylate cyclase, 44
activation
by BAY41-2272, 294
natriuretic peptides and, 295
NO and, 212, 487
penile erection and, 295
receptors linked to, 42, 44
Guinea worm (*D. medinensis*), 687, 688
therapy, 688, 689
Gut, *see* Gastrointestinal tract; Intestine
Guvacine, 470
Gynaecological uses, prostanoids, 235
Gyrase inhibitors, *see* Topoisomerase inhibitors

H

$H_1/H_2/H_3$ receptors, *see* Histamine H_1 receptor *etc.*
Habituation, 595, 596–7
mechanisms, 596–7
see also Dependence
Haem, 331
NO and, 211
Haem polymerase inhibition, plasmodial, 629, 673, 677
Haematinics, 331–6
Haematological reactions, drug-induced, 735–6
Haemodynamics
drugs interactions concerning, 721
renal, eicosanoid effects, 363
Haemoglobin, 331
carboxylated, 602
NO and, 211–12
see also Globin; Methaemoglobin
Haemoglobinopathies, gene therapy, 741, 743
Haemolysis and haemolytic anaemia, 330
drugs causing, 716, 735–6
primaquine, 681, 716
Haemophilia A (classical haemophilia), 318
Haemophilia B, 318
Haemopoiesis, 330–9
growth factors in, *see* Growth factors
megaloblastic, *see* Megaloblastic haemopoiesis and anaemia
Haemorrhage/bleeding
drugs causing
fibrinolytic, 328
injectable anticoagulants, 320
oral anticoagulants, 323
oesophageal varices, 293
postpartum, 443
subarachnoid, cerebral vasospasm following, reducing, 283
uterine, HRT-related, 435
Haemosiderin, 331, 332
Haemostasis, 314–29
definition, 314
drugs preventing/treating, *see* Anticoagulants; Antiplatelet drugs; Fibrinolysis, drugs increasing
drugs promoting (and coagulation), 315, 318–19, 322, 328–9
salicylate-induced disturbances, 251
Haemozoin, 673
Hageman factor (factor XII), 316
bradykinin synthesis and, 238
Half-life, 115
in plasma, *see* Plasma
Hallucinations
5-HT pathways and, 482
drugs causing, *see* Psychotomimetic drugs
in schizophrenia, 525
Halofantrine, 676, 679, 682
Haloperidol, 294, 529, 530
as antiemetic, 374
Halothane, 507, 510
disadvantages/toxicity, 111, 154, 507, 509, 510, 727, 736
metabolism, 509
Hapten, 228, 735
Harmful effects, *see* Adverse reactions
Hashimoto's thyroiditis, 424
Hashish, *see* Cannabis
Headache
migrainous, *see* Migraine
with nitrovasodilators, 281
Healing, 77, 229
Heart, 264–84
autonomic effects on, 123, 127
β-adrenoceptors, 163, 170, 273
binding studies, 10
catecholamine actions, 170, 273

conduction slowing/block, 267–8
treatment, 172
contraction, *see* Contraction
ectopic beats, *see* Ectopic beats
function, 272–84
drugs affecting, 272–84
physiology of, 264–72
general anaesthetic actions, 506
ischaemic disease, *see* Coronary artery disease
muscarinic receptors, *see* Muscarinic ACh receptors
output, 268
with inhalation anaesthetics, 508
rate, 264–8, 268
adrenoceptors and, 170
catecholamine/adrenoceptor agonist effects, 170, 273
glycoside effects, 278
muscarinic antagonist effects, 146
rhythm, 264–8
abnormal/disturbed, *see* Dysrhythmias
glycoside effects, 278
Heart attack, *see* Myocardial infarction
Heart block, *see* Heart, conduction slowing/block
Heart failure, 269, 300–2
drugs causing, 175
drugs used in, 279, 281, 300–2
β-agonists, 279, 302
digoxin, 279, 302
glucagon, 385
organic nitrates, 281, 302
sites of action, 300
pathogenesis, 269, 300
Heart muscle, 62
contraction, 62
excitation and, coupling, 63
see also entries under Myocardial
Heart Protection Study, 310
Heat production, *see* Thermogenesis
Heavy metals, teratogenicity, 734
Helicobacter pylori, 370
treatment, 371–2
Helminths, 687–92
drugs acting on, *see* Anthelminthic drugs
types, 687–8
see also specific (types of) helminth
Helper T cells, *see* $CD4^+$ helper lymphocytes
Hemicholinium, 154
Henderson–Hasselbach equation, 92
Henle's loop, *see* Loop of Henle
Heparan sulfate, 317
Heparin (and low-molecular weight heparin), 317, 319–21, 322
actions/effects
mechanism, 320
unwanted, 320
administration and pharmacokinetics, 320
in myocardial infarction prevention, 271
in plasma, compartmentalisation, 103
Hepatic function/metabolism/toxicity etc., *see* Enterohepatic circulation; Liver
Hepatitis B/C, interferon, 664
Her2/neu, monoclonal antibody to, 706
Heredity, *see entries under* Genetic
HERG channels, 61
Heroin, *see* Diamorphine
Herpes simplex virus, 662
Herpes viruses (in general)
as gene vectors, 741, 742
therapy, 627, 662
Heterotropic interactions in autonomic nervous system, 128
Hexamethonium, 148, 148–9
adverse effects, 148–9
High density lipoproteins, 307, 309
transport, 308
Hill–Langmuir equation, 15
Hirudin, 321
Hirugen, 321
Histamine, 229–31, 485
actions, 230–1
CNS, 485, 486
gastric, 230, 369
as neurotransmitter, 485
nociception/itching, 570
receptors, 229, 229–30
central, 485, 486
classification, 229
see also specific types (below)
release/secretion, 229
catecholamine inhibiting, 171
morphine-induced, 577–8
storage, 229
synthesis, 229
Histamine H_1 receptor, 9, 229, 230
cardiovascular, 230
central, 485, 486
Histamine H_1 receptor agonists, 230
Histamine H_1 receptor antagonists, 229, 230, 252–4
antipsychotics as, 529, 532
clinical use, 253
antiemetics, 253, 373, 375
asthma, 348
interactions, 719
pharmacokinetics, 253
pharmacological actions, 252–3
CNS, 253
unwanted effects, 253
Histamine H_2 receptor, 9, 229
agonists, 230
antagonists, 229, 230
gastric acid secretion inhibition, 370, 372
central, 485, 486
gastric, 369
Histamine H_3 receptor, 9, 485
agonists, 230
antagonists, 230
central, 485, 486
Histamine H_4 receptor, 229
Histocompatibility antigens, *see* Major histocompatibility complex
Histogenesis, drugs affecting, 732–3
History of pharmacology, 2–5
20th C., 3–4
pre-20th C., 2
HIV, 657–9
CD4 T cell binding, 241
drugs targeting, 242
as gene vector, disabled version, 741, 742
HIV disease (and AIDS), 657–9
CD4 T cells in, 658
drugs in, *see* Antiretroviral agents
gene therapy, 744
opportunistic (secondary) infections, 659
HLA, *see* Major histocompatibility complex
HMG (3-hydroxy-3-methylglutaryl-CoA reductase inhibitors; statins), 310–11
actions, 310
anabolic, 453
adverse effects, 311
withdrawal due to, 311, 750
clinical uses, 311
in peripheral vascular disease, 303
pharmacokinetics, 311
trials, 310
Hoe 140 (icatibant), 238, 239
Homeopathy, 3
Homocysteate, 462
Homocysteine, methionine synthesis from, 335–6
Homotropic interactions in autonomic nervous system, 128
Homovanillic acid formation, 476
Hookworms, 687
therapy, 688, 689
Hormone(s)
adrenal, *see* Adrenal steroids
in bone remodelling/metabolism, 446, 447, 449–50
collecting tubules in kidney and actions of, 358, 359
of endocrine system, pancreatic islet, 380–4
gastrointestinal tract, 367
role, 368, 369, 381
tumours secreting, 705
glucose regulation by, 386
as neural mediators, 199
neuropeptides and peripherally-acting, distinction, 200
peptide, nasal sprays, 100
pituitary, 404–11
in reproduction, 429–39
tumours dependent on, 730
see also Endocrine system; Neuroendocrine system; Preprohormones; Prohormones *and specific hormones*
Hormone replacement therapy, (post)menopausal (=oestrogens), 432, 434–5, 451
beneficial effects, 435
unwanted effects, 435, 730
Hormone-responsive elements, 44
Hormone therapy, cancer, 698, 704–5
prostate, 437, 438, 705
Horn, *see* Dorsal horn; Ventral horn
Human chorionic gonadotrophin, 431, 438
Human immunodeficiency virus, *see* HIV
Humoral factors/control
airways/respiration, 340
coronary flow, 270
immune response, *see* Antibody
Hunt, Reid, 136
Huntingtin, 501
Huntington's disease, 497
defects/pathogenesis, 497, 498, 501
therapy, 501
Hydatid disease (echinococcosis), 687
therapy, 689
Hydralazine, 295
adverse effects, 295
clinical uses, 295
heart failure, 302
in hypertension, 295
Hydrocarbons, aromatic, receptor for, 110
Hydrochlorothiazide, 363
dose-response curves, 357
Hydrocortisone (cortisol), 411, 412
in asthma, 349
pharmacokinetics, 418
Hydrogen peroxide–thyroperoxidase complex, 421, 422
Hydrolytic reactions, 109
Hydromorphone, 580
Hydroxocobalamin, 335
administration and pharmacokinetics, 336
clinical use, 335
Hydroxyapatite, 452
Hydroxycarbamide, 704
6-Hydroxydopamine, 176, 178, 476, 478
amphetamine and effects of, 588
5-Hydroxyindoleacetic acid (5-HIAA), 185
behaviour and mood and, 537
Hydroxylation, ring, of tricyclic antidepressants, 544
3-Hydroxy-3-methylglutaryl-coenzyme A reductase inhibitors, *see* HMG-CoA reductase inhibitors
Hydroxyprogesterone, 434
11-β-Hydroxysteroid dehydrogenase, 419
5-Hydroxytryptamine (serotonin; 5-HT), 184–92, 480–2
anxiety and, 523
biosynthesis/degradation, 185, 480–1
in CNS, 184, 480–2
depression and, 536, 537
formation/storage/release, 480–1
function, 481–2
schizophrenia and, 527
distribution, 184–5, 481
effects/actions/role, 132, 185–6, 190–2, 481–2
migraine, 191–2
nociception, 186, 570, 572
in neurotransmission, 130
transporter proteins, 132
uptake inhibitors, *see* 5-Hydroxytryptamine (re)uptake inhibitors
5-Hydroxytryptamine receptor(s) (in general/unspecified), 186–90
antagonists, H_1-receptor antagonist as, 253
antipsychotic affinity for/action at, 482, 529, 532
classification/subtypes, 186–8
see also specific subtypes below
in CNS, 186, 188, 481
drugs (in general) acting on, 187
LSD action, 527, 592
5-Hydroxytryptamine receptor type-1, 186, 188
in CNS, 481
ergot alkaloid as antagonist and partial agonists of, 189–90

5-Hydroxytryptamine receptor type-1, *continued*
type-1A, 187, 188, 481
type-1A agonists, 187, 188, 523
as anxiolytics, 482, 517, 523
unwanted effects, 523
type-1A antagonists, 187
type-1B, 187, 481
agonists/antagonists, 187
type-1C ('so-called'), *see* 5-Hydroxytryptamine receptor type-2
type-1D, 187, 481
agonists, 186, 187, 188
agonists, in migraine, 192, 193, 482
antagonists, 187
partial agonist, in migraine, 192
5-Hydroxytryptamine receptor type-2 ($5HT_2$), 186–7, 188
antagonists (non-selective/unspecified), 188, 193
antidepressants as, 541
in carcinoid syndrome, 192
in migraine, 192, 193
in CNS, 482
partial agonists (non-selective/unspecified), 193
type-2A, 187
agonists/antagonists, 187
atypical antipsychotic affinity for, 527
genetic polymorphism, 534
type-2B, 187
agonists, 187
type-2C (old classification = $5HT_{1C}$), 186
agonists/antagonists, 187
5-Hydroxytryptamine receptor type-3 ($5\text{-}HT_3$), 187, 187–8, 188
agonists, 187
antagonists, 187
as antiemetics, 373, 375, 700, 707
as anxiolytics, 482, 524
in CNS, 481
5-Hydroxytryptamine receptor type-4 ($5\text{-}HT_4$), 187, 188
agonists, 187
as prokinetics, 188, 376
antagonists, 187
CNS, 481
5-Hydroxytryptamine receptor type-5 ($5\text{-}HT_5$), 187
5-Hydroxytryptamine receptor type-6 ($5\text{-}HT_6$), 187
5-Hydroxytryptamine receptor type-7 ($5\text{-}HT_7$), 187
agonists/antagonists, 187
5-Hydroxytryptamine/noradrenaline reuptake inhibitors
as antidepressants, 540
as anxiolytics, 524
as appetite suppressants, 402
5-Hydroxytryptamine (re)uptake inhibitors
non-selective, by tricyclic antidepressants, 540, 542
selective (SSRIs), 482, 540, 544–5
actions, 540
as anxiolytics, 524
as appetite suppressants, 402
in obesity, 402
pharmacokinetics, 540, 545
unwanted effects, 540, 545
selectivity of inhibition by various antidepressants, 543
5-Hydroxytryptophan metabolism, 185, 480
Hydroxyurea, 704
25-Hydroxyvitamin D_3, 450
Hymenolepis nana, 687
Hyoscine (scopolamine), 145, 147
clinical uses, 147
antiemetic, 373
learning/memory and effects of, 484
Hyperactivity (and attention deficit) disorder, 589
Hyperaldosteronism
primary (Conn's syndrome), 411, 418
secondary, 411
Hyperalgesia, 563, 563–4
Hyperbola, rectangular, occupancy–drug concentration relationship producing, 16
Hypercalcaemia, 451
management, 363, 451, 452
Hypercholesterolaemia, 309
familial, 311, 717
NO and, 215
Hyperforoin (in St John's Wort), 541, 547
Hyperglycaemia
adrenoceptor and β-blocker effects, 175
in diabetes, 385
rebound, with insulin, 388
glucocorticoid-induced, 417
Hyperkalaemia with ACE inhibitors, 297
Hyperlipidaemia/hyperlipoproteinaemia, *see* Dyslipidaemia
Hyperphosphataemia, 451
Hyperplasia, prostatic (prostatic hypertrophy), 173, 437
Hyperpyrexia/hyperthermia
malignant, *see* Malignant hyperthermia
MAO inhibitor–pethidine interaction causing, 547
with salicylates, 251
Hyper-reactivity/hyper-responsiveness, bronchial, in asthma, 342
see also Bronchoconstriction
Hypersensitivity (allergic) reactions, 228, 735–6
drugs causing, 735–6
antipsychotics, 532–3
heparin, 321
penicillins, 641, 735
type I (anaphylactic/immediate), *see* Anaphylactic reactions
type II (cytotoxic antibody-dependent), 228, 735, 736
type III (immune complex-mediated), 228, 735, 736
type IV (delayed-type/cell-mediated), 228, 735, 736
see also Allergy
Hypertension, 298–300
arterial, 298–300
antidepressants causing, 547
diabetes co-existing with, 386
drugs treating, *see* Antihypertensives
oral contraceptives and, 440
pathophysiology, 298–9
portal, 293
Hyperthermia, *see* Hyperpyrexia
Hyperthyroidism (thyrotoxicosis), 424, 425–7
drug-induced, 424
drug therapy in, 425–7
oral anticoagulant potentiation in, 322
signal transduction affected in, 718
Hypertrophic pyloric stenosis, 216
Hyperuricaemia (and gout), 254–5, 366
Hypnotics, *see* Anxiolytic agents
Hypnozoites, plasmodial, 673, 675
drugs acting against, 680
Hypoaldosteronism, heparin-induced, 321
Hypocalcaemia, 451
treatment, 453
Hypoglycaemia
with β-blockers, 175, 175–6
glucagon in, 385
with insulin, 385, 388
with sulfonylureas, 389–90
Hypoglycaemic agents, oral, 387, 388–92
clinical uses, 391
Hypokalaemia with loop diuretics, 363
Hypokinesia in Parkinson's disease, 497
levodopa effects, 500
Hypoperfusion, *see* Shock
Hypophosphataemia, 451
Hypotension
antipsychotic-induced, 529
levodopa-induced, 500
loop diuretics causing, 363
MAO inhibitors causing, 546
morphine-like drug-induced, 578
postural/orthostatic, *see* Postural hypotension
Hypothalamic—pituitary—adrenal axis function
glucocorticoid effects, 416
testing, *see* Dexamethasone suppression test
Hypothalamus
dopamine in, 476
in energy/weight/food intake regulation, 394, 395
glucocorticoids feedback effects, 416
hormones of (in pituitary regulation), 405, 406
Hypothermia, clearance in, 717
Hypothyroidism, 424–5, 427
oral anticoagulants affected in, 322
sensitivity to drugs altered in, 717
therapy, 427
Hypovolaemia, 302
ADH secretion in, 410
causes, 302
loop diuretics, 363

I

Ibresartan, 204
Ibuprofen, 245
Alzheimer's disease, 496
interactions, 719
Icatibant, 238, 239, 569
Idarubicin, 703
Idazoxan, 173
Idiosyncratic reactions, 89, 716–17
with antipsychotics, 532–3
Ifenprodil, 466
Ifosfamide, 699
IGFs, *see* Insulin-like growth factors
Imatinib, 44, 706, 708
Imidazoles, *see* Azoles; Benzimidazoles
Imidazoline receptor agonist, hypertension, 300
N-Iminoethlyl-L-lysine, 214
Imipenem, 642–3
Imipramine, 178, 181, 540, 548
analgesic effects, 583
chemical aspects/structure, 542
metabolism, 543
unwanted effects, 539
Immune complex-mediated (type III) hypersensitivity, 229, 735, 736
Immune responses/reactions, 218–27
to cancer, enhancement, 709
cell-mediated, 226–7
azathioprine suppressing, 258
drugs suppressing, *see* Immunosuppressant drugs
humoral, *see* Antibody
to inflammation, 218–27
innate/non-adaptive, 218, 218–22
mediators, *see* Mediators
to nematode infection, 688
specific/adaptive/acquired, 222–7
effector phase, 223–4, 224
induction phase, 223, 224–5
therapeutic manipulation, 241–2
unwanted, 228
to viral infection, 655–6
circumvention by virus, 656–7
HIV, 657–9
therapies aimed at, 663–4
see also Autoantibodies; Autoimmune disease
Immunisation, *see* Immunoglobulins; Vaccination
Immunogens, drugs as, 735
Immunoglobulins
receptor, soluble domain, clinical use, 206
therapeutic use (passive immunisation), 241
in antiviral therapy, 663
see also Antibody
Immunological mechanisms of drug allergy, 735–6
Immunomodulators (immunostimulants) in antiviral therapy, 663–4
see also Biological response modifiers; Immunotherapy
Immunophilins, 23, 258
Immunostimulants, *see* Immunomodulators
Immunosuppressant drugs, 257–60
actions/effects, 225, 257–9
glucocorticoids, 258, 416–17, 418
mechanisms, 225, 257–9
unwanted, 258, 259
clinical use, 257
autoimmune disease, 228
pharmacokinetics, 258, 259
Immunosuppression
ethanol-induced, 605
opioid-induced, 578
Immunotherapy
atopic disease, 241
cancer, 709
see also Biological response modifiers; Immunomodulators

Implants
of drugs, *see* Intramuscular injection; Subcutaneous implants
impregnated coatings, 105
Impotence, *see* Erection, dysfunction
in situ hybridisation, 200
Incontinence, urinary, 568
Indapamide, 363
Indinavir, 661
Individual variations in drug effects/responses (pharmacokinetic and pharmacodynamic variation), 712–23
genetic factors (=pharmacogenomics), 5, 714–15
NSAIDs, 250
Indometacin, 245
Alzheimer's disease, 496
interactions, 719
Induction
of anaesthesia
with inhalational anaesthetics, 507–8
with intravenous anaesthetics, 511–12
of enzymes, 109–10, 720
Infections, 620–92
in diabetes aetiology, 386
gene therapy, 744, 745
glucocorticoid-suppressed responses to, 317
in HIV disease, opportunistic, 659
see also specific (types of) infection
Infertility treatment, 437
Infiltration anaesthesia, 617
Inflammation, 217–41
airway, in asthma, 344–5
chronic, 229, 240
drugs suppressing, *see* Anti-inflammatory drugs
mediators, *see* Mediators
neurogenic, 240, 564
reaction/response, 217–28
acute, 217–28
outcome, 228–9
systemic, 227–8
unwanted, 228
Inflammatory bowel disease, 99, 377–8
Infliximab, 241, 256, 257
Influenza, 663
Informed consent, 86
Inhalation, administration by, 100
anaesthetics, *see* Anaesthetics, general
in asthma
β_2-agonists, 345–6
cromoglicate, 349
glucocorticoids, 348
muscarinic antagonists, 347
Inheritance, *see entries under* Genetic
Inhibitory postsynaptic potential in cholinergic transmission, slow, 142
Injected drugs, 100–1
Injury, glucocorticoid-suppressed responses to, 417
Ink family, 72
Innervation, *see* Nervous system
Inositol phosphates (phosphoinositides), 36–8, 39, 41
inositol (1,3,4,5)-tetraphosphate, 37–8
inositol (1,4,5)-trisphosphate, 37
receptors, 53, 54
smooth muscle contraction and, 64
intracellular calcium and, 37–8
lithium action and, 548
Inotropic effects
β-adrenoceptor agonists, 279
catecholamines, 170
Insomnia treatment, 519
see also Anxiolytic agents
Insulin, 200, 380–4, 386, 387–8
actions/effects, 282–4, 386
on food intake and body fat, 382, 395, 397
long/longer-term, 383–4, 384
mechanism, 384
unwanted, 385, 388
in brain, 200
pharmacokinetics, 387–8
preparations/formulations, 387–8
delayed/prolonged absorption, 101, 387, 388
quinine stimulating release, 678–9
resistance, 387
routes of administration, 387
synthesis/secretion, 380, 380–1
oral hypoglycaemics stimulating, 389, 390
Insulin-dependent (type 1/juvenile-onset) diabetes mellitus, 386–7
amylin agonist in, 385
Insulin-like growth factors (somatomedins), 407
bone remodelling and IGF-1, 448
Insulin glargine, 388
Insulin lispro, 387–8
Insulin receptor, 384
Insulin receptor substrate proteins, 384
Integrase, 630
Integrins, 73
Integrons and antibacterial resistance, 630
Intellect, *see* Cognition
Interactions, drug, 718–22
see also specific drugs
Interferons, 240–1, 663–4
clinical use, 241
antiviral, 664
cancer, 706
pharmacokinetics, 664
Interleukin(s)
in asthma, 342, 344
in immune response, 224
Interleukin-1, in immune/inflammatory response, 218–19
Interleukin-1 receptor, soluble, 260
Interleukin-1 receptor antagonist, recombinant, 260
Interleukin-2
in immune response, 224, 225
treatment affecting/aimed at, 257, 258
treatment using, cancer, 706
International normalised ratio (warfarin), 321
Interneurons, cholinergic, 483
Interstitial cell-stimulating hormone, 405, 435
Intestinal roundworms, 687
Intestine/bowel
cancer, aspirin reducing risk of, 250
drug absorption from, 98–9
5-HT in, 184
action, 185–6
inflammatory bowel disease, 99, 377–8
motility, *see* Motility
spasm, suppression, 148, 377
see also Gastrointestinal tract
Intracellular fluid compartment, 101, 102
Intracranial pressure, raised, osmotic diuretics with, 365
Intramuscular injection, 100
antipsychotics, 533
medroxyprogesterone, 441
Intraocular pressure, raised, *see* Glaucoma
Intrathecal injection, 101
Intrauterine device, levonorgestrol-impregnated, 441
Intravenous injection, 100
general anaesthetics, *see* Anaesthetics, general
regional anaesthesia, 617
Intrinsic factor, 333, 335
deficiency, 333
Introns, 203
Invasiveness, tumour, 695–6
Iodide, 426–7
oxidation, 421
plasma
concentration, thyroid function and, 422–3
thyroid follicle cell uptake, 421, 422
Iodination of thyroglobulin, 421, 422
Iodine, 426–7, 427
in hyperthyroidism, use, 426–7
radioactive, *see* Radioiodine
Ion(s), *see also* Anions; Cations; Electrolyte balance *and specific ions*
Ion channels, 23, 26–8, 29–32, 45–7, 55–62
anaesthetic effects, 504–5
blockers (of permeation), 24
examples, 24
glycine receptor, 472
NMDA receptor, 465, 466
non-depolarising neuromuscular blockers as, 150
as drug targets, 45–7
excitability and, 55–62
as G-protein targets, 38–9
gating, *see* Gating
ligand-gated (receptors linked to ion channels), *see* Ligand-gated ion channels
modulators, examples, 24
mutations, 62
in nociception/pain sensation, 567, 583
as drug targets, 583
pharmacology, 47
selectivity, 45
structure, 46–7
voltage-gated, *see* Voltage-gated ion channels
see also specific ion channels
Ion transport
epithelial, 66–8
in loop of Henle, 357
organic ions in kidney, 361
Ionisation of drugs, 92–3, 112
Ionotropic receptors, *see* Ligand-gated ion channels
IP (PGI_2) receptors, 234
Ipecacuanha, 373
Ipratropium, 100
clinical uses, 147, 347
asthma, 145, 148, 347
chronic obstructive pulmonary disease, 350
Iproniazid, 538, 545
unwanted effects, 546, 727
Ipsapirone, 523
Iralukast, 236
Iressa, 708
Irinotecan, 704
Iron, 331–3
chelation, 333
clinical uses, 332
deficiency, 331
anaemia of, therapy, 332
distribution, 331, 332
preparations/administration, 332–3
turnover/balance, 331–2
unwanted effects, 333
Iron-dextran, 333
Iron-sorbitol, 333
Irritant(s)/irritant substances
nociceptive nerve endings and, 567–8
tobacco smoke, 602
Irritant receptors, airway, 341
Ischaemia
Ca^{2+} antagonists preventing damage in, 283
cerebral/brain, 493–4
excitotoxicity and, 493–4
NO and, 488
see also Stroke
myocardial/heart, *see* Coronary artery disease; Myocardial ischaemia
Islet amyloid peptide, *see* Amylin
Islet cell, pancreatic, hormones secreted by, 380–4
Isocarboxazid, 541
Isoenzymes, P450 mono-oxygenase, 107–8
Isoflurane, 507, 510–11
adverse effects, 507, 511
Isoniazid (isonicotinic acid), 649–50, 715
pharmacokinetics, 650
genetic influences, 715
resistance (tuberculosis), 650
unwanted effects, 650, 715, 727
Isoprenaline (isoproterenol), 162, 179
propranolol and, competitive antagonism, 12
Isoproterenol, *see* Isoprenaline
Isorbide mononitrate, 280, 281
Isotretinoin, adverse cardiovascular effects, 309
Ispaghula husk, 375
Itching and histamine, 230
Itraconazole, 668, 669
mechanism of action, 628
unwanted effects, 669
IUD, levonorgestrel-impregnated, 441
Ivermectin, 691
see also Avermectins

J

Jacksonian epilepsy, 551
Jak, 44
Jaundice with antipsychotics, 532

Juxtaglomerular apparatus (incl. nephron), 352–3
aldosterone secretion and, 358
loop of Henle in, 355

K

Kainate
epileptogenicity, 553
neurotoxicity, 491
receptors, 463, 465, 466
agonists/antagonists, 465
functional role, 466–7
Kala azar, 683
Kallidin, 238
nociception and, 569
Kallikrein, 238
Kanamycin, 651
Kaolin, 377
κ-opioid receptors, 574
antagonists, 204
opioid drug and peptide selectivity for, 575
role, 574, 575
Kernicterus, 714, 719
Ketamine, 469, 512, 513–14, 592
adverse effects, 512, 514, 527
analgesic action, 583
NMDA receptors and, 466, 469
Ketanserin, 188
Ketoacidosis, diabetic, 385
Ketoconazole, 668, 668–9
steroidogenesis and, 413
terfenadine and, avoidance, 720
unwanted effects, 668–9
Ketolides, 652
Ketotifen, 188
Kidney, 352–66
ADH/vasopressin actions, 358, 410
ANP role, 272
drugs (in general) acting on, 362–5
sites of action, 355, 356, 357, 358
excretion via, 111–17
age effects, 713–14
drugs affecting, 362–5, 721–2
drugs and metabolites, 111–17
of organic molecules, *see* Organic molecules
failure
acute, osmotic diuretics in prevention of, 365
chronic, osteodystrophy of, 452
function, 252–62
structure, 352–62
toxicity, 728–9
ACE inhibitors, 297, 729
aminoglycosides, 645
amphotericin, 668
ciclosporin, 258, 729
cytotoxic drugs, 698
lithium, 549
NSAIDs, 249–50, 728–9
xanthine actions, 346
Kinases, *see* Cyclin-dependent kinases; Protein kinases
Kindling model (epilepsy), 552–3, 553
Kinin(s), 65, 220, 238–9, 569
nociception and, 569, 570–1
Kininases, 239
Knock-ins and knock-outs, 85, 200
Kuru, 501
Kynurenic acid, 469

L

L-dopa, *see* Levodopa
L-NAME, 214
L-NMMA, *see* N^G-Monomethyl-L-arginine
L-type Ca^{2+} channels
cardiac function and, 264
dihydropyridines blocking, 23, 52
L1 (deferiprone), 333
Labetalol, 173, 181
Labour
induction and augmentation, 235, 443
preterm, delay, 443
third stage management, 443
Lacrimation
muscarinic agonist effects, 144
muscarinic antagonist effects, 146
Lactacystin, 685
β-Lactam antibiotics and ß-lactamases, *see under* Beta
Lactation, 408
with antipsychotics, 532
oxytocin effects, 441
prolactin and, 408, 431
Lactulose, 375, 375–6
Lamivudine, 660–1
Lamotrigine, 558, 559
mechanism of action, 553, 558
unwanted effects, 558
Langerhans, islets of, hormones secreted by, 380–4
Lansoprazole, 370
Larva migrans, *see Ankylostoma*; Toxocariasis
Latanoprost, 146, 235
glaucoma, 146
Law, cannabis use, 610
Law of mass action, 15
Laxatives, 375–6
LD_{50}, 89
Lead (metal), fetal toxicity, 734
Lead compounds
finding, 748–9
optimisation, 749
Learning, cholinergic pathways and, 484
see also Memory
Leflunomide, 257
Legislation, cannabis, 610
Leishmaniasis, 672, 683–4
Lemakalim, 294
Lennox–Gastaut syndrome, 552
Lenograstim, fungal infections, 670
Leprosy, 651–2
Leptazol (pentylenetetrazole), 552, 585, 586, 587
Leptin, 170, 395
function/role, 395, 396, 398
in obesity
pathophysiology, 399
therapeutic use (pegylated leptin), 402
receptors, 395, 399, 400
Lethal dose (LD_{50}), 89
Leucocytes (white blood cells)
glucocorticoid effects, 416
in inflammation, 219
see also specific types of leucocytes
Leucopenia with antipsychotics, 533
Leukaemias
monoclonal antibody therapy, 44, 706
tretinoin, 706
Leukotriene(s), 231, 235–6
actions, 235–6
cysteinyl, *see* Cysteinyl leukotrienes
metabolism, 235
synthesis, 233, 235–6
Leukotriene receptors, 236
antagonists, 236–7
actions, 347
clinical use, 236, 347–8
pharmacokinetics, 347
unwanted effects, 347
Leuprorelin, 437
Levamisole, 690–1
anthelminthic action, 628, 690–1
unwanted effects, 691
Levobupivacaine, 616
Levodopa (L-dopa), 104, 499–500
intestinal absorption, 98
in parkinsonism, 499, 499–500
therapeutic effectiveness, 499
unwanted effects, 480, 499–500
Levofloxacin, 647
Levonorgestrel
in combined pill, 439
intrauterine device impregnated with, 441
postcoital, 441
subcutaneous implants, 441
Lewy bodies and Parkinson's disease 498–9
Lexipafant, 238
Leydig cells, 435
Lidocaine (lignocaine), 276, 615
adverse effects, 276, 615
pharmacokinetics, 616
use, 625
dysrhythmias, 274, 275, 276
neuropathic pain, 583
Ligand, 8
specificity of binding to target, *see* Specificity
Ligand-gated ion channels (ionotropic receptors; receptor-operated channels), 23, 26–8, 29–32
Ca^{2+} channels, 52–3
examples, 27
gating, 30–1, 46, 47
glutamate receptors as, 473
structure, 27, 28, 29–30
Lignocaine, *see* Lidocaine
Limbic/mesolimbic system
dopamine and, 476, 596, 600
reward and, 596
Lincosamides, 646–7
Linezolid, 647
Linitript, 402
Liothyronine, 427
Lipase
glucocorticoids and, 416
lipoprotein, fibrate effects, 311
pancreatic, inhibition, 401
Lipid (fat)
diffusion through, 92, 92–4
metabolism
cAMP in regulation of, 36, 37
drug toxicity involving peroxidation, 726
ethanol effects, 604–5
insulin effects, 382
solubility in, 92
anaesthetics, 504, 507
see also Lipophilic drugs
Lipid-lowering drugs (drugs affecting lipoprotein metabolism), 309–13
site of action, 308
Lipid mediators, *see* Eicosanoids
Lipocortin, 231, 415
Lipolysis, agents enhancing, 402
Lipophilic drugs, metabolism, 106
Lipoplexes as gene vectors, 741
Lipopolysaccharide (LPS; endotoxin), 218, 635–7
macrophages binding, 221
thrombosis and, 317
Lipoprotein
drugs affecting metabolism of, *see* Lipid-lowering drugs
high blood levels, *see* Dyslipidaemia
transport in blood, 307–9
Lipoprotein lipase, fibrate effects, 311
Lipoprotein(a), 308, 327
Liposomes
drugs in, 105
as gene vectors, variants of, 741
Lipoxins, 231, 236
Lipoxygenase(s), 231
5-lipoxygenase, 235–7
inhibitors, 237
products, 235–7
5-Lipoxygenase-activating protein (FLAP), 235
Lisinopril, 296
Lisuride, 500
Lithium, 548, 548–9
actions/effects, 37, 548–9
mechanism, 548–9
unwanted/toxic/side-effects, 359, 549, 722
interactions, 722
pharmacokinetics, 548–9
Liver
blood flow, drug interactions and, 721
cancer, oral contraceptives and, 440
disease, oral anticoagulants affected, 322
metabolism in
of drugs, age affecting, 714
insulin effects, 382
see also P450 mono-oxygenase system
toxicity, 727
allergic mechanisms, 736
chloroform, 509
ethanol, 604

fluconazole, 668
halothane, 111, 510, 727, 736
ketoconazole, 667
MAO inhibitors, 546
paracetamol, 111, 252, 727–8
thiazolidinediones/glitazones, 390, 391
valproate, 558
see also Enterohepatic circulation
Loa loa, 687
therapy, 689, 690
Loading dose, 115
Lobeline, 147, 149
Local anaesthetics, *see* Anaesthetics, local
Locomotor system, *see* Motor system
Locus ceruleus, noradrenergic pathways in, 475, 566
opioid dependency and, 579
Loewi, Otto, 122–3
Lomustine, 700
Long Q–T interval, *see* Q–T prolongation
Long-term depression, 467, 468
NO and, 487–8
Long-term potentiation, 467, 468, 469
NO and, 447–8
Loop diuretics, 362–3, 365
actions/effects, 360, 362–3
on potassium balance, 360
sites/mechanisms, 356, 357
unwanted, 363
clinical uses, 363
pharmacokinetics, 362–3
Loop of Henle, 352, 355–6, 359
ascending limb, 356
descending limb, 355
Loperamide, 572
as anti-motility agent, 377
Loratidine, 253
in asthma, 348
Lorazepam, 517
as antiemetic, 707
pharmacokinetics, 520
Lormetazepam, 517
Losartan, 204, 297, 297–8
Lovastatin, 310
Low-density lipoprotein
atherogenesis and, 307, 309
receptors, pravastatin increasing synthesis, 310
transport/metabolism, 307, 308
Low-density lipoprotein-cholesterol, drugs decreasing plasma levels, *see* Lipid-lowering drugs
LQT channels, 61
LSD, *see* Lysergic acid diethylamide
Lumefantrine, 682
Lungs
chronic obstructive disease, *see* Chronic obstructive pulmonary disease
smoking adversely affecting, 601
see also Airway; Respiratory system
Lupus-like syndrome, 736
Luteinising hormone, 405, 438
in females
actions, 430, 431
progestogens (in combined pill) inhibiting release, 439
secretion, 430
GnRH in regulation of release, 437
in males (ICSH), 405, 435
LY333531, 392
Lymphocytes, 221, 222–3
β-agonist effects, 171
see also B-cell; Natural killer cells; T-cell
Lymphoma, therapy, 242, 706, 745
Lysergic acid, derivatives, 189
Lysergic acid diethylamide (LSD), 188, 586, 591–2
actions, 591–2
at 5-HT receptors, 527, 592
adverse effects, 592
Lyso-PAF, 231, 237

M

M receptors, *see* Muscarinic ACh receptors
McNA343, 138
Macrolides, 646, 647
new derivatives, 642
resistance, 646
mechanisms, 532
S. aureus, 632
Macrophage(s), 221, 226–7
atherogenesis and, 307
glucocorticoid effects, 416
in immune/inflammatory response, 221, 225
activation by Th1 cells, 226–7
leukotriene effects, 236
Macrovascular disease in diabetes, 386
Macula densa cells, 354, 358
Magnesium (ions)
loop diuretics and, 362, 363
NMDA receptors and, 466, 468
Magnesium aluminium silicate, 377
Magnesium hydroxide
as antacid, 371
as laxative, 375
Magnesium sulfate as laxative, 375
Magnesium trisilicate, 371
Magnocellular forebrain nuclei, cholinergic pathways, 483
Major histocompatibility complex (MHC; HLA in humans)
NK cells and, 222
peptide/antigen association with, 226
Malaria, 673–82
drugs in, *see* Antimalarial agents
epidemiology, 673, 674
new therapeutic approaches, 685
parasite, *see Plasmodium*
quartan, 676
tertian
benign, 676
malignant, 675–6
transmission, prevention, 680
vaccine, 685
Males
contraceptive drugs, 441
ethanol-induced feminisation, 604
neurohormonal control of reproductive system, 435–6
Malignant hyperthermia, 54, 154, 717
halothane-induced, 154, 510
Malignant tumours, *see* Cancer
Malnutrition, alcoholics, 604
see also Nutrient deficiency
Mammary gland, *see* Breast; Lactation
Mania, 535
depression and, *see* Bipolar affective disorder
Mannitol, 364
MAP (mitogen-activated protein) kinase, 42, 69
Maprotiline, 540
Marijuana, *see* Cannabis
Marimstat, 78
Marine triglycerides, 313
Marketing, phase IV studies after, 750
Mast cells, 220, 226
antibodies and, 226
histamine release, 229
opioid-induced, 577–8
histamine storage, 229
Matrix, extracellular, growth factors and cell interactions with, 73–4
Matrix metalloproteinases, 74
inhibitors
endogenous (TIMPs), 74
exogenous, therapeutic uses, 78, 708
Maximum tolerated dose, 89
Mazindol, 402
MCP-1, 241, 657
MDMA, *see* Methylenedioxymethamphetamine
Measurement in pharmacology, 80–90
toxicity, *see* Adverse reactions
see also Bioassay *and specific tests*
Mebendazole, 688
Mebeverine, 377
Mecamylamine, 483, 599
animal studies of nicotine dependence, 600–1
use, 603
Meclizine, 373
Medial forebrain bundle
dopaminergic pathways, 476
noradrenergic neurons, 475
Median eminence and dopaminergic neurons, 476
Mediators, chemical (peripheral), 64–6, 121–261
in asthma, 342–4, 345
in CNS, 457–8, 458, 462–89
exhaustion, desensitisation associated with, 20–1
of inflammation/immune response, 229–41, 564
bradykinin, 239
cell-derived, 222
eicosanoids, 234–5, 236–7
in healing/repair/chronic inflammation, 229
PAF, 237–8
plasma-derived, 219–20
substance P, 564, 571
in nervous system, *see* Neuromodulators; Neurotransmitters
in nociception, *see* Nociception
release, 64–6
vascular (incl. endothelial derived mediators), 286–92
in coronary flow control, 270
platelet-activating, 323
in shock, 302
in shock, antagonists of, 303
see also specific (types of) mediators
Medroxyprogesterone, 434
in cancer, 705
intramuscular, 441
Medulla
brainstem (medulla oblongata)
anaesthesia-induced paralysis, 505
area postrema/chemoreceptor trigger zone, vomiting and, 188, 372–3
renal, counter-current mechanisms, 352, 356, 359–60
Mefenamic acid, 245
unwanted effects, 249
Mefloquine, 676, 679, 682
pharmacokinetics, 679
resistance, 679
unwanted effects, 679
Megaloblastic haemopoiesis and anaemia, 333
treatment, 335
Megazol, 684
Megestrol, 705
Meglumine antimonate, 683
Meissner's plexus, 367
Melanocortins (melanocyte-stimulating hormone), 405, 409–10
Melanocyte-stimulating hormone, 405, 409–10
Melanocyte-stimulating hormone release-inhibiting factor, 405
Melanocyte-stimulating hormone releasing factor, 405
Melarsoprol, 684
Melatonin, 485–6
receptors, 485–6
use, 87, 485
Meloxicam, 245
Melphalan, 699
Memantine, 469
Membranes, cell (bacterial)
antibiotics with difficulties in penetrating, 637
outer membrane, *see* Outer membrane
plasma membrane, 621
drugs acting on, 627–8
Membranes, cell (human)
electrically excitable, *see* Excitation
fluidity, anaesthesia and, 504
transport/movement across, 91–5, 133
Memory
cholinergic pathways and, 484
loss, *see* Amnesia
Memory cells, 224
Men, *see* Males
Menadiol sodium diphosphate, 319
Menopause, HRT, *see* Hormone replacement therapy
Menorrhagia, 442
Menstrual cycle, 430–1
disorders, prostaglandin role, 442
Mental illness, *see* Psychotropic drugs *and specific mental disorders*
Mephenesin, 561
Meprobamate, 517, 559
Meptazinol, 582

Mepyramine, 230, 253
  interactions, 719
Mequitazine, 253
Mercaptopurine, 623, 715
  azathioprine metabolised to, 111, 258
  in cancer chemotherapy, 702
    mechanism of action, 623
  interactions, 254, 721
Mercury, fetal toxicity, 734
Merozoite, plasmodial, 673, 675
Mesalazine (5-aminosalicylic acid), 99, 378
Mescaline, 586, 591–2
Mesocortical pathways and dopamine, 476
Mesolimbic system, *see* Limbic system
Meta-analysis, 88
Metabolic acidosis with salicylates, 251
Metabolic alkalosis with loop diuretics, 363
Metabolism (bacterial), drugs affecting, 622–9, 637–52
Metabolism (humans)
  catecholamine and adrenoceptor agonist effects, 170–1
  degradative, *see* Degradative metabolism
  in diabetes, deranged, 385–6
  of drugs, 106–11, 715–16
    age affecting, 714
    degradative, *see* Degradative metabolism
    drugs inhibiting, 322
    and elimination in two-compartment pharmacokinetic model, 117
    ethanol effects, 606
    first-pass, 110
    genetic influences, 715–16
    phase I/II, 107, 107–9
    plasma concentration and variations in rate of, 118
    stereospecific inhibition of, 107, 721
    see also specific drugs
  glucocorticoid effects, 413, 415–17
    unwanted, 417
  growth hormone effects, 407
  insulin effects, 382–3
  oestrogen effects, 432
  salicylate effects, 251
  thyroid hormone effects, 423
Metabolites
  active and/or toxic, drugs producing, 111
    see also Pro-drugs
  renal excretion, 111–17
  see also Antimetabolites *and specific metabolites*
Metabotropic receptors, *see* G-protein-coupled receptors
Metal(s), heavy, teratogenicity, 734
Metalloproteinases, *see* Matrix metalloproteinases
Metaphase, 72
Metastases, 696
Metformin, 388, 391
Methacholine, 143, 144
Methadone (and methadone series of morphine-like drugs), 573–4, 575, 580, 581–2
Methaemoglobin formation with organic nitrates, 281
Methamphetamine, 587
Methanol metabolism/toxicity, 607
Methaqualone, 517
Methicillin, 631
  nephrotoxicity, 728
Methicillin-resistant staphylococci, 631, 632–3, 636
Methimazole, 425
  carbimazole conversion to, 425–6
  pharmacokinetics, 426
Methionine
  in paracetamol poisoning, 252, 728
  synthesis
    from homocysteine, 335–6
    nitrous oxide inhibiting, 510
Methiothepin, 188
Methotrexate, 701
  in cancer, 623
    in combination regimes, 707
  intrathecal, 101
  mechanism of action, 701, 702
  receptor/binding, 8
  resistance, 701
  rheumatoid disease, 256
  salicylates interactions, 720
  unwanted effects, 701, 727
Methoxamine, 179
Methoxsalen, 731
Methoxyflurane, 509, 510, 511
3-Methoxy-4-hydroxy-mandelic (VMA) acid synthesis/secretion, 168
3-Methoxy-4-hydroxyphenylglycol (MHPG) and depression, 537
15-Methyl$PGF_{2\alpha}$ (carboprost), 442, 443
β-Methylamino-alanine, 491
N-Methyl-D-aspartate receptors, *see* NMDA receptors
Methylation reactions, 109
Methylcellulose, 375, 377
Methylcobalamin, 335
Methyldopa, 176, 178, 181, 475
  haemolysis caused by, 735–6
  in hypertension, 300
Methylenedioxymethamphetamine ('ecstasy'; MDMA), 587
  harmful effects, 589
(R)-α-Methylhistamine, 230
Methylmalonyl-CoA isomerisation to succinyl-CoA, 336
3-Methylmorphine, *see* Codeine
Methylphenidate, 177, 587
  in attention deficit/hyperactivity disorder, 589
1-Methyl-4-phenyl-1,2,3,6-tetrahydropyridine (MPTP), 497–8
Methylprednisolone, 412
  actions/effects, 412
    antiemetic, 375
Methyltetrahydrofolate, 334
  conversion to tetrahydrofolate, 335–6
α-Methyltyrosine, 164, 176, 178, 181
  amphetamine and effects of, 588
Methylxanthines, *see* Xanthines
Methysergide, 188, 189, 193, 482
  in carcinoid syndrome, 192
  in migraine, 190, 192, 193
  unwanted effects, 189, 190, 193
Metoclopramide actions
  antiemetic, 374, 480
    in cancer chemotherapy, 707
  prokinetic, 98, 188, 376
Metolazone, 363
Metoprolol, 180, 276
  in heart failure, 302
Metronidazole, 683
  alcohol interactions, 721
  in amoebiasis, 683
  in bacterial infections, 649
    H. pylori eradication, 371
  in leishmaniasis, 683
  pharmacokinetics, 683
  in trichomoniasis, 684
  unwanted effects, 683
Metyrapone, 413
Mexiletine, 615
MHC, *see* Major histocompatibility complex
Mibefradil, 282
  angina, 282
Micafungin, 670
Miconazole, 668, 669
Microangiopathy, diabetic, 386
Microsomal enzymes
  age-related differences, 714
  ethanol metabolism, 606
  see also P450 mono-oxygenase system
Microspheres, 104
  as gene vectors, 741, 742
Microtubules as drug targets, 628
  anticancer drugs, 704
  helminths, 628, 688
Microvascular disease in diabetes, 386
Midazolam, 512, 514, 517
  in anaesthesia, 512
  pharmacokinetics, 520
  unwanted effects, 512
Mifepristone, 235
  misoprostol combined with, as abortifacient, 442–3
Migraine, 190–2
  drug management, 191–2, 193
    acute attack, 193
    ergot alkaloids, 190
    prophylactic, 193
    sumatriptan, 192, 193, 482
  pathophysiology, 190–1
Milk production, *see* Lactation
Milrinone, 279, 295
Miltefosine, 683
Mineral(s), bone, turnover, 448–9
Mineralocorticoids, 418–19
  actions/effects of, 418–19
    mechanism, 418–19
  clinical use, 419
  synthesis/release, 418
    deficient (Addison's disease), 411, 418
    excess (Conn's syndrome), 411, 418
  see also Adrenal steroids
Minimal alveolar concentration (MAC), anaesthetics, 504
Minimum effective dose, 89
Minocycline, 643, 647
  pharmacokinetics, 644
  spectrum of activity, 643
  unwanted effects, 644
Minoxidil, 294
Mirtazapine, 539, 541, 547
Misoprostol, 442
  uses
    as abortifacient (combined with mifepristone), 441–2
    gastrointestinal, 249, 372
Mitochondria
  apoptosis and, 76
  proteins uncoupling oxidative phosphorylation, 397
Mitogen-activated protein (MAP) kinase, 42, 69
Mitomycin, 627, 703
  mechanisms of action, 627, 703
  toxicity, 703
Mitosis, 72
Mitotane, 705
Mitoxantrone (mitozantrone), 703
Mivacurium, 151
Mixed function oxygenase/oxidase system and ethanol, 606
  see also P450 mono-oxygenase
MK801, *see* Dizocilpine
Moclobemide, 541, 546
Models, experimental/animal, 84–5
  Alzheimer's disease, 495, 496
  anxiety, 516
  depression, 538
  drug dependence, 596
  epilepsy, 552–3
  nicotine dependence, 600–1
  obesity, 395
  Parkinson's disease, 478
  see also Transgenic animals
Molecular techniques
  neuropeptides, 199–200
  receptor proteins, 26
  see also DNA technology
Molgramostim, 336, 338
  in cancer chemotherapy, 707
  in fungal infections, 670
Monoamine(s), in CNS, 474, 476–82, 485
  in depression pathogenesis, 536–8
  receptors, chronic antidepressant treatment downregulating, 539
  uptake, antidepressants inhibiting, 538, 539–45
    measurement, 538
Monoamine oxidase, 109, 545–6
  5-HT deamination by, 185
  MAO-A and MAO-B, 545–6
  MPTP metabolism by, 497
  role, 546
    catecholamine/monoamine degradation by, 167, 476
Monoamine oxidase inhibitors (MAOIs), 178, 538, 541, 545–6
  actions/effects, 541
    measurement, 538
    mechanisms, 546
    unwanted/toxic, 541, 546–7
  chemical aspects, 546
  clinical use
    depression, 546

Parkinson's disease, 498, 500
interactions with other drugs/foods, 546–7, 718–19
pharmacokinetics, 541
SSRIs combined with, unwanted effects of, 545
tricyclic antidepressants combined with, unwanted effects of, 547
Monobactams, 631, 642, 643
unwanted effects, 643
Monoclonal antibodies (therapeutic use), 241–2
as antiplatelet drugs, 241, 325
in cancer therapy, 44, 706, 708
labelled, 708
as immunosuppressants, 257, 259–60
to respiratory syncytial virus, 242, 664
in rheumatoid disease, 241, 242, 256–7
see also Antibody
Monocyte, 221
Monocyte chemoattractant protein-1 (MCP-1), 241, 659
N^G-Monomethyl-L-arginine (L-NMMA), 214
in diabetes, vasoconstrictor responses to, 216
therapeutic use, 214
Mononuclear cells
in acute inflammation, 221
in chronic inflammation, 229
Mono-oxygenases, *see* Mixed function oxygenase; P450 mono-oxygenase system
Monoxidine, 300
Montelukast, 236, 347
Mood
alterations/disturbances, *see* Affective disorders
5-HT and, 482
noradrenaline and, 475
Mood-stabilising drugs, 548–9, 556
Morphine
actions/effects, 575–8
anti-motility, 377, 577
mechanisms/sites, 566, 575–6
unwanted, 580, 581
analogues, 572
assay of analgesic action, 84
dependence, 578–9, 597
pharmacokinetics, 579–81
partitioning into body fat, 96
structure, 572
tolerance, 578–9, 597
uses, 580
biliary spasm, 378
Morphine-like drugs (narcotics; opiates; synthetic opioids), 572–84
abuse, 595
actions/effects, 575–8
mechanisms, 566, 575–6
unwanted, 580, 581
chemical aspects/structures, 572, 573
clinical uses, 580
anti-motility, 376, 377, 577
antitussive, 350, 577
biliary spasm, 378
diarrhoea, 377
dependence, 578–9, 597
pharmacokinetics, 579–81, 580
synthetic, 572, 573–4
tolerance, 578, 578–9, 597
Mosquito bite prevention, 676
Motility
gastrointestinal, 375–7
absorption affected by, 98
drugs decreasing, *see* Antimotility agents
drugs increasing, *see* Prokinetic agents
5-HT increasing, 185–6
uterine, 441
Motion sickness, 148, 373
treatment, 148, 373
Motor nerve fibres
ACh release, 126
endplate, *see* Neuromuscular junction
Motor neuron disease, progressive form, 493
Motor (locomotor) system
dopamine and, 476
drugs affecting
amphetamines, 478–9, 587–8
antipsychotics, 477, 478, 529, 531–2
ethanol, 603–4
extrapyramidal, *see* Extrapyramidal motor system
see also Dyskinesia; Hypokinesia; Movement disorders
Mouth, drugs taken by, *see* Oral administration
Movement disorders
in Huntington's disease, 501
in Parkinson's disease, 497
drug-induced, 499–500
Moxifloxacillin, 652
Moxonidine, 300
MPTP (1-Methyl-4-phenyl-1,2,3,6-tetrahydropyridine), 497–8
μ-opioid receptors, 574
opioid drug and peptide selectivity for, 575
role, 574, 575
Mucosa, gastrointestinal
damage
ethanol, 604
NSAIDs/cyclo-oxygenase inhibitors, 248–9, 370
protection
drugs enhancing, 372
endogenous mechanisms, 368
Mucus, gastric secretion, 368, 369
Multidrug regimens (combination therapy)
cytotoxic drugs, 707
leprosy, 651
tuberculosis, 649
Multidrug resistance
in cancer, 95, 707
reversal, 709
in malaria, 677
Multiple sclerosis, cannabis, 561
Muscarine, 122, 136, 144
Muscarinic ACh receptor(s), 34
ACh actions, 136–7
airway, 340–1
autonomic nervous system effects related to types of, 127
distribution, 127
brain, 483
M_1 (neural), 138, 340–1
M_2 (cardiac-type), 138, 139, 140, 273, 341
gastric acid secretion and, 369
M_3, 138, 139, 341
M_4, 138, 139
M_5, 138, 139
Muscarinic ACh receptor agonists (parasympathomimetics), 138, 139, 143–5, 148
clinical use, 145
effects, 144–5
structure–activity relationships, 143–5
Muscarinic ACh receptor antagonists (anticholinergics; antimuscarinics; parasympatholytics), 139, 145–7, 148
actions/effects, 146–7
antidepressants as, 542
antipsychotics as, 529, 532
clinical uses, 147, 148, 347
antiemetic, 373, 375
antimotility, 376–7
antispasmodic, 377
asthma, 347
Parkinson's disease, 148, 499, 500
H_1-receptor antagonists as, 254
Muscimol, 471
Muscle
anthelmintic site of action, 629
contraction, *see* Contraction
insulin effects, 382
relaxants
centrally acting, 560–1
in general anaesthesia, 506
peripherally acting, *see* Neuromuscular junction
smooth, *see* Smooth muscle
spasm, *see* Spasm
striated
cardiac, *see* Heart muscle
skeletal, *see* Skeletal muscle
tone, *see* Tone
see also Intramuscular injection, *entries under* Myo- *and specific muscles*
Muscle-type nicotinic ACh receptors, 137, 138
Mutagenesis, 729–30
biochemical mechanisms, 729
conditional, 86
site-directed, *see* Site-directed mutagenesis
teratogenesis and, overlap, 731
tests for mutagenicity, 730–1
Mutations
antibiotic resistance, 629, 632
frame-shift, agents inducing, 625, 628
individual variations in response and, 715
ion channel, 62
knock-in/knock-out, 85, 200
receptors, and disease, 48
single gene, disorders due to, 743
Myasthenia gravis, 48, 159–60, 717
anticholinesterases in, 159–60
Mycobacterial infections, 649–52
Mycophenolate mofetil, 258–9
Mycoses, *see* Fungal infections
Mydriatics (pupillary dilators), 146, 148
Myeloid leukaemia, chronic, monoclonal antibody therapy, 44, 706
Myelosuppression/bone marrow depression
anaemia caused by, 330
anticancer agents, 697, 707
chloramphenicol, 645
Myenteric plexus, 367
Myocardial cells, *see* Myocytes
Myocardial contraction, *see* Contraction
Myocardial infarction/damage (heart attack), 271–2
action potential with, 268
dysrhythmias following, 265, 267
oral contraceptives and, 440
prophylaxis, 271
secondary, 311
therapy, 271–2
antiplatelet agents, 324, 325, 326
streptokinase, 325
trials, 88, 88–9
Myocardial ischaemia
effects, 271
pain of, *see* Angina
preconditioning effect, 269
Myocardial oxygen availability and consumption, 269, 270–2
Myocardial 'stunning', 269
Myocardial viability, 269
Myoclonic seizures, therapy, 556
Myocytes, cardiac
action potential, *see* Action potential, cardiac
death in myocardial infarction, 271
drugs directly affecting, 272
Myometrium in pregnancy, 441
see also Uterus
Myosin, 62
myocardial, 269
Myosin light chain, 64
Myosin light chain kinase, 64
Myosin phosphatase, 64
Myositis, fibrate-induced, 311
Myxoedema, 424

N

N-demethylation of tricyclic antidepressants, 544
N-type Ca^{2+} channels, 52
Nabilone, 609
antiemetic effects, 375
Nabumetone, 245
NAD and ethanol, 606
Nafarelin, 437
Naftifine, 670
Nalidixic acid, 627, 648
Nalorphine, 575, 582
Naloxone, 204, 575, 581, 582–3
cannabinoid antagonism, 375
clinical use, 582
mechanisms of action, 566
Naltrexone, 204, 575, 583
in alcohol withdrawal, 608
Nandrolone, 437
Naproxen, 245
Narcolepsy, 589
Narcotics/narcotic analgesics, *see* Morphine-like drugs

Nasal decongestion, 172
Nasal sprays, 100
Nateglinide, 390
Natriuretic drugs, *see* Diuretics
Natriuretic peptides, 272, 295, 359
 atrial, *see* Atrial natriuretic peptide
 C-, 286
 cardiac, 272
 clinical use, 295
 renal actions, 359
Natural killer cells, 222, 223
 in adaptive immune response, 223
 in inflammatory response, 222, 223
 in innate immune response, 222
 in viral infection, 656
  evasion, 656, 657
Nausea, *see* Antiemetic drugs; Vomiting and nausea
Necator americanus, 687
 therapy, 689
Necrosis, 490
 in myocardial infarction, 271
 toxic reactions causing, 725
  renal papillary necrosis, 728
Nedocromil sodium, 349
Nelfinavir, 661
Nematodes, *see* Roundworms
Neomycin, 645
Neonates/newborns
 chloramphenicol cautions, 645
 metabolism of drugs in, 714
 opioid cautions, 579
 premature, kernicterus, 714, 719
 renal excretion/function in, 713
Neoplasms, *see* Cancer; Tumours
Neostigmine, 23, 156, 157
 clinical uses, 159, 160
Nephritis, interstitial, 728
Nephrogenic diabetes insipidus, X-linked, 717
Nephrons, 352–62
 drugs acting on, 362–5
  directly, 362–4
  indirectly, 364–5
  site of action, 355
 structure/function, 352–62
Nephropathy, analgesic, 728–9
Nephrotic syndrome, effects on drugs of, 717
Nephrotoxicity, *see* Kidney
Nerve
 conduction block by local anaesthetics, 614
 local blockade, 615, 617
 terminals/endings
  adrenoceptors at, 170
  5-HT action on, 186
  nociceptive, chemosensitivity, 567–70
  noradrenergic, drugs acting on, 176–82
  presynaptic, *see* Presynaptic terminals
  see also Neurotransmission; Synapse
 see also Axon reflex; Neuron
Nerve growth factor
 in Alzheimer's disease treatment, 497
 apoptosis prevention, 491
 nociception and, 564
Nervi erigentes, 125
Nervous system
 anaesthetic effects, 505–6
 in gastrointestinal tract, 367
 NO role, 212
 pain sensation, 562–72
 peptides in, *see* Peptides
 plasticity, *see* Neuroplasticity; Synapse, plasticity
 in reproductive system control, *see* Reproductive system
 see also Autonomic nervous system; Central nervous system; Enteric nervous system; Neuroendocrine system; Peripheral nervous system
Netilmicin, 645
Neural muscarinic (M_1) receptors, 138, 340–1
Neural transplantation in Parkinson's disease treatment, 500–1
Neurodegeneration and neurodegenerative disorders, 490–502
 cholinergic neurons and, 484
 inhibitors of neurodegeneration, 496–7
 mechanisms, 459, 490–3
 NO and, 488
 seizures and, 553
 smoking, protective effects, 602
Neurodevelopmental disorder, alcohol-related, 605
Neuroendocrine mediators, 199
Neuroendocrine system
 monoamine pathways and
  depression and, 537–8
  dopaminergic pathways, 480
 reproductive system and, *see* Reproductive system, neurohormonal control
Neurofibrillary tangles, 494, 495
Neurogenic disorder, migraine as, 191
Neurogenic inflammation, 240, 564
Neurohormonal regulation, *see* Neuroendocrine system
Neurohypophysis (posterior pituitary), 410–11
Neurokinin A, 341, 570–1
 biosynthesis, and gene splicing, 203
 distribution, 571
Neurokinin receptors (NK receptors), *see* Tachykinins
Neuroleptanalgesia, 512
Neuroleptic drugs, *see* Antipsychotic drugs
Neuroleptic malignant syndrome, 533
Neurological disorders, vitamin B_{12} deficiency-related, 333
 see also Central nervous system
Neuromodulators (neuroregulators) and neuromodulation, 122, 130, 133
 in CNS, 458
 definition, 130
 in nociception, 570–2
Neuromuscular junction (motor endplate), 141
 ACh at, 140
  action, 31, 140, 141
  release, 140
 anticholinesterase effects at, 158
 blockers of transmission at, in helminths, 690, 691
 blockers of transmission at, in humans (muscle relaxants), 143, 149–54
  aminoglycoside use with, paralysis caused by, 645
  side-effects, 151, 153–4
 desensitisation at, 20
 in myasthenia gravis, 159
Neuron(s)
 afferent, *see* Afferent nerves
 in autonomic nervous system, 123–6
  in gastrointestinal regulation, 367
  postganglionic, *see* Postganglionic neurons
  preganglionic, *see* Preganglionic neurons
 in CNS
  glial cells as 'inexcitable neurons', 458
  glutamate and glutamine transport, 464
  interconnections, 459
 death, mechanisms, 490–3
 degeneration, *see* Neurodegeneration
 in inflammatory reaction, 221–2
 NO effects, 213
 peptidergic, in hypothalamus, 405–6
 uptake (uptake 1) of catecholamines by, 167, 168, 169
  inhibitors, 178, 181, 182
Neuronal NOS, 213, 486, 487
 endogenous inhibitor, 214
Neuropathic pain, 556, 566–7
 therapy, 583, 615
Neuropathy, diabetic, 386
Neuropeptide(s), *see* Peptides
Neuropeptide Y, 128, 130, 132, 200
 energy balance and food intake and, 395, 397
 neurotransmission involving, 132, 200
Neuroplasticity, 563–4
 see also Synapse, plasticity
Neuroprotection
 adenosine and, 195
 drugs enhancing, 493
  Parkinson's disease, 500
Neurosteroids, 471
Neurotoxicity
 of excitatory amino acids, *see* Excitotoxicity
 lithium, 549
 organophosphates, 158
 see also Central nervous system
Neurotoxins
 ACh release inhibited by, 155
 Parkinson's disease-like state induced by, 497–8
Neurotransmission (synaptic transmission), 65–6, 122–97, 462–89
 in autonomic nervous system, 126
 basic steps in, 133
 in CNS, 457–8, 462–89
  anaesthetic effects, 505
  excitatory amino receptor antagonist effects, 468
  long-term depression and potentiation, *see* Long-term depression; Long-term potentiation
 general principles and interactions in, 126–32
 NO role, 212
Neurotransmitter(s), 122–97, 462–89
 in autonomic nervous system, 126
 in CNS, 458, 462–89
  amino acids as, *see* Amino acids
  in depression, role, 536–8
  in schizophrenia, 526–7
 histamine as, 485
 neuropeptides compared with, 200
 in nociceptive pathway, 570–2
 peptides as, 199
 release, mechanisms/regulation, 65–6, 128
 removal, defective, 126
 supersensitivity to, with denervation, 126–8
 termination of action, 131–3
 transport, *see* Transport
 see also specific transmitters
Neurotrophic factors/neurotrophins, 458
 apoptosis prevention, 491
 epileptogenesis and, 553
Neutral endopeptidase inhibitors, 295, 300
Neutropenia, CSF use in, 338
Neutrophils, 220, 221
 absence in circulation, *see* Agranulocytosis
 colchicine effects, 255
 glucocorticoid effects, 416
 in inflammation, 221
 leukotriene effects, 236
Nevirapine, 661
New drugs, *see* Development
Newborns, *see* Neonates
NF-κB, *see* Nuclear factor-κB
NGF, *see* Nerve growth factor
Niclosamide, 690
Nicorandil, 281–2, 294
Nicotinamide adenine dinucleotide (NAD) and ethanol, 606
Nicotine
 actions/effects, 136, 142, 147, 148, 149, 599
  harmful, 601–2, 602
  historical observations, 122
  protective (neurological), 602
 dependence, 600–1
  treatment, 602–3
 pharmacokinetics, 599–600
 replacement therapy, 602
 tolerance, 600–1
 see also Smoking
Nicotinic ACh receptors, 137
 ACh actions, 136–7
 agonists, 147, 149
  analgesic actions, 583
  depolarisation block with, 142
  as ganglion stimulants, 147
  in nicotine dependence, 602
 antagonists/blockers, 149
 CNS, 483, 484
 galantamine effects, 130
 in myasthenia gravis, 48, 159, 717
 nicotine addiction and, 600–1
 pain and, 484
 in presynaptic regulation, 128–30
 structure, 29–30
 types, 137, 138
Nicotinic acid (and derivatives), 310, 312
Nifedipine
 angina, 282
 dysrhythmic effects, 283
 vasodilatory effects, 293
Nifurtimox, 684
Nigrostriatal tract/pathway/neurons
 destruction, effects, 478

dopamine in, 476
in Parkinson's disease, 497
Nikethamide, 586
Nikkomycins, 670
Nimodipine in subarachnoid haemorrhage, 283
Nimorazole, 683
Nipecotic acid, 470
Nitazoxanide, 691
Nitrates (endogenous), urinalysis, 214
Nitrates (organic nitrates/nitrites; nitrovasodilators), 279–81, 298
actions, 280–1
mechanisms, 281
in myocardial infarction, 272
unwanted, 281
clinical uses, 281
angina, 281
biliary spasm, 378
heart failure, 281, 302
pharmacokinetics, 281
sublingual administration, 99–100, 281
tolerance, 281
Nitrazepam, 517
Nitric oxide (NO), 66, 128, 130, 208–16, 239–40, 286, 487–8
actions/effects, 132, 212–13, 239–40
airways, 341
cardiac muscle, 280–1
CNS, 486, 487–8
in inflammation, 221, 239
in nociception, 564
vascular, 208, 212, 213, 286, 298, 317
clinical conditions involving, 214–15
clinical use, 212, 213
of NO-NSAIDs, 260
degradation/carriage, 210–12
donors of, 213
organic nitrates, 213, 281
penile erection and, 295
potentiation, 214
production (and its regulation), 137, 209–10, 239
ACh and, 137, 288
inhibitors, 213–14, 240
Nitric oxide synthase (NOS), 209–10
constitutive, 209, 210, 341
inducible, 209, 239, 341
pathology, 210
inhibitors, 213–14, 240
neuronal, *see* Neuronal NOS
N^G-Nitro-L-arginine methyl ester (L-NAME), 214
Nitrofurantoin, 649
Nitrogen mustards, 627, 699–700
Nitroglycerine, *see* Glyceryl trinitrate
7-Nitroindazole, 214
Nitroprusside, 215, 294–5
S-Nitrosoglutathione, 212, 213
Nitrosoureas, 627, 700
Nitrous oxide (N_2O), 503, 507, 510, 511
toxicity, 507, 510
Nitrovasodilators, *see* Nitrates
Nizatidine, 370
NK receptors, *see* Tachykinins
NMDA receptors, 46, 52–3, 463, 465, 466
agonists, 465
antagonists, 465, 466
psychotic symptoms with, 527
synaptic transmission and, 468
channel blockers, 465, 466
epilepsy and, 552, 553
ethanol and, 603
excitotoxicity/neurotoxicity and, 53, 491
nociception and, 564
phencyclidine and, 466, 469, 593
special features, 466
Nociceptin, 199, 572
Nociception, 562–72
chemical mediators, 567–70
adenosine, 195, 572
ATP, 485, 570
5-HT, 186, 570, 572
definition, 563, 567
pathways of, 562–72
modulation in, 563–6
opioid actions, 576
Nocistatin, 572
Noise analysis (receptor operated ion channels), 31
Non-adrenergic non-cholinergic transmission/mediators, 130
airways, 341
Non-depolarising blocking drugs, 149–52
depolarising drugs compared with, 153
effects, 150
unwanted effects, 150
mechanism of action, 150
pharmacokinetics, 150–1
Non-Hodgkin's lymphoma, therapy, 242, 706, 745
Non-insulin-dependent (type 2/maturity-onset) diabetes mellitus, 386, 387
insulin in, 388
oral hypoglycaemics, 390, 391, 392
Non-nucleoside reverse transcriptase inhibitors, 661, 662
Non-steroidal anti-inflammatory drugs (NSAIDs; COX inhibitors), 231–4, 244–52
actions/effects, 244–50
in Alzheimer's disease, 496
analgesic, 246, 250
anti-inflammatory, 231–4, 247, 250
anti-pyretic, 235, 246, 250
cancer prevention and treatment, 708–9
in dysmenorrhoea, 442
in kidney, 362
mechanism, 247
as myometrial relaxants, 443
unwanted, *see subheading below*
ADH actions affected by, 410
COX-2 selective, 245, 249, 252, 370, 709
interactions, 719
NO-releasing moiety coupled to, 260
unwanted/harmful effects, 247–50, 252
gastrointestinal, 248–9, 370
renal, 249, 728–9
Nootropic drugs, Alzheimer's disease, 496
Noradrenaline (norepinephrine), 124, 126, 162, 176–82, 179
actions/effects, 179, 475–6
central, 475–6, 572
historical observations, 122
tests of potentiation in periphery by antidepressants, 538
unwanted effects, 179
ATP and, cotransmission involving, 131
in CNS, 475–6
depression and, 536, 537
function, 475–6, 572
metabolism, 168
in nociception, 572
pharmacokinetics, 179
release, 165–6
drugs affecting, 176–8, 180, 181
regulation, 128, 165–6, 292
storage, 165
drugs affecting, 165, 176, 177, 181
synthesis, 164–5
drugs affecting, 164, 165, 181
transporter protein, 132, 167
turnover, 165
uptake, 166–7
uptake inhibitors, 178–82, 181
selective (antidepressants), 540
selectivity of inhibition by various antidepressants, 543
by tricyclic antidepressants, 542
see also 5-Hydroxytryptamine/noradrenaline reuptake inhibitors
Noradrenergic neurons, 164, 176–82
central, 475, 566
opioid dependence and, 579
drugs affecting, 176–82, 179–81
actions, 179–81
neuron-blocking drugs, 177, 178
unwanted effects, 179–81
uses/function, 179
Noradrenergic transmission and pathways, 161–83
CNS, 475
physiology, 164–8
Nordazepam, 520
Norepinephrine, *see* Noradrenaline
Norethisterone, 434
in combined pill, 439
Norfloxacin, 627, 647
pharmacokinetics, 648
S. aureus resistance, 632
Norgestrel, 434
Nortriptyline, 540
chemical aspects/structure, 542
therapeutic window, 544
Nose, *see entries under* Nasal
NSAIDs, *see* Non-steroidal anti-inflammatory drugs
Nuclear factor-κB, 219, 413
aspirin and, 247
inhibition and inhibitors, 260, 413
receptor activator of (RANK), 448
Nuclear receptors (regulating transcription), 27, 29, 44–5
adrenal steroid, *see* Adrenal steroids
sex steroid, 432
structure, 27, 28, 44
Nucleic acid synthesis, 625–7
bacterial, 625–7
agents interfering with, 627
viral, 655
agents interfering with, 627, 660–1, 662–3
see also DNA; RNA
Nucleosides, 192–6
as reverse transcriptase inhibitors, 660–1, 662
see also Base; Purines; Pyrimidines
Nucleotides, 192
cyclic, *see* AMP; Cyclic nucleotides; GMP
synthesis, inhibitors, 625
see also Antisense strategies; Base; Single-nucleotide polymorphisms; Trinucleotide repeat diseases *and specific nucleotides*
Nucleus, cell, steroid receptors, *see* Steroids
Nucleus accumbens
dopaminergic pathways in, 476, 579
habituation/dependence and, 596–7
nicotine, 600
opioid, 579
Nucleus basalis of Meynert, cholinergic pathways, 483
Nucleus reticularis paragigantocellularis and nociception, 565–6
Number needed to treat, 90
Nutrient deficiency, haemopoiesis affected by, 330
see also Diet; Food; Malnutrition
Nystatin, 628, 669

O

Obesity, 394–403
definition, 394
health impact, 397–9
pathophysiology, 399–401
pharmacological approaches, 401–2
appetite suppressants, *see* Appetite suppressants
β_3-agonists, 170, 173, 392, 402
currently available, 402–3
potential, 402
Obstetrics, *see* Pregnancy
Occupancy (of receptors by drug), 15, 16
by agonists, 13–14
with reversible vs. irreversible competitive antagonists present, 16
Octreotide, 384
acromegaly, 385, 407
gastrointestinal tract hormone-secreting tumours, 705
migraine, 192
Ocular pharmacology, *see* Eye
Oculomucocutaneous syndrome, 176
Oedema
cerebral, osmotic diuretics, 365
in heart failure, 269
NSAIDs reducing, 247
Oesophageal varices, bleeding, 293
Oesophagitis, reflux, 369, 370
Oestradiol, 432
Oestriol, 432

Oestrogen(s), 431–2
  actions/effects, 431, 432
    anti-androgenic, 437
    on bone, 450
    mechanisms, 432
    in pregnancy, 431
    unwanted, 433
  clinical use, 433, 451
    cancers, 705
    in HRT, *see* Hormone replacement therapy
    in oral contraceptives, *see* Oral contraceptives
  pharmacokinetics, 433
  preparations, 432–3
  production/synthesis, 431
    menstrual cycle, 430–1
    sites of drug action, 432
  see also Anti-oestrogens
Oestrogen-progestogen combined pill, 439
  beneficial effects, 439, 440
  unwanted/adverse effects, 439–40
Oestrogen receptors, 432
  modulators, selective (SERMs), 432, 451
Oestrone, 432
Ofloxacin, 647
  pharmacokinetics, 648
Oil(s), fish, 313
Oil:gas partition coefficient of anaesthetics, 506, 507
Oil:water partitioning, anaesthetics, 504
Olanzapine, 529
Oligonucleotides, antisense, *see* Antisense strategies
Olsalazine, 99, 378
Omapatrilat, 295, 300
ω-3 marine triglycerides, 313
Omeprazole, 370
  pharmacokinetics, 371
On–off effect, levodopa, 500
Onchocerca volvulus infection/onchocerciasis, 687
  therapy, 689, 691
Oncogenes, 694, 729
  therapeutic targeting of signalling pathway, 708
Oncotic pressure, 354
Ondansetron, 188, 373
  as antiemetic, 373, 481
    in cancer chemotherapy, 700, 707
  as anxiolytic, 482, 524
Ondine's curse, 340
One (single) compartment model of pharmacokinetics, 114–16
ONYX-015, 709
Oocyst, plasmodial, 675
Ophthalmological pharmacology, *see* Eye
Opiates, *see* Morphine-like drugs
Opioid(s)
  definition, 572
  endogenous (opioid peptides), 128, 571–2
    actions/effects, 570
    biosynthesis/precursors, 203, 572
    selectivity for receptor subtypes, 575
  exogenous, *see* Morphine-like drugs
Opioid receptors, 574–5
  agonist(s), 575
    partial, 575, 582
    pure, 575
  agonists–antagonists, mixed, 575, 582
  antagonists, 103, 204, 575, 582–3
  opioid drug and peptide selectivity for, 575
  orphan receptor resembling, 199, 572
Opium, 572
Opportunistic infections in HIV disease, 659
Opsonin (C3b), 220, 221
Oral administration, 98
  see also specific (types of) drugs
Oral anticoagulants (coumarins etc.), 321–3
  administration and pharmacokinetics, 321–2
  interactions, 322
  mechanism/site of action, 321–2
  non-drug factors potentiating or lessening effects of, 322
  unwanted effects, 323
Oral contraceptives, 439–41
  combined, *see* Oestrogen—progestogen combined pill
  pharmacokinetics /interactions, 440–1
  postcoital/emergency, 441
Oral hypoglycaemics, *see* Hypoglycaemic agents
Oral rehydration, 376
Orexigenic factors, 396
  orexins, 199, 396
Organ(s)
  growth and development (organogenesis), drugs affecting, 731–2
  transplantation, *see* Transplant
Organelles as antibiotic targets, 628–9
Organic molecules, excretion, 355, 361
  drugs altering, 365–6
Organic nitrates, *see* Nitrates
Organophosphates, 153, 157
  clinical use, 153
  unwanted effects (and poisoning), 158
    antidote, 158
Orlistat, 401, 402
Orphan receptors, 44
  opioid-like, 199, 572
Orthostatic hypotension, *see* Postural hypotension
Osmolality, plasma, ADH release and, 410
Osmotic diuretics, 364–5
Osmotic laxatives, 375–6
Osmotic pressure, 354
  gradient, 355
    in renal medulla, 360
Osteoblasts
  bone remodelling and, 446–8
  glucocorticoid effects, 416
Osteoclasts
  bone remodelling and, 446–8
  glucocorticoid effects, 416
Osteodystrophy of chronic renal failure, 452
Osteoid, 446
Osteomalacia, 451
Osteopenia, 451
Osteoporosis, 451, 452–3
  glucocorticoid-induced, 417
  heparin-induced, 321
  therapies
    calcium salts, 453
    new, 452–3
Osteoprotegerin, 448
  clinical use, 453
Osteoprotegerin ligand, 448
Ototoxicity, aminoglycosides, 645
Ouabain, 278
Outcome, clinical, measures, 88, 89
Outer membrane of bacteria, 622, 635–7
  antibiotics with difficulties in penetrating, 637
Ovarian cancer and oral contraceptives, 440
Ovarian stimulation, *see* Ovulation, induction
Overview analysis, 88
Ovulation, induction
  by clomiphene, 434
  by gonadotrophins, 438–9
Oxalizidonones, 647
Oxamniquine, 690
Oxazepam, 517
  pharmacokinetics, 520
Oxcarbazepine, 555, 557
Oxidase, mixed function, *see* Mixed function oxygenase
Oxidation
  ethanol, 606
  glucose, glucagon effects, 385
  iodide, 421
  by non-P450 enzymes, 109
  by P450 enzymes, 108
Oxidative phosphorylation, proteins uncoupling, 397
Oxidative stress, 493
  drug-induced, 726, 727–8
  Parkinson's disease and, 499
Oxitropium, 347
Oxotremorine, 138, 144
Oxprenolol, 174
Oxybutinin, 146
Oxygen, myocardial, availability and consumption, 269, 270–2
Oxygen radicals, free/reactive, *see* Free radicals
Oxygenase, mixed function, *see* Mixed function oxygenase
Oxyntic cells, acid secretion, 368
Oxytetracycline, 643
Oxytocics (myometrial stimulants), 441–2, 443
Oxytocin, 410, 441–2
  actions/effects, 441–2
    behavioural, 431
    unwanted, 442
    uterine, 441–2
  in brain, 200
  clinical uses, 443
  pharmacokinetics, 442
  receptor antagonist, 443

P

P-glycoprotein, 95
  anticancer drug resistance and, 707
  antimalarial drug resistance and, 677
P-type Ca^{2+} channels, 52
P_1 receptors, *see* Adenosine receptors
P_{2x} receptors (AMP/ADP/ATP), 46, 194–5, 195–6
  blockade/antagonism, 196
  distribution, 195
    brain, 485
  P_{2x3}, 570
  subtypes, 195–6
P_{2y} receptors (AMP/ADP/ATP), brain, 485
p21, 72
p53
  in apoptosis, 76
  cell cycle and, 73
  gene (*p53*), in cancer therapy, 709
P450 mono-oxygenase system, 106, 107–9
  biological variation in expression/regulation, 108–9
  example substrates/drugs, 108
  inhibition, 109, 720
  nature and classification of enzymes, 107–8
  paracetamol overdose and, 720
  theophyllines and, 347
  warfarin and, 322
  see also Mixed function oxygenase system
Pacemaker activity in cardiac tissue, 265, 267
  abnormal, 268
Paclitaxel, 704
PAF, *see* Lyso-PAF; Platelet-activating factor
Paget's disease of bone, 451, 452
Pain, 562–84
  anandamide and, 488
  anginal, *see* Angina
  chronic, 563, 581
  drug management, *see* Analgesics
  gate control theory, 564–5
  local anaesthetics blocking sensation of, 614
  mechanisms of sensation, 562–72
  neuropathic, *see* Neuropathic pain
  nicotinic ACh receptors and, 484
  postoperative, 581
  spontaneous, 563
Paired helical filaments, 495
Palivusamab, 241, 664
Pamidronate, 451
Pancreas, 380–93
  B/β-cell, *see* B-cell
Pancreatic lipase inhibition, 401
Pancreatic polypeptide, 380
Pancuronium, 149, 150, 151
  unwanted effects, 150, 151
Panic disorder, 515
Pantoprazole, 370
Papaverine in erectile dysfunction, 444
Papillary necrosis, renal, 728
Paracetamol (acetaminophen), 245
  actions, 251–2
    unwanted/adverse, 111, 251–2, 720, 727–8
  pharmacokinetics, 251
  treatment of poisoning, 252, 728
Paracrine system, gastrointestinal tract, 367
Paraherquamide, 691
Parallel line assays, 82
Paralysis
  aminoglycoside-induced, 645
  anaesthesia-induced, 505

depolarising drug-induced (incl. suxamethonium), prolonged, 153, 154
non-depolarising drug-induced (curare and derivatives), 149–50
Paraoxon, 727
Parasites
definition, 620
host–parasite interactions, 672–3
protozoan/metazoan, *see* Helminths; Protozoa
see also specific types
Parasympathetic nervous system, 124
airway, 340, 340–1
anatomy, 125
cardiac, 273
gastrointestinal, 367
physiology, 125, 126
cotransmitters, 132
postsynaptic nerve terminals, 140
sympathetic and, relationship/opposition, 125–6
see also Autonomic nervous system
Parasympatholytics, *see* Muscarinic ACh receptor antagonists
Parasympathomimetics, *see* Muscarinic ACh receptor agonists
Parathion, 156, 157, 158
Parathyroid hormone (parathormone; PTH), 448, 449–50
in osteoporosis, use, 452–3
Paravertebral chain of sympathetic ganglia, 123
Parietal cells, acid secretion, 368
Parkin gene mutations, 497, 498
Parkinson's disease/parkinsonism, 497–501
dopamine in
drugs inducing release, 499, 500
loss/deficiency, 497
replacement therapy, 499
dopamine receptors in, 497
agonist use in treatment, 500
D_2 receptor mutant causing condition resembling Parkinson's disease, 478
drug-induced, 497
pathogenesis/pathophysiology, 478, 497–8
smoking and, 602
treatment of, 499–501
amantadine, 500, 663
muscarinic antagonists in, 148, 499, 500
prophylactic antiemetics in, 102, 500
Paroxetine, 540, 544
Paroxysmal depolarising shift, 553
PARs, *see* Protease-activated receptors
Partial seizures, 551, 556
Particle size and intestinal absorption, 98
Partition coefficient, 92
anaesthetics, 506, 507
Partitioning of drugs
into fat and other tissues, 96–7
anaesthetics, 96, 504, 506, 507, 512
pH and, 93–4
see also Compartments
Patch, *see* Transdermal routes
Patch-clamp recording, 31, 45
Pathogen-associated molecular patterns (PAMPs), 218, 221
Pathophysiology in animal models of disease, 85
PCPA, 480, 482
Pectin, 377
Pefloxacin, 648
Pelvic splanchnic nerves (nervi erigentes), 125
Penciclovir, pro-drug of, 104, 663
Penicillamine, 256
unwanted actions, 256, 297
Penicillin(s), 639–41
aminoglycoside combined with, 645
β-lactamase-resistant, 641, 643
broad-spectrum, 641, 643
clinical uses, 641
discovery/development, 639–40
extended-spectrum, 641, 643
mechanism of action, 624, 640
pharmacokinetics, 641
blood–brain barrier, 102
excretion/elimination, 111, 112
probenecid interactions, 112, 255, 721
resistance mechanisms, 631
spectrum of activity, 640–1
types, 640–1
unwanted effects, 641
allergy/hypersensitivity, 641, 735
Penicillin-binding protein/sites, 640
Penicillin G, *see* Benzylpenicillin
Penicillin V (phenoxymethylpenicillin), 640
Penicilloylpolylysine, 735
Penis, erection, *see* Erection
Pentamidine, 684
leishmaniasis, 683
P. carinii pneumonia, 682
pharmacokinetics, 684
toxoplasmosis, 685
trypanosomiasis, 684
unwanted effects, 684
Pentazocine, 574, 575, 580, 582
Pentobarbital, 523
Pentostatin, 702, 703
Pentylenetetrazole (leptazol), 552, 585, 586, 587
Peptic cells, 368
Peptic ulcers (gastric/duodenal)
NSAID-associated, 248–9, 370
pathogenesis, 368, 369
H. pylori, 370, 371
prostanoid in prevention of, 235
treatment, 148, 369, 370–2
Peptide(s) (as drugs), 205–6
clinical applications, 205
nasal sprays, 100
Peptide(s) (as neural mediators/neuropeptides), 198–207, 240
in airway regulation, 341
diversity within families, 203
in energy balance regulation, 395
in inflammation, 222, 240
neurotransmitters compared with, 200
in nociception, 570–2
therapeutic use, 583
physiological roles, 200–1
neurotransmission, 128, 130, 132
precursors, 202
receptor antagonists, 204–5
regulation (of synthesis/release), 201, 202
structure, 198–9
trafficking and secretion, 204
types, 199
see also specific peptides
Peptide(s) (as vascular mediators), 286–7
Peptide antibiotics, resistance mechanisms, 632
see also Glycopeptide antibiotics
Peptide–MHC complex (in immune response), 226
Peptidergic neurons in hypothalamus, 405
Peptidoglycan, bacterial, 218, 621, 635
synthesis, 623–4
drugs inhibiting, 624
Peptidomimetics, 199
Peptoids, 204
Pergolide, 500
Periaqueductal grey and pain, 565
Pericytes, 91
Perindopril, 296
Peripheral nervous system, 122–97
in coronary blood flow regulation, 270
divisions, 123–6
see also specific divisions
NO role, 212
noradrenaline transport/metabolism, 168
Peripheral vasculature
disease, 303–4
smoking and, 601
resistance, drugs affecting, 286
Periphery
cannabis effects, 609
dopamine receptors, 478
hormones acting in, distinction from neuropeptides, 200
indirectly acting sympathomimetic amine effects, 178
mediators, *see* Mediators
nicotine effects, 599
noradrenaline in, 168
tests of potentiation of effects by antidepressants, 538
Permeability coefficient, 92
Permethrin, 676
Pernicious anaemia, 333
treatment, 335
Peroxidation, lipid, 726
Peroxisome proliferation-activated receptors (PPARs), 45
activation and agonism
fibrates, 311
thiazolidinediones, 390–1
energy expenditure and obesity and, 397, 399–400
Peroxynitrite generation, NO and, 487
Pertussis toxin, 35
Pethidine, 580, 581
MAO inhibitor interactions with, 547
pharmacokinetics, 580
partition in aqueous compartments, 94
unwanted effects, 580, 581
uses, 580, 581
biliary spasm, 378
obstetrics, 579
Petit mal, *see* Absence seizures
pH (acidity/alkalinity)
drug movement/distribution related to, 92–4
local anaesthetic activity and, 613–14
urinary, *see* Urine
see also Acid–base balance
Phaeochromocytomas (chromaffinomas), 173
Phages, 630–1
Phagocytosis of bacteria, 226
Pharmacodynamic(s)
definition, 114
individual variations in, *see* Individual variations
interactions affecting, 718, 718–19
phase I studies establishing, 749
Pharmacoeconomics, 5, 81
in phase III studies, 750
Pharmacoepidemiology, 5, 81
Pharmacogenetics (genetic factors in individual variation), 5, 714–15
Pharmacogenomics, 5
Pharmacokinetic(s), 91–119
assessment
in clinical development (phase I studies), 749
in preclinical development, 749
definition, 114
individual variations in, *see* Individual variations
interactions affecting, 718, 719–22
models, 114–18
see also individual parameters
Pharmacokinetic antagonism, 18
Phase I reactions, 107, 107–9
Phase I studies, 749
Phase II depolarisation block, 143
Phase II reactions, 107, 109
Phase II studies, 749
Phase III studies, *see* Clinical trials
Phase IV studies, 750
Phenacetin, nephrotoxicity, 728–9
Phenanthrene derivatives, morphine as, 572
Phenanthrene-methanol, 679
Phencyclidine, 469, 513, 527, 586, 592–3
actions, 592–3
NMDA receptors, 466, 469, 593
Phenelzine, 541, 545
unwanted effects, 541, 546
Phenindione, 321
Phenobarbital, 557–8
as antiepileptic, 557, 560
mechanisms of action, 554, 557
pharmacokinetics, 556, 560
unwanted effects, 558
warfarin interactions, 18
Phenothiazines, 373–4, 528
clinical uses
antiemetic, 373–4
schizophrenia, 528
unwanted effect, 532
Phenotype in animal models of disease, 85
Phenoxybenzamine, 173, 180
phaeochromocytoma, 173
Phenoxymethylpenicillin, 640
Phentolamine, 173, 180
erectile dysfunction, 444

Phenylakylamines, 282
Phenylbutazone
plasma protein binding, 96
warfarin interactions, 720
Phenylephrine, 179
priapism, 444
Phenylethanolamine *N*-methyl transferase (PNMT), 165
Phenylpiperidines, 573
Phenytoin, 555, 557, 560, 719
as analgesic, 583
as antidysrhythmic, 276
as antiepileptic, 560
mechanisms of action, 554
interactions, 719
isoniazid, 650
pharmacokinetics, 118, 555, 719
genetic influences, 715
unwanted effects, 555, 556–7, 727, 734
Phobias, 515
Phocomelia, thalidomide, 733
Pholcodine, 350, 577
Phorbol esters and protein kinase, 38
Phosphate
abnormal levels, 451
bone mineral, 446
metabolism, 449
metabolism (other than bone), 449
Phosphatidylinositol(s), lithium effects on metabolism of, 548
Phosphatidylinositol (4,5)-bisphosphate, 37
Phosphodiesterase(s), 36
Phosphodiesterase inhibitors, 295
in asthma, 346
selective, 295
PDEIII (and cardiovascular effects), 279, 295
PDEV, in erectile dysfunction, 295, 444
Phosphoinositides, *see* Inositol phosphates
Phospholipase(s), site of action, 232
Phospholipase A_2 and arachidonate metabolism, 231
Phospholipase C, 36, 36–8, 41
and eicosanoid synthesis, 234
Phospholipids
bacterial membrane, as drug targets, 627–8
mediator (eicosanoid) derivation from, 231
structure, 232
Phosphonoformate (foscarnet), 627, 663
Phosphoramidon, 288
Phosphorylation, 42–4
oxidative, protein uncoupling, 397
receptors, 42–4
desensitisation and, 20
G-protein-coupled receptors, 39
see also Protein kinases
Physical dependence, 595–6
morphine-like drugs, 578, 579
nicotine, 601
see also Withdrawal syndrome
Physicochemical factors affecting intestinal absorption, 99
Physiological adaptation, drug effect diminution due to, 21
Physiological antagonism, 19
Physostigmine (eserine), 123, 147, 156, 157
arousal by, 483
in tricyclic antidepressant CNS toxicity control, 544
Phytomenadione, *see* Vitamin K
Picosulfate, sodium, 376
Picrotoxin, 471, 585, 586, 587
Pilocarpine, 143, 144, 146
Pimozide, 529
PIN (endogenous nNOS inhibitor), 214
Pinocytosis, 92
Pinworm (in USA), *see Enterobius vermicularis*
Pioglitazone, 390, 391, 392
Piperazine (and derivatives), 629, 690
Piracetam, 470, 496
Pirbuterol, 346
Pirenzepine, 145–6, 147
gastrointestinal effects, 146
Piretanide, 362
Piroxicam, 245
Pituitary, 404–11
anterior, *see* Adenohypophysis
antipsychotic effects, 532
dopamine and, 476, 480
posterior, 410–11
see also Hypothalamic–pituitary–adrenal axis
Pizotifen, 188, 193
migraine, 192, 193
pK_a, 93
movement/transport of drugs and, 93
intestinal absorption, 98
of various drugs, 95
Placebos, 88
Plant derivatives, anticancer, 698, 704
Plaque, atheromatous, 307
Plasma
compartmentalisation in, 103
half-life in, 115
age affecting, 713, 714
NSAIDs, 245
inflammatory mediators derived from, 219–20
iodide, *see* Iodide
osmolality, ADH release and, 410
pH, drugs increasing/reducing, 93
proteins in
binding to, 96
osmotic pressure and, 354
Plasma cells, 224, 225
Plasma membrane, *see* Membrane
Plasmepsins I/II, 685
Plasmids
antibiotic resistance and, 629–30, 630, 631, 632
vaccination using, 741, 742
Plasmin, 328
Plasminogen, 308, 327–8
Plasminogen activator(s), 308, 327
tissue, *see* Tissue plasminogen activators
Plasminogen activator inhibitor-1, 317
Plasmodium spp.
falciparum, 673, 675–6, 676
antifolates, 680
chloroquine resistance, 677
halofantrine, 679
lumefantrine, 682
mefloquine (and mefloquine resistance), 679
pyonaridine, 682
qinghaosu compounds, 681
quinine, 678
life cycle, 673–5
malariae, 676
ovale, 676
8-aminoquinolines, 680
vivax, 673, 676
8-aminoquinolines (incl. primaquine) and resistance, 680, 681
chloroquine resistance, 677
halofantrine, 679
mefloquine, 679
pyonaridine, 682
sulfonamides and sulfones, 680
see also Malaria
Platelet(s), 194, 222, 323–7
ADP and, 194
aggregation/adhesion and function/activation, 323–7
drugs impairing, *see* Antiplatelet drugs
ethanol effects, 605
prostanoid involvement, 235
glycoprotein IIb/IIIa receptor antagonists, *see* Glycoprotein IIb/IIIa receptor antagonists
5-HT action on, 186
in inflammation, 222
PAF and, 237
see also Thrombocytopenia; Thrombocytopenic purpura
Platelet-activating factor (PAF), 231, 236–7
antagonists, 236–7
in inflammation, 237
sources/synthesis, 237
see also Lyso-PAF
Platelet factor 4 and thrombosis risk with heparin, 320–1
Platinum-based cytotoxic drugs, 700–1
Pneumocystis carinii pneumonia, 682
Poisons, *see* Toxins *and specific poisons*
Polarisation, *see* Depolarisation; Repolarisation
Polyamines and NMDA receptors, 466
Polycyclic aromatic hydrocarbons, 110
Polydypsia in diabetes, 385
Polyene antibiotics, 628
Polyglutamates, folate in form of, 334, 335, 701
Polymixins, 627, 649
Polymorphisms, 715
Polymorphonuclear cell/leucocyte, *see* Granulocyte
Polyuria
in diabetes, 385
lithium-induced, 549
Porphyria, hepatic, drug-induced, 716–17
Portal hypertension, 293
Posaconazole, 670
Posatirelin, 402
Positron emission tomography, receptor distribution, 10
Postcapillary venules in inflammation, 218–19, 230
Postganglionic neurons/fibres, 123
parasympathetic, 123, 125, 126
sympathetic, 123, 126
Postjunctional structures/events, *see entries under* Postsynaptic
Post-marketing surveillance, 750
Postmenopausal women, HRT, *see* Hormone replacement therapy
Postoperative pain, 581
Postpartum haemorrhage, 443
Postsynaptic/postjunctional modulation, 130
Postsynaptic/postjunctional potentials in cholinergic transmission
excitatory, *see* Excitatory postsynaptic potentials
slow inhibitory, 142
Postsynaptic/postjunctional responsiveness, increased, 126
Postsynaptic/postjunctional structures
ACh actions, 148, 149–54
parasympathetic nerve, 140
Post-translational modification/events
of glutamic acid residues, *see* Glutamate residues
peptide diversity via, 203
Post-traumatic stress disorder, 515
Postural (orthostatic) hypotension
antipsychotics causing, 532
ganglion blocking drugs causing, 149
levodopa causing, 500
nitrates causing, 281
tricyclic antidepressants causing, 543
Potassium, 360–1
balance/transport (in kidney), 360–1
extracellular, glycoside interactions with, 279
loss/depletion/lowering, 360–1
aldosterone causing, 419
diuretics reducing, *see* Potassium-sparing diuretics
drugs causing, 358, 360
glucocorticoids causing, 416
loop diuretic-induced, 363
permeability, postsynaptic modulation and, 130
raised levels, with ACE inhibitors, 297
release, with suxamethonium, 153
Potassium canrenoate, 364
Potassium ion(s)
cardiac muscle cell action potential and, 265
electrical excitability and, 56
renal transport, 353
aldosterone effects, 358, 419
see also Sodium pump
Potassium ion channels, 60–2
activators, 281–2, 294
in angina, 281–2
vasodilatory effects, 294, 298
anaesthetics and, 504
blockers, sulfonylureas as, 61, 389
G-protein-coupled receptors and, 38
inwardly rectifying K^+ channels, 60, 61–2
mutations, 62
islet B-cells, 380–1
mutations (channelopathies), 62
in renal collecting tubule, 358
in shock, 302
types, 60, 61–2
ATP-sensitive K^+ channels, *see* ATP-sensitive K^+ channels
calcium-activated K^+ channels, 46, 60, 61
inwardly rectifying K^+ channels, *see subheading above*
two-pore domain K^+ channels, 60, 62, 504

voltage-gated K^+ channels, 60, 61
Potassium-sparing diuretics, 361
clinical use, 364
pharmacokinetics, 364
unwanted effects, 364
Potency, relative, 82
Potency ratio, 82–3
Potentiation, long-term, *see* Long-term potentiation
Power of trial, 87
Poxviruses, immune response subversion, 656
PP cells, 380
PPACK, 321
PPADS, 196
PPARs, *see* Peroxisome proliferation-activated receptors
PQRST trial, 312
Practolol, 173–4, 180
toxicity, 174, 176, 180
Pradimicin, 670
Pralidoxime, 158, 159
Pramipexole, 500
Pramlintide, 385
Pravastatin, 310
trials, 310
Praziquantel, 689–90
Prazosin, 173, 180
Preclinical development, 747–9
Prednisolone, 412
in asthma, 349
Pre-erythrocytic (exo-erythrocytic) stage of malarial life cycle, 673, 675
Pregabalin, 560
Preganglionic neurons/fibres, 123
parasympathetic, 123, 125
sympathetic, 123
Pregnancy, 714
iron requirements, 331
pharmacokinetics in, 714
smoking in, 601–2
termination, drugs used for, 235, 434, 443
see also Labour
Pregnenolone, 413
Prekallikrein, 238
Pre-load, 269, 285
reduction, 302
Premature labour, delay, 443
Premature neonates, kernicterus, 714, 719
Premedication, anaesthetic, 148
Prenylation, 34
Preprodynorphin (=preproenkephalin B), 203, 572
Preproenkaphalin, 203, 572
Preprohormones, 202
Preproinsulin, 380
Prepro-opiomelanocortin (POMC), 203, 572
Presenilin, 495
Presynaptic modulation, 121–2
of ACh release, 128, 140–1
Presynaptic terminals, receptors
adrenoceptors, 176–7
autoreceptors, 128
noradrenaline release and, 165
Presystemic metabolism, 110
Preterm labour, delay, 443
Prevertebral ganglia, 123–5
Priapism, 444
Prilocaine, 615
pharmacokinetics, 616
unwanted effects, 615, 616
Primaquine, 680–1, 682
in malaria, 676, 677, 680
resistance, 681–2
in *P. carinii* pneumonia, with clindamycin, 682
pharmacokinetics, 681
in trypanosomiasis, 684
unwanted effects, 681, 716
Primidone, 555, 558
Prinzmetal's (variant) angina, 271
Prion disease, 501
Probenecid, 254, 366
excretion of drugs/metabolites affected by, 112
interactions, 366
aspirin, 251
penicillins, 251, 366, 721–2
Probucol, 310, 312–13
Procainamide, 274, 275, 276
Procaine, 615
discovery, 612
sulfonamide interactions, 638
unwanted effects, 615
Procaine penicillin, 101
Procarbazine, 703–4
Procaspase-9, 76
Prochlorperazine as antiemetic, 374
Procholecystokinin, 203
Procoagulant and haemostasis-promoting drugs, 315, 318–19, 322, 328–9
Pro-drugs, 23, 104, 111
of aciclovir, 104, 663
of 5-aminosalicylic acid, 99
of gabapentin, 560
of penciclovir, 104, 663
Prodynorphin, 203
Proflavine, 625
Progenitor cells, haematopoietic, *see* Stem and progenitor cells
Progesterone
actions/effects, 431, 432
in pregnancy, 431
release (in menstrual cycle), 431
Progesterone-like drugs, *see* Progestogens
Progestogens, 434
actions/effects, 434
anti-androgenic, 437
mechanisms, 434
unwanted, 434
clinical use, 434
cancer, 705
in combined oral contraceptive pill, 439
as parenteral contraceptive, 441
as progestogen-only pill, 440
pharmacokinetics, 434
preparations, 434
see also Antiprogestogens
Proglumide, 368
Proguanil, 679–80, 681, 682
in malaria, 623, 676, 677, 679–80, 682
atovaquone, 681
structure, 680
Prohormone(s), 202
Prohormone convertase, 202
Proinsulin, 380
Prokinetic agents (gastrointestinal motility increasing-drugs), 374, 376
5-HT_4 agonists as, 188
Prolactin, 405, 407–8
actions, 405, 408, 432
lactation, 408, 431
production/secretion, 407–8
dopamine and, 480
drugs affecting, 407, 408, 480, 532
regulation, 407–8
Prolactin release-inhibiting factor, 405
Prolactin releasing factor, 405, 407
Proliferation, cell, 69–74
pathophysiological implications, 77
cancer, 77, 694–5
therapeutic implications, 77–8
Promethazine, 253, 373
as antiemetic, 373
as antipsychotic, 528
Promoters, tumour, 730
Prontosil, 637–8
Propantheline, 377
Prophase, 72
Propofol, 512, 513
Propranolol, 173, 174, 180
in asthmatics, danger, 175, 347
clinical uses, 180
alcohol withdrawal, 608
dysrhythmias, 274, 276, 277
hyperthyroidism, 427
migraine, 193
post-myocardial infarction, trial, 88
ethnicity and response to, 712
intestinal absorption, 98
isoprenaline and, competitive antagonism, 12
metabolism, ethnic differences, 712–13
pharmacokinetics, 180
side-effects, 180, 193
Propylthiouracil, 425, 426, 427
Prostacyclin (PGI_2), 234
action, 234, 235
gastric, 368
uterine, 442
vascular, 235, 286, 317
receptors, 234
synthesis, 234
synthetic, *see* Epoprostenol
Prostaglandin(s), 128, 231, 442
biosynthesis, 231
inhibition by NSAIDs, 247
clinical use (incl. analogues), 442
gastric role, 368, 370
historical aspects, 231
in inflammation, 234–5
anti-inflammatory role, 235
pro-inflammatory role, 234–5
nociception and, 569
renal effects, 361
unwanted effects, 442–3
uterine effects, 442
Prostaglandin D_2
action, 234
vasodilatory, 235
receptors, 234
Prostaglandin E_1, synthetic forms and analogues, *see* Alprostadil; Gemeprost; Misoprostol
Prostaglandin E_2
actions, 235
gastric, 368
in inflammation, 234
uterine/obstetric, 442
vasodilatory, 235
clinical use, *see* Dinoprostone
receptors, 234
Prostaglandin $F_{2\alpha}$
analogue (carboprost), 442, 443
receptors, 234
uterine effects, 442
Prostaglandin I_2 *see* Prostacyclin
Prostanoids, 231, 233–5
actions
gastrointestinal, 235
in inflammation, 233–5
renal, 361–2
vascular, 235, 286, 442
biosynthesis, 234
inhibition by NSAIDs, 237
catabolism, 233
clinical uses, 235
receptors, 234
see also Prostaglandin; Thromboxane
Prostate
cancer, endocrine therapy, 437, 438, 705
hyperplasia/hypertrophy, benign, 173, 437
Protamine sulfate, 320
Protease-activated receptors (PARs), 33
thrombin and, 317
Protease inhibitors, 661, 662
Protein(s)
anaesthetic activity and, 504–5
bacterial synthesis, 625
antibiotics affecting, 625, 626, 643–7
as drugs, 205–6
clinical applications, 205
fungal synthesis, agents acting on, 670
as mediators, 198–207
metabolism
in diabetes, deranged, 385
glucocorticoid effects, 416
growth hormone effects, 407
insulin effects, 382
phosphorylation, *see* Phosphorylation
plasma, *see* Plasma
as targets for drug binding, 8, 22–3
see also Binding; Peptides *and specific types of protein targets*
Protein C, 317
activated, 317
clinical use, 303, 317
resistance to, 317

Protein kinase(s)
cAMP-dependent, 36
receptors linked to (and related receptors), 27, 42–4
structure, 27, 28
see also Phosphorylation *and specific kinases*
Protein kinase A, 39
Protein kinase C, 38, 39
activation, 38
inhibitor, 392
Proteoglycans, extracellular matrix, 73
Proteosome inhibitors, 685
Prothrombin (factor II), 316
conversion to thrombin, 316, 318
factor Xa interactions, 318
Prothrombin time, oral anticoagulants and, 321
Protirelin, 406, 422
Proton-pump inhibitors, 370
clinical use, 372
Proto-oncogenes, 694, 729
see also Oncogenes
Protozoal diseases, 672–86
drugs used, 676–86
host–parasite interactions, 672–4
Proximal tubules
diuretics acting on, 365
secretion into, 112
Pruritus (itching) and histamine, 230
Pseudocholinesterase (butyrylcholinesterase), 155–6, 159
Pseudohypoparathyroidism, 718
Pseudomembranous colitis (with *C. difficile*), 647
treatment, 99, 647
Pseudomonas aeruginosa, antibiotic insusceptibility, 637
Psilocin and psilocybin, 586, 591–2
Psoralens, toxicity, 731
Psychedelic drugs, *see* Psychotomimetic drugs
Psychiatric disorders, drugs used with, *see* Psychotropic drugs *and specific mental disorders*
Psychoactive drugs, *see* Psychotropic drugs
Psychodysleptics, *see* Psychotomimetic drugs
Psychological dependence (craving), 596
cocaine, 589
modification/diminishing, 598
alcoholism, 608
morphine-like drugs, 578
Psychological effects/changes
cannabis, 610
levodopa, 500
vigabatrin, 559
see also Psychotropic drugs
Psychomotor epilepsy, 551
Psychomotor stimulants, 460, 486, 585, 587–91
abuse, 595
actions, 587–8
mechanisms, 586
definition, 460
Psychosis, amphetamine-induced, 588
Psychostimulants, *see* Psychomotor stimulants
Psychotomimetic drugs (psychedelics; psychodysleptics; hallucinogens), 460, 585, 586, 591–3
abuse, 585
cannabis as, 609
definition/categorisation, 460, 591
mode of action, 586
Psychotropic drugs, 459
classification, 460–1
see also Psychological effects *and specific (types of) drugs*
Pteroylglutamic acid, *see* Folic acid
Puberty, familial precocious, 718
Pulmonary function/disease etc., *see* Airway; Lungs; Respiration
Punishment and anxiety, 516
Pupillary constriction
morphine-like drugs and, 577
muscarinic agonists and, 144–5
Pupillary dilation, muscarinic antagonists, 146, 148
Purgatives, 375–6
Purines, 192–6, 485
analogues, 623, 702–3
as anticancer agents, 623, 702–3
as antifungal agents, 623
in CNS, 485, 486
receptors, *see* Adenosine; P_{2x} receptors; P_{2y} receptors
synthesis/production
anticancer agents affecting, 701
folate involvement, 334
in gout, excess, 254
see also Bases; Nucleosides
Puromycin, 684
Purpura, thrombocytopenic, 323
PXR (nuclear receptors), 45
Pyloric stenosis, hypertrophic, 216
Pyonaridine, 682
Pyrantel, 690
Pyrazinamide, 650–1
Pyrexia, *see* Fever; Hyperpyrexia
Pyridostigmine, 157, 167
Pyrimethamine, 639, 679
in malaria, 623, 676, 677, 680
and sulfadoxine, 623, 680
structures, 680
in toxoplasmosis, with sulfadiazine, 685
unwanted effects, 680, 731
Pyrimidines
analogues, as anticancer agents, 701–2
folate involvement in synthesis, 334

Q

Q-type Ca^{2+} channels, 52
Qinghaosu (artemesinin), 676, 681, 682
Q–T prolongation, 275–6
drugs causing, 275
terfenadine with ketoconazole, 720
tricyclic antidepressants, 543
hereditary, 62, 275–6
see also LQT channels
Quality of life (in clinical outcome), 88
Quantal responses in bioassays, 83
Quetiapine, 529
Quinidine
antidysrhythmic actions, 274, 275, 276
digoxin interactions, 720
Quinine, 676, 678–9, 682
actions, 678
in malaria, 678, 679, 682
resistance, 679
pharmacokinetics, 678
plasma protein binding, 96
unwanted effects, 678–9
Quinoline(s), 677–9, 680–1
in malaria, 676
new derivatives, 685
structures, 678
Quinoline-methanols, 678–9
Quinolones (incl. fluoroquinolones), 627, 647–8
clinical use, 648
mode/site of action, 627
new, 652
pharmacokinetics, 648
resistance
mechanisms, 631–2, 632
S. aureus, 632
spectrum of activity, 648
unwanted effects, 648
Quinupristin, 646, 647

R

R plasmids and r genes, 630
Rabeprazole, 370
Race, variations in response due to, 712–13
Raclopride, 526
Radioactive drugs, binding studies, 10
Radioiodine, 425, 427
adverse effects, 424
uses, 425
in thyroid cancer, 705
Radioisotope–antibody conjugates, 708
Raf, 42
Raf-1 inhibitor, 708
Raloxifene, 432, 451–2
Ramipril, 296
peripheral vascular disease, 303
RAMPs (receptor activity modifying proteins), 40
Randomisation in clinical trials, 86, 87
stratified, 87
Randomised controlled trials, 86
Ranitidine, 370
pharmacokinetics, 370
RANK, 448
RANTES, 241, 657
Raphe nucleus
5-HT-containing neurons, 481
pain and, 565
Rapid eye movement sleep and benzodiazepines, 519
Ras, 42
in cancer therapy, targeting, 708
insulin and, 384
Ravuconazole, 670
Raynaud's disease, 304
Rb, 70
Reabsorption in kidney
chloride, thiazide effects, 363
sodium, 256, 354–5, 359, 361
drugs affecting, 358, 360, 363, 365
solutes (in general), *see* Solutes
urate, drugs inhibiting, 366
urea, 359, 360
water, 353, 354–5, 359
Reboxetine, 540
Receptor(s), 8, 9–18, 18–19, 22–3, 24, 47–8
activation, 9, 17–18
constitutive, 14–15
affinity of drug for, 9
agonists, *see* Agonists
antagonists, *see* Antagonists
binding of drugs to, *see* Binding
block, antagonism by, 18–19
change in, 20
classification/types/families, 9, 26–45
subtypes, 29
concentration of drug at, 15–16
control of expression, 47–8
definition, 8
desensitisation/tachyphylaxis, *see* Desensitisation
disease and, 48, 717–18
drug interactions with, 9–18
quantitative aspects, 15–18
heterogeneity, 29
ion channels operated by, *see* Ligand-gated ion channels
isolation and cloning, 26
loss of, 20
mutations, 48
occupancy by drug, *see* Occupancy
orphan, *see* Orphan receptors
proliferation, 126
signal transduction mechanisms, *see* Signalling pathways
spare (= receptor reserve), 15
structure, 27, 28, 29
two-state model, 17, 18
virus, 655
see also specific (types of) receptors
Receptor activity modifying proteins, 40
Rectangular hyperbola, receptor occupancy—drug concentration relationship producing, 16
Rectum
administration via, 100
cancer, aspirin prophylaxis, 250
Red cells, *see* Erythrocytes
Redox properties, P450 enzymes, 108
5α-Reductase inhibition by finasteride, 437
Reduction reactions, 109
P450 enzymes, 108
Re-entry rhythms, 267, 267–8
Reflux oesophagitis, 369, 370
Regional anaesthesia, intravenous, 617
Regulatory authorities, evaluation by, 750
Rehydration, oral, 376
Reinforcement, positive and negative, 595
REM sleep and benzodiazepines, 519
Remacemide, 469
Removal of drugs, *see* Elimination

Remoxipride, 529
Renal function etc., *see* Kidney
Renin, 290
  inhibitors, 296
  secretion/release, 290, 358
    inhibitors, 296
Renin–angiotensin(–aldosterone) system, 290–2, 358, 418
  blood pressure and, 298
  inhibition, 296–8
    in heart failure, 301
Repaglinide, 390
Repair processes, 77, 229
Repolarisation, cardiac muscle, 265
  partial, 265
Reproductive system, 429–45
  neurohormonal control
    females, 429–30
    males, 435–6
  toxicity tests, 730
    see also Teratogens
  see also Pregnancy
Reprotelol, 346
Reserpine, 176, 178, 181
  depression induced by, 176
    tests of antidepressant antagonism of, 538
  schizophrenia positive symptoms controlled by, 526
Resin(s), bile acid-binding, 312
Resiniferatoxin, 568
Resistance (to drugs), 19, 620
  to anthelminthics, 691
  to antibacterials, *see* Antibacterial drug
  to antimalarial agents, 677, 679, 681–2, 681–2
  to cytotoxic agents, 706–7
    mechanisms, 706–7
    multidrug, *see* Multidrug resistance
    reversal, 709
  see also specific agents
Respiration
  disorders, 341–50
  general anaesthetic effects, 506
  regulation, 340–1
Respiratory alkalosis with salicylates, 251
Respiratory depressants, morphine-like drugs as, 577
Respiratory distress syndrome, adult, NO therapy, 213
Respiratory stimulants, 585–7
Respiratory syncytial virus, monoclonal antibody therapy, 242, 664
Respiratory system, 340–51
  adrenoceptor agonists effects, 172
  leukotriene actions, 236
  see also specific parts
Response to drug
  genetic factors in, *see* Pharmacogenetics; Pharmacogenomics
  receptor occupancy related to, 13–14
  see also Dose–response curves
Response to treatment in animal models of disease, 85
Reteplase, 328
Retina
  rods, 32
  sildenafil adverse effects, 444
Retinoblastoma gene/protein, 70
Retinoic acid in development, 44–5
Retinoids, *see* Vitamin A derivatives
Retroviruses, 627
  drug therapy, *see* Antiretroviral agents
  as gene vectors, 739–41, 742
  replication, 655
Reverse transcriptase, 627, 655
  inhibitors, 627
Reward (pathways), 595, 596
  alcohol-induced, reducing, 608
  dopaminergic, 480, 596, 600
  nicotine-induced, 600
Reye's syndrome, 251
Rhabdomyolysis, fibrate-induced, 311
Rheumatoid disease (arthritis etc.), 255–7
  drug therapy, *see* Antirheumatoid agents
Rhodopsin, 32, 33
Ribavirin, 663
Ribosomes, bacterial, 625
Rickets, 451
Rickettsiae, antibiotic choice, 637
Ridrogel, 327
Rifampi(ci)n, 650
  clinical use
    leprosy, 652
    tuberculosis, 650
  interactions, 720, 721
  mechanism of action, 627, 650
  pharmacokinetics, 650
    biliary excretion, 114
  resistance
    mechanisms, 632
    S. aureus, 632
  unwanted effects, 650
Rifamycin, action, 627
Riluzole, 493
Rimantadine, 663
Ring hydroxylation, tricyclic antidepressants, 544
Ringworm (tinea), 666, 667
Risk, determining, 89–90
Risperidone, 529
Ritonavir, 661
Ritrodine, 443
Rituximab, 241, 706
Rivastigmine, 496
RNA, structure, 625
mRNA
  insulin effects, 384
  splicing
    peptide family diversity due to, 203
    receptor diversity due to variations in, 29
  synthesis, *see* Nucleic acid synthesis; Transcription
  translation
    in bacteria, 625
    modification after, *see* Post-translational modification
RNA polymerase inhibitors
  antibacterial, 627, 650
    resistance, 632
  anticancer, 625–7, 703
RNA viruses, 654–5
  diseases caused, 654–5
  replication, 655
  see also Retroviruses
Rods (bacteria), antibiotics choice, 636
Rofecoxib, 245, 252, 370
Rosiglitazone, 390, 391, 392
Rotenone, 498
Roundworms (nematodes), 687
  common, *see Ascaris lumbricoides*
  immune response, 689
  intestinal, 687
  therapy, 688, 689, 690, 691
  tissue, 687
Routes of administration, *see* Administration
Ryanodine receptors, 53, 54
  malignant hyperthermia and, 54, 154, 717

S

S-phase, 69
  regulators in, 72
Saclofen, 472
Sacral outflow of parasympathetic nervous system, 125
Safety (of drugs/therapy)
  establishing, 725
    in phase I studies, 749
  gene therapy, 743
  see also Adverse reactions
St John's Wort, 541, 547
Salbutamol, 179
  in asthma, 346
  in chronic obstructive pulmonary disease, 350
  as myometrial relaxant, 443
Salcatonin, 452
Salicylate(s), 250–1
  interactions
    methotrexate, 720
    uricosuric agents, 251, 366
  pharmacokinetics, 250
  poisoning, 251
  unwanted effects, 250–1
  see also 4-Aminosalicylic acid; 5-Aminosalicylic acid; Bismuth subsalicylate
Salicylate–sulfapyridine combination, *see* Sulfasalazine
Salicylism, 251
Saline purgatives, 375
Salivation
  muscarinic agonist effects, 144
  muscarinic antagonist effects, 146
Salmeterol, 346
Salmonella typhimurium and Ames test, 730
Salt
  overload, treatment, 363
  renal handling
    in distal convoluted tubules, 358
    excretion, drugs increasing, *see* Diuretics
  see also specific salts/ions
Sample size, trials, 87–8
Saquinavir, 661
Sarafotoxin S6c, 289–90
Saralasin, 297
Sarcoplasmic reticulum, Ca^{2+} channels, 54
Saturation (zero-order) kinetics, 117–18
  carrier-mediated transport, 94
  phenytoin, 118, 556
Saxitoxin (STX), 616–17
Scandinavian Simvastatin Survival Study, 310
Scatchard plot, 16
Schild equation/plot, 17
  linear plot, 18
Schistosomiasis (bilharzia), 687
  immune response to *S. mansoni*, 688
  therapy, 689, 690
Schizogony, 673
Schizont, plasmodial, 673, 675
  drugs acting on, 677–9
    for acute attacks, 676
    for radical cure, 676
Schizophrenia, 525–34
  amphetamine syndrome resembling, 588
  cannabis and, 610
  dopaminergic pathways and, 479
  drug therapy, *see* Antipsychotic drugs
  nature/aetiology/pathogenesis, 525–7
  positive and negative symptoms, 525
    antipsychotic effects, 634
Schlemm, canal of, muscarinic agonist actions, 145
Scopolamine, *see* Hyoscine
Scrapie, 501
Second messengers, *see* Signalling pathways
Secretases (α/β/γ), 495
  inhibitors, 496
Secretin/glucagon receptor family, 33
Secretions
  exocrine, *see* Exocrine gland
  gastric, *see* Gastric acid secretion; Gastric secretion
  paracrine, gastrointestinal tract, 368
Sedation
  antipsychotic, unwanted, 529, 532
  benzodiazepines, 519
  H_1-receptor antagonists, 253
  phenobarbital, 558
  tricyclic antidepressant, unwanted, 543
Sedatives, *see* Anxiolytic agents
Seizures/convulsions
  drug therapy, *see* Antiepileptic drugs
  drugs inducing (convulsants), 552, 585–7
    mode of action, 586
  types, 550–2
Selective oestrogen receptor modulators (SERMs), 432, 451
Selective serotonin reuptake inhibitors, *see* 5-Hydroxytryptamine (re)uptake inhibitors, selective
Selegiline, 498, 500
Senna, 376
Sensitivity to drugs, age-related, 714
  see also Supersensitivity
Sensory nerves and migraine, 191
Sensory receptors, airway, 341
Sensory transmission and 5–HT, 482
Sepsis (and septic shock)
  activated protein C in, 317
  NO role, 215

NOS synthase inhibitors in, 240
Septohippocampal pathway and learning/memory, 484
Septohippocampal nucleus, cholinergic pathways, 483
Sequential trials, 88, 89
D-Serine, 466
Serine hydrolases, 155–6
Serotonin, *see* 5-Hydroxytryptamine
Serotonin syndrome, 545
Sertindole, 529
Sertoli cells, 435, 436
Sertraline, 540, 544
appetite suppressant, 402
7-transmembrane receptors, *see* G-protein-coupled receptors
Sevoflurane, 507, 510, 511
adverse effects, 507
Sex steroids/hormones, 131–3
actions/effects, 432
behavioural, 431
as anticancer agents, 705
production/secretion, 431–2
adrenal, 411
in cancer therapy, inhibition, 705
sites of drug action, 432
receptors, 432
Sexual behaviour, sex hormone effects, 431
Sexual dysfunction, males, *see* Erection, dysfunction
SH2-domain proteins, 42
of insulin receptor substrate proteins, 284
Shingles, 662
Shock, 302–3
anaphylactic, *see* Anaphylactic reactions
causes, 302
septic, *see* Sepsis
Sibutramine, 401, 401–2, 402
actions, 401–2
pharmacokinetics, 401–2
unwanted effects, 402
Side-effects of drugs, *see* Adverse reactions
σ-opioid receptors, 574
Sigmoid curve, receptor occupancy–drug concentration relationships, 16
Signalling pathways and signal transduction (and second messengers)
adrenoceptors and, 162, 163
airway, 340
antidepressant effects, 539
apoptosis, 75
cancer cells, 695
diseases influencing, 718
dopamine receptors and, 479
G-protein-coupled receptors, 33–5, 36–8
G-protein-independent, 41
kinase-linked receptors, 42, 42–3
growth factors and, 70, 78
5-HT receptors and, 187
insulin and, 383, 384
leptin and, 395
lithium and, 548
nociceptive neurons, 567, 568
peptides and, 198
thrombin and, 317
Sildenafil, 212, 215, 295, 444
mechanism of action, 444
pharmacokinetics/interactions, 444, 718
unwanted effects, 444
Simvastatin, 310
in peripheral vascular disease, 303
trials, 310
Single compartment model of pharmacokinetics, 114–16
Single-nucleotide polymorphisms, 715
Sinoatrial (SA) node, 265
Sinus bradycardia, 148
Site-directed mutagenesis
G-protein-coupled receptors, 32
ligand-gated ion channels, 30
Skeletal muscle (non-cardiac striated muscle), 62
β-adrenoceptors in, 163
agonist effects, 171
contraction, 62
excitation and, coupling, 63
fasciculations with suxamethonium, 153
neuromuscular junction, *see* Neuromuscular junction
relaxants
centrally acting, 560–1
peripherally acting, *see* Neuromuscular junction
rigidity in Parkinson's disease, 497, 500
spasm, 560–1
Skin
anxiety and electrical conductivity of, 516
application to
for local effect, 100
for transdermal delivery, *see* Transdermal routes
autonomic nervous system, 127
reactions
with antipsychotics, 533
with NSAIDs, 249
see also Oculomucocutaneous syndrome *and entries under* Subcutaneous
Skin test for anaphylactic hypersensitivity, 735
Sleep, 519
benzodiazepine-induced, 519
5-HT and, 482
see also Narcolepsy
Sleeping sickness, African, 684
Slow excitatory effects of chemical mediators, 130
Slow excitatory postsynaptic potential, cholinergic transmission, 142
Slow inhibitory postsynaptic potential, cholinergic transmission, 142
Slow phase of elimination, 117
Slow reacting substance of anaphylaxis, 235–6
Slow-release/sustained-release preparations, 98–9, 101
antipsychotics, 533
Slow wave sleep, benzodiazepine effects, 519
Smoking (tobacco; cigarettes), 598–603
cessation, weight gain, 599
effects, 599
beneficial, 602
harmful, 601–2
epidemiology, 598
see also Nicotine
Smooth muscle, 62–3
ADH effects, 410
adrenoceptor receptors in, 163
agonists of, effects, 170
airway, *see* Airway
bradykinin effects, 239
cAMP-dependent protein kinase, 36
contraction, *see* Contraction
histamine effects, 230
5-HT effects, 196
morphine-like drug effects, 577, 578
motility, *see* Motility
muscarinic receptor agonist effects, 144
muscarinic receptor antagonist effects, 146
PAF actions, 237
PGE_2 actions, 234
relaxation, regulation, 64
spasm, *see* Spasm
uterine, *see* Uterus
vascular, *see* Vascular system
Smooth muscle-type muscarinic ACh (M_3) receptors, 138, 139, 341
SNAREs, 66
Sodium (ions)
electrical excitability and, 56
retention, glucocorticoids causing, 412, 416
transport, 68
epithelial, 67
transport, renal, 255, 256, 353, 354–5, 361
aldosterone effects, 358
atrial natriuretic peptide and, 272, 359
drugs affecting, 358, 360, 362, 363
see also Salt
Sodium chloride, renal handling, 358, 360
loop diuretic effects, 362
prostaglandin effects, 362
Sodium ion channels, 59–60
blockers/modulators, 57–9, 60, 612–18
amiloride as, 67
antidysrhythmic actions, *see* Antidysrhythmic drugs, class I
antiepileptics as, 554, 555
local anaesthetics as, 613–14
toxins as, 59, 60, 616–17
use-dependence block, 57–9, 275, 614
voltage-dependence block, 57–9
in renal collecting tubule, 358
voltage-gated, 46, 59–60
drugs affecting gating, 618
of electrically excitable membranes, 57–9
Sodium ion/hydrogen ion exchanger, 355, 358, 419
Sodium pump (Na^+/K^+-ATPase)
cardiac, glycoside actions, 278, 279
renal, 256, 355, 359, 360
Sodium salts of drugs, *see specific drugs e.g.* Salicylate
Solubility
anaesthetics, 504, 506
in lipid, *see* Lipid; Lipophilic drugs
Solutes, reabsorption, 353
loop diuretic effects, 362
Somatic efferent pathways, 123
Somatomedins, *see* Insulin-like growth factors
Somatorelin (GHRF), 405, 406, 407
Somatostatin (growth hormone-release inhibiting factor), 405, 406
actions/effects, 385, 406
unwanted, 406
as analgesic, 583
analogue, *see* Octreotide
secretion, 380, 385
Somatotrophin, *see* Growth hormone
Somatropin, 407
Sordarins, 670
Sotalol, 277
antidysrythmic action, 274, 275, 277
with probucol, avoidance, 313
South American trypanosomiasis (*T. cruzi*), 684, 685
Spasm (skeletal muscle), 560–1
Spasm (smooth muscle)
biliary, 378
bradykinin causing, 239
bronchial, *see* Bronchoconstriction
intestinal, suppression, 148, 377
PAF as, 237
vascular, *see* Vasospasm
Specificity of drug/ligand binding, 8–9
G-protein-coupled receptors, 38
Spectinomycin, 645
Spermine and spermidine and NMDA receptors, 466
Spinal anaesthesia, 617
Spinal cord
morphine actions at level of, 576
nicotine actions at level of, 599
pain sensation and, 564–5
Spinothalamic tract, pain sensation and, 564–5
Spiperone, 188
Spirochaetes, antibiotic choice, 637
Spironolactone, 358, 364, 419
actions/effects, 358, 364
unwanted, 364
clinical uses, 300, 364
pharmacokinetics, 364
potassium loss reduced with, 361
Splanchnic nerves, pelvic (nervi erigentes), 125
Spongiform encephalopathy, transmissible, 501
Sporocyst, plasmodial, 675
Sporozoites, plasmodial, 673, 675
SR141716A, 609
Src-homology 2 domain, *see* SH2-domain proteins
Standard(s), in bioassays, 82
'Standard' treatment in trials, 86
Stanozolol, 437
Staphylococci
antibiotic choice, 636
antibiotic resistance, 631, 632–3
methicillin-resistant, 631, 632–3, 636
Starling mechanism, 269
Stat, 44
Statins, *see* HMG-CoA reductase inhibitors
Status asthmaticus, *see* Asthma
Status epilepticus, 100, 520, 555, 558
Stavudine, 661
Steady-state concentration, 88
Stem and progenitor cells, haemopoietic, 336
CSF effects, 337–8
Stents coated with drugs, 105
Sterculia, 375
Stereoselectivity, 107
of inhibition of drug metabolism, 107, 721

Stereotyped behaviour with amphetamines, 588
Steroid(s)/steroid hormone(s)
adrenal, *see* Adrenal steroids; Androgens; Mineralocorticoids
anabolic, 437
cardiotonic, *see* Glycosides, cardiac
delaying absorption, 101
interactions, 721
receptors (cytoplasmic and nuclear), 44, 413–14
corticosteroid agent affinity, 412
obesity and, 400
sex hormones, 432
in reproduction, *see* Sex steroids
sex, *see* Sex steroids
see also Neurosteroids
Stevens–Johnson syndrome, 735
azoles causing, 669
Stibogluconate, sodium, 683
Stilboestrol (diethylstilboestrol)
teratogenicity, 733
vaginal cancer and, 433
Stimulant(s), CNS, *see* Psychomotor stimulants; Respiratory stimulants; Seizures, drugs inducing
Stimulant purgatives, 376
Stomach, *see entries under* Gastric
Stones, biliary, *see* Gallstones
Storage granules/vesicles, 65
Streptogramins, 646
Streptokinase, 328
in myocardial infarction, 325
Streptomycin
S. aureus resistance, 632
tuberculosis, 651
Striated muscle, *see* Heart muscle; Skeletal muscle
Stroke (cerebrovascular accident), 493–4
dipyridamole in prevention of, 325
fibrinolytic-related risk, 328
oral contraceptives and, 440
pathophysiology (ischaemic stroke), 493–4
therapy, 494
Stroke volume, ventricular, 268
Stroke work, ventricular, 269
Strongyloides stercoralis (threadworm = US term), 687
therapy, 688, 689, 691
Strychnine, 473, 585–7
actions of, 473
Subarachnoid haemorrhage, cerebral vasospasm following, 283
Subarachnoid injection, 101
Subcutaneous implants of steroid hormones, 101
levonorgestrel, 441
Subcutaneous injection, 100
Sublingual administration, 99–100
organic nitrates, 99, 281
Submucous plexus, 367
Substance P, 130, 132, 341, 570
antagonists, 201
development, 648
nociceptive transmission and, 565
biosynthesis, and gene splicing, 203
capsaicin causing release, 568
distribution, 571
role
in inflammation, 564, 571
in neurotransmission, 132
in nociception and pain sensation, 564
vomiting caused by injection of, 375
Substance abuse, *see* Drug abuse
Substantia gelatinosa, 564–5
Substantia nigra
destruction, effects, 478
dopaminergic neurons in, 476
Succinyl CoA, methylmalonyl CoA isomerisation to, 336
Succinylcholine, *see* Suxamethonium
Sucralfate, 372
Sufentanil, 573, 581
Sulconazole, 669
Sulfadiazine, 638
in toxoplasmosis, with pyrimethamine, 685
Sulfadimidine, 638
Sulfadoxine
in malaria, 680
pyrimethamine and, 623, 680
structure, 680
Sulfamethoxazole, 638
Sulfamethoxazole–trimethoprim, *see* Co-trimoxazole
Sulfametopyrazine, 638
Sulfanilamide, 638
mechanism of action, 638
Sulfapyridine–salicylate combination, *see* Sulfasalazine
Sulfasalazine (sulfapyridine–salicylate [5–ASA] combination), 638
inflammatory bowel disease, 377–8
rheumatoid arthritis, 255
Sulfhydryl groups (-SH), free
of ACE inhibitors, toxicity associated with, 297
drug-induced modification, 726
nitrates and depletion of, 281
Sulfinpyrazone, 366
interactions with aspirin, 251, 366
myocardial infection, 324
reinfarction trial, 88–9
as uricosuric, 254, 366
Sulfonamides, 637–9
as antibacterials, 638–9
mechanism of action, 638
interactions, 719
pharmacokinetics, 638–9
plasma protein binding, 96
resistance, 638
mechanisms, 632
S. aureus, 632
structures, 638
unwanted effects, 639
Sulfonylureas, 23, 389–90, 391
actions/effects, 389
on K^+ channels, 61, 389
mechanisms, 389
unwanted, 389–90
clinical use, 390
interactions, 390
pharmacokinetics, 389
receptor, 46
Sulindac, 245
unwanted effects, 249
Sulpiride, 529
antidepressant action, 533
Sumatriptan, 186, 193, 292
in migraine, 192, 193, 482
Superoxide anion
drug-induced generation, 726
NO reacting with, 487
Superoxide dismutase, 493
mutation, 493
Supersensitivity to neurotransmitters with denervation, 126–8
Suppressor cells, *see* $CD8^+$ T cells
Supraventricular tachycardia
adenosine, 196, 277
verapamil, 277
Suramin, 193, 196, 684
trypanosomiasis, 684
unwanted effects, 684
Surface anaesthesia, 617
Surgery, postoperative pain, 581
Surgical anaesthesia, 505
Surveillance, post-marketing, 750
Survivin, 78
Sustained release preparations, *see* Slow-release preparations
Suxamethonium (succinylcholine), 149, 151, 152
fasciculations with, 153
pharmacokinetics, 151
genetic influences, 716
unwanted effects/dangers, 151, 153, 154, 717
Sweat glands
ACh effects, 137
muscarinic agonist effects, 144
muscarinic antagonist effects, 146
SXR (nuclear receptors), 45
Sympathectomy, chemical, 176
Sympathetic nervous system, 123–5
airway, 340, 341
anatomy, 123–5
cardiac, 273
gastrointestinal, 367
parasympathetic and, relationship/opposition, 125–6
physiology, 122–3, 123–5, 126, 127
cotransmitters, 132
historical perspectives, 122–3
insulin release, 382
main effects, 127
neuropathic pain, 566–7
vascular effects
blood pressure regulation, 298
vasoconstriction mediation, 295
see also Autonomic nervous system
Sympathomimetic amines
directly acting, *see* Adrenoceptor agonists
indirectly acting, 177–8, 180
MAO inhibitor interactions with, 546
mode of action, 177–8
pharmacokinetics, 180
structure–activity relationships, 177–8
unwanted effects, 180
Symport systems, 354, 355, 356
Synapse, 66
cholinergic
anticholinesterase effects at, 158
electrical events in transmission at, 141–3
ganglionic, *see* Ganglion
plasticity, 458
glutamate receptors and, 467–8
see also Exocytosis; Neurotransmission *and entries under* Postsynaptic; Presynaptic
Synaptic cleft, 140
Synaptic vesicles, glutamate storage, 463
Synaptobrevin, 77
Synaptotagmin, 77
Syntaxin, 77
Synuclein gene mutations, 497, 498
Systemic lupus erythematosus, autoimmune syndrome resembling, 736
Systemic responses to inflammation, 227–8

T

T-cells/lymphocytes, 223
in asthma, 342, 343
ciclosporin effects, 258
cytotoxic/CD8+, *see* $CD8^+$ T cells
glucocorticoid effects, 416
helper, *see* $CD4^+$ helper lymphocytes
in induction phase of immune response, 224–5
in protozoal invasion, 672
surface proteins, as drug targets, 257
T-type Ca^{2+} channels, 52
cardiac function and, 265
Tachycardia/tachyarrhythmia, 265
supraventricular, *see* Supraventricular tachycardia
Tachykinins, 570–1
biosynthesis, 203
distribution, 571
receptors (NK), 571
antagonists, 375, 571, 748
Tachyphylaxis, *see* Desensitisation
Tacrine, 496
Tacrolismus, 258
Taenia spp., 687
therapy, 689, 690
Tafenoquine, 676, 680
'Taming' effects, benzodiazepines, 518
Tamoxifen, 433, 705
in breast cancer, 705
Tamsulosin, 173, 180
benign prostatic hyperplasia, 437
Tapeworms (cestodes), 687
therapy, 689, 690
Tar, tobacco, 602
Tarceva, 708
Tardive dyskinesia with antipsychotics, 531–2
Targets for drug action, 8, 22–47
in drug development, *see* Development
see also Binding; Receptors *and specific targets*
Tau, 495
Taxanes, 704
3TC (lamivudine), 660–1

Tegaserod, 188
Teicoplanin, 648
Telomerase, 694–5
Telophase, 72
Temazepam, 517
Temperature, *see* Fever; Hyperpyrexia; Hypothermia; Thermogenesis
Tenoxicam, 245
Tension, twitch, glycosides affecting, 278
Teratogens, 731–4
cannabis/THC, 610
cocaine, 590
mechanisms of action, 731–3
mutagens as, 731
tests for, 730, 731, 733
see also Fetal development
Terazosin, 173
in prostatic hyperplasia, 437
Terbinafine, 669–70
Terbutaline, 179
in asthma, 346
Terfenadine, 253
interactions, with ketoconazole, 720
toxicity, 111
Teripatide, 432
Terlipressin, 411
Test(s), *see* Bioassay; Measurement *and specific tests*
Test group in trials, 86
Testosterone, 436–7
actions/effects, 436
mechanisms, 436
derivatives, 434
pharmacokinetics, 436–7
preparations, 436
secretion, 435
synthesis, 437
Tetanic fade, 150, 153
Tetanus toxin, 473, 585
Tetracaine (amethocaine), 615
pharmacokinetics, 616
Tetracosactide, 408
Tetracycline(s), 643–4, 647
H. pylori eradication, 371
interactions, 718
with iron, 332
in malaria, 676, 681
mechanism of action, 643
pharmacokinetics, 644
absorption, 99, 644
partitioning into tissues, 97
resistance mechanisms, 632, 643–4
spectrum of activity, 643–4
unwanted effects, 644
Tetraethylammonium, 160
K^+ channels blocked by, 61
Tetrahydrocannabinol (THC), 586, 608, 608–9
actions/effects, 609
adverse, 610
analgesic, 583–4
Tetrahydrofolate, metabolism
humans, 334, 335–6
methotrexate effects, 701, 702
microbial, 622
Tetrodotoxin (TTX), 59, 60, 616–17
TGF-β, tamoxifen effects, 433
Th1 and Th2 cells, 224
in cell-mediated immune response, 226–7
responses to disease, 224
asthma, 342, 343
protozoal infection, 672
see also CD4$^+$ helper lymphocytes
Thalassaemia, gene therapy, 743
Thalidomide, 733
toxicity, 89, 731, 733
Thapsigargin, 54
Thebaine derivatives, 574
Theobromine, 346
Theophylline (1,3-dimethylxanthine), 346–7, 348, 590
as central stimulant, 590, 591
clinical use, 347, 591
as adenosine antagonists, 278, 346
asthma, 347
interactions, 348
ciprofloxacin, 648
pharmacokinetics, 347
unwanted effects, 346–7
Therapeutic efficacy/effectiveness in clinical trials, 84, 86
Therapeutic index, 89
Thermogenesis, 396–7
progesterone and, 431
Thiabendazole, 688
unwanted effects, 688–9
Thiazide diuretics (and related drugs), 363–4, 365
actions/effects, 360
on potassium balance, 363
sites, 358
unwanted, 363–4
clinical uses, 363
hypertension, 300, 363
osteoporosis, 453
pharmacokinetics, 363–4
Thiazolidinediones (glitazones), 390–2
actions/effects, 390
mechanisms, 390–1
unwanted, 391–2
clinical use, 392
interactions, 393
pharmacokinetics, 391
Thienamycin and blood–brain barrier, 102
Thienopyridine derivatives, 325
Thiethylperazine as antiemetic, 374
Thiopental, 512–13, 523
actions/effects, 512
unwanted, 512, 513
pharmacokinetics, 512–13
partitioning into body fat, 96, 512
Thioperamide, 230
Thioridazine, 529, 532
Thiorphan, 583
Thiotepa, 700
Thioureylenes, 425–6
Thioxanthines, 528
Thoracolumbar sympathetic outflow, 123
Thought disorder in schizophrenia, 525
Threadworm
UK term, *see Enterobius vermicularis*
USA term, *see Strongyloides stercoralis*
3TC (lamivudine), 660–1
Thrombin (factor IIa), 33, 317
agonists (incl. modified thrombin), 321
formation, 316, 318
inhibitors, 320
role, 317
Thrombocyte, *see* Platelet
Thrombocytopenia (drug-induced), 736
heparin-induced, 320
Thrombocytopenic purpura, 323
Thromboembolism/thromboembolic disease
oestrogen-related risk, 432, 435
oral contraceptives and, 440
raloxifene-related risk, 451
Thrombolysis, *see* Fibrinolysis
Thrombomodulin, 317
Thrombophilias, 317
Thromboplastin time, activated partial, 320
Thrombopoietin, 336, 338
Thrombosis, 319–23
definition, 314
heparin-related risk, 320–1
treatment/prevention, 315, 319–27, 328
see also Anticoagulants; Antiplatelet drugs; Fibrinolysis, drugs increasing
see also Thromboembolism
Thromboxane(s), 231
synthesis, 234
inhibitors, 327
Thromboxane A_2
receptors, 234
antagonists, 327
synthesis, 234
Thromboxane(s), 231
Thrombus
arterial, 314–15
definition, 314
venous, 315
Thymidylate (deoxythymidylate) synthesis (from deoxyuridylate), 334
inhibition, 622
by antimetabolites, 701, 701–2
Thymoleptics, *see* Antidepressants
Thyroglobulin, 421
tyrosine residues, iodination, 421, 422
Thyroid, 421–8
cancer, therapy, 705
dysfunction/disease, 424–7
drug sensitivity affected by, 717
drugs causing, 424
drugs treating, 425–7
oral anticoagulants affected in, 322
see also Hyperthyroidism; Hypothyroidism
function, regulation, 422–3
site of drug action in, 422
Thyroid hormone(s), 421–8
actions/effects, 423–4
mechanism, 424
unwanted, 427
clinical use, 427
disorders of, *see* Thyroid, dysfunction
metabolism/transport, 424
secretion/release, 421–2
synthesis/storage, 421
Thyroid-stimulating hormone (thyrotrophin; TSH), 405, 422
actions, 405, 422
production/release, 422
Thyroperoxidase–H_2O_2 complex, 421, 422
Thyrotoxicosis, *see* Hyperthyroidism
Thyrotrophin, *see* Thyroid-stimulating hormone
Thyrotrophin-releasing hormone, 405
actions/effects, 405, 406
analogues, *see* Posatirelin; Protirelin
Thyroxine (T_4)
actions/effects, 422, 423–4
mechanism, 424
clinical use, 427
interactions with colestyramine, 99
metabolism/transport, 424
synthesis/storage/secretion, 421–2
Thyroxine-binding globulin, 424
Tiagabine, 560
mechanism of action, 554, 560
Tibolone, 435
Ticarcillin, 641
Ticlopidine, 325
Timolol, 146, 277
antidysrhythmic action, 277
glaucoma, 100, 146, 175
Tinea, 666, 667
Tinidazole, 683
in amoebiasis, 683
in trichomoniasis, 684
Tioconazole, 669
Tioguanine, 623, 702
Tiredness (fatigue) with β-blockers, 176
Tirofiban, 325
Tissue factor, 316
Tissue inhibitors of matrix metalloproteinases (TIMPs), 74
Tissue plasminogen activators, 327
clinical use, 328, 494
TNF, *see* Tumour necrosis factor
Tobacco, *see* Nicotine; Smoking
Tobramycin, 645
Tocainide, 615
Tocolytics (myometrial relaxants), 443
α-Tocopherol as anti-oxidant, 493
Tolbutamide, 389
plasma protein binding, 96
Tolerability in phase I studies, 749
Tolerance, 19, 21, 595
alcohol, 607–8
amphetamines, 588–9
benzodiazepines, 522
cannabis, 609–10
LSD, 592
methylxanthines, 591
morphine-like drugs, 578, 578–9, 597
nicotine, 600–1
organic nitrates, 281
Toll receptors, 218
Tolmetin, 245

Tolteradine, 146
Tone, muscle
and coordination, benzodiazepine effects, 519
vascular smooth, control, 286–92
see also Dystonia
Tonic–clonic seizures (grand mal), 551
Topical application
for local effect, 100
for systemic effects, *see* Transdermal routes
Topiramate, 560
Topoisomerase inhibitors
antiprotozoal, 685
topoisomerase I, anticancer, 704
topoisomerase II (DNA gyrase), 647–8
antibacterial, 627, 647–8, 704
anticancer, 627
Topotecan, 704
Torsades de pointes, 275, 277
probucol and risk of, 313
Toxic epidermal necrolysis, 735
Toxic goitre, diffuse, 424
Toxic metabolites of drugs, 111
Toxic nodular goitre, 424
Toxicity, *see* Adverse reactions
Toxins
bacterial, G-proteins and, 35
Ca^{2+} channels acted on by, voltage-gated, 52
conjugated to antibodies, 206
Na^{+} channels acted on by, 59, 60, 616–17
neurological, *see* Neurotoxins
see also specifically named toxins
Toxocariasis (visceral larva migrans), 688
therapy, 689
Toxoplasmosis, 684–5
host–parasite interactions, 672
Trafficking, *see* Transport
Tramadol, 580, 583
Trandolapril, 296
Tranexamic acid, 328, 328–9
Tranquilisers
major, *see* Antipsychotic drugs
minor, *see* Anxiolytic agents
Transcellular fluid compartment, 101, 102
Transcobalamins, 335
Transcription (of DNA)
agents interfering with
antibacterial, 627
anticancer, 703
glucocorticoid effects, 413–15
mineralocorticoid effects, 419
receptors regulating, *see* Nuclear receptors
Transdermal routes (patches), 100
nicotine, 602
organic nitrates, 281
Transduction in bacteria, 630–1
Transferrin, 332
Transformation, bacterial, 631
Transforming growth factor-ß
bone remodelling and, 448
tamoxifen effects, 433
Transgenic animals, 85–6, 200
acetylcholinesterase-overexpressing, 484
Alzheimer's disease model, 495, 496
drug dependence, 598
erythropoietin expression in, 741, 742
nicotine dependence, 600
Parkinson's disease model, 478
seizures, 552
Translation, RNA, *see* RNA
Translocation of drugs, *see* Transport
Transmitters, *see* Neurotransmission; Neurotransmitters
Transplant
neural, in Parkinson's disease treatment, 500–1
rejection (allograft), prevention, 257
monoclonal antibodies, 241, 242
Transport (translocation; trafficking)
by carrier molecules, *see* Carrier molecules
drugs and metabolites, 91–7
renal, 112
ion, epithelial, 66–8
lipoproteins in blood, 307–9
neurotransmitters, 132–3
noradrenaline, 132, 167
renal, 359–60, 360–1
in collecting tubules/ducts, 358
in distal tubules, 356
drugs and metabolites, 112
in loops of Henle, 356
in proximal tubule, 354–5
Transposons and antibiotic resistance, 630
Tranylcypromine, 541, 545
Trastuzumab, 706
Traveller's diarrhoea, 376
Trazodone, 541
metabolite (= tramadol), 580, 583
Trematodes, *see* Flukes
Tremor, Parkinson's disease, 497
Tresulphan, 700
Tretinoin, chemotherapy, 706
Trials, clinical, *see* Clinical trials
Triamcinolone, 412
Triamterene, 364
actions/effects, 358, 361, 364
on potassium balance, 361
unwanted, 364
pharmacokinetics, 364
Triazolam, 517, 518
withdrawal effect, 522
Tribavirin, 663
Trichiniasis (*T. spiralis*), 687, 688
therapy, 689
Trichloroethylene, 511
Trichomoniasis, 684
Trichuris trichiura, *see* Whipworm
Tricyclic antidepressants, 539–42
actions/effects, 178, 540, 542–3
analgesic, 583
measurement, 538
mechanisms, 542
in migraine, 192
chemical aspects, 542
interactions, 543–4
pharmacokinetics, 544
unwanted/toxic effects, 542
in combinations with MAO inhibitors, 547
Triethylcholine, 154
Trifluoroacetylchloride, 736
Trifluoroperazine, 529
as antiemetic, 374
Triglycerides, ω-3 marine triglycerides, 313
Triiodothyronine (T_3)
actions/effects, 422, 423–4
mechanism, 424
metabolism/transport, 424
synthesis/storage/secretion, 421–2
synthetic (liothyronin), 427
Trilostane, 413, 705
Trimetaphan, 148, 149
Trimethadione, 555, 558
Trimethobenzamide, 374
Trimethoprim, 639
interactions, 719
mechanism of action, 622–3, 639
in *P. carinii* pneumonia, with dapsone, 682
pharmacokinetics, 639
resistance
mechanisms, 632
S. aureus, 632
structure, 638
sulfamethoxazole and, *see* Co-trimoxazole
unwanted effects, 639
Trinucleotide repeat diseases, 510
Triplet (trinucleotide) repeat diseases, 501
Troglitazone, 390
unwanted effects, 390
Trophozoites
amoebic, 682–3
plasmodial, 673
Tropicamide, 145, 147
Tropisetron, 188, 373
Troponin, 62
myocardial troponin complex, 269
Trypanosomiasis, 672, 684
new approaches to therapy, 685
Tryptophan, metabolism, 185, 480
depression and, 537
Tryptophan hydroxylase, 185, 480
Tuberculin reaction, 228
Tuberculoid leprosy, 651
Tuberculosis, 649–51
therapy, *see* Antituberculosis drugs
Tuberohypophyseal system, dopaminergic neurons, 476, 480
Tubocurarine, 141, 149, 150, 151, 152, 483
unwanted effects, 150, 151
Tubules (renal), 112–13, 354–60
collecting, *see* Collecting tubules
diffusion across, 112
distal, *see* Distal tubules
function, 112–13, 354–60
drug effects on, 721–2
drug handling, 112–13
proximal, *see* Proximal tubules
Tubulin, colchicine binding, 255
Tumour(s)
brain, gene therapy, 744
hormone-dependent, 730
malignant, *see* Cancer; Carcinogenesis
pituitary hormone-secreting, 407
see also specific sites/types
Tumour necrosis factor-α
in immune/inflammatory response, 218–19
monoclonal antibodies targeting, in rheumatoid arthritis, 241, 242, 256–7
obesity and, 399
Tumour necrosis factor receptor family and apoptosis, 76
Tumour suppressor genes, 694, 729
Tumours, gastrointestinal tract hormone-secreting, 705
Twitch tension, glycosides affecting, 278
Two-compartment model of pharmacokinetics, 116–17
2+2 bioassay, 83
Two-pore domain K^{+} channels, 60, 62, 504
Two-state model for receptors, 17, 18
Type I and II error, 87, 89
Tyramine, 177, 178, 180
MAO inhibitors and ingestion of, 546, 546–7, 719
L-Tyrosine, 164
Tyrosine hydroxylase, 164
inhibition, 164, 176, 181
Tyrosine kinase
inhibitors, cancer, 44, 706, 708
receptors linked to, 42, 69
Tyrosine residues of thyroglobulin, iodination, 421

U

UCP1/2 (proteins uncoupling oxidative phosphorylation), 397
UDP glucuronyl transferase, 109
UK Prospective Diabetes Study, 387
Ulcer(s), peptic, *see* Peptic ulcers
Ulcerative colitis, 377–8
Uncoupling proteins 1/2 (UCP1/2), 397
Unknowns in bioassays, 82, 83
Unwanted effects, *see* Adverse reactions
Urea transport, 359, 360
Uric acid, 365–6
secretion/excretion, 365–6
drugs increasing, *see* Uricosuric agents
drugs inhibiting, 366
synthesis inhibitors, *see* Xanthine oxidase inhibitors
see also Gout
Uricosuric agents, 255, 366
interactions, with aspirin/salicylates, 251, 366
Uridine diphosphate-glucuronyl transferase, 109
Urinary incontinence, 568
Urine
concentration, 359
mechanisms, 356
flow, drugs altering, 722
glucose in, in diabetes, 385
nitrate/cGMP analysis, 214
pH
drugs altering, 365–6, 722
effects, 93
Urodilatin, 359
Urokinase, 327
Ursodeoxycholic acid, 378
Urticaria with antipsychotics, 532

Use-dependence channel block, 57–9
  Ca^{2+} channels, 282
  Na^{+} channels, 57–9, 275, 614
Uterus, 441–3
  bleeding from, with HRT, 435
  contraction (myometrium), 441
    drugs causing (oxytocics), 441–2, 443
  motility, 441
  relaxants (myometrium), 443

V

V (vasopressin; ADH) receptors, 293, 358–9, 410
Vaccination
  with DNA, 741, 742
  fungal infections, 670
  parasites
    helminths, 691
    malaria, 685
Vaginal cancer and stilboestrol, 433
Vagus
  glycosides increasing activity, 278
  physiology, 122–3, 274
Vagusstoff, 122–3
Valaciclovir, 104, 663
Valproate, 554, 556–7, 559
  as antiepileptic, 560
    mechanisms of action, 553, 558
  as mood stabiliser, 548
  pharmacokinetics, 560
  unwanted effects, 556–7, 734
Valsartan, 204, 298
Vancomycin, 648–9
  aminoglycoside combined with, 645
  clinical use, 99, 649
  mechanism of action, 624
  pharmacokinetics, 648–9
  resistance, 652
    S. aureus, 632–3
  unwanted effects, 649
Vanilloid receptor, 46, 467–8
  agonists/activators, 568–9
    anandamide, 488
Vanillylmandelic acid (VMA;
    3-Methoxy-4-hydroxy-mandelic acid)
    synthesis/secretion, 168
Variation(s)
  biological
    in bioassays, 83
    in P450 enzyme expression and regulation, 108–9
  individual, *see* Individual variations
Varicella-zoster virus, 662
Varices, oesophageal, bleeding, 293
Vasa rectae, 352, 359
Vascular beds, individual, drugs affecting resistance, 286
Vascular endothelial growth factor (VEGF), 74
  therapeutic use, 77
Vascular system (blood vessels; cardiovascular system), 285–305
  ACh effects, 137
  adrenoceptor antagonist actions/uses, 174, 175
  airway, regulation, 340
  anaesthetic actions
    general, 506
    local, unwanted, 616
  autonomic effects on, 127
  Ca^{2+} channel blocker effects, *see* Calcium channel blockers
  development of new vessels, *see* Angiogenesis
  diabetes-related disorders, 386
  effects of drugs on, 286
  endothelium, *see* Endothelium
  ergot alkaloid effects, 189
  ethanol effects, 604
  gene transfer, 744
  histamine actions, 230
  5-HT effects, 186
  in inflammation, 218–19, 219–20
  leukotriene actions, 236
  local anaesthetic effects, 616
  mediators/metabolites involved in coronary blood flow regulation, 270
  migraine as disorder of, 190–1
  muscarinic agonist actions, 144
  nephron, 352–3
  NO role, 208, 212, 213, 286, 298, 317
  oestrogen actions/effects, 432
    oral contraceptive pill, 440
  peripheral, *see* Peripheral vasculature
  prostanoid actions, 235, 286, 442
  smoking adversely affecting, 601
  smooth muscle
    calcium antagonist effects, 283
    contraction, *see* Contraction
    relaxation, drugs causing, 302
    relaxation, mediators causing, 286, 287
    tone, control, 286–92
    see also Vasoactive drugs; Vasoconstriction; Vasodilation; Vasodilator drugs
  sulfonylurea adverse effects, 390
  xanthine actions, 346
    unwanted, 346, 347
Vasoactive drugs, 292–309
  clinical uses, 298–304
    shock, 303
  directly-acting, 292, 293–5
  indirectly-acting, 292, 295–8
  see also Vasoconstrictor drugs; Vasodilator drugs
Vasoactive intestinal peptide, 130, 132, 200
Vasoactive mediators, *see* Mediators, vascular
Vasoconstriction
  angiotensin II-mediated, 292
  coronary, mediators of, 270
  dopamine-induced, 294
  endothelin-mediated, 289, 290, 293
  ergotamine-induced, 189
  fingers, 304
  intracranial, in migraine, 191
  L-NMMA-induced, 214, 216
  sympathetic control, 295
Vasoconstrictor drugs, 292, 292–3
  clinical uses, 293
Vasodilation
  ACh causing, 137
  adenosine causing, 195
  bradykinin causing, 239
  cannabis causing, 609
  coronary vessel
    Ca^{+} antagonist-induced, 283
    organic nitrate-induced, 280
    physiological factors causing, 270
  diuretics causing
    loop, 363
    thiazide, 363
  dopamine causing, 132, 294
  ethanol causing, 604
  in inflammation, 219
  local anaesthetics causing, 616
  in menorrhagia, 442
  nitrates (organic) causing, 280
  prostanoids causing, 235, 286, 442
  in shock, 302
  see also Arteriolar dilatation; Venodilation
Vasodilator drugs, 292, 293–8
  in angina, 280
  Ca^{2+} antagonists as, 283
  in cardiac failure, 302
  in hypertension, 298–300
  in Raynaud's disease, 304
  types, 298
    directly acting, 293–5
    indirectly acting, 295–8
  unknown mechanism of action, 295
Vasopressin, *see* Antidiuretic hormone
Vasospasm
  cerebral, following subarachnoid haemorrhage, reducing, 283
  coronary, 271, 280
Vaughan Williams' classification of antidysrhythmics, 273
Vectors for gene therapy, 739–41
Vecuronium, 149, 150, 151
  biliary excretion, 114
  unwanted effects, 150, 151
VEGF, *see* Vascular endothelial growth factor
Venlafaxine, 540
Venodilation with loop diuretics, 362
Venous thrombus, 315
Venous tone, drugs affecting, 286
Ventilation, alveolar, inhalation anaesthetics, 508
Ventral horn, nicotine action, 599
Ventral tegmental area and opioid dependence, 579
Ventricle
  dysrhythmias
    post-myocardial infarction, 265
    therapy, 275
    tricyclic antidepressants causing, 543
  function, 269
    curves, 268, 269
    stroke volume, 268
    see also After-load; Pre-load
Venules, postcapillary, in inflammation, 218–19, 230
Verapamil
  actions, 282
    adverse, 283, 284
    vasodilatory, 293
  clinical uses
    angina, 282
    dysrhythmias, 274, 276, 277, 278, 283
  digoxin interactions, 720
Veratridine, 60
Very low density lipoproteins, 307, 309
  fibrates effects, 311
  transport, 307, 308
Vesamicol, 140, 154
Vesicular transporter, 132–3, 133
  noradrenaline, 167
Vigabatrin, 558, 559, 560
  mechanism of action, 470, 553, 556, 558
  pharmacokinetics, 560
  unwanted effects, 558, 560
Vinblastine, 704
  actions, 628, 704
  toxicity, 704
Vinca alkaloids, 704
  ADH effects of, 410
  mechanism of action, 628, 704
  unwanted effects, 359, 704
Vincristine, 704
  actions, 628, 704
  in combination regimes, 707
  toxicity, 704
Vinorelbine, 704
Vinyl ether, 511
VIP (vasoactive intestinal peptide), 130, 132, 200
Virchow's triad, 314
Viruses, 620–1, 654–5
  in diabetes aetiology, 386
  drugs acting against, *see* Antiviral agents
  function, 655
  gene therapy against, 745
  as gene vectors, 739–41, 742
    safety, 743
  host interactions with, 655–7
  immune responses to, *see* Immune responses
  life cycle, 655
  replication, 655
  structure, 654
  types (and their diseases), 654–5
  see also Phages
Viscera, autonomic effects on, 127
Visceral larva migrans, *see* Toxocariasis
Visual disturbances, sildenafil, 444
Vitamin A derivatives (retinoids)
  adverse affects
    dyslipidaemia, 309
    teratogenicity, 734
  in chemotherapy, 706
Vitamin B_{12} (cobalamins; extrinsic factor), 333, 335–6
  actions, 335–6
  administration/use, 336
  deficiency, 333, 336
  pharmacokinetics, 336
  synthesis, 335
Vitamin C, *see* Ascorbic acid
Vitamin D, 450, 452
  actions, 448, 450
  clinical use, 452

pharmacokinetics, 452
synthesis/metabolism, 450
unwanted effects, 452
Vitamin D_2, 450, 450
Vitamin D_3 (cholecalciferol), 453
Vitamin E as anti-oxidant, 493
Vitamin K (phytomenadione), 318
administration, 318–19
warfarin and, 321
antagonists (warfarin as), 321, 719
clinical use, 319
drugs decreasing availability, 322
drugs inhibiting reduction, 321, 322
mechanism of action, 319
pharmacokinetics, 318
Vofopitant, 375
Voltage-clamp technique, 45
Voltage-gated ion channels, 23
Ca^{2+} channels, *see* Calcium channels
gating, 46, 47
K^+ channels, 60, 61
Na^+ channels, *see* Sodium ion channels
NMDA receptors and, 468
structure, 46
three functional states, 57
Volume, blood, *see* Blood volume; Hypovolaemia
Volume expansion and anaesthesia, 504
Volume of distribution, 103–4
pharmacokinetic models and, 114–15
Volume replacement/restoration, *see* Fluid replacement
Vomiting (emesis) and nausea, 372–5
control, 188, 372–3
drugs inducing (emetogenic substances)
apomorphine, 102
clinical use, 373
cytotoxic drugs, 698, 707
levodopa, 500
morphine-like drugs, 577
drugs preventing/stopping, *see* Antiemetic drugs
see also Motion sickness
von Willebrand factor (and disease), 317
Voriconazole, 670

W

Wakefulness and 5-HT, 482
Wall, cell
bacterial, 621
Gram-positive vs negative bacteria, 635–7
synthesis, 623–4
synthesis inhibitors, 624
fungal, agents acting on, 670
Ward–Romano syndrome, 276
Warfarin, 321–3
actions/effects
mechanisms, 319
unwanted, 323, 734
administration, 321–2
interactions, 322–3, 719
aspirin, 251, 322
bile acid-binding resins (incl. colestyramine), 99, 312
phenobarbital, 18
phenylbutazone, 720
raloxifene, 452
rifampicin, 720, 721
stereoselectivity and, 721
vitamin K, 321, 721
non-drug factors potentiating or lessening effects of, 322
pharmacokinetics, 18, 96, 321–2
elimination/excretion, 112
see also Oral anticoagulants
Water, body
balance (fluid balance)
in diarrhoeal illness, maintenance, 376
drugs increasing excretion, *see* Diuretics
renal control, 353, 354–5, 359, 362
distribution, 101–4
overload, treatment, 363
see also Fluid; Oil:water partitioning
Water channels, 359
Weight, body
control, 394–6
gain
with antipsychotics, 532
excess, *see* Obesity
with MAO inhibitors, 546
with smoking cessation, 599
hypothalamus in regulation of, 394, 395
Well-stirred compartments, 91, 114
West of Scotland Coronary prevention Study, 310
Whipworm (*T. trichiura*), 687
therapy, 689, 691
White blood cells, *see* Leucocytes
WHO classification of hyperlipoproteinaemia, 309
'Wind-up' phenomenon, 564
Withdrawal (abstinence) syndrome
alcohol, 608
alleviating, 598
benzodiazepine, 522, 558
cocaine, 589
nicotine, 601
opioid, 578, 579
precipitated by naloxone, 581, 583
Wolff–Parkinson–White syndrome, 277
Women, *see* Females
Worms, *see* Helminths
Wuchereria bancrofti, 687, 688
therapy, 689, 690, 691

X

Xanthine(s)/methylxanthines, 196, 346–7, 348, 586, 590–1
actions/effects, 196, 346, 590–1
adenosine receptor antagonism, 196, 278, 346, 485, 590
central stimulant, 590–1
mechanisms, 346, 586
unwanted, 346–7
clinical use, 347, 591
in asthma, 347
pharmacokinetics, 347
Xanthine oxidase, 109
Xanthine oxidase inhibitors, 254
interactions, 721
Xenon, anaesthetic properties, 510
Xipamide, 363

Y

Y27632, 293
Yohimbine, 173, 180
in erectile dysfunction, 444

Z

Zafirlukast, 236, 347
Zalcitabine (ddC; dideoxycytidine), 660
Zanamivir, 663
Zaprinast, 212
Zero-order kinetics, *see* Saturation kinetics
Zidovudine (azidothymidine; AZT), 104, 660
mechanism of action, 627
pharmacokinetics, 660
resistance to, 660
unwanted effects, 660
Zileuton, 236
Zinc fingers, 44
glucocorticoid receptors, 415
Zinc suspensions, insulin, 387
delayed absorption, 101
Zollinger–Ellison syndrome, 369
Zolpidem, 517
Zona glomerulosa, 418
Zonula occludens, 354, 356, 359